Manual of Dietetic Practice

Third Edition

Revised and Edited by Briony Thomas
in conjunction with the British Dietetic Association

Blackwell
Science

© 1988, 1994, 2001 by
Blackwell Science Ltd
Editorial Offices:
Osney Mead, Oxford OX2 0EL
25 John Street, London WC1N 2BS
23 Ainslie Place, Edinburgh EH3 6AJ
350 Main Street, Malden
  MA 02148 5018, USA
54 University Street, Carlton
  Victoria 3053, Australia
10, rue Casimir Delavigne
  75006 Paris, France

Other Editorial Offices:

Blackwell Wissenschafts-Verlag GmbH
Kurfürstendamm 57
10707 Berlin, Germany

Blackwell Science KK
MG Kodenmacho Building
7-10 Kodenmacho Nihombashi
Chuo-ku, Tokyo 104, Japan

Iowa State University Press
A Blackwell Science Company
2121 S. State Avenue
Ames, Iowa 50014-8300, USA

First Edition published 1988
Reprinted 1989
Second Edition published 1994
Reprinted 1994 (twice), 1995, 1996, 1997, 1998, 1999
Third Edition published 2001
Reprinted 2002

Set in Garamond
by Gray Publishing, Tunbridge Wells, Kent
Printed and bound in Great Britain by
MPG Books, Bodmin, Cornwall

The Blackwell Science logo is a
trade mark of Blackwell Science Ltd,
registered at the United Kingdom
Trade Marks Registry

DISTRIBUTORS

Marston Book Services Ltd
PO Box 269
Abingdon
Oxon OX14 4YN
(*Orders:*   Tel: 01235 465500
                Fax: 01235 465555)

USA and Canada
Iowa State University Press
A Blackwell Science Company
2121 S. State Avenue
Ames, Iowa 50014-8300
(*Orders:*   Tel: 800-862-6657
                Fax: 515-292-3348
                Web   www.isupress.com
                email: orders@isupress.com

Australia
Blackwell Science Pty Ltd
54 University Street
Carlton, Victoria 3053
(*Orders:*   Tel: 03 9347 0300
                Fax: 03 9347 5001)

A catalogue record for this title
is available from the British Library

ISBN 0-632-05524-3

Library of Congress
Cataloging-in-Publication Data
is available

For further information on
Blackwell Science, visit our website:
www.blackwell-science.com

Contents

Contents

Contributors

Editorial steering group

Loretta Cox (Hon. Chairman British Dietetic Association)
Dr Briony Thomas (Editor)
Dr Jacki Bishop
Catherine Collins
Carole Middleton MBE
Diane Talbot

Principal author

Dr Briony Thomas BSc PhD SRD *Nutrition and Dietetic Consultant, Surrey.*
(Address for correspondence c/o The British Dietetic Association)

Major contributors

Ursula Arens BSc SRD *Nutrition Scientist, London*

Dr Jacki Bishop PhD SRD RPHNutr DipADP *Senior Lecturer in Dietetics, University of Surrey*

Gillian Bonner BSc SRD *Research Dietitian, Warneford Hospital, Oxford*

Dr Alison Brady BSc PhD SRD *Audit Officer, British Dietetic Association, Birmingham*

Jane Butler BSc SRD *Paediatric Dietitian, St Mary's Hospital, London*

Alison Coates BSc SRD *Paediatric Dietitian, Royal Hospital for Sick Children, Edinburgh*

Catherine Collins BSc SRD *Chief Dietitian, St George's Hospital, London*

June Copeman SRD *Senior Lecturer, Faculty Health & Social Care, Leeds Metropolitan University*

Lyndel Costain SRD *Consultant Dietitian and Nutritionist, Birmingham*

Jeanette Crosland MSc SRD *Accredited Sports Dietitian, Preston*

Barbara Dobson SRD *Research Fellow, Centre for Research into Social Policy, Loughborough University*

Rachael Donnelly SRD *Senior Dietitian, Guy's and St Thomas' NHS Trust, London*

Revd Phyllis Eaton SRD *Senior Dietitian, City Hospital, Birmingham*

Jo Farrington SRD *Senior Dietitian, Health Promotion Centre, Halifax*

Margaret Gellatly Cert Ed, DipDiet, BSc SRD *Formerly District Dietitian, Mid-Essex Health Authority. Vice-President and Honorary Dietary Advisor PWSA (UK)*

Carole Glencorse BSc SRD *Senior Dietitian, John Radcliffe Hospital, Oxford*

George Hartley BSc MPhil SRD *Chief Renal Dietitian, Freeman Hospital, Newcastle*

Cathy Hodgson BSc SRD *Chief Dietitian, King's College Hospital, London*

Lee Hooper SRD *Research Associate in Evidence Based Care and Systematic Review, The Cochrane Suite, University Dental Hospital of Manchester.*

Karen Hyland SRD *Chief Dietitian, Edgware Community Hospital, Edgware*

Dr Susan Jebb PhD SRD *Head of Nutrition and Health, MRC Human Nutrition Research, Cambridge*

Angie Jefferson BSc SRD *Consultant Nutritionist, Bracknell, Berks*

Ian Jones SRD *Senior Dietitian, The Royal London Hospital*

Nicola Kerr BSc SRD *Senior Dietitian, Southern General Hospital, Glasgow*

Caroline King BSc SRD *Chief Dietitian (Paediatrics), Hammersmith Hospital, London*

Julie Leaper BSc SRD *Senior Dietitian, The General Infirmary, Leeds*

Dr Angela Madden BSc SRD *Lecturer in Human Nutrition and Dietetics, School of Health and Sports Science, University of North London*

Carole Middleton BSc SRD MBE *Chief Dietitian, St James' University Hospital, Leeds*

Fiona Moor BSc SRD *Senior Dietitian, Derbyshire Royal Infirmary, Derby*

Carole Noble SRD *Senior Dietitian, The Royal Edinburgh Hospital*

Lorna Rapoport BSc SRD *Specialist Dietitian, Health Behaviour Unit, University College London Medical School*

Dr Russell Roberts MB BChir MRCP *Specialist Registrar in Renal Medicine, Freeman Hospital, Newcastle upon Tyne*

Diane Talbot SRD Dip ADP *Community Development Dietitian, Leicestershire Nutrition and Dietetic Service, Leicestershire and Rutland NHS Healthcare Trust*

Denise Thomas SRD *Chief Dietitian, St James' Hospital, Portsmouth*

Alison Thomson BSc SRD *Senior Dietitian, Gartnaval General Hospital, Glasgow*

Kate Trotter SRD *Chief Dietitian, The Maudsley Hospital, Denmark Hill, London*

Anthony Twist BSc SRD *Dietitian, The Robert Jones and Agnes Hunt Orthopaedic and District Hospital NHS Trust, Oswestry, Shropshire*

Janet Warren SRD *Dept of Nutrition and Dietetics, John Radcliffe Hospital, Oxford*

Richard Wilson BSc SRD *Director of Nutrition and Dietetics, King's College Hospital, London*

Tanya Wright BSc SRD *Chief Dietitian, Stoke Mandeville Hospital, Bucks*

Other contributors

Sue Acreman SRD *Chief Dietitian, Velindre NHS Trust, Cardiff*

Nuzhat Ali BSc SRD *Dietitian, London*

Julie Ashton SRD *Senior Dietitian, Cookridge Hospital, Leeds*

Christine Baker SRD *Specialist Dietitian, Birmingham Heartlands Hospital, Birmingham*

Dr Alison Boyd BSc SRD *Dept of Nutrition and Dietetics, Royal Hospitals Trust, Belfast*

Hilary Bradshaw BSc SRD *Oxford Lipid Metabolism Group, Radcliffe Infirmary, Oxford*

Fran Bryan SRD *Chief Dietitian, Dept of Nutrition and Dietetics, City General Hospital, Stoke-on-Trent*

Verona Bryant SRD *Community Dietitian, South West London Community NHS Trust*

Jane Calow BSc SRD *Senior Dietitian (Mental Health), Towers Hospital, Leicester*

Judith Carpenter BSc SRD *Senior Dietitian, Southern Derbyshire NHS Trust*

Christine Carter BSc SRD *Senior Dietitian, Great Ormond Street Hospital, London*

Ka-Yee Chan SRD *Dietitian, Tokyo*

Dr Wynnie Chan BSc PhD *Formerly Nutrition Scientist, British Nutrition Foundation*

Usha Chappiti BSc SRD *Senior Dietitian, Guy's and St Thomas' Hospital Trust*

Lisa Cooper BSc SRD *Community Dietitian, St Catherine's Hospital, Birkenhead*

Sue Durrant SRD *Chief Dietitian, St Richard's Hospital, Chichester*

Denise Ellis BSc SRD *Senior 1 Community Dietitian, Dolgellau & Barmouth District Hospital, Dolgellau*

Fiona Ford SRD *Research Dietitian, Department of Obstetrics, University of Sheffield*

Dr Gary Frost PhD SRD *Head of Nutrition and Dietetics, Hammersmith Hospital, London*

Surinder Ghatoray BSc SRD *Diabetes Specialist Dietitian, Birmingham Heartlands Hospital*

Farhat Hamid SRD *Chief Dietitian, Wembley Hospital, Middlesex*

Lesley Tompkins SRD *Chief Dietitian, Leeds General Infirmary*

Rosemary Hoskin SRD *Horizon NHS Trust, Harperbury Hospital, Radlett*

Shereen Huth BSc SRD *Senior Dietitian, Southend Hospital, Westcliff on Sea*

Sarah Jean-Marie BSc SRD *Community Dietitian, St Ann's Hospital, Tottenham*

Ruth Kander BSc SRD *Renal Dietitian, St George's Hospital, London*

Karen Lake SRD *Senior Dietitian, Manor House, Aylesbury*

Deborah Lazarus BSc SRD *Specialist Dietitian for Mental Health, Chase Farm Hospital, Enfield, Middlesex*

Julie Lees SRD *Cancer Services Project Manager, Greenwich Hospital, London*

Norma McGough BSc SRD *Formerly Head of Diet Information Services, Diabetes UK*

Sheila Merriman SRD FRSH DipADP RNutr *Head of Nutrition and Dietetic Service, St Andrew's Hospital, Northampton*

Helen Molyneux MSc BSc SRD *Specialist Dietitian, Community Rehabilitation Team, Dewsbury Health Care NHS Trust, West Yorkshire*

Kathryn Morton SRD *Chief Dietitian, Lever Chambers Centre for Health, Bolton*

Alison Morton BSc SRD *Senior Dietitian, Seacroft Hospital, Leeds*

Julie Nedin BSc SRD *Chief Dietitian, Singleton Hospital, Swansea*

Dr Susan New BA MSc PhD RPHNutr *Lecturer in Nutrition, University of Surrey, Guildford*

Tracey Parkin SRD *Senior Dietitian, Portsmouth Diabetes Centre*

Gail Pollard SRD *Specialist Dietitian, Newbury Day Centre, Newbury*

Jane Power BSc SRD *Dietitian, Wrexham Maelor Hospital, Wrexham*

Dympna Pearson SRD *Senior Dietitian, Leicester & Rutland Healthcare, Leicester*

Brenda Purnell BSc SRD *Community Dietitian, Lever Chambers for Health, Bolton*

Helen Reilly BSc SRD *Nutrition and Dietetic Dept, Birmingham Heartlands Hospital*

Dr Carrie Ruxton BSc SRD PhD *The Sugar Bureau, London*

Helen Storer BSc SRD, Dip ADP *Dietetic Services Manager, Nottingham City Primary Care NHS Trust*

Dr Stephen Taylor PhD SRD *Senior Dietitian, Nutrition and Dietetics, Frenchay Hospital, Bristol*

Aruna Thaker BSc SRD *Community Dietitian, South West London Community NHS Trust*

Dimple Thakrar BSc SRD *Community Dietitian, Astley Bridge Health Centre, Bolton*

Sue Thurgood SRD *Senior Dietitian, Royal London Homoeopathic Hospital, London*

Bernice Tighe SRD *Diabetes Dietitian, Birmingham Heartlands Hospital*

Avni Vyas BSc SRD *Clinical Epidemiology Unit, University of Manchester*

Sunita Wallia SRD *Community Dietitian, Gartnavel Royal Hospital Glasgow*

Elizabeth Waters BSc SRD *Chief Oncology Dietitian, Clatterbridge Centre for Oncology*

Sheridan Waldron SRD *Dietetic Manager, Leicester Royal Infirmary NHS Trust*

Sue Wolfe SRD *Chief Dietitian, St James' University Hospital, Leeds*

Jane Wood BSc SRD *Senior Dietitian, Weston Park Hospital, Sheffield*

Hayley Wordsworth BSc SRD *Senior Oncology Dietitian, Churchill Hospital, Oxford*

Deborah Wyles SRD *Community Dietitian, St Luke's Hospital, Bradford*

The following specialist, interest and advisory groups of the British Dietetic Association:

- Burns Interest Group
- Community Nutrition Group (CNG)
- Diabetes Management and Education Group (DMEG)
- Dietitians in HIV and AIDS (DHIVA)
- Dietitians in Neurological Therapy (DINT)
- Dietitians in Primary Care
- Ethical and Professional Advisory Panel (EPAP)
- Gastroenterology Interest Group
- Multi-cultural Nutrition Group (MNG)
- Mental Health Group (MHG)
- Nutrition Advisory Group for Elderly People (NAGE)
- Nutritionists in Industry
- Oncology Group
- Paediatric Group
- Parenteral and Enteral Nutrition Group (PENG)
- Renal Nutrition Group
- UK Dietitians' Cystic Fibrosis Interest Group
- UK Heart Health and Thoracic Dietitians

Acknowledgements

Gaynor Bussell *Press Office, Medical Research Council, London*

Helen Brown *Lead Practitioner in Dietetics, Lifespan Healthcare NHS Trust, Cambridge*

Rebecca Capener *Nutritionist, Nutricia Clinical Care*

Pauline Cotterill *Membership Co-ordinator, British Dietetic Association, Birmingham*

Jane Eaton *Professional Affairs Officer, British Dietetic Association, Birmingham*

Simon Forrester *Information & Business Officer, British Dietetic Association, Birmingham*

Azmina Govindji *Consultant Nutritionist and Dietitian, Pinner, Middlesex*

Stuart Hayton *Chairman Primary Care Group of CNG*

Anne Heughan *Van den Bergh Foods*

Dr Anthony Holland *Department of Psychiatry, University of Cambridge*

Julie Holt *Food and Health Adviser, Lever Chambers Centre for Health, Bolton*

Sharran Howell *Nutrition Services Division, Fresenius Kabi*

Dr Janet Lambert *Chairman Nutritionists in Industry*

Val Jacob *Renal Dietitian, Northern General Hospital, Sheffield*

Jackie Lewin *Dietitian, SHS International Limited, Liverpool*

Anita MacDonald *Dietetic Manager, The Children's Hospital, Ladywood Middleway, Birmingham*

Michele Mackintosh *Community Nutrition and Diet Therapist, Ayrshire Central Hospital*

Carol Martin *Company Nutritionist, Tesco*

Karen McKittrick *Clinical Nutrition Services, SHS International*

Ailish Miranda *Clinical Dietetic Specialist, Nestlé Clinical Nutrition*

Judy More *Chairman Paediatric Group*

Sarah Nolan *Nutrition Manager, Van den Bergh Foods Ltd*

Elaine Riordan *Dietetic Services Manager, Novartis Consumer Health*

Christine Russell *Head of Nutrition, Nutricia Clinical Care*

Vanessa Shaw *Paediatric Dietitian, Great Ormond Street Hospital for Children, London*

Karen Shukla *Dietetic Manager, Basildon Hospital, Basildon*

Janet Stelling *Nutritional Advisor, SMA, Maidenhead*

Rae Ward *Formerly Dietetic Consultant, The Coeliac Society*

The Coeliac Society

Diabetes UK

Foreword

Once again I have the great pleasure of writing the Foreword to the *Manual of Dietetic Practice*, on this occasion the third edition. Although it is published on behalf of the British Dietetic Association, under the auspices of an editorial steering group, Dr Briony Thomas as Editor has made an enormous contribution. She has received help and advice from numerous experts in their fields and some of the writing has been done by others, but on the whole she has done a major part of the writing herself. In this way she has been able to provide more uniformity in style and depth of coverage. The contents are divided into six sections and I am overwhelmed by the thoroughness of the coverage. I have tried to find something that was missing and failed!

In recent years dietetics has assumed a much higher profile and all the caring professions, including doctors and nurses, require a basic knowledge of nutrition. I anticipate that this manual will find its way onto many shelves and into many libraries across the English-speaking world. There is now much greater appreciation that the maintenance of health and prevention of disease in closely linked to good nutrition and the role of the dietitian has become increasingly important. The British Dietetic Association can be proud of this manual and its outstanding editor for a major contribution to the knowledge of nutrition

Dame Barbara Clayton DBE
Honorary Research Professor in Metabolism, University of Southampton, Honorary President, British Dietetic Association.

Introduction

First published in 1988, the *Manual of Dietetic Practice* is a comprehensive guide to the principles and practice of dietetics across its entire spectrum – from health promotion to disease management. This is the third edition. The book aims to equip the student or novice dietitian with the solid foundations on which skills and expertise can be built, to provide dietitians moving into a new area of practice with the basic knowledge from which specialist skills can be developed, to update those returning to the profession after a career break with changes in practice and to act as a point of reference for all dietitians.

Unlike many other textbooks, the *Manual of Dietetic Practice* is not just a collection of chapters on isolated topics but a cohesive whole, with considerable interlinking between different subject areas. The text is divided into six main parts: General dietetic principles and practice, Foods and nutrients, Nutritional needs of population subgroups, Dietetic management of disease, Dietetic management of acute trauma, and Appendices.

The text has been completely revised to reflect the many advances in both nutritional knowledge and dietetic practice that have occurred in recent years. Healthcare is increasingly required to be patient centred, multidisciplinary in nature, evidence based, compatible with national standards, clinically effective and subject to audit and evaluation. As a result, the role of the dietitian has moved a long way from simply dispensing a particular diet for a particular disorder. While principles of care can be standardised, the way in which they are applied has to vary to take account of individual needs, problems, habits, lifestyle, associated health risks and readiness to change. In order to provide effective care, the dietitian has to exercise considerable clinical judgement in deciding how a specific set of circumstances may most appropriately be managed. This requires more than just nutritional knowledge. The modern-day dietitian has to be able to make a global risk assessment when setting nutritional goals, have an understanding of human behaviour in order to achieve dietary change, acquire the interviewing and counselling skills necessary for meaningful dialogue between patient and professional, and have the ability to evaluate whether objectives have been achieved. The contents of this edition reflect these changes in practice and include new topics such as achieving behavioural change, nutritional risk assessment, clinical effectiveness and healthcare ethics. More extensive coverage is also provided on problems such as undernutrition, dysphagia, dementias and neurorehabilitation.

This edition of the *Manual of Dietetic Practice* has been compiled in a different way to its predecessors. In order to provide greater consistency in terms of format and depth of coverage, much more of the writing has been carried out by one person (myself) rather than large numbers of different people, but with greater involvement of the British Dietetic Association's Specialist and Interest groups as well as individual experts. Many people have therefore played a part in the creation of this book. Some have had a major role in the revision of existing chapters or writing new ones. Others have played a smaller but no less essential part by providing information, advice or comments during the various stages of manuscript preparation. All have been crucial to the creation of the final product and I am enormously grateful to everyone who has provided assistance. Hopefully everyone who has contributed in some way has been acknowledged. If I have inadvertently missed anyone out, I sincerely apologise.

Many thanks are also due to the editorial steering group consisting of Loretta Cox, Jacki Bishop, Carole Middleton, Diane Talbot and Catherine Collins who have been a constant source of help and advice. I am also indebted to the British Dietetic Association for its continued support for this project and for the ever-willing assistance of John Grigg and other members of staff. Sincere thanks also to Richard Miles at Blackwell Science for his unfailing patience and good humour in the face of manuscript delays and ruined timetables, and to all those involved in the highly efficient final production and printing of the book.

This book has had a long gestation period. I very much hope its arrival lives up to expectations.

Briony Thomas

SECTION 1
General dietetic principles and practice

1.1   Diet, health and disease

Food is essential for health and survival. Without sufficient energy and nutrients, the body's ability to function normally is impaired. If the body is starved completely, life can only be sustained for a matter of weeks.

During the twentieth century, much was learnt about the role of nutrients in maintaining health, and the requirements for them to prevent deficiency diseases such as scurvy, pellagra and anaemia. In recent years it has become clear that diet also plays an aetiological role in the development of many life-threatening conditions associated with ageing, especially cardiovascular disease, stroke and cancer, as well as those causing significant morbidity such as constipation, obesity, osteoporosis and dental caries.

It is also being increasingly acknowledged that 'health' is more than just the absence of disease. Good health requires both physical and mental well-being and hence encompasses quality of life. Improving health requires consideration of issues such as education, employment, housing, poverty and social isolation, as well as dietary objectives and healthcare provision.

1.1.1   The global perspective

There are still many differences in the health problems of the poorer parts of the world and those of more affluent areas. In less developed regions, famine and chronic undernutrition remain a constant threat, mortality from infectious diseases, particularly the acquired immunodeficiency syndrome (AIDS) and tuberculosis (TB) is high, and childbirth still poses considerable risks to mother and child. Ninety-eight per cent of all deaths in children under the age of 15 years occur in the developing world (Murray and Lopez 1997).

In Britain, life expectancy has doubled since the midnineteenth century as a result of improvements in hygiene, safety and infection control. In 1841, 25% of children died before the age of 5 years, often from diseases such as scarlet fever, typhoid and whooping cough; in the population as a whole, one-third of deaths resulted from TB (ONS 1997). By the end of the twentieth century, these problems had drastically reduced in scale but new ones had emerged to take their place. Coronary heart disease (CHD) and cancer had become the major causes of death, with the UK having one of the highest CHD mortality rates in the world, many of the deaths occurring at a relatively young age. Stroke also accounted for significant mortality and morbidity. There was also growing realization that much of this mortality and morbidity was attributable to diet and lifestyle factors and hence preventable. The consumption of energy-dense diets, high in saturated fat and low in fibre and micronutrients, coupled with a sedentary lifestyle and use of tobacco, impact on many aspects of the process of atherogenesis, thrombogenesis or carcinogenesis, either directly or via their influence on other risk factors such as obesity, hypertension, hyperlipidaemia and diabetes.

It has also become apparent that within the UK there are major inequalities in health (and in healthcare provision), particularly between the richest and poorest sections of the population (Editorial 1997; Acheson 1998). Mortality and morbidity is greatest in those who are least advantaged, especially people from lower socioeconomic groups, some minority ethnic groups and those living in particular regions of the country, much of it attributable to adverse diet and lifestyle influences. There is increasing recognition that, in order to improve the health of the nation as a whole, the needs and problems of its most vulnerable sectors have to be addressed.

Not surprisingly, as developing countries acquire some of the less desirable aspects of the Western lifestyle, the prevalence of heart disease, stroke, cancer and diabetes in other parts of the world is also beginning to rise. Globally, as life expectancy increases, the prevalence of these diseases is expected to increase dramatically (WHO 1997).

1.1.2   Diet and health

A healthy diet has to fulfil two objectives:

1 It must provide sufficient energy and nutrients to maintain normal physiological functions, and permit growth and replacement of body tissues.
2 It must offer the best protection against the risk of disease.

Meeting the needs for energy and nutrients

Energy

The fundamental need of the human body is for a supply of energy. Without this, it will die within weeks. Most of this energy is derived from the metabolism of carbohydrate, fat and protein, the amount of energy released being measured in kilocalories (kcal) or kilojoules (kJ). Fat is the most energy-dense nutrient, providing 9 kcal (37 kJ) per gram. Protein (4 kcal or 17 kJ) and carbohydrate (3.75 kcal or 16 kJ) each provide less than half this amount of energy per gram. Other dietary constituents such as alcohol (7 kcal or 29 kJ) can also be a source of energy.

Because the body's priority for energy is so high, if insufficient energy is obtained from the diet it will start to 'cannibalize' its own tissues in order to meet energy needs. Initially it will make use of its fat stores but, as the energy deficit increases, muscle and other tissues will be broken down and used as a fuel supply.

Carbohydrate, protein and fat

Dietary carbohydrate (sugars and starches) is rapidly broken down to glucose and is the most readily available source of energy to the body. Dietary fat is a concentrated form of energy and also provides essential fatty acids necessary for the construction of cell membranes and many other functions. Protein provides amino acids which are essential for the growth and continuous replacement of body tissues and enzymes. However, in conditions of energy shortage, the body's need for a source of energy will take precedence and protein will be used as a fuel supply rather than for anabolic purposes.

Vitamins, minerals and trace elements

Many different substances are required by the body for the operation of enzyme systems, transport mechanisms, structural synthesis and regulatory processes. Most are only required in very small or even trace amounts. None provides energy so they cannot sustain life alone, but without vitamins, minerals and trace elements, metabolism will be impaired, body systems will malfunction, disease may result and life can be threatened.

Dietary fibre ('non-starch polysaccharide')

These terms refer to the unabsorbed residues of plant food, their value being in the fact that they are not absorbed (although components of them can be fermented to volatile short-chain fatty acids in the colon and used as a source of energy). Dietary fibre is not a uniform substance but a mixture of plant materials, the effects of some of which have yet to be evaluated. It is, however, clear that dietary fibre helps to maintain normal bowel function, increases the satiety value of a diet and may influence the absorption of nutrients and, indirectly, their metabolic effect.

Fluid

Fluid is also a vital component of a healthy diet; without fluid, survival time is limited to a matter of a few days, or even hours. Chronic dehydration can result in a number of ill-effects such as constipation, increased risk of renal stone formation and mental confusion. Acute dehydration (e.g. due to severe vomiting or diarrhoea) is life-threatening.

The requirements and function of each of these dietary constituents are discussed in more detail in Section 2 of the Manual. Dietary requirements for health and disease prevention are set out in Dietary Reference Values for the UK (DH 1991) (see Section 1.3, *Dietary reference values*, and Appendix 6.2).

Offering the best protection against disease

Since the mid-twentieth century, the emphasis on the type of diet needed to prevent disease has undergone a considerable change. In the 1940s and 1950s, the primary aim in the UK was to prevent nutritional deficiency. During World War II when food supplies were limited, rationing ensured nutritional adequacy for everyone. As food supplies improved in the post-war years, nutritional messages still emphasized the need for sufficiency, and a healthy diet was considered to be one containing plenty of protein-rich foods such as meat, fish, eggs and dairy foods. The needs of infants and children were especially targeted with the introduction of welfare vitamins, free school milk and school meals of an obligatory nutritional standard.

In recent years, it has become evident that 'sufficiency' has become 'surplus' for much of the population and that a high-protein, high-fat diet is not appropriate for long-term health. There is now broad consensus (WHO 1990; DH 1991, 1994a, 1998) that the type of diet which minimizes the risk of chronic disease is one which:

- has an energy content which is appropriate for body weight. Both underweight and overweight increase the risk of morbidity and mortality
- contains a relatively small proportion of this energy in the form of saturated fat. Most dietary fat should be composed of monounsaturates, together with sufficient *n*-6 and *n*-3 polyunsaturates
- contains a relatively high proportion of its energy in the form of starchy carbohydrate (and a low proportion as refined sugars)
- has a high fibre content, derived from both cereal foods and fruit, vegetables and pulses
- is relatively low in sodium and high in potassium
- is balanced in overall terms. The impact of diet on all aspects of health, not just one or two, has to be borne in mind. For example, measures to reduce saturated fat intake to prevent CHD should not inadvertently reduce the intake of iron or calcium and hence increase the risk of anaemia or osteoporosis.

1.1.3 Dietary targets for health

Numerical dietary targets for the UK population were first set out in the 1984 Committee on Medical Aspects of Food Policy (COMA) report on Cardiovascular Disease (DHSS 1984) and in the National Advisory Committee of Nutrition Education (NACNE) guidelines (NACNE 1983). The 1991 COMA report on Dietary Reference Values (DH 1991) forms the basis of current guidelines, together with some subsequent additional recommendations from the COMA report *Nutritional aspects of cardiovascular disease* (DH 1994a). These targets are summarized in Table 1.1.

The figures are population targets and are not necessarily what each person should consume. They simply represent changes in dietary composition which, if achieved on a population basis, would result in a significant

Table 1.1 Dietary targets for the UK population

	Recommended intake (DH 1991)	Current intake[1] (Gregory et al. 1990)	Change required
Total fat	< 35% energy	40% energy	Decrease (by 12%)
Saturated fat	11% energy	17% energy	Decrease (by 35%)
Monounsaturated fat	13% energy[2]	12% energy	No change[2]
Polyunsaturated fat	6.5% energy	6% energy	No further increase
n-3 polyunsaturates	0.2 g/day (minimum)	0.1 g/day	Intake of long-chain n-3 fatty acids should be at least doubled[4]
Trans fatty acids	2% energy	2% energy	No further increase
Total carbohydrate	50% energy	44% energy	Increase (by 13%)
Starches	33% energy	27% energy	Increase (by 22%)
Sugars (non-milk extrinsic sugars)	11% energy	17% energy	Decrease (by 35%)
Protein	< 15% energy	14% energy	No increase
Fibre (non-starch polysaccharide)	18 g/day[3]	12 g/day[3]	Increase (by 50%)
Salt (or equivalent as sodium)	6 g (2.4 g)[4]	9 g (3.6 g)	Decrease (by 33%)

[1]Mean rounded figures for men and women, excluding the energy contribution from alcohol.
[2]Monounsaturates may comprise a higher proportion of dietary energy provided that intake of saturates remains low and total energy intake does not exceed requirement (RCP 2000).
[3]Figures expressed as NSP, derived from DH (1991). The recommended daily intake has been estimated to be equivalent to 24 g when estimated by the AOAC method, i.e. that now used on most food labelling (see Section 2.5, *Dietary fibre*).
[4]DH (1994a, COMA report, *Nutritional aspects of cardiovascular disease*).

improvement in the nation's health. Individuals within the population have varying needs, and a diet of this composition is not necessarily suitable for those who are old, young or ill. Nevertheless, most people would benefit if the composition of their diet moved in the direction of these targets.

Recently, there has been a slight shift away from numerical targets in favour of food-based guidelines, in particular the 'Mediterranean diet', i.e. a diet high in fruits, vegetables, legumes and whole grains, and also containing fish, nuts and low-fat dairy products (RCP 2000). A diet of this type is considered to have valuable cardioprotective and other properties (see Section 4.21, Cardiovascular disease). Since most of the fat in the Mediterranean diet is derived from monounsaturated sources and relatively little from saturated fat, it is also suggested that the total proportion of fat energy can be higher than the current dietary target of <35% energy without detriment. In practice, however, many people still need to reduce their total fat and energy intake because they are overweight.

1.1.4 The UK diet

Sources on information on the UK diet

National information about the diet of the UK population is obtained from two main sources: the National Diet and Nutrition Survey (NDNS) and the National Food Survey (NFS).

The National Diet and Nutrition Survey Programme

This is a rolling programme of surveys which provides comprehensive nutritional information on a representative group of about 2000 subjects drawn from a particular age band of the population. Each survey includes weighed assessments of dietary intake in conjunction with anthropometric, biochemical and physiological measures of

nutritional status together with socioeconomic and demographic data.

To date, the programme has published reports on:

- children aged 1½–4½ years (Gregory *et al.* 1995; Hinds and Gregory 1995)
- young people aged 4–18 years (Gregory *et al.* 2000; Walker *et al.* 2000)
- adults aged 16–64 years (Gregory *et al.* 1990)
- adults aged 65 years and over (Finch *et al.* 1998; Steele *et al.* 1998).

The National Food Survey

This is an annual survey of household food consumption and expenditure carried out in about 8000 randomly selected households. The householder keeps a 7-day record of the quantity, type and cost of all food entering the home for human consumption. Since 1992, information on confectionery, alcoholic and soft drinks purchased for consumption inside and outside the home, and meals purchased outside the home has also been collected. The NFS does not directly measure food intake, only the food available for consumption, and makes no attempt to assess the distribution of food consumed by different members of a household. It is therefore not an accurate measure of the nutrient intake of individuals. The strength of the NFS is that it has been carried out continuously for over 50 years and is an invaluable marker of food-purchasing trends (Derry and Buss 1984).

Additional government information on the level of some micronutrients, contaminants, additives, pesticide residues and toxicants in the average UK diet is also provided by The Total Diet Study (TDS). Based on information derived from the NFS, foods representing the average UK diet are purchased from a variety of retail outlets in different regions of the UK and analysed for constituents considered to be of current interest or concern such as lead or selenium. The findings are published as Food Surveillance Information Sheets and available via the Food Standards Agency website.

Current nutrient intake of the UK population

The NDNS adult survey (Gregory *et al*. 1990; MAFF 1994) showed that the average UK diet tends to be high in fat, saturated fat and sugars, and low in starch and fibre (Table 1.2). While there are absolute differences in intake between the genders as a result of their different energy needs, proportional intakes as a percentage of dietary energy are very similar. There are significant socioeconomic and regional differences, with marked trends towards the highest intakes of fat and lowest intakes of fibre being found in people from the most deprived groups.

Further analysis (MAFF 1994) showed that there is a wide gap between recommended intake and actual consumption. Only 14% of the study population met the target intake for fat (<35% food energy intake) and fewer than 3% met the target for saturated fat (11% food energy). About 12% met the target for non-milk extrinsic sugars. Over one-quarter of the men achieved the target intake for fibre but fewer than 6% of women, largely because they consumed less energy, and hence less food in general. Some of those who met the fat targets often did so by consuming diets high in sugar or alcohol. Virtually none of the population sample met all of the targets.

Recent trends in UK food and nutrient intake

The National Food Survey (MAFF 1999) shows that, in absolute terms, the amount of fat consumed has fallen

considerably since the late 1980s (from 93 g/day in 1988 to 75 g/day in 1998). Saturated fat consumption has also fallen (from an average of 38.3 g/day in 1988 to 29.3 g/day in 1998). However, because total energy intake has also fallen significantly over the same period, percentage fat energy intake has only fallen slightly, from 42% in 1988 to 39% in 1998. The percentage of energy from saturated fat has only declined from 17% to 15%. Although in the right direction, both percentages still exceed recommended targets. Little if any progress has been made towards the target intakes for fibre and non-milk extrinsic sugars. Intakes of total carbohydrate and protein remain largely unchanged.

This relatively static nutritional profile of British diet masks considerable changes in the types of foods consumed. NFS data show that people now consume less red meat, whole milk, spreading and cooking fats, but more poultry, low-fat milks and low-fat spreads than they did a generation ago. At the same time, the consumption of carbohydrate in the form of bread and potatoes has also decreased, although this has been offset by an increased intake of breakfast cereals, rice, pasta and cakes. While consumption of fruit (especially bananas) has increased, much of this is attributable to a dramatic rise in the consumption of fruit juice. In contrast, consumption of green vegetables has hardly changed.

Eating habits and meal patterns have also altered. The desire to spend less time shopping, preparing, cooking and even eating food means that people eat fewer traditional meals within the home and more food in snack form, on the move or outside the home. Advances in food technology and the advent of the domestic freezer and microwave make it increasingly easy to prepare 'instant' meals. At the same time, people have become less physically active, both at home and at work. Labour-saving devices are available for household chores; the television and home computer often dominate leisure time; the car is used for journeys which before might have been made on foot or by bicycle. Many types of occupation now involve electronics rather than physical effort, e.g. machinery may be operated from a control panel instead of manually; security may be monitored by watching a closed-circuit TV screen rather than on foot.

The net result of this is that it has become easier to eat a diet which no longer balances nutritional needs. Diets tend to:

- **Provide too much energy relative to energy needs.** Lower levels of physical activity reduce the requirement for energy but the ready availability of pleasant-tasting but perhaps energy-dense, fat-rich and sugar-rich foods and snacks means that energy needs are easily exceeded.
- **Lack variety.** Paradoxically, despite the enormous increase in choice of foods available, lack of variety is a problem in many diets. In the past, food choice tended to be governed by what was available, and the seasonality of food production tended to ensure that a variety of foods would be eaten throughout the year. Nowadays,

Table 1.2 Mean energy and nutrient intakes of the UK population (Gregory *et al*. 1990)

Average daily intake	Men (*n* = 1087)	Women (*n* = 1110)
Energy (kcal [MJ])	2450 (10.3)	1680 (7.05)
Fat (g)	102.3	73.5
Saturated fatty acids (g)	42.0	31.1
Trans fatty acids (g)	5.6	4.0
Carbohydrate (g)	272.0	193.0
Total sugars (g)	115.0	86.0
Protein (g)	84.7	62.0
Dietary fibre (Southgate)[1] (g)	24.9	18.6
% Fat energy[2]	40.4%	40.3%
% Saturated fat energy[2]	16.5 %	17%
% Carbohydrate energy[2]	44.7%	44.2%
% Protein energy[2]	14.1%	15.2%

[1]These figures (measured by the Southgate method) are considerably higher than measurements of NSP by the Englyst method from which current dietary reference values (DRVs) are derived. Gregory's figures should be interpreted in the context of a recommended daily intake of 30 g dietary fibre/day, rather than the current DRV of 18 g NSP/day (DH 1991).
[2]Excluding alcohol.

people can more easily choose food on the basis of what they like or fancy. Some people choose to eat the same few favourite foods most of the time.

- **Lack fresh foods**. Especially fruit and vegetables (Billson *et al.* 1999). Less time for food preparation means that meals are often something quick and easy derived from a carton, packet or can, possibly high in fat, sugar and salt. Ready meals may be eaten without accompanying vegetables (other than chips).

These are often key issues to be addressed in order to improve the nutritional composition of the diet.

Changes needed to achieve dietary targets

Achieving the recommended dietary targets will require considerable changes in the dietary habits of the nation (Bingham 1991; DH 1994a), typically necessitating:

- a 50% increase in the consumption of potatoes and bread
- fruit and vegetable intake being doubled
- full-fat milk and dairy products being replaced by reduced/low-fat alternatives
- saturated fat spreads and cooking fats being replaced by low-fat spreads or monounsaturated oils
- all meat being lean meat
- the consumption of two portions of fish per week, one of which should be oily fish
- a 50% reduction in the consumption of biscuits, cakes, chips and snacks, sweets and soft drinks.

How these objectives can be achieved in practice is discussed in Section 1.2 (Healthy eating).

1.1.5 The health of the UK nation

In the UK, data on mortality and morbidity are collected by the Office of National Statistics (ONS) and health trends are monitored and published in a series of annual reports from the Chief Medical Officer. Since 1991, these have also been accompanied by an annual Health Survey for England which assesses a number of health parameters in a nationally representative sample of the population. In the early surveys, the sample size was confined to about 3000 people but from 1993 this was expanded to about 16 000 so that socioeconomic and regional variations could be included in the analysis. Each Health Survey has a 'core' component to obtain information on, for example, body weight, blood pressure, prescribed medications, tobacco use and alcohol consumption, plus one or more additional modules on a subject of special interest such as cardiovascular disease or the health of children and young people.

The first Health Survey for England (White *et al.* 1993) revealed that the health of the UK population left much to be desired. Almost half of the adult population was overweight and 13% of men and 16% of women could be classified as obese. Over two-thirds of the population had a raised blood cholesterol level and one-sixth had a

blood pressure which exceeded 160 mmHg (systolic) or 95 mmHg (diastolic). Exercise levels were low. Only 12% of men and 11% of women had none of the main risk factors for cardiovascular disease (smoking, raised blood pressure, raised blood cholesterol and lack of physical activity). Similar concerns have been found in other parts of the UK, particularly in Scotland.

Subsequent surveys have shown that, in many respects, the health of the nation has not greatly improved and in some instances worsened. By 1998 (DH 1999a) the prevalence of overweight and obesity had significantly increased, with 17.3% of men and 21.2% of women having a body mass index (BMI) between 30 and 40, the worst in Europe. Alcohol consumption in women had increased and young people were more likely to have adverse drinking habits with respect to amount and frequency. Only 37% of men and 25% of women were taking the recommended levels of physical activity (i.e. at least 30 min of activity of moderate intensity 5 days per week). The overall prevalence of smoking had remained much the same, a fall in the prevalence in older age groups being counterbalanced by an increase in younger age groups. The 1998 Health Survey (DH 1999a) also highlighted major differences in the health parameters between socioeconomic groups, with an increasing prevalence of obesity, hypertension and smoking as income declined.

1.1.6 Strategies to improve the nation's health

The *Health of the Nation* strategy

In 1992, in response to the clear need for a national strategy to improve the nation's health (Smith and Jacobsen 1988), the Government launched its *Health of the Nation* (HoN) initiative (DH 1992). A similar document was produced in Scotland (Scottish Office 1993). The HoN strategy was designed to promote health as well as preventing disease, i.e. it aimed to improve the quality of life as well as its longevity, 'not just by adding years to life but also by adding life to years' (DH 1992). It identified five priority areas for action: coronary heart disease and stroke; cancers; mental health; HIV/AIDS and sexual health and accidents. Targets were set in terms of reductions in incidence or mortality rates, and in the prevalence of some risk factors associated with them (e.g. obesity, hypertension, physical inactivity or smoking). Timescales by which they were to be achieved were also set. Specific dietary targets were to reduce total and saturated fat energy to <35% and <11%, respectively, by the year 2005. Task forces were created to translate these targets into realistic action plans.

The Nutrition Task Force

A Nutrition Task Force (NTF) was formed in October 1992 to consider how the dietary objectives necessary to meet the HoN targets, particularly in respect of cardiovascular disease and stroke, might be achieved. In 1993 a Physical Activity Task Force was created to work with the NTF to develop strategies to achieve the targets on obesity.

The NTF's action plan, *Eat Well!* (DH 1994b), listed 12 priorities areas to be tackled (such as nutrition educational material, labelling, food advertising, nutrition guidance for caterers, and the training of healthcare professionals) and 16 project teams were formed to tackle them. Several excellent reports were produced by NTF project teams (see Further Reading). The NTF was disbanded in 1995, with some aspects of its work being devolved to areas of the community to ensure its continuing progress. Its final report, *Eat Well II*, was published in the following year (DH 1996).

A similar group to the NTF, the Scottish Diet Action Group (SDAG), was set up in Scotland in 1994 to develop an action plan in response to the diet and health issues identified in the Scottish Diet Report, and published its multiagency action plan 2 years later (Scottish Office/DH 1996).

Effectiveness of the Health of the Nation strategy

Overall, the HoN programme had mixed success. The House of Commons Public Accounts Committee (1997) which monitored the targets reported that encouraging progress had been made in 11 of the 27 target areas and that 'good' results had been achieved on CHD, stroke and some cancers. However, the committee was dismayed by the lack of progress in others and the fact that in three areas the desired trend was moving in the opposite direction, i.e. the prevalence of obesity, alcohol consumption in women and tobacco use by teenagers.

Some health professionals consider that the HoN targets were unrealistic. Obstacles to achieving them were considered to be an over-ambitious timescale, lack of resources, inability to influence socioeconomic factors linked to health, difficulties in persuading people to change their eating habits and lack of effectiveness of national health campaigns (Cheung *et al.* 1997).

Current public health initiatives

A change in government in 1997 led to a re-evaluation of the way of in which the health needs of the population were to be met. The White Paper *The New NHS: Modern, Dependable* (DH 1997) introduced a number of National Health Service (NHS) reforms designed to provide better and uniform quality of care. Separate White Papers for health reform in Scotland (*Designed to Care: Renewing the NHS in Scotland*) and Wales (*Putting Patients First: The Future of the NHS in Wales*) were published. Some of the new initiatives set up as a result are summarized in Table 1.3. The ways in which desired health objectives should be met and health inequalities overcome were also reconsidered.

Table 1.3 Recent initiatives to improve healthcare and health provision in the UK (DH 1997)

Clinical governance	A quality initiative to improve standards of care throughout the whole of the health service. It includes action to ensure that risks are avoided, mistakes openly investigated and lessons learned with systems in place to ensure continuous improvements in care
Commission for Health Improvement (CHI)	A national body to monitor care standards and clinical services (England/Wales)
Health Action Zones	These aim to tackle specific health problems in particular parts of the country by means of innovative interorganizational schemes. Eleven health action zones were set up in 1988 and a further 15 in 1999, in some of the most deprived parts of the country
Health Improvement Programme (HImP)	A Health Authority-led action programme to improve, and reduce inequalities in, health and healthcare within a particular area. It involves NHS Trusts, Primary Care Groups and other primary care professionals working in partnership with the local authority and voluntary groups. A HImP considers how the national priorities in terms of CHD and stroke, cancer, mental health and accidents should be tackled in the context of local health needs and problems (e.g. whether the local population has a high proportion of older adults, people from ethnic minorities, single parents, or a high prevalence of drug and alcohol abuse). It also shows how National Service Frameworks (see below) are to be implemented at local level
National Institute for Clinical Excellence (NICE) (England/Wales)	Produces clinical guidelines based on clinical and cost effectiveness. In Scotland, the Scottish Health Technology Assessment Centre (SHTAC) which assesses the cost-effectiveness of treatments and drugs, and the Scottish Intercollegiate Guidelines Network (SIGN) which produces evidence-based guidelines, together perform a similar function to NICE
National Service Framework (NSF) (England/Wales)	National Service Frameworks set national standards and define service models for health promotion, disease prevention, diagnosis, treatment, rehabilitation and care. They aim to ensure that the best standards of care are available in all parts of the country and reduce variations in service quality. By 2000, NSF for Mental Health and CHD had been published and others such as for Diabetes and Older People were in preparation
Primary Care Groups (PCG) (England) Local Health Groups (LHG) (Wales) and Local Health Care Co-operatives (LHCC) (Scotland)	Local groups of GPs and community nurses who work with their health authority to determine healthcare strategy and priorities within a particular area Primary Care Trusts (PCTs) which incorporate some of the responsibilities of health authorities are a further development

Table 1.4 Health targets for the UK population (DH 1999b)

Priority Area	Parameter	Target by 2010
Cancer	Deaths from cancer in people under 75 years	Reduce by at least one-fifth
CHD and Stroke	Deaths from CHD and Stroke in people under 75 years	Reduce by at least two-fifths
Accidents	Deaths from accidents	Reduce by at least one-fifth
Mental Health	Deaths from suicide	Reduce by at least one-fifth

CHD: coronary heart disease.

Saving Lives: Our Healthier Nation

In July 1999 *Saving Lives: Our Healthier Nation* (OHN), a Government action plan for tackling poor health, was published (DH 1999b). It aims to:

* improve the health of the population as a whole by increasing the length of people's lives and the number of years spent free from illness
* improve the health of the worst off in society and to narrow the health gap.

Four priority areas necessary to meet these goals were identified – cancer, CHD and stroke, accidents and mental health – which together account for over 75% deaths in people under the age of 75 years. The Government's aim is to prevent 300 000 unnecessary and untimely deaths between now and the year 2010 by achieving the targets summarized in Table 1.4. The Health Development Agency (HDA), derived from the former Health Education Authority (HEA), has been set up to play a central part in implementing OHN.

The main difference from its HoN predecessor is that OHN stresses the need for initiatives at a local level, taking local health needs into account, and the development of interactive partnerships between care providers, support services and communities. It also aims to improve health by tackling the issues which impact on health, such as poor housing, poverty, unemployment, crime, poor education and family breakdown.

OHN gives no specific dietary targets but focuses more on initiatives which will help achieve diet and lifestyle objectives, e.g. healthy eating within schools, safer travel to school (to encourage exercise and decrease car use), improved shopping access for people living in deprived neighbourhoods, health skills training for parents of the most disadvantaged young children, and the promotion of breast feeding.

In conjunction with other recent healthcare reforms, the government hopes that the OHN will make a real impact on inequalities in health and healthcare, especially among the most disadvantaged members of society.

Text written by: Briony Thomas

Useful addresses

Ministry of Agriculture, Fisheries and Food (MAFF)
Ergon House, c/o Nobel House, 17 Smith Square, London SW1P 3JR
Consumer helpline: 0345 573012
Website: www.maff.gov.uk

Department of Health (DH)
Richmond House, 79 Whitehall, London SW1A 2NL
Tel: 020 7210 4850
Website: www.doh.gov.uk

Food Standards Agency (FSA)
England: Room 6/21, Hannibal House, PO Box 30080, London SE1 6YA
Scotland: St Magnus House, 6th Floor, 25 Guild Street, Aberdeen AB11 6NJ
Wales: 1st Floor, Southgate House, Wood Street, Cardiff CF10 1EQ
Northern Ireland: 10B and 10C Clarendon Quay, Clarendon Dock, Clarendon Road, Belfast BT1 3BW
Website: www.foodstandards.gov.uk

Health Development Agency (formerly the Health Education Authority)
Trevelyan House, 30 Great Peter Street, London SW1 2HW
Tel: 020 7222 5300
Website: www.hda-online.org.uk
Many publications and resources formerly produced by the Health Education Authority are still available from Marston Book Services.
Tel: 01235 465565

Health Promotion England (continuing some of the public education work of the former Health Education Authority)
50 Eastbourne Terrace, London W2 3QR
Website: www.hpe.org.uk

Further reading

Nutrition Task Force Reports
Catering
Department of Health. *Healthy Catering Practice*. London: DH, 1993.
Department of Health. *Nutrition Guidelines for Hospital Catering*. London: DH, 1995.
Department of Health. *Nutrition Guidelines for Hospital Catering: A Checklist for Audit*. London: DH, 1996.

School-meal providers
Department for Education and Employment. *Eating Well at School: Dietary Guidance for School Food Providers*. London: Department for Education and Employment, 1997.
> *Part 1. Guidance for Governors and Head teachers in Schools which do not manage their own School Meals Contract.*

Part 2. Guidance for Policy Makers in Local Education Authorities and Schools which manage their own School Meals Contracts.

Part 3. Guidance for Catering Contract Managers and Caterers in Schools.

Nutrition education

Department of Health. *Nutrition and Health: A Handbook for NHS Managers.* London: DH, 1994.

Guidelines for Education Materials:

Department of Health. *The Health of the Nation. Core Curriculum for Nutrition in the Education of Health Professionals.* Nutrition Task Force Project Team on Nutrition Education and Training for Health Professionals. London: HMSO, 1994.

Department of Health. *Guidelines on Educational Materials Concerned with Nutrition.* A Report by the Nutrition Task Force. London: DH, 1996.

Department of Health. *Nutrition for Medical Students: Nutrition in the Undergraduate Medical Curriculum.* London: DH, 1996.

Low income

Department of Health. *Low Income, Food, Nutrition and Health: Strategies for Improvement.* A Report by the Low Income Project Team for the Nutrition Task Force. London: DH, 1996.

Obesity and Physical activity

Department of Health. *Obesity: Reversing the Increasing Problem of Obesity in England.* London: DH, 1995.

Department of Health. *More People, More Active, More Often: Physical Activity in England: A Consultation Paper.* London: DH, 1995.

References

Acheson D. *Inequalities in Health: An Independent Inquiry.* London: The Stationery Office, 1998.

Billson H, Pryer JA, Nichols R. Variation in fruit and vegetable consumption among adults in Britain. An analysis from the dietary and nutritional survey of British adults. *European Journal of Clinical Nutrition* 1999; **53**: 946–952.

Bingham S. Dietary Aspects of a Health Strategy for England. *British Medical Journal* 1991; **303**: 353–355.

Cheung P, Hungin APS, Verrill J *et al.* Are the Health of the Nation's targets attainable? Postal survey of general practitioners' views. *British Medical Journal* 1997; **314** April: 1250–1251.

Department of Health. Report of the Panel on Dietary Reference Values of the Committee on Medical Aspects of Food Policy (COMA). *Dietary Reference Values for Food Energy and Nutrients for the United Kingdom.* Report on Health and Social Subjects 41. London: HMSO, 1991.

Department of Health. *Health of the Nation: A Strategy for Health in England.* London: HMSO, 1992.

Department of Health. Report of the Cardiovascular Review Group of the Committee on Medical Aspects of Food Policy (COMA). *Nutritional Aspects of Cardiovascular Disease.* Report on Health and Social Subjects 46. London: HMSO, 1994a.

Department of Health. *Eat Well!: An Action Plan from the Nutrition Task Force to Achieve the Health of the Nation Targets on Diet and Nutrition.* London: DH, 1994b.

Department of Health. *Eat Well II: A Progress Report from the Nutrition Task Force on the Action Plan to Achieve the Health of the Nation Targets on Diet and Nutrition.* London: DH, 1996.

Department of Health. *The New NHS: Modern, Dependable.* London: The Stationery Office, 1997.

Department of Health. Report of the Working Group on Diet and Cancer of the Committee on Medical Aspects of Food and Nutrition Policy (COMA). *Nutritional Aspects of the Development of Cancer.* Report on Health and Social Subjects 48. London: The Stationery Office, 1998.

Department of Health. *Health Survey for England: Cardiovascular Disease 1998.* Vol. 1. *Findings.* Erens B, Primatesta P (Eds). London: The Stationery Office, 1999a.

Department of Health. *Saving Lives: Our Healthier Nation.* London: The Stationery Office, 1999b.

Department of Health and Social Security (DHSS). Committee on Medical Aspects of Food Policy (COMA). *Diet and Cardiovascular Disease.* Report of Health and Social Subjects 28. London: HMSO, 1984.

Derry BJ, Buss DH. The British National Food Survey as a major epidemiological resource. *British Medical Journal* 1984; **288**: 765–767

Editorial. Health inequality: the UK's biggest issue. *Lancet* 1997; **349**: 1185.

Finch S, Doyle W, Lowe C *et al. National Diet and Nutrition Survey: People Aged 65 Years and Over.* Vol. 1. *Report of the Diet and Nutrition Survey.* London: The Stationery Office, 1998.

Gregory J, Foster K, Tyler H, Wiseman M. *The Dietary and Nutritional Survey of British Adults.* London: HMSO, 1990.

Gregory JR, Collins DL, Davies PSW *et al. National Diet and Nutrition Survey: Children Aged 1½ and 4½ Years.* Vol. 1. *Report of the Diet and Nutrition Survey.* London: HMSO, 1995.

Gregory J *et al. National Diet and Nutrition Survey: Young People aged 4 to 18 Years.* Vol. 1. *Report of the Diet and Nutrition Survey.* London: The Stationery Office, 2000.

Hinds K, Gregory JR. *National Diet and Nutrition Survey: Children aged 1½ to 4½ years.* Vol. 2. *Report of the Dental Survey.* London: HMSO, 1995.

House of Commons Committee of Public Accounts. *Health of the Nation: A Progress Report.* London: The Stationery Office, 1997.

MAFF. *The Dietary and Nutritional Survey of British Adults – Further Analyses.* London: HMSO, 1994.

MAFF. *National Food Survey 1998. Annual Report on Food Expenditure, Consumption and Nutrient Intakes.* London: The Stationery Office, 1999.

Murray CJL, Lopez AD. Mortality cause for eight regions of the world: Global Burden of Disease Study. *Lancet* 1997; **349**: 1269–1276.

National Advisory Committee of Nutrition Education (NACNE). *Proposals for Nutritional Guidelines for Health Education in Britain.* London: Heath Education Council, 1983.

Office of National Statistics (ONS). *The Health of Adult Britain.* London: The Stationery Office, 1997.

Royal College of Physicians. *2000 Consensus Statement: Dietary Fat, the Mediterranean Diet and Lifelong Good Health.* London: RCP, 2000.

Scottish Office, Home and Health Department. *The Scottish Diet: Report of a Working Party to the Chief Medical Officer for Scotland.* Edinburgh: The Scottish Office, 1993.

Scottish Office/Department of Health. *Eating for Health, A Diet Action Plan.* Edinburgh: HMSO, 1996.

Smith A, Jacobsen B. *The Nation's Health: A Strategy for the 1990s*. London: King Edward's Hospital Fund, 1988.

Steele JG, Sheiham A, Marcenes W, Walls AWG. *National Diet and Nutrition Survey: People Aged 65 Years and Over*. Vol. 2. *Report of the Oral Health Survey*. London: The Stationery Office, 1998.

Walker A *et al*. *National Diet and Nutrition Survey: Young People Aged 4 to 18 years*. Vol. 2. *Report of the Oral Health Survey*. London: The Stationery Office, 2000.

White A *et al*. *Health Survey for England 1991: A Survey Carried out by OPCS on Behalf of the Department of Health*. London: HMSO, 1993.

World Health Organization (WHO). Diet, nutrition and the prevention of chronic diseases. A report of the WHO Study Group on Diet, Nutrition and Prevention of Noncommunicable Diseases. *Technical Report Series* 797. Geneva: WHO, 1990.

World Health Organization (WHO). *Conquering Suffering, Enriching Humanity*. 1997 Annual Report of the World Health Organization. Geneva: WHO, 1997.

A healthy diet is one that provides sufficient energy and nutrients to prevent deficiency but also helps to optimize health and reduce the risk of disease. The composition of a diet which helps to achieve these objectives is discussed in Section 1.1 (Diet, health and disease). This section discusses how these compositional targets can be realized in practice.

1.2.1 Translating dietary targets into food intake

Dietary targets for the population are usually set in numerical terms such as a desirable proportion of dietary energy intake (e.g. < 35% fat energy) or a quantitative target to be either achieved or not exceeded (e.g. >18 g non-starch polysaccharide or <6 g salt/day; see Section 1.1.3). While quantitative targets are invaluable for health professionals and people who plan food supplies, they are only of limited value to the general public who eat 'foods' rather than 'nutrients'.

Following publication of the first quantitative UK dietary targets in the 1980s (NACNE 1983; DHSS 1984),

attempts to interpret what these meant in terms of food consumption led to many different messages from the media, advertising industry and health professionals. Undue emphasis was often placed on foods which were either 'good' or 'bad' and little attention was paid to overall dietary balance. Inconsistent messages as to what should, or should not, be eaten led to increasing confusion and the impression that experts were constantly changing their minds (NDC/MORI, 1992). Guidance was also often negative in overtone, with much emphasis on denial of popular foods but with few appealing alternatives being suggested. Healthy eating came to be regarded as something worthy but joyless – a form of penance to be observed from time to time, before resuming a pleasurable diet.

In an attempt to redress the misinformation and negativity, the Ministry of Agriculture, Fisheries and Food (MAFF) and the Health Education Authority (HEA) issued general guidelines on healthy eating for the general public (*Eight Guidelines for a Healthy Diet*, MAFF 1991, revised 1997) (Table 1.5). These were useful and remain valid, but the Nutrition Task Force set up as part of the Health of the

Table 1.5 Eight guidelines for a healthy diet

1. **Enjoy your food**
   Eating should be a pleasant aspect of life. Healthy eating does not mean that some foods are banned and that others are obligatory. It just means getting a better balance of foods in the diet in order to maximize health and minimize the risk of disease
2. **Eat a variety of different foods**
   The greater the variety of foods eaten, the more likely it is that the diet will contain all the essential nutrients, especially vitamins and minerals, necessary for health
3. **Eat the right amount to be a healthy weight**
   Being overweight leads to many health problems. It places greater stress on bones and joints, raises blood pressure and cholesterol level, worsens any breathing difficulties and increases the risk of developing diabetes, heart disease and stroke. Eating the right diet and being physically active help to maintain correct body weight
4. **Eat plenty of foods rich in starch and fibre**
   Contrary to what many people think, foods such as bread and potatoes are not 'fattening' but provide important nutrients such as B vitamins and fibre, are filling without providing too much fat or energy, and are relatively cheap. These foods should be a major part of every diet
5. **Eat plenty of fruit and vegetables**
   These foods are not only major sources of nutrients such as vitamin C and dietary fibre but also provide important antioxidant nutrients which may help to protect against heart disease and cancer. Everyone should eat at least five portions of fruit and vegetables every day
6. **Don't eat too many foods that contain a lot of fat**
   Eating too much fat tends to raise blood cholesterol level and increases the risk of obesity and heart disease. Most people would benefit from eating less fat, particularly spreading fats such as butter and margarine, cooking fats and fried foods, dairy fats in full-fat milk and cheese, meat fat and foods containing these types of fat such as pastry and pies
7. **Don't have sugary foods and drinks too often**
   These foods are fine as occasional treats but too many of them will increase the likelihood of the diet being too high in energy and too low in essential nutrients. Frequent intake of sugar-rich foods also causes tooth decay
8. **If you drink alcohol, drink sensibly**
   While modest amounts of alcohol are not harmful to most people, and may even have health advantages in some circumstances, regularly exceeding safe drinking limits (3–4 units/day for men; 2–3 units/day for women) incurs progressive health risks.

Based on guidelines issued by MAFF (1991, revised 1997).

Nation initiative (see Section 1.1.6) concluded that more specific guidance on food choice was also needed. Their focus studies showed that people found it difficult to perceive what eating 'less saturated fat' or 'more fibre' meant in terms of food choice. In order to do so, people needed to know which foods contain them, and general knowledge on this subject tended to be poor or inaccurate. While the advent of nutrition labelling had made it easier to discover this information, most people were still unable to interpret the figures given in the context of whether the amount present is 'a little' or 'a lot'.

As a result, a National Food Guide was developed (Hunt *et al.* 1995a, b; Gatenby *et al.* 1995) as a joint initiative between MAFF, DH and the HEA on behalf of the Nutrition Task Force. The aim was to provide a model which would help people understand what healthy eating means in terms of food choice and which could also be used as a nationwide teaching model so that healthy eating messages would always be consistent. The end result, called *The Balance of Good Health*, was launched in July 1994 (HEA 1994). Supporting material for educators and communicators was also produced.

1.2.2 The national food guide: *The Balance of Good Health*

Many countries (e.g. the USA) have used a food pyramid as a conceptual guide to dietary balance (USDA 1992). Following consumer trials, the UK opted for a pictorial model of a tilted plate with divisions of varying sizes, each representing one of five food groups to show the types and proportions of foods in a well balanced and healthy diet (Fig. 1.1). Guidance is also given on the approximate number of servings of each food group which should be consumed each day (Table 1.6). Because different people need different amounts of food, a 'serving' is a relative amount rather than a precisely quantified one. A young active adult will obviously need larger serving sizes than a young child or elderly person. The point is that the *proportion* of different types of foods in the diet should always be approximately the same.

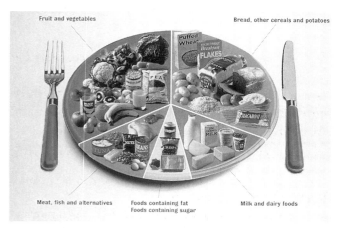

Fig. 1.1 *The Balance of Good Health*. Reproduced with permission from the Health Education Authority (HEA 1994).

The food group model conveys some important messages:

1 It attempts to change the traditional perception that a meal has to be centred around protein-rich foods such as meat, fish, cheese or eggs. Instead, starchy foods and fruit and vegetables should form a much larger proportion of food intake.
2 Healthy eating does not mean that some foods must be eaten while others are banned. It is simply a question of proportion. Over a period of time, some types of foods should be eaten more often, others less often.
3 A healthy diet has plenty of scope for flexibility; it is not confined to the same foods every day.
4 Overall dietary balance is important. No food contains every single nutrient required, so people need to eat a mixture of foods to obtain them all. It is the balance of this mixture, i.e. 'the diet' that has implications for health.

The Balance of Good Health model has many advantages:

• It is flexible enough to be applicable to all age-groups from toddlers to elderly people and all levels of energy and nutrient requirements. (It is not intended for use in children under the age of 2 years.)
• It can be used to assess dietary adequacy. Comparing the proportion of food groups in an individual's diet with the recommended proportion can indicate the likelihood of nutritional problems (see Section 1.5, Dietary assessment).
• It can be used as a basis for dietary modification. The mismatch between the actual and ideal proportion of food groups in an individual's diet reveals the type of dietary changes that need to be made (see Section 1.6, Dietary modification).
• Food choice guidance can be targeted towards individual needs or desired therapeutic objectives. A person who is overweight can be encouraged to make low-fat, low-energy density choices; a person with a small appetite or who is undernourished can be guided towards more nutrient-dense foods. High-fibre food choices can be recommended to the constipation sufferer; the person at high risk of cardiovascular disease (CVD) can be strongly advised to include oily fish among their choices from the 'Meat, fish and alternatives' group; someone with anaemia might be encouraged to include more red meat.
• Although not specifically intended for use in people with special dietary needs, it can often be used as a basic framework for therapeutic dietary guidance. It is sometimes overlooked that people who develop one disorder are not immune from the chronic diseases associated with ageing, e.g. someone with coeliac disease can still develop coronary heart disease; someone with diabetes can suffer an osteoporotic fracture. A global approach to health is important. Although the focus of advice given to, for example, the coeliac patient will be the avoidance of gluten, that advice should be given in the context of a diet which is balanced in terms of overall composition and protective for long-term

Table 1.6 Suggested proportions of different food groups in *The Balance of Good Health* (HEA 1994)

Food group	Foods included	Amount to be consumed	Principal nutrients provided
Bread, cereals and potatoes	Bread, rolls, crispbread, muffins, scones, pikelets, chapattis, pitta bread Breakfast cereals Pasta Rice Potatoes	• About one-third of the total volume of food eaten • For most people about 4–6 servings/per day • This is probably more than people currently consume	Carbohydrate Fibre (particularly insoluble fibre) B vitamins Some calcium and iron
Fruit and vegetables	All types of fruit and vegetables (except potatoes – see above), e.g. fresh, frozen, canned, dried, juices	• About one-third of the total volume of food eaten • A minimum of 5 portions per day • This is more than most people usually eat	Vitamin C Carotenes and other antioxidants Folates Fibre (especially soluble fibre) Potassium
Milk and dairy products	Milk Cheese Yoghurt Fromage frais Crème fraiche	• About one-sixth of the total volume of food intake • 2–3 servings per day of e.g. 1/3 pint of milk, one carton yoghurt, small piece (40 g) hard cheese	Calcium Protein Riboflavin Vitamins A and D (full-fat produce only)
Meat, fish and alternatives	Meat Poultry Offal Fish Meat and fish products Eggs Liver and kidney Pulses (beans and lentils) Nuts	• Up to about one-sixth of the total volume of food consumed • About 2 servings per day	Protein Iron B vitamins Zinc Magnesium
Fat-rich and sugar-rich foods	*Fat-rich foods* Butter, margarines and fat spreads Cooking fats and oils Pastry, e.g. pies, flans, sausage rolls Fried foods Savoury snacks, e.g. crisps Cream Rich sauces; fatty gravy Mayonnaise and salad dressings *Sugar-rich foods* Cakes Biscuits Puddings Ice-cream Chocolate and confectionery Soft and fizzy drinks	• These foods should ideally comprise no more than about one-twelfth of total food intake • This is less than most people usually consume	Some vitamins and essential fatty acids but often in conjunction with considerable quantities of fat, sugar and/or salt

health. Giving dietary advice in terms of suitable food choices from the *Balance of Good Health* food groups can help to achieve this.

There are some difficulties with *The Balance of Good Health* because not all foods fit neatly into one group. Composite foods such as casseroles, pies, pizza and pasta dishes may contain elements from most or all of the groups. Foods such as certain types of cheese or meat products can be regarded as a 'fat-rich' choices as well as those from their designated food groups. People also find it confusing that potatoes are, for nutritional reasons, grouped with bread and cereals when they consider them to be a 'vegetable'. However, evaluation studies showed that the general concept is easy to understand and implement (Hunt *et al.* 1995b).

Guidance on food choices in *The Balance of Good Health*

Points which may be relevant to guidance on food choice are summarized below.

Bread, cereals and potatoes

Many people still perceive these foods to be 'fattening' and need to be reassured that the opposite is true: they provide a lot of bulk without too many calories. Their energy content only increases substantially when fat is added to them (e.g. potatoes become chips or fat is thickly spread on bread). Suggesting the use of thicker slices of bread can be a useful way of boosting carbohydrate intake without increasing fat consumption.

In most cases, addition of fat should be discouraged (e.g. minimal amounts spread on bread or used in cooking). The converse may apply to people requiring a more energy-dense diet (e.g. elderly people with small appetites).

Wholemeal bread, brown rice and wholegrain cereals can be encouraged to increase fibre intake, increase dietary satiety value or alleviate constipation. These choices may be less suitable for children or for people with poor energy intake.

Many breakfast cereals are fortified with micronutrients and can be a valuable dietary source of folate, other B vitamins and iron. They are also a good choice as a snack food, particularly for hungry teenagers.

Fruit and vegetables

In practice, most people need to double their intake of fruit and vegetables and consume about 400 g (approximately 1 lb) per day. A useful rule of thumb to aim for is at least five servings a day (excluding potatoes), sometimes referred to in health promotion campaigns known as 'Give me 5' or '5 a day'.

Although, in general, guidance on portion size should not be too prescriptive, Williams (1995) has provided clarification on what might be considered to constitute 'a portion' of fruit or vegetables. These typically equate to an edible weight of 80 g, e.g. a large slice of melon or pineapple, one apple, a wine glass of fruit juice, a bowl of salad, two serving spoonfuls of green or root vegetables, three serving spoons of peas or sweetcorn, or three serving spoons of stewed or canned fruit. However, these should be adjusted for age and activity level: active men should have larger portions and children smaller ones.

Processed foods with only a small fruit/vegetable content (e.g. fruit cake, fruit yoghurt, vegetable soups and fruit-flavour soft drinks) should not count towards the five-a-day total. It is also suggested that only one of the five portions should be in the form of fruit juice, because even unsweetened fruit juice has high content of non-milk extrinsic sugars.

People should be encouraged to consume as wide a variety of fruit and vegetables as possible. Healthy adults should avoid consuming them with added fat (e.g. buttered or fried vegetables, cream with fruit). Yoghurt or fromage frais is a good accompaniment to fruit as a dessert. Vegetables should not be overboiled to avoid destruction of water-soluble vitamins such as vitamin C or folates.

The use of fruit, either fresh or dried, as a snack food should be encouraged.

Milk and dairy foods

Healthy adults should choose reduced-fat or low-fat varieties (e.g. skimmed or semi-skimmed milk, low-fat yoghurt). These products contain the same amounts of calcium, protein and riboflavin as their full-fat equivalents but less fat and energy. Because of their lower energy density, and also lower content of fat-soluble vitamins A and D, reduced-fat products are not suitable for young children, some elderly people or those who are nutritionally depleted. Children over 2 years can be given semi-skimmed milk provided that they are eating a diverse and adequate diet. Skimmed milk is not suitable for children under 5 years of age

Hard and other full-fat cheeses (e.g. Cheshire, Stilton, Brie) have a high fat (and energy) content and should be used sparingly by those who need to reduce their energy intake. Conversely, cheese is a valuable food for those who need to increase their energy intake (e.g. chronically ill people with small appetites).

Butter and cream, which are almost exclusively comprised of fat, are classified as fat-rich foods and not included in this group.

Meat, fish and alternatives

These foods are important but should not predominate dietary intake.

Meat Meat and meat products contribute a high proportion of fat to the average diet, but lean meat itself (i.e. the muscle tissue) contains relatively little fat, and about half of it is monounsaturated in composition. Lean meat is also a concentrated source of protein and micronutrients, particularly haem iron. It is the consumption of the storage fat surrounding the muscle fibres (visible fat or marbling) which significantly increases fat intake and needs to be avoided. Mixtures of lean meat and fat (e.g. minced beef) and many meat products also have a high fat content and these types of food choice may need to be reduced.

Poultry This is commonly assumed to contain less fat than red meat but this only applies to the white meat (e.g. breast meat) eaten without any skin or visible fat deposits. Darker meat (e.g. leg muscle) has a higher fat content, and a chicken joint eaten with its skin can provide a considerable quantity of fat and energy.

Offal Liver and kidney are relatively low in fat and are rich sources of haem iron. They are also relatively cheap foods but not always popular.

Fish White fish is low in fat (unless fried) and a valuable source of the antioxidant selenium.

Oily fish (e.g. herrings, mackerel, pilchards, sardines, salmon) These foods are an important part of a cardio-protective diet as they contain long chain n-3 polyunsaturated fatty acids which have anti-thrombotic properties. Most people should eat these foods once or twice a week. Oily fish are also one of the few dietary sources of vitamin D.

Eggs Although these contain dietary cholesterol, this is not a significant concern unless eggs are consumed in unusually large amounts (several per day) or by people with certain rare lipid disorders. Within the normal range of intake, dietary cholesterol has little effect on blood cholesterol. Eggs should always be well cooked to minimize the risk of salmonella poisoning.

Pulses (beans and lentils)   These have a low glycaemic index and provide soluble fibre and many minerals and trace elements as well as protein. They can be useful to help to compensate for a smaller quantity of lean meat being used in a casserole or other composite dish. Baked beans or canned kidney beans are an acceptable and convenient form of pulses for many people.

Fat-rich and sugar-rich foods

These foods are not devoid of nutrients and in some diets, particularly those of adolescents, may even account for a significant proportion of micronutrient intake (Gibson 1993). It is also unrealistic to expect people to avoid these foods altogether. They add palatability and convenience to a diet and, used sensibly, can form part of a balanced healthy diet.

The point to get across in healthy eating messages is that these foods can provide a lot of fat and sugars relative to the amount of essential nutrients that they contain. Many of them also contribute significant amounts of salt to the diet. For a diet to be balanced, fat-rich and sugar-rich foods therefore need to comprise the smallest proportion of the diet and not, as is so often the case, the largest.

Products which are low/reduced in fat, sugar, energy or salt may be useful alternative choices for some people. People should be aware of the difference between the two terms and that products which are labelled as 'reduced' may still have an appreciable content of that nutrient (see Section 2.11.2 in Food and nutrition labelling).

Spreading fats   Butter and margarine (both hard or soft margarine) have the same (high) fat and energy content (approximately 80% fat by composition). Fat spreads (e.g. sunflower spread) typically contain about 70% fat. Many products (often called 'light' or 'extra light') have a lower fat content than this (typically about 60% or 40%, respectively). Hard margarines have a higher content of saturated and *trans* fatty acids than those marketed as high in monounsaturates or polyunsaturates.

For healthy adults, the best choice of a fat to spread on bread is a reduced- or low-fat spread (40–60% fat), and those rich in monounsaturates (olive oil based) are probably preferable to those derived from polyunsaturates. Salt-reduced varieties are also available. Some products have added buttermilk for extra flavour; this does not increase the fat content.

Cooking fats   Use of these should be kept to a minimum. Vegetable oils should always be used in preference to animal fats such as lard or dripping. Olive oil is a rich source of monounsaturates; sunflower, safflower and corn oils are high in *n*-6 polyunsaturates. Rapeseed and soya oils contain most *n*-3 linolenic acid (see Section 2.3 Dietary fat and fatty acids).

Additional considerations

Supplementary guidance

To help to achieve particular dietary manipulations (e.g. reduction in intake of energy, fat or salt, or an increase in fibre), guidance on food choice can be supplemented with additional advice on food preparation and cooking methods (Table 1.7).

Meal pattern

Meal pattern is also an important component of healthy eating, and regularly spaced meals rather than 'feast or famine' is more likely to result in a diet which is varied and balanced. Consumption of breakfast may be particularly important and may be beneficial in terms of satiety (Wyon *et al.* 1997), cognitive performance (Dye *et al.* 2000), nutritional adequacy (Nicklas *et al.* 1998), nutritional status (Preziosi *et al.* 1999) and obesity (Ortega *et al.* 1998). People who consume breakfast, especially breakfast cereals, tend to have higher intakes of micronutrients such as riboflavin, folate, vitamin B_6, vitamin D, iron and calcium (Gregory *et al.* 1990) and cereal fibre (Emmett *et al.* 1993), and lower intakes of non-milk extrinsic sugars (Gibson 2000).

1.2.3 Achieving healthy eating

Achieving permanent beneficial change in an individual's dietary habits is notoriously difficult. In order to do so, the many influences on dietary behaviour have to be considered, barriers to change explored and behavioural techniques to overcome them applied (see Sections 1.6, Dietary modification, and 1.7, Achieving behavioural change).

The Institute of European Food Studies (IEFS 1997) pan-European survey on consumer attitudes to food, nutrition and health showed that people are aware of healthy eating messages. 'Trying to eat healthily' was cited as one of the five main influences on food choice (along with quality, price, taste and family constraints). The benefits of healthy eating in terms of fitness, weight control and the prevention of disease were also well understood. Lack of knowledge was not commonly cited as a barrier to change (Kearney and McElhone 1999).

However, surveys of dietary intake and health parameters suggest that, in the UK population, awareness and knowledge of the messages have not yet resulted in changes which are likely to be significant in terms of health (see Sections 1.1.4 and 1.1.5 in Diet, health and disease). Many barriers to dietary change exist and may include:

- *Lack of perception of the need for change*: the pan-European study showed that 70% of people already regard their diet as healthy and not in need of further change (Kearney *et al.* 1997). Many had made some attempt, for example, to eat more fruit and vegetables or fewer fatty foods and regarded these measures as being sufficient even if, in reality, the changes made were small.
- *Negative attitudes towards healthy eating*: Margetts *et al.* (1998) found that people who had not changed their dietary habits were more likely to believe that healthy foods were just another fashion, or expensive; they were also less likely to care about what they ate. Nearly three-quarters of them believed that that 'experts never agree about what foods are good for you'.

Table 1.7 Additional guidance which can be given to help to achieve specific dietary objectives

Reducing fat intake
- Avoid frying foods; grill, bake, boil, casserole or steam instead
- Use minimal amounts of cooking oil to lubricate cooking pans. Non-stick baking parchment is useful for lining baking trays and tins
- Avoid adding fat to cooked foods, e.g. butter/margarine on vegetables or to pasta
- Remove all visible fat from meat, and skin and fat deposits on chicken
- Drain or skim fat from mince and casseroles
- Make smaller quantities of leaner meat go further by either cooking it with foods such as vegetables, kidney beans, butter beans or lentils, or serving it with larger helpings of vegetables, rice, potatoes or pasta
- Use a reduced-fat/low-fat spread
- Use semi-skimmed or skimmed milk instead of full-fat milk, and choose low/reduced-fat dairy products
- Keep hidden sources of fat to a minimum. Particular foods to watch are pastry, pies, biscuits, cakes and meat products. Choose lower fat alternatives when available. Mashed potato toppings can be a good alternative to pastry
- If you eat chips, choose low-fat, oven-baked types
- Limit high-fat snacks such as crisps and similar products

Reducing salt/sodium intake
- Avoid adding salt directly to food
- Use minimum amounts of salt in cooking. Try leaving it out of recipes altogether (the difference may not even be noticed) and only add a pinch of salt (rather than a teaspoonful) to vegetable cooking water. Boost flavour by using more herbs, spices, mustard, onion, garlic or lemon juice
- Use fewer processed convenience foods from cans, jars, packets or cartons. Choose reduced-salt versions if available. Use more fresh or unprocessed foods instead
- Avoid highly salted foods, e.g. cheese, crisps and savoury snacks, salted foods (e.g. salted peanuts), smoked fish, preserved sausage (e.g. salami), yeast extracts

Salt substitutes may be helpful for those who find it difficult to adjust to eating less salt-tasting food, but are not necessary for most people. Because of their high potassium content, these products are contraindicated for people with renal disorders

Increasing fibre intake
- Eat more wholemeal bread or high-fibre white bread
- Eat more wholegrain breakfast cereals or those which contain bran or oats
- Eat more brown rice or wholewheat pasta
- Eat more fruit and vegetables
- Use more pulse vegetables, e.g. peas, beans and lentils; add to casseroles or composite dishes
- Use some wholemeal flour in baking, e.g. a 50:50 mixture of wholemeal and white flour

These changes should be introduced gradually; a sudden large increase in fibre consumption can result in distension and flatulence. Additional fluids will also be necessary

---

- *Lack of time*: busy lifestyles and irregular work patterns were often cited as barriers to healthy eating, especially among younger respondents and those with a higher level of education (Kearney and McElhone 1999).
- *Problems with taste and acceptability*: people may feel that healthy eating is less enjoyable or that it requires them to 'give up all their favourite foods' (Kearney and McElhone 1999).
- *Cost*: healthy eating is often perceived to be expensive because it is associated with costly foods such as lean meat, fish and fresh fruit. People tend to overlook the fact that many of the foods which are encouraged such as pasta, rice, bread and potatoes are relatively cheap. Nor need healthy food choices always incur greater cost: an apple costs no more than a bar of chocolate or bag of crisps; a glass of milk can be cheaper than a glass of cola; the cheaper plainer breakfast cereals are better choices than more expensive sugar-coated varieties; baked potatoes cost no more than chips. Nevertheless, cost can still be a significant barrier to change to some sectors of the population, especially those on low incomes. If the diet contains a high proportion of cheap meat products, sausages, chips, hard margarine, etc., it is difficult to make healthier changes without spending

more money. For those in deprived circumstances, there are also likely to be many other socioeconomic and psychological constraints on healthy eating such as lack of access to shops with the widest choice of foods and lowest prices, poor food storage and cooking facilities, and problems stemming from stress and low morale (see Section 3.8, People in low-income groups).

Similar barriers to change may also exist with other aspects of lifestyle behaviour such as increasing the level of physical activity, which may be an adjunct to dietary advice. The pan-EU survey on physical activity found that 47% people considered that they did not need to increase their levels of physical activity, irrespective of their current activity level (Vaz de Almeida *et al.* 1999).

Achieving healthy eating therefore requires far more than dispensing dietary advice. Identifying and helping people to overcome real or perceived barriers to change is essential. Misunderstandings of what is involved still persist and need to be addressed. The role of the health educator is not to tell people what to do, but to ask them what they think it is possible to achieve and guide them as to how this can be done. Advice given needs to be personally relevant taking social, economic and lifestyle factors into account (see Section 1.6.3 in Dietary modification). Targets for change should be positive (stressing what people can, rather what they cannot, do) and attainable for that particular person. For some people, a few simple goals (e.g. increasing the number of portions of fruit and vegetables per day) will have most impact; too many messages can be seen as unachievable and hence more likely to be abandoned.

Healthy eating guidance for the population is most likely to be cost-effective if it is targeted at the groups who would benefit most from dietary change. People least likely to be eating a healthy diet are younger, low-income families and people who smoke (Margetts *et al*. 1998); these groups are also known to have the greatest health problems (see Section 1.1, Diet, health and disease). Since the barriers to change in these groups may be different from those in other sectors of the population in terms of socioeconomic, educational or cultural factors, the nutrition messages conveyed may also need to reflect this if they are to have an impact on health (Margetts *et al*. 1997).

1.2.4 Sensible use of alcohol
Health implications of alcohol

Within a population there is a U-shaped relationship between alcohol consumption and all-cause mortality, with those drinking between 8 and 14 units/week having the lowest risk (Doll *et al*. 1994). Modest regular consumption of alcohol is associated with a lower risk of death from coronary heart disease (CHD), possibly as a result of beneficial effects on high-density lipoprotein (HDL) level and fibrinolytic factors (Marmot and Brunner 1991; Hendriks *et al*. 1994). However, all-cause mortality starts to increase at 21 units/week for men and 14 units/week in women and CHD risk increases considerably in men whose consumption exceeds 40 units/week (Doll *et al*. 1994).

Once ingested, alcohol is rapidly absorbed, particularly if the stomach is empty, and circulates in the blood before being metabolized in the liver to provide energy. There is considerable individual variation in the rate at which it is metabolized but, on average, it takes about an hour for the body to dispose of 1 unit (8 g) of alcohol. Alcohol is metabolized more slowly in women, which is why they are more susceptible to both the intoxicating effects of alcohol and long-term damage.

In the short term, excessive amounts of alcohol can be acutely toxic to the individual as well as potentially dangerous to others as a result of the loss of co-ordination or self-control, and behavioural change which may be of an aggressive or violent nature. In the long term, continued heavy drinking causes liver damage and can result in cirrhosis, pancreatitis and some cancers. Heavy alcohol abuse in pregnancy can cause fetal abnormalities and mental retardation.

Recommended sensible drinking limits

In the UK, 1 unit is defined as 8 g alcohol and is roughly equivalent to the alcohol content of one measure of spirits, one small glass of wine or half a pint of beer (but see below). Based on evidence of morbidity and mortality associated with alcohol use, the recommended maximum levels of alcohol consumption were originally set at no more than 21 units/week for men and 14 units/week for women. Following growing evidence that the health implications of occasional sessions of heavy drinking (e.g. all 21 units consumed in one evening) differed from the same amount of alcohol consumed over the course of a week, it was recommended that maximum intakes should be expressed on a daily basis, rather than per week (Royal Colleges 1995). The Government's Inter-Departmental Working Group on Sensible Drinking (DH 1995) therefore formulated new benchmarks for sensible drinking. The recommendations are:

- Maximum daily intakes should not exceed 3–4 units/day in men and 2–3 units/day in women. Men who consistently drink than 4 units/day and women more than 3 units/day incur progressive health risks.
- Heavy sessional drinking and intoxication should be avoided. If they do occur, alcohol should be avoided for 48 h to allow full recovery.
- The risk of CHD in men over 40 years and postmenopausal women may be reduced by drinking 1–2 units/day.
- Women who are pregnant, or planning a pregnancy, are advised to drink no more than 1–2 units, once or twice a week and to avoid intoxication. More recently, the Royal College of Obstetricians and Gynaecologists (1999) has suggested that alcohol intake during pregnancy should not exceed 1 unit/day (see Section 3.1.2 in Pregnancy).

There is evidence that, in the UK, these limits are often exceeded (DH 1999). In 1998, 39% of men were found to be consuming more than 4 units/day and 21% women more than 3 units/day. Although women less commonly exceeded the safe drinking limit, their level of alcohol consumption over the previous decade had risen markedly while that in men had remained relatively static. The prevalence of alcohol consumption among young people is also a matter of concern; over a quarter (27%) of 11–15 year olds admit to consuming alcohol.

Using the unit system

Units are a convenient way of expressing the amount of alcohol in different drinks. One unit of alcohol is approximately equal to:

- one single pub measure of spirits (25 ml)*
- one measure of sherry or fortified wine (50 ml)
- one small glass of table wine (100 ml)
- half a pint of standard strength beer, lager or cider.

* In England and Wales. In Scotland a pub measure will provide 1¼ units of alcohol, in Northern Ireland 1½ units.

The unit system is a simple and easy way for people to keep track of their alcohol consumption. However, some pitfalls may need to be pointed out:

- *Variation in serving size*: the specified measures (e.g. a glass of wine) are those typical of drinks sold in pubs and restaurants. Those dispensed at home may be considerably more generous.
- *Variation in alcoholic strength*: beers and lagers vary considerably in alcoholic strength and this, coupled with the fact that many are sold in cans containing considerably more than half a pint, can easily lead someone to underestimate the number of alcohol units consumed. Standard strength beer or lager contains 3.5% alcohol by volume (ABV). Many products have a higher strength than this and extra-strong lager or special brews of beer can contain as much as 9% ABV. Some of these may be sold in 440 ml cans, i.e. over ¾ pint (½ pint = 284 ml), so the contents may provide 4 units of alcohol and not, as may be assumed, 1 unit. Young adults in particular are likely to make this mistake and not realize that drinking two or three cans of such products is equivalent to 8–12 measures of spirits. The alcoholic strength must, by law, be declared on the label of alcoholic drinks, and beer/lager drinkers should be encouraged to take note of this information.
- *Low-alcohol drinks*: these are not always as low in alcohol as may be assumed. Some are virtually alcohol free (0.05% ABV) but most 'low' alcohol beers, lagers and ciders have about one-third of the alcohol content (1.2% ABV) of the standard product. Some low-alcohol wines are about half as strong as ordinary table wine. People may assume that all these products have a negligible alcohol content and that it is safe to drive after consuming them; this may not be the case.

Text written by: Briony Thomas

Useful addresses

Health Development Agency (formerly the Health Education Authority)
Trevelyan House, 30 Great Peter Street, London SW1 2HW
Tel: 020 7222 5300
Website: www.hda-online.org.uk
Many publications and resources formerly produced by the Health Education Authority are still available from Marston Book Services, Tel: 01235 465565

Health Promotion England (continuing some of the public education work of the former Health Education Authority)
50 Eastbourne Terrace, London W2 3QR
Website: www.hpe.org.uk

References

Department of Health. *Sensible Drinking*. Report of an Inter-Departmental Working Group. London: DH, 1995.

Department of Health. Statistics on alcohol: 1976 onwards. *Statistical Bulletin* 1999; **24** (October): 1–46.

Department of Health and Social Security (DHSS). Committee on Medical Aspects of Food Policy (COMA). *Diet and Cardiovascular Disease*. Report of Health and Social Subjects 28. London: HMSO, 1984.

Doll R, Peto R, Hall E *et al*. Mortality in relation to consumption of alcohol: 13 years' observations on male British doctors. *British Medical Journal* 1994; **309**: 911–918.

Dye L, Lluch A, Blundell JE. Macronutrients and mental performance. *Nutrition* 2000; **16**: 1021–1034.

Emmett PM, Symes CL, Heaton KW. The contribution of breakfast cereals to non-starch polysaccharide intakes in English men and women. *Journal of Human Nutrition and Dietetics* 1993; **6**: 217–222.

Gatenby SJ, Hunt P, Rayner M. The National Food Guide: development of dietetic criteria and nutritional characteristics. *Journal of Human Nutrition and Dietetics* 1995; **8**: 323–334.

Gibson SA. Consumption and sources of sugars in the diets of British schoolchildren: are high sugar diets nutritionally inferior? *Journal of Human Nutrition and Dietetics* 1993; **6**: 355–371.

Gibson SA. Breakfast cereal consumption in young children: associations with non-milk extrinsic sugars and caries experience: further analysis of data from the UK National Diet and Nutrition Survey of children aged 1.5–4.5 years. *Public Health Nutrition* 2000; **3**: 227–232.

Gregory J, Foster K, Tyler H, Wiseman M. *The Dietary and Nutritional Survey of British Adults*. London: HMSO, 1990.

Health Education Authority (HEA). *The Balance of Good Health. Introducing the National Food Guide*. London: HEA, 1994.

Hendriks HFJ, Veenstra J, Velthuis-te Wierik EJ *et al*. Effect of moderate dose of alcohol with evening meal on fibrinolytic factors. *British Medical Journal* 1994; **308**: 1003–1006.

Hunt P, Rayner M, Gatenby S. A National Food Guide for the UK? Background and development. *Journal of Human Nutrition and Dietetics* 1995a; **8**: 315–322.

Hunt P, Gatenby S, Rayner M. The format for the National Food Guide: performance and preference studies. *Journal of Human Nutrition and Dietetics* 1995b; **8**: 335–351.

Institute of European Food Studies (IEFS). Pan-EU survey of consumer attitudes to food, nutrition and health. Strain JJ (Ed.). *European Journal of Clinical Nutrition* 1997; **51** (Suppl 2): S1–S58.

Kearney JM, McElhone S. Perceived barriers in trying to eat healthier – results of a pan-EU consumer attitudinal survey. *British Journal of Nutrition* 1999; **81** (Suppl 2): S133–S137.

Kearney M, Gibney MJ, Martinez JA *et al*. Perceived need to alter eating habits among representative samples of adults from all member states of the European Union. *European Journal of Clinical Nutrition* 1997; **51** (Suppl 2): S30–S35.

Margetts BM, Martinez JA, Saba A *et al*. Definitions of 'healthy' eating: a pan-EU survey of consumer attitudes to food, nutrition and health. *European Journal of Clinical Nutrition* 1997; **51** (Suppl 2): S23–S29.

Margetts BM, Thompson RL, Speller V, McVey D. Factors which influence 'healthy' eating patterns: results from the 1993 Health Education Authority health and lifestyle survey in England. *Public Health Nutrition* 1998; **1**: 193–198.

Marmot M, Brunner E. Alcohol and cardiovascular disease: the status of the U-shaped curve. *British Medical Journal* 1991; **303**: 565–568.

Ministry of Agriculture, Fisheries and Food (MAFF). *Eight Guidelines for a Healthy Diet*. London: MAFF, 1991 (revised 1997).

National Advisory Committee of Nutrition Education (NACNE). *Proposals for Nutritional Guidelines for Health Education in Britain*. London: Heath Education Council, 1983.

National Dairy Council/MORI. *Food and Health: What does Britain Think?* London: NDC, 1992.

Nicklas TA, Myers L, Reger C *et al*. Impact of breakfast consumption on nutritional adequacy of the diets of young adults in Bogalusa, Louisiana: ethnic and gender contrasts. *Journal of the American Dietetic Association* 1998; **98**: 1432–1438.

Ortega RM, Requejo AM, Lopez-Sobaler AM *et al*. Difference in breakfast habits of overweight/obese and normal weight schoolchildren. *International Journal for Vitamin and Nutrition Research* 1998; **68**: 125–132.

Preziosi P, Galan P, Deheeger M *et al*. Breakfast type, daily nutrient intakes and vitamin and mineral status of French children, adolescents and adults. *Journal of the American College of Nutrition* 1999; **18**: 171–178.

Royal College of Obstetricians and Gynaecologists. *Alcohol Consumption in Pregnancy*. London: RCOG, 1999.

Royal Colleges of Physicians, Psychiatrists and General Practitioners. *Alcohol and the Heart in Perspective: Sensible Limits Reaffirmed*. London: Royal College of Physicians, 1995.

US Department of Agriculture. *The Food Guide Pyramid*. Hyattsville, MD: USDA's Human Nutrition Information Service, 1992.

Vaz de Almeida MD, Graca P, Afonso C *et al*. Physical activity levels and body weight in a nationally representative sample in the European Union. *Public Health Nutrition* 1999; **2** (1A): 105–113.

Williams C. Healthy eating: clarifying advice about fruit and vegetables. *British Medical Journal* 1995; **310**: 1453–1455.

Wyon DP, Abrahamsson L, Jartelius M, Fletcher RJ. An experimental study of the effects of energy intake at breakfast on the test performance of 10-year old children in school. *International Journal of Food Science and Nutrition* 1997; **48**: 5–12.

1.3 Dietary reference values

Dietary reference values (DRVs) reflect the nutritional needs of a particular population and provide a yardstick against which the nutritional adequacy of diets can be assessed. They are a useful guide to the nutritional requirements of healthy people and a valuable tool for the dietitian. However, they can be misused and it is important to understand their nature and purpose.

Many national and international bodies have set dietary reference standards (Table 1.8). Originally, the primary aim of these standards was to help to prevent nutritional deficiency and ensure nutritional adequacy within a population. Standards were therefore set in terms of the amount of a nutrient which would meet the requirements of virtually everyone within a defined population. These figures were usually known as recommended daily amounts or recommended dietary allowance (RDA), terms which are still in use in many countries and, for example, in European labelling legislation.

However, sole use of the RDA as a dietary reference standard has two main limitations:

1 Because an RDA covers the needs of virtually everyone, it overestimates the needs of many. In more affluent societies, it is becoming increasingly apparent that while nutrient deficiency remains a problem in some sectors of the population, surplus intakes lead to health problems for many others.
2 It tends to be assumed that the term 'recommended' means the same as 'required'. This is not the case. The nutrient 'requirement' is the amount sufficient to meet individual needs and prevent deficiency. The amount 'recommended' is a generous allowance which includes a safety factor to take account of individual variability.

Newer reference standards therefore attempt to take account of the relationships between diet and the development of chronic disease, and consider nutrient needs for optimum health rather than to prevent deficiency alone.

1.3.1 UK dietary reference values

Dietary reference standards have been in use in the UK since the 1960s (DHSS 1969, 1979), initially confined to one set of figures in the form of recommended daily amounts (RDA) (or recommended daily intakes – RDI). Because of the limitations outlined above, when the UK reference standards were fully revised (DH 1991), they were significantly broadened to include a set of standards for use in different applications. The umbrella term for these standards is dietary reference values (DRVs).

Definitions

DRVs are based on the assumption that, within a population, individual variability in requirement for nutrients is based on a normal distribution and that the requirements of 95% of people lie within 2 standard deviations of the mean. Dietary reference values are therefore based on estimates of this mean (average requirements) and the values which are either 2 standard deviations above or below this figure (Fig. 1.2).

DRVs comprise:

- *Estimated average requirement (EAR)*: this is the average requirement for a nutrient by a particular group of people. Individual requirements will vary from this mean; about half will require more than this EAR, and half less.

Table 1.8 National and international dietary reference standards

Country	Dietary reference standards
Australia/New Zealand	*Recommended Dietary Intakes for use in Australia* (National Health and Medical Research Council 1991)
Canada	*Nutrition Recommendations: The Report of the Scientific Review Committee* (Health and Welfare Canada 1990)
European Union	*Nutrient and Energy Intakes for the European Community* (Commission of the European Communities 1993)
UK	*Dietary Reference Values for Food Energy and Nutrients for the United Kingdom* (DH 1991)
USA	*Recommended Dietary Allowances* (National Academy of Sciences 1989) *Dietary Reference Intakes for Calcium, Phosphorus, Magnesium, Vitamin D and Fluoride* (National Academy of Sciences 1997)
WHO	*Energy and Protein Requirements* (WHO 1985) *Diet, Nutrition and the Prevention of Chronic Diseases* (WHO 1990)

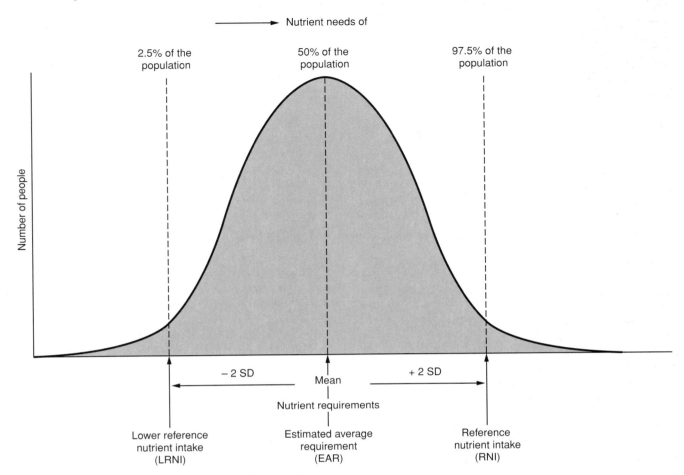

Fig. 1.2 Derivation and definition of dietary reference values.

- *Reference nutrient intake (RNI)*: this is the amount that will meet the requirements of virtually every healthy person within a group. It is therefore more than most people will actually need. This figure is equivalent to the previous RDA value and is defined as the level of nutrient requirement which is 2 standard deviations above the EAR. Assuming a normal population distribution, this covers the needs of at least 97.5% of the population. If an individual is consuming the RNI of a nutrient, they are unlikely to be deficient in that nutrient.
- *Lower reference nutrient intake (LRNI)*: this aims to define minimum nutrient requirements and is set at two standard deviations below the EAR. This amount will only be sufficient for the small percentage of the population (about 2.5%) with low needs and will not be enough for most people. Individual intakes below the LRNI are likely to be inadequate.
- *Safe and adequate intake*: this term is used to indicate the intake of a nutrient for which there is not enough information to estimate the distribution of requirements within a population (typically some vitamins and trace elements). A safe intake is one which is considered to be adequate for most people's needs but not so high as to cause undesirable effects.

Derivation of dietary reference values for specific nutrients

DRVs have been set for energy, protein, fat, sugars, starch, non-starch polysaccharide (NSP) and many vitamins, mineral and trace elements, although not all have DRVs consisting of an EAR, RNI and LRNI. It is clearly inappropriate to set a RNI (covering the needs of 97.5% of the population) for energy because such an amount would far exceed the needs of most people and, if consumed, would be detrimental to energy balance and health. The DRV for energy is therefore only set as an EAR. The DRVs for the main energy-yielding nutrients such as fat, carbohydrate, sugars and starch are also expressed in terms of averages as a percentage of food energy.

Energy

EARs for energy are based mainly on estimates of energy expenditure. In adults, EAR for energy = basal metabolic rate (BMR) × physical activity level (PAL). BMR was calculated from prediction equations derived by Schofield *et al.* (1985) (see Annex 2 in the DRV Report; DH 1991) using average weights for different age bands (e.g. those for adults aged 16–64 years were taken from a 1980 OPCS survey of 10 000 people in this age range). Individuals may vary from these averages.

The factors for PALs were defined as: 1.4, inactive men and women (this applies to most people in the UK); 1.6, moderately active women; 1.7, moderately active men; 1.8, highly active women; and 1.9, highly active men.

The calculated EARs are presented in a range of age bands for each gender. Increments are also added for the last trimester of pregnancy and for lactation.

EARs for infants and young children are derived from a combination of average weights and observed intakes.

Because it is an average, half of a population is expected to require more than the EAR for energy, and half less. In practice, a body weight which is in accordance with the ideal remains the best indication for the individual that requirements for energy expenditure are adequately balanced by energy intake.

Protein

Dietary reference values for protein are based on estimates of the amount needed to maintain nitrogen balance. The DRVs also make allowance for the fact that only about 70% of protein consumed is incorporated into body tissue.

Protein DRVs are expressed in terms of the EAR and RNI. Incremental amounts are added to these figures for pregnancy and lactation. It is recommended that protein intakes do not exceed twice the RNI.

The protein EAR and RNI figures assume that the needs for energy are met; if this is not the case, protein will be preferentially used as an energy source. They also assume that the protein consumed is of high biological value (see Section 2.2, Protein).

Fats and carbohydrate

These nutrients cannot be given EARs or RNIs in absolute terms because there is no specific requirement for them (other than for small quantities of linoleic and alpha-linolenic acid) and they do not cause specific signs or symptoms of deficiency or toxicity. However, because it is recognized that the proportion of these nutrients in the diet have health implications, dietary reference values are given in the form of the percentage of dietary energy which should be derived from these nutrients.

The DRVs for fat recommend the percentage of dietary energy which should be derived from:

- saturated fatty acids
- monounsaturated fatty acids
- *cis*-polyunsaturated fatty acids (as *n*-3 and *n*-6 fatty acids)
- *trans* fatty acids
- total fat.

These percentage figures are recommended averages for a population and vary according to whether the diet contains alcohol or not. They also assume that protein comprises 15% of dietary energy intake (which is typical of average UK intake, although higher than the RNI for protein).

Recommended minimum intakes of essential fatty acids (*n*-3 and *n*-6), and maximum intake of *cis*-polyunsaturated fatty acids are also given.

The DRVs relating to dietary carbohydrate recommend the percentage of dietary energy from:

- non-milk extrinsic sugars
- intrinsic and milk sugars and starch
- total carbohydrate.

Non-starch polysaccharides/dietary fibre

By definition, 'dietary fibre' is not a 'nutrient' and hence no specific requirement can exist, although the importance of this dietary component is not in doubt. However, because there is still much debate regarding the terminology, analysis and physiological significance of this complex group of compounds, recommendations regarding intake are fraught with difficulty. Nevertheless, a DRV for a specifically defined form of dietary fibre (NSP as analysed by the method of Englyst and Cummings 1988) is given in terms of a recommended average intake for the adult population. Recommended individual minimum and maximum levels of NSP intake are also given.

It should be noted that these figures may not be comparable with 'dietary fibre' figures estimated by other methods (e.g. as declared on food labels) (see Section 2.5, Dietary fibre).

Minerals and vitamins

For most vitamins and minerals, DRVs are given as the EAR, RNI and LRNI.

Insufficient information was available for establishing the distribution of requirement for pantothenic acid, biotin, vitamin E, vitamin K, manganese, molybdenum, chromium and fluoride, and guidance on safe intakes is given instead.

DRVs for sodium take account of the facts that current intakes greatly exceed need and that lower intakes may help to reduce blood pressure levels in the UK population. An EAR was not set and the RNI for sodium is much lower than the typical UK intake. Similar but converse reasoning applied to potassium; its beneficial role in promoting sodium excretion was acknowledged and the RNI for potassium is thus higher than the usual UK intake.

Summary tables of UK DRVs are provided in Appendix 6.2, but the full publication (DH 1991) sets out the details of all DRVs and is required reading for dietitians. The Department of Health's *Dietary Reference Values: A Guide* (Salmon, 1991) is also helpful for understanding how the values were derived and how they should be used.

1.3.2 Using dietary reference values

DRVs are based on the normal distribution of nutritional requirements within a population and take account of variation as a result of:

- gender
- age

- physiological status: pregnancy and lactation
- growth.

However, DRVs do not take account of differences in nutritional needs as a result of:

- illness, trauma or metabolic stress
- malabsorption
- nutritional deficiency states
- genetic abnormalities affecting nutrient requirements (e.g. for folate; Molloy *et al.* 1997).

DRVs therefore reflect the needs of healthy people and may not be appropriate in many clinical circumstances.

Use of DRVs in individuals also requires caution. DRVs reflect the nutritional needs of groups of people, and the nutritional needs of individuals within this group will vary. Within a population, the nutritional requirements of individuals form a continuum but where on that continuum a particular individual lies will be unknown. It is therefore impossible to determine whether an individual's needs are being met on the basis of a DRV. It is only possible to assess the degree of probability that an individual's needs will or will not have been met. If the EAR for a nutrient is being consumed, there is about a 50% chance that needs will be met. If intake is at or above the RNI, it is highly likely that needs are being met (and probably exceeded). If intake is below the LRNI, it is highly unlikely that sufficient is being consumed, unless that person is part of the 2.5% of the population with unusually low requirements.

Similarly, DRVs cannot be used in isolation to estimate the nutritional requirements of a particular individual and additional means of doing this are required (see Section 1.10, Estimating nutritional requirements). DRVs are, however, a useful baseline from which individual needs can be determined taking other factors into account.

Other factors which need to be considered when using DRVs are:

- *Not everything consumed is absorbed.* While more than 90% of ingested carbohydrate, fat and protein is absorbed, the percentage absorption of micronutrients, particularly minerals, can be much less. DRVs recognize this to some extent. For example, the fact that only about 15% of dietary iron is absorbed is built into DRV calculations to reflect the amount of iron that needs to be consumed in order for iron requirements to be met. However, DRVs are unable to take into account the many other factors which can influence bioavailability such as the amount consumed, body stores, the presence or absence of other nutrients or dietary constituents, the form of the nutrient (e.g. haem or non-haem iron) and the food source from which it is derived (e.g. calcium from milk has a higher bioavailability than that from cereals). These factors may have considerable influence on whether a dietary intake is adequate or inadequate.

  Conversely, DRVs (particularly for micronutrients) do not apply to diets administered by the parenteral route because no absorptive losses will occur and the required intake will be much closer to the actual metabolic requirement.

- *DRVs assume that requirements for other nutrients are met.* An apparent adequacy of one nutrient may in reality be an inadequacy if another nutrient essential for its absorption or utilization is lacking.

- *DRVs are not infallible.* DRVs are based on the best evidence available at a particular point in time (e.g. dietary intakes needed to maintain circulating enzyme levels or to prevent signs or symptoms of deficiency or disease). Comprehensive data are still lacking in respect of some nutrients and hence there are uncertainties and differences in DRVs between different countries. As more scientific information emerges, and knowledge about the relationships between diet and disease advances, DRVs are reviewed and possibly changed. For this reason, and as their name implies, DRVs should be regarded as a point of reference rather than as a definitive set of values valid for all time.

Text revised by: Briony Thomas

References

Commission of the European Communities. *Nutrient and Energy Intakes for the European Community*. Reports of the Scientific Committee for Food, 31st series. Luxembourg: Office for Official Publications of the European Communities, 1993.

Department of Health (DH). *Dietary Reference Values for Food Energy and Nutrients for the United Kingdom. Report of the Panel on Dietary Reference Values of the Committee on Medical Aspects of Food Policy*. Report on Health and Social Subjects 41. London: HMSO, 1991

Department of Health and Social Security (DHSS). *Recommended Intakes of Nutrients for the UK*. Report on Public Health and Medical Subjects No. 120. London: HMSO, 1969.

Department of Health and Social Security (DHSS). *Recommended Daily Amounts of Food Energy and Nutrients for Groups of People in the United Kingdom*. Report by the Committee on Medical Aspects of Food Policy. Report on Health and Social Subjects 15. London: HMSO, 1979.

Englyst HN, Cummings JH. An improved method for the measurement of dietary fibre as the non-starch polysaccharides in plant foods. *Journal of the Association of Official Analytical Chemists* 1988; **71**: 808–814.

Health and Welfare Canada. *Nutrition Recommendations: The Report of the Scientific Review Committee*. Ottawa: Canadian Government Publishing Centre, 1990.

Molloy AM, Daly S, Mills JL *et al.* Thermolabile variant of 5,10-methylenetetrahydrofolate reductase associated with low red cell folates: implications for folate intake recommendations. *Lancet* 1997; **349**: 1591–1593.

National Academy of Sciences, Food and Nutrition Board. *Recommended Dietary Allowances*, 10th edn. Washington, DC: National Academy Press, 1989.

National Academy of Sciences, Food and Nutrition Board. *Dietary Reference Intakes for Calcium, Phosphorus, Magnesium, Vitamin D and Fluoride*. Washington, DC: National Academy Press, 1997.

National Health and Medical Research Council. *Recommended Dietary Intakes for use in Australia*. Canberra: Australian Government Publishing Service, 1991.

Salmon J. *Dietary Reference Values: A Guide*. London: HMSO, 1991.

Schofield WN, Schofield C, James WPT. BMR – review and prediction. *Human Nutrition: Clinical Nutrition* 1985; **39** (Suppl): 1–96.

World Health Organization. *Energy and Protein Requirements*. Technical Report Series 724. Geneva: WHO, 1985.

World Health Organization. *Diet, Nutrition and the Prevention of Chronic Diseases*. Technical Report Series 797. Geneva: WHO, 1990.

1.4 Food composition tables

1.4.1 National food tables

UK food tables

In the UK, the primary source of information on the nutritional composition of foods is McCance and Widdowson's *The Composition of Foods* and its associated series of supplements (Table 1.9). These publications are continually being updated as part of a rolling process of food analysis conducted jointly by the Royal Society of Chemistry (RSC) and the Ministry of Agriculture, Fisheries and Food (MAFF).

The current (fifth) edition of *The Composition of Foods* (Holland *et al*. 1991a) has been published as a single volume and is widely used as the standard reference source on the nutrient content of UK foods. However, it should be appreciated that, while convenient, the single-volume edition does not contain the complete set of data available, nor necessarily the most recent analytical information on some groups of foods (Black and Paul 1999). The most comprehensive and up-to-date information is contained within the separately published supplements (Table 1.9), and a complete collection of these should be regarded as the definitive UK food tables. As well being available in printed format, the data are available in electronic form, sometimes in conjunction with dietary analysis software programs.

Specialist food tables have been produced for food manufacturers for food labelling purposes (RSC 1992) using the conversion factors which are compatible with the EC Directive on Nutrition Labelling of Foodstuffs (EC 1990). Compositional data on foods commonly consumed by South Asians in the UK have recently been published by the Aga Khan Health Board (Judd *et al*. 2000) and usefully complement *The Composition of Foods*.

Other sources of food compositional data which have been derived from *The Composition of Foods* include the *Manual of Nutrition* (MAFF 1995) and *Nutrient Content of Food Portions* (Davies and Dickerson 1991). Although useful as a quick reference source or rule-of-thumb guide, these publications are not adequate for detailed dietary investigations because they only include a limited range of foods.

Some nutrient analysis software programs, particularly those designed for use in schools or within a general practice setting, use abbreviated data derived from the main food tables. These also need to be used with caution. Figures for groups of foods may be either averaged or confined to a few selected possibilities; thus, for example, data for 'meat' may be confined to just a few possible choices from the hundreds cited in the main food tables. Dietary estimates based on such generalized figures can be very misleading.

Food tables used in other countries

In order to be useful and accurate, food tables need to reflect the foods consumed in the culture in which they are used. *The Composition of Foods* is therefore really only applicable to the food consumption of people living in the UK. Many other countries produce national food

Table 1.9 UK food tables and supplements

Main compilation of food tables: McCance and Widdowson's *The Composition of Foods*, 5th edn (Holland *et al*. 1991a)
Supplements comprising the entire food table database.

Edition of *The Composition of Foods*	Supplement no.	Title (authors)
4th edition	1	*Amino Acid Composition and Fatty Acid Composition* (Paul *et al*. 1980)
	2	*Immigrant Foods* (Tan *et al*. 1985)
	3	*Cereals and Cereal Products* (Holland *et al*. 1988)
	4	*Milk Products and Eggs* (Holland *et al*. 1989)
	5	*Vegetables, Herbs, and Spices* (Holland *et al*. 1991b)
5th edition	1	*Fruit and Nuts* (Holland *et al*. 1992a)
	2	*Vegetable Dishes* (Holland *et al*. 1992b)
	3	*Fish and Fish Products* (Holland *et al*. 1993)
	4	*Miscellaneous Foods* (Chan *et al*. 1994)
	5	*Meat, Poultry and Game* (Chan *et al*. 1995)
	6	*Meat Products and Dishes* (Chan *et al*. 1996)
	7	*Fatty Acids* (MAFF 1999)

compositional tables and dietary investigations carried out in other parts of the world should use the appropriate local data.

1.4.2 Using food compositional data and tables

Food tables are an extremely valuable resource but it is important to understand their limitations and some of the pitfalls associated with their use.

Understanding the derivation of food table data

Before using any set of food tables, it is essential to read the introduction explaining how the values in the tables have been derived. This is particularly important if compositional data from other sources (e.g. food tables from other countries, food labelling information or data obtained by direct analysis) is used alongside standard food table data, because the definition and expression of the nutrients may not be the same. The following factors should be considered.

The analytical methodology

Different analytical techniques can be used to obtain estimates of the same nutrient.

At the beginning of the twentieth century, food analysis consisted of determining the percentage of water, fat, nitrogen and ash (minerals) in a food. Protein content was derived by multiplying the percentage of nitrogen by 6.25. Carbohydrate content was estimated 'by difference', i.e. the summed percentages of the other constituents subtracted from 100. This figure included the contribution from any dietary fibre present, as well as errors from the other analyses.

As chemical analysis methods became more sophisticated, it became possible to determine different types of sugars (glucose, fructose, galactose, sucrose, maltose, lactose and oligosaccharides) and complex carbohydrates (dextrins, starch and glycogen), amino acids and fatty acids, as well as individual minerals and vitamins. However, much commercial food analysis (e.g. for nutrition labelling purposes) is still carried out using simpler analytical techniques.

The use of different methodology can result in different estimates of nutrient content, for example:

- *Carbohydrate*: this may be determined as monosaccharide equivalents, actual weights or 'by difference'. Monosaccharide equivalents, the usual form of expression in UK food tables, result in slightly higher estimates of carbohydrate content (due to the fact that disaccharides and polysaccharides gain water when hydrolysed) than when expressed as actual weight (as on food labels).
- *Dietary fibre*: different methods of analysis give different estimates of fibre or non-starch polysaccharide content. The method derived by Englyst (Englyst and Cummings 1988) is considered to give the most representative

estimate of biologically useful 'fibre' as it measures 'non-starch polysaccharides', i.e. cellulose and both the soluble and insoluble non-cellulosic polysaccharides. The Association of Official Analytical Chemists (AOAC) method (based on that of Southgate 1969), commonly used by the food industry, gives much higher estimates of fibre content, particularly for cereal foods, because it includes lignin (or substances measuring as lignin) and enzymatically resistant starch.

- *Vitamins*: many vitamins are composites of substances with variable degrees of activity and either some or all of these may be quoted depending on the type of analysis performed. For example, vitamin A may be expressed as retinol and beta-carotene separately, or as retinol equivalents. Different units may also be used, e.g. micrograms or International Units (IU).

Conversion factors used to calculate data

The conversion factors used to calculate the energy yield or nutrient content may vary.

There are several differences between factors used in *The Composition of Foods* and those required for food labelling declarations in accordance with the 1990 EC Directive on Nutrition Labelling. For example:

- *Energy*: in UK food tables, carbohydrate is assumed to have an energy yield of 3.75 kcal (16 kJ) per gram; on food labels, a factor of 4 kcal (or 17 kJ) per gram is used.
- *Protein*: for food labelling purposes, protein content is derived by multiplying the nitrogen content in all foods by 6.25. UK food tables use specific conversion factors for different types of food.

The sampling procedure

Since compositional data are only derived from a sample of foods, their accuracy depends on how closely this sample represents the composition of all those available for consumption. The UK food tables are designed to be as representative as possible. Significant numbers of food samples are taken, foods for analysis are purchased from different retail outlets and pooled before analysis, 'market share' information is used to assess which brands of a particular type of food are included, and recipes are chosen to be as similar as possible to those used in the normal domestic setting. Other sources of food compositional data may not be based on such high standards.

How recently the data were compiled

Food compositional data need to be regularly updated because:

- The nutritional composition of staple foods can change with time. Particularly marked changes have occurred in the fat content and composition of meat in recent years. Selective breeding has produced leaner animals and changes in feeding techniques have reduced both intra-muscular (invisible) fat and visible fat stores. Modern butchery techniques also tend to remove a greater proportion of carcass fat. As a result, the content of fat in meat and its fatty acid profile have changed considerably. The fat content of pork has been reduced by about 35% since the late 1960s and that of beef and lamb by about 15% and 10%, respectively.

- Farming methods change. Changes in the level of usage of nitrate fertilizers or animal feeding practices can affect the composition of the end food product.
- The range of manufactured foods continually increases. New products are developed, old ones reformulated (perhaps to contain less fat or sugar), and processing techniques and fortification practices change.
- Cooking methods may change, e.g. greater use of microwaving or stir-frying.
- New foods may be imported, e.g. exotic fruits and vegetables.
- More accurate methods of analysis are developed.

The use of analytical data prepared many years before will considerably increase the likelihood of inaccuracies in dietary estimations. The most detailed dietary assessment will have serious inaccuracies if it is calculated from a food table database that is several decades out of date. Conversely, in some circumstances (e.g. the analysis of dietary information obtained many years before) it may be necessary to use compositional data which were contemporary at the time in order to obtain realistic figures of nutrient intake.

It is particularly important that those engaged in dietary survey work are aware of the implications of using data from the different editions and supplements of *The Composition of Foods*, and these have been extremely well explained by Black and Paul (1999). For example, data for meat, fish and miscellaneous foods in the single-volume 5th edition of *The Composition of Foods* were transferred from the 4th edition and have now been superseded by subsequent revisions published in supplement form. There are also some differences in code numbers between different editions which can have implications in computerized analysis.

Because data for food tables are updated on a rolling basis, it is important to know which data have been incorporated into any nutrient analysis programmes purchased and to ensure that such data are updated as necessary, or appropriate for the purpose for which they are to be used.

Limitations of food table data

Food tables will always have some limitations as a result of the following factors.

Variability between foods consumed and food table values

Even when great care has been taken in the compilation of food table data, it must be borne in mind that the resultant values will be 'typical' of a particular food but that there will still be some variation from foods actually consumed. This is particularly likely in respect of micronutrient content, which may be affected by:

- the soil in which it was grown (e.g. this can markedly affect selenium content);
- the use of food fortification in some but not all brands of a particular food (e.g. folate or iron added to breakfast cereals);
- the use of food additives which are also nutrients, e.g. beta-carotene (colour) or vitamin C (antioxidant);
- the duration and conditions of storage before being eaten (e.g. water-soluble vitamin content will reduce with time);
- the way in which the food is cooked (some vitamins and minerals may be lost).

It should also be noted that in food table analyses, vegetables will usually have been cooked in distilled water and without added salt. This means that the measured content of sodium, chloride and calcium (present in tap water) will be much lower than is likely in the typical domestic setting.

In terms of dietary significance, the relative importance of any differences between theoretical and actual nutrient composition decreases as the number of foods consumed during the day increases. Thus, for instance, in a typical African diet where only a few foods may be eaten during the day (maybe three to five), and where individual foods vary widely in their water content, food table values will be unlikely to be a good reflection of true nutrient intake (Cameron and van Staveren 1988). In Western diets where many different food items are eaten, agreement will be closer, although there will still be some differences; comparisons between the nutrient content of diets calculated from food tables and determined by direct analysis have been shown to vary by between 2 and 20% (Bingham 1987). For the purposes of metabolic studies based on the consumption of very few foods, or where extreme precision is required, duplicates of the actual foods concerned must be prepared for direct laboratory analysis.

Lack of information on bioavailability

Bioavailability is defined as the proportion of a nutrient capable of being absorbed, and hence available to the human body. The bioavailability of a particular nutrient can vary according its source of origin (e.g. calcium in milk is absorbed better than calcium in bread), its chemical form (e.g. haem iron is better absorbed than non-haem iron), the presence of binding agents consumed at the same time (e.g. phytates in cereal foods can reduce calcium absorption), its level of intake and physiological factors (e.g. percentage absorption may be increased in states of nutritional depletion) (Bender 1989). Since these interactions are so variable, UK food tables take no account of bioavailability and the nutrient content given in the food table is the amount present in the food. The only exception is that allowance has been made for the reduced activities of the different forms of three of the vitamins (13-*cis* retinol, carotenes other than beta-carotene, and tocopherol fractions other than alpha-tocopherol). When using other food tables it is worth checking whether any of the nutrient values have been modified to take account of their bioavailability.

Error associated with the use of food table data

Coding errors

In addition to inherent error in the food table data, additional error may be introduced into nutrient analysis programmes in a number of ways:

- Missing nutrient values in food composition tables may be treated as zero values during calculation, resulting in an underestimation of nutrient intake (missing values in the UK food tables are flagged with an 'N' to indicate that there may be significant quantities of a nutrient present but no reliable information on the amount is available).
- There may not be a suitable code for the food consumed or an inappropriate code may be chosen.
- There may be incorrect entry of food code numbers into the computing system.
- Errors can occur in the measurement, recording and estimation of food weights.

Nutrient intakes should never be reported with a greater apparent precision than that of the published values.

Errors of interpretation

Food tables are useful to help identify 'good' and 'poor' food sources of nutrients but are not always used for this purpose in an appropriate way. While scanning an eye down a column of nutrient content per 100 g will identify foods which are concentrated sources of a given nutrient, this does not necessarily mean that they are *significant* sources of that nutrient. The contribution which a particular food makes to nutrient intake depends on:

- the concentration of nutrient in the food (content per 100 g)
- the amount of the food consumed (portion size)
- the frequency with which that food is consumed (whether daily, weekly, monthly or never).

Thus, for example, a food such as parsley is a highly concentrated source of vitamin C but is unlikely to be a significant dietary source because it is usually used only infrequently and in minute quantities, if at all. In contrast, potatoes are a much less concentrated source of vitamin C but, because they are a regular and significant feature of most diets, usually make a major dietary contribution to vitamin C intake.

When giving dietary advice, it should never be forgotten that, however valuable a food may be as a source of a nutrient, it will make no contribution to dietary intake if it is never eaten.

Text revised by: Briony Thomas

References

Bender AE. Nutritional significance of bioavailability. In Southgate DAT, Johnson IT, Fenwick GR (Eds) *Nutrient Availability. Chemical and Biological Aspects*. Special publication No. 72, pp. 3–9. Cambridge: Royal Society of Chemistry, 1989.

Bingham S. The dietary assessment of individuals: methods, accuracy, new techniques and recommendations. *Nutrition Abstract and Reviews* 1987; **57**: 705–742.

Black AE, Paul AA. McCance & Widdowson's Tables of Food Composition: origins and clarification of the fifth edition. *Journal of Human Nutrition and Dietetics* 1999; **12**: 1–5.

Cameron ME, van Staveren WA. *Manual on Methodology for Food Consumption Studies*. Oxford: Oxford University Press, 1988.

Chan W, Brown J, Buss DH. *Miscellaneous Foods: Fourth Supplement to The Composition of Foods*, 5th edn. Cambridge: Royal Society of Chemistry/MAFF, 1994.

Chan W, Brown J, Lee SM, Buss DH. *Meat, Poultry and Game: Fifth Supplement to McCance and Widdowson's The Composition of Foods*, 5th edn. Cambridge: Royal Society of Chemistry/MAFF, 1995.

Chan W, Brown J, Church SM, Buss DH. *Meat Products and Dishes: Sixth Supplement to McCance and Widdowson's The Composition of Foods*, 5th edn. Cambridge: Royal Society of Chemistry/MAFF, 1996.

Davies J, Dickerson J. *Nutrient Content of Food Portions*. Cambridge: Royal Society of Chemistry, 1991.

Englyst HN, Cummings JH. An improved method for the measurement of dietary fibre as the non-starch polysaccharides in plant foods. *Journal of the Association of Official Analytical Chemists* 1988; **71**: 808–814.

Holland B, Brown J, Buss DH. *Fish and Fish Products: Third Supplement to McCance and Widdowson's The Composition of Foods*, 5th edn. Cambridge, Royal Society of Chemistry/MAFF, 1993.

Holland B, Unwin ID, Buss DH. *Cereals and Cereal Products: Third Supplement to McCance and Widdowson's The Composition of Foods*, 4th edn. Cambridge: Royal Society of Chemistry/MAFF, 1988.

Holland B, Unwin ID, Buss DH. *Milk Products and Eggs: Fourth Supplement to McCance and Widdowson's The Composition of Foods*, 4th edn. Cambridge: Royal Society of Chemistry/MAFF, 1989.

Holland B, Welch AA, Unwin ID *et al. McCance and Widdowson's The Composition of Foods*, 5th edn. Cambridge: Royal Society of Chemistry/MAFF, 1991a.

Holland B, Unwin ID, Buss DH. *Vegetables, Herbs, and Spices: Fifth Supplement to McCance and Widdowson's The Composition of Foods*, 4th edn. Cambridge: Royal Society of Chemistry/MAFF, 1991b.

Holland B, Unwin ID, Buss DH. *Fruit and Nuts: First Supplement to McCance and Widdowson's The Composition of Foods*, 5th edn. Cambridge: Royal Society of Chemistry/MAFF, 1992a.

Holland B, Welch A, Buss DH. *Vegetable Dishes: Second Supplement to McCance and Widdowson's The Composition of Foods*, 5th edn. Cambridge: Royal Society of Chemistry/MAFF, 1992b.

Judd PA, Kassam-Khamis T, Thomas JE. *The Composition and Nutrient Content of Foods Commonly Consumed by South Asians in the UK*. London: Aga Khan Health Board for the United Kingdom, 2000.

Ministry of Agriculture Fisheries and Food (MAFF). *Manual of Nutrition*, 10th edn. Reference Book 342. London: HMSO, 1995.

Ministry of Agriculture, Fisheries and Food (MAFF). *Fatty Acids: Seventh Supplement to McCance and Widdowson's The Composition of Foods*, 5th edn. Cambridge: Royal Society of Chemistry/MAFF, 1999.

Paul AA, Southgate DAT, Russell J. *Amino Acid Composition (mg per 100 g Food) and Fatty Acid Composition (g per 100 g Food): First Supplement to McCance and Widdowson's The Composition of Foods*, 4th edn. London: HMSO/Cambridge: Royal Society of Chemistry, 1980.

Royal Society of Chemistry. *Food Labelling Data for Manufacturers*. Cambridge: RSC, 1992.

Southgate DAT. Determination of carbohydrates in foods. II. Unavailable carbohydrates. *Journal of Food Science and Agriculture* 1969; **20**: 331–335.

Tan SP, Wenlock RW, Buss DH. *Immigrant Foods: Second Supplement to McCance and Widdowson's The Composition of Foods, 4th edn*. London: HMSO/Cambridge: Royal Society of Chemistry, 1985.

1.5 Dietary assessment

It is impossible to know precisely what a free-living individual eats. Dietary intake is inherently variable and no method can assess food intake accurately enough and for long enough without in itself altering eating behaviour. Even the most detailed assessment of dietary intake is at best a snapshot in time which, like a photograph, bears some relation to reality but by no means reveals the whole picture.

Dietary assessment is therefore just that – an assessment, not an exact measurement. The quality, and hence value of the assessment, depends largely on the skills of the assessor. These in turn depend on a clear understanding of the purpose of the assessment, the ways in which this can be done and the limitations of the information obtained.

1.5.1 Methods of dietary assessment

Dietary assessment methods can be divided into those which measure:

- current food intake (by weighed or unweighed food records)
- past food intake (recall methods)
- typical food intake (estimates of food consumption frequency).

In clinical practice, dietary assessment may require elements of all three.

Recording current dietary intake

This requires keeping a contemporary record of everything consumed over a specified period.

Weighed dietary intake record

Prior to its consumption, every item is accurately weighed or measured and the amount recorded, usually for a period of 5–7 days. Traditionally this has been done by providing subjects with a set of scales and a notebook for recording the results. People have to be taught how to weigh a meal on to their normal plates and record the cumulative weights together with adequate descriptions of brand names and recipes of composite foods. Any leftover food also has to be weighed and deducted from the original portion weight. However, the advent of electronic scales with integrated recording facilities has simplified this procedure considerably. Other innovations such as bar-code data entry (Anderson *et al*. 1999a) and integrated dietary analysis (Nelson *et al*. 1997) are also streamlining the transcription and nutritional analysis of the data obtained.

A number of problems are associated with weighed dietary record keeping:

- It disrupts normal life. People find it awkward and inconvenient to have to carry recording equipment with them all day, and may be embarrassed or reluctant to use it outside the home.
- People may be tempted to alter, either consciously or subconsciously, their dietary intake in favour of foods which are easier or less messy to weigh. Alternatively, people may guess the weights of items (especially drinks or snacks) which are inconvenient to weigh.
- It requires a certain level of intellectual ability to understand what is required and dexterity to use the equipment. This limits its use in some sectors of the population, e.g. people with learning or physical disabilities or a poor command of the English language.
- Subjects usually need to be followed up during the record-keeping process to make sure that they have understood the recording technique and are applying it correctly. This requires resources in terms of personnel.
- The recording equipment (particularly if electronic) can be costly and beyond the resources available for small studies or routine dietetic work.

The weighed dietary record is often referred to as the 'gold standard' of dietary assessment and undoubtedly is the most 'accurate', i.e. gives the most precise quantitative measurement of intake. However, its influence on eating habits means that it may not always be the most 'valid', i.e. truly reflecting what someone normally eats. Its invasiveness and complexity mean that it is not appropriate for all types of subject and, in survey work, this can introduce an element of bias. It is, however, the best tool for research purposes and detailed dietary investigations.

Unweighed/semi-quantitative dietary intake record

This is an adaptation of the weighed dietary intake method in which food and drink consumed is quantitatively described as accurately as possible, but using household measures or description of portion sizes. It still requires a considerable degree of co-operation from subjects and a certain level of literacy skills but, because it is less invasive, tends to be more acceptable. While a certain amount of quantitative accuracy will be lost, there may be gains in terms of subject participation and compliance. Tape-recorded food records have been used to make the recording process simpler, although there is evidence that some people, especially children or those who are obese, provide less accurate records using this approach (Lindqvist et al. 2000).

The major problem with this method is interpretation of portion sizes. Subjects need to be encouraged to give as accurate a description as possible – perhaps in comparison with other items, e.g. the size of a piece of cheese in relation to a matchbox, or potatoes in relation to the size of an egg. Subjects can also be shown how to find the net weight or volume recorded on the label of prepackaged food, and state what proportion of the product was consumed. Accuracy can be enhanced if the record is discussed with a dietitian making use of replica food models or quantified pictures of food portion sizes (see Estimating food portion size below).

The lower level of precision makes the unweighed record less suitable than the weighed record for research purposes, particularly in large-scale or multicentre trials where different personnel evaluating portion sizes will introduce additional error and bias. However, its simplicity and acceptability make it a useful tool for clinical practice particularly when qualitative, rather than quantitative aspects of the diet need to be assessed, e.g. meal patterns, dietary variety, representation of different food groups or food–symptom associations.

Recalling past intake

This involves asking a subject to recall in as much detail as possible everything consumed in the previous 24 hours, or perhaps longer. This approach has the advantage of not directly influencing food choice, which is always a risk with contemporary record-keeping. The method is also quick and simple to perform and places a minimal burden on the subject. In the USA, 24-hour recalls conducted over the telephone have been shown to be an adequate way of obtaining data for national food consumption surveys (Casey et al. 1999).

Its disadvantages are:

- The method depends on memory and the reliability of this varies. Recalled intake nearly always underestimates actual dietary intake and the method may be of little value in children or elderly people, particularly if the latter are confused or suffering memory impairment.
- Fabrication of dietary intake (perhaps to impress the observer) is a possibility, although invention is surprisingly difficult to sustain under close questioning and usually detectable.
- Assessment is confined to a short period. Intake over the previous 24 hours may not be typical of usual intake and will not reflect daily variations. Longer periods of recall are fraught with inaccuracies; most people find it impossible to remember everything that they consumed two or more days ago.

The 24-hour recall is rarely sufficient on its own to provide a quantitative estimate of nutrient intake, but can reveal major imbalances or obvious dietary inadequacies, or highlight areas of concern which need further exploration. The main value of the 24-hour recall in the clinical setting is that it is a useful starting point for further exploration. It can set the scene in terms of meal pattern and the types of food consumed which can then be used as a basis for more detailed discussion.

Attempting to evaluate past food intake using distant recall (e.g. foods consumed many years previously such as during childhood) is fraught with problems of bias, as reports of past intake are greatly influenced by current levels of intake (Friedenreich et al. 1992) and people also recall their intake of some foods better than others (Dwyer and Coleman 1997). Information obtained using this approach should always be regarded with caution.

Estimating typical food intake

Food Frequency Questionnaires (FFQs)

These assess the frequency and level of consumption of foods and attempt to assess 'typical' food intake over a longer timescale than is possible with short-term recording or recall methods. The FFQ may thus be an important tool in the assessment of the relationships between diet and disease (Willett 1998).

Foods are listed in a questionnaire format or a multiple-response grid, and subjects attempt to estimate how often each food is consumed. A common format comprises up to 10 categories ranging from 'never' via 'once a month or less' to 'six times per day'. A modification of this approach is the 'picture-sort', where participants sort cards containing names or pictures of foods in categories of consumption frequency (Kumanyika et al. 1997). Since the information is in a standardized format, it is computer readable and hence quick and economical to analyse in large-scale studies.

The questionnaire can be either self-administered or completed by an interviewer, depending on the nature of the study and the resource implications. FFQs administered with nutritionist input may be more accurate than those which are self-administered but increase the cost of using this method (Caan et al. 1999).

Although it is possible to calculate energy and nutrient intake from FFQ data, the method is less suitable for estimating the intakes of individuals. For example, when compared with urinary urea excretion measurements, the FFQ has been shown to be capable of assessing the mean protein intake of a group but to be much less accurate in respect of individual protein intake or changes in intake (Pijls et al. 1999). The FFQ is, however, a useful way of classifying individuals, e.g. into tertiles or quintiles of intake within a population, and is therefore a useful tool in epidemiological studies (Kassam-Khamis et al. 1999; Kroke et al. 1999; Jain et al. 1996).

Another major use of the FFQ is to explore broad dietary patterns and intake of specific foods or groups of foods. Questionnaires can be targeted to explore dietary concerns in particular sectors of the population such as minority ethnic groups (Coates and Monteilh 1997; Teufel 1997) or children and adolescents (Rockett and Colditz 1997; Blum *et al.* 1999; Robinson *et al.* 1999). Alternatively, the focus of a FFQ can be on a particular aspect of a diet such as consumption of fruit and vegetables, or foods rich in iron.

This application of the FFQ has also been incorporated into dietary risk assessment tools designed to identify specific dietary behaviours (e.g. risk factors for cardiovascular disease; Olendzki *et al.* 1999) or for more general application in primary care (Calfas *et al.* 2000; Little *et al.* 2000). People who would benefit from dietary change can be targeted and given appropriate counselling. These simple food-based checklists can, if validated, have a useful place in data collection, monitoring and audit. They do not, however, provide a sophisticated or accurate nutritional assessment and should not be used as such.

A further developing modification of the FFQ technique, particularly in the USA, is the construction of indices of dietary quality. These involve the calculation of scores to reflect aspects such as dietary variety, dietary balance, nutritional adequacy and post-counselling dietary change (e.g. the Dietary Diversity Score, Overall Variety Score, Nutrient Adequacy Score (Kant and Graubard 1999) or the Recommended Food Group Change Score, Total Food Group Change Score, Nutrient Improvement Score (Alexy *et al.* 1999)). However, while attractive in concept, this approach is not without problems and any such index requires careful validation (Kant and Graubard 1999).

The main problems associated with FFQs are:

- Knowing which foods to include. The accuracy of the assessment depends on the number of foods in the list. A typical FFQ is composed of about 150 food items but this is only a fraction of the 5000 or so food items available in the Westernized food supply (DH 1998). However, completing even a 150-food FFQ requires a considerable amount of time and effort from the participants; FFQs which are longer than this soon become impractical in terms of subject co-operation. Choice of foods to be included in a FFQ therefore has to be made with care.
- Completing a FFQ requires an ability to think abstractly and some people find this easier than others (Field *et al.* 1999).
- Like all unweighed assessment methods, its accuracy is dependent on an evaluation of portion size. With discrete items (e.g. a piece of fruit, a biscuit, a carton of yoghurt) this is less difficult, but assessing consumption of foods of variable portion size (e.g. meat, salad, cake, pies, puddings) is more problematical.
- People may be tempted to give the answers which they think are 'correct' or 'desirable', e.g. more fruit and vegetables or fewer cakes and biscuits than is really the case.
- Frequency of food intake is related to total food (and energy) intake. This can lead to distortions, particularly if FFQ data are used to assess the degree of dietary 'balance' or 'healthiness'. For example, people who eat a lot of food in general may well have a high consumption of fruit and vegetables but may also consume more fat and sugar and be overweight.

1.5.2 General aspects of dietary assessment

Error

Error is inherent in dietary assessment. This does not make the procedure valueless, but the likely nature and extent of error must be considered when choosing an assessment method and interpreting the results (Beaton *et al.* 1997).

Errors can occur as a result of a method of dietary assessment not being sufficiently:

- accurate (e.g. portion sizes being estimated or recorded inaccurately by the subject)
- reliable (e.g. owing to invention, omission or distortion on the part of the subject)
- representative of usual food habits (e.g. the recording period may be too short)
- unbiased (e.g. some subjects may not be willing or able to provide the necessary information).

Error may also be introduced by the investigator as a result of:

- incorrect coding of data (e.g. a food being coded wrongly, or perhaps twice by mistake)
- inappropriate analysis of data (e.g. limitations of food table data, see Section 1.4)
- incorrect interpretation (e.g. as a result of a limited choice of questions in a FFQ)
- differences between investigators in the way in which they apply or interpret a particular assessment method.

These are particularly important considerations in epidemiological studies. Errors always blur the picture between apparent and genuine dietary intake, and weaken associations between diet and other variables. If the errors are not randomly distributed (e.g. particular types of subjects underreport their intakes, or particular investigators provide less reliable information than others) they can also introduce bias and can create an apparent relationship when in reality none exists. Bias can also be introduced by the choice of the method itself, e.g. the inability or refusal of some types of subjects to complete a 7-day weighed record or a detailed FFQ. A detailed review of nutritional epidemiology can be found in Willett (1998).

Validity

The validity of different methods of dietary assessment (i.e. how closely they assess the truth) has often been evaluated using the 7-day weighed food record as a basis for comparison. However, the 7-day weighed record, while quantitatively more accurate than any other method, has its own elements of error and cannot be regarded as an infallible determinant of dietary intake (see Weighed records, above). All methods of dietary assessment are in reality different estimates of an unknown (Thompson and Byers 1994).

Comparisons between different methods show that recall methods tend to produce lower estimates of intake than contemporary record-keeping, probably because memory is involved (Kroke *et al.* 1999). Comparisons between FFQs and dietary records are more variable and have been reported to produce both higher (Coates and Menteilh 1997) and lower (Caan *et al.* 1999; Forman *et al.* 1999) mean intakes. Since the dietary record may be more 'accurate' but the FFQ may be more 'representative', it is perhaps arguable which can best reflect true dietary intake.

Biomarkers are a better way of assessing the validity of dietary assessment methods (Bingham *et al.* 1995; Bingham and Day 1997). Energy intake can be validated by comparison with estimates of energy expenditure derived from doubly labelled water measurements; and protein intake can be compared with 24- hour urinary nitrogen excretion (Black *et al.* 1997). The 24-hour urinary excretion of sodium and potassium can be used as a marker of dietary sodium and potassium intake (Dyer *et al.* 1997). FFQs have been validated by comparing estimates of intake of *n-3* fatty acids with levels stored in adipose tissue (Andersen *et al.* 1999b), or intake of antioxidant vitamins with measured plasma levels (Bodner *et al.* 1999). However, biomarkers are not available for every nutrient; for example, none exists to evaluate total fat or carbohydrate intake (Bingham and Day 1997).

Under-reporting

Validation using biomarkers has revealed evidence that dietary records, and probably all methods of dietary assessment, underestimate true dietary intake, particularly energy intake (Black *et al.* 1993). Furthermore, this does not occur uniformly across a population but is more likely to occur in some subgroups than others, particularly women and people who are overweight or trying to lose weight (Briefel *et al.* 1997). This introduces significant bias into dietary surveys (Price *et al.* 1997; Blundell 2000).

As well as under-reporting (i.e. recording less than was actually eaten), underestimation may also result from undereating (i.e. consuming less during the study period than is usually the case). Goris *et al.* (2000) showed that both of these factors greatly influence the records of overweight people; comparison with biomarkers showed that a group of obese men reduced their habitual food intake by 26% and failed to record 12% of what they ate. Significant under-reporting of fat intake (but not protein or carbohydrate) was also observed.

Blundell (2000) explores some of the psychological issues which may underlie this phenomenon and suggests that dietitians (and nutrition scientists) underestimate the unwillingness of individuals to reveal to others what they regard as highly personal information, or even admit to behaviour which they know to be undesirable (e.g. consuming foods rich in fat or sugar). Furthermore, the complexities involved in making an accurate record of dietary intake, a process which requires motivation, attention, perception, memory, mathematical ability and perhaps a perceived need for truthfulness, should not be overlooked.

Duration of recording period

Variability determines the length of time over which dietary information needs to be obtained in order to obtain a meaningful assessment of intake. People do not eat the same foods every day (within-person variability) and everyone eats a different diet (between-person variability). For an individual, estimated intake on a single day is unlikely to take sufficient account of daily variation, or to be able to distinguish between genuine differences in nutrient intake between different individuals. However, an estimate based on a single day can be sufficient to provide a meaningful mean intake of a group because individual variations (i.e. whether someone's intake is higher or lower than usual on that day) will tend to cancel each other out.

A minimum of 7 days is considered necessary to assess the energy and protein intakes of individuals to within ± 10% standard error (Bingham 1987). A shorter timescale may be adequate in people with very stable eating habits, but those with highly variable food habits will require longer. To assess the intake of other nutrients, many more days of recording may be necessary, particularly if the nutrient is derived from relatively few foods in the diet. For example, 36 days of recording may be required to assess vitamin C intake to within ± 10% of the true intake.

In practice, continuous recording periods of more than a few days are counterproductive because subjects tire of the recording procedure and the quality of the record-keeping tends to deteriorate or is abandoned altogether. A more acceptable approach is to make repeated short assessments of, for example, 2–3 days' duration on several separate occasions. If meal pattern or food consumption rather than absolute nutrient intake is the primary focus of interest, a single, short recording period may be sufficient.

Estimating portion size

Inaccurate estimation of portion size can be a major source of error. This can be reduced in unweighed recording methods by encouraging subjects to make use of net weights recorded on packaged foods or using other descriptive measures, e.g. the number of 'egg-sized' potatoes consumed. For recall methods, portion size can be estimated with the help of replica food models or by photographs such as those in *Food Portions Sizes: A Photographic Atlas* (Nelson *et al.* 1997). The latter was developed by MAFF for use in dietary surveys but is also a valuable resource in the clinical setting. It contains a series of eight photographs of 76 foods ranging in portion size from the 5th to the 95th centile of portion sizes observed in the Dietary and Nutritional Survey of British Adults (Gregory *et al.* 1990). Many of the foods included are those which are particularly difficult to quantify in terms of household measures, e.g. spaghetti, mashed potato or the thickness of fat spread on bread. Additional photographs show tin sizes, crockery and cutlery sizes and fluid volumes.

Evaluation studies of the food atlas showed that, in general, the method of estimating food portion size by photographs was capable of estimating nutrient intake to within ± 7% of the nutrient content actually consumed (Nelson *et al.* 1996). However, small portion sizes tended to be overestimated and large portion sizes underestimated; butter and margarine intake also tended to be overestimated by photographic assessment. People with a body mass index (BMI) > 30 underestimated portion size more than people with a BMI < 25.

Directories of food portion sizes (MAFF 1993) can be used to make quick approximate estimates of intake but are obviously much less accurate.

1.5.3 Dietary assessment in clinical practice

Assessment of the current, recent or usual dietary intake of an individual is an essential component of assessing nutritional status (see Section 1.8) or nutritional risk (see Section 1.9) and as a basis for providing dietary guidance (see Section 1.6) or nutritional support (see Section 1.11). The way in which this is done depends on the clinical circumstances, the characteristics of the person being investigated (e.g. age, ethnic background, cognitive ability) and the purpose of the assessment, which may be to:

- assess overall dietary balance and meal pattern
- identify the level of consumption of specific foods, or groups of foods
- obtain a quantitative estimate of energy and/or nutrient intake
- identify nutritional deficiencies or surpluses
- identify food-related symptoms
- assess the risk of malnutrition
- monitor compliance with dietary advice.

In the clinical setting, information is often required immediately, and has to be obtained in a short timescale and with limited resources. In many instances this can be achieved by obtaining a 'dietary history' whereby, by means of questioning, a picture of typical food intake is built up. An approach based on the 24-hour recall, 'What did you eat and drink yesterday?' can be a good starting point. Depending on the level of quantification required, typical portion sizes of foods consumed can be established using replica food models or a photographic atlas (see above). Further questioning can then help establish a 'typical' day's intake by ascertaining the:

- degree of daily variation in both terms of quantity of food eaten and type of food
- differences between weekdays and weekends
- influence of work pattern on eating habits, e.g. shift work, business entertaining, frequent travel
- meals eaten out
- social aspects, e.g. whether food is eaten as part of formal family meals, as a snack on the move or in front of the television.

Good counselling skills are needed to elicit useful information. Most people are sensitive about their food intake, especially if they are overweight, and a non-judgemental approach from the dietitian is essential. Searching questions may need to be asked about consumption of items such as biscuits, confectionery and other snack foods, since people tend to assume that dietitians will 'disapprove' of such items so are reluctant to admit to eating them. Conversely, patients may be tempted to exaggerate their consumption of foods such as fruit or wholemeal bread to create a better impression. Indirect questions focusing on shopping habits, e.g. 'how often do you buy...?' or 'which brands of biscuits do you buy...?' can sometimes help to provide clues to actual consumption levels.

Patients can be prompted to remember things that may be overlooked (such as between-meal snacks or drinks), but leading questions should be avoided. For example, asking someone 'What did you eat for breakfast?' conveys the expectation that breakfast will have been eaten; the patient may therefore be tempted to invent 'a slice of toast' to avoid seeming inadequate. The question 'What was the first thing you ate yesterday?' is more likely to reveal that this was a chocolate bar on the way to work.

This information provides an overall picture of dietary balance and likely nutritional adequacy. Comparing the proportion of different food groups in the diet with that recommended in *The Balance of Good Health* can quickly identify major imbalances (e.g. lack of fruit and vegetables; over-representation of fat-rich foods) (see Section 1.2.2 in Healthy Eating). It also highlights the type of dietary changes that are likely to be needed in terms of food choice.

Depending on the individual and clinical circumstances, other influences on current food intake, and their impact and duration, may need to be considered. These may include:

- appetite level
- symptoms affecting food intake, e.g. nausea, vomiting, pain
- eating or swallowing difficulties
- treatment affecting food intake, e.g. drugs, radiotherapy, surgery
- difficulties with shopping or cooking
- socioeconomic factors, e.g. low income, housing conditions
- psychological factors, e.g. depression, anxiety, apathy, recent bereavement
- self-imposed food exclusions or modifications (e.g. avoidance of foods due to intolerance, or use of liquidized diets for dysphagia).

Other diet-related and lifestyle factors which may need to be taken into account include:

- physical activity level
- use of alcohol
- use of tobacco
- prescribed medications
- use of dietary supplements.

Concerns over intake of a particular nutrient (e.g. iron) may need to be explored in more depth (e.g. the level of consumption of haem/non-haem iron-containing foods and dietary influences on iron absorption such as vitamin C, fibre or zinc supplements).

In order to consider the impact on nutritional status, dietary information may need to be considered in conjunction with clinical, anthropometric, biochemical or haematological factors (see Section 1.8).

Dietary assessment should also take a global view of health. Assessment of a person diagnosed with one disorder (e.g. hyperlipidaemia) should not be confined only to those parameters which have a direct influence (e.g. dietary fat intake) but also take account of dietary factors which impact on associated risks (e.g. cardiovascular disease). Nor should general health risks (e.g. that of osteoporosis from a low calcium intake) be overlooked. Therapeutic dietary measures will only be of optimum benefit if the overall diet is balanced.

Other dietary assessment methods also have applications in the clinical setting and some examples of these are given in Table 1.10. Contemporary dietary record-keeping is rarely appropriate for initial clinical assessment because of the timescale involved. Dietary records may, however, be a useful adjunct to baseline assessment to investigate food-related symptoms (e.g. certain types of food intolerance or, in the diabetic patient, unexplained episodes of hypoglycaemia). They may also be useful to monitor the effectiveness of dietary treatment (e.g. in relation to pancreatic enzyme replacement therapy in the patient with cystic fibrosis) or to monitor compliance with dietary advice (e.g. a patient may be asked to keep a 3-day dietary record prior to a dietetic consultation or an annual review). Periods of dietary record-keeping can also sometimes be a useful part of treatment, e.g. patients trying to achieve weight control may find that dietary records can help act as a brake on eating, or highlight when episodes of binge eating are most likely to occur.

As well as providing information about dietary adequacy and being a useful diagnostic tool, it should not be forgotten that dietary assessment is a fundamental requirement for dietary modification and the provision of dietary advice (see Section 1.6). Dietary guidance is only likely to result in dietary change if it has personal relevance to an individual; it therefore needs to be based on that person's usual eating habits and take account of the influences on them. Time spent by a dietitian making a realistic assessment of these factors is ultimately a good investment.

Text written by: Briony Thomas

Table 1.10 Practical applications of different methods of dietary assessment

Method of assessment	Principal uses	Examples of uses
Weighed food records	When an accurate quantified measure of nutrient intake is required	• Detailed investigation of individual dietary intake • Assessing the mean and range of nutrient intake within a population • Investigating relationships between nutrient intake and other parameters • Specialized research studies
Unweighed food records	When quantification, although relevant, is less important than identifying meal pattern and food choice When the loss of quantitative accuracy is outweighed by the advantages of a method which is acceptable to the subject and cheap to administer	• Assessing dietary balance, e.g. comparing food intake with *The Balance of Good Health* • Investigating relationships between food intake and symptoms (e.g. due to food intolerance, or hypoglycaemic episodes in diabetic patients) • Assessing dietary compliance (e.g. that the diet of a treated coeliac patient remains gluten free) • Investigating food habits (e.g. exploring parental concerns that their child 'doesn't eat anything')
24-hour recall	As a quick baseline assessment of meal pattern and food choice	• A starting point for investigation of dietary inadequacies or poor food habits
Food Frequency Questionnaires	To identify nutritional problems as a result of inappropriate food choice To identify consumption of foods consumed infrequently which may not be apparent from short-term food records (e.g. consumption of oily fish) To categorize individuals, e.g. into tertiles or quintiles of intake within a population	• To investigate relationships between diet and disease in large-scale prospective studies • Assessing food choices (e.g. consumption of iron-rich foods) • Monitoring the effectiveness of healthy eating guidance (e.g. increased consumption of fruit and vegetables) • As a cross-check against other methods of dietary assessment (e.g. a 5-day food record) • As a component of nutritional risk assessment (e.g. lack of fruit and vegetables, iron-containing foods, oily fish)

Further reading

2nd International Conference on Dietary Assessment Methods. Proceedings of a symposium. Boston, Massachusetts, January 22–24, 1995. *American Journal of Clinical Nutrition* 1997; **65**: 1097S–1368S.

References

Alexy U, Sichert-Hellert W, Kersting M *et al*. Development of scores to measure the effects of nutrition counselling on the overall diet: a pilot study in children and adolescents. *European Journal of Nutrition* 1999; **38**: 196–200

Anderson AS, Maher L, Ha TK *et al*. Evaluation of a bar-code system for nutrient analysis in dietary surveys. *Public Health Nutrition* 1999a; **2**: 579–586.

Andersen LF, Solvoll K, Johansson LR *et al*. Evaluation of a food frequency questionnaire with weighed records, fatty acids, and alpha-tocopherol in adipose tissue and serum. *American Journal of Epidemiology* 1999b; **150**: 75–87.

Beaton GH, Burema J, Ritenbaugh C. Errors in the interpretation of dietary assessments. *American Journal of Clinical Nutrition* 1997; **65**: 1100S–1107S.

Bingham S. The dietary assessment of individuals; methods, accuracy, new techniques and recommendations. *Nutrition Abstract and Reviews* 1987; **57**: 705–742.

Bingham SA, Day NE Use of biomarkers to validate dietary assessments and the effect of energy adjustment. *American Journal of Clinical Nutrition* 1997; **65**: 1130S–1137S.

Bingham SA, Cassidy A, Cole T *et al*. Validation of weighed records and other methods of dietary assessment using the 24 hour urine technique and other biological markers. *British Journal of Nutrition* 1995; **73**: 531–550.

Black AE, Prentice AW, Goldberg GR *et al*. Measurement of total energy expenditure provide insights into the validity of dietary measures of energy intake. *Journal of the American Dietetic Association* 1993; **93**: 572–579.

Black AE, Bingham SA, Johansson G, Coward WA. Validation of dietary intakes of protein and energy against 24 hour urinary nitrogen and doubly-labelled water energy expenditure in middle-aged women, retired men and post-obese subjects: comparisons with validation against presumed energy requirements. *European Journal of Clinical Nutrition* 1997; **51**: 405–413.

Blum RE, Wei EK, Rockett HR *et al*. Validation of a food frequency questionnaire in Native American and Caucasian children 1 to 5 years of age. *Maternal and Child Health* 1999; **3**: 167–172.

Blundell JE. What foods do people habitually eat? A dilemma for nutrition, an enigma for psychology. *American Journal of Clinical Nutrition* 2000; **71**: 3–5.

Bodner C, Godden D, Brown K *et al*. Antioxidant intake and adult-onset wheeze: a case–control study. Aberdeen WHEASE Study Group. *European Respiratory Journal* 1999; **13**: 22–30.

Briefel RR, Sempos CT, McDowell MA *et al*. Dietary methods research in the third National Health Nutrition Examination Survey: underreporting of energy intake. *American Journal of Clinical Nutrition* 1997; **65**: 1210S–1214S.

Caan BJ, Lanza E, Schatzkin A *et al*. Does nutritionist review of a self-administered food frequency questionnaire improve data quality? *Public Health Nutrition* 1999; **2**: 565–569.

Calfas KJ, Zabinski MF, Rupp J. Practical nutrition assessment in primary care settings. A review (1). *American Journal of Preventive Medicine* 2000; **18**: 289–299.

Casey PH, Goolsby SL, Lensing SY *et al*. The use of telephone interview methodology to obtain 24-hour dietary recalls. *Journal of the American Dietetic Association* 1999; **99**: 1406–1411.

Coates RJ, Monteilh CP. Assessments of food-frequency questionnaires in minority populations. *American Journal of Clinical Nutrition* 1997; **65**: 1108S–1115S.

Department of Health. Report of the Working Group on Diet and Cancer of the Committee on Medical Aspects of Food and Nutrition Policy (COMA). *Nutritional Aspects of the Development of Cancer*. Report on Health and Social Subjects 48, p. 75. London: The Stationery Office, 1998.

Dwyer JT, Coleman KA. Insights into dietary recall from a longitudinal study: accuracy over four decades. *American Journal of Clinical Nutrition* 1997; **65**: 1153S–1158S.

Dyer A, Elliott P, Chee D, Stamler J. Urinary biochemical markers of dietary intake in the INTERSALT Study. *American Journal of Clinical Nutrition* 1997; **65**: 1246S–1253S.

Field AE, Peterson KE, Gortmaker SL *et al*. Reproducibility and validity of a food frequency questionnaire among fourth to seventh grade inner-city school children: implications of age and day-to-day variation in dietary intake. *Public Health Nutrition* 1999; **2**: 293–300.

Forman MR, Zhang J, Nebeling L *et al*. Relative validity of a food frequency questionnaire among tin miners in China: 1992/93 and 1995/6 diet validation studies. *Public Health Nutrition* 1999; **2**: 301–315.

Friedenreich CM, Slimani N, Riboli E. Measurement of past diet: review of previous and proposed methods. *Epidemiological Review* 1992; **14**: 177–196.

Goris AHC, Westerterp-Plantenga MS, Westerterp KR. Undereating and underreporting of habitual food intake in obese men: selective underreporting of fat intake. *American Journal of Clinical Nutrition* 2000; **71**: 130–134.

Gregory J, Foster K, Tyler H, Wiseman M. *The Dietary and Nutritional Survey of British Adults*. London: HMSO, 1990.

Jain M, Howe GR, Rohan T. Dietary assessment in epidemiology: comparison of a food frequency and a diet history questionnaire with a 7-day food record. *American Journal of Epidemiology* 1996; **143**: 953–960.

Kant AK, Graubard BI. Variability in selected indexes of overall diet quality. *International Journal for Vitamin and Nutrition Research* 1999; **69**: 419–427.

Kassam-Khamis T, Nanchalal K, Mangtani P *et al*. Development of an interview-administered food-frequency questionnaire for use amongst women of South Asian ethnic origin in Britain. *Journal of Human Nutrition and Dietetics* 1999; **12**: 7–19.

Kroke A, Klipstein-Grobusch K, Voss S *et al*. Validation of a self-administered food-frequency questionnaire administered in the European Prospective Investigation into Cancer and Nutrition (EPIC) Study: comparison of energy, protein and macronutrient intakes estimated with the doubly labeled water, urinary nitrogen, and repeated 24-h dietary recall methods. *American Journal of Clinical Nutrition* 1999; **70**: 439–447.

Kumanyika SK, Tell GS, Shemanski J *et al*. Dietary assessment using a picture-sort approach. *American Journal of Clinical Nutrition* 1997; **65**: 1123S–1129S.

Lindqvist CH, Cummings T, Goran MI. Use of tape-recorded food records in assessing children's dietary intake. *Obesity Research* 2000; **8**: 2–11.

Little P, Barnett J, Kinmonth AL *et al*. Can dietary assessment in general practice target patients with unhealthy diets? *British Journal of General Practice* 2000; **50**: 43–45.

Livingstone MBE, Prentice AM, Strain JJ *et al*. Accuracy of weighed dietary records in studies of diet and health. *British Medical Journal* 1990; **300**: 708–712.

Ministry of Agriculture Fisheries and Food (MAFF). *Food Portion Sizes*. 2nd edn. Compilers: Mills A, Sejal P. London: The Stationery Office, 1993.

Nelson M, Atkinson, Darbyshire S. Food photography 2. Food photographs for estimating portion size and nutrient content of meals. *British Journal of Nutrition* 1996; **76**: 31–49.

Nelson M, Atkinson M, Meyer J, on behalf of the Nutritional Epidemiology Group UK. *Food Portion Sizes. A Photographic Atlas*. London: MAFF, 1997.

Olendzki B, Hurley TG, Hebert JR *et al*. Comparing food intake using the Dietary Risk Assessment with multiple 24-hour recalls and the 7-day dietary recall. *Journal of the American Dietetic Association* 1999; **99**: 1433–1439.

Pijls LT, de Vries H, Donker AJ, van Eijk JT. Reproducibility and biomarker-based validity and responsiveness of a food frequency questionnaire to estimate protein intake. *American Journal of Epidemiology* 1999; **150**: 987–995.

Price GM, Paul AA, Cole TJ, Wadsworth ME. Characteristics of the low-energy reporters in a longitudinal national dietary survey. *British Journal of Nutrition* 1997; **77**: 833–851.

Robinson S, Skelton R, Barker M, Wilman C. Assessing the diet of adolescent girls in the UK. *Public Health Nutrition* 1999; **2**: 571–577.

Rockett HRH, Colditz GA. Assessing diets of children and adolescents. *American Journal of Clinical Nutrition* 1997; **65**: 1116S–1122S.

Teufel NI. Development of culturally competent food-frequency questionnaires. *American Journal of Clinical Nutrition* 1997; **65**: 1173S–1178S.

Thompson FE, Byers T. Dietary assessment resource manual. *Journal of Nutrition* 1994; **124**: 2245S–2317S.

Willett W. *Nutritional Epidemiology – Monographs in Epidemiology and Biostatistics*. New York: Oxford University Press, 1998.

1.6 Dietary modification

Dietary modification is the core of dietetic practice and requires enormous skill. The role of the dietitian is far removed from the layperson's image of someone who hands out standard diet sheets for standard diseases. People, and their needs and problems, are infinitely variable and no two situations requiring dietetic intervention will be exactly the same. The skill of the dietitian lies in assessing individual needs and problems and deciding how, in those particular circumstances, they may best be addressed. Increasingly, the role of the dietitian is seen as being that of an 'enabler', i.e. someone who helps people to make the necessary changes, rather than a 'dictator' who instructs people what to do.

Dietary advice may take many different forms:

- It may be targeted at patients, clients, carers or the general public, or to educate other health professionals.
- It may be delivered via direct one-to-one contact, direct contact with a small or large group of people, or indirect contact with the general public (e.g. via the media).
- It may be very simple (e.g. aiming to increase consumption of fruit of vegetables) or very complex (e.g. management of renal failure).
- It may be provided in a verbal, written, audiovisual or interactive format, or a combination of these.

1.6.1 Rationale for dietary modification

Whatever the type of advice given, it must be based on sound scientific reasoning. The importance of 'evidence-based practice' in all areas of healthcare has been emphasized in recent years (see Section 1.17, Professional practice). However, in the field of dietetics, 'evidence' in the form of unequivocal proof is hard to obtain. The blueprint model of the randomized controlled trial, used to evaluate drug versus placebo, does not lend itself readily to dietary studies in humans. In a drug trial people either do, or do not, take a drug; in a dietary study everyone consumes a diet of some sort and the composition of this diet is variable and impossible to standardize in free-living people. Furthermore, unlike a drug, a diet is not a single entity but a variable mixture of interrelated components where changes to one aspect directly affect others, thus making evaluation difficult. Dietary studies in laboratory animals are easier to control but the findings may not be relevant to humans. Other types of study such as prospective or case–control studies can provide valuable information but because of the timescale and size required for meaningful results are extremely costly to carry out.

Justification for dietary manipulation therefore usually has to be based on a combination of:

- *scientific rationale*: reasoned expectation based on a knowledge of nutrition, physiology, anatomy and biochemistry
- *scientific evidence*: presented in the literature or at symposia
- *clinical experience*: knowledge acquired via direct experience, or from the experience of others, of the effectiveness of different types of treatment
- *clinical judgement*: considering all relevant factors in a particular situation and deciding what course of action and level of intervention may be most appropriate in that situation.

Dietary interventions are undertaken on the basis that they will be of benefit. It is also vital to ensure that they do not inadvertently cause harm. Altering one aspect of the diet invariably affects another and hence an overall view has to be taken of the likely consequences. Increasing the consumption of one nutrient (such as iron) can impair the absorption and precipitate a deficiency of others (such as zinc). Fat restriction may reduce energy intake, which may be advantageous in some circumstances (e.g. obesity) but harmful in others (e.g. undernutrition). Dietary measures which may reduce the risk of one disease could also increase the risk from another (on a population basis, abstinence from alcohol could reduce the risk of pancreatic cancer but increase the risk of heart disease). The risk–benefit equation must always be borne in mind.

1.6.2 Types of dietary modification

The purpose of dietary modification may be:

- to achieve a nutrient profile which offers greater health benefits
- to correct a dietary deficiency or surplus
- to avoid the consumption of a particular dietary component
- to produce specific metabolic or clinical effects
- to obtain symptom relief.

This may necessitate either qualitative or quantitative dietary adjustments, or both.

Qualitative methods

Wherever possible, people should be given dietary advice in terms of adjustments to food choice and meal pattern rather than in nutritional terms such as 'carbohydrate' or 'calories' (Wearne and Day 1999). This has two advantages:

1 People eat foods, not nutrients, and obviously find it easier to understand advice given in terms of 'choose low-fat dairy products' rather than 'eat less saturated fat'.
2 It is easier to ensure that the diet is balanced overall and that there is not undue focus on one dietary component to the detriment of others.

There are various ways in which this can be done but *The Balance of Good Health* model (HEA 1994) for healthy eating is a good basis for many types of dietary advice (see Section 1.2.2 in Healthy eating). Not only is it suitable for the general population but, by modifying the suggested choices within each of the food groups, it can be targeted at particular client groups within the population, e.g. elderly people or those on low incomes or from particular ethnic groups.

Increasingly, *The Balance of Good Health* model is also being used for those requiring therapeutic dietary advice. Dietary adjustments to achieve an increase in decrease in particular nutrients can be achieved by altering the balance of food groups within the diet, the number of portions per day from each group and appropriate food choices within those food groups. For example, guidance to increase iron intake to correct anaemia can emphasize the need for sufficient choices from the 'meat and alternatives' and 'bread and cereals' groups, highlight particularly good (iron-rich) food choices within those groups, and encourage plenty of choices from the 'fruit and vegetables' group in order to ensure sufficiency of vitamin C. The advantage of this approach is that therapeutic guidance in given within the context of overall healthy eating. Dietary changes designed to boost iron intake, for example, do not create other dietary imbalances (e.g. a high fat intake as a result of an increased consumption of meat).

For the same reason, the model is also increasingly being used as a basis for dietary management in more complex disorders such as diabetes, hyperlipidaemia or coeliac disease in conjunction with additional guidance on other relevant dietary aspects (e.g. timing of meals, use of alcohol, foods that need to be avoided). Disease states should not be managed in total isolation without regard to their possible interaction with others. For example, the dietary management of hyperlipidaemia should not be exclusively confined to manipulation of blood lipid levels; it also needs to include cardioprotective dietary measures to reduce the associated high risk of cardiovascular disease. It should also not be overlooked that people with one disorder can still be at the same risk as the rest of the population from unrelated disorders associated with ageing such as heart disease, cancers or osteoporosis.

Quantitative methods

Dietary guidance quantified in terms of kilocalories or grams of carbohydrate per day is now rarely used in the management of disorders such as obesity or diabetes. Qualitative advice focusing on food choice and dietary balance is not only just as effective but also, being more acceptable to the patient, more likely to be followed.

However, some types of therapeutic dietary manipulation necessitate quantified restriction or regulation of the consumption of specific nutrients, for example dietary treatment of phenylketonuria or chronic renal failure, or in the provision of enteral or parenteral nutrition support. As with any type of dietary manipulation, it is important to ensure that the focus on certain dietary components does not result in neglect of other nutritional parameters relevant to health or growth.

Levels of nutrients in a quantified diet are usually determined by considering individual nutritional requirements and the clinical indications in terms of biochemical, physiological or symptomatic parameters. Alternatively, a statistical definition of 'low' or 'high' intake can be made based on figures which are more than 2 standard deviations away from average consumption (Bingham 1979).

Where there is no biochemical or other yardstick, then a 'low X' diet usually implies a level which is as low as is practicable and acceptable in terms of usual eating patterns. Generally accepted target nutrient levels for therapeutic regimens will be found in the relevant clinical sections of this book.

Constructing quantified diets

Quantified therapeutic diets regulate nutrient intake by controlling the types and amounts of foods in the diet. The level of control varies according to the dietary objectives and clinical circumstances and may be achieved by:

- total regulation of nutrient intake specified by a fixed menu plan or quantified intake of an enteral/parenteral feed
- partial control of nutrient intake by using an exchange system which delivers a fixed amount of nutrient per food portion
- partial control of nutrient intake by regulating food consumption frequency.

Total regulation: This approach is usually only appropriate in situations where nutritional intake needs to be closely regulated and monitored, usually in seriously ill people receiving artificial nutritional support.

Exchange systems: The quantity of a food containing a specified amount of a particular nutrient (e.g. 50 mg phenylalanine) is defined, and intake of that nutrient is regulated by specifying the number of these exchanges that may be consumed each day. This method has in the past been used for a number of dietary regimens where the disease is monitored by biochemical parameters, e.g. protein exchanges in the management of renal disease or liver failure, or carbohydrate exchanges in the management of diabetes. However, exchange systems are now rarely used for these disorders, either because treatment objectives have changed (protein restriction is rarely considered necessary in renal and liver disease) or because the exchange system is now seen as an inappropriate and unnecessarily restrictive way of achieving the objective (i.e. glycaemic control in the case of diabetes). Exchange systems are now usually only used in the management of disorders where strict quantitative regulation is imperative (e.g. phenylketonuria).

Regulation via food consumption frequency: Foods are graded according to their energy or nutrient content per portion and control is exercised by regulating the frequency with which different foods are consumed. Foods with a low content of a particular nutrient may be permitted *ad libitum*, while those with a high content of the nutrient may need to be excluded altogether; the number of portions of foods with a moderate content of the nutrient can be specified.

Increasingly, a less prescriptive approach is being adopted whereby foods are similarly stratified but guidance on food choice is given along the lines of 'best choices', 'good choices' and 'occasional treats only'. This allows a more negotiated set of dietary targets, agreed between the client and dietician, where clients select from a number of options their favoured way of achieving dietary change.

1.6.3 Giving dietary advice

The purpose of giving dietary advice is to achieve dietary change. No matter how appropriate the advice or how sophisticated its delivery, if that advice is not followed it will be of no benefit to the individual.

The difficulties involved in achieving dietary change should not be underestimated (Hunt and Hillsdon 1996). Eating is not an adjunct to life (like taking medicine) but an integral part of lifestyle. Individual food habits evolve slowly over a long period and become deeply ingrained. Asking someone to change their food habits is therefore asking them to change their way of life and, since most people find this disruptive, it will tend to be resisted. The more this disruption can be kept to a minimum, the more likely change is to occur.

Dietary guidance therefore has to be appropriate for individual needs and circumstances if it is to have any chance of being implemented. Some of the general aspects which need to be considered are outlined below. Behavioural strategies to help to achieve dietary change are discussed in detail in Section 1.7.

In order to change food habits it is vital to understand the influences on them. People need to eat food in order to obtain the nutrients needed for health and survival, but this fact is only a small component of food choice and for some people it plays no part at all. In general, people eat the foods they eat because:

- they like them
- they are available
- they are affordable
- they have always eaten them
- they are convenient
- they provide comfort
- they are given them.

These choices will have been influenced by factors such as:

- cultural background
- religious or ethical beliefs
- taste preferences
- income
- occupation and lifestyle
- state of health
- social conventions
- family and peer-group pressures
- advertising
- knowledge and beliefs about food and diet
- habit and familiarity.

In order to change the dietary habits which have evolved in response to these influences, the conditions outlined below have to be met.

Motivation

Because making dietary change is disruptive, people will only do so if they are convinced it is justified. People therefore need to be told why change is necessary and what the benefits from change will be.

It is not usually difficult to motivate the patient suffering from a disease state where:

- Dietary measures will result in immediate and tangible benefit in terms of symptom relief, e.g. alleviating the effects of short bowel syndrome or coeliac disease.
- Dietary measures are seen as essential adjunct of treatment, e.g. to prevent hypoglycaemic attacks in the diabetic patient treated with insulin.
- People are anxious to prevent recurrence of a life-threatening event, e.g. myocardial infarction or allergen-induced anaphylaxis.

However, even in these patients, the level of motivation will decline in time, particularly if the penalties for non-compliance are not immediately obvious, e.g. the diabetic patient may not feel any worse with a fasting blood glucose level of 10 mmol/l rather than 7 mmol/l; coeliac patients may discover that they can 'get away with' eating small amounts of gluten-containing foods without apparent ill-effects. Yet, in both instances, cumulative pathological damage will still occur. Patients therefore need to be 're-motivated' at intervals by being reminded of the importance of the treatment goals in order to prevent long-term ill-effects.

Motivation is much more difficult to achieve, and much more volatile, if patients are asked to make changes for the purpose of distant events which may or may not occur, e.g. health benefits in later life in terms of prevention of cardiovascular disease, cancer or osteoporosis. People are being asked to make major changes to their lifestyle with no guarantee of ultimate benefit; the dietary advisor cannot promise that eating a particular diet will prevent a particular disease in later life, only that it may reduce the risk. While the health professional may feel that the argument in favour of dietary change is compelling, the individual may be less convinced; the theoretical rewards may seem a poor return for the practical effort involved. Assessing the degree of 'readiness to change' is a vital component of health promotion advice; it is pointless, and sometimes even counterproductive, for a health professional to provide detailed dietary guidance before an individual is at the point on the stages of change cycle where they will be receptive to it (see Section 1.7, Achieving behavioural change).

Knowledge and understanding

Even if people are ready to make dietary change, they can only do so if they know what changes they have to make. The nutritional objectives therefore have to translated into guidance which the recipient can understand and implement.

How this is done will differ in every situation. The facts have to be explained in terms (and possibly even a language) which people can understand. In general, this means explaining change in terms of food choice and meal planning rather than in terms of nutrients and scientific jargon (Secker and Pollard 1995; DH 1996; Perkins 2000).

People have to be given an appropriate amount of information. Some people will require one or two very simple dietary messages, while others will appreciate a much more detailed explanation.

The way in which the message is put across is also important. Some people acquire knowledge via written information but others will assimilate more from information delivered in an audiovisual or interactive form. Some require one-to-one tuition, while others may feel less threatened and respond more positively in a group setting.

The dietetic advisor may also have to correct misinformation. People are bombarded with dietary messages from many sources, including television, newspapers, magazines, diet books, advertising and the opinions of friends and family, much of it conflicting, confusing and often wrong. The impact of this information can be considerable (Margetts *et al.* 1998).

Acceptability

Even if someone is motivated to make dietary changes and knows how to do so, these changes will only occur in practice if they are acceptable to that individual (Glanz 1985; Contento *et al.* 1995). Any form of dietary guidance has to consider:

- *Food preferences*: people will not eat foods that they do not like or that the rest of the family will not eat.
- *Food constraints*: people will not eat foods that are not acceptable for cultural, religious or ethical reasons.
- *Food availability*: people cannot buy foods if they are not on sale in the places where they shop.
- *Income*: people on low incomes may not be able to afford certain foods or many be reluctant to experiment with unfamiliar ones.
- *Practicality*: the suggested changes must not pose too great a burden in terms of time, effort or complexity.

The key to providing acceptable dietary advice is dietary assessment (see Section 1.5). Whether advising individuals or groups of people, it is essential to have some measure of their needs, problems and customary eating habits to provide the starting point for dietary change.

Achievability

Targets for dietary change must be achievable. Few people will revolutionize their eating habits overnight; for most, dietary modification will be a gradual process of adjustment.

'Desired objectives' are not necessarily the same as 'reasonable targets'. It may be desirable that someone consumes a diet containing 50% energy from carbohydrate and less than 35% from fat, but this goal may be well beyond an individual's capacity or willingness to change, at least in the short term. A few simple dietary changes which shift the diet in the right direction may be a more appropriate target in the first instance.

It is important to start from where people are, not where one might like them to be. Making unrealistic expectations of the dietary change required will be counterproductive because, if targets are out of reach, people will become discouraged and probably abandon their efforts altogether.

Setting achievable goals is therefore a balance between clinical objectives and dietetic judgement.

It is essential to:

- *Identify the most important objectives* and concentrate on those. It is far better for people to make one or two significant alterations to their diet than none at all.
- *Set realistic targets*. Achieving a series of short-term goals is more likely to lead to long-term change.
- *Work with existing food habits*, not against them. Focus on changes that are compatible with existing food habits, not totally alien to them.
- *Give positive advice*. Emphasize suitable foods and alternative choices rather than just foods that need to be avoided.
- *Not expect too much too quickly*. Permanent change takes time.

Support

Permanent dietary change is highly unlikely to result from a single dietetic encounter. In the group setting, dietary information may heighten awareness or stimulate interest, but further intervention is likely to be necessary for significant change to occur. Dietary advice given to individuals nearly always needs to be followed up to assess its impact, reinforce motivation, expand knowledge and evaluate progress.

Good explanatory literature, food lists and other educational tools may be helpful, but on their own are not enough. Unexpected diagnosis of a condition such as diabetes or cancer can leave people feeling dazed or distressed and unable to take much in during an initial consultation with a dietitian. If the dietary advice is complex, further explanation may be needed. Questions may occur to people some time after the consultation. Motivation may fade and need reinforcement. Problems may arise. People should always have a contact point for further advice and many will require regular follow-up.

Communication

The way in which dietary advice is given will have a marked influence on its effectiveness. Individual needs and problems can only be identified and overcome if there is a relationship between client and advisor which promotes a climate of interactive dialogue, disclosure and trust (HEA 1997). In order to achieve this, dietitians need to have an understanding of human behaviour and good counselling skills (Gable 1997). These aspects of dietetic practice are discussed in Section 1.7 (Achieving behavioural change).

Text revised by: Briony Thomas

References

Bingham SA. Low residue diets: a reappraisal of their meaning and content. *Journal of Human Nutrition* 1979; **33**: 5–16.

Contento J, Balch GI, Bronner YL *et al.* The effectiveness of nutrition education and implications for nutrition education policy, programs, and research: a review of research. *Journal of Nutrition Education* 1995; **27** (6, Special Issue).

Department of Health. *Guidelines on Educational Materials Concerned with Nutrition*. A report by the Nutrition Task Force. London: DH, 1996.

Gable J. *Counselling Skills for Dietitians*. London: Blackwell Science, 1997.

Glanz K. Nutrition education for risk factor reduction and patient education: a review. *Preventive Medicine* 1985; **14**: 721–752.

Health Education Authority. *The Balance of Good Health. Introducing the National Food Guide*. London: HEA, 1994.

Health Education Authority. *Health Promotion Interventions to Promote Healthy Eating is the General Population – A Review*. London: HEA, 1997.

Hunt P, Hillsdon M. *Changing Eating and Exercise Behaviour. A Handbook for Professionals*. Oxford: Blackwell Science, 1996.

Margetts BM, Thompson RL, Speller V, McVey D. Factors which influence 'healthy' eating patterns: results from the 1993 Health Education Authority health and lifestyle survey in England. *Public Health Nutrition* 1998; **1**: 193–198.

Perkins L. Developing a tool for health professionals involved in producing and evaluating nutrition education leaflets. *Journal of Human Nutrition and Dietetics* 2000; **13**: 41–49.

Secker J, Pollard R. *Writing Leaflets for Patients – Guidelines for Producing Written Information*. Edinburgh: Health Education Board for Scotland, 1995.

Wearne SJ, Day MJ. Clues for the development of food-based dietary guidelines: how are dietary targets being achieved by UK consumers? *British Journal of Nutrition* 1999; **81** (Suppl 2): S119–S126.

1.7 Achieving behavioural change

1.7.1 Context

Dietetics originated as a hospital-based profession with the traditional dietetic interview being based firmly on the medical consultation model which uses advice giving and direct persuasion to encourage people to change their behaviour (Hunt 1995). For this purpose, dietitians are trained how best to prescribe appropriate diets and to teach and advise people about the important dietary changes that they need to make (see Section 1.6, Dietary modification). They translate scientific and medical decisions relating to food and health into terms which everyone can understand (British Dietetic Association 1997).

This professional-led persuasive approach assumes that people will already be motivated enough to act on the information given, partly due to the credibility of the professional giving the advice and partly in response to the health risk. Although this information component is important, it is by no means the only factor affecting change in dietary behaviour. It is generally accepted now that increasing knowledge alone does not necessarily change behaviour (Glanz 1985; Shepherd and Stockley 1987; Thomas 1994). Likewise, nutritional intervention studies have demonstrated that the dissemination of information alone is not very effective in bringing about behavioural change (Contento *et al*. 1995).

Whereas nutrition education has focused on *what* changes to make, within the field of psychology there is a focus on *how* to help people to make behaviour changes. Brownell and Cohen (1995a, b) emphasize that psychological factors are paramount in setting the stage for dietary change. Recent reviews recommend that nutrition education and healthy eating interventions should have a clearly stated theoretical basis, incorporating effective models of communication and behaviour change and adopting a behaviourally based approach which includes active involvement of individuals in the change process (Contento *et al*. 1995; HEA 1997). Behavioural strategies have been developed in various areas of healthcare in an attempt to increase effectiveness, but there remain a number of practitioner barriers to applying these behaviour change interventions. These include inadequate knowledge of behaviour change principles and methods, a deficit in counselling and behaviour change skills, negative attitudes towards those clients who appear not to want or be able to change and organizational barriers (Goldstein *et al*. 1998). These barriers can lead to lack of success with interventions, which in turn leads to reduced motivation and confidence in practitioners (Grueninger *et al*. 1995).

For dietitians to become true 'dietetic counsellors' it is essential for them to be trained in both the behavioural and motivational aspects of human behaviour. For the dietetic advice given to be effective, dietitians need to help clients increase their motivation to change and develop self-management skills to implement the proposed changes.

Following a survey of dietetic practice, Gilboy (1994) observed that although dietitians have made changes in their practice since the early 1980s that have changed their roles from dietary educators to dietary counsellors, they still lag behind the ideal in the use of adherence-enhancing counselling practices needed for behaviour change. Increasingly, dietitians themselves have highlighted the need for counselling skills and behaviour change training (Isselman *et al*. 1993; Rapoport 1998). In a British Dietetic Association working group survey examining structure and content of pre-registration education and training for dietitians, respondents perceived counselling skills as largely absent in courses (Rogers and Judd 1996). Subsequently, the British Dietetic Association/Council for Professions Supplementary to Medicine Dietitians Board Joint Working Party has recommended that more emphasis is placed on developing skills in communication and counselling (Judd *et al*. 1997).

As an introduction to the subject, the following subsections:

- outline the requirements for an optimal dietetic interview and describe the interpersonal or counselling skills which need to underpin the therapeutic relationship;
- consider the clinical challenges which face dietitians, together with key strategies for dealing with these. A thorough grounding in these skills will optimize the chances of dietitians becoming effective behaviour change agents in addition to nutrition educators;
- present guidelines for the intervention process and consider their implications for dietetic practice and training. Although the majority of behaviour change examples given in this chapter are applied to weight management as the literature is well established in this area, these strategies can be modified for application in all areas of dietetic practice.

1.7.2 The dietetic interview: the framework

'Dietary counselling' in its widest context incorporates an approach which has many of the components of the counselling process. In counselling the agenda is set by clients, and the counsellor listens and helps them to explore their own feelings and needs. This process enables clients to feel empowered to make decisions to help them live in a more satisfying and resourceful way. In dietary counselling, the specific aim is to change behaviour to manage disease or improve risk factors for overall health. Working in a client-centred way means dietitian and client work collaboratively as partners in solving problems related to dietary and lifestyle change. Egan's (1998) 'skilled helper model' provides a useful framework for helping clients effectively manage their eating-related problems and engage in constructive change. The model describes three stages:

1 Establishing the current scenario
2 Establishing the preferred scenario and goal setting
3 Action stage.

The process involves a combination of the use of good interpersonal communication skills for exploration of issues, information gathering, advice giving and application of appropriate behaviour change strategies (see below).

Client-centred helping

Traditionally, dietitians have been trained to give information and advice in a one-way relationship in which the helper is in the powerful position of being the expert in control of the situation (Gable 1997). Using a client-centred helping approach means that the dietitian exerts less control. This involves a redistribution of power, a two-way relationship whereby the dietitian supports clients to find out what is best for them, thereby allowing them to gain a sense of self-regulation and control. The view is that clients have the 'expertise' about themselves and that the aim of an interview is to explore clients' thoughts, feelings and beliefs about a behaviour. The traditional role of advice giving, teaching and instructing still has a place at the point when clients are ready to receive it, as part of a menu of approaches rather than the only available one.

Core conditions

It is no easy task to identify the best counselling method or the most effective style. Reviews, however, show that perhaps the single most important factor for an effective helping relationship is the possession of good interpersonal skills (Najavits and Weiss 1994). Regardless of theoretical orientation, there seems to be an emphasis on the clinician's need to possess core qualities which are linked to helping (Rogers 1951). These consist of:

- *Genuineness*: being as freely, sincerely and deeply oneself as possible, being who one really is without any front.
- *Acceptance*: this means demonstrating to clients that they are accepted with no strings or conditions attached, whether or not one likes them and regardless of who they are and what they have done.
- *Empathy*: feeling and sensing what the client may be thinking and feeling, and then sharing it with them.

The development of these core conditions provides an essential psychological environment and foundation for the acquisition and application of all strategies for achieving dietary change. The ability to apply these core conditions develops with experience, increasing self-awareness and a rigorous approach to self-evaluation. Developing and maintaining these conditions requires ongoing commitment and development on the dietitian's part.

The physical environment in which the interview takes place must also be considered. Ideally, the interview should take place in a suitable room with comfortable chairs, as many distractions as possible removed, and ensuring that interruptions do not occur.

Guiding principles

Three key principles underpin work using basic therapeutic counselling skills (Egan 1998):

- *Client responsibility*: people are responsible for their own actions and need to be given the freedom to make their own decisions and choices. Clients have the right to choose whether to explore concerns about their behaviour and whether or not to change.
- *Social influence*: the dietitian hopes to influence the thinking and behaviour of clients, but recognizes that outside influences may have a greater impact on clients' behaviour.
- *Collaboration*: working in true collaboration with clients involves a process in which clients and dietitians work *together* on the same side to identify goals and methods of achieving them. A collaborative relationship helps to resolve the tension between addressing both clients' and the dietitian's agenda.

Establishing a helping relationship

Fundamental to all relationships where behaviour change is the desired outcome, is the nature of the helping relationship itself. Establishing a helping relationship where clients feel comfortable is the first goal of the initial interview. Clients invariably come to a dietetic consultation with their own set of expectations and concerns. It is important that these are explored at the outset before the main purpose of the interview is addressed.

The helping relationship needs to be underpinned by the appropriate use of good counselling skills. At all stages it is crucial that the dietitian resists the urge to tell clients what to do, but instead practises effective listening, reflecting and summarizing skills. This facilitates the process of clients seeing themselves as capable agents of control rather than helpless victims in a situation beyond their control.

1.7.3 The dietetic interview: core counselling skills

It is important to clarify that what is being considered here is the integration of counselling skills into professional dietetic practice, distinct from the use of counselling skills by a trained counsellor for other ends than dietary and lifestyle change. Counselling skills as used in dietetic practice are specific interpersonal communication skills used in the helping relationship between client and dietitian to achieve a specific health-related aim. They are critical tools to help engage clients in the change process. Within this process, building on this foundation, more specific behaviour change strategies can then be selected and applied (see below).

What follows is a brief overview of the core generic skills which could be used in a dietetic interview with clients. These skills need to be learnt and practised to be used effectively.

Initial contact

The initial contact should be friendly and inviting, with an introduction being made by the dietitian to put clients at ease and allow them to settle. The opening sentences combined with the use of suitable body language demonstrate to clients that the dietitian is ready to listen to them. It is important to let clients know how much time is available for the session. The initial task is to establish the purpose of the interview and the desired outcome, paying appropriate attention to both clients' and the dietitian's agenda.

Open invitation to talk

The dietitian asks questions to help clients clarify their thoughts or feelings. Open questions invite clients to talk and can be used at various points of the interview, e.g. 'How have things been since we last met?', or 'where would you like to start?'

Closed questions elicit a specific answer, e.g. yes or no, and are often used to check whether the dietitian has understood the client's story, e.g. 'did you find that difficult?', or 'does your daughter live near you?'

'Why' questions (e.g. 'why do you feel the need to do that?') should be used with caution. Although they appear to be open, clients may feel they have to justify themselves in their response, and therefore may become defensive. The tone of voice used by the dietitian is paramount when asking 'why' questions.

Active listening

Attending behaviour

Listening is the most basic helping skill and it is demonstrated by using attending behaviour which includes making good but varied eye contact to communicate, appropriate body language and verbal following. It is important for clients to feel that they are being listened to, attended to and understood. A relaxed natural posture and gestures communicate that full attention is being given to clients. Verbal following involves responding to what clients have said whilst staying with the topic.

Minimal encouragers

Minimal encouragers help to keep clients talking whilst giving focus and direction to the session. They are small indicators to clients that the dietitian is with them. Examples of verbal minimal encouragers include: 'yes', 'uh-huh', 'go on'. Verbal following (repeating the last word or phrase clients have said) is also a minimal encourager. Silence can be a very valuable minimal encourager. It allows clients time to think, feel and express. Talking too much before being given a mandate to do so is a common mistake made by health professionals. Once the goal for change has been identified, the dietitian might need to impart the relevant information.

Paraphrasing

Paraphrasing means repeating the essence of what clients have just said. This conveys empathy and that the dietitian is closely following their story. For example:

> Client: 'If there are biscuits in the cupboard, I just can't keep away from them. I don't know what to do about it'
> Dietitian: 'You are unsure of what action to take to keep you away from the biscuits.'

Paraphrasing emphasizes the content of clients' stories, and demonstrates to clients genuine interest, understanding and acceptance on the part of the dietitian.

Reflection

Reflecting involves feeding back and mirroring feelings alluded to by clients. Reflection of this kind demonstrates to clients that their feelings have been understood, and that these are accepted and worthy. For example:

> Client: 'I feel that my world has been blown apart by this news.'
> Dietitian: 'It sounds as though you feel devastated by this.'

It is important that the intensity of the feeling is understood, so clarification in a tentative way is essential if the dietitian is not entirely sure that the feeling and its intensity have been correctly interpreted.

Summarization

Summarization is an attempt to condense the essence of the conversation and feed this back to clients. In addition, it serves to check that the dietitian has fully understood what has been said. This can best be achieved by prefixing summarization with 'have I got this right…'. Summarization can be used at the start of a new session, during an interview to move the interview forward, or at the end of an interview.

Concreteness

Concreteness is particularly useful when clients are being vague and using words such as 'everything', 'it' and 'always'. Clients should be asked to clarify such words, otherwise the dietitian may not understand what clients are actually referring to.

Concreteness means encouraging clients to talk as concretely and specifically as possible about their situation.

Concreteness can be directed to behaviour, thoughts and feelings. The dietitian can ask clients to clarify their story by asking concrete open questions, for example: 'what happened exactly?' or 'can you give me an example of that?', and by using concrete paraphrases and reflections.

Ending the interview

When the allotted time is coming to an end, the dietitian should refer to this and begin to summarize what has taken place during the interview. It is important that closing sentences are clear and that new issues are not introduced and dealt with in a hurried way at this stage. It is better to arrange to discuss any new issues in detail at a subsequent interview.

Immediacy or role explanation

Clients may have expectations which the dietitian cannot or does not want to meet. For example, clients may want the dietitian to provide instant solutions to their problems or want to befriend the dietitian. If the dietitian continues to use counselling skills to reflect and paraphrase the situation, he or she may appear to be agreeing to meet these expectations. In such a situation, the dietitian needs to discuss and clarify the situation with clients so that unrealistic expectations are not perpetuated.

1.7.4 Applying behavioural change strategies to clinical challenges

Behaviour change models and theories can be used as helpful guides to why and how people change behaviour. They provide methods of categorizing reality from a particular perspective and a foundation for applying skills, but none can be perfect as reality and people are infinitely varied. All models should therefore be viewed as flexible guides rather than absolute realities. Although there has been an increasing interest in models of health behaviour (Shumaker *et al.* 1998), there are no thoroughly reliable models of why people adopt new behaviours. The Prochaska and DiClemente stages of change model (Fig. 1.3) is currently one of the most popular (Prochaska and DiClemente 1986) and its application in dietetic practice has been described in detail (Hunt and Hillsdon 1996). The application of brief behaviour strategies to change health behaviour is also being developed (Rollnick *et al.* 1999).

The model describes a series of six stages through which individuals pass when making lifestyle changes:

- precontemplation
- contemplation
- preparation
- action
- maintenance
- relapse.

Prochaska and DiClemente found that these stages occur naturally without formal intervention in people who make successful changes. The dietitian's task then is to facilitate a natural change process. Successful outcome can be defined as moving clients around the cycle of change. People normally go around the cycle several times before achieving a stable change.

As different processes are at work at each stage, the dietitian needs to employ different strategies depending on where clients are in the cycle of change. To ensure that strategies are appropriately matched to the individual's stage of change, it is important to establish a client's readiness to change and location in the change process before proceeding with the intervention. This helps to avoid resistance which can occur when inappropriate strategies for a particular stage of change are applied. For example, attempting directly to persuade someone who is uninterested in, or ambivalent about, change is likely to lead to some form of resistance and indeed can increase it. The 'You really need to cut your fat intake down...' is likely to result in the counterproductive 'Yes, but...' response from clients. More appropriate strategies for someone who is uninterested in change are discussed below.

The first challenge in the process of change is motivational. Motivation can be understood as a person's present stage of readiness for change. People often may not be highly motivated to change their dietary behaviour in the first place and, secondly, once they have started treatment they often stop midway. This has led to a growing interest in methods to motivate clients who are reluctant to change. Motivational interviewing (MI) consists of a range of therapeutic strategies to motivate people to work through ambivalence about behaviour change, build commitment

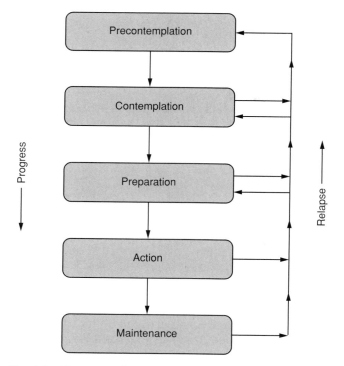

Fig. 1.3 The stages of change model.
Reproduced with permission from S. Rollnick.

and reach a decision to change if appropriate (Miller and Rollnick 1991; Rollnick *et al.* 1992). MI strategies are most appropriate in the precontemplation and contemplation stages of change, although ambivalence often persists or re-emerges during the action stage. MI strategies are therefore useful throughout the process, providing a motivational foundation for cognitive and behavioural strategies.

Cognitive and behavioural approaches offer key methods to help people to build confidence and make continued and sustained behaviour change (Wing, 1992; American Psychological Association 1995; Wilson, 1995). Behavioural approaches help clients identify unhelpful behavioural patterns and develop ways of modifying these. Cognitive strategies aim to help clients identify and then change underlying thoughts, ideas and beliefs which might be maintaining their undesirable behaviour. Effective nutritionally related self-help manuals based on these strategies have been developed in a range of areas, most notably for use with clients in obesity and eating disorders (Treasure and Schmidt 1993; Cooper 1995; Brownell 1997) as well as treatment manuals for health professionals (Fairburn *et al.* 1993; Wolfe 1996).

Table 1.11 summarizes the key challenges which face dietitians at each stage of change. The key behaviour change strategies for each clinical challenge, which can help to move the client successfully on to the next stage of change, are discussed below.

Encouraging the possibility of change (*Precontemplation*)

People who are not aware of the fact that they have a problem do not think seriously about changing, even though others might recognize the need. These people seldom present for treatment. Dietitians may be confronted with a precontemplator, for example in hospital when they receive a referral for lipid lowering where the person has not made the decision to consult the dietitian. The task of the dietitian at this stage is to create doubt or concern in the client about their health or their unhealthy behaviour. Motivation for change can only begin when a person perceives a discrepancy between where they are and where

Table 1.11 Main clinical challenges at each stage of change

Stage of change	Key clinical challenge
Precontemplation (not interested in change)	To encourage the possibility of change
Contemplation (thinking about change)	To tip the balance in favour of change
Preparation (preparing to change)	To explore options for change and choose the best course of action
Action (making changes)	To help people make changes successfully
Maintenance (maintaining change)	To consolidate changes achieved
Relapse (relapsing)	To prevent lapses from becoming relapses

they would like to be. Clients in this stage of change need information and feedback to raise awareness of the problem and the possibility of change. Launching in to giving advice to clients at this stage is likely to be met with resistance.

People will be motivated to change their lifestyle when they know what problems are caused by their behaviour and are concerned about these problems, whilst at the same time they feel positive about themselves and competent to make a change (Van Bilsen 1991). A combination of four key elements is required:

- knowledge (of the problems caused by their behaviour)
- concern (about these problems)
- self-esteem
- competence (self-efficacy).

When a person who is unaware of having a problem becomes more aware, this can be accompanied by a lowering of self-esteem as they realize that they have been doing something to themselves which has endangered their health. Care therefore has to be taken to build self-esteem as awareness is increased.

Overall, an individual's progress may be blocked by various factors including a lack of awareness of their problem, a lack of concern about the problem, a low self-esteem or their lack of faith in their ability to implement the required changes (low self-efficacy). Raising client awareness in these domains will make change more likely. For example, clients who are not concerned about their behaviour, and are unaware of its impact are unlikely to feel the need for change. Using MI techniques, the dietitian can elicit self-motivational statements from the client, i.e. things that clients say which are signs of knowledge, self-esteem, concern or competence. The application of MI techniques provides the opportunity for clients to develop all of these areas to an equilibrium where they are ready to consider change and ultimately acquire the confidence in their ability to make successful changes.

Tipping the balance in favour of change (*Contemplation*)

A person who is thinking about change may realize that there is a problem and that change is needed. However, although some thought may have been given to the potential gains and losses if change were made, the actual decision to change has not yet been made. This sort of ambivalence is a normal part of human behaviour. Clients often express a desire to change which is not matched by their actions. In this situation, the dietitian's role is to encourage clients to explore their ambivalence about changing their behaviour without pressurizing them to change. By carrying out what, in MI terms, is known as a decisional balance, the dietitian can help clients to weigh up the personal advantages and disadvantages of changing a specific behaviour against those of no change (Hoyt and Janis 1975; Rollnick *et al.* 1992). This process helps to build motivation for change.

For example, where clients like eating chips, the dietitian could firstly explore what they like about it (e.g. tasty, enjoyable) and what concerns them about continuing to do so (e.g. weight gain, hyperlipidaemia). They could also consider the advantages (e.g. weight loss, lower lipids) and disadvantages of eating fewer chips (e.g. food less enjoyable). This process can be done verbally or on paper (Table 1.12). A decision not to change is a viable option as it may be better for clients not to start to make changes if they are not really ready. Alternatively, if they have already tried and failed many times, a further half-hearted attempt and failure might reinforce an already low self-esteem.

As unhelpful eating behaviours are often underestimated, encouraging clients to start self-monitoring as soon as possible helps to demonstrate the extent of the problem and can thereby sometimes increase readiness for change (see Self-monitoring, below).

Exploring options for change and choosing the best course of action (*Preparation*)

A person who is still weighing up the options for change will eventually decide either to make active changes or not to go any further. The task for the dietitian at this stage is to recognize that a window of opportunity is open and that it is time for action. If a commitment to change has been made with clients it is helpful to explore the advantages and disadvantages of implementing a whole range of change options. The task is not so much to motivate change but to help clients to determine a suitable course of action. Common perceived barriers include lack of cooking skills, lack of food-storage or cooking facilities, low income, other financial priorities than food and health, food preferences, and social and time constraints.

Making changes to eating habits usually means changing long-established habits related to shopping, cooking and eating. When changes to lifestyle are being planned, clients can help themselves to be more successful by thinking it through beforehand. This can help by drawing their attention to problems or difficulties that they may be able to sort out in advance and it makes revising the plan easier if they know clearly what they are expecting of themselves. There are things which can be done before trying to make changes to make it more likely that the change will be successful. From an early stage it is also helpful to encourage clients to consider alternatives to current unhelpful behaviour, the need to reward themselves for successful changes and strategies for maintaining changes.

For example, strategies to overcome barriers encountered in weight management which can be explored with the clients include:

- planning meals and shopping in advance so that appropriate foods are available to eat regularly
- planning eating times daily in advance
- carrying around suitable snacks
- having suitable snacks available in the car, fridge or desk at work

Table 1.12 The decisional balance

Advantages of change	Disadvantages of change
Advantages of no change	Disadvantages of no change

- asking a friend, partner or workmate to change at the same time, or to be encouraging
- avoiding tasting when cooking, as this may result in overeating
- avoiding unnecessary exposure to food and leftovers.

It is important to address the difficulties and barriers related to change and to allow clients to generate solutions to perceived barriers themselves. This helps to increase their sense of confidence, competence and self-esteem and to emphasize that there is no single right option for change, rather it is a question of experimenting to find what works best for them. Any information should be presented neutrally, with the responsibility and decision for change being placed firmly with the client. Once each option for change has been explored, a client's favourite will probably emerge. At this point it is necessary to discuss the option in terms of its appropriateness.

Setting behavioural goals

Setting appropriate behavioural goals is key to achieving a successful outcome. Setting an unrealistic goal can set clients up for failure and may lead to blame being attributed to personal shortcomings rather than the shortcomings of the treatment. It can also lead to both the client and the dietitian undervaluing what they do achieve.

It is important to encourage clients to think about what changes they are willing to make and allow them to lead the discussion, rather than telling them what to do. Clients need to focus on the small steps towards achieving any goal. Good goals can be defined by the acronym SMART:

- *Specific*: e.g. for a goal of wanting to eat less fat: 'I will spread fat more thinly on my bread'.
- *Measurable*: e.g. 'I'm going to eat *five* portions of fruit and vegetables each day'.
- *Achievable and realistic*: setting realistic goals means aiming for something that can be achieved and then working up gradually to what might be desired. A client who eats two bars of chocolate each day could start by cutting down to one chocolate bar per day.
- *Relevant to the goal of treatment*: if the aim of treatment is to decrease fat intake, clients need to concentrate on eating foods which are low in fat.

• *Time specific*: setting a goal to be achieved within an agreed time-frame.

For a goal to make a difference in the time set to achieve it, it needs to be as far reaching as possible. For example, if the main goal is to reduce fat intake, the main dietary source of fat intake needs to be identified and reduced to a level that will make a difference. If fried foods are eaten daily, an appropriate weekly goal may be to use fat-free methods of cooking. This would have a bigger effect than a goal of, for instance, not eating doughnuts if these are only consumed once a fortnight.

Only two or three specific, realistic and achievable changes should be chosen. These may be further divided into a series of smaller steps towards the larger goal. Successful negotiation of each of the smaller steps gives clients a sense of achievement to keep them motivated in the longer term.

Once the precise nature of the goal has been agreed and ways of implementing it have been explored with the client, it is helpful to summarize this by completing a change plan (Table 1.13). The examples given are for someone on a lipid-lowering diet, but the plan can be modified for many conditions and to suit particular clients. Although not all elements of the plan would necessarily be used in every dietetic interview, it is important to remember that even when the dietary advice is essential to preserve life (e.g. nut allergy, short bowel syndrome), strategies to support implementation of the required changes will still be required.

Helping people to make successful changes (*Action*)

This is the stage that is traditionally most heavily emphasized by health professionals who often assume that each person they treat is immediately ready for this active change process. In this stage, clients take action to bring about a particular change. Once they start to make changes, they tend to re-evaluate whether the change is worth the effort. At this point it becomes important to work with clients on how best to implement changes and develop strategies for coping with temptations to return to old behaviour. The following strategies are fundamental for behaviour change and they can be adapted for application in a wide range of conditions.

Stimulus control

Stimulus control consists of changing the environment to decrease exposure to triggers or stimuli which make unhelpful behaviour likely to happen, or increase exposure to triggers/stimuli which make the desired new behaviour likely to happen. A number of triggers, both internal (e.g. feelings, thoughts, beliefs), and external (events and situations), can start a behaviour happening. Although the examples below refer mainly to weight management, triggers causing unhelpful behaviours in any set of circumstances may need to be identified and a strategy designed to influence clients' behaviour in a positive direction.

A range of strategies is available for modifying *external* triggers:

• limiting the opportunities for seeing tempting foods other than at meal times, e.g. put things away in cupboards, don't shop when hungry;
• removing oneself from the food which triggers over-eating;
• taking a route home which does not involve passing a tempting food shop, baker or confectioner;
• always making sure that there are suitable foods (e.g. fruit and vegetables) available at home to avoid being tempted to eat less suitable foods if hungry;
• not buying or only occasionally buying tempting, calorie-dense foods such as chocolates, cakes and crisps;
• if tempted by food that is not part of the plan, distracting oneself from food by doing something incompatible with eating.

Strategies for modifying *internal* triggers include:

• Asking in response to an urge to eat: 'am I really hungry?' Urges to eat or cravings need to be distinguished from hunger. The former are psychological triggers to eating and distinct from physical hunger, which is the real need to eat. Real hunger often needs to be responded to, but various strategies can be learned to overcome psychological urges. Urges or cravings are sometimes described as being like waves: they build and build until they are at their peak, but then break on the shore and fade away within 15–30 minutes. An urge or craving can be withstood by doing something incompatible with eating until it has faded away.
• Making a list of alternative activities that make it impossible to give in to urges (e.g. walking, reading a novel, phoning a friend, cleaning the car, planning a holiday, running, painting, having a relaxing massage or bath, or

Table 1.13 The change plan

The main reasons I want to change are: (e.g. to lower my cholesterol)
The changes I am prepared to make are: (e.g. change to skimmed & semi-skimmed milk)
The steps I will take to implement the change are: (e.g. change my daily order with the milkman, bring skimmed milk powder with me to work)
I will start making the change: (e.g. tomorrow)
I will ask for help from: (e.g. my husband)
I will ask them to: (e.g. praise me for making so much effort to change my diet)
Situations that might make change difficult: (e.g. going to friends)
My plans for coping with difficult situations are: (e.g. practise saying no, warn friend)
I will judge my success by: (e.g. my feeling better, more in control of my eating, eating healthier foods, reduction in cholesterol, weight loss)
When I achieve the change, I will tell myself: (e.g. how well I am doing with my change plan)
I will reward myself for being successful with: (e.g. some special bath oils)

practising a relaxation exercise). When faced with an urge, do something from this list.

- Sometimes mood changes can be due to other worries, for example being depressed about one's job or long-term effects of illness. These need to be addressed and it may be necessary to refer the client for more in-depth counselling or therapy. Careful consideration needs to be given to when this is appropriate and how such referral should be made.

Learned self-control

In the short term, clients can avoid situations which lead to inappropriate eating through reducing exposure to these triggers. In the longer term, they need to have a plan to respond to triggers in a way that does not lead to a lapse in eating behaviour.

Over a period of time, clients with overeating problems can be guided to expose themselves gradually for longer periods to foods which trigger an urge to overeat. They can learn to resist and tolerate the associated discomfort. Exposure to a trigger food first results in a dramatic increase in the urge to eat, but this reduces over 5–30 minutes. As clients learn to resist the temptation to eat, their self-confidence increases. Learned self-control strategies include:

- setting homework assignments over a period of weeks of gradual exposure to a trigger food, progressing through the least difficult foods to the most difficult;
- practising relaxation strategies to manage emotional disturbances.

Self-monitoring

As clients often have difficulty identifying what triggers their unhelpful eating behaviours, self-monitoring using a diary is a key part of both the assessment and treatment. It involves systematic observation and recording of target behaviours, i.e. the external (people, events, places) and internal (feelings, thoughts) conditions which trigger lapses from the planned behaviour. Although clients often do not report their dietary intake accurately, the prime purpose of self-monitoring is to increase clients' self-awareness of their own behaviour and to highlight new problems. This forms an essential basis for planning and monitoring change. The self-monitoring process in itself has also been shown to be beneficial in changing food intake, albeit in the short term.

Self-monitoring can be used, for example, to identify:

- time of eating
- what person was doing prior to eating
- place of eating
- with whom eating occurs
- how the person felt
- what thoughts went through a person's head.

Difficulty in keeping to the self-monitoring process suggests that unresolved motivational issues exist and need to be addressed before the more active phase of the treatment can be effective.

Rewarding and reinforcing desired behaviours

The frequency with which a positive behaviour occurs can be increased or decreased by what happens after it. For example, if a person has become very ill after eating a certain food, it is unlikely that they will want to eat that food again for some considerable time. In contrast, a positive experience, such as praise from a friend after eating a food on the dietary plan, makes it more likely that a person will repeat this behaviour at another time.

Once dietary goals have been established, dietitians need to help clients to identify ways to reward themselves on a regular basis when they have achieved the desired change. Suitable rewards may be doing enjoyable leisure-time activities and hobbies, being with favourite people, buying small things that they want, or doing what they find relaxing or fun (Holli and Calabrese 1998). When clients reward themselves, this reinforces the new behaviour, thus making it more likely to happen again. Clients should also be encouraged to focus on what they have achieved, however small, and mentally congratulate themselves for every small step taken. The importance of this cannot be underestimated as clients frequently focus on their failures without acknowledging their achievements.

If pleasurable and rewarding eating habits are those which are to be changed, new and pleasurable non-food rewards will need to be established. Care should also be taken that where eating changes are being made, they are as pleasurable as possible for them to be self-reinforcing. If clients enjoy eating chocolate and biscuits it is important that they find substitutes which they find enjoyable, e.g. raisins on crumpets with low-sugar jam. It is helpful to explain to clients that it may take time to learn to enjoy these alternative foods.

Consolidating changes achieved (*Maintenance*)

From the moment when clients actively start to make changes and achieve desired outcomes, they face the challenge of maintaining these. This requires another set of skills and a consolidation period of at least 6 months. Addressing this vital element is often neglected in current dietetic practice. Once preoccupation with a possible relapse disappears, clients step out of the cycle of change as the new behaviour becomes a permanently established feature of their lifestyle. To maximize the chances of this being achieved, the therapeutic focus needs to be on preventing lapses as well as continuing to apply all of the relevant strategies developed in the planning and action stages of change.

The most likely outcome for anyone who tries to change their diet is relapse (Marlatt and Gordon 1985). A lapse can be defined as a one-off deviation from a new eating behaviour, a mistake or a slip; a relapse is often defined as a string of lapses that occur over a short period; a collapse is a complete return to previous eating behaviours (Brownell 1997).

Everybody who attempts to change their behaviour occasionally finds that they have eaten something which does not fit in with their plan. These one-off slip-ups, or lapses, often lead to feelings of guilt, which make a person more susceptible to other slips. This may result in relapse and can eventually lead to them abandoning their changes altogether, with a return to previous patterns. To avoid this, it is important to guide clients into a new understanding: how they think about lapses will determine the outcome. An explanation of the nature of the change process, of lapses and of their management can help:

- Lapses do not come out of the blue, they are usually triggered.
- High-risk situations (ones which present an increased and significant risk of returning to old behaviours) are triggered by internal states (e.g. anxiety, boredom, anger, loneliness) or external events (e.g. social situations, passing a bakery, smell of good food). Successful coping is achieved by changing triggers to prevent eating inappropriate foods and by learning how best to manage in high-risk situations.
- Change is an ongoing process. The goal is an ongoing evolving journey rather than the outcome alone. Every small change in behaviour is a step in the right direction and a sign of important progress.
- Lapses are a natural and accepted part of change. Eating the wrong food is a slight error, a slip and not a personal failure.
- Lapses are educational and can be useful in that they provide important information about what triggers lapse and relapse.
- It takes many lapses to relapse.
- Even if clients completely abandon their change plan, all is not lost; motivational strategies can be used to remotivate them if appropriate.

Collaboratively, the dietitian can work with clients to identify what triggers lead to a lapse so that plans can be made in advance to prevent them, rather than just relying on willpower. A list of coping strategies can be established which can be accessed when necessary, akin to a first-aid plan.

This stage of change is an opportunity to review progress to date, with both its positive and negative effects. The aim is to help clients to increase their confidence for coping with unavoidable lapses.

Preventing lapses from becoming relapses (*Relapse*)

Clients who have relapsed or collapsed after a succession of lapses generally return to weighing up the advantages and disadvantages of change. At this stage, clients who have been unsuccessful at coping with high-risk situations may view themselves as failures. Dietitians need to help clients to see the causes of the relapse as attributable to controllable external factors and help them to renew their commitment to, and confidence about, change. Otherwise, clients can be encouraged to return if and when they feel ready.

Successful behaviour change includes careful management of lapses when they do occur. However, the way in which clients cope once having lapsed can affect whether a lapse becomes a relapse or not. The following six steps can be offered to clients to help them to cope with a lapse and prevent it becoming a relapse:

- *Stop*: go away from the situation to a safe place to think about what has happened.
- *Say*: it's not a catastrophe. One error does not mean the end of the world.
- *Learn*: what was going on before the lapse? Analyse the situation to see why it happened.
- *Plan*: what can be done in the same situation to avert another lapse? Use the information from above to plan in advance to reduce the risk of it happening again. Decide what can be done immediately to stop the slip becoming a fall. Put these strategies into practice at once.
- *Be positive*: has anything really changed? Review personal goals and motivation for change.
- *Ask*: is there anything that can be done to balance up the slip? For example, do some extra exercise. (It is not recommended that clients skip a subsequent meal as a result of a lapse, as this in itself can trigger overeating.)

Changing negative cognitions

The way in which a person thinks about a lapse often determines what they do next and whether lapse leads to relapse. Thoughts can both trigger and suppress behaviours. For example, thinking 'I've slipped up and blown it completely, I may as well not bother any more' is likely to make the person eat more and lead to relapse or even collapse. In contrast, thinking a more helpful thought, such as 'it's a shame that I've slipped, I'll do some extra exercise to compensate, and think about ways to stop myself slipping again', gives a greater chance of returning to the eating plan and stopping the slip becoming a fall. Thoughts can be like traps: they can knock a person off their agreed course of action and they tend to make the situation worse, not better. Clients can be helped to identify their negative thoughts which frequently arise in a situation and to decrease or replace these with helpful, coping thoughts.

Where more pervasive unhelpful ways of looking at the self, the world or the future exist, the dietitian may need to refer clients to other agencies to enable change.

Support across all stages of change

As well as needing support from the dietitian and other health professionals to change, the importance of support from other sources across all stages of change cannot be underestimated. Clients' family members, friends and colleagues can play key roles in helping them to change and thereby improving all treatment outcomes. An individual's environment can make it more or less easy for them to change. Ideally, dietitians should include family members in consultations wherever possible and encourage them to participate in dietary and lifestyle changes. Leaflets can be produced for family members explaining to them how they can support the person making the changes. For example, with clients following a cholesterol-lowering diet, the medical problem and benefits of changing their diet can be described to relatives who can be encouraged to:

- think of alternative gifts and treats to buy the person instead of chocolates or cakes;
- think about changing their diet too, as everyone can benefit from a healthier diet;
- try not to tease the person or belittle their efforts or tell them 'go on just once won't hurt', remembering that the friend or relative is changing what they eat because they value their health;
- reinforce and congratulate the person for changes made and encourage them to stick to the changes.

Alternatively, for an undernourished person, relatives and friends can be encouraged to:

- offer tempting treats to the person;
- avoid offering large portions if they have a small appetite;
- congratulate the person for every small amount they eat;
- try not to pressurize the person to eat prepared food if they do not feel like it;
- reinforce positive thoughts about the return of health.

1.7.5 Implications for dietetic practice

Guidelines for the dietetic intervention process

Traditional dietary advice giving is a central part of the overall therapeutic process but, as shown in Table 1.14, its use is limited without the support of the other behaviour change strategies.

Table 1.14 The intervention process

- Work at establishing core qualities (empathy, acceptance, genuineness) as well as professional competence
- Create an appropriate environment
- Establish a helping relationship
- Review client's view of problem
- Assess readiness to change: explore costs and benefits of change/staying the same
- Assess degree of medical/psychosocial risk
- If ready for change: review rationale and objectives for recommended diet and explore client's concerns. Discuss importance of maintaining changes made
- Assess diet and follow by giving appropriate advice
- Discuss and negotiate possible options for change
- Set goals
- Plan how to make a change successfully by modifying triggers
- Consider coping in high-risk situations
- Encourage social support
- Monitor progress. Agree future follow-up arrangements with client. Revise goals in the light of progress, dietary and activity diaries, changes in physiological, biometric and psychological measures

Time constraints

Many dietitians feel under pressure to see large numbers of patients and some may feel that they do not have adequate time to apply behaviour change strategies. Dietitians need to find the balance between size of caseload and clinical effectiveness. If insufficient time is allocated to meet each client's needs, then, behavioural change is less likely to be achieved and the dietitian's effectiveness is likely to be diminished. Dietitians may need to have the confidence to limit the size of their caseload so that they can be effective in their job, rather than accepting every referral and compromising quality for quantity. Nonetheless, a dietitian who applies behaviour change strategies skilfully can optimize effectiveness within even a very restricted time allocation.

A dietitian acting as a behaviour change agent will develop the skill to move between advice giving and a range of other behaviour change strategies as appropriate. Within an intervention, whether advice giving precedes or follows other behaviour change strategies will depend on the nature of the problem. Where the consequences of a condition may be long term, for example obesity and hyperlipidaemia, a range of behaviour change strategies might precede advice giving. In other cases, the first line of action may need to be advice giving to support implementing immediate dietetic change to prevent a life-threatening situation, for example anaphylactic shock with nut allergy. Nonetheless, the need for help with applying long-term coping strategies remains crucial in these situations even though introduction to more sophisticated strategies may come after the advice giving rather than before.

Although the point at which different behaviour change strategies are introduced varies in different dietetic situations, good communication and counselling skills are necessary at first contact and in *every* encounter between dietitian and client.

Training needs and practice issues

Nutrition education has traditionally focused on what dietary changes to make. Psychological methods focus on increasing skills to enhance motivation and support people through the process of making successful changes. Given that a dietitian's role is to ensure that people make nutrition-related behavioural changes, the integration of these two fields of information and skills seems to be a prerequisite for optimal training. The foundation for all behaviour change methods is likely to be a generic training in counselling skills. At present, few dietitians have received in-depth training in psychological skills in general, and cognitive and behavioural strategies in particular. Training in these areas need to be integrated into undergraduate training as well as offered at postgraduate level. In the current climate in the health service, where evidence-based practice is crucial for all practitioners with the emphasis on improved quality of care with measurable outcomes, the need to enable dietitians to act effectively as behaviour change agents is compelling (DH 1997). It may also be helpful for dietitians to consider working collaboratively with other clinicians who have expertise in behaviour change methods in cases which do not respond solely to dietetic management.

Text written by: Lorna Rapoport with additional contributions from Judith Carpenter and Dympna Pearson

References

American Psychological Association. Training and dissemination of empirically-validated psychological treatments: report and recommendations. *Clinical Psychologist* 1995; **46**: 3–23.

British Dietetic Association. Puzzled about qualifying as a dietitian? In *The BDA has the Answers* (Leaflet). British Dietetic Association, Birmingham, 1997.

Brownell KD. *The Learn Programme for Weight Control*. Dallas, TX: American Health Publishing Company, 1997.

Brownell KD, Cohen LR. Adherence to dietary regimens 1: An overview of research. *Behavioral Medicine* 1995a; **20**: 149–154.

Brownell KD, Cohen LR. Adherence to dietary regimens 2: Components of effective interventions. *Behavioral Medicine* 1995b; **20**: 155–164.

Contento J, Balch GI, Bronner YL *et al*. The effectiveness of nutrition education and implications for nutrition education policy, programs, and research: a review of research. *Journal of Nutrition Education* 1995; **27** (6, Special Issue).

Cooper PJ. *Bulimia Nervosa and Binge-eating. A Guide to Recovery*. Robinson Publishing, 1995.

Department of Health. *The New NHS, Modern and Dependable*. London: The Stationery Office, 1997.

Egan G. *The Skilled Helper: A Problem Management Approach to Helping*, 6th edn. USA: Brooks/Cole Publishing Co., 1998.

Fairburn CG, Marcus MD, Wilson GT. Cognitive–behavioural therapy for binge eating and bulimia nervosa: a comprehensive treatment manual. In Fairburn CG, Wilson GT. (Eds) *Binge Eating: Nature, Assessment and Treatment*, pp. 361–404. New York: Guilford Press, 1993.

Gable J. *Counselling Skills for Dietitians*. London: Blackwell Science, 1997.

Gilboy MB. Compliance-enhancing counselling strategies for cholesterol management. *Journal of Nutrition Education* 1994; **1**: 228–232.

Glanz K. Nutrition education for risk factor reduction and patient education: a review. *Preventive Medicine* 1985; **14**: 721–752.

Goldstein MG, DePue J, Kazura A, Niaura R. Models for provider–patient interaction: applications to health behaviour change. In Shumaker SA, Schron EB, Ockene JK, McBee WL (Eds) *The Handbook of Health Behaviour Change*, pp. 85–113. New York: Springer, 1998.

Grueninger U, Duffy F, Goldstein M. Patient education in the medical encounter: how to facilitate learning, behaviour change and coping. In Lipkin MJ, Putnam S, Lazare A (Eds) *The Medical Interview: Clinical Care, Education, Research*, pp. 122–133. New York: Springer, 1995.

Health Education Authority. *Health Promotion Interventions to Promote Healthy Eating in the General Population – A Review*. London: HEA, 1997.

Holli BB, Calabrese RJ. *Communication and Education Skills for Dietetics Professionals*. Baltimore, MD: Williams & Wilkins, 1998.

Hoyt MF, Janis IL. Increasing adherence to a stressful decision via a motivational balance-sheet procedure: a field experiment. *Journal of Personality and Social Psychology* 1975; **31**: 833–839.

Hunt P. Dietary counselling: theory into practice. *Journal of the Institute of Health Education* 1995; **33**: 4–8.

Hunt P, Hillsdon M. *Changing Eating and Exercise Behaviour. A Handbook for Professionals*. Oxford: Blackwell Science, 1996.

Isselmann MC, Deubner LS, Hartman M. A nutrition counselling workshop: integrating counselling psychology into nutrition practice. *Journal of the American Dietetic Association* 1993; **93**: 324–326.

Judd PA, Butson S, Hunt P *et al*. Pre-registration education and training for dietitians. Report and recommendations from the British Dietetic Association/CPSM Dietitians Board Joint Working Party, February 1996. *Journal of Human Nutrition and Dietetics* 1997; **10**: 157–162.

Marlatt GA, Gordon JR. *Relapse Prevention: Maintenance Strategies in Addictive Behavior Change*. New York: Guilford Press, 1985.

Miller WR, Rollnick S. *Motivational Interviewing: Preparing People to Change Addictive Behaviour*. New York: Guilford Press, 1991.

Najavits LM, Weiss RD. Variations in therapist effectiveness in the treatment of patients with substance use disorders: an empirical review. *Addiction* 1994; **89**: 679–688.

Prochaska JO, DiClemente CC. Towards a comprehensive model of change. In Miller WR, Heather N (eds), *Treating Addictive Disorders: Processes of Change*, pp. 3–27. New York: Plenum, 1986.

Rapoport L. Integrating cognitive behavioural therapy into dietetic practice: a challenge for dietitians. *Journal of Human Nutrition and Dietetics* 1998; **11**: 227–237.

Rogers A, Judd P. Current and future training for dietitians in the UK – results of the BDA pre-registration working group survey. *Journal of Human Nutrition and Dietetics* 1996; **9**: 387–411.

Rogers CR. *Client-centered Therapy*. Boston, MA: Houghton Mifflin, 1951.

Rollnick S, Heather N, Bell A. Negotiating behaviour change in medical settings: the development of brief motivational interviewing. *Journal of Mental Health* 1992; **1**: 25–37.

Rollnick S, Mason P, Butler C. *Health Behavior Change*. Edinburgh: Churchill Livingstone, 1999.

Shepherd R, Stockley L. Nutrition knowledge, attitudes, and fat consumption. *Journal of the American Dietetic Association* 1987; **87**: 615–619.

Shumaker SA, Schron EB, Ockene JK, McBee WL. (Eds). *The Handbook of Health Behavior Change*. New York: Springer, 1998.

Thomas J. New approaches to achieving dietary change. *Current Opinion in Lipidology* 1994; **5**: 36–41.

Treasure J, Schmidt U. *Getting Better Bit(e) by Bit(e)*. Hove: Lawrence Erlbaum Associates, 1993.

Van Bilsen HP. Motivational interviewing; perspectives from the Netherlands, with particular emphasis on heroin-dependent clients. In Miller WR, Rollnick S (Eds) *Motivational Interviewing: Preparing People to Change Addictive Behaviour*, pp. 214–224. New York: Guilford Press, 1991.

Wilson GT. Behavioural approaches to the treatment of obesity. In Brownell KD, Fairburn CG (Eds) *Eating Disorders and Obesity. A Comprehensive Handbook*, pp. 479–485. New York: Guilford Press, 1995.

Wing RR. Behavioural treatment of severe obesity. *American Journal of Clinical Nutrition* 1992; **55**: 545S–551S.

Wolfe BL (Ed.). *The Lifestyle Counselor's Guide for Weight Control*. Dallas, TX: American Health Publishing Company, 1996.

1.8 Assessment of nutritional status

Assessment of nutritional status means determining the extent to which an individual's nutritional needs have been, or are being, met. It is a fundamental component of dietetic practice and may be undertaken to:

- identify the existence and degree of severity of malnutrition
- identify those likely to benefit from nutritional support
- determine the goals of nutritional therapy and the level of nutritional support required
- provide a basis from which subsequent treatment can be planned
- monitor the progress of those receiving nutritional support.

There is no single or standard way of assessing nutritional status. Nutritional status is a dynamic entity reflecting physiological requirements, nutritional intake, body composition and function, and all these aspects have to be considered and the findings interpreted in conjunction with one another. The parameters investigated and the methods used to evaluate them will vary according to individual circumstances (Charney 1995) but may need to include:

- clinical considerations
- physical considerations
- dietary considerations
- anthropometric considerations
- biochemical and haematological considerations.

Very simple assessment may be sufficient to identify early signs of malnutrition, but more detailed investigation may then be needed to assess the level of nutritional support required. Different and more complex methods may be required to determine and monitor the nutritional status of those who are seriously ill (Jeejeebhoy 1998; Ge *et al*. 1998).

Various assessment tools have been developed, which may be disease-specific (Stall *et al*. 1996), age-specific (Boosalis and Stiles 1995) or simple tools such as the Mini Nutritional Assessment designed to identify those at risk of malnutrition and which can be predictive of mortality and hospital cost (Vellas *et al*. 1999) (see Section 1.9, Assessment of nutritional risk). However, no assessment tool is appropriate for all circumstances.

1.8.1 Clinical considerations

These can alert to the possibility of nutrient deficiencies. Acute or chronic illness, injury or surgery have consider-

able impact on nutritional status, both directly (due to the effects of the disease or injury itself) and indirectly (via possible effects on food intake). These effects may include:

- Increased nutrient requirements due to
  - fever
  - the metabolic response to trauma
  - the metabolic costs of repairing tissue damage
  - sepsis;
- Increased nutrient losses via
  - vomiting
  - diarrhoea
  - renal excretion
  - haemorrhage
  - wound or fistula exudates;
- Impaired nutrient digestion and absorption
  - Lack of digestive enzymes, e.g. pancreatitis
  - Loss of absorptive surfaces, e.g. gastric or intestinal resection, coeliac disease.

These effects are likely to be compounded if the illness or injury impairs intake of food and fluids (see Dietary considerations, below). Associated drug therapy may further affect nutrient intake, absorption, metabolism and excretion (see Section 2.12, Drug – nutrient interactions).

1.8.2 Physical considerations

Simple observation of the patient may reveal physical signs and symptoms which may result from disease but may also be indicative of nutritional depletion:

- *Physical appearance*: emaciation, pale complexion and hair loss are features of chronic undernutrition. Loose clothing, rings or dentures may indicate more recent or rapid weight loss. Sunken eyes, dry mouth and reduced skin elasticity are indicative of dehydration.
- *Mobility*: weakness and impaired movement may result from loss of muscle mass. Weakened, immobile people are likely to have difficulties with procuring, preparing or even eating food.
- *Mood*: apathy, lethargy and poor concentration are features of undernutrition and also exacerbate disinterest in food. Confusion can also be a sign of dehydration.
- *Breathlessness*: can be a symptom of anaemia, and can make it more difficult to eat.
- *Pressure sores and poor wound healing*: may reflect impaired immune function as a consequence of undernutrition and associated vitamin deficiencies, or lack of mobility.

- *Oedema*: may reflect underlying disease, or heart failure secondary to prolonged protein or thiamin deficiency.

1.8.3 Dietary considerations

These should focus on the extent to which dietary intake is likely to have met nutritional needs. Factors which need to be assessed include:

- current food and fluid intake
- duration and severity of any changes in appetite and oral intake
- the presence of factors which may be affecting food and fluid intake.

These findings then need to be interpreted in the context of the individual's nutritional requirements.

Assessing current intake

The way, and depth, in which current intake is assessed will depend on the nature of the enquiry (see Section 1.5, Dietary assessment). In most cases, a picture of current dietary intake in terms of meal pattern, food choice and overall balance can be obtained by careful questioning of either the patient or their carer (see Section 1.5.3). Particular aspects can then need to be explored further if specific deficiencies seem likely.

In those who are hospitalized or in residential care, it may be relevant to find out how much food is actually being consumed, as distinct from being served to the patient. With patients who are unable to self-feed, it is important to establish how much time is available for administering food and fluids (particularly at weekends when staff cover may be low) and the provision for recording and monitoring the amounts consumed.

Assessing recent changes in intake

As well as current intake, it is important to identify recent alteration in food intake such as:

- changes in appetite
- changes in meal pattern
- changes in food choice or food consistency.

The greater the extent and duration of these, the greater the likelihood of nutritional imbalance or depletion.

Identifying factors which may be affecting food and fluid intake

Factors which may be having a chronic but significant nutritional impact include:

- difficulties with buying, preparing or cooking food as a result of poor mobility or feeling unwell;
- apathy or disinterest in food as a result of depression, anxiety, social isolation or illness;

- confusion or memory loss, e.g. in patients with dementia;
- adverse effects of illness or drug treatment, e.g. nausea, vomiting, diarrhoea;
- physical problems affecting eating, e.g. poor dentition, dry mouth, sore or painful mouth, orofacial surgery;
- swallowing difficulties resulting in a limited choice or amount of food being consumed;
- repeated medical investigations or treatments requiring fasting or dietary change.

Other factors such as alcoholism, deprived social or economic circumstances, or recent discharge from hospital may also be relevant (Edington 1999).

Considering nutritional requirements

These need to be taken into account in order to determine whether nutritional intake is likely to have met nutritional needs. Nutritional requirements are primarily determined by age, gender, level of physical activity and growth (see Section 1.10, Estimating nutritional requirements) but may change significantly as a result of illness, trauma or malabsorption (see Clinical considerations, above).

1.8.4 Anthropometric considerations

Anthropometry is the means by which body composition can be assessed in living people. Anthropometric parameters reflects both health and nutritional status and can predict performance, health and survival. The WHO report (1995) provides guidelines on the use of anthropometry within different population and age groups.

For practical purposes body composition can be considered to be comprised of lean body mass, fat stores and body water. Ways in which these can be measured are summarized in Table 1.15. Some anthropometric measurements assess just one of these components, others a combination of them.

In clinical practice, body composition can be assessed by measurements of body weight, adiposity, muscle mass, electrolyte levels and water content. Sophisticated techniques used in clinical research include dual-energy X-ray absorptiometry (DEXA), multiple frequency bioimpedance analysis (BIA), computed axial tomography (CAT), magnetic resonance imaging (MRI), nuclear magnetic resonance (NMR) spectroscopy, neutron inelastic scattering and gamma-ray resonance.

Table 1.15 Anthropometric measurements of body composition

Protein status	Fat stores	Body water
Mid-arm muscle circumference (MAMC)	Triceps skinfold thickness	Bioelectrical impedance
Grip strength	Body mass index (BMI)	Biochemistry
Nitrogen balance		Fluid balance charts
Plasma proteins		Rapid weight change
Plasma urea		Girth (ascites)
		Pitting oedema

Body weight

Although being underweight or overweight adversely influences morbidity and mortality, body weight is a crude indicator of body composition, since it includes measurement of lean tissue, fat and fluid – the latter influenced by short-term fluid balance. However, change in body weight is an important indicator of nutritional status.

Percentage weight loss

In the absence of oedema or ascites, unexpected weight loss over a period of weeks or months is an important indicator of nutritional depletion, and the percentage of body weight lost has significant prognostic value:

$$\% \text{ Weight loss} = \frac{(\text{Usual weight kg} - \text{Actual weight kg})}{\text{Usual weight kg}} \times 100$$

The significance of weight loss as a percentage of pre-illness weight has been defined (Heymsfield and Matthews 1994) as:

<5% weight loss	Not significant (unless likely to continue)
5–9% weight loss	Only of clinical significance if rapid, or if malnutrition is clearly present
10–20% weight loss	Clinically significant; nutritional support indicated
>20% weight loss	Severe; aggressive nutritional support indicated.

However, these percentages should be interpreted in term of the rapidity of weight loss; a 5% weight loss over 3 months is of greater concern than if it has occurred over 12 months. Rapid weight loss over a few days reflects changes in fluid balance rather than body tissue.

Sequential measurements of weight

Isolated comparisons of body weight with reference tables of ideal body weight (Metropolitan Life 1983) are rarely used, as the standards relate to the healthy American population and are of little clinical value.

However, sequential body weight measurements taken at weekly (or fortnightly) intervals, using admission weight or first weight assessment as a baseline measurement, are a simple and useful way of monitoring nutritional status, unless significant fluid retention is present. Oedema or ascites has been estimated by Mendelhall (1992) to contribute between 1 and 14 kg of measured weight (see Table 4.17 in Section 4.13, Liver and biliary disease).

Adiposity

Body mass index (BMI)

BMI reflects body fat stores and has important predictive value in terms of morbidity and mortality in those classified as underweight or obese (de Onis and Habicht 1996).

BMI is calculated as: $\dfrac{\text{weight kg}}{(\text{height m})^2}$.

A ready reckoner of BMI is given in Appendix 6.3.

BMI can be interpreted as follows:

<16	Severely underweight
16–19	Underweight
20–25	Normal range
26–30	Overweight
31–40	Obese
>40	Morbidly obese.

However, it should be borne in mind that these cut-off levels are to some extent arbitrary and based on data derived from young, healthy adults. A BMI value may have different prognostic significance in different age groups, particularly elderly people (Beck and Ovesen 1998). Adult BMI reference ranges are also not appropriate for children (see Adiposity in children, below).

BMI has widespread application but needs to be used with caution in people who have a distorted fluid balance (oedema, ascites or dehydration), a high proportion of muscle mass (e.g. athletes and body builders) or enforced immobility (e.g. tetraplegia).

BMI may be difficult to determine accurately if facilities for measuring weight and height are not available. Weight may be difficult to measure in people who are bed-bound or in a wheelchair, particularly in the domestic setting where specialist weighing equipment is not available. Height cannot be measured directly in people unable to stand unaided or who have spinal curvature.

In some circumstances, estimates of weight and/or height may be sufficient for the purposes of assessing nutritional status. Weight can be assessed visually, perhaps in conjunction with information about that person's usual weight. People often know their height with a reasonable degree of accuracy.

In the older adult, the use of height for BMI calculation fails to take into account the loss of height with increasing age or osteoporosis, and the regression equation fails to consider the loss of fat-free mass associated with ageing. Using an alternative parameter such as knee height compensates for age-related changes (Roubenoff and Wilson 1993). Arm demispan can also be used when spinal curvature, infirmity or mental confusion prevents direct measurement of, or enquiry about, height (Bassey 1986). Knee height and demispan measurement techniques, and height conversion formulae are given in Table 1.16.

Demiquet and Mindex

Alternative indices to the BMI based on weight and demi-span (rather than height) have been derived for use in elderly people (Lehmann et al. 1991).

In men over 64 years, the Demiquet can be used:

$$\text{Demiquet} = \frac{\text{Weight kg}}{(\text{Demispan m})^2} .$$

In women over 64 years, the Mindex is considered more suitable. This is defined as:

$$\text{Mindex} = \frac{\text{Weight kg}}{\text{Demispan m}} .$$

Table 1.16 Estimation of height from knee height or demispan

Knee height

With the leg flexed so that the thigh and calf create a right angle, the fixed blade of a knee height caliper is placed under the heel and the sliding blade moved down to rest on the top of the knee, about 5 cm behind the knee cap. The knee height is then read from a scale to the nearest 0.1 cm. Height is calculated using the following formulae (Cameron Chumlea 1985):

Men   19–59 years: Height cm = (Knee height cm $\times$ 1.88) + 71.85
        60–80 years: Height cm = (Knee height cm $\times$ 2.05) + 59.01

Women   19–59 years: Height cm = (Knee height cm $\times$ 1.86) − (age years $\times$ 0.05) + 70.25
        60–80 years: Height cm = (Knee height cm $\times$ 1.91) − (age years $\times$ 0.17) + 75.00

Demispan

Demispan can be measured using one of two methods:
1. From the centre of the sternal notch in the midline, to the tip of the middle finger with the arms outstretched (Kwok and Whitelaw 1991).
or
2. From the second finger web to the midline chest.

Height is calculated from either of the following formulae:
Kwok and Whitelaw (1991):
   Adult males: Height cm = (Demispan cm $\times$ 1.40) + 57.8
   Adult females: Height cm = (Demispan cm $\times$ 1.35) + 60.1

White *et al.* 1993:
   Men: Height cm = (1.2 $\times$ demispan) + 71
   Women: Height cm = (1.2 $\times$ demispan) + 67

Because Demiquet and Mindex are independent of stature, they can be useful in studies of elderly people where the use of BMI based on height may be questionable (Smith *et al.* 1995). Tables showing the percentile distribution of Demiquet and Mindex in the elderly population are given in Appendix 6.4, although the limitations of these reference data (which are based on relatively small population samples) should be borne in mind (Bannerman *et al.* 1997).

Skinfold thickness

The relationship between subcutaneous fat and total body fat can be exploited by measuring skinfold thickness at specific sites to estimate adiposity (Durnin and Womersley 1974). Skinfold thickness is measured by pinching a fold of skin with subcutaneous fat between a pair of Harpenden skinfold calipers (Table 1.17).

The most accurate estimates of adiposity require skinfold measurements at a number of sites, usually the triceps, biceps, subscapular and iliac crest. In clinical practice, and especially in the bed-bound patient, triceps skinfold thickness alone is most commonly used as an indicator of body fat stores and, in conjunction with mid-arm circumference (see below), can be a useful way of evaluating body

Table 1.17 Procedure for measurement of skinfold thickness

In order to minimize measurement error, three separate readings should be taken and averaged. All measurements on a particular individual should be made by the same person.

Triceps skinfold
Measurement should be made on the *non-dominant* arm. This should be bent at a right-angle. The length from the tip of the acromion process on the scapula to the olecranon process of the ulna is measured and the midpoint marked. With the arm hanging loosely by the side, the skinfold at the midpoint level on the back of the arm over the triceps muscle is picked up between the thumb and forefinger of the left hand. The calipers are placed on the skinfold just below the fingers, the fingers are removed and a reading is taken 2–3 seconds later.

Biceps skinfold
As for the triceps, but over the biceps muscle on the front of the arm.

Subscapular skinfold
Measurement is made about 2.5 cm in and below the angle of the scapula towards the midline and at an angle of approximately 45 degrees to the spine along the natural line of skin cleavage.
Alternatively, the skinfold is picked up just below the tip of the right scapula. The natural potential crease which is lifted to form this fold runs at an angle of about 45 degrees downwards from the spine.

Suprailiac skinfold
This is measured midway between the anterior superior iliac spine crest and the lowest point of the ribs, horizontal to the floor, or just above the iliac crest in the midaxillary line.
Alternatively, the vertical skinfold can be picked up immediately above the anterior superior iliac spine in the midaxillary line.

composition in patients with ascites or peripheral oedema, or who cannot be weighed. However, it should be noted that loss of body weight results in non-proportional changes in muscle and fat stores at different sites (Katch and Hortobagyi 1990). Patients with liver disease and alcoholism have vastly reduced arm circumference measurements compared with normal controls (Thuluvath and Triger 1994).

Selected reference values of triceps skinfold thickness in a normal adult population (Bishop *et al.* 1981) are given in Appendix 6.4.

Problems associated with measurement of skinfold thickness include:

- *Measurement error*: since subcutaneous fat is compressible when the full pressure of the caliper is applied, the observed reading initially falls rapidly and is then followed by a slow drift downwards. It is therefore difficult to know precisely when the reading should be taken. As a result, it takes time and practice to acquire a measurement technique which gives reproducible recordings, and even then these measurements may differ substantially from those made on the same person by other observers.
- *Measurement difficulties*: the correct anatomical site is difficult to establish and in some cases the site may be inaccessible due to burns, bandages, etc. The jaws of the calipers may not be wide enough to encompass the fat fold in people who are grossly obese.
- *Errors due to individual variation in fat distribution*: although the relationship between subcutaneous fat and total body fat is relatively constant, there are variations between individuals, or within an individual, at different points in time. In particular, the relationship of skinfold thickness to total body fat changes with age; as people grow older a greater proportion of body fat is deposited internally rather than subcutaneously.
- *Population differences in body fat distribution*: people of Afro-Caribbean origin tend to have more visceral and upper-body fat deposition than Caucasians (Zillikens and Conway 1990; Conway *et al.* 1995). Asian adults have also been shown to have more upper-body subcutaneous fat and a higher body fat:BMI ratio than Caucasian adults, a difference more pronounced in women (Wang *et al.* 1994).
- *Insensitivity*: body fat has to change by several kilograms before this is detectable by skinfold thickness measurements. This, therefore, limits the value of the technique as a short-term monitoring tool. However, serial measurements of triceps skinfold thickness, for example, can be a useful way of monitoring long-term clinical status.

Waist circumference

Despite its simplicity, waist circumference has been shown to be an accurate indicator of central obesity and to have valuable prognostic value in terms of health risks from adiposity (Ashwell *et al.* 1996). A standard technique for measurement of waist circumference has been described by WHO (1995). This requires that the waist should be measured with the patient standing and in gentle expiration at a level midway between the lowest rib and the iliac crest. The advantage of this method is that it uses a bony landmark and there is little scope for error provided the patient can be partially undressed. Moreover, waist measurement does not need to be adjusted for height in order to assess body fat or fat distribution.

A single waist measurement can be used to predict those with a BMI >25 (Lean *et al.* 1995). Waist measurements >94 cm in men, and >80 cm in women were predictive of this level of obesity, with only 2% of the 2000-strong cohort being misclassified using this criterion.

Alternative predictive formulae based on the ratio between waist and hip circumference measurements have been devised and may be predictive of heart disease and mortality risk (Hseih and Yoshinaga 1995; Cox and Whichelow 1996) but appear to have little advantage over the simpler technique of measuring waist circumference alone. In addition, measurement of hip circumference is less acceptable to subjects as accurate measurement requires removal of clothing.

Other techniques, such as DEXA, can also be used to determine intra-abdominal fat content (Treuth *et al.* 1995).

Muscle mass

Mid-arm circumference (MAC)

Measurement of the circumference of the non-dominant arm midway between the shoulder and elbow can be used as a simple determinant of muscle mass. Reference values for MAC (derived from an American population; Bishop *et al.* 1981) are given in Appendix 6.4.

Mid-arm muscle circumference (MAMC)

An estimate of skeletal muscle mass can be derived from measurement of mid-arm circumference (MAC) and triceps skinfold thickness (TSF) using the formula:

MAMC cm = MAC cm − (TSF mm × 0.314).

Standards for interpreting the MAMC are given in Appendix 6.4.

Dynamometry (grip strength)

Grip strength can be a useful index of muscle function (Griffith and Clark 1984). Subjects are asked to grip a handgrip dynamometer with the non-dominant hand and three separate measurements are made. The mean value obtained is expressed as a percentage of the standard (Appendix 6.4). Values which are below 85% of normal may indicate protein malnutrition.

The technique is limited by the fact that grip strength may be affected by debility, age and familiarity with the technique (ability improves with repeated use) and cannot be used by those with arthritis or who are seriously ill. It can be useful for measuring functional muscle status in those on long-term nutritional support.

Body composition

Bioelectrical impedance analysis (BIA)

Portable bioelectrical impedance (BIA) analysers are increasingly popular as a field or bedside method of measuring body composition. Most incorporate sophisticated software to interpret the measurements.

BIA is based on the principle that lean tissue, with its high water and electrolyte content, is highly conductive to electrical current, whereas fat tissue is more resistant. By measuring the change in voltage when a small current is passed through electrodes placed on specific parts of the body, a measurement of total body water (TBW) can be made. Fat-free mass (FFM) can be estimated from TBW by assuming that it comprises 73% of the body's water content. Body fat can be determined by subtracting the estimate of FFM from total body weight.

Although BIA measurements are extremely accurate, errors can arise as a result of:

- Inaccuracies in the measurement of body weight.
- The assumed hydration of the fat-free mass: although relatively constant in the healthy population, significant variation can occur in subjects with abnormalities of water balance.
- Variation in body geometry: the contribution of different segments of the body to whole-body impedance is assumed to be relatively standard. For example, an arm is assumed to contribute 46% of total body impedance and the body trunk 10%. Significant individual variation in body shape and fat distribution may distort these conversion factors.

BIA can be useful for assessing nutritional status in seriously ill patients where anthropometric methods are less suitable and a greater level of precision is required. Sequential BIA measurements may be used as a way of monitoring hydration status in the critically ill. However, the measurements are of limited use in patients with grossly abnormal fluid balance (e.g. severe dehydration, ascites). BIA can be used to monitor changes in body composition in patients during refeeding (Pencharz and Azcue 1996).

Specialized methods of measuring body composition

Body composition can be ascertained with considerable precision by techniques such as densitometry, radioisotope dilution, MRI or DEXA. However, these are highly specialized procedures requiring complex equipment and their use tends to be confined to the research or diagnostic setting.

1.8.5 Biochemical and haematological considerations

Profound nutritional depletion has physiological effects which can alter clinical chemistry. However, biochemical and haematological measurements have only limited value in the assessment of nutritional status as many of these parameters are dynamic and change on a daily basis, compensated by homoeostatic mechanisms or influenced by underlying disease. Clinical chemistry can be useful to monitor nutritional support, particularly in those who are critically ill (see Section 1.13, Artificial nutritional support).

Vitamins, minerals and trace elements

Serum levels of trace elements are of limited value as indicators of nutritional inadequacy because body stores of elements such as iron and zinc must be severely depleted before circulating levels are affected. Compensatory homoeostatic mechanisms may mask nutrient deficiencies until an advanced stage of depletion. Conversely, metabolic or physical stress can influence serum levels of micronutrients or their biochemical markers (Singh *et al.* 1991)

Hydration status and serum electrolytes

Iatrogenic, dietetic and clinical causes can all influence these factors. Refer to Sections 1.13.2 (Enteral feeding) and 5.2 (Intensive care) for further details.

Serum proteins

Synthesis of serum proteins such as albumin and transferrin is compromised in protein-energy malnutrition, and levels of these proteins have traditionally been used as markers of nutritional depletion. However, non-nutritional factors such as trauma, sepsis, dehydration, disease states and drug therapy can influence plasma levels to a greater extent than nutritional factors. These parameters therefore need to be interpreted with caution.

Serum albumin has a long half-life of 21 days so will not reflect recent changes in nutritional intake (Klein 1990). Its potential to fall by more 20 g/l over a few days when a patient is severely stressed demonstrates its relatively minor role in acute disease (Gabay and Kushner 1999). Total protein levels in plasma are maintained as the liver produces acute-phase proteins of greater physiological significance (such as haptoglobulin, caeruloplasmin and C-reactive protein). Normal albumin levels in severe anorexia nervosa have been reported.

Serum transferrin has a shorter half-life than albumin (8–10 days) and may be a more sensitive marker of nutritional status, but it is also influenced by metabolic or septic stress. In addition, transferrin is an iron-transport protein so will be markedly affected by changes in iron status, e.g. anaemia, use of iron supplementation, severe blood loss or blood transfusion.

Rapid turnover proteins such as thyroxine binding prealbumin (with a half-life of 2–3 days) and retinol binding protein (half-life 12 hours) are much more sensitive to protein depletion but are also extremely sensitive to changes in metabolic stress and disease (Casati *et al.* 1998).

1.8.6 Monitoring nutritional status

A variety of techniques is available for monitoring nutritional status in the clinical situation. Suitable methods and the frequency of deployment are summarized in Table 1.18.

1.8.7 Assessing nutritional status in children

Great care is needed when assessing the nutritional status of children, particularly neonates. Although the general principles of assessment of nutritional status – clinical, physical, dietary, anthropometric and biochemical/haematological considerations – apply to children as well as adults, the ways in which these are assessed and the standards used to interpret them may differ significantly (Zemel *et al*. 1997). More details can be found in specialist textbooks of paediatric dietetics such as that of Shaw and Lawson (2001).

Growth

Progression of growth is an important parameter to be considered and can be assessed in terms of height and weight or, in infants, weight and head circumference in relation to reference standards for age. New reference standards (Freeman *et al*. 1995) which take account of the upward shift in the average weight and height of children in recent decades have now replaced the Tanner and Whitehouse data compiled in the 1950s and 1960s. Centile charts containing nine centile curves showing the distribution of height, weight or head circumference in relation to age have been produced by the Child Growth Foundation (1993).

Centile charts need to be used with care. An isolated measurement on a centile chart does not necessarily mean a great deal; there is considerable variability in normal height, weight or rate of growth and it is only a measurement that falls above the 99.6th or below the 0.4th centile which is a matter of concern (Cole 1994). Deviation of growth from a centile line is more indicative of impaired growth and a growth curve which crosses a centile line between two annual measurements (e.g. crossing from the 25th to the 9th centile) warrants further investigation. A growth curve which crosses a centile line over a period of 2 years (i.e. three annual assessments) is an indication for further assessment a year later and subsequent referral if necessary.

To minimize the risk of errors and misinterpretation, it is particularly important that all anthropometric measurements in children are made accurately (Sardinha *et al*. 1999):

- *Weight*: infants or toddlers should be weighed naked on a self-calibrating or regularly calibrated scale. Older children should be weighed with a minimum of clothing.
- *Height*: Standing height should be measured against a vertical measure with the child's heels, buttocks and shoulder blades touching the vertical and the head positioned in the Frankfurt plane (an imaginary line from the centre of the ear hole to the lower border of the eye socket). Below the age of 18 months, supine length should be measured by the child lying on its back with its head, facing upwards in the Frankfurt plane, being held against a fixed headboard while a moveable footboard is brought up to the heels.
- *Head circumference* measurements in infants should be taken from midway between the eyebrows and the hairline at the front of the head and the occipital prominence at the back.

Table 1.18 Monitoring nutritional status

Assessment parameter	How	When
Weight	Weight charts Nursing kardex Prior outpatient clinic records	Initial assessment Weekly or fortnightly
Weight history	Medical notes, dietetic notes, patient or carer recall	Initial assessment
Height, demispan, knee height	Stadiometer, patient's own knowledge, tape measure, knee height measurer	Once only
Drug and medical history	Relevant notes, pharmacy chart	Every 2–3 days acutely, weekly long-term.
Diet history	Interview, food-frequency questionnaire, food diary	At assessment, then at considered intervals thereafter
Food and fluid intake charts	Food intake chart Fluid balance notes	Initial 3 days, then dependent on patient's condition
Clinical biochemistry	Medical notes	Daily, or weekly review, depending on the patient
Social history	Dietetic record cards	Initial assessment, and thereafter as required
Nutrition risk score tool	Nutrition risk score Medical notes	Long-term – monthly
General review/discussion with nurse	Nurse/carer record in notes Observation in nursing notes	Initial review and ongoing review

Growth impairment can occur for a variety of reasons, not all of which have a nutritional basis. The influence of genetic, pathological and psychological factors has to be considered alongside information from dietary enquiry before the cause and significance of growth failure can be established.

Adiposity in children

BMI changes with age as children grow, and adult parameters of BMI are thus inappropriate. However, BMI reference curves have now been devised for children in the UK (Cole *et al*. 1995) and BMI centile charts for use in boys and girls from birth to 20 years have been produced by the Child Growth Foundation.

Percentile monitoring is a useful way of identifying excessive weight gain at an early stage before the problem becomes harder to correct. Children who exceed the 98th centile should be considered overweight and in need of remedial measures.

There are important differences in height, weight and BMI between children from different ethnic groups (Chinn *et al*. 1996) and a summary of how centile charts should be interpreted in these population subgroups can be found in the SIGN guidelines (1996).

Text revised by: Briony Thomas and Catherine Collins

Useful addresses

Child Growth Foundation
2 Mayfield Avenue, London W4 1PW

SIGN (Scottish Intercollegiate Guidelines Network)
Royal College of Physicians, 9 Queen Street, Edinburgh EH2 1JQ

Anthropometry Resource Center
Website: www.odc.com/anthro

References

Ashwell M, Cole TJ, Dixon AK. Ratio of waist circumference to height is strong predictor of intra-abdominal fat. *British Medical Journal* 1996; **313**: 559–560.

Bannerman E, Reilly JJ, MacLennan WJ *et al*. Evaluation of validity of British anthropometric reference data for assessing nutritional state of elderly people in Edinburgh: cross sectional study. *British Medical Journal* 1997; **315**: 338–341.

Bassey JE. Demispan as a measure of skeletal size. *Annals of Human Biology* 1986; **13**: 499–502.

Beck AM, Ovesen L. At which body mass index and degree of weight loss should hospitalized elderly patients be considered at nutritional risk? *Clinical Nutrition* 1998; **17**: 195–198.

Bishop CW, Bowen PE, Ritchley SI. Norms for nutritional assessment of American adults by upper arm anthropometry. *American Journal of Clinical Nutrition* 1981; **34**: 2530–2539.

Boosalis MG, Stiles NJ. Nutritional assessment in the elderly: biochemical analyses. *Clinical and Laboratory Science* 1995; **8**: 31–33.

Cameron Chumlea W. Estimating stature from knee height for persons 60 to 90 years of age. *Journal of the American Geriatric Society* 1985; **33**: 116–120.

Casati A, Muttini S, Leggieri C *et al*. Rapid turnover proteins in critically ill ICU patients. Negative acute phase proteins or nutritional indicators? *Minerva Anesthesiologica* 1998; **64**: 345–350.

Charney P. Nutrition assessment in the 1990s: where are we now? *Nutrition in Clinical Practice* 1995; **10**: 131–139.

Child Growth Foundation. *Child Growth Standards*. London: Child Growth Foundation, 1993.

Chinn S, Cole TJ, Preece MA, Rona RJ. Growth charts for ethnic populations in the UK. *Lancet* 1996; **437**: 839–840.

Cole TJ. Do growth centile charts need a face-lift? *British Medical Journal* 1994; **308**: 641–642.

Cole TJ, Freeman JV, Preece MA. Body Mass Index reference curves for the UK, 1990. *Archives of Disease in Childhood* 1995; **73**: 25–29.

Conway JM, Yanovski SZ, Avila NA *et al*. Visceral adipose tissue differences in black and white women. *American Journal of Clinical Nutrition* 1995; **61**: 765–771.

Cox BD, Whichelow MJ. Ratio of waist circumference to height is better predictor of death than body mass index. *British Medical Journal* 1996; **313**: 1487.

de Onis M, Habicht JP. Anthropometric reference data for international use: recommendations from a World Health Organization Expert Committee. *American Journal of Clinical Nutrition* 1996; **64**: 650–658.

Durnin JVGA, Wolmersley J. Body fat assessed from total body density and its estimation from skinfold thickness: measurements on 481 men and women aged from 16 to 72 years. *British Journal of Nutrition* 1974; **32**: 77–97.

Edington J. Problems of nutritional assessment in the community. *Proceedings of the Nutrition Society* 1999; **58**: 47–51.

Freeman JV, Cole TJ, Chinn S *et al*. Cross-sectional stature and weight reference curves for the UK, 1990. *Archives of Disease in Childhood* 1995; **73**: 17–24.

Gabay C, Kushner I. Acute-phase proteins and other systemic responses to inflammation. *New England Journal of Medicine* 1999; **340**: 448–454.

Ge YQ, Wu ZL, Xu YZ, Liao LT. Study on nutritional status of maintenance hemodialysis patients. *Clinical Nephrology* 1998; **50**: 309–314.

Griffith CDM, Clark RG. A comparison of the 'Sheffield' prognostic index with forearm muscle dynamometry in patients from Sheffield undergoing major abdominal and urological surgery. *Clinical Nutrition* 1984; **3**: 147–151.

Heymsfield SB, Matthews D. Body composition: research and clinical advances. *Journal of Parenteral and Enteral Nutrition* 1994; **18**: 91–103.

Hseih SD, Yoshinaga H. Abdominal fat distribution and coronary heart disease risk factors in men – waist/height ratio as a simple and useful predictor. *International Journal of Obesity* 1995; **19**: 585–589.

Jeejeebhoy KN. Nutritional assessment. *Gastroenterology Clinics of North America* 1998; **27**: 347–369.

Katch FI, Hortobagyi T. Validity of surface anthropometry to estimate upper-arm muscularity, including changes with body mass loss. *American Journal of Clinical Nutrition* 1990; **52**: 591–595.

Klein S. The myth of albumin as a measure of nutritional status *Gastroenterology* 1990; **99**: 1845–1846.

Kwok T, Whitelaw MN. The use of armspan in nutritional assessment of the elderly. *Journal of the American Geriatric Society* 1991; **39**: 492–496.

Lean MEJ, Han TS, Morrison CE. Waist circumference as a measure for indicating need for weight management. *British Medical Journal* 1995; **311**: 158–161.

Lehmann AB *et al*. Normal values for weight, skeletal size, body mass indices in 890 men and women over 65 years of age. Table 3, Deciles for weight for skeletal size, weight and demispan. *Clinical Nutrition* 1991; **10**: 18–23.

Mendenhall CL. Protein-calorie malnutrition in alcoholic liver disease. In Watson RR, Watzl B (Eds) *Nutrition and Alcohol*, pp. 363–384. Boca Raton: CRC Press, 1992.

Metropolitan Life. *Metropolitan Life Insurance Company Statistical Bulletin* 1983; **64**: 1–9.

Pencharz PB, Azcue M. Use of bioelectrical impedance analysis measurements in the clinical management of malnutrition. *American Journal of Clinical Nutrition* 1996; **64**: 485S–488S.

Roubenoff R, Wilson PW. Advantage of knee height over height as an index of stature in expression of body composition in adults. *American Journal of Clinical Nutrition* 1993; **57**: 609–613.

Sardinha LB, Going SB, Teixeira PJ, Lohman TG. Receiver operating characteristic analysis of body mass index, triceps skinfold thickness, and arm girth for obesity screening in children and adolescents. *American Journal of Clinical Nutrition* 1999; **70**: 1090–1095.

Shaw V, Lawson M. *Clinical Paediatric Dietetics*. Oxford: Blackwell Science, 2001.

SIGN (Scottish Intercollegiate Guidelines Network). *Obesity in Scotland*, pp. 52–53. Edinburgh: SIGN, 1996.

Singh A, Smoak BL, Patterson KY *et al*. Biochemical indices of selected trace minerals in men: effect of stress. *American Journal of Clinical Nutrition* 1991; **53**: 126–131.

Smith WD, Cunningham DA, Paterson DH, Koval JJ. Body mass indices and skeletal size in 394 Canadians aged 55–86 years. *Annals of Human Biology* 1995; **22**: 305–314.

Stall SH, Ginsberg NS, DeVita MV *et al*. Comparison of five body-composition methods in peritoneal dialysis patients. *American Journal of Clinical Nutrition* 1996; **64**: 125–130.

Thuluvath PJ, Triger DR. Evaluation of nutritional status by using anthropometry in adults with alcoholic and nonalcoholic liver disease. *American Journal of Clinical Nutrition* 1994; **60**: 269–273.

Treuth MS, Hunter GR, Kekes-Szabo T. Estimating intra-abdominal adipose tissue in women by dual-energy X-ray absorptiometry. *American Journal of Clinical Nutrition* 1995; **62**: 527–532.

Vellas B, Guigoz Y, Garry PJ *et al*. The Mini Nutritional Assessment (MNA) and its use in grading the nutritional state of elderly patients. *Nutrition* 1999; **15**: 116–122.

Wang J, Thornton JC, Russell M *et al*. Asians have lower body mass index (BMI) but higher percent body fat than do whites: comparisons of anthropometric measurements. *American Journal of Clinical Nutrition* 1994; **60**: 23–28.

White A, Nicolaas G, Foster K *et al*. *Health Survey for England 1991*. London: HMSO, 1993.

World Health Organization. *Physical Status: The Use and Interpretation of Anthropometry*. Report of a WHO Expert Committee. Technical Report Service 854. Geneva: WHO, 1995.

Zemel BS, Riley EM, Stallings VA. Evaluation of methodology for nutritional assessment in children: anthropometry, body composition and energy expenditure. *Annual Reviews in Nutrition* 1997; **17**: 211–235.

Zillikens MC, Conway JM. Anthropometry in blacks: applicability of generalized skinfold equations and differences in fat patterning between blacks and whites. *American Journal of Clinical Nutrition* 1990; **52**: 45–51.

1.9 | Assessment of nutritional risk

The prevalence of malnutrition among people in hospitals and institutions and among vulnerable sections of the community is a considerable cause for concern (see Section 1.11, Undernutrition). Given the consequences to patient health and recovery highlighted in the King's Fund Report (Lennard-Jones 1992), early identification and correction of malnutrition is essential (McWhirter and Pennington 1994; Lennard-Jones *et al*. 1995). It is also important to assess those who are at risk of being malnourished so that measures can be taken to prevent its onset before it becomes clinically significant (Blackburn and Ahmad 1995).

At the other end of the scale, overnutrition and obesity are also major health risks requiring identification and intervention.

1.9.1 The need for nutritional risk assessment

The King's Fund Report highlighted the importance of nutrition as an integral component of healthcare and proposed that nutritional status should be a standard component of patient assessment and monitoring procedures. Yet a survey by Lennard-Jones *et al*. (1995) showed that even the most basic nutritional assessment of newly admitted hospital in-patients may be haphazard or non-existent. In this study, carried out in 70 UK hospitals, 454 ward nurses and 319 junior doctors were questioned about the last patient they had admitted. Only two-thirds of patients had been asked about recent food intake, and enquiries about recent weight loss had only been made by 53% of nurses and 73% of doctors. Answers to these questions had been recorded in the notes on 52–82% of occasions. Weight was recorded by 63% of nurses but only 11% measured height (mainly because no facilities for measuring height were available). Most doctors and nurses who failed to ask about nutrition did so because they believed it to be unimportant.

In the community setting, the situation may be even worse. General lack of awareness of the prevalence and hazards of undernutrition or overweight means that these problems may not be identified until they are well advanced, particularly among the elderly sector of the population. Residential and nursing homes are a particular area of concern; care staff are often young, part-time and unskilled, and there may be heavy reliance on the use of agency staff for qualified nursing cover. As a result, there tends to be lack of continuity of care and less likelihood of emerging nutritional problems being noticed.

Lack of nutritional knowledge by medical, nursing and care staff is part of the problem and better nutrition education of health professionals is still an area which needs to be addressed. But even if awareness of nutrition is heightened, it is equally important that health professionals and carers know what to look for, are able to look for it and can assess the significance of what they find. Assessment of nutritional status is a complex procedure (see Section 1.8, Assessment of nutritional status) requiring both time and dietetic expertise, and these resources are in short supply. Dietitians have the expertise but it is neither practical nor cost-effective for them to assess the nutritional status of every patient admitted to hospital, and they are unlikely to come into direct contact with many of those at risk in the community until after problems have developed. Identification of people with, or at risk of, malnutrition therefore requires the assistance of other health professionals, but few doctors, nurses or care staff will have either the time or the expertise to make detailed nutritional assessments.

The solution to this problem is nutritional risk assessment (more commonly known as nutritional screening) – a simple, quick yet reliable means of identifying those likely to have or develop nutritional problems who can then be referred for more detailed assessment and possible nutritional intervention (Lennard-Jones *et al*. 1995; BDA 1999). Repeated use of such a screening tool at regular (e.g. weekly) intervals as a routine part of every patient's care plan can also be a valuable way of monitoring the nutritional status of patients and identifying any emerging problems.

This assessment procedure needs to be a component of the standard nursing admission process; if left as an *ad hoc* arrangement, time constraints will result in some patients being overlooked. Hospitals that have a nutrition support team are more likely to have appropriate nutritional risk-assessment procedures than those that do not (Daniels and Wright 1997). In the primary care setting, nutritional screening can be incorporated into standard health reviews or be a component of nursing care plans.

Effective nutritional screening not only detects undernutrition but can also be a valuable means of highlighting obesity. As well as having its own health risks, obesity can also mask severe tissue wasting during periods of illness; any patient with a rapid or prolonged decline in nutritional status can be at risk of associated complications and can require nutritional support, regardless of current body weight.

As well as measures being in place to identify those at nutritional risk, it is equally important that there is a system which ensures that appropriate action is taken when necessary. A study by Reilly *et al.* (1995) showed that in about two-thirds of hospital in-patients identified as being at 'moderate risk' of malnutrition, and almost one-third of those at 'high risk', no action was taken to prevent a deterioration in nutritional status.

All patients or clients identified at being at nutritional risk need to be referred to a dietitian for more detailed assessment of nutritional status (see Section 1.8) and, if necessary, nutritional support (see Sections 1.12, Oral nutritional support, and 1.13, Artificial nutritional support).

1.9.2 Nutrition screening tools

In recent years various nutrition screening tools have been developed to help facilitate the process of risk assessment. These attempt to categorize an individual's level of risk by means of a scoring or grading system applied to a number of indicators of nutritional status, such as changes in body weight, appetite and dietary intake.

The problem with nutrition screening tools is that those which identify nutritional risk with the greatest degree of accuracy tend to be the most complex and difficult to administer, and hence the least suitable in terms of time, practicality or cost. Some of the first nutrition screening tools to be devised, such as the Likelihood of Malnutrition Index (LMI) (Weinsier *et al.* 1979) and the Prognostic Nutritional Index (PNI) (Mullen *et al.* 1980), used a combination of anthropometric, clinical and biochemical/haematological parameters to construct an index of undernutrition. Although they were shown to have predictive value in terms of risk of post-operative complications or prolonged hospital stay, their cost and complexity limited their use as routine assessment tools. Subsequent screening tools, such as the Subjective Global Assessment (SGA) (Detsky *et al.* 1987) or Nutrition Risk Index (Wolinsky *et al.* 1990), were less dependent on laboratory measurements and focused more on indicators such as changes in body weight or dietary intake, but even these had limited practical application because of the training required to obtain reproducible results and the time taken for their completion.

Since then there have been many attempts to develop nutrition screening tools which find a better balance between effectiveness and ease of use. Many have not been validated or published and none is ideal for every situation. However, a number of screening tools designed for specific circumstances such as on hospital admission (Reilly *et al.* 1995; Goudge *et al.* 1998), or in primary care (Hickson and Hill 1997; Ward *et al.* 1998), or targeted at particular sections of the population such as elderly people (Guigoz *et al.* 1996; Vellas *et al.* 1999) or clients with learning disabilities (Bryan *et al.* 1998) have been shown to have considerable value. Recently a screening tool for adults at risk of malnutrition has been developed by BAPEN (2000).

Current consensus is that, in order to be effective, a nutrition screening tool needs to be:

- quick and simple to administer
- sensitive enough to identify individuals at risk
- appropriate for the client group being screened
- capable of being used by non-dietetic staff
- reproducible when used by different observers
- able to guide non-dietetic staff into taking appropriate action for the findings recorded.

The types of question asked depends to some extent on the population being screened, but in most instances should attempt to identify:

- unintended weight loss (e.g. 5–10% weight loss in the previous 2–3 months)
- impaired food intake (e.g. due to reduced appetite or physical difficulties with eating and/or swallowing)
- increased nutritional requirements (e.g. pyrexia, trauma, sepsis)
- increased nutritional losses (e.g. diarrhoea, malabsorption)
- current body weight and adiposity (e.g. weight, height, BMI).

Much of this information can be derived from four simple questions (Lennard-Jones *et al.* 1995):

- Have you unintentionally lost weight recently?
- Have you been eating less than usual?
- What is your normal weight?
- How tall are you?

Relatives and carers may be able to answer these questions if the patient is too ill to do so.

However, even these questions may be not appropriate for all client groups. For example, stroke patients may have been fit and well on the day before admission and nutritional risk assessment will need to focus more on the nutritional implications of the effects of the stroke (e.g. dysphagia, degree of paralysis).

A different, less historical, questioning format may also be needed if nutritional screening is used as a means of monitoring progress and identifying emerging problems while in hospital or institutional care, or living at home. Changes in body weight, food intake and physiological function may need to be the primary focus.

The development and use of nutrition screening tools is an active area of development and undoubtedly a wider range of validated nutrition screening tools will become available in the future. In the meantime, it is vital that those which are currently available are not used indiscriminately but applied only in the specific circumstances for which they were designed. In many instances, a screening tool which is more appropriate for the needs and risks of a particular population group will need to be devised. In order to assist this process, the British Dietetic Association (1999) has produced detailed guidance on how such tools can be constructed.

Text written by: Briony Thomas

Acknowledgements: Helen Reilly, Sheila Merriman, Michele Mackintosh, Helen Molyneux.

Further reading

Reilly HM. Screening for nutritional risk. *Proceedings of the Nutrition Society* 1996; **55**: 841–853

References

Blackburn GL, Ahmad A. Skeleton in the hospital closet – then and now. *Nutrition* 1995; **11** (Suppl): 193–195.

British Association for Parenteral and Enteral Nutrition (BAPEN). *Screening Tool for Adults at Risk of Malnutrition*. Maidenhead: BAPEN, 2000.

British Dietetic Association. *Nutrition Screening Tools*. Professional Development Committee, Briefing Paper No. 9. Birmingham: BDA, 1999.

Bryan F, Jones JM, Russell L. Reliability and validity of a nutrition screening tool to be used with clients with learning difficulties. *Journal of Human Nutrition and Dietetics* 1998; **11**: 41–50.

Daniels A, Wright J. Hospitals with Nutrition Support Teams are more likely to have a Nutritional Assessment Policy and ward nurses who identify at risk patients than those who do not. *Proceedings of the Nutrition Society* 1997; **56**: 254A.

Detsky AS, McLaughlin JR, Baker JP *et al*. What is subjective global assessment of nutritional status? *Journal of Parenteral and Enteral Nutrition* 1987; **11**: 8–13

Goudge DR, Williams A, Pinnington LL. Development, validity and reliability of the Derby Nutritional Score. *Journal of Human Nutrition and Dietetics* 1998; **11**: 411–421

Guigoz Y, Vellas B, Garry PJ. Assessing the nutritional status of the elderly: The Mini Nutritional Assessment as part of the geriatric evaluation. *Nutrition Reviews* 1996; **54**(1, Part 2): S59–65.

Hickson M, Hill M. Implementing a nutritional assessment tool in the community: a report describing the process, audit and problems encountered. *Journal of Human Nutrition and Dietetics* 1997; **10**: 373–377.

Lennard-Jones JE. *A Positive Approach to Nutrition as Treatment*. London: King's Fund Centre, 1992.

Lennard-Jones JE, Arrowsmith H, Davison C *et al*. Screening by nurses and junior doctors to detect malnutrition when patients are first assessed in hospital. *Clinical Nutrition* 1995; **14**: 336–340.

McWhirter JP, Pennington CR. Incidence and recognition of malnutrition in hospital. *British Medical Journal* 1994; **308**: 945–948.

Mullen JL, Busby GP, Matthews DC *et al*. Reduction of operative morbidity and mortality by combined pre-operative and post-operative nutritional support. *Annals of Surgery* 1980; **192**: 604–613.

Reilly HM, Martineau JK, Moran A, Kennedy H. Nutritional screening – evaluation and implementation of a simple Nutrition Risk Score. *Clinical Nutrition* 1995; **34**: 269–273.

Vellas B, Guigoz Y, Garry PJ *et al*. The Mini Nutritional Assessment (MNA) and its use in grading the nutritional state of elderly patients. *Nutrition* 1999; **15**: 116–122.

Ward J, Close J, Little J *et al*. Development of a screening tool for assessing risk of undernutrition in patients in the community. *Journal of Human Nutrition and Dietetics* 1998; **11**: 323–330.

Weinsier RL, Hunker EM, Krundieck CL, Butterworth CE. Hospital malnutrition: a prospective evaluation of general medical patients during the course of hospitalization. *American Journal of Clinical Nutrition* 1979; **32**: 418–426.

Wolinsky FD, Coe RM, McIntosh WMA *et al*. Progress in the development of a nutritional risk index. *Journal of Nutrition* 1990; **120** (Suppl 11): 1549–1553.

1.10 Estimating nutritional requirements

Nutritional requirements need to be known in order to assess or monitor the adequacy of nutrient intake and for the provision of nutritional support.

Dietary reference values (DRVs; DH 1991) provide guidance on the nutritional needs of particular groups of the healthy population but have limited application to individuals (see Section 1.3, Dietary reference values). Within a population, individual requirements will vary and the needs of a specific individual will be unknown. Furthermore, DRVs reflect the needs of healthy people and take no account of the effect of factors such as pyrexia, infection, sepsis, metabolic trauma or malabsorption on nutritional requirements. Yet in clinical dietetic practice, it is very often the nutritional needs of the unwell individual which need to be determined.

DRVs can provide some yardstick as to the level of energy and nutrients required, but additional means of estimating the needs of a particular individual are likely to be needed, particularly if artificial nutritional support is required. The way in which nutritional requirements are determined will depend on the purpose for which the information is needed, the clinical circumstances and the level of precision required.

1.10.1 Energy requirements

Sufficient energy provision prevents the progressive weight loss associated with loss of body fat and protein stores proportional to the cumulative energy deficit. Unintentional weight loss is associated with an increase in morbidity and mortality across many clinical conditions and so is a major consideration in estimating requirements (see Section 1.11, Undernutrition). Overfeeding should also be avoided, to minimize the immediate derangements in biochemistry (hypercapnia, hypertriglyceridaemia and fatty liver) and in the longer term to prevent obesity. Maintenance or restoration of body weight to fall within the ideal weight range [body mass index (BMI) 20–25] may be the goal, but may not be appropriate or achievable in some clinical conditions. The dietitian should be empathetic to the needs of the patient.

Several methods are available for calculating energy requirements. The preferred technique for determining a patient's energy requirement in the clinical setting would be to use indirect calorimetry (Ireton-Jones and Jones 1998; Glynn *et al*. 1999). However, the cost of the metabolic equipment necessary to do this, and the time available to use it, prevent this from being a practical consideration in most hospitals. Estimations and prediction equations are therefore used instead. Each method takes into account a variety of influencing factors on which to base an estimation of a patient's energy needs. Age, gender, activity and body weight are common variables considered in prediction equations which, together with estimates for growth, tissue repair and unusual energy losses (e.g. due to pyrexia), form the basis of energy prediction. These equations are merely estimations of a patient's energy needs. Actual needs may be more or less than the figure produced.

Estimating energy requirements from body weight

Although relatively imprecise, a clinically useful method of calculating energy requirements is to allocate an arbitrary allowance of energy based on weight and clinical condition. Adult energy requirements are between 25 and 35 kcal/kg (Bagley 1996; Glynn *et al*. 1999), with the higher value reserved for pyrexia or extreme sepsis. A baseline value of 25 kcal/kg body weight should maintain weight in most clinically unstressed patients.

Estimating energy requirements from prediction equations

Basal metabolic rate estimation using Schofield equations

Schofield equations (Schofield 1985) can be used to predict the basal metabolic rate (BMR) of healthy adults using the patient's gender, age, height and weight (or weight alone). Schofield equations are in common use (McAtear and Wright 1996), often in conjunction with the Elia nomogram (Elia 1990) to estimate energy expenditure in clinical conditions (see Appendix 6.5).

The original Schofield equations (Schofield 1985) were derived from a study group of some 5000 healthy adults. The equations were subsequently modified by the COMA Panel on Dietary Reference Values (DH 1991) to make them more applicable to the UK population; some data from developing nations were excluded and additional equations for people over the age of 75 years, based on Italian data, were incorporated. Ready reference tables of BMR based on these modified equations can be found in Appendix 6.5. The Schofield equations are given in Table 1.19.

The procedure for estimating energy requirements using Schofield and Elia is:

Table 1.19 Schofield formulae for estimating basal metabolic rate from body weight (W = body weight in kg)

(a) Original Schofield equations (Schofield 1985)

Males	BMR	Females	BMR
Age (years)	kcal/day	Age (years)	kcal/day
15–18	$17.6W + 656$	15–18	$13.3W + 690$
18–30	$15.0W + 690$	18–30	$14.8W + 485$
30–60	$11.4W + 870$	30–60	$8.1W + 842$
> 60	$11.7W + 585$	> 60	$9.0W + 656$

Note that the Schofield data provide no estimate to treat the 75+ population group as a separate entity, unlike the COMA DRV Report 1991, which also includes values for the over-75s derived from Italian data (see below).

(b) Modified Schofield equations (DH 1991)

Males	BMR		Females	BMR	
Age (years)	kcal/day	MJ/day	Age (years)	kcal/day	MJ/day
10–17	$17.7W + 657$	$0.074W + 2.754$	10–17	$13.4W + 692$	$0.056W + 2.898$
18–29	$15.1W + 692$	$0.063W + 2.896$	18–29	$14.8W + 487$	$0.062W + 2.036$
30–59	$11.5W + 873$	$0.048W + 3.653$	30–59	$8.3W + 846$	$0.034W + 3.538$
60–74	$11.9W + 700$	$0.0499W + 2.930$	60–74	$9.2W + 687$	$0.0386W + 2.875$
75+	$8.4W + 821$	$0.0350W + 3.434$	75+	$9.8W + 624$	$0.041W + 2.610$

A ready reckoner of BMR derived from these equations can be found in Appendix 6.5.
Crown copyright material is reproduced with the permission of the Controller of Her Majesty's Stationery Office.

1 *Estimate BMR for healthy adults.* This can be done using one of the formulae in 1.19. or by using the ready reference table in Appendix 6.5.
2 *Adjust for stress using the Elia nomogram* (Appendix 6.5).
3 *Add a combined factor for activity and diet-induced thermogenesis*:

Bedbound, immobile	+ 10%
Bedbound, mobile or sitting	+ 15–20%
Mobile, on ward	+ 25%

Limitations of the Schofield equations include overestimation of energy requirements in young adults of North European, Australian and American descent (Piers *et al*. 1997), and dubious validity when used with obese clients (Tverskaya *et al*. 1998). The nomogram used alongside the Schofield equation is also not without its critics. Elia has cast doubt recently over the need for increased energy provision in disease states. He questioned the early methods used to calculate energy requirements and also cites new medical and surgical techniques which decrease caloric needs (Elia 1995).

Estimation of basal energy expenditure using the Harris–Benedict equation

Although devised in 1919, the Harris–Benedict equation is still widely used as a method of estimating basal energy requirements for clinical and research purposes. A recent review of the data and methodology on which it was based concluded that the equation remains valid and reasonable, although not error free (Frankenfield *et al*. 1998).

The equation is derived from multiple regression analysis of the gender, age, height and weight of 239 *healthy* volunteers. It estimates basal energy expenditure (BEE), i.e. the energy expended by a fasting subject at rest in a 'thermoneutral' environment (i.e. an ambient room temperature), and so excludes the energy contribution from dietary-induced thermogenesis, pyrexia, activity or exercise. The BEE is usually assumed to be equivalent to the BMR, although in reality it overestimates this by about 5% (Frankenfield *et al*. 1998).

Estimation of BEE by the Harris–Benedict equation is calculated as:

Males (kcal/24 hours) = $66.5 + (13.8W) + (5H) - (6.8A)$
Females (kcal/24 hours) = $655 + (9.6W) + (1.8H) - (4.7A)$

where W = weight in kg, H = height in metres, A = age in years

Stress factors of between 1.0 and 1.5 can be added to the BEE calculated from the Harris–Benedict equation to obtain an estimate of resting energy expenditure (REE), which can be a more accurate reflection of actual energy needs (Seale 1995). However, assigning stress factors is arbitrary and subject to the whim of the investigator. Dietitians should use their own judgement to decide on energy needs for particular clinical circumstances.

Estimating energy requirements from dietary reference values

Lack of data necessary for the predictive formula often requires the dietitian to 'guesstimate' a value into the chosen equation, thus compromising accuracy. Although the estimated average requirements (EARs) for energy are specific to gender, age and normal weight range in a section of the population rather than in an individual (DH 1991), they may provide an estimate of energy requirements when unable to measure a patient's weight or height, or when obesity would confound other equations (see Energy requirements in obese patients, below). Use of these values in hospitalized patients would require some modification of the physical activity level (PAL) component of estimated energy requirement. The process would be:

1 Determine appropriate EAR for energy from DRVs for UK population.
2 Remove or amend PAL of 1.4, to adjust for decrease in activity for hospitalized patients.
3 Adjust for stress using Elia or other nomogram, if relevant.
4 Add combined factor for activity and diet-induced thermogenesis (as above).

Estimating energy requirements in specific disease states or clinical circumstances

Several nomograms exist to include the metabolic requirements associated with disease (Wilmore 1977; Long 1984; Elia 1990), yet their rigid categories often compromise their use in clinical practice. Where possible, dietitians should use evidence of indirect calorimetry on specific clinical conditions as a gold standard, provided that the evidence in the paper is robust, or other equations relevant to their area of work, such as the Seashore (1984) equation for children in the intensive treatment unit (ITU) or the World Health Organization equations (1984) for adolescents (cited in Ringwald-Smith et al. 1999).

Resting energy expenditure in critical illness

Whilst the Schofield and the Harris–Benedict equations (derived from data on healthy subjects) can, with the use of appropriate factors, be applied in clinical circumstances, the Ireton-Jones formulae were developed specifically for estimating the energy expenditure of critically ill patients (Ireton-Jones and Jones 1998). These equations appear in Section 5.2 (Intensive care), although they – along with other prediction equations – are not infallible:

> A patient may require more calories than his measured energy expenditure to assure that weight gain and repletion of nutritional status occurs, whereas an obese patient or a patient with similar fluid and substrate limitations may tolerate fewer calories than would be predicted or measured by indirect calorimetry... Clinical judgement must be used by the dietitian or other clinician in converting energy expenditure into energy requirements (Ireton-Jones and Jones 1998).

Estimating energy requirements in obese patients

The level of energy provision to the obese subject is controversial, with much debate whether the subject should be fed to actual body weight (ABW), ideal body weight (IBW) or some intermediate weight (Ireton-Jones and Turner 1991; Glynn et al. 1999).

Feeding to ABW provides energy intakes that sustain obesity, and may precipitate the metabolic effects of overfeeding such as hyperglycaemia and respiratory distress, especially in those with concurrent sleep apnoea syndrome (Cutts et al. 1997; Klein et al. 1998).

Conversely, feeding to IBW in obese patients will promote weight loss and should be clinically beneficial (Amato et al. 1995), but may compromise glucose tolerance and wound healing. Energy provision should achieve a balance between the conservation of lean body mass and weight maintenance.

It has been proposed that an 'obesity-adjusted' weight be used when determining energy requirements. Several adjustments to a patient's ABW have been suggested:

Obesity-adjusted weight (kg)
$$= IBW + \frac{(ABW - IBW)}{4} \text{ (Cutts et al. 1997)}$$

or

Obesity-adjusted weight (kg)
$$= \frac{(IBW + ABW)}{2} \text{ (Amato, 1995)}$$

These figures can be substituted into the chosen equation to achieve a better estimation of caloric requirements, although a generic 18–21 kcal/kg ABW will permit safe weight loss.

Estimating energy requirements in depleted patients

Weight gain should only be attempted in clinically stable patients, who will tolerate the metabolic stresses potentially imposed by overfeeding. Critically ill patients and those with cachexia are unlikely to gain weight until the acute phase/cytokine response is ameliorated by clinical intervention. Energy provision should be modest and provide for weight maintenance until the patient is more stable. Addition of a further 500–1000 kcal/day in addition to predicted requirements, or feeding to desirable rather than actual weight (or a point mid-range if this difference is greater than 15–20 kg) should promote weight gain.

1.10.2 Nitrogen/protein requirements

Unlike excess energy, surplus protein cannot be stored so there is a minimum daily requirement to protect the body's structural proteins (e.g. muscle), visceral proteins (e.g. internal organs, serum transport proteins) and immune competence.

Protein is the only macronutrient that contains nitrogen, and hence protein requirements or provision are often considered in terms of nitrogen. Approximately 16% of protein is nitrogen, so grams of nitrogen can be converted to grams of protein by multiplying the nitrogen value by 6.25.

Traditionally, the protein content of parenteral feeds is expressed in nitrogen, and the energy contribution from this nitrogen source is excluded from stated energy content of the feed on the basis that this separation permits 'protection' of the protein source from utilization for energy (assuming that carbohydrate and fat provision is adequate). This outdated mode of expression is unique to parenteral nutrition, and appears unlikely to change in the near future.

Measurement of protein turnover requires the collection and analysis of body losses that contain nitrogen, and so have ultimately required protein in their manufacture. Nitrogen losses can be measured in urine, faeces or skin losses, or from routes associated with surgery (such as fistulae, stoma losses, drains, burns exudate or ascites). Serum albumin is neither a marker of nutritional status nor protein turnover (Klein 1990; Vanek 1998).

Nitrogen/protein requirements can be assessed in a number of ways and these are outlined below.

Estimating protein requirements from dietary reference values

The reference nutrient intake (RNI) for protein for the average adult is 0.75 g/kg body weight per day (DH 1991). Proportionally more is required by those who have to meet physiological requirements for growth and the RNIs for these groups of the population can be found in tables of DRVs (see Appendix 6.2).

Using ABW as a basis for determining protein requirements will overestimate protein needs in people who are obese. It is therefore recommended that in obese individuals with a BMI >30, approximately 75% of the estimated protein requirement determined from ABW be given. If BMI >40, only 65% of the estimated protein requirements should be provided.

Historically, any trauma or sepsis was predicted to increase the metabolic need for protein, hence the arbitrary recommendations such as those of Elia (1990) (Table 1.20). In reality, the judicious use of antibiotics, pain control and sedation alleviates the teleological response to trauma, thus reducing metabolic demands. For those patients with sepsis or a profound immune response, a positive nitrogen balance is impossible to achieve, even at levels of protein provision in excess of 2 g/kg body weight per day. Many of these 'hypermetabolic'

patients may not tolerate high protein intakes because of concurrent clinical conditions such as renal or liver impairment.

The use of very low protein diets in the management of renal or hepatic failure has lost favour, as protein turnover will be met in these individuals through catabolism of their own protein stores if dietary protein is inadequate.

Estimating protein requirements from measuring nitrogen losses from the body

A more precise estimate of nitrogen needs can be obtained by measuring daily nitrogen losses from the body via urine, faeces, fistulae or drain losses, or burn exudates, although in practice this is difficult to achieve.

Urinary nitrogen excretion can be estimated by measuring urinary urea nitrogen (UUN) excretion from a 24-hour urine sample. Nitrogen excretion in grams is approximately equal to:

$$\text{g urinary urea excreted in 24 hours} \times \frac{28^*}{60} \times \frac{6^\dagger}{5}$$

*The molecular weight of urea is 60, of which 28 parts are nitrogen.
†Assumes that 80% of the total urinary nitrogen is urea.

For practical purposes this formula can be condensed to:

$$\frac{\text{Nitrogen excretion in g}}{\text{per 24 hours}} = \frac{\text{mmol urinary urea per 24 hours}}{30}$$

or

$$\text{g protein lost per 24 hours} = \frac{\text{mmol urinary urea excreted in 24 hours}}{5}.$$

Problems associated with urinary urea measurement

UUN is a commonly used tool to determine protein needs. Urea is a byproduct of protein metabolism, and measurement of UUN can give an indication of nitrogen losses. Approximately 80% of total urinary nitrogen is urea nitrogen, the remaining 20% nitrogen being comprised of urinary creatinine, creatine, small molecular weight amino acids and other compounds.

Urea production is influenced by liver failure, sepsis, starvation or stress, thus urinary urea is an insensitive and unreliable measure of nitrogen loss in clinically unstable patients, and often reflects a lag time in response to changes in therapy (e.g. diuretic use). The ratio of total urea nitrogen:urinary urea nitrogen is not constant, varying with the degree of stress, the course of an illness, or with different disease states (Konstantinides et al. 1991). In such circumstances, UUN can represent between 10–90% of urinary nitrogen losses. Measurement of total urinary nitrogen is therefore a superior method, but is technically difficult and beyond the resources of most hospital biochemistry departments.

Nitrogen requirements are difficult to assess in renal failure, as urine production may be variable or absent. The

Table 1.20 Protein requirements for adults in conditions of trauma or metabolic stress (derived from Elia 1990)

Energy status	Nitrogen (g/kg/day)[1]	Protein (g/kg/day)[1]
Normal	0.17 (0.14–0.20)	1 (0.87–1.25)
Hypermetabolic		
(+5–25%)	0.20 (0.17–0.25)	1.25 (1.0–1.5)
(+25–50%)	0.25 (0.20–0.30)	1.5 (1.25–1.87)
(>50%)	0.30 (0.25–0.35)	1.87 (1.56–1.87)
Depleted	0.30 (0.2–0.4)	1.87 (1.25–2.5)

[1]Mean (range).

equation below can be used for anuric patients, and estimates the rate of urea nitrogen production from changes in serum urea concentrations:

$$\text{g urea nitrogen/day} = [(\text{Urea 2} - \text{Urea 1}) \times \text{wt} \times 0.6 + (\text{wt gain} \times \text{Urea 2})] \times 0.028$$

where Urea 1 = serum urea at start of period (mmol/l); Urea 2 = serum urea at end of period (mmol/l); 0.6 = factor to estimate total body water; wt = weight in kg.

Nitrogen losses from faeces and exudates are difficult to measure. Fistulae contents can be sent for analysis if volumes are significant enough to cause concern.

Nitrogen–energy ratios

Traditionally, ratios of nitrogen to energy needs in different metabolic states were used to ensure optimum nutrient intake for specific clinical conditions. This concept has lost favour, and current practice is to calculate energy and protein requirements independently.

1.10.3 Fluid requirements

Although not a nutrient as such, the maintenance of fluid balance is an important factor in physiological homoeostasis. The provision of sufficient fluid ensures an optimal internal milieu for regulating digestion, absorption, metabolism and excretion, yet fluid provision is often inadequate in the clinical setting. Maintenance of fluid balance is vital for renal, cardiovascular and respiratory function (Lipp *et al*. 1999).

Estimating basic fluid requirements

Guidelines for estimating fluid requirements are summarized in Table 1.21.

Estimating fluid requirements by assessing fluid status

It is possible to titrate a patient's fluid input against their daily fluid losses. In general, fluid input should be 500–750 ml greater than urinary losses to compensate for fluid losses via lung and skin evaporation (i.e. insensible fluid losses). This volume may increase in hot weather, or if the patient has pyrexia or burns. Significant fluid losses also occur with vomiting or diarrhoea, enterocutaneous fistula, ileostomy or recent colostomy, or losses from

Table 1.21 Estimation of normal fluid requirements (Todorovic and Micklewright 1997)

Fluid requirements	ml/kg body weight/day
Maintenance levels: 18–60 years	35
>60 years	30
Additional losses due to fever	+ 2– 2.5 ml per 1°C rise in temperature above 37°C
Other losses	Individual assessment

Table 1.22 Daily volume of external secretions

Secretion	Volume (l/24 hours)
Pancreatic juice	0.5–1
Bile	0.5–1
Ileostomy (adapted)	0.5
Ileostomy (newly formed)	Variable (0.5–5)
Colostomy	0.1–0.2
Diarrhoea	Variable (0.5–3)
Insensible skin losses	0.5
Visible sweat, per °C	0.5

drains. Stoma losses are easily monitored, but for patients with fistulae or diarrhoea, the amount of extra fluid loss is less easily quantified. The daily volume of external secretions is shown in Table 1.22.

Serum biochemistry, urine output and central venous pressure (CVP) monitoring can be used to estimate hydration status.

Dehydration

This concentrates the extracellular fluid, reflected as hypernatraemia, uraemia and an increased serum haemoglobin. If sodium and urea rise concurrently, dehydration should be suspected even in the presence of tissue fluid overload (e.g. due to pulmonary or generalized oedema). Symptoms of dehydration include headache, mild confusion, postural hypotension, fatigue, thirst, and concentrated, dark urine (assuming liver function tests are normal) (Kleiner 1999). Skin turgor is also reduced – skin pinched on the back of the hand fails to 'spring back'; this is called 'skin tenting'.

Dehydration with raised urea may occur without raised sodium levels if patients are losing both sodium and fluid, yet are having a low sodium diet (a frequent occurrence in patients with rampant diarrhoea on most UK enteral feeds). Provision of both fluid and sodium will be required. A negative fluid balance may benefit patients with cerebral oedema or fluid overload associated with cardiac and renal dysfunction. Fluid balance and the regulatory mechanisms governing fluid balance may all be disturbed by illness or trauma.

Iatrogenic use of aggressive diuretic therapy to reduce peripheral oedema often results in a 'clinically dry' or 'crispy' person with vascular dehydration and fluid-overloaded tissues. There is little point in providing a low sodium feed or increasing fluid intake in such patients if diuretic therapy is not reduced.

Fluid overload

This is unlikely in health, and is a consequence of cardiac, hepatic or renal disorders, or the psychiatric condition psychogenic polydipsia.

1.10.4 Electrolyte requirements
Sodium

In the presence of normal renal function and fluid balance, the basic requirement for sodium is 1.0 mmol Na^+/kg body weight (60–100 mmol/day).

Sodium requirements can be increased by:

- *Pyrexia*: this will also increase fluid requirements (see above) and sodium should be added to this extra fluid at the rate of 15 mmol/100 ml additional fluid (e.g. the content of normal saline intravenous fluid).
- *Fistulae/small bowel losses*: gastrointestinal secretions contain 130–150 mmol Na/l. Large volume losses will require replacement of sodium and water. If enteral replacement increases gastrointestinal output, intravenous fluid correction is recommended.
- *Hyponatraemia*: in the absence of fluid overload, low serum sodium levels should be corrected. Chronic hyponatraemia is common with increasing age, and in postmenopausal women is associated with major morbidity and mortality. Fluctuations in sodium concentration as a result of fluid overload or dehydration affect brain function, which is less able to tolerate fluctuations in fluid pressure across its cells (Preston 1997). Sodium supplementation rather than fluid restriction is necessary to normalize serum levels (Ayus and Arieff 1999). For patients with renal failure, oedema, ascites or SiADH (stress-induced syndrome of inappropriate antidiuretic hormone), a fluid restriction may also be used as part of their treatment.

An estimate of the amount of the additional sodium required to correct hyponatraemia can be obtained by using the formula:

$$(140 - \text{measured serum sodium}) \times 0.2 \times \text{body wt in kg}.$$

Sodium can be administered within intravenous fluids, as salt or salt tablets, or as intravenous ampoules added to the enteral feed (see Section 5.2, Intensive care). Rapid correction of hyponatraemia or hypernatraemia can cause permanent and severe damage to the pontine area of the brain. Correction of serum sodium, in either direction, should not exceed 6–10 mmol/day (Arieff 1991).

Potassium

The basic requirement for potassium is 1.0 mmol/kg body weight (50–100 mmol/day). For intravenous feeding, 1–1.5 mmol/kg per day, or 5 mmol/g nitrogen, may be required and as much as 7 mmol/g nitrogen if serum potassium levels are less than 3.5 mmol/l or if refeeding severely malnourished patients.

Additional potassium may be required when serum potassium is low and may be estimated by using the formula:

$$(4.0 - \text{measured serum potassium mmol/l}) \times 0.4 \times \text{body wt in kg}.$$

Iatrogenic hypokalaemia is commonly due to use of potassium-losing diuretics. Prediction of potassium requirements should be assessed in the context of whether the same level of diuresis is to continue.

Unlike sodium, serum potassium is largely unaffected by large gastrointestinal losses, as the potassium content of gastrointestinal secretions is in the region of 5–15 mmol K/l.

Calcium

Total plasma calcium is a measure of both ionized and non-ionized calcium (the latter being calcium bound to albumin, citrate or phosphate), thus if plasma albumin is low, total calcium will also appear low. The biochemistry value for 'corrected calcium' takes into account the reduction in circulating calcium secondary to low circulating protein levels, and is the value to use.

Plasma pH will influence calcium binding. In acidosis, less calcium is albumin bound and more exists in the ionized form. Calcium balance is influenced by hormonal and biochemical factors including parathyroid hormone (PTH), calcitonin and calcitriol (the active metabolite of vitamin D).

Hypocalcaemia can manifest itself as neuromuscular symptoms (muscle spasms, tetany) or cardiac dysrhythmias (bradycardia or ventricular tachycardia).

Causes of hypocalcaemia include:

- surgical hypoparathyroidism (thyroid or surgery proximal to the thyroid)
- acute pancreatitis and malabsorption syndromes (intraluminal soap formation with dietary fats)
- sepsis
- hypomagnesaemia
- hypophosphataemia
- alkalosis or infusion of citrated blood
- drug interactions.

Hypercalcaemia can be secondary to:

- diabetes insipidus or other polyuric states
- thiazide diuretics
- hyperphosphataemia
- hyperparathyroidism
- Addison's disease
- malignancy
- prolonged immobility
- oversupplementation with calcium, vitamin A or D supplements.

Magnesium

Only 1% of magnesium is found within the plasma, with the remainder being located in the skeleton and intracellular fluid. Magnesium has an integral role in more than 300 enzymatic reactions, especially those related to energy release.

Hypomagnesaemia

Muscle weakness and cramps, hypertension and cardiac arrhythmias including cardiac spasm are all symptoms of hypomagnesaemia. Causes include:

- inadequate magnesium intake
- increased intestinal losses of magnesium (diarrhoea, laxative abuse, fistula losses)
- increased renal excretion of magnesium secondary to diuretic therapy
- changes in magnesium distribution (pancreatitis, plasmapheresis, thermal injury).

Hypermagnesaemia

This is a common occurrence secondary to:

- renal failure (acute or chronic)
- adrenal insufficiency
- administration of excessive oral or intravenous magnesium
- peripheral vasodilatation (with clinical manifestations such as drowsiness, respiratory depression, hypotension and bradycardia with possible cardiac arrest).

Phosphorus

Phosphorus is primarily an intracellular ion and so plasma levels may not reflect body stores. Intestinal uptake can be reduced by some medications or malabsorption. Maintenance of normal phosphate levels requires sufficient dietary provision and efficient renal conservation mechanisms as the kidneys are the major route of excretion of phosphate.

Hypophosphataemia

This can occur secondary to:

- respiratory alkalosis
- diabetic ketoacidosis
- insulin or adrenalin use
- refeeding syndrome
- excessive antacid use causing intestinal binding of phosphate.

Symptoms of hypophosphataemia include muscle weakness (especially related to respiratory depression), central nervous system depression and cardiomyopathy, and in the absence of the above conditions can be treated by phosphate supplementation.

Hyperphosphataemia

This can occur secondary to:

- renal failure
- chemotherapy
- overzealous intake of milk or phosphate supplements
- excessive use of phosphate-containing bowel-cleansing solutions (e.g. Fleet Phospho-soda, De Witt).

Tetany and muscle spasms are early indications of hyperphosphatemia, with precipitation of calcium phosphate in soft tissue a long-term concern.

1.10.5 Micronutrient requirements

Even if energy and nitrogen needs are met, tissue maintenance and/or repletion cannot occur in the presence of micronutrient deficiency. Clinical requirements are normally prescribed according to DRVs and normal clinical practice.

Absolute requirements for individual vitamins, minerals or trace elements prove difficult to determine in the presence of sepsis, metabolic stress, trauma or conditions which may alter circulating and stored levels of micro-nutrients as a teleological response to physical trauma or disease.

Assessment of micronutrient adequacy should be considered in the context of:

- the disease process
- drug therapy
- increased or decreased fluid losses from different sites
- concurrent medical therapy (e.g. dialysis).

Text revised by: Catherine Collins and Briony Thomas

References

Amato P, Keating KP, Quercia RA *et al*. Formulaic methods of estimating caloric requirements in mechanically ventilated obese patients: a reappraisal. *Nutrition in Clinical Practice* 1995; **10**: 229–230.

Arieff AI. Treatment of symptomatic hyponatremia. *Critical Care Medicine* 1991; **19**: 748–751.

Ayus JC, Arieff AI. Chronic hyponatremic encephalopathy in postmenopausal women: association of therapies with morbidity and mortality. *Journal of the American Medical Association* 1999; **281**: 2299–2304.

Bagley SM. Nutrition needs of the acutely ill with acute wounds. *Critical Care Nursing in North America* 1996; **8**: Issue 2.

Cutts ME, Dowdy RP, Ellersieck MR *et al*. Predicting energy needs in ventilator-dependent critically ill patients: effect of adjusting weight for oedema or adiposity. *American Journal of Clinical Nutrition* 1997; **66**: 1250–1256.

Department of Health. *Dietary Reference Values for Food Energy and Nutrients for the UK*. Report of the Panel on Dietary Reference Values of the Committee on Medical Aspects of Food Policy. Report on Health and Social Subjects 41. London: HMSO, 1991.

Elia M. Artificial nutritional support. *Medicine International* 1990; **82**: 3392–3396.

Elia M. Changing concepts of nutrient requirements in disease: implications for nutritional support. *Lancet* 1995; **345**: 1279–1284.

Frankenfield DC, Muth ER, Rowe WA. The Harris–Benedict studies of human basal metabolism: history and limitations. *Journal of the American Dietetic Association* 1998; **98**: 439–445.

Glynn CC, Greene GW, Winklet MF *et al*. Predictive versus measured energy expenditure using limits-of-agreement analysis in hospitalised, obese patients. *Journal of Parenteral and Enteral Nutrition* 1999; **23**: 147–154.

Harris JA, Benedict FG. *A Biometric Study of The Basal Metabolism in Man*. Publication No. 279. Washington DC: Carnegie Institution of Washington, 1919.

Ireton-Jones CS, Jones JD. Should predictive equations or indirect calorimetry be used to design nutrition support regimens? *Nutrition in Clinical Practice* 1998; **13**: 141–145.

Ireton-Jones CS, Turner WW. Actual or ideal body weight: which should be used to predict energy expenditure? *Journal of the American Dietetic Association* 1991; **91**: 193–195.

Klein S. The myth of serum albumin as a measure of nutritional status. *Gastroenterology* 1990; **99** (6): 1845–1846.

Klein CJ, Stenek GS, Wiles CE *et al*. Overfeeding macronutrients to critically ill adults: metabolic complications. *Journal of the American Dietetic Association* 1998; **98**: 795–806.

Kleiner SM. Water: an essential but overlooked nutrient. *Journal of the American Dietetic Association* 1999; **99**: 200–206.

Konstantinides FN, Konstantinides NN, Li JC *et al*. Urinary urea nitrogen: too insensitive for calculating nitrogen balance studies in surgical clinical nutrition. *Journal of Parenteral and Enteral Nutrition* 1991; **15**: 189–193.

Lipp J, Lord LM, Scholer LH. Fluid management in enteral nutrition. *Nutrition in Clinical Practice* 1999; **14**: 232–237.

Long CL. The energy and protein requirements of the critically ill patient. In Wright RA, Heymsfield S (Eds) *Nutritional Assessment*, pp. 157–181. Boston, MA: Blackwell Scientific Publications, 1984.

McAtear C, Wright C. *Dietetic Standards for Nutritional Support*. Birmingham: British Dietetic Association, 1996.

Piers LS, Diffey B, Soares MJ *et al*. The validity of predicting the basal metabolic rate of young australian men and women. *European Journal of Clinical Nutrition* 1997; **51**: 333–337.

Preston RA. *Acid–Base, Fluids and Electrolytes made Ridiculously Simple*. Miami, FL: MedMaster, 1997.

Ringwald-Smith K, Williams R, Mackert P *et al*. Comparison of energy estimation equations with measured energy expenditure in obese adolescent patients with cancer. *Journal of the American Dietetic Association* 1999; **99**: 844–848.

Schofield WN. Predicting basal metabolic rate, new standards and a review of previous work. *Human Nutrition: Clinical Nutrition* 1985; **39C** (Suppl): 5–41.

Seale JL. Energy expenditure measurements in relation to energy requirements. *American Journal of Clinical Nutrition* 1995; **62** (Suppl): 1042S–1046S.

Seashore JH. Nutritional support of children in the intensive care unit. *Yale Journal of Biology and Medicine* 1984; **57**: 111–134.

Todorovic VE, Micklewright A (Eds). *A Pocket Guide to Clinical Nutrition*, 2nd edn. Parenteral and Enteral Nutrition (PEN) Group of the British Dietetic Association. Birmingham: British Dietetic Association, 1997.

Tverskaya R, Rising R, Brown D, Lifshitz F. Comparison of several equations and derivation of a new equation for calculating basal metabolic rate in obese children. *Journal of the American College of Nutrition* 1998; **17**: 333–336.

Vanek VW. The use of serum albumin as a prognostic or nutritional marker and the pros and cons of i.v. albumin therapy. *Nutrition in Clinical Practice* 1998; **13**: 110–122.

Wilmore DW. *The Metabolic Management of the Critically Ill*. New York: Plenum, 1977.

1.11 Undernutrition and the principles of nutritional support

Although protein-energy malnutrition ('undernutrition') among people in UK hospitals was identified in the mid-1970s (Bistrian *et al.* 1974; Hill *et al.* 1977), it is clear that this remains a common and often unrecognized problem, and that its contribution to patient morbidity and mortality continues to be underestimated (Lennard-Jones 1992; McWhirter and Pennington 1994; Potter *et al.* 1995).

The problem of undernutrition is not confined to people in hospital. Within the community, up to 10% of people with cancer or other chronic diseases may be significantly malnourished (Edington *et al.* 1996) and many elderly people are also at high risk of undernutrition (Finch *et al.* 1998). As a result, people are commonly admitted to hospital in a state of nutritional depletion. McWhirter and Pennington (1994) found that 40% of 500 consecutive hospital admissions could be considered to be malnourished. In a recent study conducted in four hospitals in England, Edington *et al.* (2000) found that one in every five patients admitted was malnourished, a figure which is almost certainly an underestimate since it does not include those who were too ill on admission to be assessed. Kelly *et al.* (2000) estimated that malnutrition in acute hospital admissions goes unrecognized in 70% of cases.

Once in hospital, undernutrition is likely to get worse. Of the 500 patients in the McWhirter and Pennington study, two-thirds of those who were reassessed on discharge had lost weight. A study on a random sample of 150 in-patients found approximately half of them to be at either moderate risk (23.5% patients) or high risk (26.1%) of malnutrition (Reilly *et al.* 1995). The prevalence and level of risk may be even higher among high-dependency medical, surgical, geriatric or paediatric patients (Larsson *et al.* 1990; Moy *et al.* 1990; Silk *et al.* 1994; Edington *et al.* 1997). Since illness and hospitalization are frequently associated with negative energy balance, deterioration in nutritional status is almost inevitable unless action is taken to prevent it (Klipstein-Grobusch *et al.* 1995).

1.11.1 Consequences of undernutrition

Undernutrition primarily results from an inadequate intake of dietary energy and its principal feature is loss of body weight, by depletion of body fat stores, and muscle wasting. However, because energy intake is so closely correlated with nutrient intake, energy deficiency is likely to result in an inadequate intake of many important nutrients, particularly vitamins, minerals and trace elements. As a result the effects of undernutrition are not confined to loss of body tissue alone but produce widespread metabolic, physiological and functional effects as the body attempts to adapt to the conditions of starvation and nutritional deficiencies. The effects may include:

- impaired immune function and hence increased susceptibility to infection and sepsis (Neumann *et al.* 1975; Chandra and Kumari 1994; Lesourd 1995). Infection will further impair a malnourished state;
- delayed wound healing (Casey *et al.* 1983; Dickhaut *et al.* 1984; Haydock and Hill 1986; Ondrey and Hom 1994);
- increased risk of pressure sores, particularly due to loss of cushioning from fat stores (Allcock *et al.* 1994; Bergstrom 1997);
- muscle wasting and weakness which may affect:
  - *respiratory function*: impaired respiratory muscle strength makes it difficult for a patient to cough and expectorate effectively, thus increasing the risk of chest infection (Windsor and Hill 1988a). It may also prove more difficult to wean a patient from artificial ventilation (Benotti and Bistrian 1989)
  - *cardiac function*: this may be impaired, resulting in reduced cardiac output and risk of heart failure (Heymsfield *et al.* 1978)
  - *mobility*: weakness of skeletal muscles delays a return to full mobility (Bastow *et al.* 1983). Reduced mobility increases the risk of thromboembolism and bedsores (Holmes *et al.* 1987);
- altered structure of the small intestine which may result in malabsorption (Stanfield *et al.* 1965; Mehta *et al.* 1984);
- increased risk of postoperative complications (Windsor and Hill 1988b);
- apathy and depression leading to loss of morale and reduced will to recover (Theologes 1978);
- general sense of weakness and illness which impairs appetite and physical ability to eat and hence tends to perpetuate and worsen the state of undernutrition (Silk *et al.* 1994).

As a result, undernutrition causes considerable morbidity, delays recovery and increases the risk of mortality (Larsson *et al.* 1990; Potter *et al.* 1995); a body mass index (BMI) at or below the 15th percentile has been shown to be a significant and independent predictor of mortality in seriously ill patients (Galanos *et al.* 1997). The economic cost in terms of increased need for nursing care and extended hospitalization is also considerable (Reilly *et al.* 1987; Robinson *et al.* 1987; Lennard-Jones 1992).

There is clear evidence that correcting undernutrition has many benefits (Potter *et al*. 1998). Improvement in body weight and anthopometric parameters has been shown to be associated with improvement in immune function (Dionigi *et al*. 1988; Chandra 1992), wound healing (Haydock and Hill 1987) and muscle function (Whittaker *et al*. 1990; Rana *et al*. 1992; Fiatarone and Evans 1993), and in clinical outcomes such as recovery time (Bastow *et al*. 1983; Delmi *et al*. 1990; Larsson *et al*. 1990) and incidence of postoperative complications (Veterans Affairs Total Parenteral Nutrition Co-operative Study Group 1991). In addition to these clinical benefits, substantial cost savings result from reduced length of stay (Forman 1996; Treber and Harris 1996; Tucker and Miguel 1996).

1.11.2 Causes of undernutrition

Undernutrition is the consequence of a nutritional intake that does not meet nutritional needs as a result of one or more of the following:

- decreased dietary intake
- increased nutritional requirements
- impaired ability to absorb or utilize nutrients.

Undernutrition is usually of insidious onset resulting from a chronic shortfall between intake and requirements over a period of weeks or months. However, in conditions of acute metabolic stress (e.g. burns patients) where nutritional demands are high, utilization is disturbed and oral intake is likely to be compromised, nutritional depletion can occur rapidly and be severe.

Many factors can impair dietary intake :

- difficulties with shopping, preparing, cooking or eating food due to illness or lack of mobility;
- reduced appetite as a result of the effects of illness or associated anxiety or depression;
- symptoms associated with a disease or its treatment, e.g. nausea, vomiting, sore mouth, abdominal discomfort, diarrhoea;
- disinterest in food as a result of social isolation, significant life change (such as bereavement) or mental illness;
- inadequate or unappetizing meals (Stephen *et al*. 1997) or the provision of culturally inappropriate food (McGlone *et al*. 1996) (see Section 1.16, Food service in hospitals and institutions);
- repeated fasting for diagnostic or treatment procedures;
- difficulties with eating or chewing, e.g. due to ill-fitting dentures or poor oral hygiene;
- swallowing difficulties;
- difficulty with self-feeding (e.g. due to disability, immobilization or disorders such as Parkinson's Disease) or inadequate help given to those unable to self-feed;
- sedation, semiconsciousness or coma.

In the hospital or institutional setting these problems may be compounded by the fact that nutritional considerations may receive little attention from medical and nursing staff.

Lack of awareness of the prognostic significance of undernutrition, and lack of knowledge among doctors and nurses regarding its assessment and management (Nightingale and Reeves 1999) may mean that it is neither looked for nor taken into account when treatment priorities are being set. In particular, there may be failure to:

- identify those with, or at risk of, nutritional depletion;
- identify nutritional requirements, especially when these are increased as a result of pyrexia, surgery or injury;
- provide food of an appropriate composition and consistency;
- encourage its consumption: food will be of no benefit if it is not eaten. People may be served meals which are placed out of reach, require too much effort to eat or cannot be finished before being taken away (see Section 1.16, Food service in hospitals and institutions);
- monitor what is consumed: if meals are cleared away by ward assistants, there may be no mechanism by which nursing staff are made aware of food or fluids which remain unconsumed. Even if plate wastage is recorded, this may not take account of food lost as a result of spillage or being thrown around (which may be significant in people with neurological or behavioural disorders). In some circumstances, direct observation of food and fluid consumption is essential;
- identify those whose nutritional needs are not being met;
- correct inadequate intake.

A report by the King's Fund centre clearly identified the need for nutrition to be regarded as an integral aspect of 'treatment' and for better training of junior doctors in this respect (Lennard-Jones 1992).

1.11.3 Identification of undernutrition

Early identification of undernutrition is important. Since the onset is often insidious, it can remain unnoticed until it has become quite severe. Correcting the physical and psychological consequences of undernutrition can take a long time, particularly in patients who are metabolically stressed (e.g. post-trauma or surgery), where the catabolic nature of metabolism will inhibit tissue restitution.

There is no universally accepted definition of 'undernutrition' or of its classification in terms of severity. Its existence is usually based on the presence of one or more parameters such as:

- significant and/or rapid unintended weight loss (see Section 1.8.4)
- low BMI (see Section 1.8.4)
- evidence of depletion of muscle mass (e.g. mid-arm circumference below the 15th percentile) (see Section 1.8.4)
- evidence of poor food intake (see Section 1.5, Dietary assessment).

The criteria used to define undernutrition in terms of these parameters can vary. Unintended weight loss may be assessed solely in terms of the extent of body weight loss, either in absolute amounts or as a percentage of usual body weight (e.g. > 5kg or >10% pre-illness weight). Alternatively, the degree of weight loss may be interpreted in the context of the timescale over which this has occurred (e.g. > 5% weight loss within 3 months).

Similarly, different levels of BMI may be used as criteria of undernutrition. Ranges and cut-off points used to define the normal or the ideal are derived from measurements made on healthy young individuals and are neither age nor disease-specific. The prognostic significance of a particular level of BMI may therefore vary between different client groups. A BMI <20 is usually considered to be evidence of underweight and indicative of undernutrition, but higher cut-off points may be more appropriate for some subjects; Beck and Ovesen (1998) found that a BMI < 24 may be clinically significant in elderly people.

The cut-off points used to define undernutrition may also vary according to whether they are used in isolation or in combination with other risk parameters; for example, Kelly *et al.* (2000) defined undernutrition as BMI <18.5 or BMI 18.5–20 with unintended weight loss >3 kg in the previous 3 months.

Some form of simple nutritional screening process should be a routine part of clinical assessment on admission to hospital or residential care home, or in the primary care setting. The use of nutrition screening tools for this purpose is discussed in Section 1.9 (Assessment of nutritional risk). The parameters assessed will depend on the nature of the client population being screened and on the personnel carrying out the screening process (e.g. whether medical, nursing or other care staff), but those which are most likely to be used as indicators of nutritional risk are:

- changes in body weight (possibly by visual assessment if scales are not available)
- changes in appetite or food intake
- the presence of gastrointestinal symptoms
- the presence of metabolic stress.

Nutritional screening should also be a routine part of continuing care in order to identify those whose nutritional status is deteriorating.

The screening process will only be of value if the findings are acted upon. Clear guidance therefore needs to be provided on how the information should be used. This will need to include:

- documentation of the findings and action taken
- the action process for those identified as various levels of risk
- the criteria for dietetic referral
- how the situation is to be monitored
- procedures for repeat screening.

Local protocols should drawn up to ensure that these objectives are achieved (BDA 1999). In the hospital setting, this may be under the remit of the nutrition support team (Daniels and Wright 1997). In the primary care setting, nutritional screening can be incorporated into standard health reviews or be a component of nursing care plans.

If nutritional concerns or problems are highlighted, patients should be referred to a dietitian for more detailed evaluation of the extent or risk of nutritional depletion (see Section 1.8, Assessment of nutritional status). Particular attention should be paid to:

- *dietary aspects*: adequacy of current intake, recent changes in food intake, and existence of factors likely to impair food intake;
- *clinical aspects*: presence of factors likely to increase nutrient requirements, presence of factors likely to increase nutrient losses, acute or chronic disease affecting the gastrointestinal tract, and use of drugs which affect food intake or nutrient utilization;
- *physical aspects*: signs of muscle wasting, emaciation or oedema, presence of pressure sores or evidence of dehydration;
- *anthropometric aspects*: degree and rapidity of any unintended weight loss, BMI, and evidence of muscle wasting (e.g. reduced mid arm muscle circumference or grip strength);
- *psychological aspects*: depression, anxiety or apathy, social isolation, and poverty

The nature and extent of these problems will determine the way in which undernutrition is managed or averted.

1.11.4 Management of undernutrition

While there is universal acceptance that undernutrition is deleterious, some clinicians remain to be convinced of the benefits of nutritional support (other than when there is a clear clinical need for enteral or parenteral feeding). This stems in part from misunderstanding over the meaning of the term 'nutritional support' and the assumption that the only alternative to enteral or parenteral nutrition is the use of commercial supplements. This is not the case: while supplements have a role in the management of some cases of undernutrition, they are by no means necessary in every patient. The first step is always to consider whether nutrient needs can be met via ordinary foods and beverages. It is only when this option is obviously inadequate or inappropriate that other measures need to be considered.

In practice, nutritional support can be regarded as a graded process of increasing levels of intervention:

- improving energy and nutrient intake from ordinary foods
- fortifying the energy and nutrient content of ordinary foods
- sip feed and others forms of supplementation
- enteral nutrition
- parenteral nutrition.

These methods are not mutually exclusive. Sip feed supplements may be useful as an occasional substitute for food on days where the patient feels particularly unwell or unable to eat; in some clinical circumstances overnight enteral feeding may be a useful accompaniment to normal daytime eating. Even when parenteral nutrition is indicated, some feeding via the enteral route (e.g. overnight) may be possible and should be considered unless specifically contraindicated (Pennington 1996).

The measures taken to prevent or correct undernutrition depend on the level of risk or severity, the factors which have led to its development in a particular patient and the accessibility of the gastrointestinal tract as a feeding route (Fig. 1.4). The route, type and level of nutritional support therefore have to be determined on an individual basis. Dietitians are uniquely qualified to provide such guidance.

Detailed guidance on oral and artificial nutrition support can be found in Sections 1.12, 1.13 and 1.15.

1.11.5 Monitoring progress

With any nutritionally compromised or at-risk patient, it is essential that patient is reviewed at regular intervals to assess the effectiveness of the nutritional support strategy.

In those maintaining an oral intake, this may need to be assessed in terms of:

- weight loss, stabilization or gain
- changes in nutritional (and fluid) intake: quantity, type, variety
- effectiveness of remedial suggestions for alleviating problems with food intake
- improvement in bowel function, skin condition or other symptoms indicative of undernutrition
- compliance with advice given in terms of food choice or fortification
- compliance with recommended use of supplements.

People who are severely malnourished should be assessed weekly. Monthly assessment may be sufficient for those with milder undernutrition (see Section 1.8, Assessment of nutritional status).

Patients receiving artificial nutritional support (enteral or parenteral nutrition) will require more sophisticated monitoring procedures encompassing factors such as fluid balance, nitrogen balance, electrolyte status and bowel pat-

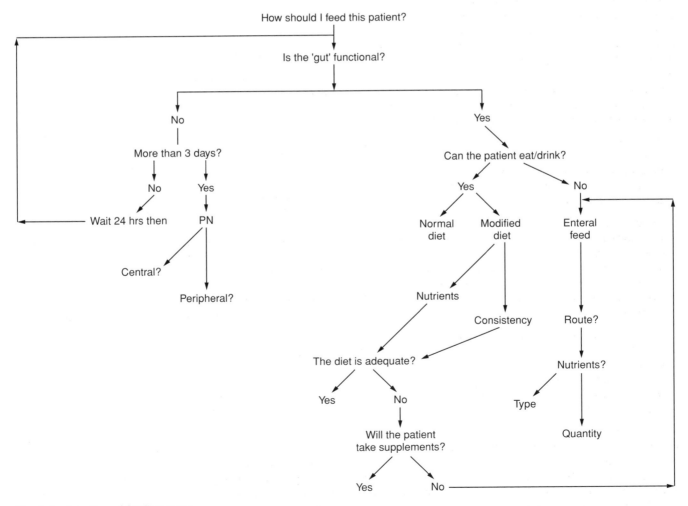

Fig. 1.4 Selection of feeding route.

tern changes. In some circumstances these may need to be monitored on a daily basis (see Sections 1.13 and 1.15).

As a result of the monitoring process, the type or level of support may need to be adjusted, dietary guidance amended or reinforced and new progress targets set.

Text written by: Briony Thomas

Useful address

King's Fund Centre, 11–13 Cavendish Square, London W1M 0AN

Further reading

ASPEN Board of Directors. Guidelines for the use of parenteral and enteral nutrition in adult and paediatric patients. *Parenteral and Enteral Nutrition* 1993; **17** (4, Suppl).

British Dietetic Association. *Malnutrition in Hospitals*. Position Paper. Birmingham: BDA, 1996.

Green CJ, on behalf of the Council of the British Association for Parenteral and Enteral Nutrition (BAPEN). Existence, causes and consequences of disease-related malnutrition in the hospital and the community, and clinical and financial benefits of nutritional intervention. *Clinical Nutrition* 1999; **18** (Suppl 2): 3–28.

Nuffield Trust. Maryon-Davis A, Bristow A (Eds). *Managing Nutrition in Hospital: A Recipe for Quality*. London: Nuffield Trust, 1999.

Plester CE. *Organisation of Nutrition Support in Hospitals*. BAPEN Working Party Report. Maidenhead: BAPEN, 1994.

References

Allcock N, Wharrad H, Nicolson A. Interpretation of pressure sore prevalence. *Journal of Advanced Nursing* 1994; **20**: 37–45.

Bastow MD, Rawlings J, Allison SP. Benefits of supplementary tube feeding after fractured neck of femur: a randomised controlled trial. *British Medical Journal* 1983; **287**: 1581–1592.

Beck AM, Ovesen L. At which body mass index and degree of weight loss should hospitalized elderly patients be considered at nutritional risk? *Clinical Nutrition* 1998; **17**: 195–198.

Benotti P, Bistrian B. Metabolic and nutritional aspects of weaning from mechanical ventilation. *Critical Care Medicine* 1989; **17**: 181–185.

Bergstrom NI. Strategies for preventing pressure ulcers. *Clinics in Geriatric Medicine* 1997; **13**: 437–454.

Bistrian BR, Blackburn GL, Hallowell E, Heddle R. Protein status of general surgical patients. *Journal of the American Medical Association* 1974; **230**: 858–860.

British Dietetic Association. *Nutrition Screening Tools*. Briefing Paper. Birmingham: BDA, 1999.

Casey J, Flynn WR, Yao JST. Correlation of immune and nutritional status with wound complications in patients undergoing vascular operations. *Surgery* 1983; **93**: 822–827.

Chandra RK. Effect of vitamin and trace element supplementation on immune responses and infection in elderly subjects. *Lancet* 1992; **340**: 1124–1127.

Chandra RK, Kumari S. Effects of nutrition on the immune system. *Nutrition* 1994; **120**: 207–210.

Daniels A, Wright J. Hospitals with Nutrition Support Teams are more likely to have a Nutritional Assessment Policy and ward nurses who identify at risk patients than those who do not. *Proceedings of the Nutrition Society* 1997; **56**: 254A.

Delmi M, Rapin C-H, Bengoa J-M *et al*. Dietary supplementation in elderly patients with fractured neck of femur. *Lancet* 1990; **335**: 1013–1016.

Dickhaut SC, DeLee JC, Page CP. Nutritional status: importance in predicting wound-healing after amputation. *Journal of Bone and Joint Surgery* 1984; **66**(1): 71–75.

Dionigi R, Zonta A, Dominioni L *et al*. The effects of total parenteral nutrition on immunodepression due to malnutrition. *Annals of Surgery* 1988; **185**: 467–474.

Edington J, Kon P, Martyn CN. Prevalence of malnutrition in patients in general practice. *Clinical Nutrition* 1996; **15**: 60–63.

Edington J, Kon P, Martyn CN. Prevalence of malnutrition after major surgery. *Journal of Human Nutrition and Dietetics* 1997; **10**: 111–116.

Edington J, Boorman J, Durrant ER *et al*. Prevalence of malnutrition on admission to four hospitals in England. *Clinical Nutrition* 2000; **19**: 191–195.

Fiatarone MA, Evans WJ. The etiology and reversibility of muscle dysfunction in the aged. *Journal of Geriatrics* 1993; **48**: 77–83.

Finch S, Doyle W, Lowe C *et al*. *National Diet and Nutrition Survey: People Aged 65 Years and Over*. Vol. 1. *Report of the Diet and Nutrition Survey*. London: The Stationery Office, 1998.

Forman H. Relationship of malnutrition and length of stay in the hospital. *Journal of the American Dietetic Association* 1996; **96** (Suppl): A29.

Galanos AN, Pieper CF, Kussin PS *et al*. Relationship of body mass index to subsequent mortality among seriously ill hospitalized patients. SUPPORT Investigators. The Study to Understand Prognoses and Preferences for Outcome and Risks of Treatments. *Critical Care Medicine* 1997; **25**: 1962–1968.

Haydock DA, Hill GL. Impaired wound healing in surgical patients with varying degrees of malnutrition. *Journal of Parenteral and Enteral Nutrition* 1986; **10**: 550–554.

Haydock DA, Hill GL. Improved wound healing response in surgical patients receiving intravenous nutrition. *British Journal of Surgery* 1987: **74**: 320–323.

Heymsfield SB, Bethel RA, Ansley JD *et al*. Cardiac abnormalities in cachectic patients before and during nutritional repletion. *American Heart Journal* 1978; **95**: 584–594.

Hill GL, Blackett RL, Pickford I *et al*. Malnutrition in surgical patients. An unrecognised problem. *Lancet* 1977; **i**: 689–692.

Holmes R, Macchiano K, Jhangiani SS *et al*. Combating pressure sores – nutritionally. *American Journal of Nursing* 1987; **87**: 1301–1303.

Kelly IE, Tessier S, Cahill A *et al*. Still hungry in hospital: identifying malnutrition in acute hospital admissions. *Quarterly Journal of Medicine* 2000; **93**: 93–98.

Klipstein-Grobusch K, Reilly JJ, Potter JM *et al*. Energy intake and expenditure in elderly patients admitted to hospital with acute illness. *British Journal of Nutrition* 1995; **73**: 323–340.

Larsson J, Unosson M, Ek A-C *et al*. Effect of dietary supplement of nutritional status and clinical outcome in 501 geriatric patients – a randomised study. *Clinical Nutrition* 1990; **9**: 179–184.

Lennard-Jones JE. *A Positive Approach to Nutrition as a Treatment*. London: King's Fund Centre, 1992.

Lesourd B. Protein undernutrition as the major cause of decreased immune function in the elderly: clinical and functional implications. *Nutrition Reviews* 1995; **53**: S86–S94.

McGlone PC, Dickerson JWT, Davies GJ. Provision of Asian foods in hospital. *Proceedings of the Nutrition Society* 1996; **55**: 74A.

McWhirter JR, Pennington CR. Incidence and recognition of malnutrition in hospital. *British Medical Journal* 1994; **308**: 945–948.

Mehta HC, Saini AS, Singh H. Biochemical aspects of malabsorption in marasmus. *British Journal of Nutrition* 1984; **5**: 1–6.

Moy RJD, Smallman S, Booth IW. Malnutrition in a UK children's hospital. *Journal of Human Nutrition and Dietetics* 1990; **3**: 93–100.

Neumann CG, Lawlor GL, Steihms ER *et al*. Immunologic responses in malnourished children. *American Journal of Clinical Nutrition* 1975; **28**: 89–104.

Nightingale JM, Reeves J. Knowledge about the assessment and management of undernutrition: a pilot questionnaire in a UK teaching hospital. *Clinical Nutrition* 1999; **18**: 23–27.

Ondrey FG, Hom DB. Effects of nutrition on wound healing. *Otolaryngology – Head and Neck Surgery* 1994; **110**: 557–559.

Pennington CR. *Current Perspectives on Parenteral Nutrition in Adults*. BAPEN Working Party Report. Maidenhead: BAPEN, 1996.

Potter JM, Klipstein K, Reilly JJ, Roberts MA. The nutritional status and clinical course of acute admissions to a geriatric unit. *Age and Ageing* 1995; **24**: 131–136.

Potter J, Langhorne P, Roberts M. Routine protein energy supplementation in adults: systematic review. *British Medical Journal* 1998; **317**: 495–501.

Rana SK, Bray J, Menzies-Gow N *et al*. Short-term benefits of postoperative oral dietary supplements in surgical patients. *Clinical Nutrition* 1992; **11**: 337–344.

Reilly HM, Martineau JK, Moran A, Kennedy H. Nutritional screening – Evaluation and implementation of a simple Nutrition Risk Score. *Clinical Nutrition* 1995; **34**: 269–273.

Reilly JJ, Hull SF, Albert N *et al*. Economic impact of malnutrition: a model system for hospitalized patients. *Journal of Parenteral and Enteral Nutrition* 1987; **12**: 372–376.

Robinson G, Goldstein M, Levine GM. Impact of nutritional status on DRG length of stay. *Journal of Parenteral and Enteral Nutrition* 1987; **11**: 49–51.

Silk DBA, Cottam TK, Neilsen MS *et al*. Organisation of Nutrition Support in Hospitals. BAPEN Working Party Report. Maidenhead: BAPEN, 1994.

Stanfield JP, Hutt MSR, Tunnicliffe K. Intestinal biopsy in kwashiorkor. *Lancet* 1965; **ii**: 519–523.

Stephen AD, Beigg CL, Elliot ET *et al*. Food provision, wastage and intake in medical, surgical and elderly hospitalized patients. *Clinical Nutrition* 1997; **16** (Suppl 2): 4.

Theologies A. Origins of anorexia in neoplastic disease. *American Journal of Clinical Nutrition* 1978; **31**: 1104–1107.

Treber LA, Harris MA. Effect of early nutrition intervention on patient length of stay. *Journal of the American Dietetic Association* 1996; **96** (Suppl): A29.

Tucker HN, Miguel SG. Cost containment through nutrition intervention. *Nutrition Reviews* 1996; **54**: 111–121.

Veterans Affairs Total Parenteral Nutrition Co-operative Study Group. Perioperative total parenteral nutrition in surgical patients. *New England Journal of Medicine* 1991; **325**: 525–532.

Whittaker JS, Ryan F, Buckley PA, Road JD. The effects of refeeding on peripheral and respiratory muscle function in malnourished chronic obstructive pulmonary disease patients. *American Review of Respiratory Diseases* 1990; **142**: 283–286.

Windsor JA, Hill GL. Risk factors for post-operative pneumonia: the importance of protein depletion. *Annals of Surgery* 1988a; **208**: 209–214.

Windsor JA, Hill GL. Weight loss with physiologic impairment: a basis indicator of surgical risk. *Annals of Surgery* 1988b; **207**: 290–296.

1.12 Oral nutritional support

The term 'nutritional support' does not just mean the use of supplements or enteral/parenteral nutrition (see Section 1.11.4, Management of undernutrition). Chronic undernutrition usually results from poor food intake and, in most instances, improving nutritional intake via ordinary foods and beverages is the first step in the process of providing nutritional support. For many people with mild undernutrition (or identified as being at risk of undernutrition) simple dietary advice focused on food quality and quantity (or measures which ensure better food provision) may be sufficient to correct or avert the problem (Gall *et al.* 1998). Specific guidance to help in alleviating problems such as nausea or dry mouth may also result in considerable improvements in oral intake. If food intake is particularly poor, food enrichment measures may help improve nutrient density. Some people may need further support in the form of sip feed and other supplements. Only a few will require artificial nutritional support in the form of enteral or parenteral nutrition (see Sections 1.13 and 1.15).

1.12.1 General dietary guidance to improve food intake

The first nutritional objectives for anyone with a poor food intake are to:

- increase the frequency of consumption of foods and fluids
- increase the energy and nutrient content of foods and fluids consumed.

Increasing the frequency of consumption

People should be encouraged to consume some form of nourishment at frequent intervals, e.g. every 2–3 hours throughout the day. This might be:

- a small meal
- a snack (e.g. a sandwich, yoghurt, biscuits, crackers and cheese, fruit)
- a nourishing drink (e.g. milk-based).

Patients should be encouraged to regard 'eating' as being as important as any other treatment or medication they are receiving, and a positive step that they can take to help recovery. (Medical and nursing staff sometimes need to be reminded of this too.)

Increasing the energy and nutrient content of foods and fluids consumed

Energy- and nutrient-dense foods

Patients should be encouraged to consume foods which provide concentrated sources of energy and nutrients in a relatively small volume. Good choices are:

- lean meat
- fish (tinned fish such as pilchards or sardines are particularly useful)
- cheese (especially grated)
- eggs
- full-fat yoghurt
- double cream
- full-cream, evaporated or condensed milk
- butter and full-fat spreads (or margarine)
- jams and preserves, honey, peanut butter, chocolate spread.

Snack foods such as cakes, biscuits, pastries, chocolate and crisps can also be useful additional sources of energy in people with poor food intake. However, it is important that these are not used in a way which impairs intake of more nutrient-dense foods, e.g. by being consumed just before a meal.

Nourishing drinks

As much as possible, people should be encouraged to consume drinks that are better sources of nourishment than just tea or coffee. Suitable suggestions are:

- milky drinks (e.g. cocoa, drinking chocolate, malted milk drinks, coffee made with milk)
- milk-based supplement drinks (e.g. Build-up, Complan, Recovery)
- soup (especially condensed or 'cream of' varieties)
- fruit juices (or drinks enriched with vitamin C)
- sugar- or glucose-containing fizzy or soft drinks.

Maintenance of oral hygiene is essential if refined carbohydrates are consumed at frequent intervals.

It is important that people with a poor food intake consume a diet which is 'healthy' in terms of supplying all the energy and nutrients required. However, for those who do not feel much like eating or cannot cope with large volumes of food, this does not mean a low-fat, high-fibre 'healthy-eating' diet, because people are unlikely to be able to eat sufficient of it to meet their needs. Sometimes it is necessary to explain this to carers who feel that a diet containing butter, cream, sugar-rich foods and drinks, etc., is 'unhealthy'.

It is also essential to ensure that people are able to obtain the type of diet they need. Those living in the community should be encouraged to make full use of local support services (e.g. social services, home helps, meals on wheels, day-care facilities) which can provide practical help in terms of shopping, cooking or meal provision and perhaps also reduce the social isolation of those who live alone.

1.12.2 Dietary guidance for problems affecting food intake

Many factors can impair food intake and it is important that any such problems are identified and alleviated as much as possible. Sometimes quite simple dietary suggestions can result in a considerable improvement in nutrient intake.

Loss of appetite

Loss of appetite is a common consequence of the physical and psychological effects of illness and, sometimes, the side-effects of its treatment. Factors such as feeling unwell, pain, tiredness, worry and depression can markedly suppress the desire to eat, and the anorexic patient needs support and encouragement in order to do so. This problem is often best tackled by a team approach so that the different skills of team members can be used to identify the underlying causes of the anorexia and alleviate its effects.

Helpful dietary suggestions may include:

- Eat most at times of day when appetite is best.
- Make eating as easy as possible. Make use of ready-to-eat or convenience foods which are easy to prepare (e.g. microwaveable ready meals).
- Serve food in manageable portions. The sight of a large pile of food is off-putting.
- Do not hurry over meals. Eat slowly, chew food well and relax for a short while between courses and after each meal.
- Eat anything which is particularly fancied.
- Do not fill up with liquids before or during meals. Have them at least half an hour beforehand or at the end of a meal.
- A short walk before a meal may help appetite.
- If alcohol is allowed, a small tot before a meal (such as a glass of sherry), or a glass of wine with a meal, can stimulate appetite. This strategy may be particularly helpful with elderly people.
- Do not let cooking smells linger in the house.
- If a main meal cannot be faced, have a snack instead (e.g. a sandwich, cheese on crackers). Alternatively, have some nourishment in liquid form, e.g. a chilled milky drink, soup or supplement drink.

Tiredness or difficulty in preparing meals

Some people are able to eat if food is placed in front of them but, if they live alone, find it difficult to make the effort to prepare food for themselves due to debility, feeling unwell or just lack of interest in food. Encourage people to:

- Ask for and accept help. Neighbours and friends are often pleased to be asked to help out with shopping, cooking and other chores.
- Make use of convenience foods, e.g. canned or packet soups, canned fruit, instant desserts, ready meals, breakfast cereals.
- Make use of good days and better times during the day to eat most and prepare meals and snacks to eat later or put in the freezer.
- Consume nourishing drinks such as milky drinks or milk-based supplements (Build-Up, Complan, Recovery).

Early satiety

Stomach resection, abdominal tumours or radiotherapy to the upper abdominal area often result in people feeling full when they have only consumed a small quantity of food. Helpful suggestions may include:

- Eat smaller meals and snacks more often.
- If a two-course meal is too much, have puddings between meals, e.g. canned fruit with added custard, cream or evaporated milk, ice-cream, full-fat yoghurt, mousses or instant desserts.
- Avoid drinking fluids with meals or for an hour beforehand. Have something to drink as soon as is comfortable after a meal.
- Avoid fatty, greasy or 'rich' foods.

Chronic nausea and vomiting

These can occur for numerous reasons as they are a consequence of many disease states as well as being common side-effects of drug treatment and radiotherapy.

If nausea and vomiting are severe and food cannot be faced at all, people should be encouraged to consume small amounts of nourishing liquids as often as possible. Sipping drinks through a straw may be helpful. In some cases, antiemetics may be necessary.

As people feel better, more solid foods should gradually be introduced. Helpful advice may include:

- Eat anything which is fancied.
- Make use of times when nausea is least to eat or prepare foods to eat later in the day.
- Try to avoid cooking smells or letting them linger in the house. Make use of convenience foods which create little smell when cooked, or ask someone to cook something for you in their kitchen.
- Avoid fatty and fried foods.
- Avoid drinks with meals and serve food relatively dry (unless on a modified consistency diet). Between meals, sip cold drinks at intervals or slowly through a straw.
- Do not lie down immediately after eating.
- Cold foods (e.g. cold meat, cheese and sandwiches)

may be better tolerated than hot foods as they have less smell.

- Savoury foods and drinks may be more acceptable than sweet-tasting items.
- Ginger-flavoured drinks and foods may help, e.g. ginger ale, ginger beer, ginger biscuits, ginger tea.
- Early-morning nausea may be alleviated by dry carbo-hydrate-based foods, e.g. unbuttered toast, cream crackers, plain biscuits.

Taste changes

Radiotherapy to the mouth and throat and some types of chemotherapy result in changes in taste sensation. These can cause loss of taste or changes in taste.

Loss of taste (mouth blindness)

The following measures may enhance the flavour of food:

- Choose foods full of flavour and aroma.
- Use plenty of seasonings, especially herbs and spices, e.g. basil, oregano, sage, black pepper, garlic.
- Add soup or sauce mixes to savoury dishes such as mince and casseroles.
- Try sharp-tasting foods and drinks that are refreshing, e.g. fresh fruit, boiled sweets, mints, lemonade, fruit juice, tonic water, citrus fruits.
- Lemon juice in water before food may be helpful.
- Enhance the flavour of salads and vegetables by adding onion, orange or lemon juice or vinaigrette dressings.
- Marinate food to enhance flavour (e.g. in wine, beer or cider, or fruit juice).

Changes in taste

A common side-effect of chemotherapy and some types of radiotherapy is that foods may taste metallic, bitter or even unpleasant. Other taste sensations may be heightened, for example, sweet-tasting foods may suddenly taste unbearably sweet. Helpful guidance may include:

- Avoid any food which tastes unpleasant.
- Allow hot food to cool a little before eating; high temperature can accentuate an unpleasant taste sensation.
- If meat tastes unpleasant try alternatives such as fish, eggs, cheese and dairy products. Cold meats may taste better than hot meats. Marinading can also be helpful.
- If bitterness is a problem, avoid foods sweetened with saccharine, which can exacerbate this sensation.
- If food tastes metallic, a gargle of lemon juice in water before eating may be helpful.
- If excessive sweetness is a problem, this can be offset by adding lemon juice or diluting drinks with soda or min-eral water. Adding spices such as ginger, nutmeg or cin-namon to desserts and puddings may also reduce the sensation of sweetness. Sharper fruit flavours (e.g. grape-fruit, rhubarb, gooseberry) may be more acceptable than blander types.
- If excessive saltiness is a problem, avoid packet soups, gravy and sauces or add a pinch of sugar to them before

they are served. Avoid bacon, ham and other types of preserved or canned meat and obvious sources of salt such as salted nuts or crisps.

Dry mouth (xerostomia)

This is a common consequence of damage to the salivary glands, usually as a result of surgery or radiotherapy to the head and neck region. The resulting lack, or even absence, of saliva makes mastication and swallowing dif-ficult. People should be encouraged to:

- make meals moist with the use of gravy, sauces, butter, cream or evaporated milk;
- avoid very dry foods such as biscuits or toast;
- sip drinks frequently, particularly with meals;
- suck items which help stimulate saliva flow, e.g. boiled sweets, fruit pastilles, pineapple chunks, grapefruit seg-ments, ice cubes (perhaps flavoured with lemon juice or made from fruit juice);
- choose sharp-tasting foods such as those flavoured with lemon, grapefruit, gooseberry or rhubarb.

Many patients receiving radiotherapy to the head and neck region proceed to develop sore mouths during their treat-ment programme. In this case, the last two recommenda-tions will not be applicable since these food items will exacerbate the soreness.

Lack of saliva can predispose to tooth decay and hence good oral hygiene should be encouraged in all patients. Artificial saliva sprays, gels or salivary stimulant pastilles are prescribable for dry mouth associated with radiotherapy and some other conditions.

Sore or painful mouth

This may result from infection, inflammation or ulceration of the oral areas making eating painful and difficult. Stom-atitis and mucositis may follow radiotherapy in the head and neck area or as a side-effect of some cytotoxic drugs. Dietary guidance is to:

- eat soft, moist foods by adding sauces, gravy, custard, etc. Some foods may be easier to eat if they are mashed or liquidized;
- avoid very dry or rough-textured foods, e.g. toast, raw vegetables, cereal bars or crisps;
- avoid foods and drinks at extremes of temperature. Very hot or very cold items can exacerbate pain;
- avoid salty or highly spiced foods, e.g. salted crackers, salted nuts, crisps, pepper, chilli, curry powder and soy sauce;
- avoid tart beverages, e.g. pure orange juice, grapefruit juice. Consuming other drinks through a straw may be soothing.

It is also important to ensure that these patients are receiv-ing effective pain control so that their food intake is not compromised more than necessary. Appropriate mouth care is also essential.

Swallowing difficulties (dysphagia)

Swallowing difficulties may seriously compromise nutritional intake and it is important that dysphagia is properly assessed and managed. This is discussed in detail in Section 4.3 (Dysphagia).

1.12.3 Food enrichment

In addition to the general measures to improve food intake described above, some people may benefit from food-enrichment strategies which boost the nutrient content of foods and beverages without significantly affecting their volume, and hence the patient's ability to consume them.

Enrichment using ordinary foods

Suitable ways of doing this are to:

- make fortified milk by adding 4 tablespoons of skimmed milk powder to 1 pint of milk. This fortified milk can then be used throughout the day in drinks, on cereals or to make custard, milk puddings, etc.;
- add grated cheese to soup, savoury dishes, mashed potato;
- add evaporated milk to milk or fruit-based desserts;
- add double cream to soup, mashed potato, sauces or desserts;
- add butter (or margarine) to vegetables, pasta, scrambled egg and during cooking;
- add jam, syrup or honey to breakfast cereals, milk puddings or other desserts;
- add sugar or glucose to foods or drinks. Glucose powder is less sweet than table sugar, so more can be added without creating an unacceptable level of sweetness, but it is much more expensive.

Proprietary enrichment supplements

Foods and drinks can also be fortified with proprietary modular energy and protein supplements. These are ACBS prescribable for certain conditions and examples of currently available products are given in Appendix 6.7.

Some supplements in powdered form are best incorporated into foods by being dissolved in a small volume of liquid and then added to prepared food or drink such as soft drinks, soups, sauces or milk puddings. However, newer, more soluble powders can usually be added directly to foods and drinks without problems. Liquid energy supplements can be mixed with double cream, frozen and used as a type of ice-cream.

Experimentation may be necessary to discover the amount that can be added without impairing texture and flavour.

It is also important that recommended dosage levels are not exceeded to avoid creating new problems such as diarrhoea, or renal problems in elderly people as a result of excessive protein loads.

1.12.4 Sip feed and other supplements

If sufficient energy intake cannot be achieved via normal foods, proprietary supplements can be a useful addition to the diet and can improve clinical outcome (Bolton *et al.* 1990, 1992; Larsson *et al.* 1990).

Some types of nutritional supplement can be purchased directly from chemists or supermarkets (e.g. Build-Up, Recovery, Complan). These are usually in powdered form and are made up with milk to provide sweet, neutral or savoury drinks; natural flavoured products can also be used to fortify other foods. Some are also available in a ready-to-drink form. They are not nutritionally complete (as they are lacking in trace elements) but they provide a more concentrated source of nutrients than a milky drink alone.

Many types of sip feed supplements are also available which are ACBS prescribable for severe undernutrition as detailed in the Monthly Index of Medical Specialities (MIMS) or the British National Formulary (BNF). Many, but not all, are nutritionally complete, come in a ready-to-drink form in cartons or cups and can be sipped at intervals throughout the day, or if necessary as a meal replacement. Some are milk based; others are formulated with a fruit or yoghurt base for those who have tired of the taste of milk. Some are designed to meet higher energy needs or particular clinical indications (e.g. people with malabsorption or renal disease). Prescribable supplements in the form of soups or desserts are also available.

One potential problem with nutritional supplements is that few, if any, of the products currently available are suitable for vegans or people who strictly follow Vegetarian Society guidelines. Most supplements contain vitamin D derived from wool fat, and milk derivatives such as whey or caseinates which have been extracted from milk using animal rennet. Some of the newer yoghurt-based supplements contain animal gelatine. People who are strict vegetarians because of religious constraints may be able to obtain exemption from the usual dietary restrictions on the grounds of ill-health. However, those who follow a vegan or strict vegetarian diet for ethical reasons may be less prepared to compromise their principles.

Guidance on the range of products available is given in Appendix 6.7. Detailed compositional details of all currently available products can be found in MIMS or BNF, or obtained directly from the manufacturers.

Use of prescribable supplements

Prescribed supplementary products are costly to the National Health Service and it is important that they are not used unnecessarily. There has been concern at the rate at which the prescription of supplements has increased in recent years and their accelerating proportion of local drugs budgets. While invaluable for some patients when used appropriately, auditing procedures have shown that these products are often prescribed without any involvement of a dietitian and with no attempt made to improve oral nutritional intake by conventional dietary means

(McCombie 1999). In hospitals, particularly where catering budgets are tight, supplements may be regarded as an easier option than providing high nutrient density meals or extra snacks. In the primary care setting, general practitioners may routinely prescribe supplements to anyone considered to be malnourished, usually in response to a request by a district or palliative care nurse rather than a dietitian. The need for these products may not be properly assessed and their effectiveness once prescribed may be poorly monitored. As a result, their usage is often inappropriate or unnecessary (McCombie 1999). A systematic review evaluating the value of oral nutritional supplements used in the community setting highlights the need for better guidelines regarding their use (Stratton and Elia 1999).

Supplementation should only be considered when dietary measures alone have proved to be, or clearly will be, insufficient to sustain or improve oral intake. Supplements should always be regarded as an addition to normal food and not a substitute for it. They can also be used to enrich ordinary foods; they do not always have to be consumed as a drink. Only on days when food cannot be faced at all should supplements be regarded as an alternative form of nutrition (and at such times they are a very valuable source of nutrients). Patients should always be given simple written guidance on both general dietary aspects and the use of supplements.

Prescribed usage may range from one to three supplements per day which, depending on the type of product used, may provide between 250 and 900 kcal/day. People should be encouraged to consume supplements at intervals throughout the day but not immediately before meals to avoid impairing appetite. Sip feeds may be need to be texturally modified for those with dysphagia (see Section 4.3, Dysphagia).

It is important that wastage is avoided and that compliance with supplement use is monitored. Compliance is very dependent on factors such as appetite and taste (Bolton *et al*. 1990, 1992) and ideally patients or clients should have the opportunity of sampling different products before one of them is prescribed. If this is not possible, pharmacists should be asked to dispense a prescribed product in a range of flavours (if available) and repeat prescriptions can then be made up according to patient preference. One week's supply may be appropriate to begin with until an acceptable product is found. If one particular product is unappealing or taste fatigue sets in, an alternative formulation can be tried. Once established on an acceptable supplement, supplies can be prescribed monthly. Local delivery arrangements (possibly operated by community pharmacists) may be available for patients with transport difficulties.

The patient's progress and use of supplements should be monitored and as the patient's nutritional status improves or goals of treatment are reached, supplement intake can be gradually reduced and perhaps discontinued.

After 6 months, all patients prescribed supplements should have a detailed dietary review to assess overall dietary adequacy and necessity for supplementation.

When patients maintained on supplements are moved from secondary care into the primary care setting, it is important that hospital dietitians liaise with community dietetic services regarding treatment aims, dietary advice given and follow-up arrangements.

Because dietetic services are thinly spread and unable to oversee the management of every individual in need of oral nutritional support, dietitians currently have an important role as educators of medical and nursing staff, particularly those in the primary care sector, regarding dietary measures which can be taken to improve oral intake and the circumstances in which supplements may be beneficial.

Text written by: Briony Thomas

Acknowledgement: The British Dietetic Association's Nutrition Advisory Group for Elderly People (NAGE).

Useful resources

The British Dietetic Association's Nutrition Advisory Group for Elderly People (NAGE) produces a number of resources for either patients/carers or health professionals to help people with poor appetites. Current details of availability can be obtained from the British Dietetic Association's website at www.bda.uk.com or by contacting the Association directly.

References

Bolton J, Shannon V, Smith V *et al*. Comparing the short-term and long-term palatability of six commercially available oral supplements. *Journal of Human Nutrition and Dietetics* 1990; **3**: 345–350.

Bolton J, Abbott R, Keily M *et al*. Comparison with three oral sip feed supplements in patients with cancer. *Journal of Human Nutrition and Dietetics* 1992; **5**: 79–84.

Gall MJ, Grimble GK, Reeve J, Thomas SJ. Providing fortified meals and between-meal snacks significantly increases energy intake of hospital patients. *Proceedings of the Nutrition Society* 1998; **57**: 94A.

Larsson J, Unosson M, Ek A-C *et al*. Effect of dietary supplement of nutritional status and clinical outcome in 501 geriatric patients – a randomised study. *Clinical Nutrition* 1990; **9**: 179–184.

McCombie L. Sip feed prescribing in primary care: an audit of current practice in Greater Glasgow Health Board, Glasgow, UK. *Journal of Human Nutrition and Dietetics* 1999; **12**: 210–212.

Stratton RJ, Elia M. A critical, systematic analysis of the use of oral nutritional supplements in the community. *Clinical Nutrition* 1999; **18** (Suppl 2): 29–84.

1.13 Artificial nutritional support and enteral feeding

Undernutrition in hospital patients is neither new nor rare, occurring in some 40–55% of hospitalized patients, with up to 12% being severely undernourished (Gallagher-Allred *et al*. 1996), incurring increased hospital costs of 35–75% compared with well-nourished patients (Chima *et al*. 1997) (see Section 1.11, Undernutrition). Improving clinical outcomes of malnourished patients can only be achieved when appropriate nutrition intervention is given, yet prospective, randomized controlled trials on the clinical benefits of nutrition support are ethically suspect, time consuming, expensive and difficult to conduct (Woo *et al*. 1994).

Oral nutritional support measures (see Section 1.12) can improve outcome but, if oral intake remains compromised or is contraindicated, artificial nutritional support in the form of enteral or parental feeding becomes necessary. Nutritional supplementation shows consistently improved changes in body weight and anthropometry compared with controls, but there are insufficient data to confirm influence on mortality (Potter *et al*. 1999). The benefits of nutritional support in terms of maintaining or improving nutritional status and other clinical parameters have been well documented and are discussed in Section 1.11 (Undernutrition). Readers are also directed to the excellent review by Green (1999).

1.13.1 Principles of artificial nutritional support

The dietitian's role in artificial nutritional support

The dietitian is uniquely placed to give guidance and recommendations regarding nutritional support (ADA 1997). In the past there has been considerable variation in the practice of artificial nutrition support (Payne-James *et al*. 1992) and standards for its provision produced by the British Association for Parenteral and Enteral Nutrition (BAPEN) are a useful development (Sizer *et al*. 1996). The development and implementation of local policies also help to ensure efficient and effective nutritional support (Main and Morrison 1998). In the UK, national dietetic standards for nutritional support have been set by the Parenteral and Enteral Nutrition Group of the British Dietetic Association (PENG 1996).

A well co-ordinated approach can maximize the effectiveness and reduce complications of artificial nutrition support. The composition and mode of operation of nutrition teams will vary according to local needs, but dietitians should be key members (Silk *et al*. 1994). Clearly delineated roles for each team member prevent conflict and overlap. Formal nutrition teams can take up a great deal of time and require considerable co-ordination, and a less structured team approach, or multi-disciplinary nutrition strategy committee, may reap similar benefits.

Assessment for artificial nutritional support

Nutrition support should be tailored to the clinical state and the perceived best outcome of the patient. Readers are directed to Section 1.8 (Assessment of nutritional status) for details of assessment techniques, and Section 1.10 (Estimating nutritional requirements) for estimating nutritional needs based on clinical status.

Ethics of withholding or withdrawing nutrition

Enteral feeding is often delayed until it is thought that the patient will make some form of recovery, despite the fact that aggressive early nutrition intervention will improve clinical outcomes. For patients who present *in extremis* (e.g. brainstem CVA), feeding is obviously not indicated. However, the issue of continuing to feed severely ill patients who have a poor but not hopeless prognosis is less clear. Nutrition support per se will not keep unresponsive patients alive if regular nursing, chest physiotherapy and antibiotic therapy are discontinued. Withdrawal of these therapies in tandem with food and fluid reduction all hasten the terminal event.

A recent observational study reported that clinical interventions perceived as more artificial, scarce or expensive were withdrawn earlier from terminal patients. From earliest to latest, the order of treatment withdrawal was blood products, haemodialysis, vasopressors, mechanical ventilation, total parenteral nutrition, antibiotics, intravenous fluids and tube feedings (Asch *et al*. 1999).

Consistency of treatment and transparency of clinical issues discussed with the next of kin are important dietetic factors. If patients are being actively treated then it is appropriate to assert that nutritional support also be provided (Rabeneck *et al*. 1997). Dietitians should be guided by their own judgement if there is no department policy regarding the issue of feeding.

A comprehensive overview of the legal position in the UK regarding the withholding and withdrawing of life-prolonging medical treatment, including nutritional support, has been provided by the British Medical Association (1999) and Luttrell (1999). Ethical aspects of artificial feeding and hydration are discussed further in Sections 1.19 (Healthcare ethics) and 4.39 (Terminal illness and palliative and care).

Monitoring of artificial nutritional support

Close liaison with nursing colleagues is vital when initiating and monitoring enteral nutrition. The use of a proforma to document nutrition feed schedules is associated with a greater proportion of feed being delivered.

Regular patient monitoring should be used to assess whether a patient is achieving sufficient intake compared with previously determined goals (Baker *et al.* 1982). Adequacy of nutrition intervention can be reviewed in the context of:

- nutritional requirements for the current clinical condition
- nutrient intake: prescribed versus delivered (Robertson 1990)
- tolerance/capability of maintaining current route and prescribed intake
- current weight/recent history of weight loss
- level of nutrition support required (aggressive or palliative)
- clinical chemistry – biochemistry and haematology results (Sizer *et al.* 1996)
- fluid balance: short-term (24 hours) and longer term balance, taking into account the influence of pyrexia (Kleiner 1999)
- concurrent drug therapy
- complications that are associated with feed or route of administration.

The frequency and choice of monitoring depends on the clinical condition and stability. Monitoring frequency may be more intense at the start of treatment than at a later stage, but should continue throughout the episode of care. The dietitian should act on any necessary changes as a result of monitoring, and ensure that these are carried out effectively. These should be clearly documented on the patient record card (BDA 1996).

Electrolyte status

Electrolyte imbalances reflect clinical condition or drug therapy. Low-sodium and low-electrolyte feeds are available for electrolyte restriction secondary to renal or hepatic insufficiency. These feeds are inappropriate in iatrogenic dehydration, where additional fluid rather than electrolyte restriction will correct hypernatraemia and uraemia (Preston 1998).

The electrolyte content of the feeding regimen should be stated on the feeding chart. Additional electrolytes can be added to the feed from ampoules intended for injection (see Section 5.2, Intensive care), as oral forms often coagulate feeds and increase the risk of feeding-tube obstruction. Sterile intravenous electrolytes can be safely added to the enteral feed, thus reducing the need for additional intravenous fluids.

Mineral status

Clinical measurement of trace elements and minerals is expensive, incurs delayed analysis (as most samples need to be sent to outside laboratories) and rarely indicates nutritional status as levels are often influenced by stress (Singh *et al.* 1991).

Anthropometric monitoring

Many techniques are available to measure body composition, and these are discussed in Section 1.8.4). Measurements such as mid-arm muscle circumference measurement (MAMC), hand-grip dynamometry and bioelectrical impedance analysis may be irrelevant in circumstances where declining parameters reflect deteriorating clinical condition rather than nutritional status (e.g. MAMC measured in paralysed patients).

1.13.2 Enteral feeding

Feeding enterally is superior to the parenteral route in terms of physiology, immunology and cost, and has numerous clinical advantages such as helping to maintain normal intestinal function and structure (McClave *et al.* 1999). Mechanical obstruction, prolonged ileus and cardiovascular instability are the only absolute contraindications to enteral nutrition (Kirby and Teran 1998). Guidelines on the management of enteral nutrition in the adult patient have been produced by the BAPEN (McAtear *et al.* 1999).

Routes of enteral feeding

The route and level of enteral feeding are decided on an individual basis according to the clinical indications, treatment plan and nutritional state of the individual patient.

Enteral feed may be delivered:

- directly into the stomach (gastric feeding) via orogastric or nasogastric tube, gastrostomy or oesophagostomy;
- beyond the stomach (postpyloric feeding) via a nasoduodenal/nasojejunal tube or jejunostomy.

Gastric feeding routes

Nasogastric feeding This is usually used for short-term nutritional support (<14 days) or in the longer term when other options such as gastrostomy feeding are contraindicated.

A fine-bore nasogastric tube with integral guidewire (stylet) is inserted transnasally into the stomach. Patients with facial trauma may have a nasogastric tube placed through the mouth to bypass suspected nasal damage. Polyvinyl chloride (PVC) tubes are recommended for short-term feeding (<10 days); more expensive, durable polyurethene tubes may be more suitable for longer-term feeding. In practice, both tubes become dislodged with similar frequency and, although feasible, polyurethane tubes are rarely repassed owing to discoloration or loss of the guidewire for reinsertion. Fine-bore feeding tubes are 6–9 FG (French gauge: the external circumference of the tube measured in millimetres).

Patients at risk of pulmonary aspiration are usually intubated with a rigid wide-bore (10–18 FG) nasogastric tube (Ryles or Levin's tube). Complications associated with wide bore tubes are well known (nasal erosion, oesophageal ulceration) but, despite this, should be considered an initial feeding route, with conversion to a fine-bore tube once successful gastric emptying is established. Planned aspiration of gastric contents is possible with a fine-bore tube, but residual removal is slow and tends to be incomplete (Metheny et al. 1986). It is prudent for patients with large and variable aspirates unable to protect their airway to continue feeding via a wider lumen tube.

To confirm the length of tube required before placement:

1 Place the tip of the tube at the highest point of the central ribcage (the xiphoid sternum).
2 Pass the tube behind the ear, over the top of the ear and to the tip of the nostril, and mark this position.
3 Placement of the enteral tube to the position of the nostril mark will ensure that the tube is in the stomach.

Before feeding commences it is vital to establish that the tube is positioned in the stomach and not the lungs. Any or all of the following methods can be used:

• With the tube length *half* inserted, placing the luer end of the tube in a glass of water. If the tube is in the trachea or bronchus, violent water bubbling will occur on patient exhalation. (This should be done before the tube is fully sited, as air flow in the lower bronchus is limited and the results will not be as obvious.)
• Aspirating liquid from the tube and checking that the contents are acidic with pH/litmus strips.
• Injecting air into the tube and listening for borborygmi with a stethoscope over the stomach.
• X-ray confirmation: this tends to be carried out if there is any doubt over the position of the tube. All enteral feeding tubes are radio-opaque and will show up on X-ray. The guidewire is usually removed beforehand so that there is no risk of its subsequent removal displacing the feeding tube. (If a guidewire is not removed within 5 minutes of flushing water or aspirating stomach contents, the internal lubricant may be lost and its later removal may dislodge the tube.)

Tube placement should be reconfirmed following violent coughing fits, vomiting, or other potential causes of displacement.

Gastrostomy feeding A gastrostomy is the creation of an artificial tract between the stomach and the abdominal surface for intragastric feeding and is commonly used for long-term enteral support. The gastrostomy can be placed endoscopically, surgically or radiologically, although the latter technique has a higher complication rate. The use of Foley catheters as a feeding gastrostomy may cause duodenal obstruction (Tibbitts and Sorrell 1999). Marking the tube at skin surface ensures that the optimal position of the bulb in the antrum of the stomach is maintained.

Percutaneous endoscopic gastrostomy (PEG) can be placed at a day-care endoscopy unit, so reducing costs compared with other placement methods. The gastric bumper may be compressible, in which case removal at a later stage is possible percutaneously and without repeat endoscopy.

Formation of an abdominal stoma is unsuitable for patients with frank ascites, sepsis, or in those who have previously had extensive gastric surgery. It is possible to gastrostomy feed whilst pregnant (Godil and Chen 1998; Serrano et al. 1998). Prophylactic antibiotic 'stat' dose at placement minimizes the risk of subsequent stoma tract infection (Rey et al. 1998).

Tract formation occurs within a few hours, with administration of sterile water or dextrose saline becoming possible 4–6 hours postplacement. Feed introduction is usually between 10 and 24 hours post-insertion. Serous fluid loss around the stoma site during the first 24 hours is common, and can be treated with a dry dressing. Once the oozing has reduced, the gastrostomy should remain uncovered to minimize the risk of skin infection.

There are two forms of replacement gastrostomy tube:

• a 'balloon gastrostomy'; a catheter with an end balloon that is inflated with sterile water or saline to hold the tip against the gastric wall following percutaneous insertion;
• a 'button' gastrostomy, which has an extension tube detachable from the stoma for a more discreet skin surface appearance, and so is a popular choice for children. The extension tube is attached for periods of feeding, and detached once feeding is complete. 'Button' kits are available in different stoma lengths to allow for individual variation in the depth of tissue between the gastric mucosa and the skin surface. Each kit comes with a measuring device, to measure the depth of stoma and select the most appropriate button kit, and an obdurator, which is used to elongate the gastric bumper for insertion and removal purposes. Removal of button gastrostomies without endoscopic retrieval requires an obdurator.

Post-pyloric feeding routes

Nasoduodenal or nasojejunal feeding A feeding route bypassing the stomach overcomes the problem of gastric stasis and subsequent risk of aspiration. Paradoxically, those patients more likely to require jejunal feeds are often less able to have a tube placed jejunally because of limited endoscopic access, or reluctance to create a gut stoma in a septic individual.

Fine-bore duodenal tubes (usually 100–120 cm length) are endoscopically or radiologically placed beyond the ligament of Treitz. A dual-lumen tube may be placed for simultaneous gastric aspiration and jejunal feeding.

Gastrojejunostomy Post-pyloric feeding access can be obtained in a patient with an established gastrostomy access by the insertion of an extension device that threads through the existing gastrostomy lumen, and is captured intragastrically using an endoscope to facilitate jejunal placement. A dedicated gastrojejunostomy combination must be used, as basic gastrostomies cannot house jejunal extensions.

Jejunostomy A jejunostomy creates a stomal tract between the jejunum and the abdominal surface, and is usually a form of needle catheter jejunostomy (NCJ). Jejunostomy insertion is indicated when major gastrointestinal or hepatobiliary surgery necessitates postpyloric feeding (e.g. oesophagogastrectomy), or if the clinical condition increases likelihood of gastric stasis secondary to ileus or pseudoileus (e.g. acute pancreatitis). A feeding jejunostomy should be considered if gastric feeding has failed, and may provide a useful route to use to avoid parenteral nutrition. It is not uncommon for general surgeons to place nasogastric tubes as feeding jejunostomies. This practice is not recommended as tubes frequently block or become dislodged, and they possess no skin retention device like dedicated stoma devices.

Unlike the stomach and large bowel, small intestine motility returns within a few hours of surgery (Sax 1996) and a jejunostomy can be used for feeding within 12 hours.

A whole-protein feed should be well tolerated in jejunostomy feeding. However, if there is pancreatic or biliary insufficiency, or if the jejunostomy has been sited in the lower small bowel, a peptide-based or elemental feed is indicated. Feed usually commences at a low volume (20–30 ml/hour), increasing in 30–50 ml increments 4–6 hourly until the optimal feeding rate is achieved.

Enteral feed formulae

Enteral feeding formulae can be categorized into:

- whole-protein (polymeric) feeds, including disease-specific feeds
- elemental/peptide feeds.

A summary of enteral feeding products currently available in the UK can be found in Appendix 6.7.

Whole-protein (polymeric) feeds

These require an intact gut for their digestion and absorption.

Constituents of whole-protein feeds

- *Protein*: the protein source is usually derived from milk or hydrolysed casein, although soya protein formula is available for those with milk protein intolerance.
- *Carbohydrate*: this is usually in the form of maltodextrin, glucose, sucrose or corn syrup solids.
- *Dietary fibre*: This may be added to feed as soy polysaccharides or fructo-oligosaccharides (FOS). Soy polysaccharide comprises approximately one-third insoluble fibre and so is inadequate to alleviate constipation. There is little evidence to support improvement of bowel function or increased transit time with fibre-containing feeds compared with fibre-free equivalent in children or adults (Kapadia *et al*. 1995; Tolia *et al*. 1997). However, FOS may be beneficial for maintaining gut

ecology and function, rather than promoting bowel transit time. Fermentation of these soluble fibres to short-chain fatty acids may help establish good colonic physiology and function, but can also cause bloating and abdominal distension. The increased viscosity of fibre-containing feeds requires that they are administered via a tube of 1.5 mm internal diameter or greater, with pump assistance.

- *Fat*: the fat source is usually a vegetable oil derivative, although many feed companies are now reblending fats to alter the ratio of omega-3:omega-6 polyunsaturated fatty acids (PUFA), and increase the monounsaturated fat content. Omega-3 PUFA may be provided by the use of rapeseed (canola) oil, or fish oils to provide eicosapentaenoic acid (EPA) and docosahexaenoic acid (DHA) directly. Provision of omega-3 PUFA can down-regulate the inflammatory response by reducing arachidonic acid (omega-6 PUFA) metabolites, but the mechanism to convert omega-3 PUFA to the active EPA and DHA is impaired in the severely ill.
- *Vitamin, mineral and electrolytes*: all current UK suppliers of enteral feeds provide 100% of the reference nutrient intake (RNI) for micronutrients (excluding sodium and potassium) in a modest volume of feed (usually within 1–1.8 l of standard enteral feed). Current levels of fortification in some products are likely to change following the introduction of the Medical Food Regulations (2000) to implement the EC Directive on Dietary Foods for Special Medical Purposes (EC 1999).

Types of whole protein feeds

These can be categorized as:

- *Standard adult and paediatric formulae*: these provide 1 kcal/ml and are suitable for the majority of patients. They are available with and without fibre. Paediatric versions contain less protein, lower levels of fat-soluble vitamins and more calcium than adult formulae.
- *High-energy adult and paediatric formulae*: these provide between 1.2 and 2 kcal/ml and are useful for patients on fluid restriction, or with increased nutritional requirements such as burns. The electrolyte and protein content of these feeds is variable. Fibre-containing, energy-dense feeds are also available.
- *Disease-specific enteral formulae*: a variety of enteral feeds is provided by companies to encompass the continuum of clinical problems. However, dietitians should consider the usage of specific products within the context of the patient's clinical picture, and not take the manufacturer's recommended client group as the sole indication for use. Disease-specific feeds include:
  - *Renal feeds*: these contain reduced amounts of sodium, potassium and phosphate. The protein content is variable, providing similar or lower protein:calorie ratios compared with standard feeds. Energy-dense versions for fluid restriction are available, with subtle modification of other nutrients, e.g. higher water-soluble vitamin content to allow for intradialytic losses.

- *Low sodium feeds*: these are standard feeds with the sodium content reduced to around 10–15 mmol/l. Clinical hypernatraemia is often secondary to dehydration, and so the use of a standard feed (providing 35–40 mmol Na/l) still provides less sodium per litre than plasma levels. As uptake of water from the gut is dependent on the Na:glucose ratio, absorption of a very low sodium feed across a gradient into a plasma sodium of >145 mmol/l is rarely successful, with the resulting diarrhoea contributing further to hypernatraemia. Correction of hypernatraemia should be at a rate of no more than 6–10 mmol/l per day, to minimize brain damage (Arieff 1991).
- *Respiratory feeds*: these contain a higher percentage energy content from fat, which reduces the amount of carbon dioxide produced from feed metabolism, and may be useful in patients with respiratory failure. Avoidance of overfeeding is as clinically significant as the choice of feed in respiratory failure (Malone 1997). This topic is further discussed in Section 5.2 (Intensive care).
- *Immune feeds*: these feeds contain variable amounts of specific amino acids or fats, together with altered levels of specific micronutrients which have an immune benefit attributed to them. The additional nutrients added to such feeds include glutamine, arginine, dietary nucleotides, fish oils, beta-carotene and FOS. They are more expensive than standard feeds, although evidence is accumulating that they may benefit postsurgical or septic patients (Heys *et al.* 1999) (see Section 5.2, Intensive care).

Elemental/peptide feeds

These provide nitrogen in the form of free amino acids or peptides and are indicated in the presence of severe maldigestion or malabsorption.

The majority of patients can tolerate whole protein feeds, even in the presence of some degree of gut malfunction. However, with severe gut impairment a predigested formula may be indicated. Appropriate use of these feeds may reduce the requirement for parenteral nutrition (Hamaoui *et al.* 1990). The absorption of peptide feeds is superior to elemental solutions and may reduce the incidence of osmotic diarrhoea (Adibi 1990). There appears to be no clinical benefit in using peptide feed rather than whole protein feed in patients with Crohn's disease (Verma *et al.* 2000; see Section 4.10, Inflammatory bowel disease).

Drug–nutrient interactions

Enteral feeding may interfere with the dosage, presentation and action of many drugs. Crushing oral preparations to pass down a tube may compromise their activity. Some medications are not available in syrup form, and those in a sorbitol syrup base may induce diarrhoea in enterally fed patients given as little as 10 g sorbitol daily. Drugs should not be added to the feed infusion, as this may alter the stability of the medication and introduce a potential route of contamination into the enteral feed. Common drugs such as ciprofloxacin (Cohn *et al.* 1996), penicillin, sucralfate and theophylline all bind to the feed and/or have altered absorption kinetics, so should be administered during a rest period.

Oral phenytoin given with enteral feed forms complexes with calcium and protein, thus reducing its absorption by almost 80%, and reducing serum levels below therapeutic range. Feed should be halted for at least 1 hour pre- and post-dose. If this is not possible, then intravenous phenytoin administration should be considered.

Drugs such as cimetidine, aluminium hydroxide, chlorpromazine, lithium, metaclopromide and potassium chloride syrups are all physically incompatible with enteral feeds (Engle and Hannawa 1999).

Soy protein formulae may sequester warfarin, and the use of any enteral feed will antagonize warfarin therapy secondary to vitamin K content.

Complications of enteral feeding

Common complications associated with particular enteral feeding routes are summarized in Table 1.23.

Aspiration

Delayed gastric emptying (gastroparesis) may be a function of disease and its management, starvation, or intrinsic gastric disease such as the gastroparesis of diabetic neuropathy. Regurgitation of stomach contents and aspiration into the lungs can cause asphyxia; small amounts increase the risk of pneumonia. Aspiration risk increases with residual volumes of 200 ml or above (McClave *et al.* 1992), and

Table 1.23 Summary of complications associated with particular enteral feeding routes

Common complications	Enteral feeding route			
	Nasogastric	Nasojejunal	Gastrostomy	Jejunostomy
Aspiration	•	•	•	
Reflux	•	•	•	
Tube blockage	•	•		•
Tube displacement	•	•		
Intraperitoneal leakage			•	•
Gut infections		•		•
Candida tube occlusion			•	
Dumping syndrome		•		•
Secretory diarrhoea	•			

so elective aspiration of the gastric feeding tube 4-hourly is recommended to establish tolerance.

Aspiration risk for gastrostomy feeding is the same as for nasogastric feeding, and the initial placement may further interfere with the propulsive migratory motor complexes (MMCs) that assist gastric emptying.

Failure to establish gastric emptying is not a reason for immediate intravenous nutritional support. Reduced feed rate and the concurrent use of prokinetic agents should establish adequate emptying. Failing this, post-pyloric feeding should be considered.

If aspiration is a risk:

- Confirm the gastric position of the tube regularly.
- Elevate the head and upper body by at least 30 degrees and maintain this position during feeding and for 1 hour following feeding.
- Use prokinetic agents to stimulate gastric emptying such as metaclopromide, propulsid, erythromycin, domperidone or cyclazine.
- Consider a postpyloric feeding route. Jejunostomy feeding with aspiration of gastric contents by a nasogastric tube is the only safe way to prevent feed aspiration (Elpern 1997).

Diarrhoea

Diarrhoea is a common occurrence in enterally fed patients and is rarely attributable to the enteral feed. Prolonged use of antibiotics (especially third-generation cephalosporins and aminoglycosides) permits *Clostridium difficile* overgrowth and subsequent diarrhoea (Bliss *et al*. 1998). Enteral administration of magnesium or electrolytes can cause osmotic catharsis. Osmolality of the feed is rarely an issue, and feed dilution exacerbates the problem.

Measures which may help alleviate diarrhoea include:

- stool sample analysis to exclude pathogenic bacteria overgrowth
- use of probiotics and prebiotics (soluble fibre-containing feeds and/or a source of commensile *lactobacillus/ bifidobacterium* spp. bacteria in yoghurt or capsule form)
- prophylactic administration of *Saccharomyces boulardii* capsules (Bleichner *et al*. 1997)
- reduction in infusion rate of postpyloric feed
- converting to bolus feed from continuous feeding in intragastric infusions (Bowling *et al*. 1994)
- reviewing the need for and choice of antibiotic
- use of a peptide feed if malabsorption is suspected
- bile acid sequestrants (e.g. cholestyramine) if bile salt diarrhoea is suspected

Tube blockage

The small internal diameter (1–2 mm) of fine-bore tubes increases the risk of occlusion. The most common cause is coagulation of feed by drug syrups or suspensions combined with inadequate tube flushing, or obstruction by particles of crushed oral medications. Occasionally the coagulated feed may solidify around the tube externally, forming a hardened mass of feed and drug known as a bezoar, which increases in size over time and may eventually lead to gastrointestinal obstruction (Taylor *et al*. 1998).

Tube occlusion risk can be minimized by:

- flushing with water at regular intervals
- flushing tube with water following drug administration
- using drugs in syrup or linctus form rather than crushed tablets.

Several anecdotal methods are recommended to clear a blocked tube, ranging from lemonade or cola to pineapple juice (which contains bromelain, a weak protease) and alcoholic spirits. Pancreatic enzymes are effective, and can unclog a feeding tube within 10–20 minutes (Marcaud and Stegall 1990). Adding the contents of a Pancrex V (nonenteric coated enzyme replacement therapy) capsule to 1–2 ml water and injecting down the blocked tube is usually successful. Tube clearance should never be considered using the stylet alone, as tube perforation could occur.

Gastrostomy tube occlusion is less likely as tube sizes are larger (usually 14–20 FG). A common cause of tube blockage and fracture is *Candida* fungal overgrowth, which is usually transmitted during endoscopic placement. If this is suspected, the only effective action is to replace the gastrostomy.

Problems common to stoma feeding

Stoma site complications include leakage, exit-site infections, necrotizing fasciitis, pneumoperitoneum, intra-abdominal abscesses and problems with self-care secondary to poor placement (Hanlon 1998).

Small-bowel bacterial overgrowth secondary to lack of stomach acid can be minimized by the aseptic technique when setting up a jejunostomy feed. Regular assessment of the stoma site and enteral nutrition are important in the long term, with protocols if necessary to ensure continuity of care in the community.

Enteral feed delivery

Period of feeding

The period of feeding should be clearly stated on the feeding regimen, with nursing fluid balance charts used to confirm administration. Timing of feed should include feed breaks to encompass the psychosocial aspects of feeding, together with the influence on other clinical involvement, e.g. physiotherapy. Overnight feeding may supplement an inadequate daytime oral intake, but overnight fluid volume should be considered in the context of whether the patient has a urinary catheter.

Infusion rate

Bolus feeding Bolus feeding involves the delivery of 100–300 ml of feed over a 10–30 minute period several times per day. Administration is usually by syringe, using the syringe barrel as a funnel to allow the feed to infuse using gravity. Water can then be added to the barrel to flush the tube.

Intragastric bolus feeding may be useful in the agitated patient who dislodges feeding equipment and it also reduces secretory diarrhoea (Bowling *et al.* 1994), but fluctuations in carbohydrate supply may prove problematic in the diabetic patient.

Gravity feeding Patients may be continuously drip-fed by adjusting the roller clamp on the giving set. This involves calculating the drip rate, and adjusting it to administer the prescribed volume in a set time. This method of feed administration is more time-consuming and less accurate than pump-assisted feeding.

Continuous feeding Continuous feeding requires a feeding pump and pump set for administration, and if ready-to-hang formulae are not used, the additional cost of a feed reservoir. The cost of 'plastics' for enteral feeding can be reduced by contract pricing, and there is a move towards hospital-community contracts to provide cost-effective enteral nutrition.

Intermittent continuous feeding for periods of 8–20 hours promotes antibacterial conditions in the gut, as gastric pH drops below 2.5 if feed delivery is interrupted for periods of 4 hours or more. The substantial rest period allows for feed to 'catch up' if it has been interrupted during the day, and also allows an overnight break for those without urinary catheterization, who may otherwise experience nocturia and interrupted sleep.

Microbiological aspects of enteral feeding

Enteral feeds provide an ideal growth medium for microbial contamination, and so should be handled cleanly. There is much evidence in laboratory conditions of the ability to contaminate feed by handling (Anderton and Nwoguh 1991; Beatie *et al.* 1996) but little published evidence in the clinical environment. Readers are reminded that normal food and diets are not sterile, and that low counts of non-pathogenic bacteria are clinically unimportant. To cause food poisoning, a significant number of pathogenic bacteria must be present. Bacterial growth within the feed can be minimized by practices such as:

- limiting the 'hanging time' of the feed to a maximum of 24 hours
- replacement of the reservoir and giving set daily
- aseptic addition of substances to feed if necessary (e.g. sterile water, intravenous electrolytes).

These practices are sufficient for patients with normal gastric function. Additional care should be taken with jejunal feeds, in patients with achlorhydria and immunosuppressed patients, as the lack of gastric acidity and impaired immune function may increase infection risk. Preparation techniques demonstrated to reduce the bacterial contamination risk include:

- priming the feeding set on an alcohol-treated metal tray
- spraying the bottle opener and top with 70% alcohol
- wearing non-sterile disposable gloves
- filling the feeding reservoir with feed for up to 24 hours' use rather than only 4 hours (Patchell *et al.* 1998).

Inadvertent intravenous administration of enteral feed

Gravity and pump administration sets are clearly marked 'not for intravenous use', but the availability of dual-option luer ends increases the risk of connection to an intravenous line. Parenteral administration of an enteral feed causes septic shock. Two or more emergency cycles of plasmapheresis may improve the chances of recovery (Ong and Soo 1997).

Home enteral feeding

Home enteral feeding is an expanding area of nutritional support (Ireton-Jones *et al.* 1997), with the majority of home enteral-fed patients having stroke or head and neck cancer (McNamara *et al.* 2000). The dietitian's role in the discharge into the community of patients on nutritional support is integral to the process. Local policies and procedures should be in place for training, discharge planning and monitoring of the patient (Elia *et al.* 1994).

Pressure on hospital beds often leads to early discharge of enterally fed patients, so it is important that patients are reviewed regularly during the initial period to ensure that optimal nutrition support is achieved. Patient support groups, such as Patients on Intravenous and Nasogastric Therapy (PINNT), are useful for some patients.

Enteral feeds in the community are available on prescription, but the feed equipment ('plastics') is financed by the community budget (usually the district nurse budget or nursing home if the patient is a resident). Determination of who pays for the plastics must be confirmed before the patient is discharged. Most UK feed companies provide training, delivery of feeds and equipment, and servicing of pumps to community patients.

In planning a home discharge, the dietitian should (Elia *et al.* 1994):

- Follow the local policy/procedure for enteral feeding discharge (if there is one).
- Contact the general practitioner regarding feed prescription and any concerns regarding nutrition support and clinical monitoring.
- Contact the district nurse/nursing home regarding specific plastics needs, and budget codes allocation for payment of plastics used.
- Contact the referring dietitian or healthcare professional in the home area taking responsibility for care provision regarding nutritional concerns and biochemical and physical monitoring.
- Ensure that the patient/carer is familiar with management of the feeding tube, clean handling and administration of feed, repeat prescriptions, and feed and plastics home delivery processes.
- Liaise with patient/carer and other relevant individuals to design a suitable feeding regimen, taking into consideration normal home routines and patient/carer preferences, and provision of written information related to nutrition support.

- Provide contact numbers of relevant professionals, and useful numbers (local feed company representative or helpline) so that help can be obtained if required.

Weaning from enteral nutrition

Once the patient recovers sufficiently to achieve a safe swallow (i.e. is not at risk of aspirating food or fluid into the lungs) weaning from feed can be considered. Feeding can be continued in conjunction with an oral diet, but halting the feed for a time may encourage more of an appetite. If the feed is halted, the rate can be increased later to compensate, or the feed can continue to provide less than 100% of predicted requirements if energy status is not a problem.

Care should be taken to ensure that patients do not become dehydrated during the weaning schedule. If necessary, feed can be given as a bolus during the day if meal consumption is inadequate, with continuous administration overnight. Increasing the overnight feed rate in a patient without urinary catheterization should be avoided to prevent nocturia and interrupted sleep pattern. Concentrated feed can be administered at a lower volume, with fluid balance made up during the day enterally or orally.

Text revised by: Catherine Collins, Briony Thomas and Lisa Cooper

Acknowledgement: The British Dietetic Association's Parenteral and Enteral Nutrition Group (PENG).

Useful addresses

American Society for Enteral and Parenteral Nutrition
Website: www.clinnutr.org

British Association for Parenteral and Enteral Nutrition (BAPEN)
PO Box 922, Maidenhead, Berks SL6 4SH

King's Fund Centre
11–13 Cavendish Square, London W1M 0AN

Parenteral and Enteral Nutrition Group (PENG)
c/o The British Dietetic Association, 5th Floor, Elizabeth House, 22 Suffolk Street Queensway, Birmingham B1 1LS

Patients on Intravenous and Nasogastric Therapy (PINNT)
c/o Mrs Carolyn Wheatley, PO Box 3126, Christchurch, Dorset BH23 2XS
Tel/Fax: 01202 481625

Further reading

BAPEN (British Association of Parenteral and Enteral Nutrition) publications:
- BAPEN. *Current Perspectives in Enteral Nutrition*. Maidenhead: BAPEN, 1999.
- Elia M, Cottee S, Holden C *et al*. *Enteral and Parenteral Nutrition in the Community*. BAPEN Working Party Report. Maidenhead: BAPEN, 1994.

- McAtear CA, Arrowsmith H, McWhirter J *et al*. *Current Perspectives on Enteral Nutrition in Adults*. BAPEN Working Party Report. Maidenhead: BAPEN, 1999.
- Pennington CR. *Current Perspectives on Parenteral Nutrition in Adults*. BAPEN Working Party Report. Maidenhead: BAPEN, 1996.
- Silk DBA, Cottam TK, Neilsen MS *et al*. *Organisation of Nutrition Support in Hospitals*. BAPEN Working Party Report. Maidenhead: BAPEN, 1994.
- Sizer T, Russell CA, Wood S *et al*. *Standards and Guidelines for Nutritional Support of Patients in Hospitals*. BAPEN Working Party Report. Maidenhead: BAPEN, 1996.
- Wood S, Shaffer J, Wheatley C. *Home Parenteral Nutrition*. BAPEN Working Party Report. Maidenhead: BAPEN, 1995.

PENG (Parenteral and Enteral Nutrition Group of the British Dietetic Association) publications:
PENG. *Dietetic Standards for Nutritional Support*. Birmingham: British Dietetic Association, 1996.
PENG. *Adult Enteral and Parenteral Nutrition. Guidelines for Dietitians in Training*. Birmingham: British Dietetic Association, 1996.
PENG. *A Pocket Guide to Clinical Nutrition*, 2nd edn. Micklewright A, Todorovic V (eds). Birmingham: British Dietetic Association, 1997.

References

Adibi SA. Physiological significance and practical application of peptide transport in human intestine. *Nutrition* 1990; **6**: 267–268.

American Dietetic Association (ADA). Position Paper. The role of registered dietitians in enteral and parenteral nutrition support. *Journal of the American Dietetic Association* 1997; **97**: 302–304.

Anderton A, Nwoguh CE. Bacterial colonisation of enteral feeding tubes. *Journal of Human Nutrition and Dietetics* 1991; **4**: 273–280.

Arieff AI. Treatment of symptomatic hyponatremia. *Critical Care Medicine* 1991; **19**: 748–751.

Asch DA, Faber-Langendoen K, Shea JA, Christakis NA. The sequence of withdrawing life-sustaining treatment from patients. *American Journal of Medicine* 1999; **107**: 153–156.

Baker JP, Detsky AS, Wesson DS *et al*. Nutritional assessment: a comparison of clinical judgement and objective measurements. *New England Journal of Medicine* 1982; **306**: 969–972.

Beatie T, Anderton A, White S. Aspiration of gastric residuals – a cause of bacterial contamination of enteral feeding systems? *Journal of Human Nutrition and Dietetics* 1996; **9**: 105–115.

Bleichner G, Blehaut H, Mentec H, Moyse D. *Saccharomyces boulardii* prevents diarrhea in critically ill tube-fed patients. A multicenter, randomized, double-blind placebo-controlled trial. *International Care Medicine* 1997; **23**: 517–523.

Bliss DZ, Johnson S, Savik K *et al*. Acquisition of *Clostridium difficile* and *Clostridium difficile*-associated diarrhea in hospitalized patients receiving tube feeding. *Annals of Internal Medicine* 1998; **129**: 1012–1019.

Bowling TE, Raimundo AH, Grimble GK *et al*. Colonic secretory effect in response to enteral feeding in humans. *Gut* 1994; **35**: 1734–1741.

British Dietetic Association/Dietitians Board. *Guidance on Standards for Records and Record Keeping*. Birmingham: BDA, 1996.

British Medical Association. *Witholding or Withdrawing Life-prolonging Medical Treatment. Guidelines for Decision Making*. London: BMA Publications, 1999.

Chima C, Barco K, Dewitt ML *et al*. Relationship of nutritional status to length of stay, hospital costs, and discharge status of patients hospitalised in the medicine service. *Journal of the American Dietetic Association* 1997; **97**: 975–978.

Cohn SM, Sawyer MD, Burns GA *et al*. Enteric absorption of ciprofloxacin during tube feeding in the critically ill. *Journal of Antimicrobial Chemotherapy* 1996; **38**: 871–876.

Elia M, Cottee S, Holden C *et al*. *Enteral and Parenteral Nutrition in the Community*. BAPEN Working Party Report. Maidenhead: BAPEN, 1994.

Elpern EH. Pulmonary aspiration in hospitalized adults. *Nutrition in Clinical Practice* 1997; **12**: 5–13.

Engle KK, Hannawa TE. Techniques for administering oral medications to critical care patients receiving continuous enteral feed. *American Journal of Health-System Pharmacy* 1999; **56**: 1441–1444.

European Community (EC). Commission Directive on Dietary Foods for Special Medical Purposes. 1999/21/EC of 25 March 1999. *Official Journal of the European Communities* 1999; L91/29–L91/35.

Gallagher-Allred C, Voss AC, Finn SC, McCamish MA. Malnutrition and clinical outcomes: the case for medical nutrition therapy. *Journal of the American Dietetic Association* 1996; **96**: 361–366.

Godil A, Chen YK. Percutaneous endoscopic gastrostomy for nutrition support in pregnancy associated with hyperemesis gravidarum and anorexia nervosa. *Journal of Parenteral and Enteral Nutrition* 1998; **22**: 238–241.

Green CJ on behalf of the Council of the British Association for Parenteral and Enteral Nutrition (BAPEN). Existence, causes and consequences of disease-related malnutrition in the hospital and the community, and clinical and financial benefits of nutritional intervention. *Clinical Nutrition* 1999; **18** (Suppl 2): 3–28.

Hamaoui E, Lefkowitz R, Olender L *et al*. Enteral nutrition in the early postoperative period: a new semi-elemental formula versus total parenteral nutrition. *Journal of Parenteral and Enteral Nutrition* 1990; **14**: 501–507.

Hanlon MD. Preplacement marking for optimal gastrostomy and jejunostomy tube site locations to decrease complications and promote self-care. *Nutrition in Clinical Practice* 1998; **13**: 167–171.

Heys SD, Walker LG, Smith I, Eremin O. Enteral nutritional supplementation with key nutrients in patients with critical illness and cancer: a meta-analysis of randomized controlled clinical trials. *Annals of Surgery* 1999; **229**: 467–477.

Ireton-Jones C, Orr M, Hennessy K. Clinical pathways in home nutrition support. *Journal of the American Dietetic Association* 1997; **97**: 1003–1007.

Kapadia SA, Raimundo AH, Grimble GK *et al*. Influence of three different fiber-supplemented enteral diets on bowel function and short-chain fatty acid production. *Journal of Parenteral and Enteral Nutrition* 1995; **19**: 63–68.

Kirby DF, Teran JC. Enteral feeding in critical care, gastrointestinal diseases, and cancer. *Gastrointestinal Endoscopy Clinics of North America* 1998; **8**: 623–643.

Kleiner SM. Water: an essential but overlooked nutrient. *Journal of the American Dietetic Association* 1999; **99**: 200–206.

Luttrell S. Editorial. End of life decisions. Withdrawing or withholding life-prolonging treatment. *British Medical Journal* 1999; **318**: 1709–1710.

McAtear CA, Arrowsmith H, McWhirter J *et al*. *Current Perspectives on Enteral Nutrition in Adults*. BAPEN Working Party Report. Maidenhead: BAPEN, 1999.

McClave SA, Snider HL, Lowen CC *et al*. Use of residual volume as a marker for enteral feeding intolerance: prospective blinded comparison with physical examination and radiographic findings. *Journal of Parenteral and Enteral Nutrition* 1992; **16**: 99–105.

McClave SA, Snider HL, Spain DA. Preoperative issues in clinical nutrition. *Chest* 1999; **115**: 64S–70S.

McNamara EP, Flood P, Kennedy NP. Enteral tube feeding in the community: survey of adult patients discharged from a Dublin hospital. *Clinical Nutrition* 2000; **19**: 15–22.

Main BJ, Morrison DL. Development of a clinical pathway for enteral nutrition. *Nutrition in Clinical Practice* 1998; **13**: 20–24.

Malone AM. Is a pulmonary enteral formula warranted for patients with pulmonary dysfunction? *Nutrition in Clinical Practice* 1997; **12**: 168–171.

Marcaud SP, Stegall KS. Unclogging feeding tubes with pancreatic enzyme. *Journal of Parenteral and Enteral Nutrition* 1990; **14**: 198–200.

Medical Food (England) Regulations 2000. Statutory Instrument 2000/845. London: The Stationery Office, 2000.

Metheny NA, Eisenberg P, Spies M. Aspiration pneumonia in patients fed through nasoenteral tubes. *Heart and Lung* 1986; **15**: 256–261.

Ong BC, Soo KC. Plasmapheresis in the treatment of inadvertent intravenous infusion of an enteral feeding solution. *Journal of Clinical Apheresis* 1997; **12**: 200–201.

Parenteral and Enteral Nutrition Group of the British Dietetic Association (PENG). *Dietetic Standards for Nutritional Support*. Birmingham, British Dietetic Association, 1996.

Patchell CJ, Anderton A, Holden C *et al*. Reducing bacterial contamination of enteral feeds. *Archives of Disease in Childhood* 1998; **78**: 166–168.

Payne-James JJ, De Gara CJ, Grimble GK *et al*. Artificial nutrition support in hospitals in the United Kingdom – 1991. Second national survey. *Clinical Nutrition* 1992; **11**: 187–192.

Potter J, Langhorne P, Roberts M *et al*. Routine protein energy supplementation in adults: systematic review. *British Medical Journal* 1999; **317**: 495–501.

Preston RA. *Acid–Base, Fluids and Electrolytes Made Ridiculously Simple*, 3rd edn. Miami, FL: MedMaster, 1998.

Rabeneck L, McCullough LB, Wray NP. Ethically justified, clinically comprehensive guidelines for percutaneous endoscopic gastrostomy tube placement. *Lancet* 1997; **349**: 496–498.

Rey JR, Axon A, Budzynska A *et al*. Guidelines of the European Society of Gastrointestinal Endoscopy (ESGE). Antibiotic prophylaxis for gastrointestinal endoscopy. *Endoscopy* 1998; **30**: 318–324.

Robertson SM. How much of the prescribed volume of enteral feed does the hospitalized patient actually receive? *Journal of Human Nutrition and Dietetics* 1990; **3**: 165–170.

Sax HC. Early nutritional support in critical illness is important. *Critical Care Clinics* 1996; **12**: 661–666.

Serrano P, Velloso A, Garcia-Luna PP *et al*. Enteral nutrition by percutaneous endoscopic gastrojejunostomy in severe hyperemesis gravidarum: a report of two cases. *Clinical Nutrition* 1998; **17**: 135–139.

Silk DBA, Cottam TK, Neilsen MS *et al*. *Organisation of Nutrition Support in Hospitals*. BAPEN Working Party Report. Maidenhead: BAPEN, 1994.

Singh A, Smoak BL, Patterson KY *et al*. Biochemical indices of selected trace minerals in men: effect of stress. *American Journal of Clinical Nutrition* 1991; **53**: 126–131.

Sizer T, Russell CA, Wood S *et al*. *Standards and Guidelines for Nutritional Support of Patients in Hospitals*. BAPEN Working Party Report. Maidenhead: BAPEN, 1996.

Taylor JR, Streetman DS, Castle SS. Medication bezoars: a literature review and report of a case. *Annals of Pharmacotherapy* 1998; **32**: 940–946.

Tibbitts GM, Sorrell RJ. Duodenal obstruction from a gastric feeding tube. *New England Journal of Medicine* 1999; **340**: 970–971.

Tolia V, Ventimiglia J, Kuhns L. Gastrointestinal tolerance of a pediatric fiber formula in developmentally disabled children. *Journal of the American College of Nutrition* 1997; **16**: 224–228.

Verma S, Brown S, Kirkwood B, Gaiffer MH. Polymeric versus elemental diet as primary treatment in active Crohn's disease: a randomized, double-blind trial. *American Journal of Gastroenterology* 2000; **95**: 735–739.

Woo J, Ho SC, Mak YT *et al*. Nutritional status of elderly patients during recovery from chest infection and the role of nutritional supplementation assessed by a prospective randomized single-blind trial. *Age and Ageing* 1994; **23**: 40–44.

1.14 Enteral feeding in paediatric patients

The general principles and practice of enteral feeding are discussed in detail in Section 1.13.2 (Enteral feeding). This section highlights some of the issues to be considered when paediatric patients need to be enterally fed. For more detailed information, the reader is referred to *Clinical Paediatric Dietetics* (see Further Reading).

1.14.1 Basic considerations of enteral feeding in paediatric patients

Nutritional support in children requires a number of different considerations to those in adults:

Nutritional needs for growth

In children, estimations of energy and nutrient requirements have to allow for normal growth as well as all other metabolic needs (including any metabolic consequences of illness or injury). The nutritional requirements of a child can vary widely with age and circumstances and no single standard commercially available feed will be appropriate for the nutritional needs of all paediatric patients.

Problems resulting from nutritional deficiency are most likely to occur in infancy. Infants and children have fewer body reserves of all nutrients, particularly energy, than adults. For example, an adult has sufficient energy stores for approximately 90 days and a full-term infant for about 32 days, but a preterm infant may only have sufficient for 5 days (Heird 1977). If an infant or child is unable to feed orally, it is more imperative that nutritional support is started quickly.

Interruption of normal feeding development

Normally during infancy and early childhood, new feeding skills are being learnt and developed. If an infant or young child is tube-fed for any length of time during this critical period and no oral food or drink is consumed, it may adversely affect and delay normal feeding behaviour. In paediatrics it is therefore vital, wherever possible, that oral consumption at some level is encouraged.

Effects of malnutrition

In infants and children, poor nutritional support may result not only in growth failure and inadequate growth, but also in immunodeficiency, apathetic and withdrawn behaviour, widespread gastrointestinal dysfunction, reduced muscle power and myocardial dysfunction (Booth and MacDonald 1990).

1.14.2 Indications for enteral feeding in paediatric patients

There are five broad indications for enteral feeding in children:

Inadequate energy and nutrient intake

Anorexia associated with chronic illness, and inability to eat adequate quantities of food, are common problems in children. Categories of patients requiring enteral feeding include infants with breathing difficulties associated with respiratory and cardiac disorders, and infants and children with orofacial malformations and oral–motor incoordination, where normal sucking and chewing mechanisms are impaired (Stapleford 1989). Children with degenerative disease who can no longer eat or drink, and children with chronic illnesses such as malignancy, cystic fibrosis and renal disease are also frequently enterally fed.

Increased nutritional requirements

Many infants and children with chronic or severe illnesses have a need for extra nutrients, particularly energy, but owing to the anorexia associated with their disease are unable to meet their nutritional requirements by normal eating. Disease states where this commonly occurs include liver disease, cystic fibrosis and congenital heart disease. However, tube feeding is normally only initiated when a child struggles to gain weight and grow adequately on an oral diet after appropriate dietary advice. In many cases, the feed is given as an overnight continuous infusion so that the child can eat 'normally' during the day, and it will supply a varying percentage of the patient's nutritional needs depending on the child's clinical condition and overall appetite. It is often stated that overnight feeding will not decrease the appetite during the day (Stapleford 1989); in practice, children's intake at breakfast time is often reduced, but their appetite improves during the morning.

Disease or injury to the oesophagus

Examples in children include oesophageal injury after ingestion of caustic soda chemicals or tracheo-oesophageal fistula.

Gastrointestinal disease

Infants and children with a very short bowel following resection may absorb nutrients more efficiently if their nutrition is given as continuous enteral feed rather than as intermittent bottle feeds. In addition, enteral feeds (either elemental, semielemental or polymeric feeds) may be used in Crohn's disease to treat growth failure and induce remission of the disease (see Section 4.10, Inflammatory bowel disease). Other indications for enteral feeding are children with severe oesophageal reflux requiring continuous pump feeds, gastrointestinal malformation and/or malabsorption.

Metabolic disease

Infants and children with type 1 glycogen storage disease need a continuous enteral feed overnight to avoid hypoglycaemia.

1.14.3 Choice of enteral feed

The choice of feed is dependent upon the age, weight, activity and clinical condition of the child. There are four main categories of feeds:

- whole protein
- protein hydrolysate
- modular
- elemental.

Whole-protein feeds are used primarily for children with a normal gut, while protein hydrolysate, modular and elemental feeds are used for children with defective bowel function.

Feeding paediatric patients with normal gut function

Infants aged 0–12 months

Infants less than 4 months of age can be given either expressed breast milk (EBM) or an infant formula milk at a fluid volume of 150–180 ml/kg body weight. Infants failing to achieve adequate weight gain on full volumes of EBM or infant formula, or who are over the age of 4 months, require additional calories. Traditionally, this has been achieved using a glucose polymer. This is gradually introduced in 1–2 g/100 ml increments to a total of 10–15 g carbohydrate/100 ml (depending on the age of the infant). Further energy supplementation can be achieved by the use of fat emulsion, added in 1 g/100 ml increments to a total fat concentration of 5–6 g/100 ml.

Recently, there has been a trend towards providing additional energy by concentrating the infant formula. This has the advantage of maintaining the energy:protein ratio, which is thought to be particularly important for catch-up growth. Manipulation of feed concentration should always be supervised by a dietitian. There are some concerns about the accuracy of such feeds being made up at home and it is essential that parents are given clear written instructions.

A simpler, and possibly better, alternative to concentrating feeds is to use one of the recently developed nutritionally complete, high-energy infant feeds (Table 1.24). These provide 91–100 kcal/100 ml and are suitable for infants from birth to 12–18 months. They are available on prescription.

Children 1–6 years or 8–20 kg with normal gut function

Adult feeds are not suitable for this age group because of their high content of protein, sodium and potassium and their inappropriate vitamin and mineral profile. Paediatric feeds have therefore been formulated to meet the nutritional needs of this age group (Table 1.24). Until recently these have been based on the recommendations of the Joint Working Party of the Paediatric and Parenteral and Enteral Nutrition Groups of the British Dietetic Association (BDA 1988). These have now been superseded by the EC Directive on Dietary Foods for Special Medical Uses (EC 1999), which requires all proprietary enteral feeds (and other products classified as medical foods) to conform to defined compositional standards by November 2001. Details of the new compositional requirements can be obtained from the Infant and Dietetic Foods Association (IDFA) (the address is given at the end of this section) or directly from enteral feed manufacturers. The EC Directive expresses nutritional compositional data for products in just two age categories: below the age of 1 year, and from the age of 1 year to adulthood. The wide age band of the latter group means that, with the exception of calcium and vitamin D levels (where levels appropriate for 1–10 year olds are stated), recommended nutrient content is given as a very broad range. This makes it difficult for a dietitian to know what level within this range is appropriate for a young paediatric patient. For this reason, the 1988 paediatric feed compositional guidelines are given in Table 1.25 to provide some indication of the likely needs of patients aged 1–6, although it must be emphasized that these figures are provided for guidance only. It should also be noted that the nutritional recommendations in the EC Directive are quoted per 100 kcal, whereas the BDA (1988) guidelines are given per 100 ml feed.

Proprietary paediatric enteral feeds available are based on cows' milk for their protein source and provide either 1 kcal/ml or 1.5 kcal/ml. High energy feeds are indicated for children with raised energy requirements or for those who can only tolerate small volumes of feed. Paediatric feeds with fibre are also available.

Children over 6 years (>20 kg) with normal gut function

Any commercially available standard enteral feed is suitable for paediatric patients, as long as it is given in appropriate volumes. However, care needs to be exercised when using high-energy feeds for older children as these products have a high protein content. They may be required for overnight

Table 1.24   Products suitable for paediatric enteral feeding

Type of product	Indications	Examples
Whole-protein feeds	Infants (0–18 months or <8 kg body weight)	Infatrini (Nutricia Clinical Care) SMA High Energy (SMA)
	Children (1–6 years or 8–20 kg body weight): • Standard energy (1 kcal/ml)	Frebini Original (Fresenius Kabi) Isosource Junior (Novartis Consumer Health) Novasource Junior (Novartis Junior) Nutrini (Nutricia Clinical Care) Nutrini Fibre (Nutricia Clinical Care) Paediasure (Abbott) Paediasure with fibre (Abbott) Sondalis Junior (Nestlé Clinical Nutrition)
	• High energy (1.5 kcal/ml)	Nutrini Extra (Nutricia Clinical Care) Paediasure Plus (Abbott) Resource Junior (Novartis Consumer Health) Sondalis Junior (Nestlé Clinical Nutrition)
Protein hydrolysate feeds		Alfaré (Nestlé Clinical Nutrition) Nutramigen (Mead Johnson) PeptiJunior (Cow & Gate) Pregestimil (Mead Johnson)
Elemental/semi-elemental feeds		Elemental 028 (SHS) Elemental 028 Extra (SHS) Elemental 028 Extra Liquid (SHS) Neocate (SHS) Neocate Advance (SHS) Pepdite (SHS) Pepdite 1+ (SHS)
Modular feed components • Protein sources		Comminuted Chicken (SHS) Complete amino acid mix (SHS) Powdered protein sources such as Casilan 90 (Heinz), Maxipro (SHS), ProMod (Abbott), Protifar (Nutricia Clinical Care), Vitapro (Vitaflo)
• Carbohydrate sources (glucose polymers)		Caloreen (Nestlé Clinical Nutrition) Maxijul (SHS) Polycal (Nutricia Clinical Care) Nutrition) Polycose (Abbott) Vitajoule (Vitaflo)
• Fat sources: LCT fat emulsion		Calogen (SHS) Solagen (SHS)
MCT fat emulsion		Liquigen (SHS)
• Fat + carbohydrate		Duocal (SHS)

Data compiled 2001.
Full compositional details of these products and prescribing indications can be found in the British National Formulary or the Monthly Index of Medical Specialities (MIMS), or obtained directly from the manufacturers (for addresses see Appendix 6.9).

enteral feeds for some older paediatric patients who need a high-energy feed in a small volume. If these feeds are used, it is important to monitor overall protein intake to ensure that this is not excessive.

Feeding paediatric patients with defective bowel function

Protein hydrolysate feeds

The majority of infants and young patients with protracted diarrhoea, short bowel syndrome or cow's milk protein enteropathy who need a tube feed can usually tolerate a commercially available standard protein hydrolysate feed (Table 1.24). If additional energy is required, concentrated feeds or glucose polymers with or without LCT fat emulsion can be used as described above.

Pepdite 1+ (SHS) is a protein hydrolysate designed for children over 1 year of age. For children over 6 years of age, adult semi-elemental feeds may be used.

Modular feeds

If protein hydrolysate feeds are not tolerated, it may be necessary to use a modular feed based on separate protein,

Table 1.25 Recommended composition of paediatric enteral feeds for the 1–6-year-old age group (BDA Paediatric Group/PENG, 1988)[1]

	Nutrient	Recommended content per 100 ml feed for patients aged 1–6 years (BDA 1988)
Energy and macronutrients	Energy	100 kcal
	Protein	2.6 g
	Fat	4.0 g
	Carbohydrate	13.5 g
Minerals and trace elements	Sodium	2.5 mmol
	Potassium	2.5 mmol
	Calcium	55 mg
	Phosphorus	1.7 mmol
	Iron	0.7 mg
	Zinc	0.7 mg
	Manganese	0.1 mg
	Selenium	4 μg
	Molybdenum	5 μg
	Copper	0.1 mg
	Iodine	6 μg
	Chromium	4 μg
Vitamins	Vitamin A	35 μg
	Vitamin D	0.7 μg
	Vitamin E	0.4 mg
	Vitamin K	2 μg
	Vitamin C	3 mg
	Vitamin B_1	0.15 mg
	Vitamin B_2	0.2 mg
	Nicotinic acid	0.8 mg
	Vitamin B_6	0.09 mg
	Folic acid	12 μg
	Vitamin B_{12}	0.2 μg
	Pantothenic acid	0.3 mg
	Inositol	15 mg
	Biotin	6 μg
	Choline	15 mg

[1]These figures have now been superseded by the EC Directive on Dietary Foods for Special Medical Purposes (EC 1999) but are given here as guidance on the likely nutritional needs of 1–6 year olds (see accompanying text in *Section 1.14.3*, Children 1–6 years with normal gut function). It should be noted that the figures above are expressed per 100 ml feed, whereas the EC Directive gives recommendations in terms of per 100 kcal.

fat, carbohydrate, vitamin and mineral components so the individual ingredients and their quantities used can be adapted to meet the specific needs and tolerances of an infant and child (Table 1.24). A commonly protein source used is the product Comminuted Chicken (SHS), which is simply finely ground chicken meat in water. A variety of carbohydrates may be used, including glucose polymers, sucrose and fructose, and either a long-chain or medium-chain fat emulsion (or combination of the two) added as the fat source. A comprehensive mineral and vitamin supplement is also given.

The chief advantage of modular feeds is their flexibility; the ingredients can be changed or adjusted relatively easily. However, they are complex, require detailed calculations and accurate weighing and measuring facilities, and mistakes can be made in their calculation and preparation; it also takes several days to build the feed up to full strength. In addition, if Comminuted Chicken is given via a continuous enteral feed, the chicken fibres have a ten-

dency to block the tube. To avoid this, Comminuted Chicken can be thickened with 0.5% Nestargel, and a slightly wider bore nasogastric tube may be required.

Elemental feeds

Elemental diets are used in children with multiple food intolerance, short gut syndrome, other malabsorption syndromes and sometimes Crohn's disease. With the exception of the infant preparations Neocate and Neocate Advance (SHS), elemental preparations based on amino acids have been formulated for adults and are generally high in protein with a variable content of electrolytes, vitamins and minerals. The elemental and semi-elemental feeds such as Elemental 028 Extra (SHS) and Pepdite 1+ (SHS) contain less protein than other similar feeds and have acceptable electrolyte, vitamin and mineral profiles, but these need to be matched to the specific nutritional requirements of the individual child being fed. Elemental 028 Extra has a very high osmolality and tolerance is improved by careful introduction. Many children find these preparations unpalatable and they usually need to be given via a nasogastric tube.

1.14.4 Enteral feeding tubes and equipment

Nasogastric feeding

Either polyvinyl chloride (PVC) or polyurethane nasogastric tubes may be used. PVC tubes are generally used for short-term feeding and for children who vomit repeatedly (e.g. patients on chemotherapy or with reflux). Polyurethane tubes are usually used for longer term feeding.

Gastrostomy feeding

Gastrostomy feeding is usually considered for infants and children requiring long-term nutritional support or children who do not tolerate a nasogastric tube. The advantages are that it is more comfortable, the discomfort of frequent tube changes is avoided and the tube can be hidden by clothes. The main complications are leakage and infection around the gastrostomy site; carers therefore need to be educated regarding care of the site.

Common practice is for a percutaneous endoscopic gastrostomy (PEG) to be inserted in the first instance. This may be changed to a gastrostomy button at a later date. These low-profile devices are particularly popular with teenagers, in whom body image may be of more concern.

Enteral feeding pumps

The administration of enteral feeds which are given continuously should be controlled by an enteral feeding pump. Desirable features of a pump suitable for paediatrics include accuracy, a reliable alarm system and the delivery of feeds in 1 ml increments up to 50 ml/hour, and thereafter in 5 ml or 10 ml increments. Ideally, they should also be lightweight, portable and easy to use.

1.14.5 Home enteral feeding

Enteral nutrition for children is increasingly being given at home as the advantages of home treatment over long term hospitalization are recognized, along with the positive effect of improved nutrition in chronic disease (McCarey *et al.* 1996).

Before discharge from hospital, parents and carers need to be competent in all aspects of enteral feeding. Particular emphasis should be placed on safety during parent training. The parent's teaching programme should include familiarization with the feeding equipment, safety aspects, any preparation of special feeds and discussion of any problems that they are likely to encounter at home. The child also needs to be psychologically prepared for enteral feeding, and dolls and teddies with enteral tubes attached, photographs of other children receiving enteral feeds, colouring booklets, reward stickers and certificates are all helpful in making enteral feeding a more acceptable process (Holden 1990).

Older children requiring nasogastric feeds are usually taught and encouraged to pass their own nasogastric tube. Some prefer to remove this before going to school and repass it every night. The timing of enteral feeds should be arranged as much as possible to fit in with the child's normal routine. Information obtained from an initial dietary assessment, in respect of the child's feeding skills, feeding patterns, family routine and food tolerance, is essential for formulating an acceptable feeding plan.

In a survey of 35 patients on home enteral feeding, no major complications such as aspiration or entanglement in the tubing were found (Holden *et al.* 1991). However, problems such as nocturia, vomiting, diarrhoea, gastrooesophageal reflux and excess weight gain can occur (Booth and MacDonald 1990). It is essential that good hospital and community support is provided for infants and children on home enteral feeding, and that there is regular monitoring of growth, nutritional intake and food intolerance.

Text revised by: Alison Coates

Useful address

Infant and Dietetic Foods Association (IDFA)
IDFA Secretariat, 6 Catherine Street, London WC2B 5JJ
Tel: 020 7836 2460
Website: www.idfa.org.uk

Further reading

Hussain A, Woolfrey S, Massey J *et al.* Percutaneous endoscopic gastrostomy. *Postgraduate Medical Journal* 1996; **72**: 581–585.

Shaw V, Lawson M (Eds). *Clinical Paediatric Dietetics*, 2nd edn. Oxford: Blackwell Science, 2001.

References

Booth IW, MacDonald A. Nutrition. In Insley JA (Ed.) *Paediatric Vade Mecam*. London: Edward Arnold, 1990.

British Dietetic Association Paediatric Group/Parenteral and Enteral Nutrition Group (PENG). Report of a Joint Working Party. Birmingham: BDA, 1988.

European Community (EC). *Directive on Dietary Foods for Special Medical Purposes* (1992/21/EC), OJ L91 p29, 7.4.1999.

Heird WC. Feeding the premature infant human milk or artificial formula. *American Journal of Diseases of Children* 1977; **131**: 468–469.

Holden C. Home enteral feeding. *Paediatric Nursing* 1990; **2**: 14–16.

Holden C, Puntis J, Charlton C, Booth IW. Home enteral nutrition acceptability and safety. *Archives of Disease in Childhood* 1991; **66**: 148–151.

McCarey DW, Buchanan E, Gregory M *et al.* Home enteral feeding of children in the West of Scotland. *Scottish Medical Journal* 1996; **41**: 147–149.

Stapleford P. Formula feeding. *Paediatric Nursing* 1989; **1**: 14–16.

1.15 Parenteral nutrition

Parenteral nutrition (PN) is a method of providing nutritional support to an individual whose gastrointestinal tract is not functioning or is inaccessible. Nutrients are delivered directly into the circulatory system via a dedicated venous catheter. Parenteral nutrition is synonymous with total parenteral nutrition (TPN) – a term still used in the USA.

PN has lost favour in the treatment of conditions that were previously thought to require it, such as acute pancreatitis, paediatric and adult burns, critical care, and preoperative use in patients with mild or moderate malnutrition (Veterans Affairs Group 1991). The indications for PN are diminishing as the evidence from scientific and clinical studies of the benefits of enteral feeding continues to increase, and as the techniques for initiating enteral nutrition improve (Archer *et al*. 1996).

1.15.1 Indications for parenteral nutrition

PN should only be used when it is not possible to meet nutritional needs via the enteral route. Although PN is an essential and potentially life-saving therapy, it is expensive and carries life-threatening complications (e.g. sepsis and metabolic disorders), so must be monitored and administered correctly.

Short-term PN is indicated for:

- prolonged gastrointestinal ileus
- high-output small bowel fistula (Dudrick *et al*. 1999)
- severe pancreatitis with ileus
- acute exacerbation of inflammatory bowel disease in the small intestine (e.g. Crohn's disease)
- anastamotic breakdown following intestinal resection
- oral mucositis following chemotherapy that prevents enteral access being established.

Long-term PN, possibly at home, may be necessary for:

- intestinal atresia
- radiation enteritis
- motility disorders such as scleroderma
- short bowel syndrome
- some cancer patients.

PN can also be used as a 'top-up' form of nutrition support. Patients with short bowel syndrome who maintain energy and protein homoeostasis but have compromised enteral fat absorption can have intravenous 'top-up' of fat-soluble vitamins and essential fatty acids. 'Intradialytic' PN given whilst the patient is undergoing haemodialysis using the same vascular access may improve nutritional status and protein kinetics (McCann *et al*. 1999), but has no recorded effect on morbidity or mortality (Koretz 1999).

A meta-analysis of 26 randomized trials of 2211 patients comparing the use of PN with standard care (usual oral diet plus intravenous dextrose) in surgical and critically ill patients demonstrated that PN failed to influence the mortality rate of surgical or critically ill patients, but that the complication rate was reduced, especially in malnourished patients (Heyland *et al*. 1998).

1.15.2 The role of the parenteral nutrition team

Much has been made of the role of a formal multidisciplinary team (MDT) to manage parenteral nutrition on a clinical site and to co-ordinate PN in the community setting. Whether this team takes the role of a nutrition advisory team or nutrition steering committee to set standards of nutritional assessment, intervention and monitoring, or a more formal 'hands-on' ward-based MDT is determined by local need. Setting up the latter takes 'the courage of an explorer, the finesse of a diplomat, and the steadfastness of a saint' (Tougas 1994). Much research published in the mid-1980s demonstrated improvement in clinical outcome with the MDT approach (Hindle *et al*. 1996), but more recently, cost-effectiveness has become the more dominant issue as teams select the most appropriate feeding route, and the choice of enteral rather than parenteral nutrition is pursued more aggressively.

1.15.3 Administration of parenteral nutrition

Parenteral nutrition may be administered via either a central or peripheral vein, the choice being dictated by venous access and the choice of PN to be infused.

Peripheral catheters

These are suitable for short-term PN of up to 2 weeks (although can be administered for longer) as they avoid the clinical risks and costs of a central venous catheter (CVC). Peripheral access is via a small cannula inserted into a peripheral vein with the subsequent attachment to a short extension set, or via a fine-bore catheter inserted into an arm vein in the antecubital fossa. Thrombophlebitis (inflammation of the vein) is the main problem of peripheral feeding, and may be minimized by use of low osmotic load PN solutions, and/or reducing catheter availability for non-feed use, i.e. drug administration.

Catheters need to be managed with appropriate aseptic techniques and the veins inspected at least once a day. Catheters and cannulae should be resited if there are signs of redness or discomfort at the site. Peripheral catheters are a viable alternative to a CVC, as the use of lipid solutions can provide adequate energy without the risk of thrombophlebitis associated with hypertonic glucose solutions.

Central venous catheters

These are used for longer term PN administration if peripheral venous access is not possible, in patients who already have suitable central venous access (such as intensive-care patients) or those with unusual needs, e.g. fluid- restricted hypertonic feed. CVCs are inserted by a clinician, with X-ray confirmation of correct placement (the catheter tip should lie at the junction of the superior vena cava and right atrium) and absence of insertion-related complications (vessel puncture, pneumothorax). A variety of central catheters is available for feeding: with or without subcutaneous skin hubs, antibiotic-impregnated, single or multi-lumen. The clinical picture and personal clinician preference are the main factors deciding choice. CVCs with two, three or four lumens are being used increasingly in intensive treatment units (ITUs), particularly in patients requiring central venous pressure monitoring plus multiple drug infusions.

Peripherally inserted central catheters (PICCs)

These are a relatively new development. They are CVCs for short- to medium-term administration of PN. They can successfully administer hypertonic PN as the catheter tip lies in the superior vena cava. A variety of insertion techniques is available which can be tailored to patient and clinician preference (Anonymous 1998), thus minimizing complications such as venous thrombosis, venous damage or insertion-related phlebitis (Thompson 1999).

All intravenous nutrition must be administered through a volumetric pump with occlusion and air-in-line alarms to minimize infusion complications. Some feed lines have in-line filters to remove any particulate matter in the solution.

Most PN is administered continuously over 24 hours, but cyclical infusion may have physiological and psychological advantages. Continuous infusion is more appropriate for severely stressed patients such as those in intensive care.

1.15.4 Content of parenteral nutrition

PN may be delivered from a 3 litre bag (all-in-one or 'AIO' bag) containing the compounded daily regimen or using a multiple bottle system (individual bottles of protein, fat and carbohydrate administered via a 'piggyback' giving set),

although the latter is less popular than the AIO bag owing to the increased infection risk with multiple bottle changes, more nursing time and metabolic derangements. However, the AIO bag is not without its problems such as physical instability and the relative inability to respond quickly to changes in nutrient requirements.

An AIO bag will contain a combination of protein solution, fat emulsion, hypertonic dextrose solution, water-soluble and fat-soluble vitamins, trace elements, minerals and electrolytes and water to the desired volume.

Protein

The protein content of PN is normally expressed as grams of nitrogen – an archaic term to define protein as separate from the energy sources of carbohydrate and fat (Napolitano 1998). One gram of nitrogen is equivalent to 6.25 g protein. Nitrogen is usually supplied as a balanced mixture of crystalline amino acids, or dipeptides for the less soluble heat-labile amino acids, e.g. glutamine. Different amino-acid profile solutions are available for particular disease states.

Traditionally, nitrogen provision has been matched to urinary nitrogen excretion, but this method can overestimate nitrogen requirements and be hazardous. Most patients can be maintained with 0.2 g N/kg body weight per day. Nitrogen intake should not exceed 0.3 g N/kg body weight per day, and should be based on predicted need. Nitrogen estimation should include clinical management of the patient; for example, patients on haemodialysis may lose up to 16% of their daily protein intake in the dialysate (Kihara *et al*. 1997).

The optimum amino acid profile for parenteral nutrition remains unknown. The weight ratio of essential amino acid:total nitrogen (the E:T ratio) should be about 1:3, and the majority of solutions currently available meet this. However, some amino acids may be conditionally essential, or be necessary to improve the utilization of others:

- *Glycine* is a cheap 'filler' amino acid but is an efficient source of nitrogen. The presence of arginine with glycine prevents hyperammonaemia associated with glycine metabolism.
- *Cysteine* is unstable in PN solutions, being hydrolysed to cystine. Lack of sufficient cysteine and glutamine may contribute to reduced synthesis of glutathione manufactured from these amino acids. Low glutathione levels are associated with an increase in reactive oxygen species, free radical damage and worse clinical outcome (Fuhrman *et al*. 1999).
- *Glutamine* is a conditionally essential amino acid and an important metabolic fuel for intestinal enterocytes, lymphocytes and macrophages, and a precursor for purines and pyrimidines. Administration of dipeptide glutamine-supplemented PN improves nitrogen balance, increases cellular proliferation, decreases the incidence of infection (Powell-Tuck 1999; Sacks 1999) and shortens hospital stay in metabolically stressed patients (Griffiths *et al*. 1997).

- *Branched-chain amino acids (BCAAs: valine, leucine and isoleucine)* are metabolized by peripheral tissues rather than the liver, and may benefit patients with severe burns, sepsis or trauma. Leucine stimulates muscle protein synthesis and inhibits protein breakdown. In patients given isonitrogenous PN, a 45% BCAA-rich formula was associated with increases in prealbumin and retinal-binding protein, and lower mortality rate, but no significant difference in length of hospital stay (Garcia-de-Lorenzo *et al*. 1997). Patients with portal systemic encephalopathy have an increased ratio of aromatic to branched-chain amino acids in their blood which may influence amino-acid transport in the central nervous system and lead to the formation of false neurotransmitters. The use of BCAAs in liver failure remains controversial.

Fat

Fat emulsions are commonly long-chain triglycerides (LCTs) from soybean and/or safflower oils (providing an energy-dense yet isotonic alternative to dextrose), and essential fatty acids to maintain cell-membrane integrity and immune function.

Fat emulsions are available in a number of concentrations. For example, intralipid (KabiPharmacia) is available as 10%, 20% or 30% fat emulsions. The concentration of fat influences metabolic effect. In critically ill patients, a 30% Intralipid emulsion improves the differential serum lipid profile compared with a 10% emulsion (Kalfarentzos *et al*. 1998).

Fat normally provides between 30 and 50% of energy needs in PN, and may help to minimize the risk of hyperglycaemia and hypercarbia. In some cases (respiratory distress, peripheral feeding) fat may provide up to 60% of the energy requirements. However, as metabolism of LCTs is rate limiting, intravenous lipid may accumulate in the reticuloendothelial system, impairing the clearance of systemic bacteria and increasing susceptibility to infection (Battistella *et al*. 1997). In a clinically relevant dosage range, lipid emulsions are efficiently metabolized, even in critically ill patients with combined organ dysfunction and associated sepsis (Druml *et al*. 1998).

Medium-chain triglycerides (MCTs) are rapidly oxidized and, unlike LCT, do not require carnitine for mitochondrial membrane transportation. However, clinical trials of 50/50 MCT/LCT lipid emulsions in immunosuppressed, critically ill and liver-failure patients have failed to demonstrate a clinical advantage (Ulrich *et al*. 1996; Delafosse *et al*. 1997). Normalization of serum bilirubin appeared to be the sole clinical benefit of MCT solutions (Nijveldt *et al*. 1998).

Structured lipids containing MCTs were found to have no effect on liver-function tests or plasma triglyceride levels compared with PN containing MCT/LCT mix (Chambrier *et al*. 1999).

Addition of lipid increases the cost of PN, but the clinical benefits of reducing high glucose loads and associated hypertonic feed may offset this cost.

Loss of stability of lipid emulsions can result in irreversible lipid/water phase separation. Stability is primarily affected by pH, amino-acid composition and electrolyte content. A lower pH will destabilize the solution, whereas amino-acid solutions enhance stability via their buffering effects. Different amino-acid preparations have different effects on the stability of AIO mixtures, hence this aspect needs to be considered when formulations are changed. The presence of electrolytes, particularly divalent and trivalent cations, affects the surface charge on the droplet and may cause aggregation of the emulsion. Destabilization may also be caused by the addition of heparin.

The high content of omega-6 polyunsaturated fatty acids in lipid derived from soybean oil may contribute adversely to immunosuppressive effects and pulmonary complications, an effect minimized by appropriate fat administration (Askanazi *et al*. 1981; Furukawa *et al*. 1999). In order to avoid these complications, the rate of lipid infusion should not exceed 50 mg/kg per hour.

Carbohydrate

Glucose is a cheap energy source, but at the concentrations needed for an energy source in PN is extremely hypertonic, thus contributing to thrombophlebitis. Other previously advocated energy substrates such as fructose, sorbitol and xylitol are less likely to cause thrombophlebitis and hyperglycaemia, but their metabolism results in lactate production which can precipitate lactic acidosis. Levels of these substrates are also less easy to monitor.

The rate of glucose administration commonly used during PN of critically ill patients does not suppress endogenous gluconeogenesis or net protein loss, but markedly increases blood levels of glucose and insulin, *de novo* lipogenesis and carbon dioxide production. Increasing the proportion of fat may be beneficial, provided that lipid emulsion has no adverse effects (Tappy *et al*. 1998).

High infusion rates of glucose (> 40 kcal/kg per day, or >4 mg/kg per minute) can:

- increase CO_2 production
- aggravate impaired respiration function causing difficulties in weaning patients from artificial ventilation
- cause fatty liver secondary to hypertriglyceridaemia
- cause hyperinsulinaemia, preventing the mobilization of endogenous lipid (Schloerb and Henning 1998).

Hyperglycaemia associated with insulin resistance is common in severe trauma or sepsis.

Electrolytes

The electrolyte content of the PN bag reflects serum measurement of these electrolytes, although the amount added must concur with (lipid) stability data supplied by the PN manufacturers.

Vitamins

Guidance on the provision of vitamins during PN is provided by the American Medical Association (1979). These recommendations suggest that the required intake of water-soluble vitamins exceeds normal daily requirements in order to offset tissue losses and facilitate the synthesis of new tissue.

Vitamin losses from the PN solution may also occur in several ways:

- Vitamin A is photodegradable, with 40–98% lost over a 24-hour period.
- Amino-acid solutions with sulphite as an antioxidant will destroy most of the thiamin and one-third of the vitamin E present.
- Oxidation of ascorbate to oxalate, especially in the presence of catalysts such as copper and iron in PN bags, is implicated in neonatal formation of renal stones (nephrocalcinosis), as well as in the formation of insoluble precipitates in the PN administration sets (Rockwell et al. 1998).

Trace elements and minerals

Intravenous administration of minerals and trace elements bypasses the selective absorption that normally occurs in the gut, which markedly increases the risk of overdosage of micronutrients given intravenously.

Requirements for trace elements in critically ill and metabolically stressed patients remain poorly substantiated. Many PN patients are metabolically stressed, and the acute-phase response will alter serum levels, thus making estimation of predicted requirements impossible.

The needs of most patients can be met by standard trace element solutions devised for PN. However, these are designed to meet daily needs and make little provision for the restoration of body stores. Severely depleted or metabolically stressed patients may therefore need additional amounts of some trace elements. For example, iron-resistant anaemia secondary to copper deficiency has been reported in a patient fed PN secondary to active Crohn's disease (Spiegel and Willenbucher 1999). Other nutrient deficiencies may include selenium (deficiency resulting in cardiomyopathy) and chromium (impaired glucose tolerance factor, exacerbating hyperglycaemia).

Conversely, because normal mechanisms for preventing the absorption and excretion of surplus trace elements may be bypassed or impaired, the risk of toxicity from trace elements such as copper and manganese is high: both are excreted via the biliary tract and hence their excretion is compromised in the presence of cholestatic syndromes. Excess manganese may cause neurotoxicity.

Inadvertent delivery of trace elements from contaminated PN solutions may be substantial. Analysis of solutions used to compound PN were found to contain 12 trace element contaminants in amounts >1 μg/l (zinc, copper, manganese, chromium, selenium, boron, aluminium, titanium, barium, vanadium, arsenic and strontium). The measured concentrations of trace elements in the multi-trace element additive solution were also higher than the labelled values (Pluhator-Murton et al. 1999a).

Longer storage duration and higher storage temperature progressively reduce the deliverable concentrations of zinc, copper and manganese and other trace elements in compounded PN solutions and also trace elements present as contaminants, i.e. boron, aluminium, vanadium, titanium, barium, strontium and cobalt (Pluhator-Murton et al. 1999b).

1.15.5 Monitoring of parenteral nutrition

Baseline assessment

Initial assessment before PN commences should include:

- weight and height (to determine actual, and predict ideal body mass index)
- temperature, blood pressure and fluid balance (to predict fluid requirements)
- haematology (to consider nutritional anaemias)
- full blood count (to monitor infection)
- baseline liver-function tests.

Information on electrolytes (sodium, potassium, calcium, phosphate, magnesium), coagulation parameters (e.g. International Normalized Ratio (INR)) and trace elements should be considered, particularly in severely malnourished, stressed or clinically unstable patients. Patients with coagulopathies may require omission of Vitlipid (containing vitamin K) from the PN bag.

Anthropometry such as mid-arm circumference and triceps skinfold thickness may be considered, but the measurements must be taken in context of the clinical picture (see Section 1.8, Assessment of nutritional status).

Monitoring during parenteral nutrition

This should include:

- Standard measurements of blood pressure, temperature, pulse and respiration at least four times daily.
- Fluid balance: daily fluctuations in weight reflect changes in fluid balance, and indicate whether fluid restriction is necessary. Fluid losses through vomiting, diarrhoea or high-output fistulae may require additional fluid and electrolytes.
- Blood glucose should be measured at least twice daily for the first few days. Persistent hyperglycaemia requires concurrent sliding-scale insulin.
- The catheter site should be inspected daily for signs of infection.

Concurrent drug usage should also be considered: steroids may cause sodium retention, whilst diuretics such as frusemide will result in significant potassium losses. Vitamin K given in PN is sufficient to antagonize warfarin therapy (Camilo et al. 1998).

Unstable patients, and patients who are severely malnourished, will require frequent monitoring of serum biochemistry, usually on a daily basis (Driscoll 1996). Appropriate guidelines and standards have been set by BAPEN (Sizer et al. 1996).

Table 1.26 Suggested frequency of monitoring during parenteral nutrition (PENG 1996)

Daily	Twice weekly	Weekly	Long-term
Urea	PO$_4$	Nitrogen balance	Selenium
Creatinine	Bicarbonate	Weight[2]	Other trace elements
Na	Ionized calcium	Zinc	
K	Liver function tests	Magnesium	
Glucose	Albumin[1]		
Fluid balance			

[1]As a marker of disease state rather than nutritional status (Vanek 1998).
[2]Continued weight loss may indicate inadequate energy from PN, or optimal PN in the presence of a catabolic state, e.g. major sepsis.

The British Dietetic Association's Parenteral and Enteral Nutrition Group (PENG) has also produced summary guidance on monitoring frequency (Table 1.26).

1.15.6 Complications of parenteral nutrition

The main complications of PN are metabolic, physiological, mechanical or infectious.

Metabolic complications

These include fluid overload, hyperglycaemia and electrolyte abnormalities. Malnourished patients are at risk of developing electrolyte abnormalities during refeeding, particularly hypophosphataemia and hypokalaemia (Duerksen and Papineau 1998). PN may cause renal oxalate stones (Rockwell *et al.* 1998).

Rebound hypoglycaemia can occur after discontinuing the infusion of concentrated glucose solutions until endogenous insulin levels fall. Tapering the rate of infusion before disconnection can prevent this problem.

Physiological complications

These include a rise in serum bilirubin, secondary to reduced bilirubin binding capacity, and increasing free circulating bilirubin due to free fatty acids from the lipid emulsion competing with bilirubin for the binding sites on plasma albumin. Serum bilirubin usually normalizes on cessation of PN. Cholestatic jaundice in infants on long-term PN may progress to cirrhosis.

If hepatic changes are sufficient to give rise to clinical concern the following procedure is suggested:

- Consider whether there is a non-nutritional cause (e.g. sepsis).
- If glucose alone is being used for energy, substitute 30–50% of energy with lipid.
- If practical (i.e. in a stable patient), cyclical feeding (e.g. 12 hours out of 24 hours) can be tried.
- Reduce the total energy intake by reducing lipid or glucose, maintain nitrogen intake and monitor.

- If jaundice worsens, consider stopping feeding for 3–4 days and observe.
- If allowed, giving a small amount of oral food may be considered as this may help to reduce cholestasis.

Excess glucose will lead to fatty liver, and is accompanied by increased respiratory demands and stimulation of the sympathetic nervous system.

Cholelithiasis is common in adults and children receiving long-term PN, and is likely to be due to cholestasis in the gall bladder. Minimal oral or enteral intake may prevent this.

Polymyopathy with muscular pain and high serum creatinine and phosphate has been reported in long-term PN. This may be due to deficiency of essential fatty acids or possibly selenium. Metabolic bone disease characterized by skeletal pain and hypercalcuria may also occur with prolonged PN (Shike *et al.* 1980; McCullough *et al.* 1987), potential causes of this being excess vitamin D or aluminium intake, or a high nitrogen intake.

Administration of PN to cancer patients is associated with increased tumour cell proliferation, but the increased sensitivity of these cells to chemotherapy may mean that PN increases the effectiveness of chemotherapy in malnourished patients (Jin *et al.* 1999).

Mechanical complications

These are related to the catheter and include thrombus, occlusion or fracture. Insertion-related complications include pneumothorax or chylothorax, air embolism, cardiac arrhythmias or nerve injury (Buckley and Lee 1999). Risk of thrombus local to the catheter tip increases the longer the catheter is *in situ*. It is associated with the administration of glucose-rich hypertonic PN; thrombotic tendency is reduced by the administration of lipid emulsions. Heparin may be given concurrently as a prophylactic measure. It is not usually added to the PN as it adversely affects stability of the fat emulsion. Low-dose warfarin is usually ineffective because of PN vitamin K antagonism (Camilo *et al.* 1998).

Catheter occlusion may be due to kinking or luminal deposition of fibrin, lipid sludge or amorphous debris. This is a particular problem with lipid mixes, the tendency to which may be reduced by use of an ethanol flush, or short-term infusion of fibrinolytic/thrombolytic solutions (e.g Urokinase).

Catheter fracture is minimized by the use of connection devices or extension sets that reduce the need to clamp the catheter, and prolong its life.

Infectious complications

These may be secondary to the catheter, or other non-catheter concurrent infections.

The ability to mount an adequate immune response may be reduced in stressed patients given lipid-containing PN, as the biosynthesis of arachidonic acid from linoleic acid is inhibited, resulting in the diminished synthesis of leukotriene B$_4$ by neutrophils which may diminish chemotactic and chemokinetic signals to other leukocytes (Sane *et al.* 1999).

PN in the critically ill significantly increases the risk of *Candida* spp. infection (Borzotta and Beardsley 1999). The use of all-in-one PN bags reduces bacteraemia-related mortality compared with glass-bottle PN administration (Durand-Zaleski *et al.* 1997).

CVC-related infections can originate from endogenous skin flora, contamination of the catheter hub, contamination of the CVC from a distant site or contamination of the infusate, although the latter is rare (Krzywda *et al.* 1999). Antiseptic-impregnated CVCs in patients at high risk for catheter-related infections reduced the incidence of catheter-related sepsis and death, and provide significant saving in costs.

1.15.7 Home parenteral nutrition

The indication for home parenteral nutrition (HPN) is permanent intestinal failure, and in the UK the most frequent indication is short bowel syndrome related to Crohn's disease. In the USA and parts of Europe, the acquired immunodeficiency syndrome (AIDS) and cancer are common indications for HPN. Patients considered for PN should be referred to specialist centres with the experience and back-up facilities required.

Protocols for the training of patients requiring HPN and their carers, the recognition and management of problems are now readily available. The ability to counsel patients and relatives and the availability of a 24-hour telephone contact number are important. Research has demonstrated a reported reduction in quality of life (social, psychological and physical parameters) in patients on HPN compared with those with anatomical or functional short bowel not receiving HPN. HPN also reduced quality of life in patients with a stoma, whereas a stoma did not reduce quality of life among the non-HPN patients (Jeppesen *et al.* 1999).

HPN should be tailored to the patient. A cyclical infusion (e.g. feed is infused for 12 hours overnight at a suitably increased flow rate) may reduce hepatic abnormalities and allow greater patient mobility.

1.15.8 Weaning from parenteral nutrition

Weaning of patients should consider two possible outcome options:

- whether it is necessary for the patient to achieve full nutritional intake before discontinuing PN, or
- whether the absence of clinical symptoms is sufficient to reduce or halt PN.

Introduction of oral or enteral feed should be accompanied by a reduction in PN infusion rate to avoid both fluid overload and overfeeding with their attendant clinical sequelae. In practical terms, this can be achieved by slowing the infusion rate and using each bag for more than 24 hours, which is simpler and cheaper than compounding a series of individually modified bags.

If fluid intake is not a problem, a patient may be able to take oral or enteral fluids in addition to intravenous feed. As energy consumption increases, the amount of PN can then be reduced by an equivalent amount. Concurrent PN may not necessarily impair appetite (Reifen *et al.* 1999), although many patients express satiety when parenterally fed.

Most patients can be transferred entirely to enteral or oral feeding when intestinal tolerance of more than half of their total nutrient needs is established.

1.15.9 Future research

The use of other novel substrates such as RNA nucleotides, ornithine alpha-ketoglutarate and short-chain fatty acids is also under assessment but at present none can be recommended for routine clinical use.

Glutathione is a tripeptide of cysteine, glutamine and glycine, and is an important antioxidant against reactive oxygen species (ROS), which include superoxide and hydrogen peroxide derived from fatty acid peroxidation. The relative lack of cysteine and the variable glutamine content of PN may favour ROS production. Supplementation of PN with nutrients that promote glutathione synthesis may in future attenuate ROS-induced cell destruction (Fuhrman *et al.* 1999).

Carnitine is a trimethylamine hepatically synthesized from lysine, methionine and glycine in the presence of ascorbic acid and pyridoxine. It has an important role in the oxidation of fatty acids by facilitating their transport across the mitochondrial membrane. PN solutions contain no carnitine. Carnitine synthesis may be impaired in sick patients (Tao and Yoshimura 1980), impairing fat utilization, and its use in parenterally fed patients needs to be reviewed.

Text revised by: Catherine Collins

References

American Medical Association, Department of Foods and Nutrition. Guidelines for essential trace element preparations for parenteral use – a statement by an Expert Panel. *Journal of the American Medical Association* 1979; **241**: 2051–2054.

Anonymous. Peripherally inserted central catheters and midline catheters: 1998 product update. *Infusion* 1998; **5**: 32–38.

Archer SB, Burnett RJ, Fischer JE. Current uses and abuses of total parenteral nutrition. *Advances in Surgery* 1996; **29**: 165–189.

Askanazi J, Nordenstrom J, Rosendaum SH *et al.* Nutrition for the patient with respiratory failure: glucose vs. fat. *Anesthesiology* 1981; **54**: 373–377.

Battistella FD, Widergren JT, Anderson JT *et al.* A prospective, randomized trial of intravenous fat emulsion administration in trauma victims requiring total parenteral nutrition. *Journal of Trauma* 1997; **43**: 52–58.

Borzotta AP, Beardsley K. Candida infections in critically ill trauma patients: a retrospective case–control study. *Archives of Surgery* 1999; **134**: 657–664.

Buckley CJ, Lee SD. Placement of vascular access devices for parenteral nutrition. *Nutrition in Clinical Practice* 1999; **14**: 194–201.

Camilo ME, Jatoi A, O'Brien M *et al*. Bioavailability of phylloquinone from an intravenous lipid emulsion. *American Journal of Clinical Nutrition* 1998; **67**: 716–721.

Chambrier C, Guiraud M, Gibault JP *et al*. Medium- and long-chain triacylglycerols in postoperative patients: structured lipids versus a physical mixture. *Nutrition* 1999; **15**: 274–277.

Delafosse B, Viale JP, Pachiaudi C *et al*. Long- and medium-chain triglycerides during parenteral nutrition in critically ill patients. *American Journal of Physiology* 1997; **272**: E550–E555.

Driscoll DF. Delivery of parenteral nutritional therapy: implementation and monitoring nutrient homeostasis. *Nutrition* 1996; **12**: 834–835.

Druml W, Fischer M, Ratheiser K. Use of intravenous lipids in critically ill patients with sepsis without and with hepatic failure. *Journal of Parenteral and Enteral Nutrition* 1998; **22**: 217–223.

Dudrick SJ, Maharaj AR, McKelvey AA. Artificial nutritional support in patients with gastrointestinal fistulas. *World Journal of Surgery* 1999; **23**: 570–576.

Duerksen DR, Papineau N. Electrolyte abnormalities in patients with chronic renal failure receiving parenteral nutrition. *Journal of Parenteral and Enteral Nutrition* 1998; **22**: 102–104.

Durand-Zaleski I, Delaunay L, Langeron O *et al*. Infection risk and cost-effectiveness of commercial bags or glass bottles for total parenteral nutrition. *Infection Control and Hospital Epidemiology* 1997; **18**: 183–188.

Furhman MP, Herrmann V, Smith GS. Reactive oxygen species and glutathione: potential for parenteral nutrition supplementation? *Nutrition in Clinical Practice* 1999; **14**: 254–263.

Furukawa K, Tashiro T, Yamamori H *et al*. Effects of soybean oil emulsion and eicosapentaenoic acid on stress response and immune function after a severely stressful operation. *Annals of Surgery* 1999; **229**: 255–261.

Garcia-de-Lorenzo A, Ortiz-Leyba C, Planas M *et al*. Branch-chain amino acids in septic patients: clinical and metabolic aspects. *Critical Care Medicine* 1997; **25**: 418–424.

Griffiths RD, Jones C, Palmer TE. Six-month outcome of critically ill patients given glutamine-supplemented parenteral nutrition. *Nutrition* 1997; **13**: 295–302.

Heyland DK, MacDonald S, Keefe L, Drover JW. Total parenteral nutrition in the critically ill patient: a meta-analysis. *Journal of the American Medical Association* 1998; **280**: 2013–2019.

Hindle T, Dhoot R, Georgieva C. Clinical nutrition in NHS hospitals: a project on management by a multi-disciplinary team. *British Journal of Intensive Care* 1996; February: 61–65.

Jeppesen PB, Langholz E, Mortensen PB. Quality of life in patients receiving home parenteral nutrition. *Gut* 1999; **44**: 844–852.

Jin D, Phillips M, Byles JE. Effects of parenteral nutrition support and chemotherapy on the phasic composition of tumor cells in gastrointestinal cancer. *Journal of Parenteral and Enteral Nutrition* 1999; **23**: 237–241.

Kalfarentzos F, Kokkinis K, Leukaditi K *et al*. Comparison between two fat emulsions: Intralipid 30 cent vs Intralipid 10 cent in critically ill patients. *Clinical Nutrition* 1998; **17**: 31–34.

Kihara M, Ikeda Y, Fujita H *et al*. Amino acid losses and nitrogen balance during slow diurnal hemodialysis in critically ill patients with renal failure. *Intensive Care Medicine* 1997; **23**: 110–113.

Koretz RL. Does nutritional intervention in protein-energy malnutrition improve morbidity or mortality. *Journal of Renal Nutrition* 1999; **9**: 119–121.

Krzywda EA, Andris DA, Edmiston CE. Catheter infections: diagnosis, etiology, treatment, and prevention. *Nutrition in Clinical Practice* 1999; **14**: 178–190.

McCann L, Feldman C, Hornberger J *et al*. Effect of intradialytic parenteral nutrition on delivered *Kt/V*. *American Journal of Kidney Diseases* 1999; **33**: 1131–1135.

McCullough ML, Hsu N. Metabolic bone disease in home total parenteral nutrition. *Journal of the American Dietetic Association* 1987; **87**: 915–920.

Napolitano LM. Parenteral nutrition in trauma patients: glucose-based, lipid-based, or none? *Critical Care Medicine* 1998; **26**: 813–814.

Nijveldt RJ, Tan AM, Prins HA *et al*. Use of a mixture of medium-chain triglycerides and longchain triglycerides versus long-chain triglycerides in critically ill surgical patients: a randomized prospective double-blind study. *Clinical Nutrition* 1998; **17**: 23–29.

Parenteral and Enteral Nutrition Group of the British Dietetic Association (PENG). *Adult Enteral and Parenteral Nutrition. Guidelines for Dietitians in Training*. Birmingham: British Dietetic Association, 1996.

Pluhator-Murton MM, Fedorak RN, Audette RJ *et al*. Trace element contamination of total parenteral nutrition. 1. Contribution of component solutions. *Journal of Parenteral and Enteral Nutrition* 1999a; **23**: 222–227.

Pluhator-Murton MM, Fedorak RN, Audette RJ *et al*. Trace element contamination of total parenteral nutrition. 2. Effect of storage duration and temperature. *Journal of Parenteral and Enteral Nutrition* 1999b; **23**: 228–232.

Powell-Tuck J. Total parenteral nutrition with glutamine dipeptide shortened hospital stays and improved immune status and nitrogen economy after major abdominal surgery. *Gut* 1999; **44**: 155.

Reifen R, Khoshoo V, Dinari G. Effect of parenteral nutrition on oral intake. *Journal of Pediatric Endocrinology and Metabolism* 1999; **12**: 203–205.

Rockwell GF, Campfield T, Nelson BC, Uden PC. Oxalogenesis in parenteral nutrition solution components. *Nutrition* 1998; **14**: 836–839.

Sacks GS. Glutamine supplementation in catabolic patients. *Annals of Pharmacology* 1999; **33**: 348–354.

Sane S, Baba M, Kusano C *et al*. Fat emulsion administration in the early postoperative period in patients undergoing esophagectomy for carcinoma depresses arachidonic acid metabolis in neutrophils. *Nutrition* 1999; **15**: 341–346.

Schloerb PR, Henning JF. Patterns and problems of adult total parenteral nutrition use in US academic medical centers. *Archives of Surgery* 1998; **133**: 7–12.

Shike M, Harrison JE, Sturtridge WC *et al*. Metabolic bone disease in patients receiving long term total parenteral nutrition. *Annals of Internal Medicine* 1980; **92**: 343–350.

Sizer T, Russell CA, Wood S *et al*. *Standards and Guidelines for Nutritional Support of Patients in Hospitals*. BAPEN Working Party Report. Maidenhead: BAPEN, 1996.

Spiegel JE, Willenbucher RF. Rapid development of severe copper deficiency in a patient with Crohn's disease receiving parenteral nutrition. *Journal of Parenteral and Enteral Nutrition* 1999; **23**: 169–172.

Tao RC, Yoshimura NN. Carnitine metabolism and its application in parenteral nutrition. *Journal of Parenteral and Enteral Nutrition* 1980; **4**: 469–486.

Tappy L, Schwarz JM, Schneiter P *et al*. Effects of isoenergetic glucose-based or lipid-based parenteral nutrition on glucose metabolism, de novo lipogenesis, and respiratory gas exchanges in critically ill patients. *Critical Care Medicine* 1998; **26**: 860–867.

Thompson SE. Insertion of peripherally inserted central catheters for the administration of total parenteral nutrition. *Nutrition in Clinical Practice* 1999; **14**: 191–193.

Tougas JG. Starting a nutrition support team. Short term pain for long term gain. *Nutrition in Clinical Practice* 1994; **9**: 221–225.

Ulrich H, Pastores SM, Katz DP, Kvetan V. Parenteral use of medium-chain triglycerides: a reappraisal. *Nutrition* 1996; **12**: 231–238.

Vanek VW. The use of serum albumin as a prognostic or nutritional marker and the pros and cons of IV albumin therapy. *Nutrition in Clinical Practice* 1998; **13**: 110–122.

Veterans Affairs Total Parenteral Nutrition Co-operative Study Group. Perioperative total parenteral nutrition in surgical patients. *New England Journal of Medicine* 1991; **325**: 525–532.

1.16 Food service in hospitals and institutions

It is important to remember that 80–100% patients in hospitals and institutions depend solely on the food provided for their nutritional support (Stephen *et al.* 1997). Ensuring that the food is of good nutritional quality, is appealing to patients and is eaten is a complex and difficult challenge for the dietitian and the caring team. If dietitians do nothing else but maximize the amount of food that patients eat while in hospital, they will have achieved a great deal.

1.16.1 General issues

Malnutrition in hospitals

The provision of artificial nutrition has been the focus of much attention in recent decades and has developed considerably. It can truly be said that nutritional support is now possible in all clinical situations. Despite these advances, malnutrition in hospitals remains common (McWhirter and Pennington 1994) and is often unrecognized (Lennard-Jones *et al.* 1995) (see Section 1.11, Undernutrition).

In the hospital setting, malnutrition is malpractice and it is costly and indefensible (Tucker 1996; Reilly *et al.* 1988); managing this risk is an important part of corporate and clinical governance in the modern National Health Service (NHS Executive 1998). The clinical and management team need to recognize and act when poor food consumption compromises patient nutrition.

Public concern about food in hospitals and institutions

The public and the press are very interested in hospital food. Almost everyone has an anecdote about how a friend or relative 'starved' in hospital. Innumerable newspaper articles have voiced this public concern over the years. Many of these concerns were also highlighted in the report *Hungry in Hospital* by the Association of Community Health Councils of England and Wales (1997).

Why good-quality food service is important

Providing food in hospitals and other institutions is fundamental to the success of that organization. There are no other services delivered to every patient, every day that affect their well-being so profoundly.

Food must be eaten to be beneficial; it provides a background, basic level of nutritional care. If food service fails to nourish, the process of identifying and addressing that failure is complex and difficult (Wheatley 1999). Food service is front line and is a 'shop window' for the institution.

Patients often cannot tell the difference between good treatment and bad treatment, but they can always identify poor food.

1.16.2 Guidance and opinion in the UK

Many reports regarding food service in hospitals and institutions have been published since 1990 and a summary of their recommendations is given in Table 1.27.

The gap between guidance and implementation

At the current time, there is still a gap between the guidance available on best practice and its implementation (Kelly 1999). More research on the cost-efficiency of improving food intake in hospitals and institutions is needed. Although the work that has been published is very convincing (Larsson *et al.* 1990; Ödlund-Olin *et al.* 1996; Gall *et al.* 1998; Kondrup *et al.* 1998), it remains scarce and good practice is not widespread.

1.16.3 How to ensure that more food is eaten

Getting food eaten is the principal goal of any food service system as the nutritional value of food not eaten is nil. The dietitian must understand the principles of food service in order to achieve this goal. The process begins with menu planning.

Menu planning

The menu is the blueprint of food service and time spent in planning the menu is never wasted. Dietitians' expertise is in their knowledge of the nutritional requirements of the client group to be served and in understanding how these might be met by the food supplied.

Knowing the client group

The first step in menu planning is gathering information about the client group:

- What do they like to eat?
- What are their cultural and religious preferences?
- What are their physical needs?
- When do they like to eat?
- How do they like to eat?
- What assistance will they need with eating?

Table 1.27 Guidance and opinion on food service in the UK: a review of documents produced since 1990

Year	Organization and report title	Main recommendations
1992	Department of Health Committee on Medical Aspects of Food Policy *Nutrition of Elderly People*	• Health professionals should be made aware of the often inadequate food intake of elderly people in institutions • Effective methods of ensuring adequate nutrition need to be developed and evaluated for elderly people in hospital or institutions
1992	King's Fund (Lennard-Jones) *A Positive Approach to Nutrition as Treatment*	• Every hospital should organize its nutrition services to link management, catering and all of the clinical disciplines involved • Managers should take account of the potential cost of complications and increased hospital stay due to malnutrition when assessing the cost of nutritional support
1993	British Dietetic Association /Nutrition Advisory Group for Elderly People (NAGE) *Dietetic Standards of Care for the Older Adult in Hospital*	• The dietitian advises on nutritionally adequate food which is acceptable to the patients and appropriate to the patients' needs • The dietitian advises on hospital policies that affect nutritional care of the older adult
1993	Royal College of Nursing *Nutrition Standards and the Older Adult*	• The client has an initial assessment made of their food and fluid intake and eating and drinking patterns • The ward/unit team works towards ensuring that the organization of the ward and staff is responsive to and meets the requirements of the client in order to satisfy their eating and drinking needs • The nutritional goals set for the client and the care received are continually evaluated and revised
1993	South East Thames Regional Health Authority *Service Standards: Nutritional Guidelines: The Food Chain*	• Best-practice guidelines on hospital food service • Recommendations aiming for as much food to be eaten by patients in hospital as possible
1993	South East Thames Regional Health Authority *Service Standards: Nutritional Guidelines: Menu Planning*	• Help and advice on menu planning in the institutional setting • Recommendations aiming to ensure that an appealing and attractive menu is constructed which can be delivered and will be eaten
1993	The Patients' Association *Catering for Patients in Hospital*	• Meals should be served at times that reflect the normal eating patterns of the majority of patients • Patients should be able to order as near to the meal itself as possible • The children's menu should reflect the foods they are used to at home • Snacks should be available • There should be adequate staffing so that patients who cannot feed themselves, or who need encouragement, have the full attention of a member of staff • Staff should have responsibility to monitor and report on patients' intake of food and liquid • Nurses should collect trays from patients for monitoring of intake • There should be a regular evaluation of food and catering services, looking at quality, content and presentation
1994	British Association for Parenteral and Enteral Nutrition (BAPEN) *Organisation of Nutrition Support in Hospitals*	• All UK hospitals should have a nutrition support team • All major UK hospitals or hospital groups should appoint a nutrition steering committee • Nutrition steering committees should be responsible for setting standards for catering services, dietary supplements and nutritional support • All nutrition steering committees should appoint at least one nutrition support team to implement the standards of nutritional support they recommend
1994	Health of the Nation Nutrition Task Force *Nutrition and Health: A Management Handbook for the NHS*	• Makes suggestions for managers about how they can develop and improve nutrition services in their institution
1995	English National Board for Nurse Education (ENB) *Nutrition for Life: Issues for Debate in the Department of Education Programmes*	• Nutrition themes should be integrated through both pre-registration and continuing post-registration programmes • Every student should be able to conduct a detailed nutritional assessment of a healthy person
1995	Health of the Nation Nutrition Task Force *Nutrition Guidelines for Hospital Catering*	• Makes recommendations on the nutritional content of hospital food based on the Committee on Medical Aspects of Food Policy recommendations for **healthy individuals** • Provides guidance on best practice in food service and delivery, aiming for as much food to be eaten as possible
1996	BAPEN *Standards and Guidelines for Nutritional Support of Patients in Hospitals*	• Purchasers of healthcare should insist on standards for the organization and provision of nutrition support • There should be an interdepartmental and multidisciplinary nutrition steering committee • There should be a catering liaison group with representative caterers, doctors, nurses and dietitians
1996	BDA/Parenteral and Enteral Nutrition Group (PENG) *Dietetic Standards for Nutritional Support*	• Dietitians should actively promote the identification and treatment of protein-energy malnutrition and increase awareness of this issue among other health-care professionals • Managers of nutrition and dietetic services should ensure that resources are available for the provision of nutritional support within both the hospital and the community

Table 1.27 Continued

Year	Organization and report title	Main recommendations
1996	National Health Service Executive *Hospital Catering: Delivering a Quality Service*	• Contractors should provide meals which meet patients' dietetic and nutritional requirements • Catering procedures should comply with the Nutrition Task Force's guidelines for hospital caterers • Chefs should be trained in nutrition to meet dietary needs • Contractors should keep prescribed records to demonstrate that nutrition and dietetic requirements are monitored and met • The Trust's dietetic manager should ensure that nutrition standards are satisfactory • An annual independent audit should be conducted to show meal quality to be satisfactory and to meet patients' needs • A guide should be provided for each patient explaining the hospital's catering policies and catering services • Patients' meals should not be ordered more than two meals in advance • The catering manager's name should be made available to patients • Help should be readily available for patients where required to help them to make use of the catering service
1996	British Dietetic Association (BDA) *Malnutrition in Hospitals*	• Dietitians should be actively involved in menu planning to ensure that a nutritionally adequate diet is provided in hospital and that patients requiring special or therapeutic diets are catered for • Patients who require artificial nutritional support or a supplemented diet should have access to a dietitian • Adequate resources should be available to ensure that high-quality nutritional care, whether via the oral, enteral or parenteral route, can be delivered and monitored • Dietitians should foster close links with other healthcare professionals involved in the detection and management of malnutrition
1997	Association of Community Health Councils for England and Wales *Hungry in Hospital?*	• Concerns that patients are 'starving to death' must be investigated • Roles and responsibilities at mealtimes must be defined • Existing guidance with regard to hospital catering must be enforced
1997	Centre for Health Services Research, University of Newcastle upon Tyne (Bond) *Eating Matters*	• Meal provision should be responsive to the patients' needs • Patients should be asked for their opinions about the meals provided • Multidisciplinary and cross-departmental dietary care groups should be created • All other ward activities should stop when meals are being eaten • Audits of dietary care should be carried out regularly
1997	United Kingdom Central Council for Nursing and Midwifery (UKCC) *Responsibility for Feeding of Patients*	• Nurses have an implicit responsibility for ensuring that patients are appropriately fed
1997	British Dietetic Association *National Professional Standards for Dietitians Practising in Healthcare*	• Dietitians will liaise with catering concerning the production of food to specified nutritional standards, the development of menus (including choice), food delivery systems (in-house or outside caterers), and ensure that the food service encourages and enables the client to eat the food provided • Dietitians will be involved in documentation relating to the provision of food and its service to clients • Dietitians will advise on the provision of nutritionally adequate food specific to clients' needs and in accordance with national standards • Dietitians will ensure that catering and other staff have accurate information and receive appropriate training • Dietitians will liaise with other members of the multiprofessional team to ensure that all aspects of the individual's care are considered in the nutrition care plan
1999	The Nuffield Trust *Managing Nutrition in Hospital: A Recipe for Quality*	• Makes recommendations on the management of nutrition services to the Department of Health, NHS Executive, National Institute for Clinical Excellence (NICE), The Audit Commission, health professional bodies, research funding agencies, Health Authorities, Primary Care Groups and Hospital Trusts • Food provision should be managed as an integral component of clinical care rather than a 'hotel' function
1999	BAPEN *Hospital Food as Treatment*	• Doctors should acknowledge a responsibility for patient nutrition as an important part of overall management • The chief dietitian should have an executive not just an advisory input into the catering services • Consideration should be given to a new nutrition directorate with overall responsibility for all aspects of nutritional care • Consideration should be give to transferring the catering and nutritional care service from the hotel/facilities directorate to the clinical support and treatment service budget

Knowing what resources are available

It must be possible to deliver the menu that is being planned:

- Can it be afforded?
- Is the kitchen equipment needed available (i.e. enough oven space, crockery, cutlery, serving utensils)?
- Is the necessary staffing and expertise available?
- Are the food storage facilities sufficient?
- Are food supplies secure?
- Can the items needed be delivered in time on a regular basis?
- Can the food be distributed to the patients?

Nutrition support team and policy

Menu planning is best practised as a team. Input from the dietitian, caterer, nurse, doctor, pharmacist, speech and language therapist and patients' representative are required to bring the necessary knowledge and expertise to the planning process.

This team will be recognizable to most dietitians as the core membership of the nutrition support team. The reports of the Nuffield Trust and the British Association for Parenteral and Enteral Nutrition (BAPEN) in 1999 both recommended that such a group be formed in all hospitals or groups of hospitals to oversee the nutritional health of the in-patient population.

It is recommended that such a cross-department and interdisciplinary team develop nutritional policy for the hospital and oversee the implementation and monitoring of the effectiveness of that policy. It is further recommended that nutritional support policy should extend to the provision of food. The nutrition support team's involvement in menu planning ensures that this responsibility is executed.

Menu structure

Once the team has gathered the information on policy, patient requirements and resources, the next step is to plan the structure of the menu:

- Over how many days will the menu cycle run?
- How many meals are to be provided each day?
- Will the meals be hot or cold?
- What is the structure of each individual meal?
- Will a starter be offered?
- How many choices will be offered?
- What types of dish are to be offered (i.e. meat, fish, vegetarian, egg, cheese, salad, sandwiches, soft choices, etc.)?
- Can each item of the meal be chosen separately or is a meal to be offered as a single choice? (This is a particularly important consideration.)

Developing the structure of the menu is the most difficult part of the planning process and it is important to spend time on this stage. Regardless of the dishes offered, a menu with a poor structure will not meet the patient's needs and desires (Table 1.28).

Selection of suitable dishes

Once the structure of the menu has been determined, decisions can be made about individual dishes which will make up the menu. It is useful to put the menu structure on a large sheet of paper on the wall at this stage, write the names of the dishes available on sticker notes and assemble the menu. This visual technique allows a degree of interactivity within the planning team and highlights the way in which individual dishes complement one another. A visual prompt such as this will also bring to light any repetitions in the menu, particularly at the beginning and end of the menu cycle.

Information required for each dish

It is important to have to hand a considerable amount of information about the dishes which may be offered on the menu. Detailed information about nutritional composition, cost and availability of pre-prepared dishes, and standard recipes for dishes which are to be prepared on site, will be needed.

Nutritional information

Nutritional information required by the menu planner will depend on the requirements of the client group. A renal dietitian will be more interested in the electrolyte composition of foods offered than a dietitian responsible for care of elderly people, whose focus of interest is more likely to be food consistency and energy density.

Information about other aspects of food composition, such as whether it contains gelatin, gluten, milk, nuts or peanuts, for example, is also likely to be required. The menu planning team should agree on information requirements at an early stage in the planning process.

An increasing amount of nutritional information is demanded by a food and health-conscious public. The planning team has a duty to meet these needs; for example,

Table 1.28 Outline structure of a menu for a large hospital

Breakfast	Lunch	Supper
Fruit juice	Fruit juice	Fruit juice
Fresh fruit	Soup	Soup
Wholemeal cereal	Main meat or fish	Main meat or fish
Low-residue cereal	dish	dish
Porridge	Soft dish (suitable for those with no teeth)	Snack dish
		Soft dish
	Vegan dish	Vegan dish
Wholemeal bread	Salad	Sandwich
White bread		
	Suitable staple	Suitable staple
Butter	Mashed potato	Mashed potato
Low-fat spread		
	Vegetable 1	Vegetable 1
Boiled egg	Vegetable 2	Vegetable 2
Jam	Baked pudding	Baked pudding
Marmalade	Milk pudding	Milk pudding
	Custard	Ice-cream
Milk	Fresh fruit	Cheese and biscuits

this means knowing whether any food item on the menu contains ingredients derived from genetically modified organisms.

Ratification of the menu

Once the first draft of the planned menu has been agreed, it will need to be ratified by analysis of its nutritional composition and cost. It is recommended that nutritional analysis be carried out and interpreted by a state registered dietitian (Health of the Nation, Nutrition Task Force, 1995). The dietitian needs to be sure that the menu will meet the nutritional requirements of the client group, including the needs of those requiring modified diets. The ratification process will lead to a fine tuning of the menu, ensuring that the finished product represents the best available in terms of nutritional content, cost and practical 'deliverability'.

Publishing the menu

Once completed, the menu will need to be published. At this point the team needs to consider how patients are going make their choice from the menu. Ensuring that patients understand what is being offered encourages active participation in food choice. Food chosen by the patient is much more likely to be suitable and much more likely to be eaten.

Systems and food service

The chain of events from provisions arriving at the hospital gate to completed dishes being presented to the patient is often referred to as the 'food chain'. The best planned menu can fail at any point if the food delivery system is not robust. No one wants to eat cold food that should be hot, or which is poorly presented.

There are many new systems and technologies available to assist in the delivery of food in hospitals. Different types of food service system, together with a summary of their benefits and drawbacks, are summarized in the following three tables:

- Ways in which food can be prepared and stored (Table 1.29).
- Ways in which food can be distributed to the ward (Table 1.30).
- Methods of food service at ward level (Table 1.31).

Table 1.29 Food service systems: ways in which food can be prepared and stored

The way food is prepared and stored	Benefits	Concerns
Cook/serve 75% of hospitals in the UK prepare most food on site from fresh, raw ingredients. Increasingly, items such as pies, puddings, pre-prepared vegetables and cooked meats are used.	• Flexibility, capable of adaptation to most situations • Food preparation skills maintained on site • Recipes can be adapted quickly to meet unusual requirements • Traditional and regional variability	• Depends on a well-trained, skilled and motivated workforce • Production facilities are expensive to maintain and take up a lot of space
Cook/chill Food is cooked and blast chilled to between 0 and 4°C. Food can be stored and distributed at this temperature for up to 5 days after production. It is then reheated (regenerated) ready for food service.	• Requirement for skilled cooks is reduced • Requirement for expensive cooking equipment is reduced • Can reduce 'hot holding' of food and improve nutritional value when served • Fewer peaks and troughs in the kitchen working day • Can increase variety of food available on the menu	• Food costs increase to pay for pre-prepared food • Regeneration must be done skilfully to optimize food quality • Five-day shelf-life • Greater distribution leads to increased food-safety risks • Increased dependence on outside supplier • Some dishes are not suitable for this type of service • Less flexible service if no production facilities are maintained on site
Cook/freeze Food is cooked and quickly chilled to −18°C. Food can be stored and distributed at this temperature for periods of up to 3 months. It is then reheated (regenerated) ready for food service	• As per cook/chill • Increased shelf-life makes distribution logistics easier	• As per cook/chill • Energy costs associated with freezing, storage and regeneration
Cook/conserve Cook/chill and cook/freeze are often described as cook/conserve systems. This term is also used to describe sous vide systems. Food is cooked, sealed in an air-free, oxygen-impermeable, multilayered plastic bag. It is then chilled or frozen prior to storage and distribution. The food is then reheated (regenerated) ready for service	• As per cook/chill • Sealed package makes handling easier and safer • Increased shelf-life makes distribution logistics easier	• As per cook/chill • Increased cost of packaging

Table 1.30   Food service systems: ways in which food can be distributed to the ward

Method	Benefits	Concerns
Plated service Food is served on to the plate centrally and distributed	• Good portion control • Food-safety risks contained in one area • Fewer staff required on the ward • Tight control of waste	• Difficult to maintain food temperature and quality during distribution • Logistics of collecting data on patient choice • Difficult to cater for out-of-hours requirements • Serving staff do not know who they are serving for
Bulk food service Food is distributed in large containers and is served on to the plate at ward level	• Food choice takes place at the bedside • Food temperature and quality easier to maintain during distribution • 'You can have your gravy where you want it' • Greater flexibility in terms of portion size • Serving staff get to know the patients • Patients can participate in the food service process	• More space required at ward level • More food-handling risks at ward level • Portion control more complex • More ward-based time required • More staff required at ward level

Table 1.31   Food service systems: methods of food service at ward level

Method	Benefits	Concerns
Trayed service Food is assembled on a tray and the patient eats at the bedside or in bed	• No communal ward areas needed • Tight control of modified diets more practicable • May be preferred by patients with eating difficulties • Privacy • Suitable for bed-bound patients	• Second helpings more difficult to provide • Lack of social interaction • Monitoring of food intake more difficult • Problems unpacking some food items • If whole meal is served, parts of it may go cold
Cafeteria-style service	• More normal • Flexibility of service and portion size available at point of service • Possibility of social interactions • Food choice at point of service	• Communal eating area needed • Patients need to be mobile
Family meal service	• As above • Meal times more of an occasion, breaking up the ward day	• More food service equipment needed at ward level • Requires a degree of patient independence or increased staffing • Communal eating area needed

Ward hostesses

Dedicated staff at ward level can dramatically improve food service (Stephen *et al*. 1997). Staff whose main function is to ensure that patients are fed appropriately can make a great deal of difference to the amount of food eaten. By ensuring that all of the administration related to securing patient meal choices is carried out, liaising with the hospital kitchen in a timely manner, having time to discuss meal choices with patients and reporting food intake to nursing staff, a significant input to patients' nutritional support can be made. In addition, trained staff can implement food hygiene regulations on the ward and ensure food safety.

The eating environment

The environment and ambience on the ward can make a dramatic difference to the acceptability of food and the amount eaten. Meal times should be regarded as special

and important times in the patients' day and every effort should be made by ward staff to ensure that patients are uninterrupted and have time to enjoy their meals.

Decisions made at the time when new buildings or new food service systems are being planned can have considerable influence on the subsequent quality of food provision. Particular thought should be given to the amount of space required on wards for food preparation, service and consumption; inadequacies in these respects can ultimately affect the amount of food eaten (Bond 1997).

Food waste

Up to 40% of food provided to patients is wasted (Fenton *et al*. 1995; Edwards and Nash 1997; Stephen *et al*. 1997; Kelly 1999). We have full dustbins and empty patients! Systems for the monitoring of food waste are a valuable performance indicator and act as a proxy measure for the amount of food that is being eaten. It is important to distinguish between plate waste (i.e. where a patient has attempted to eat a meal and not eaten all of it) and trolley or tray waste (i.e. food which was surplus to requirements and was never offered to patients).

High levels of plate waste may indicate either that the patient has a poor appetite, in which case a different approach to nutrition support needs to be considered, or that the taste, presentation or temperature of the food was at fault.

High levels of tray or trolley waste indicate that there is a food delivery problem. Information on needs may be poor, meal times may be inappropriate or portion control needs to be studied more carefully.

Audit of food service

Food service is a large-scale, hospital-wide operation, and the monitoring and auditing procedures are complex. It is important at the policy-setting stage, or the contract-specification stage, that output measures are agreed which will truly reflect the quality of the service. The nutrition support team should play a pivotal role in receiving, reviewing and recommending hospital board action on these output measures. Closing the audit loop in food service is difficult and resource intensive, but it is an important part of ensuring that the food service plays its full role in the nutritional support of patients. Developments in information technology are improving the ability to capture data on a large scale and interpret it appropriately. These developments need to be applied to food service monitoring to make it operationally practicable.

1.16.4 NICE, CHI and the future of food service in the NHS

The National Institute for Clinical Excellence (NICE) has been set up in England to develop standards of best practice in healthcare (NHS Executive 1998) (see Table 1.3 and Section 1.18 Clinical effectiveness). These standards are being set out in National Service Frameworks (NSF). In the next few years, NICE Service Frameworks related to hospital treatment will include requirements for best practice in food service. The Commission for Health Improvement (CHI) is the inspection body which will enforce the Service Frameworks. CHI has as its ultimate sanction the power to dismiss the board of a Hospital Trust.

As the crucial role of food in the nutritional support of patients in hospital is recognized, the clinical team needs to be ready to use it. Food is an essential part of care and recovery, and food service needs to be accorded the care and attention it deserves.

Text revised by: Richard Wilson

Useful addresses

British Association for Parenteral and Enteral Nutrition (BAPEN)
PO Box 922, Maidenhead, Berkshire SL6 4SH

King's Fund Centre
11–13 Cavendish Square, London W1M 0AN

The Nuffield Trust
59 New Cavendish Street, London W1M 7RD

The Patients' Association
PO Box 935, Harrow, Middlesex HA1 3YJ
Tel: 020 8423 9111
Website: www.patients-association.com

References

Association of Community Health Councils for England and Wales. *Hungry in Hospital?* London: ACHCEW, 1997.

Bond S (Ed.). *Eating Matters: A Resource for Improving Dietary Care in Hospitals*. University of Newcastle Upon Tyne, Centre for Health Services Research, 1997.

British Association for Parenteral and Enteral Nutrition. *Organisation of Nutritional Support in Hospitals*. Report of a Working Party, Silk DBA (Ed.). Maidenhead: BAPEN, 1994.

British Association for Parenteral and Enteral Nutrition. *Standards and Guidelines for Nutritional Support of Patients in Hospitals*. Sizer T. (Ed.). Maidenhead: BAPEN, 1996.

British Association for Parenteral and Enteral Nutrition. *Hospital Food as Treatment*. Maidenhead: BAPEN, 1999.

British Dietetic Association. *Malnutrition in Hospitals*. Position Paper. Birmingham: BDA, 1996.

British Dietetic Association. *National Professional Standards for Dietitians Practising in Healthcare*. Birmingham: BDA, 1997.

British Dietetic Association/Nutrition Advisory Group for Elderly People (NAGE). *Dietetic Standards of Care for the Older Adult in Hospital*. Birmingham: BDA/NAGE, 1993.

British Dietetic Association/Parenteral and Enteral Nutrition Group (PENG). *Dietetic Standards for Nutrition Support*. Birmingham: BDA/PENG, 1996.

Department of Health. *The Nutrition of Elderly People*. Report of the Working Group on the Nutrition of Elderly People of the Committee on Medical Aspects of Food Policy. Report on Health and Social Subjects 43. London: HMSO, 1992.

Edwards J, Nash A. Measuring the wasteline. *Health Service Journal* 1997; November: 26–27.

English National Board for Nurse Education. *Nutrition for Life: Issues for Debate in the Department of Education Programmes*. London: ENB, 1995.

Fenton J, Eves A, Kipps M, O'Donnell CC. The nutritional implications of food wastage in continuing care wards for elderly patients with mental health problems. *Journal of Human Nutrition and Dietetics* 1995; **8**: 239–248.

Gall MJ, Grimble GK, Reeve NJ, Thomas SJ. Effect of providing fortified meals and between-meal snacks on energy and protein intake of hospital patients. *Clinical Nutrition* 1998; **17**(6): 259–264.

Health of the Nation, Nutrition Task Force. *Nutrition and Health: A Management Handbook for the NHS*. London: Department of Health, 1994.

Health of the Nation, Nutrition Task Force. *Nutrition Guidelines for Hospital Catering*. London: Department of Health, 1995.

Kelly L. Audit of food wastage: differences between a plated and bulk system of meal provision. *Journal of Human Nutrition and Dietetics* 1999; **12**: 415–424.

Kondrup J, Bak L, Stenbaek Hansen B *et al*. Outcomes from nutrition support using hospital food. *Nutrition* 1998; **14**: 319–321.

Larsson J, Unosson M, Ek AC *et al*. Effect of dietary supplement on nutritional status and clinical outcome in 501 geriatric patients – a randomised study. *Clinical Nutrition* 1990; **9**: 179–184.

Lennard-Jones JE. *A Positive Approach to Nutrition as a Treatment*. London: King's Fund Centre, 1992.

Lennard-Jones JE, Arrowsmith H, Davison C *et al*. Screening by nurses and junior doctors to detect malnutrition when patients are first assessed in hospital. *Clinical Nutrition* 1995; **14**: 336–340.

McWhirter JP, Pennington CR. Incidence and recognition of malnutrition in hospital. *British Medical Journal* 1994; **308**: 945–948.

NHS Executive. *Hospital Catering: Delivering a Quality Service*. London: Department of Health, 1996.

NHS Executive. A first class service: Consultation document on quality in the new NHS. *Health Service Circular* 1998/113. London: Department of Health, 1998.

Nuffield Trust. *Managing Nutrition in Hospital: A Recipe for Quality*, Maryon-Davis A, Bristow A. (Eds). London: Nuffield Trust, 1999.

Ödlund-Olin A, Osterberg P, Hadell K *et al*. Energy-enriched hospital food to improve energy intake in elderly patients. *Journal of Parenteral and Enteral Nutrition* 1996; **20**: 93–97.

Patients' Association. *Catering for Patients in Hospital*. Harrow: The Patients' Association, 1993.

Reilly JJ, Hull SF, Albert N *et al*. Economic impact of malnutrition: a model system for hospitalised patients. *Journal of Parenteral and Enteral Nutrition* 1988; **12**: 371–376.

Royal College of Nursing. *Nutrition Standards and the Older Adult*. London: RCN, 1993.

South East Thames Regional Health Authority. *Service Standards: Nutritional Guidelines: The Food Chain*, 1993a.

South East Thames Regional Health Authority. *Service Standards: Nutritional Guidelines: Menu Planning*, 1993b.

Stephen AD, Beigg CL, Elliot ET *et al*. Food provision, wastage and intake in medical, surgical and elderly hospitalised patients. *Clinical Nutrition* 1997; **16** (Suppl 2): 4.

Tucker H. Cost containment through nutrition intervention. *Nutrition Reviews* 1996; **54**: 111–121.

United Kingdom Central Council for Nursing and Midwifery. *Responsibility for Feeding of Patients*. London: UKCC, 1997.

Wheatley P. Report of a nutritional screening audit. *Journal of Human Nutrition and Dietetics* 1999; **12**: 433–436.

1.17 Professional practice

This section aims to encourage dietitians to think more widely about how they practise and why they do what they do. Although much of what follows focuses on patient/client-related work, the principles apply to all dietitians and should be taken into account in whatever circumstances they are working.

Every dietitian is an autonomous practitioner responsible for his or her own actions and therefore must be able to justify and explain what he or she has done. Where national or local guidelines, policies or procedures exist they should be followed, or reasons given when they have not been followed. In the event of a complaint, the person will be judged against their peers, current good practice and any guidelines that exist.

1.17.1 Code of practice

As with all professionals, there is an expectation by clients, colleagues and the public that a dietitian will adopt a certain standard of behaviour.

In the UK, on qualification dietitians are eligible to become *state registered*. Registration is currently administered by the Dietitians Board of the Council for Professions Supplementary to Medicine (CPSM). Some changes to this system are likely in the near future. Registration is a public declaration of the quality of the registrant's education, clinical training and suitability as a practitioner. It gives the public confidence in the registrant as a practitioner, and offers protection from the illegal or unprofessional activities of improper practitioners. Registration, however, is only mandatory for working in the National Health Service (NHS) or for a Local Authority Social Services department; some dietitians working in other sectors choose not to register.

As a state registered dietitian (SRD), the practitioner agrees to abide by a strict *Statement of Conduct* that influences the way in which they work. The *Statement of Conduct* prepared by the Disciplinary Committee of the Dietitians Board of the CPSM (1996) outlines the type of conduct which would be considered to be infamous conduct in a professional respect.

The American Dietetic Association has published a *Code of Ethics for the Profession of Dietetics*, which is a useful reference (ADA 1999). This outlines the commitments and obligations to client, society, self and profession. In summary, dietitians are expected to:

- conduct themselves with honesty, integrity and fairness
- recognize and exercise professional judgement within the limit of their qualification and collaborate with others, seek council and make referrals as appropriate
- protect confidential information
- provide a service with objectivity and respect for the unique needs and values of individuals
- provide a service in a manner that is sensitive to cultural differences and does not discriminate against others on the basis of race, ethnicity, creed, religion, disability, gender, age, sexual orientation or national origin.

Although a code of ethics for dietitians has not been produced in the UK, the *Statement of Conduct* (Dietitians Board 1996) together with the *National Professional Standards for Dietitians Practising in Healthcare* (BDA 1997) (Table 1.32) form a set of guiding principles for all dietitians.

1.17.2 Steps for safe practice

Dietitians now work in a wide variety of settings and apply their skills in many different ways. Traditional roles are being expanded and tasks now undertaken are much more diverse, with some of their original duties now delegated to nursing, secretarial or clerical staff and dietetic helpers or technicians. What is now considered the 'normal' role of the dietitian is quite different to that of 20 years ago. The environment within which the dietitian works (e.g. an acute hospital, the primary care sector, in schools or industry) and the nature of the work (e.g. therapeutic, health promotion, one-to-one, public health, media) dictate the role which is developed. Further insight can be gained from the British Dietetic Association's Community Nutrition Group (CNG) publication *Community Dietetics, What Do We Offer?* (BDA, CNG 1999).

Care must be taken when taking on new duties and consideration should be given to their appropriateness within an existing post, competence to undertake the new duties, level of training required to carry them out, whether these activities are covered by professional indemnity insurance, and remuneration aspects. If in doubt, advice should be sought from managers, senior colleagues or the British Dietetic Association. General guidance can also be found in the briefing paper *The Extended Role of the Dietitian* (BDA 1999).

Dietitians rarely work in isolation and recognize that they will influence most effectively by working with and through other professionals (DH 1994). Most dietitians are part of a number of unidisciplinary and multidisciplinary teams and probably function in different ways in all of them. The members of the team will vary depending on its function,

Table 1.32 National Professional Standards for Dietitians Practising in Healthcare (BDA 1997)

Standard 1	Dietitians are state registered and work within the professional code of conduct and other legislative orders
Standard 2	Dietitians engage in self-development to improve knowledge and skills in order to remain competent to practise within a framework which will include a suitable learning environment and appraisal system
Standard 3	Dietitians generate and interpret research to enhance and develop dietetic practice
Standard 4	Dietitians are committed to and promote the advancement of the profession
Standard 5	5.1 Screening/Appropriate Referral The dietitian sets up a system whereby appropriate personnel identify and refer to them those who are at nutritional risk 5.2 Developing and implementing a plan of nutritional care The dietitian formulates a nutrition care plan for referred clients 5.3 Providing a nutritionally adequate diet The dietitian gives advice to ensure that the food available to the client is nutritionally adequate, acceptable to the client and appropriate to the client's needs 5.4 Developing and implementing a nutrition intervention programme The dietitian develops and plans a programme of work to meet the needs of the client group
Standard 6	Dietitians are responsible for an explicit quality of service
Standard 7	Dietitians work co-operatively with others to integrate dietetics into overall care/services
Standard 8	8.1 Effective communication: nutrition education resources The dietitian is responsible for developing, reviewing and disseminating resources and information relating to food and health 8.2 Effective communication: education and training Dietitians implement education and training to meet the identified needs of clients

but where applicable should include the patient or client and their family or carer. Being a successful member of a team means utilizing a range of skills and requires more than contributing specialist knowledge. Teamwork is about mutual respect, trust and support. Effective collaboration improves communication and the quality of care given.

Whatever role the dietitian is fulfilling, in whatever setting, the ultimate aim is to provide the highest quality service possible with each professional performing to the best of their ability. Quality and performance have been linked together by the NHS under the umbrella of *clinical governance*. Clinical governance is defined as:

a framework through which NHS organisations are accountable for continuously improving the quality of their services and safeguarding high standards of care by creating an environment in which excellence in clinical care can flourish. [The aim is] to provide an NHS that continually improves the overall standard of clinical care, whilst reducing variations in outcomes of, and access to, services as well as ensuring that clinical decisions are

based on the most up to date evidence of what is known to be effective (NHS Executive 1998a).

Clinical governance embraces many concepts (Fig. 1.5), all of which need to be incorporated into everyday practice in order to provide what would be considered good or safe practice. Some of these aspects are covered below as part of guidance on good practice; others are explained in more detail in the Section 1.18 (Clinical Effectiveness).

1.17.3 Guidance on good practice

The following subsections provide guidance on good practice in a number of areas, but it should be noted that the list of topics covered is not exhaustive.

Referral

In order to give therapeutic advice to an individual, the dietitian first needs to be made aware of that individual.

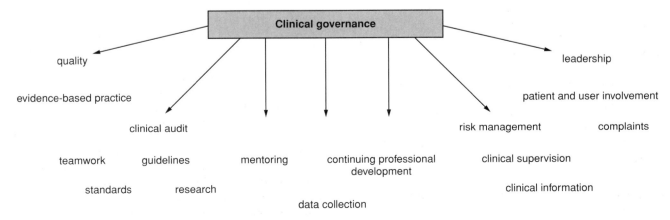

Fig. 1.5 Clinical governance.

This may be via a referral from another health professional or by the person referring themselves. The current *Statement of Conduct* does not require a formal referral system provided that a diagnosis is available.

The way in which referrals are made to the dietitian will depend on local policy and may be on a referral form, by letter, via the telephone, via the medical notes or electronically. Whichever method is used, enough information needs to be available in order to identify the patient correctly and to provide a diagnosis, a reason for the referral and sufficient medical information on which to base the dietetic treatment.

Verbal referrals should always be backed up by written information and appropriately documented. If insufficient information is available at the time of referral, this needs to be supplemented from the medical and nursing notes if they are available, any computerized records or directly from other health professionals. All information should be from a reliable, bone fide source. If the diagnosis is obtained directly from the patient, or insufficient information is available at the time of the consultation, the patient should only be given advice that will do no harm. Confirmation of the diagnosis should be sought before proceeding with more detailed treatment.

The person who provides the diagnosis and makes the referral is also a matter of local policy. These may come from a medical practitioner or alternatively from any member of the multidisciplinary team if a blanket system has been agreed and documented.

Therapeutic advice given to groups of people should be general and not specific to any one individual. When giving general nutritional advice to individuals (e.g. regarding sports nutrition) the assumption is that the person is healthy. If that person then develops a medical condition, a diagnosis from the appropriate doctor is required.

Competence to treat

Having received a referral, the dietitian should feel confident that they have sufficient knowledge and the appropriate skills to treat the case. Will treating the patient do more harm than good, or should the referral be passed to someone with more experience?

As professionals, all dietitians have a responsibility and a right to say that they are not competent to deal with a particular situation. Equally, all patients have a right to be treated by appropriately qualified staff.

If the dietitian is not competent to deal with the case but the situation is commensurate with that individual's status and a need for further education or additional skills has been identified, this needs to be incorporated into that individual's professional development plan (see *Continuing professional development*, below). It may, however, be inappropriate for that dietitian to see the patient, in which case a system should then be put in place to refer on to someone with the appropriate training. Development of a framework for assessing clinical competence through continuing professional development and clinical supervision is proposed within the profession.

Consent to treat

In most situations, advice and information are given and the person then makes an informed choice on whether to follow the advice. It is assumed that by attending an appointment or talking to the dietitian they have consented to treatment.

When the person is incapable of making an informed decision as with, for example, children or people with learning disabilities, then the decision to treat should be arrived at using local policies, where they exist. The decision should be made involving all members of the multidisciplinary care team, including relatives and friends if appropriate. Where there is conflict or doubt then the dietitian should discuss the situation with a more senior colleague or manager, either within or outside the profession. As part of a multidisciplinary team the dietitian is there to present the nutritional issues. The dietitian is also entitled to a personal view. Ultimately, however, the decision whether to treat or not should be a team decision (see Section 1.19, Healthcare ethics).

For any invasive procedure, signed consent should be obtained. This includes ensuring that the procedure, the reasons for it and any risks associated with it have been fully explained.

Treatment

Any advice or recommendations for treatment should be based on current evidence. It should always be scientific, objective, sound and without bias (see Section 1.18, Clinical effectiveness). Any commercial products used as part of the treatment should be advocated for their nutritional content and not improperly promoted.

A clear care plan should be devised which is appropriate for each individual and which includes measures for monitoring the success or otherwise of the treatment.

All professionals have an obligation to keep up to date and practise in an effective and efficient manner. *Continuing professional development* (CPD) is the process by which professionals update, maintain and enhance their knowledge and expertise in order to ensure their continuing competence to practise. At present in the UK, once qualified a dietitian does not have to prove their CPD but this is, however, one of the *National Professional Standards for Dietitians Practising in Healthcare* and will become mandatory in the near future.

According to guidelines produced by the British Dietetic Association (1998a), CPD:

- is a systematic and ongoing process
- should not be viewed as additional to normal working activities, as work itself and reflection on day-to-day practice is a learning process worthy of recognition
- formalizes experimental learning: what has been learnt should be constantly reviewed and ways sought to apply this learning to enhance the practice of the individual, their colleagues and team
- should be supported by employers and managers by

encouraging learning to take place at work and through the provision of learning opportunities
* is continuous and involves identifying development/ training needs, planning how these needs might be met, implementing a plan of action, applying learning to the job, making an assessment of the benefits of the application of that learning, identifying further needs and again planning for continued development.

Mentoring within the workplace is a process to be encouraged. It focuses on continuous learning and development within the context of that workplace and assists the individual to reach their full potential. A formal process of mentoring could be a senior 'expert' adopting a 'protégé'; less formally, it could be an established person helping the learner. Typically, mentoring in the workplace covers career enhancement for both learner and mentor, induction into the department and the politics of the department or organization (BDA 1998b).

Documentation

This is a fundamental part of the work of a dietitian. The creation, collection and recording of information – whether a note of a telephone conversation, a large report, or personal data about a specific patient or their treatment – is only as valuable as its content, and that is only of value if it can be found when needed, and then used effectively (NHS Executive 1999).

Clinical practice is knowledge driven, underpinned by the need to know how effective it is being. Managers, patients and colleagues within the profession and in other professions also need this knowledge. There is a need to produce, share and retrieve information to help to make the right decisions about clinical practice to benefit patients (NHS Information Authority 1999).

At present, most information is collected manually and hence is difficult to use effectively without a determined effort. Advances in information technology need to be utilized and exploited to provide direct benefits to patients, clients and health professionals. Within the NHS, the document *Information for Health: An Information Strategy for the Modern NHS* (NHS Executive 1998b) has been produced with the aim of ensuring that information is used to help patients to receive the best possible care. It is hoped this will be achieved by:

* improving the quality and accessibility of information for health professionals to support them in their work;
* enabling patients to be better informed about their condition;
* ensuring that planning and management of services is based on good quality information.

Information collected for management purposes should be a by-product of that collected for clinical purposes. Data need to be available, and in a suitable form, to enable analysis for the purposes of clinical governance, audit and standard setting, development of clinical guidelines and performance management. Historically, performance has been measured by the number of contacts made with a patient or client, irrespective of the quality of those contacts. Such activity data provided little useful information by which the efficacy and effectiveness of the service could be judged. More meaningful measures are likely to be developed as a result of the NHS Executive information strategy.

Patient-related documentation

This includes dietetic records, medical and nursing records, multidisciplinary case notes and patient-held records. The Electronic Health Record (a longitudinal record of a patient's health and healthcare from the cradle to the grave) and Electronic Patient Record (the record of the periodic care given mainly by one institution) are being developed. They have the advantage that they are more likely to be legible, accurate, safe, secure and available when required. They also more easily support the collection of information for management purposes.

Any documents (letters, charts, reports) written in connection with a patient are considered part of the record and copies should be kept with that record. The documentation could be paper based or computerized but the standard of record keeping remains the same and should meet the *Standards for Records and Record Keeping* (BDA/Dietitians Board 1996). These standards form part of the *Statement of Conduct*.

Records are kept to give a full, accurate and justifiable account of what has happened to, and what is planned for, the patient or client. They should include any information relevant to the care of that person. The rationale behind the chosen course of action should also be recorded. Any information given over the telephone should be fully documented. If telephone advice is routinely given, for example to nursing homes, local procedures need to be in place and adequate training given to safeguard all parties. Shoddy record keeping implies shoddy work.

Good record keeping:

1 promotes best quality patient care by:
   * facilitating continuity of care (there is an obvious treatment plan)
   * allowing communication between staff
   * avoiding duplication
   * avoiding the risk of omission
   * allowing the early detection of deviations from the norm;
2 safeguards, in the event of complaint or legal action, by providing:
   * evidence of the care given (no record, no contact)
   * reasons for decisions made;
3 contributes to the preparation of reports and statements;
4 supports standard setting and audit by collecting the evidence to contribute to research and evidence-based practice;
5 supports the appropriate management of resources.

When writing notes or letters, it should be borne in mind that a patient could request access to them and they should therefore be written in a suitable way using language that is readily understood.

When holding patient data in any form, registration with the Data Protection Registrar is required under the Data Protection Act 1998. Within the NHS this is done centrally but dietitians working privately will need to make sure they conform to the Act. The explicit consent of the individual is usually necessary before sensitive data can be processed. Data kept must also be secure. This may be as simple as keeping it in a locked place or could be password protection of all relevant systems (NHS Executive 1999).

Patient-related information contained on slides, film, video or other media is considered to be a public record and as such is covered by the same restrictions as all other records.

All documentation needs to be kept for the appropriate length of time. Detailed guidance on this can be found in the NHS Executive Health Service Circular *For the Record: Managing Records in NHS Trusts and Health Authorities* (NHS Executive 1999).

Communication

One of the strengths of a dietitian is the ability to communicate. Effective communication is stipulated in the *Statement of Conduct* (Dietitians Board 1996) and the *National Professional Standards for Dietitians Practising in Healthcare* (BDA 1997). There is an expectation that a dietitian will communicate effectively:

- with patients or clients to facilitate their making the behaviour changes required of them;
- with other health professionals to make them aware of the care being given, and hence to maximize care by avoiding duplication or omission and possible harm;
- through written, visual, audio and audiovisual communication by ensuring that all resources used by them and others are appropriate, unbiased and based on the professional consensus of scientific evidence;
- by training and educating others in all aspects of food and health to allow them to disseminate information which is based on professional consensus. Training needs to encompass knowledge and skills to facilitate food-related health gain.

Inadequate documentation and poor communication have been cited in most of the cases dealt with by the NHS Complaints Procedure and the Disciplinary Committee of the Dietitians' Board.

Caseload

An issue facing many dietitians, particularly in the NHS, is the expectation that an increasing volume of work will be undertaken within existing resources. This raises the issue of what is a 'safe' caseload. For many years this has been debated and formulae have been suggested, but because of the complexity and individuality of each situation no agreement has been reached. The variables, in addition to number, which need to be considered are:

- the clinical complexity of the caseload;
- the client group involved;
- local and national standards (dietetic, medical and multi-professional) for the level of involvement, number of appointments and frequency of review, for example The British Diabetic Association's *Recommendations for the Structure of Specialist Diabetes Care Services* (1999) or the Renal Association's *Treatment of Adult Patients with Renal Failure. Recommended Standards and Audit Measures* (1997);
- local and national clinical guidelines and protocols;
- other duties undertaken such as teaching, domiciliary visits and case conferences.

The development of National Service Frameworks for certain conditions or client groups and national clinical guidelines will also provide an indication of the type of service expected.

Ultimately, staffing levels, skill mix and the level of service provision are a management responsibility. It is, however, the responsibility of individuals to alert their manager if they are not able to meet standards or do not feel competent to deliver the service being expected of them.

Students

When involved in the training of any students, it should be remembered that any work undertaken by the student is ultimately the responsibility of the supervising dietitian. Each dietitian should therefore feel confident that the student is competent to handle the work expected and must accept responsibility for teaching, coaching, monitoring, assessing and mentoring as appropriate and in line with local policies for student training.

Local arrangements need to be made for the handling of notes in line with the Data Protection Act. Standards for record keeping need to be observed in line with the BDA/Dietitians Board *Standards for Records and Record Keeping* (1996).

Dietitians involved in training must also be competent in their own field of work and have the necessary skills to train students. Clinical supervisory skills courses specifically focused on the training of student dietitians are often organized in-house, regionally or nationally.

Non-client/freelance work

When working as a SRD, in whatever capacity, the *Statement of Conduct*, professional standards and the aim to deliver the highest quality service still apply. The nature of work may be much more varied but the fundamental principles remain the same:

- Protection of the public is paramount.
- The dietitian should be competent to undertake the work and, if not, should be prepared to pass it on to someone with more appropriate knowledge, skills and experience.
- The dietitian should be participating in continuing professional development.

- The work should be evidence based, monitored and evaluated.
- All appropriate information is collected, documented and shared with the appropriate people.
- All relevant legislation is understood and abided by.
- The dietitian communicates effectively.

Decisions on what constitutes 'acceptable work' may be much harder to make. It is important that professional independence is not compromised. Being isolated may make it difficult to consult others who have been in a similar situation but, if in doubt, discussion with peers is a good starting point.

Self-employed dietitians need to familiarize themselves with current business and legal requirements.

The Professional Approach (BDA 1996) contains useful information and advice for dietitians contemplating freelance work.

Text written by: Carole Middleton MBE

Further reading

American Dietetic Association. Standards of professional practice for dietetics professionals. *Journal of the American Dietetic Association* 1998; **98**: 83–88.

British Dietetic Association: Clinical Effectiveness Bulletins
Briefing Papers
Information Papers
Position Papers

Data Protection Act 1998. London: The Stationery Office, 1998.

Data Protection Registrar Information Line 01625 545 745.

References

American Dietetic Association. Code of Ethics for the Profession of Dietetics. *Journal of the American Dietetic Association* 1999; **99**: 109–113.

British Diabetic Association. *Recommendations for the Structure of Specialist Diabetes Care Services*. London: British Diabetic Association (now Diabetics UK), 1999.

British Dietetic Association. *The Professional Approach*. Birmingham: BDA, 1996.

British Dietetic Association. *National Professional Standards for Dietitians Practising in Healthcare*. Birmingham: BDA, 1997.

British Dietetic Association. *Continuing Professional Development for Dietitians*. Policy Paper. Birmingham: BDA, 1998a.

British Dietetic Association. *Mentoring in the Dietetic Profession*. Guidance Paper. Birmingham: BDA, 1998b.

British Dietetic Association. *The Extended Role of the Dietitian*. Briefing Paper No. 8. Birmingham: BDA, 1999.

British Dietetic Association, Community Nutrition Group. *Community Dietetics: What Do We Offer?*. Birmingham: BDA, 1999.

British Dietetic Association/Dietitians Board. *Guidance on Standards for Records and Record Keeping. Statement of Conduct*. London: Council for the Professions Supplementary to Medicine, 1996.

Department of Health. *Health of the Nation. Targeting Practice: The Contribution of State Registered Dietitians*. London: Department of Health, 1994.

Dietitians Board, Disciplinary Committee. *Statement of Conduct*. London: Council for the Professions Supplementary to Medicine, 1996.

NHS Executive. *A First Class Service: Quality in the New NHS*. London: Department of Health, 1998a.

NHS Executive. *Information for Health: An Information Strategy for the Modern NHS*. London: Department of Health, 1998b.

NHS Executive. *For the Record. Managing Records in NHS Trusts and Health Authorities*. Health Service Circular 1999/053. London: Department of Health, 1999.

NHS Information Authority. *Information for Practice. The National Information Management Agenda and You*. Bristol: NHS Information Authority, 1999.

Renal Association (Ed.). *Treatment of Adult Patients with Renal Failure. Recommended Standards and Audit Measures*, 2nd edn. London: Royal College of Physicians, 1997.

1.18 Clinical effectiveness

Improving the quality of healthcare is an important goal of all healthcare professionals. Although difficult to define in relation to health services, key components of quality in healthcare include:

- making care available to someone who needs it within a time period that is consistent with his or her clinical needs;
- providing appropriate care by making the 'best' choice of treatment or care from the available options, with the patient sharing in the decision making to the greatest extent possible;
- providing effective care that is consistent with current evidence of what works and in a correct and safe manner;
- providing acceptable care, as judged by the patient, client or patient's advocate;
- providing efficacious care that ultimately can be shown to benefit the patient or client.

In the 1960s, the Minister of Health Mr Enoch Powell suggested that some form of rationing is required in modern healthcare, as demand is potentially infinite, whereas resources are limited. As a consequence, some rationalization of healthcare is inevitable and it is necessary to prioritize and determine which treatments are the most effective in terms of both clinical efficacy and cost. At the same time, clinicians are increasingly being asked to demonstrate and promote effectiveness whilst coping with large quantities of rapidly changing, and at times apparently conflicting, evidence.

In the UK during 1997 and 1998 the Department of Health published a number of important policy documents that put quality firmly at the heart of the National Health Service (NHS) and had far-reaching implications for all healthcare professionals (DH 1997; Scottish Office 1997; Welsh Office 1998; DHSS Northern Ireland 1998). The document *A First Class Service: Quality in the New NHS* (DH 1998) outlined the government's plans for ensuring quality in the NHS by setting, delivering and monitoring quality standards.

1.18.1 What is clinical effectiveness?

Clinical effectiveness is:

The extent to which specific clinical interventions, when deployed in the field for a particular patient or population, do what they are intended to do, i.e. maintain and improve health and secure the greatest possible health gain from the available resources (DH 1996).

Or, more simply:

Doing the right thing in the right way for the right patient at the right time. This involves getting evidence of what works into everyday clinical practice and evaluating its effect in patient care (RCN 1998).

Clinical effectiveness incorporates elements of quality that have existed in healthcare services for some years and as such is not a new concept. However, the change is in seeing these individual elements as being linked and in exploiting these links to improve the quality of healthcare. It is concerned with clinical interventions that are based on the best available evidence of what works, derived where possible from rigorous research, applying these interventions and assessing their efficacy within real-life situations. It links research, the implementation of research findings through the development of clinical guidelines and standard setting, and clinical audit to provide a framework for quality improvement. This framework can be illustrated as a cycle (Fig. 1.6). In the clinical effectiveness cycle, research helps to provide the evidence that directs what to do and how to do it. It forms the basis of clinical guidelines and standard setting. The process of clinical audit then evaluates dietetic practice against these standards and, if necessary, provides the mechanism for change.

In essence, it means that what dietitians do for their clients should be supported by evidence that it works and performed in a way that means that it will work.

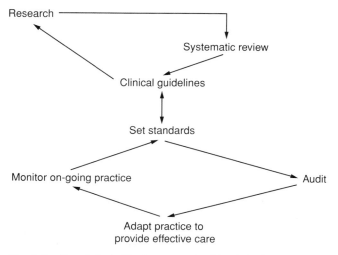

Fig. 1.6 The clinical effectiveness cycle. BDA (1997).

There are three main elements in achieving clinical effectiveness (NHS Executive 1996a). These can be applied to all areas of dietetic practice and are as follows:

- *Evidence*: tells dietitians what is the 'right thing to do'
- *Implementation*: ensures that dietitians do 'the right thing'
- *Monitoring*: demonstrates whether dietitians are 'doing the right thing right', how dietetic practice can be improved and whether a dietetic service is cost-effective.

1.18.2 What is evidence-based healthcare or evidence-based medicine?

Evidence-based healthcare/medicine is a frequently used term which is associated and often confused with clinical effectiveness. There are many definitions available in the medical literature. One defines it as being:

> ... the conscientious, explicit and judicious use of current best evidence in making decisions about the care of individual patients. The practice of evidence based medicine means integrating individual clinical experience with the best available clinical evidence from systematic research (McKibbon *et al.* 1995; National Centre for Clinical Audit 1997).

However, central to all definitions is the drive to make informed decisions based on evidence derived, wherever possible, from rigorous research and drawing upon individual clinical expertise, professional judgement and patient preferences. Good clinicians will use both individual expertise and the best available evidence, and neither alone is enough. The practice of evidence-based healthcare should promote clinical effectiveness and thereby improve the quality of health services.

1.18.3 The evidence

In order to achieve clinical effectiveness there needs to be sufficient evidence made available in such a way as to inform clinicians, patients and managers. Sources of evidence include research findings, professional recommendations based on experience and expert opinion and feedback from clients, their carers and user organizations. Data on patterns of care, population needs and the availability of resources are also needed (DH 1998). Without such information or evidence clinical effectiveness is unlikely to be achieved.

Research

Research findings are important sources of evidence since they can tell dietitians the 'right thing to do'. Where they are lacking new research must ultimately be undertaken to build up the evidence base. In the UK, the importance of research within dietetic practice is clearly stated in the British Dietetic Association's *Research Strategy* (BDA 1998) and *The National Professional Standards for Dietitians Practising in Healthcare* (BDA 1997). The BDA

publication *Getting Started in Research and Audit* (O'Kane 1998) offers a valuable guide to undertaking research. However, in order to base practice on research evidence, all the available research in a particular clinical area needs to be considered, not just part of it. To do this, literature searches must be comprehensive and systematic.

Once research papers have been identified, they need to be appraised. Critical appraisal skills are essential for weighing up the evidence to see how useful it is for decision making. Training in critical appraisal skills is widely available locally throughout the UK. In addition, the Critical Appraisal Skills Programme (CASP) offers training and has produced a number of appraisal tools (CASP/HCLU 1999). In the USA, the Department of Health and Human Services Agency for healthcare Policy and Research (AHCPR) has developed a scheme for categorizing research studies to indicate their predictive power and give ratings for the strength of the evidence (Table 1.33) (USDHHS 1993). Other workers have since adapted this scheme and variations on it can be found in the medical literature.

Unfortunately, all weigh heavily in favour of randomized controlled trials (RCTs) and do not adequately reflect qualitative research. RCTs are generally taken as the gold standard for research evidence, providing the least risk of bias in results and, therefore, the strongest evidence. Although it is important to use the best available evidence, areas of dietetic practice for which RCTs have not been carried out, or are not feasible, should not be ignored. Unlike drug trials, for which RCTs were designed, dietary studies involving free-living people can never be tightly controlled. To help overcome this, large numbers of people need to be studied. However, such trials are expensive and hence rare. In addition, the effects of diet on health can take years, or even a lifetime, to appear and RCTs are unlikely to be conducted for this long. For these reasons alone, other forms of evidence usually have to be relied on. For example, there is no definitive RCT showing that five portions of fruit or vegetables per day prevents cancer, and there never will be. However, there is now so much evidence to suggest that this measure is beneficial that it would unethical to ignore it.

Table 1.33 AHCPR classification of evidence levels (USDHHS 1993, Agency for Health Care Policy and Research)

Category of evidence
Ia   Evidence from meta-analysis of randomized controlled trials
Ib   Evidence from at least one randomized controlled trial
IIa   Evidence from at least one well-designed controlled study without randomization
IIb   Evidence from at least one other type of well-designed quasi-experimental study
III   Evidence from well-designed, non-experimental descriptive studies, e.g. comparative studies, correlation studies and case – control studies
IV   Evidence from expert committee reports or opinions or clinical experiences of respected authorities

Systematic reviews

Systematic review is an efficient scientific technique to identify and summarize evidence on the effectiveness of interventions, and to allow the generalizability and consistency of research findings to be assessed and data inconsistencies to be explored. Older style reviews are sometimes called narrative reviews. They do not usually state the methods used in their creation and may be biased by the author's beliefs. In contrast, systematic reviews clearly describe the objectives, materials and methods used and, are conducted according to explicit and reproducible methodology. They are less likely to be biased. An example of this is the famous narrative review by Linus Pauling, in which he used selective quotes from the medical literature to 'prove' his theory that large doses of vitamin C can prevent the common cold. His conclusions have since been discredited by a systematic review in the Cochrane Library (Douglas *et al.* 1999).

Systematic reviews may be descriptive (qualitative) or give some overall mathematical summary of the effect of an intervention (meta-analysis). However, systematic reviews and meta-analyses are not the same thing. A systematic review may or may not incorporate a meta-analysis. Alternatively, the trials in meta-analysis may not always be identified in a systematic way.

Good-quality systematic reviews of RCTs provide the strongest evidence for clinical effectiveness. The Cochrane Collaboration and the NHS Centre for Reviews and Dissemination are only concerned with evidence from good-quality reviews and systematic reviews, although they are not the only sources of these. The Cochrane Library is primarily interested in systematic reviews of RCTs.

It is extremely important to assess the quality of a systematic review before looking at the results and their implications for clinical practice. Greenhalgh (1997) and Oxman *et al.* (1994) have both published guides on assessing their quality.

Sources of evidence

The following are some important sources of research evidence and systematic reviews:

For research findings:

- the common bibliographic databases: MEDLINE, HEALTHSTAR, CINAHL, EMBASE
- NHS/medical/college libraries
- the National Research Register (UK)
- the National Clinical Improvement Projects Index (UK)
- publications: professional and medical journals, evidence-based medicine publications such as *Effective Health Care Bulletin* and *Effectiveness Matters* (UK).

For systematic reviews:

- the Cochrane Library
- medical databases such as MEDLINE, EMBASE
- the British Dietetic Association's list of diet-related systematic reviews

- the NHS Centre for Reviews and Dissemination Database of Abstracts of Reviews of Effectiveness (DARE).

Websites for these and other evidence sources are listed at the end of this section.

1.18.4 Implementation

If dietitians are to improve clinical effectiveness it is essential that research-based evidence is incorporated into everyday practice. This may require practitioners to change long-held patterns of behaviour and can be a difficult and complex process. Tools for translating the evidence into practice include evidence-based clinical guidelines, care pathways and care profiles, and standards. However, knowledge of a practice guideline, or some other research-based recommendation, alone is rarely sufficient to bring about changes in practice. There is a large volume of literature concerned with changing professional practice. The NHS Centre for Reviews and Dissemination has presented some of this in the form of an overview (NHS Centre for Reviews and Dissemination 1999).

Clinical guidelines

There is a great deal of interest in the development of clinical guidelines across Europe, North America, Australia, New Zealand and Africa. This interest arises from the increasing healthcare costs, unexplained variations in service delivery and drives to improve the quality of healthcare apparent in most healthcare systems. It is reflected in the large number of clinical guidelines available in the UK alone. Unfortunately, published clinical guidelines vary greatly in quality and many do not merit attention. Historically, most British guidelines have been derived from expert opinion or consensus conferences rather than scientific evidence of what works, although current interest is in developing rigorous evidence-based guidelines.

What are clinical guidelines?

In the UK, the NHS Executive defines clinical guidelines as being 'systematically developed statements which assist clinicians and patients in making decisions about appropriate treatment for specific conditions' (NHS Executive 1996b). They provide information about the care for a particular condition, including the options available, but do not replace clinical expertise. Valid guidelines, when appropriately disseminated and implemented, can lead to changes in healthcare practice, improvements in patient care and ultimately in health outcomes for patients. In short, they can help to ensure that the care clinicians give is up to date and is the 'best' that is possible. However, to realize their potential, clinical guidelines must be carefully developed, described and implemented. Key characteristics of high quality guidelines have been listed by the NHS Centre for Reviews and Dissemination (1994) and staff at the Health Care Evaluation Unit at St George's Hospital Medical School, London, have developed a clinical guideline appraisal instrument (Cluzeau *et al*. 1997).

National versus local clinical guidelines

Clinical guidelines can be developed nationally, regionally or locally, the distinction between them being in the level of specificity of information that they contain. Nationally developed guidelines generally reflect a broad statement of good practice with little operational detail. They need to be adapted for local use, so becoming 'local clinical guidelines' or, as in Scotland, 'protocols'.

Standards

Standards are statements of minimum, excellent or a range of acceptable levels of performance or results (Grimshaw and Russell 1993). The British Dietetic Association has described them as being 'agreed statements of good practice that are achievable, measurable and reviewed regularly' (BDA 1997). In addition, they should be amenable to audit and be evidence based where possible. They outline an objective and give guidance for its achievement in the form of criteria sets that specify required resources, activities and predicted outcomes. Standards can be developed locally or nationally and, by defining the quality of the service provided, they enable service quality to be developed and improved upon. They provide a basis for measuring actual clinical practice using clinical audit.

Care pathways and care profiles

Care pathways are sometimes referred to as critical pathways, multidisciplinary pathways of care, anticipated recovery pathways, care protocols, clinical pathways, integrated care pathways, collaborative care plans, care maps or clinical algorithms. Despite a lack of one accepted definition, the National Pathways Association in the UK has developed a consensus definition within its membership. They view care pathways as determining locally agreed multidisciplinary practice, based on guidelines and evidence where available, for a specific patient or client group. They form all or part of the clinical record, documenting the care given and facilitating the evaluation of outcomes for continuous quality improvement. In short, their primary function is to assist clinical staff in the day-to-day delivery of care.

Care profiles were initially called care packages and are outline descriptions of the health and social care normally provided to meet the health needs of a patient or group of patients to achieve an expected outcome to an explicit quality standard. Like care pathways they are clinical tools for use in the provision of planned clinical care. However, in contrast to care pathways, they are used less in the everyday delivery of care and more as a summary of the planned or anticipated care and the standards of care aimed for. They give less detail on the clinical tasks to be performed than do care pathways.

1.18.5 Monitoring

Clinical audit provides the ideal mechanism to monitor compliance with clinical guideline recommendations, care pathways and profiles, and standards in day-to-day practice.

Clinical audit

Clinical audit is a 'clinically led initiative which seeks to improve the quality and outcome of patient care through structured peer review whereby clinicians examine their practices and results against agreed explicit standards and modify their practice where indicated' (National Centre for Clinical Audit 1997). Whilst the outcome or result of a clinical intervention is often the primary focus for healthcare professionals, there are other aspects of clinical practice and service delivery which have a bearing on outcome. Accordingly, audit may examine aspects of service structure (the availability and organization of human and material resources required for service delivery) and process (the way in which the patient is received and managed by the service from the time of referral to the time of discharge) as well as outcome and quality of life for patients or clients. Medical audit refers to audit carried out by doctors and has been used routinely in healthcare for some time. In 1991, the Department of Health launched an initiative to encourage other professions to use similar audit methods. This became known as clinical audit and is now a widespread practice amongst dietitians. Indeed, our National Professional standards state that 'dietitians will continually assess the efficacy of their current practice by using a range of models including evaluation and audit' (BDA 1997).

The process of clinical audit involves comparing current practice against preset agreed standards, examining the findings, if necessary implementing changes to improve current practice and re-auditing to establish whether or not improvement has occurred. In this way it can be viewed as a cycle (Fig. 1.7). It is the process of making changes and re-auditing that brings about tangible improvements in practice.

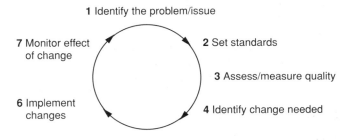

Fig. 1.7 The clinical audit cycle. From Kogan and Redfern (1995); reproduced with permission from Open University Press.

Differences between research and audit

The terms 'research' and 'clinical audit' can be confusing. Both activities involve searching published literature, working to answer a question and collecting, analysing and interpreting data. It is easy to think of them as one and the same and to use the terms indiscriminately. However, an audit project is not the same thing as a research project. The essential difference is that research answers the question 'what is the right thing to do?', whereas clinical audit answers the questions 'are we doing the right thing?', 'are we doing it well?' and 'are we doing what we think we are?' (Charny 1998).

Text written by: Alison Brady and Diane Talbot

Useful sources of evidence

Databases on the internet
The Cochrane Library (Update Software)
Website: www.update-software.co.uk

DARE (Database of Abstracts of Reviews of Effectiveness), The Health Technology Assessment (HTA) Database and The NHS Economic Evaluation Database
All can be accessed at http://nhscrd.york.ac.uk/welcome. html or on CD-ROM in the Cochrane Library

MEDLINE
Accessed via PubMed Internet site (www.ncbi.nlm.nih. gov/PubMed) or on CD-ROM in health libraries

CINAHL (Cumulative Index to Nursing and Allied Health Database)
Accessed at www.the-caa-ltd.demon.co.uk/aud2 and on CD-ROM in health libraries

AMED (Allied and Alternative Medicine Database)
Available on CD-ROM

HealthSTAR (HSTR)
Website: www.nlm.nih.gov

Health Promotion Research Internet Network
Website: www.dsg.ki.se/socmed

Evidence Based Medicine Reviews
Website: www.ovid.com

TRIP (Turning Research into Practice)
Website: www.gwent.nhs.gov.uk/trip

Outcomes Database of Structured Abstracts and Outcomes Activities Database
Website: www.leeds.ac.uk/nuffield/infoservices/UKCH-home.html

National Research Register
Website: www.doh.gov.uk/research/nrr.htm

National Clinical Improvement Projects Index
Website: http://www.nice.org.uk

Clinical Practice Guidelines Infobase
Website: www.mls.cps.bs.ca/mlsbkmk.htm

National Guideline Clearinghouse (USA)
Website: www.guidelines.gov/index.asp

Guideline
Website: www.his.ox.ac.uk/guidelines/index.html

Other useful internet sites

Netting the Evidence – A SCHARR Introduction to Evidence Based Practice on the Internet
Website: www.shef.ac.uk/uni/academic/R-Z/scharr/ir/netting.html

CHAIN (Contact Help Advice Information Network for Effective Health Care)
Website: www.nthames-health.tpmde.ac.uk/chain.htm

Critical Appraisal Resource Guide
Website: http://nzgg.org.nz/tools/resources_critical_appraisal.htm

Evidence Based Medicine Resource List
Website: www.herts.ac.uk/lrc/subjects/health/ebm.htm

Evidence Based Healthcare – A Resource Pack
Website: http://drsdesk.sghms.ac.uk/Starnet/pack.htm

Evidence Based Topics
Website: www.ohsu.edu/bicc-informatics/ebm/ebm_topics. htm

National Electonic Library for Health (NELH)
Website: www.nelh.nhs.uk

Sources of Evidence (CASPFEW)
Website: www.his.ox.ac.uk/caspfew/sources.html

Useful evidence-based healthcare publications

Bandolier
Anglia and Oxford Region Health Authority
Tel: 01865 226132
Website:www.jr2.ox.ac.uk:80/Bandolier

British Journal of Clinical Governance
(formerly *Journal of Clinical Effectiveness*)
MCB University Press
Tel: 01274 777700
Website: http://mcb.co.uk

Clinical Evidence (http://www.evidence.org), *Evidence-Based Medicine, Evidence-Based Nursing, Evidence-Based Mental Health* and *Quality in Health Care*
BMJ Publishing Group
Tel: 020 7383 6270

Effective Health Care Bulletins, Effectiveness Matters and CRD (Centre for Reviews and Dissemination) Reports
Tel: 01904 433648
Website: www.york.ac.uk/inst/crd

Health Evidence Bulletins – Wales
Website: www.uwcm.ac.uk/uwcm/ib/pep/index.html

Journal of Clinical Excellence. Radcliffe Medical Press Ltd
Tel: 01235 528820

Evidence-Based Purchasing. The NHS Executive R+D Directorate, Bristol.
Tel: 0117 928 7224

Useful addresses

Aggressive Research Intelligence Facility (ARIF)
University of Birmingham
Website: www.hsrc.org.uk/links/arif/arifhome.htm

British Library, Health Care Information Service
Tel: 01937 546039
Website: www.bl.uk

Central Health Outcome Unit
Department of Health, Wellington House, 133–155 Waterloo Rd, London SE1 8UG
Tel: 020 7972 2000

Centre for Evidence Based Medicine
University of Oxford, Nuffield Department of Clinical Medicine, Level 5, The Oxford Radcliffe NHS Trust, Headley Way, Headington, Oxford OX3 9DU
Tel: 01865 221321
Website: cebm.jr2.ox.ac.uk

Centre for Evidence Based Child Health
Department of Epidemiology and Biostatistics, Institute of Child Health, University College London, 30 Guilford Street, London WC1N 1EH
Tel: 020 7242 9789
Website: www.ich.bpmf.ac.uk/ebm/ebm.htm

Clinical Effectiveness Support Unit for Wales (CESU)
'Roseway', UHW and Llandough NHS Trust, Llandough Hospital, Penlan Road, Penarth, Vale of Glamorgan CF64 2XX
Tel: 02820 716841

Clinical Resource and Audit Group (CRAG)
Room 205, St Andrew's House, Regent Road, Edinburgh EH1 3DE
Tel: 0131 244 2345

Cochrane Library
Update Software Ltd, Summertown Pavillion, Middle Way, Summertown, Oxford OX2 7LG
Tel: 01865 513902
Website: www.update-software.co.uk or www.cochrane.org/cochrane/cdsr.htm

Critical Appraisal Skills Programme (CASP)
Institute of Health Sciences, Old Road, Headington, Oxford OX3 7LF
Tel: 01865 226730
Website: www.phru.org/casp/rct.html

Eli Lily National Clinical Audit Centre
Department of General Practice and Primary Health Care, University of Leicester Leicester General Hospital, Gwendolen Road, Leicester LE5 4PW
Tel: 0116 258 4873
Website: www.el.ac.uk/clinaudit/

King's Fund and the Health Quality Service
11–13 Cavendish Square, London W1M 0AN
Tel: 020 7307 2400/2408
Website: www.kingsfund.org.uk

National Co-ordinating Centre for Health Technology Assessment
Mailpoint 728, Wessex Institute for Health R+D, Boldrewood, University of Southampton, Southampton SO16 7PX
Tel: 023 8059 5586
Website: www.hta.nhsweb.nhs.uk

NHS Centre for Reviews and Dissemination
University of York, Helsington, York YO1 5DD
Tel: 01904 433634
Website: www.york.ac.uk/inst/crd

National Institute for Clinical Excellence (NICE)
11 Strand, London WC2N 5HR
Tel: 020 7766 9191
Website: www.nice.org.uk

School of Health and Related Research (ScHARR)
University of Sheffield, Regent Court, 30 Regent Street, Sheffield S1 4DA
Website: www.shef.ac.uk/uni/academic/R-Z/scharr/index. html

Scottish Intercollegiate Guidelines Network (SIGN)
SIGN Secretariat, Royal College of Physicians, 9 Queen St, Edinburgh EH2 1JQ
Tel: 0131 225 7324
Website: www.show.scot.nhs.uk/sign/home.htm

Systematic Reviews Training Unit
Institute of Child Health, University College London, and the Royal Free Hospital School of Medicine, 30 Guilford Street, London WC1N 1EH
Tel: 020 7242 9789
Website: www.ich.ucl.ac.uk/srtu

UK Clinical Audit Association
Room 9, Cleethorpes Centre, Wilton Road, Humberston, South Humberside DN36 4AS
Tel: 01472 210682
Website: www.the-caa-ltd.demon.co.uk

References

British Dietetic Association. *National Professional Standards for Dietitians Practising in Healthcare*. Birmingham: BDA, 1997.

British Dietetic Association. *Research Strategy*. Birmingham: BDA, 1998.

Charny M. Audit and research – untangling the ball of string. *Interchanges* 1998; **1**: 8–10.

Cluzeau F, Littlejohns P, Grimshaw JM, Feder G. *Appraisal Instrument for Clinical Guidelines*. London: St George's Hospital Medical College, 1997.

Critical Skills Appraisal Programme (CASP) and the Health Care Libraries Unit (HCLU). *Evidence-based Healthcare. An Open Learning Resource for Healthcare Practitioners*. Oxford: CASP and HCLU, 1999.

Department of Health. *Promoting Clinical Effectiveness: A Framework for Action in and Through the NHS*. Leeds: NHS Executive, 1996.

Department of Health. *The New NHS: Modern, Dependable*. London: The Stationery Office, 1997.

Department of Health. *A First Class Service: Quality in the New NHS*. London: The Stationery Office, 1998.

Department of Health and Social Services in Northern Ireland. *Fit for the Future: A New Approach*. Belfast: DHSS, 1998.

Douglas RM, Chalker EB, Tracey B. *Vitamin C for Preventing and Treating the Common Cold (Cochrane Review)*. In *The Cochrane Library*, Issue 4. Oxford: Update Software, 1999.

Greenhalgh T. Papers that summarise other papers (systematic reviews and meta-analyses). *British Medical Journal* 1997; **315**: 672–675.

Grimshaw J, Russell I. Achieving health gains through clinical guidelines. 1: Developing scientifically valid guidelines. *Quality in Healthcare* 1993; **2**: 243–248.

Kogan M, Redfern S. *Making Use of Clinical Audit: A Guide to Practice in the Health Professions*. Buckingham: Open University Press, 1995.

McKibbon KA, Wilczynski N, Hayward RS *et al*. The medical literature as a resource for healthcare practice. *Journal of the American Society for Information Science* 1995; **46**: 737–742.

National Centre for Clinical Audit. *Glossary of Terms used in the NCCA Criteria for Clinical Audit*. London: NCCA, 1997.

NHS Centre for Reviews and Dissemination. Implementing clinical practice guidelines. *Effective Health Care* 1994: **8**.

NHS Centre for Reviews and Dissemination. Getting evidence into practice. *Effective Health Care* 1999; **5** (1).

NHS Executive. *Information on Clinical Effectiveness*. Leeds: NHS Executive, 1996a.

NHS Executive. *Clinical Guidelines: Using Clinical Guidelines to Improve Patient Care within the NHS*. Leeds: NHS Executive, 1996b.

O'Kane M (Ed.). *Getting Started in Research and Audit*. Birmingham: BDA, 1998.

Oxman AD, Cook DJ, Guyatt GH. How to use an overview. *Journal of the American Medical Association* 1994; **272**: 1367–1371.

Royal College of Nursing (RCN). *Clinical Effectiveness: A Royal College of Nursing Guide*. London: RCN, 1998.

Scottish Office. *Designed to Care: Renewing the NHS in Scotland*. Edinburgh: The Stationery Office, 1997.

US Department of Health and Human Services (USDHHS). Agency for Healthcare Policy and Research. *Acute Pain Management: Operative or Medical Procedures and Trauma*. Clinical Practice Guideline No. 1. AHCPR Publication No. 92-0023. p. 107. Rockville (MD): The Agency; 1993.

Welsh Office. *NHS Wales: Putting Patients First*. London: The Stationery Office, 1998.

1.19 Healthcare ethics

The interest in and the need for ethical discussion as a part of clinical practice have arisen from new technology giving new choices in how to proceed. For instance, the flexible endoscope was introduced in 1980, making percutaneous endoscopic gastrostomy (PEG) possible. Consequently, dietetic practice in PEG feeding developed throughout the 1980s, making long-term nutritional support a more widely available option but, at the same time, raising ethical questions as to when this option is appropriate.

The dietitian working to an ethical standard is a moral agent, capable of judging right and wrong and acting for good or bad. Each dietitian brings a personal belief system when taking part in a discussion. The dietitian has the right to an opinion but not to force that opinion as the right course of action without discussion and as wide agreement as possible, preferably interdisciplinary as well as intradisciplinary.

1.19.1 Principles influencing ethical decisions

Some of the principles and terminology which are relevant to ethical decision making are outlined below.

The four principles

Four basic principles – autonomy, beneficence, non-maleficence and justice – are currently considered to underlie biomedical ethics (Table 1.34).

Ethical principles which arise from respecting a person's autonomy include confidentiality and informed consent.

Confidentiality

Information about a person belongs to that person. A dietitian may not divulge information received from a person to anyone else except in certain circumstances. The dietitian always has the option to pass on confidential medical information on the grounds of acting in the client's best interests and exercising discretion but, if challenged, the decision would have to be defended.

Informed consent

This is the ethical term for asking a patient's permission to carry out a procedure on the body. Informed consent is needed by surgeons before operating, but the principles, which are designed to respect autonomy, are equally useful in dietetic clinical practice (see Section 1.17, Professional practice). Obtaining informed consent reinforces the element of trust in the patient–practitioner relationship. Enhanced trust helps communication and can reinforce behaviour change in the best interests of the patient.

There are four requirements for obtaining informed consent:

1 The patient must be *competent* (see below) to make a decision.
2 Sufficient information must be given to understand the nature of the proposed action and its possible outcome.
3 The decision has to be voluntary, not coerced.
4 There has to be a clear decision, yes or no, made by the patient.

A form may be signed as evidence to support the patient's decision but this form, of itself, does not contain any of the four criteria necessary to informed consent. It does not

Table 1.34 The Four Principles (basic moral commitments) (based on Gillon 1986, 1994; after Beauchamp and Childress)

Principle	Meaning	Notes
Autonomy	Self-rule Ability to take responsible decisions for oneself	There has been a shift in practice from paternalism to individual rights Empowerment of a patient to control health and healthcare enhances autonomy
Beneficence	To do good	The traditional Hippocratic oath promises overall medical benefit with minimal harm
Non-maleficence	Not to harm	Dietitians 'profess' to benefit patients. Rigorous, effective ongoing education is needed to remain professional
Justice	To act fairly	This includes: *Distributive justice*: fair distribution of scarce resources. Microallocation looks at resources for individuals; macroallocation deals with populations *Rights-based justice*: respect for people's rights *Legal justice*: respect for morally acceptable law

prove that sufficient information was given in a way that the patient could understand. A patient may change a decision on what action to take, with or without a form being signed.

In an emergency, in order to save life, a treatment decision can be taken without informed consent. This also holds for the mentally ill person if that person's life is endangered. Action which is taken because the practitioner believes it will be good for the client, irrespective of what the client thinks, overrides autonomy, infringes liberty and is, at best, *paternalistic*. At worst it could be an assault.

Any non-consensual bodily contact (such as an injection or passing a nasogastric tube) is, in law, a battery or trespass. If someone holds out an arm for the injection or tolerates the passing of a nasogastric tube this can be taken as implied consent, even if not expressed in words. If there is argument, the defence of tacit consent or of *necessity* could be used. The patient will have to show that the person carrying out the procedure should have been aware of non-consent.

Competence

Competence in children

Adulthood begins at 18. Children under 18 years old are minors with fewer responsibilities for making their own choices. Legal practice currently makes a distinction between 16/17-year-old juveniles and younger children:

- 16/17 year olds can give consent if they are competent: this is deemed valid consent.
- It is acceptable for younger children to give consent provided that they are mature enough to understand the implications (e.g. 12–15 year olds asking for contraceptives). This is supported by legal precedent.

No juvenile or child has a legal right to refuse treatment. If the parents give consent, this is valid. Equally, parents are able to refuse consent if it is in the child's best interests to refuse. In cases where the child would consent but the parents refuse, the medical treatment decision will be based on the child's best interest, if necessary with application to the courts in order to proceed. If an anorexic is refusing treatment and is thought to be at risk, the patient may be made a ward of court so that treatment on an eating disorders unit can be given.

Children old enough to understand have a right to confidentiality, if they so wish, and parents should not automatically be given details, or oversee details, of the child's medical appointments.

Mental competence

There is no single definitive test to measure incompetence.

A mentally competent person is considered to have the mental capacity to be responsible for his or her own acts and omissions, and their consequences. In order to be judged competent to make a decision, there must be some evidence of decision-making ability.

An individual may be found competent to make some decisions but incompetent to make others. It is possible for a person to be capable of expressing preference for a place to live but not to be competent to sign a will. A patient detained under the Mental Health Act may be competent to decide whether to undergo surgery for a physical ailment or to participate in dietary treatment.

The Mental Health Act, 1983, allows three bases for compulsory admission. These are:

1 In the interests of the client's own health.
2 In the interests of the client's own safety.
3 For the protection of other people.

Application for admission for a person suffering from a mental disorder may be made by an approved social worker or nearest relative. Two medical recommendations are needed. For assessment, the person can be detained for up to 28 days. For treatment, detention can last for up to 6 months at a time.

For assessment in emergency, only one medical recommendation is needed but detention is permitted for no more than 72 hours.

There is an important distinction between *irrational behaviour* and *mental incompetence*. The irrational person retains responsibility for taking decisions. For example, dietitians often treat elderly, incapacitated patients who want to return home. It is logical for the dietitian to favour residential care because this is seen as a safe, monitored food supply, however, the patient has the right to make an autonomous choice. The dietitian's task is to give appropriate information on food supply for the home circumstances, not to overrule the patient's wishes, no matter how irrational they appear. Mental competence to take the decision on where to live is verified by the consultant physician and is a personal judgement which may be made after team discussion.

Proxy decision taking

In England and Scotland, as the law stands in 1999, no one, not even the next-of-kin, can make treatment decisions on behalf of an adult patient, not even when the person is unconscious or unable to make a decision due to mental incapacity. The onus is on the physician to offer treatment in the best interests of the patient.

In order to determine *best interests*, relatives and friends may be consulted to give information on the patient's wishes, previously expressed. However, note that an *advance directive* (or living will) giving written instructions on what the patient would want to happen if mentally incapacitated is not legally binding on the physician. The doctor may decide that new and extenuating circumstances override the original viewpoint of the advance directive. The choice of treatment is made by the doctor at the time when treatment is needed. The treatment will be that which, in the doctor's view, confers most benefits and least burdens on the patient.

Conscious patients can invite relatives, friends or other advisers to help them to make medical decisions, if they so wish.

1.19.2 Death and end-of-life issues

Definition of death

An individual who has sustained irreversible cessation of all functions of the entire brain including the brainstem is dead. Cell function stops at different rates in different parts of the body during death.

If all higher cortical function has been destroyed the person will be in a *persistent vegetative state* (PVS). Breathing is controlled by the brainstem, which continues to function in PVS. Therefore, the person is not dead, although lacking capacity to respond to nervous stimuli.

Is food 'care' or 'treatment'?

Food supply, including enteral feeding, is part of a general duty of care. Anyone who takes on the care of a dependant, conscious or unconscious, has a duty to see that the care is continued. Care cannot be abandoned, although the responsibilities may be handed on to someone else. Therefore, in PVS, which by definition will have persisted for more than a year, application to withdraw feeding should always be made through the Courts. The local Health Trust lawyers should deal with the application, which is made in the Family Division of the High Court. The family medical lawyers at the office of the Official Solicitor are available to discuss a case when proceedings are being considered. It is important to know who is medically in charge. Lawyers for families may also make enquiries (British Medical Association 1999).

Food can be defined as treatment if there is a therapeutic intention when a particular item is supplied. If this is done, the length of time for treatment should be decided and the clinical signs to measure the outcome of the trial agreed. If there is no improvement after the stated time then the food item, or enteral feeding, can be withdrawn on the basis that it is *futile treatment* (i.e. is without benefit). There is no obligation to continue any treatment unless it has beneficial effects for the patient.

Quality of life

Treatment and care decisions may be targeted at improving an individual's *quality of life*. Quality of life is an elusive concept. Only the client knows his or her own feelings. Therefore the client should be included in discussion of the issues. Relatives and friends may express their views but this is an opinion only, and no more than that.

In palliative and terminal care for irreversible illness, the first target is the comfort of the patient. There is no duty to force feed where the patient does not want food. The primary aim is beneficent – relief of suffering – not to impose unwanted extra burdens. Any action which will unnecessarily prolong the process of dying should be avoided. Most patients, but not all, will be most comfortable with adequate hydration, given by the most comfortable route. Some will be most comfortable without hydration but with full attention to oral hygiene. The aim should be to maintain dignity, not to prolong suffering (Dunphy and Randall 1997) (see Section 4.39, Terminal illness and palliative care).

Euthanasia

Eu-thanatos (Greek) means 'a good death'. Euthanasia is the intentional bringing about of the death of a person, either by killing or by allowing to die for the *person's own sake*. Those who hold a personal *sanctity of life* ethic will seek to preserve life against any other considerations. Some countries have laws which permit euthanasia, but in Britain it is a criminal offence.

Ethical judgements look at motives behind actions, particularly where treatments have undesirable side-effects. For instance, morphine is given for pain relief but it can kill and, in large doses, does shorten life. Tube feeding provides nourishment but may result in death from aspiration pneumonia. Provided that the primary intention was treatment and care intending net benefit to the patient, the practitioner is not guilty of murder. This is known as the *doctrine of double effect*.

1.19.3 The role of the law

Common law is built up year by year from the major decisions of judges. The legal principles which have evolved through many centuries are called precedents. These become established principles which other judges will follow in similar cases and add to as additional complexities are questioned. An example of this is the Bolam Test (All England Law Reports 1957). Mr Bolam was a patient who suffered fractures while receiving electroconvulsive therapy (ECT). He claimed that his doctor was negligent for not warning him of the risk, but the judge found that the amount of information given accorded with acceptable medical practice at that time. This judgement established a principle which has been extended to all people professing a particular skill. If a dietitian acts in a way that a recognized, responsible group of fellow professionals would rightly accept as proper, this is acceptable practice.

The All England Law Reports and similar bound case law can be consulted in any law library. Recent volumes make interesting reading on matters of feeding, treatment, care and resource distribution ('rationing' of healthcare).

Statute law is the written law made by Parliament. As well as Acts of Parliament it includes the rules made by Ministers and Secretaries of State under the authority given by an Act.

Ethical discussion will take account of statute law and of precedents. In addition, dietitians have to comply with other sources of regulations, such as National Health Service (NHS) circulars, regulations laid down by employers and requirements of regulatory bodies.

Criminal law regulates conduct between individuals and the State. *Civil law* is concerned with relationships between individuals. The European Communities Act, 1972, makes European law binding over British law.

Principles of negligence

In order to establish *negligence* it has to be proved that duty of care is breached when the reasonable standard is not followed and, as a reasonably foreseen consequence, harm occurs. The employee is rarely sued; it is usually the employer (e.g. an NHS Trust) who will be held to be vicariously liable if the *employee* is *negligent* whilst acting *in the course* of employment. However, the employer has a right of indemnity against the negligent employee.

Reasonableness is at the heart of practice, i.e. it is only possible to take account of risk if it is foreseeable.

1.19.4 Established sources of ethical debate

In order to have a foundation for ethical decision making there needs to be a structure for working towards a common consensus. This may include:

- the multidisciplinary team policy planning conference or case conference
- the hospital-based ethics committee: in Britain, these committees are sometimes limited to research ethics
- the clinical ethics committee: these are developing in some Health Trusts
- the ethics committee of professional dietetic associations: in Britain this would be the Ethical and Professional Advisory Panel (EPAP) of the British Dietetic Association
- committees of other professional bodies or organizations such as the British Medical Association or the Council for Professions Supplementary to Medicine.

1.19.5 Practical aspects

The first step in any ethical debate is to promote conversation between all the people with an interest in the situation under review. People must start talking to each other. The overall motivation of such conversation is how to enhance the common good. A wide variety of viewpoints should be included in order to reach a generally acceptable ethical consensus.

Moral discourse and legal precepts can both shed light on practice but, in deciding what is in a person's best interests, moral discourse should take precedence. The discussion will take account of precepts set by similar circumstances elsewhere, but will come to a fresh decision for the immediate situation. The term 'best interests' does not only mean medical interests; it also encompasses the whole of a person's circumstances and relationships.

Ethical method is an analytical activity comprised of a number of steps:

1 *Define the situation*: the process begins with precision. The situation needs to be clearly defined. All the facts need to be stated and all the terminology listed in words which a lay person outside dietetics can understand.

2 *Consider the options*: when the description of the particular situation is complete in all its details, the possible courses of action should be set out together with the pros and cons to support or reject each suggestion. A range of moral approaches (e.g. duty, consequence, virtue) may need to be considered as well as each of the four principles.

3 *Be prepared to support an opinion*: the four principles often conflict in a given situation so the optimum will have to be selected from the possibilities.

4 *Select the optimum*: this requires looking at the *scope* of each principle. How far does the principle apply to the immediate situation and what limits the application? For instance, in a situation involving a group of people including a young baby, the baby cannot exercise autonomy.

5 *Reach a group decision*: ultimately, a group decision based on all the evidence has to be made. The dietitian will need to be able to refer back to the details of any such discussion if the decision is subsequently questioned.

Mediation and conciliation techniques are important in reaching a decision on an individual's 'best interest' because disagreement on an issue such as feeding can be very heated.

Text written by: Revd Phyllis Eaton in association with the Ethical and Professional Advisory Panel (EPAP) of the British Dietetic Association

Useful addresses

The Association of Palliative Medicine
11 Westwood Road, Southampton SO17 1DL
Tel: 01703 672888

National Council for Hospice and Specialist Palliative Care Services
7th Floor, 1 Great Cumberland Place, London W1H 7AL
Tel: 020 7723 1639

The Office of the Official Solicitor to the Supreme Court
(Family Medical Lawyers' Department)
81 Chancery Lane, London WC2A 1DD
Tel: 020 7911 7127

Further reading

Books

Beauchamp TL, Childress JF. *Principles of Biomedical Ethics*. Oxford: Oxford University Press, 1994.

Brazier M. *Medicine, Patients and the Law*. London: Penguin, 1992.

British Medical Association. *Medical Ethics Today. Its Practice and Philosophy*. London: BMJ Publications, 1993.

Gillon, R. (Ed.). *Principles of Health Care Ethics*. Chichester: John Wiley, 1994.

Lennard-Jones JE. *Ethical and Legal Aspects of Clinical Hydration and Nutrition Support*. Maidenhead: BAPEN, 1998

Montgomery J. *Health Care Law*. Oxford: Oxford University Press, 1997.

Montgomery J. *Health Care Choices. Making Decisions with Children*. Institute for Public Policy Research, 1996.

Journals

Luttrell S. End of life decisions. Withdrawing or witholding life-prolonging treatment (Editorial) *British Medical Journal* 1999; **318**: 1709–1710.

Millard PH. Ethical decisions at the end of life. *Journal of the Royal College of Physicians* 1999; **33**: 365–367.

Rabeneck L, McCullough LB, Wray NP. Ethically justified, clinically comprehensive guidelines for percutaneous endoscopic gastrostomy tube placement. *Lancet* 1997; **349**: 496–498.

General reading

Journal of Medical Ethics

References

All England Law Reports. 1957; Vol 2, p. 118 (Legal reference: [1957] 2 AII ER 118).

British Medical Association. *Witholding or Withdrawing Life-prolonging Medical Treatment. Guidance for Decision Making*. London: BMJ Publications, 1999.

Dunphy K, Randall F. Ethical decision-making in palliative care. *European Journal of Palliative Care* 1997; **4**: 126–128.

Gillon R. Philosophical medical ethics: doctors and patients. *British Medical Journal* 1986; **292**: 466–469.

Gillon R. Medical ethics: four principles plus attention to scope. *British Medical Journal* 1994; **309**: 184–188.

SECTION 2
Foods and nutrients

2.1 Dietary energy

A fundamental need of the human body is for a supply of energy. Energy is needed for:

- the metabolic processes which sustain life
- generation of tissue (for growth and for the continuous replacement of existing tissue throughout life)
- thermoregulation (to prevent body temperature rising or falling outside a very narrow range)
- involuntary muscle movement (breathing, peristalsis, heart-muscle contraction)
- voluntary muscle movement (for physical movement of the body).

If insufficient energy is derived from dietary intake, requirements will initially be met by utilization of stored energy in the form of fat in adipose tissue. Once these reserves are depleted, lean tissue (muscle) will be used as an energy source. Prolonged inadequate energy intake in relation to requirement will result in undernutrition, which has important prognostic significance in terms of morbidity and mortality (see Section 1.11, Undernutrition). A sustained level of energy intake which results in energy surplus will result in obesity and its many associated health risks (see Section 4.17, Obesity).

2.1.1 Energy expenditure

Energy requirements are primarily determined by energy expenditure. This comprises:

- basal metabolic rate (BMR)
- physical activity
- dietary-induced thermogenesis.

Basal metabolic rate

This is the amount of energy expended by the body to maintain basic physiological functions over a period of 24 hours and is the largest component (about 60–75%) of total energy expenditure.

BMR is principally determined by body mass and therefore varies with:

- *Body weight*: Larger people have a higher BMR than smaller ones.
- *Body composition*: Adipose tissue has a lower metabolic rate than lean tissue. However, in terms of total energy expenditure, this tends to be counteracted by the fact that the energy cost of moving a body containing a high proportion of adipose tissue is greater in someone who is overweight or obese. Differences in basal or resting energy metabolism due to different degrees of adiposity can be overcome by calculating them in terms of the fat-free mass.
- *Age*: Children have a higher BMR per unit surface area than adults. Since there is a loss of lean mass with age and also a fall in the rate of cellular metabolism, older adults have a lower BMR than younger adults.
- *Gender*: Males tend to have greater body mass and hence higher BMR than females.

Genetic differences may also account for up to 10% variation in BMR between people of same gender, age, body weight and fat content.

A number of factors may influence the BMR:

- *nutritional status*, e.g. undernutrition results in an adaptive fall in BMR
- *physiological factors*, e.g. BMR rises in pregnancy and lactation
- *psychological factors*, e.g. anxiety can increase BMR
- hormonal effects, e.g. hyperthyroidism increases BMR; hypothyroidism reduces it
- *disease or trauma*, e.g. metabolic rate may be increased as a result of fever, infection, sepsis or the metabolic response to injury
- *pharmacological effects*, e.g. metabolic rate may be increased by substances such as nicotine and caffeine, or altered by therapeutic drugs
- *ambient temperature*, e.g. the effects of climate, air temperature, windchill factor or type of clothing may necessitate either increased heat production or increased heat loss in order to maintain constant body temperature; both extreme heat and extreme cold will increase BMR.

Metabolic energy is expended in the form of heat. In theory, the amount of heat produced by a fasting subject totally at rest over a given period can be used to calculate 24 hour heat production and hence BMR. However, the type of insulated respiratory chamber needed to measure BMR in this way (direct calorimetry) is complex and expensive to construct and only exists in a few specialized research centres. BMR is more easily measured by the technique of indirect calorimetry which measures oxygen consumption and, by extrapolation, metabolic heat production. The standardized way of carrying this out is in subjects immediately upon waking, in a state of complete physical rest, 13 hours after the last meal and in a thermoneutral temperature. Resting energy expenditure (REE) (sometimes called resting metabolic rate, RMR) is measured under slightly less stringent conditions, with the subject lying at rest, and produces a similar (slightly higher) estimate to the BMR.

In clinical practice, BMR is usually estimated by Schofield prediction equations (Schofield *et al.* 1985; DH 1991) (see Section 1.10.1 in Estimating nutritional requirements). Ready reference tables for BMR according to an individual's age, gender and body weight can be found in Appendix 6.5.

Physical activity

This makes a significant but variable contribution to daily energy expenditure of between 20 and 40%. Any type of physical movement requires energy. The more strenuous the activity, the more energy is required. Furthermore, the greater the mass of the body, the greater the amount of energy required to make that particular movement.

In order to estimate the energy requirements of different sectors of the population, the COMA panel on Dietary Reference Values (DH 1991) devised two factors to help to determine the contribution of physical activity to total energy expenditure:

- *physical activity ratio (PAR)*: the ratio of the energy cost of a specific activity to the BMR
- *physical activity level (PAL)*: the ratio of daily physical expenditure to BMR.

Typical PARs range from 1.0–1.4 for activities such as sitting, standing or lying down, through 2.5–3.3 while walking at a normal pace to 6.0–9.0 when jogging, skiing or playing tennis. A detailed list can be found in Annex 3 of the COMA report on Dietary Reference Values (DH 1991).

The PAL is obtained by calculating the energy cost of the various activities of varying PAR within a 24 hour period and deriving the average daily increase in energy expenditure above the BMR. PALs for groups of the population are estimated to be:

1.4: inactive men and women
1.6: moderately active women
1.7: moderately active men
1.8: highly active women
1.9: highly active men.

The majority of the UK population can be considered to be 'inactive' during both work and leisure time and assumed to have a PAL of 1.4. Multiplying the PAL by the BMR provides an estimation of the daily energy expenditure (and hence energy requirements) of groups of people according to their level of occupational or recreational activities.

Occupation can make a significant contribution to energy expenditure if it involves considerable physical activity, but this is less commonly the case in technologically advanced societies where tasks formerly requiring strenuous manual effort now tend to be carried out by machinery or electronic equipment. In the UK, the overall energy expenditure of an individual is more likely to be influenced by recreational than occupational activity. This does not necessarily mean strenuous physical activity such as digging the garden, hand-sawing or a game of squash; although these have a high energy cost while being performed, they are rarely maintained for extended periods and so may not make an enormous difference to daily energy requirements, particularly if only undertaken periodically (e.g. at weekends). During the waking hours of the day, most physical energy expenditure results from the general activities of daily living: sitting, standing or moving about. Significant increases in energy expenditure can therefore be made by generally being more active during these hours, e.g. spending less time sitting down, walking more, climbing stairs instead of using a lift, and making more journeys on foot or bicycle instead of by car.

Dietary-induced thermogenesis

Dietary-induced thermogenesis is the rise in metabolic rate (and hence heat production) which occurs following the consumption of food. The effect is complex and remains poorly understood. It used to be thought to be a consequence of protein consumption but it is now known that all elements of the diet are thermogenic. The magnitude of the effect is largely unrelated to either the type or amount of food consumed. Some variation in dietary-induced thermogenesis has been observed between obese and lean people, and with the level of physical activity, but the differences are small. In the average person, dietary thermogenesis accounts for about 5–10% of energy expenditure over a 24 hour period.

2.1.2 Energy intake
Dietary energy requirements

The dietary energy requirement of an individual is the amount required to balance energy expenditure and maintain a body mass which is optimal for good health. In healthy people of normal body weight, this is primarily determined by age, gender, daily physical activity level and any additional physiological demands as a result of the energy costs of growth, pregnancy or lactation.

In the presence of disease or metabolic stress, dietary energy requirements may be additionally increased by:

- pyrexia
- infection or sepsis
- tissue injury and subsequent repair
- increased nutrient losses via vomiting, diarrhoea, tissue exudates and glycosuria
- impaired absorption.

The implications of these influences must be considered on an individual basis according to their severity and duration.

Ways of estimating the energy requirements of either groups of people or individuals are discussed in Section 1.10.1 in Estimating nutritional requirements.

Dietary energy intake

The body's energy supply is derived from nutrients which can be oxidized to provide energy. The amount of energy released from food is expressed either as kilojoules (kJ) (or megajoules, MJ) or as kilocalories (kcal). The joule is, scientifically, the more correct way of quantifying energy. However, in dietetic practice, the kilocalorie remains the most commonly used unit of quantification, partly because the general public is far more familiar with the term (in the form of the 'calorie').

Energy-yielding nutrients in the diet are:

- protein: 4 kcal (17 kJ)/g
- carbohydrate: 3.75 kcal (16 kJ)/g
- fat: 9 kcal (37 kJ)/g
- alcohol: 7 kcal (29 kJ)/g.

Small amounts of energy may also be derived from polyols (e.g. sorbitol) in the diet and from volatile (short-chain) fatty acids absorbed from the colon following bacterial fermentation of some fibre components.

The contribution of a particular food to total energy intake is determined by:

- its energy density (kcal/100 g of food)
- the amount consumed (portion size)
- the frequency of consumption.

Energy density

Fat is the most energy-dense nutrient, with protein and carbohydrate each providing less than half the amount of energy per gram. It should be noted that alcohol is also a potentially significant contributor to energy intake. The most concentrated sources of dietary energy (kcal/100 g) therefore tend to be those containing a high proportion of fat (e.g. spreading fats and cooking oils). Conversely, the least concentrated sources of energy are foods with a high content of water, fibre and very little fat (e.g. fruit and vegetables).

Dietary energy density has important implications. A much greater quantity of a low-energy dense food is required to provide the same amount of energy as a food with a high energy density. Energy density is also a useful indicator of dietary energy provision because people tend to eat a relatively constant amount of food, whatever its energy density (Bell *et al.* 1998). Energy intake therefore tends to be directly related to the energy density of the diet. Diets of high energy density facilitate overconsumption and hence increase the likelihood that energy requirements will be exceeded (Rolls and Bell 1999).

Energy density is an important consideration in the management of both undernutrition and overnutrition. If energy intake is inadequate but, for reasons such as small appetite, early satiety or nausea, it is physically difficult for people to eat a greater quantity of food, dietary energy density needs to be increased so that more calories are supplied in a small volume of food. In these circumstances, the consumption of energy-dense foods such as butter, cheese and full-fat milk may need to be encouraged (see Section 1.12.1 in Oral nutritional support). Conversely, it is easier for people who are overweight to reduce their energy consumption by decreasing the energy density of the food consumed rather than the total quantity of food consumed, because the satiety value of the diet is more likely to be maintained (Poppitt and Prentice 1996; Rolls and Bell

2000). Dietary guidance therefore needs to focus on food choices that provide less fat (e.g. use of reduced-fat milk and low-fat spreads and milk products; less consumption of fat-rich food choices) and more fluid and fibre (e.g. greater consumption of fruit and vegetables). Table 2.1 provides some examples of foods of different energy density.

Amount consumed (typical portion size)

Energy-dense foods do not necessarily contribute large amounts of energy to the diet if eaten in small portions, for example 10–15 g portions of jam or marmalade.

Frequency of consumption

Milk contains less energy per 100 g than cream but, because it is consumed more frequently, is a more significant contributor to daily energy intake in the average diet.

Percentage energy composition

The percentage of dietary energy derived from each of the energy-providing nutrients can be calculated as follows:

% fat energy = (g fat/day × 9)/total kcal per day
% carbohydrate energy = (g carbohydrate/day × 3.75)/total kcal per day
% protein energy = (g protein/day × 4)/total kcal per day.

The percentage of dietary energy from other nutrients such as saturated fat or sugars can be calculated in a similar way using appropriate caloric conversion factors.

The percentage of energy intake derived from different nutrients has little impact on energy balance. In the short term, a reduction in % carbohydrate intake may result in changes in fluid balance and hence apparent weight loss, but reduction in fat stores will only occur when total energy intake is less than the energy requirement.

Percentage energy intake is, however, a useful indicator of overall dietary composition and its desirability in terms of long-term health. Target intakes for the main energy-providing nutrients are therefore expressed in these terms (see Section 1.1.3 in Diet, health and disease). Most of the UK population should derive a greater proportion of their dietary energy from carbohydrate (especially starchy carbohydrate) and less from fat (especially saturated fat) than is currently the case.

It is important to appreciate that percentage energy figures are interdependent and need to be considered in conjunction with one another, particularly % fat and % carbohydrate energy. The percentage of protein energy in the UK diet tends to be fairly constant and this results in a reciprocal relationship between carbohydrate and fat intake: if the percentage of energy derived from one is high (or increased), the other will be low (or decreased). For example, a diet containing 30% fat energy might be desirably low in fat but could also reflect an excessively high sugar intake which will (in mathematical terms) dilute the percentage of energy derived from fat. This effect is commonly seen in the diets of teenagers (Gregory *et al.* 2000). A diet containing a higher % fat energy might be healthier in terms of overall composition. Dietary quality should there-

Table 2.1 Altering the energy density of food choices

Food group	Lower energy density	Average energy density	Higher energy density
Cereal foods	Slice of wholemeal bread with low-fat spread	Slice of white bread with full-fat spread	Fried bread
	Pitta bread	Chappati	Paratha
		Naan	Poories
	High-fibre breakfast cereal	Plain breakfast cereal (e.g. cornflakes)	Sugar-coated breakfast cereals
	Plain boiled rice		Pilau (fried) rice
Fruit and vegetables	Fresh fruit	Fruit cooked with sugar	Fruit with pastry
		Fruit canned in natural juice	Fruit with cream
			Fruit canned in syrup
	Raw, boiled or steamed vegetables	Buttered vegetables	Fried vegetables
			Vegetables roasted in fat
Milk and dairy products	Skimmed or semi-skimmed milk	Full-fat milk	Cream
		Evaporated or condensed milk	
	'Diet' low-fat yoghurt	Standard low-fat yoghurt	Full-fat ('creamy') yoghurt
	Cottage cheese	Full-fat cheese	Cream cheese
Meat, fish and alternatives	Lean red meat	Meat with fat marbling	Visible meat fat
	Poultry breast meat	Poultry joints	Meat pies and puddings
			Fatty mince
			Poultry skin
	Fresh or frozen fish	Fish canned in oil	Fried fish
			Fish coated in batter or breadcrumbs
	Boiled or poached egg	Omelette or scrambled egg	Fried egg
			Scotch egg
			Pastry-based flans
Fat-rich and sugar-rich foods	Low-fat spreads	Reduced-fat spreads	Full-fat spreads
			Butter
			Ghee
	Dry-fried foods (no fat/oil used)	Stir-fried foods	Shallow or deep-fat fried foods
			Foods roasted in fat
	Crispbread	Sweet biscuits	Chocolate biscuits
	Savoury biscuits or crackers		Iced or filled biscuits
	Fat-free sponge cake	Plain sponge cake	Iced sponge cake
	Sugar-free gum	Pastilles	Chocolate bars
		Boiled sweets	Fudge
	Sugar-free drinks	Diluted sugar-containing drinks (e.g. squashes or cordials)	Undiluted sugar-containing drinks (e.g. lemonade, cola)

fore never be assessed by considering one percentage energy parameter in isolation.

Because percentage energy figures are interrelated, it can be very misleading to look at individual foods, or even meals, in terms of percentage energy composition since these figures will change as soon as other foods or meals are consumed. For example, the % fat energy content of a hamburger will decrease if it is consumed in conjunction with a glass of sugar-containing cola (even though the absolute amount of fat consumed is unchanged). The percentage figures will change again as soon as food intake from other meals is taken into account. A food with a high % fat energy content but containing relatively little fat in absolute terms (e.g. one biscuit) may have a negligible impact on the % fat energy content of a day's diet. A food with a low percentage of fat energy but consumed in relatively large quantities (e.g. full-fat milk) may make a significant contribution to daily % fat intake. Foods cannot therefore be classified in terms of 'healthiness' on the basis of their percentage energy content alone; their significance in terms of overall energy composition depends on how much is consumed and what else is consumed.

Sources of dietary energy in the UK diet

The main sources of energy in the UK diet are foods which are eaten in significant quantities and have a relatively low water content (such as bread, flour and other cereals) and/or a high fat content (meat and meat products, visible fats, and milk and dairy products) (MAFF 1998). Figure 2.1 shows the contributions made by different food groups to energy intakes from household food purchases in the UK (excluding soft and alcoholic drinks, confectionery and meals purchased and eaten away from the home) (MAFF 1998).

In the Dietary and Nutritional Survey of British Adults aged 16–64 years (Gregory et al. 1990), the average energy intake was 2450 kcal/day in men and 1680 kcal/day in women. These intakes are less than the estimated average requirements (EAR) for energy for these age groups, but this is not considered to indicate generalized energy inadequacy since the prevalence of obesity in the UK population is high and continuing to increase. It is more likely to reflect overestimation of energy requirements due to declining levels of physical activity.

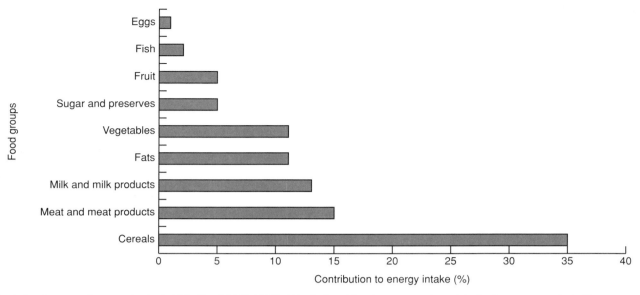

Fig. 2.1 Sources of energy in the British diet (MAFF 1998). (Alcohol and foods consumed outside the home are excluded.)

Data from the National Food Survey show that the energy content of household food has steadily declined since the late 1980s, falling from 2039 kcal/person per day in 1987 to 1788 kcal/person per day in 1997, largely as a result of a decrease in the level of consumption of fats, meat and meat products, sugar and full-fat milk (MAFF 1998). As a result of this decline in total energy intake, the percentages of energy derived from protein, fat and carbohydrate have changed relatively little over this period.

2.1.3 Energy balance

The fundamental principle of energy balance, and hence weight maintenance or weight change, is:

Energy intake = Energy expenditure ± Changes in body stores.

Intake and expenditure are not balanced on a daily or even a weekly basis but, over a period of time, weight stability depends on energy intake equalling energy expenditure. In order to achieve weight gain, energy intake must exceed energy expenditure; for weight loss, energy intake has to be less than expenditure.

For clinical purposes, energy balance can be estimated very simply by estimation of either adiposity (e.g. body mass index) or change in body weight (see Section 1.8.4 in Assessment of nutritional status).

In order to correct energy imbalance, it is not always necessary to make a numerical estimate of either energy requirements or expenditure. Irrespective of what the actual levels are, changing energy balance requires long-term adjustment in either the habitual level of energy intake or the usual level of physical activity in that individual, or both. For the purposes of dietetic intervention, assessment of an individual's usual dietary habits and lifestyle (see Section 1.5, Dietary assessment) often provides sufficient pointers to the type of changes needed. These aspects are

discussed further in Sections 1.2 (Healthy eating), 1.11 (Undernutrition) and 4.17 (Obesity).

Text revised by: Briony Thomas and Angie Jefferson

Further reading

FAO/WHO. *Energy and Protein Requirements*. Report of a Joint FAO/WHO ad hoc Expert Committee. Rome: FAO; 1997.

References

Bell EA, Castellanos VH, Pelkman CL *et al*. Energy density of foods affects energy intake in normal-weight women. *American Journal of Clinical Nutrition* 1998; **67**: 412–420.

Department of Health. *Dietary Reference Values for Food Energy and Nutrients for the United Kingdom*. Report on Health and Social Subjects 41. London: HMSO, 1991.

Gregory J, Foster K, Tyler H, Wiseman M. *The Dietary and Nutritional Survey of British Adults*. London: HMSO, 1990.

Gregory J *et al*. *National Diet and Nutrition Survey: Young People aged 4–18 years*. Volume 1: *Findings*. London: The Stationery Office, 2000.

Ministry of Agriculture, Fisheries and Food (MAFF). *National Food Survey: 1997*. London: The Stationery Office, 1998.

Poppitt SD, Prentice AM. Energy density and its role in the control of food intake: evidence from metabolic and community studies. *Appetite* 1996; **26**:153–174.

Rolls BJ, Bell EA. Intake of fat and carbohydrate: role of energy density. *European Journal of Clinical Nutrition* 1999; **53** (Suppl 1): S166–S173.

Rolls BJ, Bell EA. Dietary approaches to the treatment of obesity. *Medical Clinics of North America* 2000; **84**: 401–418.

Schofield WN, Schofield C, James WPT. Basal metabolic rate review and prediction together with an annotated bibliography of source material. *Human Nutrition: Clinical Nutrition* 1985; **39C** (Suppl 1): 1–96.

2.2 Dietary protein and amino acids

2.2.1 Function

Proteins are vital for both the structure and metabolic operation of the human body. Tens of thousands of different proteins can be found within the body, each having a different and essential role.

Protein is a major component of body tissues and about half of the body's protein is present in structural tissues such as muscle and skin in the form of myosin, actin and collagen (somatic protein). Protein is thus essential for growth and, because there is continuous turnover of body tissues, for maintenance of body structure throughout life.

In addition to their structural role, proteins have a number of other diverse functions:

- *Enzymatic function*: Many different types of enzymes are essential for the operation of the chemical processes on which body function depends. Digestive enzymes break down food into its constituent nutrients in the gastrointestinal tract; cellular enzymes catalyse and regulate metabolic processes. All enzymes are proteins.
- *Transport function*: Proteins act as carriers in blood and body fluids for many nutrients and other molecules, e.g. lipoproteins transport lipids; haemoglobin carries oxygen. Proteins also act as carriers across cell membranes and help to regulate the movement of nutrients and metabolites between the intracellular and extracellular compartments.
- *Hormonal function*: Some hormones such as insulin and thyroxine are proteins.
- *Immune function*: Antibodies are proteins synthesized by lymphocytes as part of the immune response.
- *Buffering function*: The pH of the blood has to be maintained within a very narrow range in order for the body to be able to function. Proteins such as albumin in the blood help to maintain the acid–base balance by accepting and releasing hydrogen ions as necessary.

Proteins also can, and will, be used as an energy source in conditions of energy insufficiency.

2.2.2 Structure

Proteins consist of building blocks called amino acids, all of which are composed of a nitrogen-containing amino (-NH_2) group, a carboxyl (-COOH) acid group plus a third component – a distinctive side-chain which gives each amino acid its individual properties. This side-chain may vary from being a single hydrogen atom to a complex molecule containing a benzene ring.

The amino group of one amino acid can form a link (a peptide bond) with the acid group of another amino acid to form a chain of amino acids. This is called a peptide, the length of the chain denoted by its name:

- dipeptide: 2 amino acids
- tripeptide: 3 amino acids
- oligopeptide: 4–10 amino acids
- polypeptide: >10 amino acids.

Interactions between reactive groups in the amino acid side-chains within a polypeptide chain lead to the formation of cross-links either between parts of the chain or with other chains. These cross-links give the molecule its particular shape and structure; for example, it may twist and fold to form a spherical globular structure (e.g. haemoglobin) or it may remain elongated and fibrous (e.g. collagen).

About 20 amino acids are found in nature and, just as the 26 letters of the alphabet can be arranged into an almost infinite number of words, so can these 20 amino acids be arranged to create a vast array of different proteins. Each protein is unique, with its own specific number and sequence of amino acids. Some are relatively small, containing about 50 amino acid units; most are much larger, containing hundreds or even thousands of amino acid units.

Dietary proteins are broken down by digestive enzymes into their constituent amino acids. Some will directly enter the body's pool of amino acids and be used for protein synthesis; others may be converted to other amino acids by the process of transamination (transfer of the amino group). Surplus amino acids will be deaminated, the amino group being converted to urea and excreted by the kidneys, and the remainder converted to glucose or used as a source of energy (see Protein requirements, below).

Types of amino acids

Some amino acids can be synthesized as needed by the body, while others must be provided by the diet.

Essential amino acids

These either cannot be synthesized at all by the body, or not at a fast enough rate to meet the body's needs, and are therefore termed essential (or indispensable) amino acids. Nine amino acids are essential in adults and are listed in Table 2.2. In infants, arginine is also an essential amino acid.

Table 2.2 Classification of amino acids

Requirement	Amino acid	Chemical features
Essential (indispensable)	Isoleucine	Branched-chain amino acid
	Leucine	Branched-chain amino acid
	Valine	Branched-chain amino acid
	Lysine	6-carbon chain, with basic properties
	Methionine	4-carbon chain, containing sulphur
	Phenylalanine	3-carbon chain with benzene ring
	Threonine	4-carbon chain
	Tryptophan	Contains a benzene ring
	Histidine	Has an imidazole side-chain necessary for many catalytic reactions
Semi-essential	Cysteine	A sulphur-containing amino acid synthesized from the essential amino acid methionine
	Tyrosine	Can be made from phenylalanine
Non-essential (dispensable)	Glycine	The simplest amino acid in structure
	Proline	Contains an imino group
	Glutamic acid	Also exists in an amide form as glutamine[2]
	Aspartic acid	Also exists in an amide form as asparagine[2]
	Serine	A hydroxy-amino acid
	Alanine	Non-polar, hydrophobic
	Arginine[1]	Similar in structure to lysine

[1]An essential amino acid in infants.
[2]May be conditionally essential in critically ill people.

Semi-essential amino acids

These can be synthesized from other amino acids provided that precursor amino acids are present in the diet in sufficient amounts.

Non-essential amino acids

These can normally be readily synthesized by the body from other carbon- and nitrogen-containing precursors.

Conditionally essential amino acids

These are amino acids which are normally non-essential but may become essential in circumstances when the requirement for them exceeds the body's ability to synthesize them, such as during illness or following trauma. There is increasing speculation that glutamine and arginine may be conditionally essential in critically ill people (see Section 5.2, Intensive care).

Protein quality

The biological value of dietary protein is determined by its content of essential amino acids. Proteins which contain all of the essential amino acids in amounts sufficient to meet protein synthesis are termed high biological value (HBV) proteins (sometimes termed 'complete' proteins). In general, proteins derived from animal foods such as meat, fish, poultry, eggs and milk are of high biological value. The exception is gelatin, which is an incomplete protein.

Foods which lack one or more essential amino acids are termed low biological value (LBV) protein (or 'incomplete' protein). The essential amino acid which is in shortest supply relative to the body's requirement for it is termed the limiting amino acid. Most plant proteins are, in isola-tion, incomplete but, since different types of plant proteins have different limiting amino acids, combinations of plant proteins create HBV protein mixtures. This is a cardinal principle of vegan diets (see Section 3.10, Vegetarianism and veganism). For example, the limiting amino acid in wheat is lysine, while that in pulses is methionine, but a diet containing both wheat-based foods and pulses will provide sufficient quantities of both lysine and methionine to meet requirements for protein synthesis. Protein combining is not necessary in a vegetarian diet where milk, cheese and eggs are consumed because such foods will supply adequate amounts of all essential amino acids.

2.2.3 Protein requirements

In the body, protein is constantly broken down and resynthesized, resulting in a continuous requirement for new sources of protein. The process of growth during childhood or pregnancy additionally increases the requirement for protein so that new tissues can be created. The body attempts to conserve protein as much as possible. When proteins are broken down, their constituent amino acids enter a metabolic pool. Some are recycled to make new proteins, while in others the nitrogen component is removed and the carbon skeleton used as an energy source.

The synthesis of proteins takes place throughout all cells and tissues of the body, drawing on the liver's pool of essential and non-essential amino acids as required. If non-essential amino acids are not directly available, they are made in body cells by the process of transamination (where the amino group of one amino acid is transferred to an appropriate base group, thus creating the amino acid required). This process is controlled by transaminase enzymes and the coenzyme pyridoxal-5-phosphate derived from vitamin B_6.

There is a constant dynamic interaction between amino acids entering the body and those available as a result of the continuous breakdown and resynthesis of body protein. This process of breakdown and resynthesis is known as protein turnover. Every day in the normal adult about 200–300 g protein is turned over in this way and this is equivalent to about 3–4 g protein/kg body weight per day. Protein turnover per kilogram body weight is even higher in infants and children. The rate declines with age.

About 10–15 g nitrogen is excreted each day in the urine of a healthy adult, mainly in the form of urea with smaller contributions from ammonia, uric acid, creatinine and some free amino acids. Some nitrogen is also lost in skin and faeces. The body is in nitrogen balance when nitrogen intake from the diet is equal to nitrogen output in urine, faeces and skin. Healthy adults are normally in nitrogen balance. In times of growth or increase in muscle mass, there will be a positive nitrogen balance, with more nitrogen being retained in the body than is lost. In conditions of starvation or trauma, nitrogen balance will be negative, and there will be a net loss from the body due to the breakdown of protein tissue to create an energy source.

Protein requirements are determined by measuring the amount of protein needed to maintain nitrogen equilibrium. This is not a simple procedure (see Section 1.10.2 in Estimating nutritional requirements). Nitrogen excretion in urine or faeces is not constant throughout the day or even between days. Furthermore, the urea pool in the body is large and has a 12 hour turnover, so it may take 2 days for a change in urea synthesis (i.e. nitrogen balance) to be fully reflected in the urine.

Based on nitrogen balance studies, the UK dietary references values (DRVs; DH 1991) assume that healthy adults consuming a mixed diet require 0.75 g protein/kg ideal body weight per day. An adult weighing 60 kg is therefore assumed to require 60 x 0.75 = 45 g protein/day. Additional increments are set for the additional demands of pregnancy and lactation. In the UK, protein intakes are usually well in excess of requirements, typical mean daily intakes being 84.7 g in adult men and 62.0 g in women (Gregory *et al.* 1990).

Fewer detailed studies of nitrogen balance have been performed in infants and children and their protein requirements are more uncertain. DRVs for these groups are therefore best estimates of protein intakes which will meet the variable demands of growth.

The reference nutrient intakes (RNIs) for protein for different sectors of the population can be found in Appendix 6.2.

Adaptation

Humans can adapt to a wide range of protein intake. Low protein intakes result in decreased protein turnover and, provided energy needs are met, reduced amino acid oxidation. When protein intake is high the body increases the formation of urea, with consequent loss of nitrogen in urine.

The total amount of protein in the body can also vary to a considerable degree without serious consequences for health. The body of a well-fed adult contains about 11 kg protein but up to 3 kg can be lost without significant detrimental consequences. During starvation or protein depletion, liver and visceral tissues lose protein very rapidly (by as much as 40%), while skeletal muscle loses protein more slowly. Pathological conditions such as injury, infection, cancer and diabetes can cause substantial rates of protein loss. If these losses continue they can become life threatening.

Protein deficiency

Even if dietary protein intake is theoretically sufficient, it will be inadequate for needs if energy requirements are not also met. The body's priority is for energy and if necessary it will meet this by breaking down protein, removing the nitrogen from the amino acids and oxidizing the carbon skeleton in much the same way as it derives energy from glucose or fat. Protein deficiency can therefore result from deficiency of either dietary protein or dietary energy or, as is usually the case, a combination of the two. Protein-energy malnutrition (PEM), characterized by muscle wasting and growth retardation in children, remains a major problem in developing countries. However, it can also occur in certain groups of the UK population. Severe PEM is often associated with acquired immunodeficiency syndrome (AIDS), tuberculosis, anorexia nervosa and cancer cachexia. Mild to moderate PEM is a common, but often unrecognized problem among surgical patients in hospitals and chronically undernourished elderly people and may have a considerable impact on morbidity and mortality (see Section 1.11, Undernutrition).

Protein deficiency is most likely to occur as a result of:

- failure to meet energy requirements, resulting in use of dietary and/or tissue protein as an energy source
- the catabolic response to trauma such as burns, surgery or injury, when breakdown of body protein exceeds the body's ability to replace it, resulting in a period of negative nitrogen balance
- failure to absorb or utilize dietary protein as a result of gastrointestinal disorders or liver disease
- excessive protein loss from body due to renal disease, haemorrhage or exudative losses.

Long-term deficiency of protein can result in:

- stunted growth in children
- muscle wasting, including that of the heart
- increased susceptibility to infection
- poor wound healing
- anaemia
- oedema
- fatty infiltration of the liver.

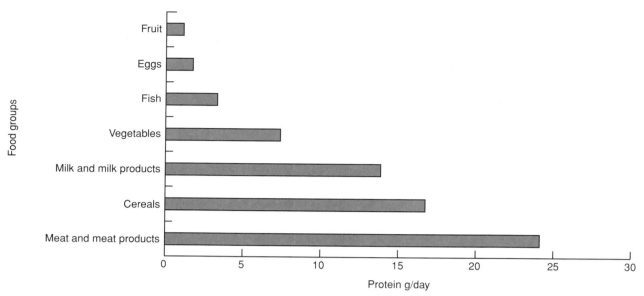

Fig. 2.2   Average contribution of foods groups to protein intakes in the UK (MAFF 1999).

Protein surplus

Since surplus protein cannot be stored by the body, over-consumption of protein offers no benefits and may have some health risks in terms of renal function (particularly in people with diabetes) and possibly demineralization of bone (DH 1991). It is therefore recommended that adults should avoid protein intakes of more than twice the RNI, i.e. 1.5 g protein/kg per day.

Although athletes may require a protein intake approaching or even exceeding this limit in order to develop and maintain their high muscle mass (see Section 3.12, Nutrition for exercise and sport), this does not necessitate a diet disproportionally high in protein-rich foods. Because the athlete's energy requirements are also extremely high, protein needs can usually be met by consuming sufficient quantities of a diet containing 12–15% protein energy. The use of amino acid supplements is not recommended as little is known about their effects, and their safety remains to be evaluated.

2.2.4 Sources of protein in the UK diet

Figure 2.2 shows the average contributions made by different food groups to protein intakes in the UK diet. HBV animal proteins provide about 60% of protein in the average UK diet, with LBV plant proteins providing the remaining 40%. Guidance on the protein content of some common foods can be found in Appendix 6.2.

Protein restriction

Protein restriction is now less commonly used in clinical practice. Where used, the level of protein restriction required will depend on the severity of the disease state and will be a compromise between the body's requirement for protein and the clinical indications. When protein intake is limited, the biological value of protein consumed is a vital consideration (see Appendix 6.2). Specially manufactured low-protein items such as breads, biscuits, crackers, flour and pasta are prescribable in specified circumstances.

Protein supplementation

An increase in protein intake may be necessary to correct chronic protein depletion and restore muscle mass following disease, injury or prolonged poor food intake. This can be achieved by increasing the proportion of protein-rich foods in the diet (e.g. milk and milk products, eggs, meat, fish, cheese and pulses) or by enriching foods with sources of protein (e.g. adding skimmed milk powder to liquid milk) (see Section 1.12.3 in Oral nutritional support). In some cases proprietary high-protein supplements may be indicated (Section 1.12.4 in Oral nutritional support). However, it should be borne in mind that most malnourished people will also require a significant increase in total energy intake in order for any additional protein to be used for anabolic purposes. If the energy supply is limited, the body's priority for a metabolic fuel source will always take precedence over that of tissue synthesis.

Text revised by: Briony Thomas and Angie Jefferson

Further reading

FAO/WHO. *Report of the Joint FAO/WHO Expert Consultation on Protein Quality Evaluation*. Rome: FAO, 1990.
FAO/WHO. *Energy and Protein Requirements*. Report of a Joint FAO/WHO ad hoc Expert Committee. Rome: FAO, 1997.
FAO/WHO/UNU. *Energy and Protein Requirements*. WHO Technical Report Series 724. Geneva: WHO: 1985.

Garlick PJ, Reeds PJ. Proteins. In Garrow JS, James WPT (Eds) *Human Nutrition and Dietetics*, 9th edn, pp. 56–76. Edinburgh: Churchill Livingstone, 1993.

Paul AA, Southgate DAT, Russell J. *Amino Acid Composition (mg per l00g food) and Fatty Acid Composition (g per 100g food): First supplement to McCance and Widdowson's The Composition of Foods*, 4th edn. London: HMSO/Cambridge: Royal Society of Chemistry, 1980.

References

Department of Health. *Dietary Reference Values for Food Energy and Nutrients for the United Kingdom*. Report on Health and Social Subjects 41. London: HMSO, 1991.

Gregory J, Foster K, Tyler H, Wiseman M. *The Dietary and Nutritional Survey of British Adults*. London: HMSO, 1990.

Ministry of Agriculture, Fisheries and Food. *National Food Survey: 1998*. London: The Stationery Office, 1999.

2.3 Dietary fat and fatty acids

2.3.1 Function

Fats are distributed universally amongst all body cells and fulfil a wide range of structural, storage and metabolic functions which include:

- supplying fuel for cells: fats are oxidized to provide energy and are the most concentrated form of dietary energy
- providing essential fatty acids
- being a carrier for fat-soluble vitamins and antioxidants
- insulating against heat loss by means of subcutaneous fat stores
- providing a protective layer around essential organs
- forming a structural component of brain tissue and the myelin sheath surrounding nerves
- forming phospholipids, the principal component of cell membranes
- being a substrate for hormone and prostaglandin synthesis
- providing a reserve supply of energy in the form of adipose tissue.

2.3.2 Chemical structure and properties

Dietary fats consist primarily of triglycerides (which comprise more than 95%) but also contain other components such as cholesterol, phospholipids, sterols and carotenoids.

Triglycerides have a glycerol backbone to which three long- or medium-chain fatty acids are attached. Fatty acids vary according to chain length and the presence and number of double bonds. The type of fatty acids present in a triglyceride determines not only the physical characteristics of the fat (such as its degree of softness or resistance to rancidity) but also its nutritional properties and physiological effects. However, irrespective of the type of fatty acids they contain, all triglycerides provide 9 kcal (37 kJ) per gram, making fat the most concentrated source of energy in the diet.

Nomenclature of fatty acids

Fatty acids are composed of a chain of carbon atoms with a methyl (CH_3) group at one end and a carboxyl group (COOH) at the other. The number of carbon atoms ranges from 4 to more than 22, but the most common chain length is 16 or 18. In nature, fats almost always only contain fatty acids with an even number of carbon atoms. The carbon atoms may be linked by single or double bonds, and this allows them to be grouped into three main types: saturated (SFA), monounsaturated (MUFA) and polyunsaturated (PUFA). A typical dietary fat contains a mixture of both saturated and unsaturated fatty acids.

About 21 different fatty acids are found in the diet in appreciable amounts, the most prevalent being palmitic, stearic, oleic, linoleic and arachidonic acids. In addition to being known by these common names, fatty acids also have a systematic name based on their structure. For example, eicosapentaenoic acid (EPA), the long-chain PUFA found in fish oils, reflects the fact that it contains 20 (*eicosa*) carbon atoms and five (*penta*) double bonds.

Increasingly, fatty acids are described by a notational system which summarizes their structure. In this scheme, the total number of carbon atoms in the fatty acid is expressed as C12, C16, etc. The total number of double bonds is then shown following a colon; for example, palmitic acid is C16:0 and linoleic acid is C18:2. The position of the first double bond is defined in relation to the methyl end of the carbon chain, with the carbon atom at the methyl end termed the omega (or *n*) carbon. Thus linoleic acid has its first double bond between the sixth and seventh carbons from the methyl end, so its full notional name is C18:2 omega-6, or C18:2 *n*6.

Common, systematic and notational names of fatty acids are summarized in Table 2.3.

Types of fatty acids

Saturated fatty acids (SFA)
These:

- contain carbon atoms linked only by single bonds
- have relatively high melting temperatures and are solid at room temperature
- are chemically stable, both within the body and when present in foods.

SFA are principally obtained from the storage fats of animals and products derived from them, e.g. meat fat, lard, dripping, milk, butter, cheese and cream. Foods of plant origin generally have a much lower content of SFA, although there are some exceptions such as coconut and palm oil. Manufactured margarines and fat spreads derived from plant oils also contain significant amounts of SFA.

SFA tend to elevate the level of low-density lipoprotein (LDL)-cholesterol, and hence total cholesterol, in blood. A high intake therefore enhances the process of atherogenesis and increases the risk of cardiovascular disease.

Table 2.3 Nomenclature of fatty acids commonly found in food

Notational name (No. of carbon atoms: No. of double bonds, location of first double bond)	Common name	Systematic name	Common natural sources
Saturated fatty acids			
4:0	Butyric	Tetranoic	
6:0	Caproic	Hexanoic	
8:0	Caprylic	Octanoic	
10:0	Capric	Decanoic	Coconut oil and dairy products
12:0	Lauric	Dodecanoic	
14:0	Myristic	Tetradecanoic	
16:0	Palmitic	Hexadecanoic	Palm oil, cottonseed oil, butter, meat fat
18:0	Stearic	Octadecanoic	Meat fat, butter, chocolate
20:0	Arachidic	Eicosanoic	Nut and seed oils
22:0	Behenic	Docosanoic	Peanut oil, peanuts
Monounsaturated fatty acids			
16:1 $n7$	Palmitoleic	9 *cis*-hexadecenoic	Cod liver oil, meat fat, fish
18:1 $n9$	Oleic	9 *cis*-octadecenoic	Olive oil, nut and seed oils, meat fat, butter, eggs, avocado
18:1 $n9$	Elaidic	9 *trans*-octadecenoic	Hydrogenated oils, fats from ruminants
20:1 $n9$		11 *cis*-eicosaenoic	Fish, peanut oil
22:1 $n9$	Erucic	13 *cis*-docosaenoic	Rapeseed, if not a low erucic acid liquid variety
Polyunsaturated fatty acids			
18:2 $n6$	Linoleic	9,12 *cis*, *cis*-octadecadienoic	Vegetable oils, nuts, lean meat, eggs
18:3 $n3$	Alpha-linolenic	9,12,15 all *cis*-octadecatrienoic	Soyabean and rapeseed oils
18:3 $n6$	Gamma-linolenic	5 *trans*, 9 *cis*, 12 *cis*-octadecatrienoic	Evening primrose oil
20:4 $n6$	Arachidonic	5,8,11,14 *cis*-eicosatetraenoic	Offal, game, lean meat, eggs
20:5 $n3$	–	Eicosapentaenoic (EPA)	Fish
22:6 $n3$	–	Docosahexaenoic	Fish, liver, egg yolk

Monounsaturated fatty acids

These:

- contain one double bond
- are usually liquid at room temperature.

The most concentrated dietary sources of monounsaturated fatty acids are olive oil and rapeseed oil. However, MUFA are present in many foods. For example, they comprise about one-third of the fatty acids in meat fat and, in softer meat fats such as lard, MUFA content exceeds that of SFA. Most of the fat present in nuts and seeds is also in the form of MUFA.

Dietary MUFA are regarded as the most beneficial type of fatty acid as they do not have a hypercholesterolaemic effect and, when substituted for SFA, lower the LDL-cholesterol level without adversely affecting high-density lipoprotein (HDL) concentration (DH 1994; Roche *et al.* 1998). Substitution with MUFA rather than PUFA also poses less risk of lipid peroxidation.

Polyunsaturated fatty acids

These:

- contain two or more double bonds
- are liquid (oils) at room temperature
- are susceptible to oxidation within foods or the body.

These fatty acids have a pivotal role in many metabolic processes. They are key components of phospholipids in membranes, involved in the regulation of cholesterol metabolism, and precursors of many vital metabolic intermediaries (eicosanoids) such as prostaglandins, leukotrienes and thromboxanes.

Polyunsaturated fatty acids are divided into two types, $n6$ (omega-6) and $n3$ (omega-3), and these have distinctly different metabolic effects. The parent fatty acids in each of these groups, linoleic acid ($n6$) and alpha-linolenic acid ($n3$), are termed essential fatty acids (EFA) because humans (and other mammals) lack the enzymes to synthesize them and therefore require a dietary source, principally from plant foods such as oils, nuts and seeds. Long-chain fatty acids derived from these essential fatty acids are precursors of many metabolic intermediaries such as prostaglandins, leukotrienes and thromboxanes, and hence have variable influences on inflammatory processes, immune response and blood clotting. Because these long-chain derivatives can be synthesized by the body, they are not 'essential' components of the diet. However, they may become so if the dietary supply of their essential fatty acid precursors is limited.

EFA and their long-chain derivatives arachidonic acid, EPA and docosahexaenoic acid (DHA) play an important role in neural development in fetal and early life, and there is increasing speculation that deficiency at this time may impair subsequent brain, optical and cortical function (see Section 3.3 Infants).

n6 Polyunsaturated fatty acids Most dietary polyunsaturated fat is in the form of *n6* fatty acids, principally linoleic acid derived from vegetable oils such as sunflower, safflower, corn, palm, groundnut, canola and soya oils.

n6 PUFA have a hypocholesterolaemic effect and their substitution for saturated fatty acids has in the past been actively encouraged in order to lower LDL and total cholesterol levels. This advice has now been moderated as a result of concerns over the possible adverse effects of excessive *n6* PUFA intake. While PUFA are effective at lowering blood LDL cholesterol, they also lower HDL-cholesterol concentration, necessary for atherogenic protection (see Section 4.23, Hyperlipidaemia). PUFA are also susceptible to metabolic oxidation, and high intakes can enhance lipid peroxidation and free radical production with potentially adverse effects in terms of atherogenesis and carcinogenesis. Dietary intake of *n6* PUFA therefore needs to be adequate but not excessive. For lipid-lowering manipulations, substituting SFA with MUFA rather than PUFA is probably preferable.

Important derivatives of linoleic acid include gammalinolenic acid (GLA) (18:3 *n6*) and arachidonic acid (AA) (20:4 *n6*). These are present in small amounts in the diet but are mainly synthesized from linoleic acid via the omega-6 pathway (Fig. 2.3). Arachidonic acid is a major component of cell structure and an important regulator of prostaglandin and leukotriene production. GLA also affects prostaglandin production and supplemental daily doses of 240–480 mg GLA/day, taken for a period of 3–4 months, may help to relieve symptoms of premenstrual mastalgia in some, although not all, sufferers (Bussell 1998).

n3 Polyunsaturated fatty acids Alpha-linolenic acid (18:3 *n3*) and its principal long-chain *n3* derivatives EPA (20:5 *n3*) and DHA (22:6 *n3*) comprise a much smaller proportion of dietary PUFA intake but have important physiological effects.

Unlike *n6* PUFA, *n3* polyunsaturated fatty acids have minimal effects on blood cholesterol levels, although in pharmacological doses can reduce fasting and postprandial triglyceride concentrations (see Section 4.23.4 in Hyperlipidaemia). The main interest in *n3* PUFA is in their ability to influence thrombotic and inflammatory function.

EPA, high concentrations of which are found in fish oils, has an anti-thrombogenic effect. Increased consumption of fish, especially oily fish, is now recognized as an important dietary protective measure against myocardial infarction (see Section 4.21, Cardiovascular disease).

Both EPA and DHA (also found in marine oils) may have the ability to alter prostaglandin production in a way that can diminish the inflammatory response. Fish oil supplements may therefore have the ability to ameliorate symptoms in inflammatory disorders such as rheumatoid arthritis or Crohn's disease, although the benefits of this remain equivocal (see Sections 4.32.2 in Arthritis and 4.10.3 in Inflammatory bowel disease).

EPA and DHA also have an important structural role in

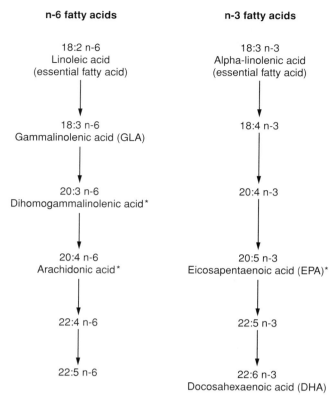

n-6 fatty acids	n-3 fatty acids
18:2 n-6 Linoleic acid (essential fatty acid)	18:3 n-3 Alpha-linolenic acid (essential fatty acid)
18:3 n-6 Gammalinolenic acid (GLA)	18:4 n-3
20:3 n-6 Dihomogammalinolenic acid*	20:4 n-3
20:4 n-6 Arachidonic acid*	20:5 n-3 Eicosapentaenoic acid (EPA)*
22:4 n-6	22:5 n-3
22:5 n-6	22:6 n-3 Docosahexaenoic acid (DHA)

*Influences the production of prostaglandins, prostacyclins, thromboxanes and leukotrienes.

Fig. 2.3 *n6* and *n3* fatty acid pathways.

brain, retinal and nervous tissue (see above).

Trans fatty acids

Double bonds in fatty acids may be in the *cis* or *trans* form. In the *cis* form the hydrogen atoms bonded to the carbon atoms at either end of the double bond are on the same side; in the *trans* form these hydrogen atoms are on opposite sides. Most dietary fatty acids contain *cis* double bonds, a characteristic which makes the fatty acid more rigid and bulky. *Trans* bonds are rare in nature, only being created in the rumen of cows and sheep, and hence only found in small amounts in milk, cheese, beef and lamb. However, *trans* fatty acids are also created during the manufacture of margarine when polyunsaturated fatty acids in liquid vegetable oils are artificially hydrogenated to create more solid spreading fats. Significant quantities of *trans* fatty acids are therefore found in margarine, some fat spreads and the many manufactured foods containing hydrogenated fat. *Trans* unsaturated fatty acids appear to be metabolized in a similar way to saturated fatty acids and are considered to have similar, potentially adverse, nutritional effects if consumed to excess.

Dietary cholesterol

Cholesterol is a wax-like substance belonging to the steroid family and has a simple chemical structure compared with the triglyceride molecule. Cholesterol is essential to life; it is a primary component of cell membranes and a substrate for the synthesis of bile acids, steroid hormones and vitamin D.

The influence of dietary cholesterol on blood cholesterol is relatively small because most circulating cholesterol is of endogenous origin (see Section 4.23.4 in Hyperlipidaemia). Significant effects of dietary cholesterol are only seen at extreme levels of intake: either as a result of an unusually high consumption of cholesterol-rich foods such as shellfish, eggs and liver, or a diet devoid of animal foods containing <300 mg cholesterol/day (Table 2.4). In most people, dietary measures which reduce intake of saturated fat will also prevent excessive consumption of dietary cholesterol.

2.3.3 Dietary fat requirements and intake

Recommended intake

There is no physiological requirement for dietary fat *per se*, only for essential fatty acids. Although estimates of requirements vary, dietary reference values (based on prevention of overt EFA deficiency) are that at least 1% dietary energy should be provided by dietary linoleic acid and 0.2% by dietary linolenic acid (DH 1991). However, there is increasing speculation that higher intakes of EFA may be necessary for optimal health.

Healthy people normally need to derive a much greater proportion of dietary energy from fat than a mere 1–2% in order for the diet to be sufficiently energy dense to meet energy needs, to obtain sufficient fat-soluble vitamins

and for dietary palatability. However, it has become increasingly apparent in recent decades that diets containing an excessive proportion of dietary fat energy, especially from saturated fat, contribute to the high prevalence of obesity, cardiovascular disease and other major health problems in Western societies (see Section 1.1, Diet, health and disease). The UK dietary reference values (DRVs) for fat are therefore expressed in terms of desirable percentages of energy which should be derived from fat and its constituent types (DH 1991) (Table 2.5).

Current intake in the UK

In the Dietary and Nutritional Survey of British Adults (Gregory *et al.* 1990), mean total fat intake was 102.3 g/day (38% energy) in men and 73.5 g/day (39% energy) in women. When the energy contribution from alcohol was excluded, this represented a mean fat energy intake of 40% for both sexes. SFA intake was 42.0 g/day in men (15.4% energy) in men and 31.1 g/day (16.7% energy) in women. Excluding alcohol, the average saturated fat energy intake of the entire group was 17%.

Current intakes of both total and saturated fat are thus well above the recommended levels of <35% and <11% energy, respectively. Although the National Food Survey (MAFF 1999) shows that the total amount of fat consumed per head of population has fallen considerably since the late 1980s (from an average 93 g/day in 1988 to 75 g/day in 1998), the accompanying fall in total energy intake means that % fat energy intake has only fallen slightly over the same period, from 42% in 1988 to 39% in 1998. Similarly, consumption of saturated fat has fallen in absolute terms from an average of 38.3 g/day per head of population in 1988 to 29.3 g/day in 1998 but % saturated fat intake has only declined from 17% to 15% (MAFF 1999). Considerable further reduction in the type and amount of fat consumed is required if the targets required for the prevention of coronary heart disease are to be met (DH 1994; Scottish Office 1996).

MUFA currently contribute about 12–13% of energy intake (Gregory *et al.* 1990). Current recommendations (DH 1991) are that this level should not change. While monounsaturates may usefully replace dietary saturated fat,

Table 2.4 Sources of dietary cholesterol

Cholesterol content	Foods
High	Liver, offal and products containing these (e.g. paté)
	Egg yolk, mayonnaise
	Fish roes
	Shellfish
Moderate	Fat on meat, duck, goose and cold cuts (e.g. salami)
	Full-fat milk, tinned milks, cream, ice-cream, cheese, butter
	Most manufactured pies, cakes, biscuits and pastries
	Meat and fish products
Low	Uncoated fish (white and oily), fish canned in vegetable oil
	Very lean meats, poultry (no skin)
	Skimmed milk, low-fat yoghurt, cottage cheese
	Bread
	Low-cholesterol margarine and fat spreads
Cholesterol-free	All vegetables and vegetable oils
	Fruit including avocado and olives
	Nuts
	Cereals, pasta (without added eggs), rice, popcorn (unbuttered)
	Egg white, meringue
	Sugar

Table 2.5 Fat intake of the UK population

	Current average UK intake[1] (Gregory *et al.* 1990)	Recommended UK intake[1] (DH 1991)
Total fat	40% energy	<35% energy
Saturated fat	17% energy	<11% energy
Monounsaturated fat	12% energy	(13%) No change
*n*6 Polyunsaturates	6% energy	(6.5%) No further increase
*n*3 Polyunsaturates	0.1 g/day	0.2 g/day (minimum)
Trans fatty acids	2% energy	<2% energy

[1]Excluding any energy contribution from alcohol.

it is also considered important to keep the overall proportion of dietary fat energy low. Recently it has been suggested that monounsaturates may beneficially make up a higher proportion of dietary energy provided that intake of saturates remains low, and total energy intake does not exceed requirement (RCP 2000). The extent to which monounsaturates should be used as a substitute for saturated fat (and as an alternative to carbohydrate energy in the management of diabetes; see Section 4.16.4 in Diabetes mellitus) is therefore largely determined by the presence or absence of obesity.

Current total intake of polyunsaturated fat is just over 6% food energy (Gregory *et al.* 1990) and, in view of the possible adverse effects of high intakes of *n*6 PUFA (see above), it is recommended that this level should not increase (DH 1991).

The ideal ratio of *n*6 and *n*3 dietary PUFA is a matter of speculation. National Food Survey data show that in 1995 the average intake of *n*6 PUFA was 10.2 g/day compared with *n*3 intake of 1.8 g/day, i.e. a ratio of just over 5:1 (MAFF 1996). Since the *n*6 and *n*3 fatty acid pathways share common enzymes (for example, *n*6 linoleic acid and *n*3 alpha-linolenic acid both compete for the enzyme delta-6 desaturase) it is likely that the balance between the two influences the type and amount of long-chain fatty acids and eicosanoids formed as a result of their metabolism. It has been suggested that diets containing a high proportion of *n*6 fatty acids relative to *n*3 fatty acids (such as may occur in vegetarian diets rich in linoleic acid-containing foods but devoid of fish and meat; see Section 3.10, Vegetarianism and veganism) could inhibit endogenous production of EPA and DHA, with possible adverse consequences (BNF 1999). A high ratio between n6 and *n*3 families of fatty acids may also influence the nature and potency of prostaglandins and leukotrienes formed,

possibly increasing the inflammatory response (BNF 1999). However, at the present time the optimal balance of dietary *n*6 to *n*3 fatty acids required for health is not known and recommendations are simply to increase the consumption of oily fish or other sources of *n*3 fatty acids (DH 1994).

Trans fatty acids currently provide about 2–3% of energy intake (4–5 g/day) (Gregory *et al.* 1990), but this proportion may be greater in people who consume large quantities of foods containing artificially hydrogenated fat such as manufactured pies, pastries, cakes and biscuits. It is recommended that *trans* fatty acid intake should not exceed 2% energy (DH 1991).

Sources of fat in the UK diet

Sources of fat and fatty acids in the average UK diet (MAFF 1999) are shown in Fig. 2.4. Although concentrated sources of fat such as oils and fat spreads are major contributors to fat intake, significant amounts are also derived from other food groups such as meat and meat products (especially the latter), milk and milk products (especially full-fat milk and cheese), and cereal foods (primarily from pastry, biscuits, cakes and puddings). In order to change fat consumption, attention therefore needs to be paid to the habitual level of consumption of these food groups and, in particular, the fat content of the food choices made from them.

For the purposes of general dietary guidance, the fat content of some typical food portions is shown in Table 2.6. More detailed information on the fat and fatty acid content of foods can be found in McCance and Widdowson's *The Composition of Foods* (Holland *et al.* 1991; MAFF 1998). In respect of processed foods, it should be noted that there may be significant differences in the fat content

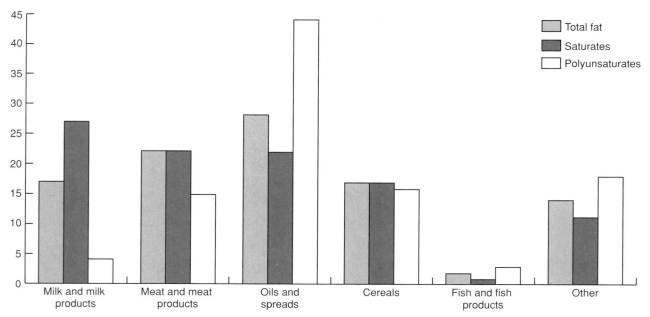

Fig. 2.4 Percentage contribution made by major food groups to total, saturated and polyunsaturated fat intakes.

Table 2.6 Approximate fat content of food portions

Food group	Very high-fat foods (>20 g/portion)	High-fat foods (10–20 g/portion)	Medium-fat foods (5–10 g/portion)	Low-fat foods (<5 g/portion)
Bread, cereals and potatoes	Pizza Pilau rice Fried rice dishes Chips, purchased or homemade	Bread thickly spread with fat Oven chips	Bread thinly spread with fat Potato salad	Bread Boiled rice Boiled pasta Breakfast cereals
Fruit and vegetables	Avocado	Fruit pies and flans Fried vegetables	Olives Coleslaw	All other fresh, frozen, stewed, dried, canned fruit[1] Fruit juices[1] Fresh, frozen, dried or canned vegetables[1]
Milk and dairy products		Double/whipping cream	Whole milk Greek yoghurt Single cream	Semi-skimmed milk Skimmed milk[1] Low-fat yoghurt Cottage cheese
	Cauliflower cheese Cheese omelette	Full-fat soft cheeses Cheddar cheese Cream cheese	Reduced-fat cheddar	Cottage cheese Fromage frais
Meat, fish and alternatives	Fatty meat or mince Poultry joint with skin Meat curries Meat pies, puddings and pasties Sausages Sausage roll, pork pie Liver sausage, patés	Red meat with fat marbling Poultry breast meat with skin Luncheon meat Beefburgers	Lean mince Poultry dark meat Corned beef	Lean red meat Poultry breast meat
	Fish canned in oil Taramasalata	Oily fish Fried fish White fish in batter Fried scampi Fish cakes	Grilled fish coated in breadcrumbs Fish fingers Fish canned in tomato sauce or brine	Grilled or baked white fish Smoked salmon
	Pastry-based flans or quiches Scotch egg	Omelette Fried egg	Boiled, poached egg	Egg white[1] Meringue[1]
		Peanuts (salted/dry roast) Chick-pea curry	Peanut butter Hummus, dahl, tofu	Baked beans
Fat-rich foods	Fried foods Pastry Pies Tarts	Thickly spread butter/fat spread Oil-based dressings Mayonnaise	Thinly spread butter/fat spread Reduced-fat mayonnaise Salad cream	Thinly spread low-fat spread (40% fat)
Sugar-rich foods		Chocolate Sponge puddings Trifle Sponge cake Fruit cake	Ice-cream Milk puddings Chocolate biscuits	Sugar[1] Jelly[1] Jams or preserves[1] Boiled sweets, pastillles, peppermints and gums[1] Plain biscuits Fatless sponge cakes

[1] Fat free or virtually fat free.

and fatty acid composition of similar products made by different manufacturers. The composition of a product may also change over a period of time as a result of fluctuations in world market prices of oils and fats and consequent product reformulation.

2.3.4 Modifying fat intake

Consuming less fat is an important aspect of dietary guidance for healthy eating, cardioprotection and weight management. In order to reduce total fat intake, the primary focus should be on curtailing consumption of sources of saturated fat. Particular emphasis should be placed on:

- avoiding obvious sources of saturated fat (e.g. by trimming visible fat, discarding poultry skin, draining off fat from cooked meat)
- using minimal amounts of fat in cooking (e.g. boiling, braising, steaming, grilling rather than frying or roasting)
- avoiding adding fats to food as much as possible (e.g. not adding butter to vegetables, reducing the amount of fat spread on bread)
- substituting foods with lower fat alternatives (e.g. skimmed or semi-skimmed milk instead of full-fat milk;

reduced-fat spread instead of butter or margarine; reduced-fat manufactured foods)
- eating fewer fat-rich foods (e.g. pastry, pies, cream, meat products, cakes, biscuits, chocolate).

It is important that such guidance is given in the overall context of a healthy diet, for example based on *The Balance of Good Health* guidelines, and does not focus on fat restriction alone. People should be encouraged to increase their intake of foods from the 'Bread, cereals and potatoes' and 'Fruit and vegetables' food groups, and also be guided towards other healthy food choices such as fish or pulses from the 'Meat, fish and alternatives' group. More detail on *Balance of Good Health* food choices and guidelines on fat restriction can be found in Section 1.2.2 and Table 1.7 in Section 1.2, Healthy eating).

People should also be encouraged to make use of nutrition labelling information to help them to choose foods containing the least fat. Many food labels now quote guideline daily amounts (GDAs) developed by the Institute of Grocery Distribution (1998) in consultation with MAFF, the Department of Health and the food industry (see Section 2.11, Food and nutrition labelling). By providing a yardstick of appropriate daily intake, GDAs help people to assess whether, for example, the amount of fat in a food is 'a little' or 'a lot'. The GDAs for fat are 95 g for men and 70 g fat for women. GDAs for saturated fat are less likely to be quoted on food labels, but people may find it helpful to know that they are 30 g for men and 20 g for women.

An increasing number of manufactured foods is being marketed as being 'low' or 'reduced' in fat. All such choices are likely to be a better option than their full-fat counterparts, but consumers should also be aware of the differences between these claims. Under current guidance regarding nutrition claims (see Section 2.11, Food and nutrition labelling), foods described as:

- *reduced fat* contain at least 25% less fat then the standard product. Although this is a significant reduction, many such products (e.g. reduced-fat sausages) will still have an appreciable fat content. Reduced-fat foods may therefore be better choices than standard products but should still only be consumed occasionally and not to excess;
- *low fat* contain <3 g fat/100 g or 100 ml. Most such products can be regarded as good food choices but they should not be considered to be 'fat free'. If consumed in large quantities, they can still make a significant contribution to total fat intake;
- *fat free* contain <0.15 g fat/100 g or 100 ml. Only these products can be regarded as having a negligible fat content.

The extent to which saturated fat should be substituted with unsaturated fats depends on clinical indications such as obesity and hyperlipidaemia. Both monounsaturates and *n*6 polyunsaturates have a hypocholesterolaemic effect, MUFA having the added advantage of doing so without adversely affecting the HDL-cholesterol level. Partial replacement of saturated fat with MUFA (such as olive oil

or fat spreads made from it) and, to a lesser extent, PUFA (derived from sunflower, soya or safflower oils) may therefore be beneficial when active cholesterol-lowering measures are indicated. Such measures may also help to improve dietary palatability. However, the high energy content of all types of oils and fat spreads should be borne in mind; liberal quantities of olive oil will not be beneficial to someone who is trying to lose weight. If weight management is a therapeutic objective, substitution of saturated fat with unsaturated fats should be kept to a minimum so that total fat (and energy) intake remains low.

More severe fat restriction (e.g. to a level of 10–40 g/day) may be indicated in clinical circumstances such as chylothorax (see Section 5.7, Chyle leakage) or certain types of fat malabsorption (see Section 4.8.2 in Malabsorption). Depending on the level of fat restriction required, such regimens will need to be composed of foods containing small or minimal amounts of fat, often in conjunction with modular supplements of carbohydrate and/or medium-chain triglycerides (MCT) (see Appendix 6.7) so that energy needs can be met. Supplementation with essential fatty acids and fat-soluble vitamins is also likely to be needed. Alternatively, proprietary low-fat feeds may be used as a partial or total dietary substitute.

Functional foods

Fat spreads containing plant sterols and stanols, and specifically designed to lower blood cholesterol (i.e. act as a 'functional' food), have recently been launched in the UK. Sterols and stanols are structurally similar to cholesterol and act by inhibiting cholesterol absorption. Even though the reduction in cholesterol absorption appears to stimulate the liver to increase cholesterol synthesis, the response is not sufficient to compensate for the reduced supply and the circulating cholesterol level falls. The cholesterol reduction is specific to LDL-cholesterol; HDL-cholesterol levels remain unchanged. Clinical trials show that regular use of a stanol- or sterol-enriched spread in place of a conventional spread can reduce total blood cholesterol level by 10–15% (Miettinen *et al.* 1995; Westrate *et al.* 1998). They may therefore be a useful adjunct to a cholesterol-lowering regimen. However, the relatively high cost of these products is, at the present time, a considerable drawback to their use (Law 2000).

Text revised by: Briony Thomas and Angie Jefferson

Further reading

FAO/WHO. *Fats and Oils in Human Nutrition*. Report of a Joint Expert Consultation. Rome: FAO, 1994.

References

British Nutrition Foundation. *n-3 Fatty acids and Health*. London: BNF, 1999.

Bussell G. Pre-menstrual syndrome and diet. *Journal of Nutritional and Environmental Medicine* 1998; **8**: 65–75.

Department of Health. Report of the Panel on Dietary Reference Values of the Committee on Medical Aspects of Food Policy (COMA). *Dietary Reference Values for Food Energy and Nutrients for the United Kingdom*. Report on Health and Social Subjects 41. London: HMSO, 1991.

Department of Health. Report of the Cardiovascular Review Group of the Committee on Medical Aspects of Food Policy (COMA). *Nutritional Aspects of Cardiovascular Disease*. Report on Health and Social Subjects 46. London: HMSO, 1994.

Gregory J, Foster K, Tyler H, Wiseman M. *The Dietary and Nutritional Survey of British Adults*. London: HMSO, 1990.

Holland B, Welch AA, Unwin ID *et al. McCance and Widdowson's The Composition of Foods*, 5th edn. Cambridge: Royal Society of Chemistry, 1991.

Institute of Grocery Distribution. *Voluntary Nutrition Labelling Guidelines to Benefit the Consumer*. Watford: IGD, 1998.

Law M. Plant sterol and stanol margerines and health. *British Medical Journal* 2000; **320**: 861–864.

Miettenen TA, Puska P, Gylling H *et al*. Reduction of serum cholesterol with sitostanol ester margarine in a mildly hypercholesterolemic population. *New England Journal of Medicine* 1995; **333**: 1308–1312.

Ministry of Agriculture, Fisheries and Food. *National Food Survey: 1995*. London: The Stationery Office, 1996.

Ministry of Agriculture, Fisheries and Food (MAFF). *Fatty Acids: Seventh Supplement to The Composition of Foods, 5th edn.* Cambridge: Royal Society of Chemistry/MAFF, 1998.

Ministry of Agriculture, Fisheries and Food. *National Food Survey: 1998*. London: The Stationery Office, 1999.

Roche HM, Zampelas A, Knapper J *et al*. Effect of long term olive oil dietary intervention on post prandial triacylglycerol and factor V11 metabolism. *American Journal of Clinical Nutrition* 1998; **68**: 552–560.

Royal College of Physicians. *2000 Consensus Statement: Dietary Fat, the Mediterranean Diet and Lifelong Good Health*. London: RCP, 2000.

Scottish Office. *Eating for Health: A Diet Action Plan for Scotland*. Edinburgh: HMSO, 1996.

Westrate JA, Meijer GW. Plant sterol enriched margarines and reduction of plasma total and LDL cholesterol concentrations in normocholesterolemic and mildly hypercholesterolemic subjects. *European Journal of Clinical Nutrition* 1998; **52**: 334–343.

2.4 Dietary carbohydrate

2.4.1 Function

Carbohydrates are an important source of energy in the human diet. All carbohydrates are ultimately converted to, and absorbed into the blood in the form of, glucose. Glucose is a vital fuel substrate for all body tissues, especially the brain, and blood glucose levels are usually maintained within tight parameters to meet fuel demands. Following the consumption of carbohydrate, blood glucose levels rise, triggering increased insulin production and increased cellular uptake of glucose. As surplus glucose is removed from the blood, insulin production declines and the blood glucose level gradually returns to its normal level. Once in body cells, glucose is oxidized as a source of energy. Glucose surplus to immediate requirement is stored as glycogen in the liver or skeletal muscles. When glycogen reserves are saturated, excess glucose is converted to fat for long-term storage in adipose tissues.

The liver has the highest concentration of glycogen at 250 mmol/kg (about 70 g carbohydrate in total), but skeletal muscle, because of its large size, has the greatest glycogen reserve of approximately 450 g carbohydrate. The size of an individual's glycogen reserves can be manipulated by specific eating and exercise behaviours (see Section 3.12, Nutrition for exercise and sport). The principal role of the liver glycogen reserve is to maintain a constant blood glucose level between meals; muscle glycogen plays a minimal role in blood glucose maintenance. As liver glycogen becomes depleted, glucose is synthesized from lactate, body fat or proteins by gluconeogenesis. During extreme carbohydrate restriction or inability to use glucose (e.g. in untreated type 1 diabetes), increased breakdown of fat results in the formation of ketones by the liver. Some will be used as a fuel source and some can be excreted in the urine, but if production is excessive or prolonged, the potentially fatal condition of ketoacidosis may develop.

Muscle glycogen reserves are used to provide fuel during periods of increased muscle activity. At rest, muscle glycogen utilization is negligible and during localized activity it is possible to deplete stores in some muscles while others remain virtually replete, e.g. during cycling, there is considerable depletion of muscle glycogen in the legs but very little in the muscles of the arms and upper body areas.

2.4.2 Structure and types of carbohydrate

Dietary carbohydrates originate from plants which synthesize them from carbon dioxide and water by the process of photosynthesis. The glucose so created is converted into other sugars and starches (to provide the plant with energy), and to cellulose and other non-starch polysaccharides (required for the plant's structure). Although, in living animals, liver and muscle contain carbohydrate in the form of glycogen, this dissipates rapidly after death and is no longer present by the time these tissues are eaten as food.

Chemically, carbohydrates are classified according to the number of saccharide units in their structure. There are four major groups of saccharides: monosaccharides, disaccharides, oligosaccharides and polysaccharides (Table 2.7). Not all can be digested and hence utilized as an energy source by the human body, although some non-digestible forms can be fermented by colonic bacteria and provide small amounts of energy. Some sugar derivatives such as sugar alcohols (polyols) such as sorbitol, xylitol and mannitol can be partly digested (providing about 2.4 kcal/g). While unavailable carbohydrates such as cellulose, hemicelluloses, pectins and mucilages (non-starch polysaccharides or 'dietary fibre') have no direct metabolic role, they are nevertheless important dietary components owing to their beneficial influences on gut function and motility (see Section 2.5, Dietary fibre (non-starch polysaccharide)).

Most available dietary carbohydrate is derived from:

- sugars, principally glucose, fructose and galactose (monosaccharides) and sucrose, lactose and maltose (disaccharides)
- starches (polysaccharides).

All these types of carbohydrate are either converted to glucose or join its metabolic pathways at some point, and are oxidized to provide the same amount of energy, i.e. 3.75 kcal (16 kJ)/g. Once absorbed, all sugars and starches are therefore indistinguishable in metabolic effect. There are, however, different health implications between them depending on their dietary origin. Starches are principally found in foods which provide other essential dietary components such as B vitamins, minerals, protein and fibre. In nature, sugars are also found in nutrient-rich foods such as fruits, vegetables and milk which provide vitamin C, beta-carotene, calcium and soluble fibre. However, humans have also developed the ability to extract sucrose from foods and use it as a sweetener, either added directly to foods and beverages or used to create foods such as cakes, biscuits or confectionery. Such foods tend to have a high content of sugars in a readily absorbable form, and also be relatively low in essential nutrients such as

Table 2.7 Classification of dietary saccharides

Class of saccharide	Type of saccharide	Digestibility	Dietary sources
Monosaccharides	Glucose	Readily absorbed and utilized	Small amounts of free glucose are present in fruit and vegetables, and larger amounts are present in honey. Manufactured foods containing commercial glucose syrups are a major source Most of the body's glucose is derived from the digestion and conversion of other saccharides
	Fructose	Well absorbed at normal levels of intake (approx. 10 g/day), but may cause osmotic diarrhoea in larger quantities, particularly in children Can be directly oxidized without being converted to glucose	Principal sugar in fruits, vegetables and honey Component of sucrose Commercial fructose syrups are used in the manufacture of some products (e.g. jams)
	Galactose	Absorbed by an active transport mechanism and rapidly converted to glucose	Not found in its free state, but as a component of lactose the principal sugar in milk and milk products
Disaccharides	Sucrose	Broken down by the enzyme sucrase to glucose and fructose which are rapidly absorbed	Table sugar Manufactured foods sweetened by the addition of sugar Foods which are naturally sweet (e.g. fruits and young vegetables)
	Lactose	Broken down by lactase to glucose and galactose. Some racial groups lose the ability to produce lactase beyond childhood, resulting in lactose intolerance	Milk and milk products
	Maltose	Converted by the enzyme maltase to glucose	Malted wheat and barley Malt extracts Beers
	Trehalose	Converted by the enzyme trehalase to glucose.	Mushrooms and edible fungi
Oligosaccharides	Raffinose Stachyose Verbascose	Composed of galactose, glucose and fructose units, but humans do not possess the enzymes to digest them. They can, however, be fermented in the colon	Peas Beans Seeds
Polysaccharides	Starch	Composed of amylase (linear molecules of 200–2000 glucose units) and amylopectin (branched-chain molecules of 10 000–1 million glucose units) Broken down by pancreatic amylase to glucose once the starch has been released from its storage granules by heat and moisture. Raw uncooked starch is poorly absorbed After heating, some types of starch also undergo retrograde conversion to a form which is resistant to amylase digestion. This 'resistant starch' can be fermented in the large intestine	The principal sources are cereal foods and potatoes Smaller amounts are present in root vegetables and unripened fruit
	Glycogen	Similar in composition to amylopectin, this is a storage form of glucose in living animals but is not present in foods derived from them	
	Non-starch polysaccharides	A heterogeneous mixture of cellulose (a polymer of glucose) and non-cellulosic polysaccharides containing a variety of hexoses, pentoses, uronic acids and other components in their structure Humans lack digestive enzymes which can break down these compounds. Some can, however, be partially broken down by colonic bacteria	Vegetables, fruits, wholegrain cereals and cereal brans, pulses
Sugar alcohols (polyols)	Sorbitol Xylitol Mannitol	These are only partially absorbed and hence provide less energy per gram than other available carbohydrates. Large amounts of polyols can cause osmotic diarrhoea	Small amounts are naturally present in a few foods (such as certain fruits) but are usually only obtained in significant quantities from manufactured foods where they have been used as a substitute for sucrose

micronutrients and fibre but relatively high in fat and energy. The COMA Panel on Dietary Sugars (DH 1989) therefore suggested that dietary sugars should be divided into two distinct groups:

- *Intrinsic sugars*: those still present within intact cells (e.g. sugars in whole fruit). The sugars present in milk (lactose and galactose) are also regarded as intrinsic sugars (despite being present in a free state) because their metabolic effects are similar to those of intrinsic sugars.
- *Non-milk extrinsic sugars (NMES)*: those present in a free, and hence readily absorbable, state as a result of being added to foods (usually in the form of sucrose) or released from disrupted cells (e.g. the sugars present in fruit purée or fruit juice).

This is a classification of convenience rather than chemistry. The sucrose present in a bar of chocolate (extrinsic) is no different from that found in an apple (intrinsic). However, the distinction is a useful one as an indicator of dietary quality. A diet with a high proportion of NMES often reflects relatively high consumption of sugar-rich food choices and low consumption of starchy cereals, fruits and vegetables. Such a diet is more likely to be inadequate in terms of overall balance (e.g. its content of dietary fat, fibre or micronutrients), have a high palatability/low satiety value thus increasing the risk of overconsumption of energy, and hence less likely to be appropriate for long-term health. Since foods and drinks containing added sugar also tend to be used as snack foods and consumed at frequent intervals throughout the day, high intake of NMES can also have implications in respect of dental caries (see Section 4.1.1 in Dental disorders).

2.4.3 Carbohydrate requirement and intake

Recommended carbohydrate intake

The amount of carbohydrate required by the body to prevent ketosis is relatively small, about 50–70 g/day. However a much greater intake of carbohydrate than this is usually desirable in order to keep the proportion of dietary energy derived from fat (particularly saturated fat) relatively low and the dietary satiety value high. Dietary reference values (DRVs) for carbohydrate are therefore expressed in percentage energy terms (DH 1991) and at levels that will help to achieve a reduction in the consumption of fat and NMES by the UK population (to help to reduce the prevalence of heart disease, obesity and dental caries). It is recommended that, in the adult diet (excluding any contribution from alcohol):

- total carbohydrate should provide about 50% energy intake
- non-milk extrinsic sugars should not exceed 11% energy intake.

Starches, intrinsic and milk sugars should therefore contribute about 39% energy intake.

These targets may not be appropriate for young children, or people with small or compromised appetites, who may require diets of greater energy density in order to meet their energy needs. Typically, infants derive about 40% of dietary energy from sugars (primarily lactose), preschool children obtain about 25–30% energy, and older children and adolescents 17–25% (DH 1989). While consumption of intrinsic sugars, especially milk, should be encouraged, consumption of NMES by these groups may well need to exceed 11% energy intake. The most important aspect is to try to ensure that NMES are obtained from sources which also provide essential nutrients, e.g. fruit juice, flavoured yoghurt or desserts, and that consumption is primarily limited to meal times.

Current carbohydrate intake

The diet of the average UK adult does not meet the recommended targets in terms of carbohydrate content. In the Dietary and Nutritional Survey of British Adults (Gregory *et al.* 1990), mean intakes of total carbohydrate were 272 g/day (44% energy) in men and 193 g/day (46% energy) in women, i.e. less than the desired 50% energy. Intake of NMES exceeded the recommended maximum of 11%, on average contributing 17% of dietary energy. Starch and intrinsic sugars together only provided 27% energy (rather than 39% energy). In men, total intake of sugars was 115 g/day (19% energy); in women it was 86 g/day (20% energy).

Sources of carbohydrate in the UK diet

In the average household diet (MAFF 1998), cereal foods are the major contributors to the intake of both starch and total carbohydrate intake. Dietary intake of sugars is derived almost equally from four main groups of foods: fruit, milk and milk products, cereals, and sugar and preserves (Fig. 2.5).

Principal dietary sources of different types of carbohydrate are summarized in Table 2.8. Guidance on the carbohydrate content of specific foods can be found in Appendix 6.2. Detailed information can be obtained from McCance and Widdowson's *The Composition of Foods* (Holland *et al.* 1991) and its various supplements (see Table 1.9 in Section 1.4, Food composition tables).

2.4.4 Alteration of carbohydrate intake

Increasing carbohydrate intake

Most of the UK population need to obtain a greater proportion of their dietary energy from appropriate carbohydrate so that their overall diet is more compatible with long-term health. In terms of food choice, this means an increased consumption of starchy foods such as bread, cereals and potatoes, together with sufficient choices from the 'Fruit and vegetables' and 'Milk and dairy products' food groups (see Section 1.2, Healthy eating).

The energy density of the food choices is also relevant. For many adults, and especially those who are overweight,

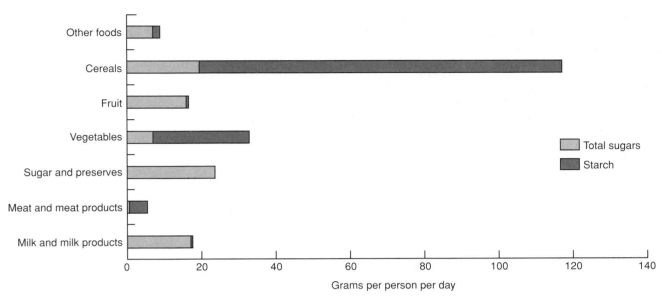

Fig. 2.5 Contribution of selected food groups to the carbohydrate content of the diet. (MAFF 1998)

Table 2.8 Principal sources of available dietary carbohydrates

Starches	Sugars		
	Intrinsic sugars	Milk sugars	Non-milk extrinsic sugars (NMES)
Bread	Whole fruit	Milk	Table sugar
Rice	Vegetables	Milk products	Honey, jam and preserves
Pasta			Fruit juices and purees
Potatoes			Manufactured foods containing added
Root vegetables			sugar or glucose/fructose syrups
Pulses, nuts and seeds			

fibre-rich sources of starchy carbohydrate (wholewheat and wholegrain products) can be encouraged to help increase dietary satiety value. In children and people with relatively high requirements but small appetites, or whose food intake is compromised as result of illness, more concentrated sources of carbohydrate may be appropriate. Food choices should be those with a more moderate fibre content, and a greater proportion of carbohydrate in the form of sugars may be desirable. If food intake is severely compromised, proprietary drinks or supplements based on glucose or liquid glucose polymers may be required (see Sections 1.12.3 and 1.12.4 in Oral nutritional support). In any instance where a high NMES intake is indicated, sufficient attention must also be paid to issues such as dental hygiene and consumption frequency in order to protect dental health (see Section 4.1, Dental disorders).

Restriction of carbohydrate intake

There are very few clinical circumstances which require restriction of total carbohydrate intake. Low-carbohydrate diets used to be a central feature of the management of diabetes but this is now no longer the case (see Section 4.16, Diabetes mellitus). Similarly, in weight loss regimens,

energy restriction is not usually best achieved by a diet low in carbohydrate because of its low satiety value (see Section 4.17, Obesity).

However, a decrease in the consumption of some types of carbohydrate is indicated in some clinical circumstances. Different carbohydrate-containing foods are digested and absorbed at different rates, so equal amounts of carbohydrate do not have equal effects in terms of glycaemia or other metabolic parameters such as insulin production or blood lipid concentration. The effect of carbohydrate on glycaemia is complex; in general, isolated sources of NMES (such as sugar-containing drinks or confectionery) are absorbed more rapidly than carbohydrate from starchy or fibre-containing foods such as cereals or fruit. However, there is considerable variability in glycaemic effect between foods of seemingly similar composition and this can be quantified in terms of the glycaemic index (GI) (the glycaemic effect of 50 g of a particular food in relation to 50 g of glucose or other carbohydrate standard) (Foster-Powell and Brand-Miller 1995; FAO/WHO 1998). Encouraging low rather than high GI food choices is therefore an important part of diabetes management and may also have application in the management of hypertriglyceridaemia and hyperinsulinaemia associated with obesity.

More details of the GI and a summary of high and low GI foods can be found in Section 4.16, Diabetes mellitus (subsection 4.16.6 and Table 4.33).

Some types of food intolerance may necessitate total or partial exclusion of specific saccharides. This may be result from:

- the lack of a digestive enzyme needed for the absorption of a disaccharide or polysaccharide (e.g. lactase deficiency causing lactose intolerance)
- an impaired ability to transport or metabolize a monosaccharide (e.g. galactosaemia).

Lactose intolerance

This is the most common form of saccharide intolerance and may result from:

- *hereditary alactasia*: an extremely rare disorder characterized by complete absence of the digestive enzyme lactase and necessitating total lactose exclusion;
- *primary lactase deficiency*: a common disorder in particular racial groups where there is a decline in lactase activity after infancy. In most cases, lactose intake only needs to be reduced to individual levels of tolerance, not excluded altogether;
- *secondary lactose deficiency*: usually a temporary disorder following gastrointestinal infection, damage or resection which results in impaired villous lactase production. It is a common accompaniment to cow's milk protein intolerance at the time of diagnosis. Lactose restriction is usually only required for a matter of weeks until either villi have regrown or the body has adapted to a reduced capacity for enzyme production.

The various types of lactose intolerance are discussed in more detail in Section 4.8.2 in Malabsorption. Practical aspects of milk exclusion can be found in Section 4.35.2 in Food exclusion in the management of allergy and intolerance.

Sucrose intolerance

Sucrose intolerance may be either primary (congenital sucrose deficiency) or secondary to severe intestinal enteropathies or infections.

Many sources of dietary sucrose are readily apparent (e.g. table sugar and obviously sweetened foods). However, most fruits, many vegetables and many manufactured (especially canned) products contain sucrose and must also be eliminated from the diet.

Secondary sucrose intolerance is likely to be accompanied by lactose intolerance, which will necessitate the additional exclusion of dietary sources of all sources of milk and lactose (see Section 4.35.2 in Food exclusion).

Starch intolerance

Primary starch intolerance is rare and results from congenital isomaltase deficiency. It is usually associated with primary sucrose intolerance and requires specialist dietetic management to ensure the exclusion of sucrose-containing foods as well as those containing:

- flour and foods containing flour (i.e. bread, cakes and biscuits)
- breakfast cereals
- cornflour (and most manufactured desserts)
- rice
- pasta
- food coated in breadcrumbs or batter
- potatoes
- many manufactured meat products (e.g. sausages, beefburgers, and meat and fish pastes).

Monosaccharide intolerances

Rare inherited disorders of metabolism such as galactosaemia or fructokinase deficiency require strict exclusion of specific monosaccharides soon after birth in order to prevent permanent brain damage. They require specialist management and further details can be found in paediatric dietetic textbooks.

2.4.5 Alternative sweeteners

Various substances are used as alternative sweeteners to sucrose. These fall into two categories:

- intense (non-nutritive) sweeteners
- nutritive (bulk) sweeteners.

Some, but not all, can be used in isolated form as table-top sweeteners, while others will only be found in manufactured foods. Compound mixtures of intense and nutritive sweeteners, sometimes in conjunction with other carbohydrates, are also marketed as sugar substitutes.

Intense sweeteners

These are compounds which have the unique property of imparting an intensely sweet flavour in minute amounts. Although some do have an energy value, their caloric contribution to a food is negligible because they are used in such small quantities. Intense sweeteners are widely used by the general public, particularly those with diabetes or obesity, as a substitute for sugar in drinks such as tea and coffee. They are also incorporated into a wide range of reduced-calorie or sugar-free products such as soft drinks, desserts and processed foods. Since they are non-cariogenic, they have an additional role as sweeteners in 'tooth-friendly' products such as sugar-free chewing gum. However, because they do not add volume to food or have the physical properties of sucrose, they cannot be used for domestic baking, e.g. to make cakes or preserves.

Intense sweeteners are classified as food additives and their use is controlled by *The Sweeteners in Foods Regulations* 1995 (and 1997 Amendments), which implement EC Directives. These specify the types of foods in which they may be used and the maximum level of usage within each category. The latter are based on the acceptable daily intake (ADI) for each compound (the amount, expressed on a body weight basis, that can be ingested daily over a lifetime without appreciable health risk). Intense sweeteners are not permitted for use in foods specifically prepared for babies and young children.

In the UK, the consumption of intense sweeteners is monitored to ensure that levels of intake do not exceed the ADI. Current trends show that most adults are unlikely to exceed the ADI for each sweetener on a regular basis. However, people who consume a lot of artificially sweetened products (especially children and people with diabetes) can have intakes that approach ADI levels, particularly in respect of saccharin and cyclamates. It is therefore advisable that people who regularly consume these products choose varieties containing different sweeteners to lessen the risk of exceeding the ADI of any one of them.

The following intense sweeteners are currently permitted within the EC.

Saccharin (E954)

Saccharin was the first available artificial sweetener and it has been used in food for more than 80 years. It is approximately 300 times as sweet as sucrose, although its sweetening intensity can vary according to its technical application.

Saccharin is cheap to use and stable to food processing and storage. It does, however, have a noticeable bitter aftertaste, particularly if heated. When saccharin is used as a sugar substitute in cooked foods (e.g. to sweeten stewed fruit or custard) it therefore has to be added at the end of any heating process. In manufactured foods, saccharin is often used in conjunction with another sweetener in order to mask its aftertaste.

In the late 1970s, concerns arose over the safety of saccharin following studies suggesting it could cause bladder cancer in rats and it was temporarily banned. However, public demand led to a moratorium on the ban and, following further safety evaluation, saccharin is now approved for use throughout Europe. In the USA, products containing saccharin are still required to carry a health warning.

The maximum ADI for saccharin is 5 mg/kg body weight per day, which for a 60 kg adult is equivalent to 20 saccharin tablets daily (less for a child). For those with a sweet tooth, this level of intake is not difficult to achieve, especially if saccharin-containing foods and drinks are consumed as well, and surveys suggest that some people, especially children, may exceed it (MAFF 1990). This risk has since been lessened by the wider availability of other intense sweeteners, many of which are used by the food industry in preference to saccharin. Nevertheless, people with a high consumption of artificially sweetened foods should be encouraged to check food labels to ensure that they do not rely solely on saccharin.

Aspartame (E951)

Aspartame has been available in the UK since 1983 and is approximately 200 times sweeter than sucrose. It is a combination of two amino acids, phenylalanine and aspartic acid, and hence has a theoretical energy value of 4 kcal/g. In practice, its minute level of consumption makes an insignificant contribution to energy intake.

Aspartame has better taste acceptability than saccharin but is much less stable. Prolonged heating causes it to break down into its constituent amino acids, with resulting loss of sweetness. It therefore tends to be used in unheated foods such as soft drinks, yoghurts and chilled desserts. It is also available as a table-top sweetener. Because of its relatively high cost, aspartame is often used by food manufacturers in conjunction with saccharin.

Aspartame has been implicated in altering mood (Renwick 1993), precipitating seizures, and producing hyperactivity and other behavioural problems in children (Walton *et al.* 1993), but these findings have not been substantiated (MAFF 1992; Tollefson and Barnard 1992; Ha and Lean 1998).

Aspartame is contraindicated for people with phenylketonuria who are unable to metabolize the phenylalanine which it contains. In the UK, foods and drinks containing aspartame contain a warning to this effect.

Acesulfame potassium (acesulfame K) (E950)

Acesulfame K has also been available in the UK since 1983. It is less sweet than other intense sweeteners (about 150 times sweeter than sucrose) and tends to produce a delayed sensation of sweetness. It is more stable to heat than aspartame, although not to all types of food processing.

Acesulfame K is synergistic with other sweeteners, intensifying their sweetness. It therefore tends to be used in combination with another sweetener such as aspartame, as this reduces the amount of sweetening compound needed with benefits in terms of product palatability and manufacturing costs.

Sodium and calcium cyclamate (E952)

Cyclamates were banned from use in the UK until 1996 because of concerns about carcinogenicity, but have now been approved for use throughout Europe. As with saccharin, the estimated ADI is relatively low (up to 1.5 mg cyclamate/kg body weight per day), and can be exceeded if consumption of products containing it (especially soft drinks) is high.

Thaumatin (E957)

Thaumatin is a protein extracted from the seeds of a West African plant and is approximately 2000–2500 times as sweet as sucrose. It is too concentrated in sweetness to be suitable for use as a table-top sweetener on its own, and is principally used as a flavour enhancer in manufactured foods, usually in combination with other sweeteners.

Neohesperidine DC (NHDC) (E959)

This is the most recently approved intense sweetener and is gaining increasing use in manufactured foods such as soft drinks, desserts, confectionery, savoury snacks and alcohol-free beer.

The non-nutritive sweetener alitame, a compound of two amino acids alanine and aspartic acid and with a sweetness 2000 times that of sucrose, has not yet been approved for use by the EC.

Bulk (nutritive) sweeteners

These are sugar substitutes which, because they are used in similar quantities to sucrose, add bulk, and some of the properties of sugar, to foods. Although, on a weight-for-weight basis, some provide less energy than sucrose, all provide some carbohydrate and energy.

Fructose is sometimes used as an alternative sweetener to sucrose because, although it has the same energy content, it is 1.5 times sweeter so less is needed for equivalent sweetness. It also used to be thought that fructose was a better alternative for diabetic patients because its metabolism does not initially require insulin. However, in the UK, isolated use of fructose is not recommended. For overweight patients, its potential energy saving is small and, in terms of diabetes, any short-term glycaemic advantage over sucrose is considered to be offset by potential adverse effects on blood lipids and other metabolic parameters. Fructose is also expensive and high intakes can result in osmotic diarrhoea.

Other types of bulk sweeteners are derivatives of carbohydrates, particularly sugar alcohols (polyols). Although many of these occur in small amounts in nature, they are classified as food additives and, like intense sweeteners, their use is controlled by the *Sweeteners in Foods Regulations*. Bulk sweeteners most commonly in use within the EC are:

- sorbitol (E420)
- mannitol (E421)
- isomalt (E953)
- maltitol (E965)
- lactitol (E966)
- xylitol (E967).

Hydrogenated glucose syrup is a commercially produced mixture of sugar alcohols, mostly maltitol.

The maximum permitted dose in foods is *quantum satis*, i.e. no numerical maximum level is specified for additive use because there is no need on safety grounds to do so. However, the additive should not be present at a level higher than is necessary to achieve the intended purpose.

Polyols are less well absorbed than other carbohydrates and can cause gastrointestinal side-effects. Individual tolerance varies and depends on dosage and previous exposure. However, stomach cramps, flatulence and osmotic diarrhoea can occur at intakes of about 30 g/day and sometimes much less, especially in children.

Because of their reduced absorption, polyols only provide 2.4 kcal/g compared with 3.75 kcal/g of other sugars. In theory, therefore, they provide less energy than sucrose but, since most are only half as sweet as sucrose, twice as much has to be consumed to create the same degree of sweetness, thus negating any energy saving.

Because their slower rate of absorption produces a smaller rise in postprandial glycaemia, polyols such as sorbitol have in the past been used as an alternative to sucrose by diabetic patients, particularly in the form of 'diabetic foods' such as chocolate, cakes and biscuits. However, as

with fructose, any small benefit in this respect is far outweighed by the many disadvantages associated with the use of either polyols or special foods containing them. The need for such products can also no longer be justified now that total dietary exclusion of sugar is no longer considered necessary for good management of diabetes (see Section 4.16.4 in Diabetes).

However, with the exception of fructose, bulk sugar substitutes are much less cariogenic than sucrose and hence have value as substitutes for sucrose in products such as sugar-free chewing gum, pastilles, mints and toothpaste. Xylitol is particularly useful in this respect as it also imparts mouth-cooling properties.

Compound sweeteners

These are commercially made products marketed as an alternative to table sugar. Most are mixtures of an intense sweetener with one or more of the following:

- a carbohydrate (e.g. saccharin + sucrose; aspartame + lactose; aspartame + maltodextrin)
- a bulk sugar substitute (e.g. saccharin + sorbitol)
- an inert filler (e.g. acesulfame K + cellulose).

Most are designed to be added to drinks or sprinkled on foods. Only a few are suitable for use in baking. They vary considerably in sweetness; some have an equivalent sweetness to sucrose, others are 10 times as sweet. As a result, their nutritional profile and sweetening power vary considerably. Although, on a spoonful basis, they will provide less energy than table sugar, the energy saving in absolute terms is often small and of questionable significance in the context of total daily energy intake.

Text revised by: Briony Thomas and Angie Jefferson

Further reading

FAO/WHO. *Carbohydrates in Human Nutrition*. Report of a Joint FAO/WHO Consultation. FAO Food and Nutrition Paper 66. Rome: FAO, 1998.

References

Department of Health. Report of the Panel on Dietary Sugars of the Committee on Medical Aspects of Food Policy. *Dietary Sugars and Human Disease*. Report on Health and Social Subjects 37. London: HMSO, 1989.

Department of Health. Report of the Panel on Dietary Reference Values of the Committee on Medical Aspects of Food Policy (COMA). *Dietary Reference Values for Food Energy and Nutrients for the United Kingdom*. Report on Health and Social Subjects 41. London: HMSO, 1991.

FAO/WHO. *Carbohydrates in Human Nutrition*. Report of a Joint FAO/WHO Consultation. FAO Food and Nutrition Paper 66, p. 85 and Table 8 in Annex 2. Rome: FAO, 1998.

Foster-Powell K, Brand Miller J. International tables of glycaemic index. *American Journal of Clinical Nutrition* 1995; **62**: 871S–893S.

Gregory J, Foster K, Tyler H, Wiseman M. *The Dietary and Nutritional Survey of British Adults*. London: HMSO, 1990.

Ha TK, Lean MEJ. Technical review: Recommendations for the nutritional management of patients with diabetes mellitus. *European Journal of Clinical Nutrition* 1998; **52**: 467–481.

Holland B, Welch AA, Unwin ID *et al. McCance and Widdowson's The Composition of Foods*, 5th edn. Cambridge: Royal Society of Chemistry/MAFF, 1991.

Ministry of Agriculture, Fisheries and Food. *Intakes of Intense and Bulk Sweeteners in the UK 1987–88*. London: HMSO, 1990.

Ministry of Agriculture, Fisheries and Food. *Sweetener intake within safe limits*. MAFF Food Safety Directorate News Release. FSD 44/92, 30 July 1992.

Ministry of Agriculture, Fisheries and Food. *National Food Survey: 1997*. London: The Stationery Office, 1998.

Renwick AG. A data derived safety (uncertainty) factor for the intense sweetener saccharin. *Food Additives and Contaminants* 1993; **10**: 337–350.

Tollefson L, Barnard RJ. An analysis of FDA passive surveillance reports of seizures associated with the consumption of aspartame. *Journal of the American Dietetic Association* 1992; **92**: 598–601.

Walton RG, Hudak R, Green-Waite RJ. Adverse reactions to aspartame: double-blind challenge to patients from a vulnerable population. *Biological Psychiatry* 1993; **34**: 13–17.

2.5 Dietary fibre (non-starch polysaccharide)

2.5.1 Definition and principal fibre components

There are many components of complex carbohydrate that are believed to resist digestion in humans and together these have been thought of as 'dietary fibre', although the term has been defined in various ways to consider analytical and physiological aspects. In practice, the chemistry of individual polysaccharides (polymers which exceed 20 sugar residues) cannot always be used to describe biological actions in the gastrointestinal tract, and some carbohydrate components which are chemically defined as starches also appear to resist digestion in humans. Attempts have been made to use functional characteristics of different polysaccharides to predict differences in physiological actions. The concept of 'soluble' and 'insoluble' fibre was developed through the assessment of solubility of components at controlled pH. This division helps in understanding the diverse physiological effects of fibre observed: soluble fibres blunt glucose and lipid absorption, whereas insoluble fibres contribute more to increased stool weight and reduced intestinal transit times. However, many variables such as the extent of fermentation in the colon, viscosity and binding capacity also affect physiological responses to the consumption of different fibre components, and it has been recommended that descriptions of fibre relating to solubility be phased out (FAO/WHO 1998). Nevertheless, for the time being, the soluble/insoluble distinction remains useful for many practical dietetic purposes.

The term 'dietary fibre' is also controversial. The UK COMA Panel (DH 1991) in their report on dietary reference values (DRVs) considered that it should become obsolete, and the term 'non-starch polysaccharide' (NSP) should be used in preference. NSPs are the major component of plant cell walls, are chemically identifiable and can be measured with precision. They consist of cellulose and non-cellulosic polysaccharides, the latter being a diverse mixture of pectins, glucans and arabogalactans, gums and mucilages containing a variety of hexoses, pentoses, and other constituents in their structure.

While the definition of NSP provides a welcome degree of precision to those trying to research the effects of this diverse group of dietary components, the term itself seems unlikely to replace 'dietary fibre' in the near future because the general public is unfamiliar with it, while most people have some concept of what is meant by dietary fibre and also encounter this term on food labelling.

2.5.2 Analysis and labelling

There are several ways in which the fibre content of foods can be measured, but the different methods can result in very different figures, depending on the fractions of fibre in the food. Analytical methods are either enzymatic–gravimetric, which measure a variety of components believed to resist digestion in the small intestine, or enzymic–chemical, which identify a chemically defined fraction of the diet, i.e. NSP. At present, UK food tables (see Section 1.4) present data on fibre content using both the Englyst method, which measures the NSP content of a food, and the Southgate method, which also measures other forms of carbohydrate not available for digestion, principally resistant starch and lignin. The Englyst method usually results in dietary fibre figures that are significantly lower than analyses by the Southgate method.

The European Commission Directive on nutrition labelling (90/496/EC) gives definitions for nutrition labelling of foodstuffs of all the major nutrients with the exception of dietary fibre. In the absence of harmonized legislation, MAFF issued guidance that the current UK definition, supported by the COMA Panel, is NSP measured by the Englyst technique, based on the premise that NSP is the major component of plant cell walls and the best index of the 'dietary fibre' concept.

MAFF proposals in May 1996 were that fibre declarations on food labelling, other than by the Englyst method, should be identified and described, to provide consumers with information to distinguish between fibre declarations based upon different non-comparable methods. However, such information was regarded as being meaningless to consumers, and in 1999 MAFF and the Department of Health (DH) proposed the adoption of the Association of Official Analytical Chemists (AOAC) international method of analysis of dietary fibre for labelling purposes (JFSSG 1999). This method is the preferred method of analysis in all other EU member states, and would ensure consistency, and hence usefulness, of information available on food labels to consumers across the EU. The AOAC international method measures a range of components in addition to NSP and produces analysis figures that are about 30% higher than analysis by the Englyst method. Formal recommendations by MAFF and DH to adopt the AOAC analysis method will require a revision (an increase by one-third) of the guidance for 'high-fibre' claims on food labels. In addition, the UK DRV for fibre intakes of 18 g NSP/day will need to be revised upwards to about 24 g/day of fibre measured by the AOAC method.

2.5.3 Physiological actions of dietary fibre

There are four principal effects of different fibre components on gastrointestinal function.

Absorption of nutrients

Viscous polysaccharides ('soluble fibre') blunt postprandial blood glucose responses, although this effect does not appear to relate to rate of gastric emptying.

Viscous polysaccharides may also reduce total blood cholesterol, specifically low-density lipoprotein (LDL)-cholesterol concentrations, although there is uncertainty about the degree to which this effect relates to a modification of the rate or site of absorption of lipids, or binding of compounds such as bile acids, and to what degree other mechanisms are involved.

Some fibre fractions, specifically phytates, bind with some minerals such as magnesium, calcium, zinc and iron, and diets habitually high in fibre and low in certain micronutrients may result in micronutrient deficiencies becoming overt, e.g. zinc deficiency in areas where unleavened wholemeal bread containing large amounts of phytic acid is a staple food. In practice, levels and types of fibre-containing foods consumed in mixed typical UK diets are unlikely to affect mineral status.

Metabolism of bile acids

Some fibre components reduce the reabsorption of bile acids in the lower part of the small intestine (ileum). The binding of bile acids reduces their enterohepatic circulation and increases losses via the faeces. Hypocholesterolaemic effects observed with diets high in some types of fibre (Brown *et al.* 1999) may relate to cholesterol in the body then being used to increase synthesis of bile acids *de novo*.

Fermentation in the large intestine

Many polysaccharide components resist digestion in the small intestine and become substrates for bacterial fermentation in the ascending large intestine. Dietary fibre has an influence on bacterial mass and enzyme activity, but appears to have little effect on the types of bacteria in the colonic flora. Short-chain fatty acids produced from bacterial fermentation are absorbed by the colonic mucosa and contribute to energy provision (mainly as acetic acid). Short-chain fatty acids (mainly as butyric acid) are also an important fuel source for the mucosal cells of the colon. The production of short-chain fatty acids influences faecal pH levels and colonic cellular proliferation and differentiation; such effects may contribute to a reduction in the risk of colorectal cancer.

Faecal weight and composition

Fibre contributes to faecal weight as a result of the amount which remains undigested and unfermented, and also through the contribution to bacterial bulk following the entry of substrate into the colon; in turn, both of these factors affect the water-holding capacity of colonic contents. For example, the increase in faecal weight following consumption of wheat bran is mostly due to an increase in undigested and unfermented residue and associated bound water, whereas that following ingestion of oat bran primarily results from an increase in bacterial bulk following its use as a substrate (Chen *et al.* 1998).

2.5.4 Intakes of dietary fibre

The average UK diet contains approximately 12 g of NSP/day (Bingham *et al.* 1990; MAFF 1998). In a survey of the diets of over 2000 British adults (Gregory *et al.* 1990), the fibre intake of men was found to vary little with age, but there was a trend towards increasing fibre consumption with age among older women, with the oldest group having a significantly higher intake than those aged 16–24 years. Women of all ages had higher intakes of fibre per unit energy than men.

The Survey of British Adults (Gregory *et al.* 1990) indicated that:

- Nearly half of total fibre intake (47%) in the UK diet came from cereal products; white bread contributed 13% of intake and all other types of bread including wholemeal contributed a further 17%.
- Vegetables were the next most important category (38% of fibre intakes), of which about one-third (12%) came from potatoes alone.
- Fruits and nuts provided 8% of fibre intake.

The COMA Panel on Dietary Reference Values (DH 1991) proposed that adult diets in the UK should contain an average of 18 g fibre (NSP)/day from a variety of foods whose constituents contain it as a naturally integrated component. There is no specific recommendation for children other than that intake should be proportionately lower. The basis for the reference value for fibre intakes relates principally to bowel habit; in the UK median stool weight is about 100 g/day, and in epidemiological studies, stool weights below 150 g/day are associated with increased risks of colon cancer and diverticular disease. The COMA Panel considered that an increase in average intakes of NSP from 12–13 g to 18 g/day would increase average stool weight by 25%, and would reduce the number of individuals with stool weights below 100 g/day. The COMA Panel saw no benefit of intakes of NSP above 32 g/day, and specifically pronounced caution with the use of unprocessed bran, especially in elderly people, as a method of increasing intake of fibre in the diet.

2.5.5 Altering fibre intake

Individuals advised to increase intake of dietary fibre will generally need to increase intake of cereal foods, and especially to replace 'refined' forms with wholemeal or wholegrain products. Some breakfast cereals contain particularly high amounts of fibre per portion. Pulses and

Table 2.9 Dietary sources of non-starch polysaccharides

Good sources (>4 g/portion)	Peas, beans, brussels sprouts, parsnips, spring greens Wholemeal, rye and granary bread Wholemeal pasta Bran-based breakfast cereals, muesli
Moderate sources (1–4 g/portion)	Most fruits, vegetables and nuts Brown and white bread Brown rice Other pasta Baked products containing wholemeal flour or dried fruit Wholewheat breakfast cereals, porridge
Poor sources (<1 g/portion)	Lettuce, marrow, grapes, canned mandarin oranges White rice, sago, cornflour, tapioca, arrowroot Plain cakes and biscuits Cornflakes, rice-based breakfast cereals

beans are a rich source of fibre, and emphasis also needs to be placed on increased intakes of fruit and especially of vegetables. Table 2.9 is a guide to good, moderate and poor sources of NSP per portion.

Sometimes temporary use is made of fibre supplements to relieve symptoms of constipation (see Section 4.11.1). Methylcellulose or ispaghula, for example, may be prescribed as drugs. General advice with the use of concentrated sources of fibre-containing products is the concomitant and plentiful intake of fluids; such guidance may be particularly important in older people prone to constipation.

People requiring a diet low in fibre will need to limit intakes of fruits and vegetables, pulses and beans, and all unrefined cereal products. In practice, some control over intakes of sources of starch will also be needed, as a proportion of starch escapes digestion in the small intestine and promotes bacterial fermentation in the large intestine, resulting in an increase in faecal weight. The main food sources of starch resistant to digestion are bananas, cooled cooked potato (for instance, eaten as potato salad), bread, beans and cornflakes. In extreme cases, low-residue diets for research purposes consist entirely of meat, cheese, eggs, fish and sugar; alternatively, a liquid formula diet may be necessary.

Text revised by: Ursula Arens

References

Bingham S, Pett S, Day KC. NSP intake of a representative sample of British adults. *Journal of Human Nutrition and Dietetics* 1990; **3**: 333–337.

Brown L, Rosner B, Willett WW, Sacks FM. Cholesterol-lowering effect of dietary fiber: a meta-analysis. *American Journal of Clinical Nutrition* 1999; **69**: 30–42.

Chen HL, Haack VS, Janecky CW *et al*. Mechanisms by which wheat bran and oat bran increase stool weight in humans. *American Journal of Clinical Nutrition* 1998; **68**: 711–719.

Department of Health. Report of the Panel on Dietary Reference Values of the Committee on Medical Aspects of Food Policy (COMA). *Dietary Reference Values for Food Energy and Nutrients for the United Kingdom*. Report on Health and Social Subjects 41. London: HMSO, 1991.

FAO/WHO. *Carbohydrates in Human Nutrition*. Report of a Joint FAO/WHO Consultation. FAO Food and Nutrition Paper 66. Rome: FAO, 1998.

Gregory J, Foster K, Tyler H, Wiseman M. *The Dietary and Nutritional Survey of British Adults*. London: HMSO, 1990.

Joint Food Safety and Standards Group. *Definition and Determination of Dietary Fibre for Nutrition Labelling Purposes*, 9 August 1999. London: JFSSG.

MAFF. *National Food Survey 1997*. London: The Stationery Office, 1998.

2.6 Vitamins

This section provides an overview of the function, requirements and sources of vitamins from a dietetic perspective. More detailed information on vitamin structure, metabolism and effects can be found in standard textbooks of nutrition.

2.6.1 General aspects

Vitamins are a diverse array of chemicals. They are required in very small quantities, usually only a few micrograms (μg) or milligrams (mg) per day, but are essential for many of the processes carried out in the body. Most vitamins cannot be made by the body, so a dietary intake is essential to prevent symptoms attributable to deficiency. While there are some exceptions, such as vitamin D (which can be made by the action of sunlight on the skin), vitamin K (which can be made by intestinal bacteria) and niacin (which can be made from the amino acid tryptophan), synthesis often cannot occur in quantities needed to meet physiological requirements, and some dietary intake remains essential.

Vitamins were usually first identified in relation to their pivotal roles in the prevention of a specific 'deficiency disease', and past research interest has been on the relationship between such defined diseases or symptoms (such as scurvy, beri-beri and pellagra) and intakes of specific vitamins. Overt deficiency diseases in relation to inadequate intakes of individual vitamins are very rare in the UK population. However, there is considerable interest within current scientific research on the possible associations between 'suboptimal' intakes of vitamins and the increased risk of adverse effects on health, including several conditions considered to have long-term multifactorial risk factors, such as some cancers and heart disease.

Vitamins are not chemically related. The classification of vitamins was originally with a letter, and once a chemical structure was identified a specific chemical name could be identified; however, it was discovered that while some vitamins were single chemicals, e.g. vitamin C (ascorbic acid), others consisted of a family of related compounds, such as vitamins A and D. Classification according to principal functions and actions in the body can be a useful way of describing roles and predicting the effects of inadequate intakes. Some vitamins, e.g. many of the B group, act as cofactors for enzymes required in energy production pathways. Other vitamins have actions that are specific to the development or maintenance of body tissues, e.g. blood (folate and vitamin B_{12}) or bone (vitamin D). In addition to such functional roles, vitamins have been described through possible effects on general systems such as the description of antioxidant functions for ascorbic acid and vitamin E.

Another form of classification of vitamins relates to their solubility in lipids or in water. The lipid-soluble (fat-soluble) vitamins are vitamins A (retinol), vitamin D (cholecalciferol), vitamin K and vitamin E (tocopherols). The B group vitamins and vitamin C (ascorbic acid) are water soluble. Such classification provides some indication to food sources, function and distribution in the body, and potential toxicity (Table 2.10).

Different methods of classification of vitamins appear to offer some benefit in terms of characterization of properties, but there are anomalies with each system, and ultimately each vitamin requires individual description to define its functional features clearly.

2.6.2 Fat-soluble vitamins

Vitamin A

Vitamin A describes the activity of retinol (preformed vitamin A) and of some of the carotenoids found in plant pigments with provitamin A activity. Beta-carotene is the most widespread carotenoid in the human diet, and 6 μg is calculated to be equivalent to the vitamin A activity of 1 μg of retinol; all other carotenoids are calculated to require, as an average figure, 12 μg to equate to the vitamin A activity of 1 μg of retinol. Many of the carotenoids in the diet have no vitamin A activity, e.g. zeaxanthin, the pigment found in sweetcorn, and lycopene, the red pigment of tomatoes.

Table 2.10 Characteristics of fat-soluble and water-soluble vitamin groups

	Fat-soluble vitamins	Water-soluble vitamins
Risk of deficiency	Very low-fat diets Conditions where fat absorption is impaired	Diets lacking variety
Stability in foods	Robust to heat and light	Various; often labile to heat and light
Storage in body	Can be large and long term	Often small; frequent, regular intakes required
Risk of toxicity	High	Low; high intakes can usually be excreted in urine

Function

Vitamin A is required for the normal development and differentiation of tissues. The effects of deficiency tend to be most apparent in rapidly dividing tissues such as those of the skin and conjunctiva and cornea of the eye. Vitamin A is also necessary for the manufacture of rhodopsin in the retina, necessary for adaptation of vision in the dark.

Requirement and intake

The reference nutrient intake (RNI) for children aged 1–10 years is 400–500 μg/day and 600 μg/day for 11–14 year olds. Over this age, it is 700 μg/day for men and 600 μg/day for women. During pregnancy daily requirement is increased by 100 μg and during lactation by 350 μg (DH 1991).

In the UK, mean intakes usually exceed these levels. The Survey of British Adults showed that average daily intakes of vitamin A (from both retinol and carotene) were 1679 μg for men and 1488 μg for women; about three-quarters was provided by retinol in the diet (Gregory et al. 1990). Only 2.5% of the adult survey sample had intakes below the lower reference nutrient intake (LRNI; 300 μg and 250 μg for men and women, respectively) although the proportion of 16–18 year olds who fell into this category ranged between 7 and 11% (for females and males, respectively) (MAFF 1994).

Sources in the UK diet

Most preformed retinol in the UK diet (Gregory et al. 1990) is derived from:

- meat and meat products (61%), relating mainly to the contribution of liver and products made using liver
- milk and dairy products (14%)
- fat spreads (13%).

Vegetables provided 70% of the carotenes in the diet, with fruit providing less than 3%. Although meat products were reported as providing 12% of the carotenes in the diet, this is attributable to the vegetable component of prepared meat dishes.

The most concentrated food sources of retinol in the diet are:

- liver and products
- kidney and offal products
- oily fish and fish liver oils
- eggs.

The most concentrated food sources of beta-carotene in the diet are:

- carrots
- red peppers
- spinach
- broccoli
- tomatoes.

Deficiency

Low vitamin A status can occur in any condition which results in significant fat malabsorption. Poor intakes can occur in young children not given supplementary vitamin A and also in people consuming long-term diets that are very low in fat, particularly if animal-source foods are also excluded.

Symptoms of deficiency can include:

- impaired night vision
- loss of integrity of skin and mucous membranes and consequent increased risk of infection.

Toxicity

Surplus amounts of vitamin A are stored in the body and excessive intakes can cause liver damage and be fatal. High intakes of vitamin A are also potentially teratogenic and concentrated sources of the vitamin such as liver and liver products should be avoided by pregnant women (see Section 3.1, Pregnancy).

Recommended maximum intakes are 9000 μg/day for adult men and 7500 μg/day for women.

Vitamin D

There are several compounds with vitamin D activity. Dietary forms are principally cholecalciferol (vitamin D_3) and ergocalciferol (vitamin D_2). Most of the vitamin D required by humans is produced by ultraviolet (UV) irradiation of the 7-dehydrocholesterol present in the skin. However, dietary intakes of vitamin D are critical where:

- there is little or no skin exposure to UV light
- conversion is reduced (such as in people with dark skin containing high levels of melanin, or in older people)
- physiological requirements are particularly high, such as in young children or during pregnancy.

Vitamins D_2 and D_3 consumed in foods are biologically inactive. A proportion of vitamin D absorbed is converted into 25-hydroxyvitamin D in the liver, which has a very small amount of biological activity; however, further conversion by the kidney into 1,25-dihydroxyvitamin D (calcitriol) then produces the active form of vitamin D.

Function

The active form (1,25-dihydroxyvitamin D) is involved in calcium homoeostasis, mainly by controlling the amount of calcium absorbed and excreted. It may also have a direct effect on bone synthesis.

Requirement and intake

The RNI for infants under the age of 6 months is 8.5 μg/day and then up to the age of 4 years is 7 μg/day (DH 1991). People in the age range 4–64 years are assumed not to require a dietary source of vitamin D, as long as there is some exposure of skin to sunlight in the summer months. Specific recommendations for dietary intakes of 10 μg/day relate to:

- people over the age of 65 years
- pregnant and lactating women

- people in situations where there is no exposure to sunlight.

The Survey of British Adults showed that average dietary intakes of vitamin D were 3.78 μg/day for men and 3.09 μg/day for women (Gregory *et al.* 1990). Intakes of vitamin D were higher in older age groups than in younger age groups. Vitamin D from food supplements provided, on average, over 10% of intake in men and over 20% of intake in women. The lower 2.5 percentile intake level was 0.51 μg for men and 0.43 μg for women.

Sources in the UK diet

Most dietary vitamin D comes from:

- margarines and fat spreads (30%)
- cereal products (24%)
- oily fish (21%).

The natural carriers of vitamin D (oily fish, meat, eggs and dairy products) provide less than 50% of total intake of vitamin D in the UK, with most coming into the diet as a result of the mandatory fortification of margarines and the fortification of other fat spreads, breakfast cereals and some dairy products. Both vitamin D_3 and vitamin D_2 are used to fortify foods, although the former appears to be more potent in terms of affecting 25-hydroxyvitamin D serum levels (Trang *et al.* 1998).

Deficiency

The risk of vitamin D deficiency in the UK population is low, but may be high in elderly people not exposed to sunlight (institutionalized or housebound), in ethnic groups where complete clothing covering is practised (usually only in adult females), and in some Asian infants and children.

Prolonged deficiency of vitamin D in children results in rickets, characterized by skeletal deformities accompanied by bone pain, muscle weakness and reduced bone growth. In adults, deficiency results in osteomalacia, the principle symptoms being bone tenderness or pain and muscle weakness.

Vitamin D deficiency may also play a contributory role in the development of osteoporosis (see Section 4.31).

Toxicity

Excessive intakes can result in hypervitaminosis D, resulting in hypercalcaemia. The risk is greatest in infants.

Vitamin E

There are eight tocopherols and tocotrienols with vitamin E activity. D-alpha-tocopherol has the highest biological potency and its activity is the standard against which other forms are compared. Synthetic vitamin E is a mixture of stereoisomers with biological activities ranging from 20 to 90% of the activity of natural vitamin E.

Function

Vitamin E is an important antioxidant and, because it is fat soluble, plays a major role in preventing oxidative damage to lipid-containing structures such as cell membranes.

Requirement and intake

The biological function of vitamin E is general rather than specific (e.g. as a cofactor for an enzyme) and hence the assessment of requirements is difficult. The COMA report on Dietary Reference Values (DH 1991) did not define RNI values for vitamin E, but stated levels of safe intake (amounts considered adequate to prevent deficiency) as:

- >4 mg/day in men
- >3 mg/day in women.

However, vitamin E requirements are influenced by dietary intakes of polyunsaturated fatty acids (PUFA); each gram of PUFA is thought to require an intake of about 0.4 mg vitamin E, so average diets containing 7% energy from PUFA would result in vitamin E requirements of 6 mg for women and 8 mg for men.

Gregory *et al.* (1990) found that average intakes of vitamin E were 11.7 mg for men and 8.6 mg for women. Supplements provided nearly 20% of average intakes in adults. The lower 2.5 percentile intake level was 3.7 mg and 2.6 mg for men and women, respectively.

Sources in the UK diet

Most vitamin E in the diet comes from fats, either directly through spreads and margarines (20%), or from foods such as fried potatoes or cereal products in which fat is a major ingredient. Meat, fish and eggs as a group provide about 20% of intake.

The most concentrated sources of vitamin E are vegetable oils, particularly wheatgerm oil (180 mg/100 ml) and sunflower seed oil (60 mg/100 ml). Olive oils are not generally rich in vitamin E. The vitamin E level in margarines is variable depending on the oils used in manufacture and whether the product is fortified; however, levels can be high.

Deficiency

Clinical deficiency of vitamin E is rare and has only been clearly identified in premature infants. However, there is increasing speculation that low vitamin E intakes increase the risk of some chronic diseases in which tissue oxidation is involved, such as coronary heart disease and some degenerative conditions such as cataracts. Population groups thought most at risk of poor vitamin E status are:

- premature infants
- people with high intakes of PUFA
- those with medical conditions resulting in the malabsorption of fat.

Toxicity

Few adverse effects have been reported from the consumption of as much as 3200 mg vitamin E/day (DH 1991) but the safety of high levels of intake remains to be established.

Vitamin K

Vitamin K is a naphthoquinone and occurs in two forms:
- K_1 (phylloquinone, present in food)
- K_2 (menaquinone, produced in the body by intestinal bacteria).

Function

Vitamin K is essential for the formation of prothrombin and other factors necessary for blood coagulation.

Requirement and intake

No RNI value for vitamin K has been defined, although dietary intakes of 1 μg/kg body weight per day are believed to be adequate for adults.

Infants are born with very low body stores of vitamin K and, since the gut is sterile at birth, production via intestinal bacterial cannot occur initially. Because such low status would put 1 in 800 babies at risk of severe bleeding within the first week postpartum, vitamin K injections or tablets are routinely given at birth.

The vitamin K contents of foods are not known with precision, and there are few reliable estimates of dietary intakes in the UK. Reports of normal diets consumed by healthy adults in the USA indicate intakes of vitamin K to be in the region of 300–500 μg/day (Olson 1988) or 100 μg/day (Booth *et al*. 1999).

Sources in the UK diet

Vitamin K is present in green leafy vegetables, e.g. spinach, broccoli, cabbage and kale. Soyabean oil and beef liver are also good sources of the vitamin, and dried seaweed appears to be a particularly concentrated source.

Deficiency

Acute deficiency of vitamin K may occur in newborn infants not given synthetic vitamin K at birth. Deficiency in adults is rare and results in prolonged blood clotting time; occurrence is possible in those with bowel disorders affecting the absorption of lipids.

Toxicity

Few adverse effects have been reported, but high intakes of non-medically prescribed supplements may not be advisable (DH 1991).

2.6.3 Water-soluble vitamins

Thiamin (vitamin B_1)

Function

Thiamin is the precursor of the coenzyme thiamin pyrophosphate, involved in the metabolism of carbohydrate, fat and alcohol. Requirements are therefore related to energy metabolism. It is not stored in the body other than in very small amounts bound to enzymes.

Requirement and intake

The RNI for thiamin is calculated on the basis of energy requirements, at 0.4 mg/1000 kcal energy intake. In practice, these result in the following RNIs (DH 1991):

- children: 0.5–0.7 mg/day
- adult men: 1.0 mg/day
- adult women: 0.8 mg/day.

There is an increase in the daily RNI in the last trimester of pregnancy by 0.1 mg, and during lactation by 0.2 mg.

The Survey of British Adults showed that average intakes of thiamin exceeded the RNIs and were 2.0 mg/day for men and 1.6 mg/day for women (Gregory *et al*. 1990). Only a small proportion (<10%) of the population had intakes below the RNI and very few below the LRNI (MAFF 1994).

Sources in the UK diet

Thiamin is widely distributed in foods. Cereal products provide about 40% of total intakes, including breakfast cereals (12%) and bread (20%). Vegetables provide a quarter of thiamin intake, whereby most comes from potatoes alone (17%). Meat and meat products provide a further 20% of intake, and milk and dairy products a further 10% (Gregory *et al*. 1990).

In the UK there is mandatory fortification of all flour other than wholemeal with thiamin, and in practice most breakfast cereals are fortified. Other concentrated sources of thiamin in the diet are:

- yeast and yeast extracts
- pork
- nuts
- pulses
- wholegrain cereal foods, e.g. brown rice and wholemeal bread.

It should be noted that there is an uneven distribution of thiamin in cereal products, with most present in outer germ layers, so without fortification, consumption of diets based on white rice and white flour result in intakes of thiamin that are low, and may be inadequate.

Deficiency

Deficiency in the UK population is most likely to occur in alcoholics, resulting in alcoholic neuropathy and Wernicke–Korsakoff syndrome.

Toxicity

Although thiamin is excreted via urine, chronic intakes of more than 3 g/day have been associated with a variety of neurological and dermatological symptoms (DH 1991).

Riboflavin (vitamin B_2)

Function

Riboflavin forms flavoproteins in the body, which are involved in metabolism with the oxidation of fatty acids and of glucose, and with the production of ATP. Riboflavin is not stored in the body, and any excess amounts are excreted unchanged in the urine.

Requirement and intake

Riboflavin RNIs (DH 1991) are:

- children: 0.6–1.0 mg/day
- adult men: 1.3 mg/day
- adult women: 1.1 mg/day.

There is an increase in the RNI during pregnancy by 0.3 mg, and lactation by 0.5 mg.

The Survey of British Adults showed that average intakes of riboflavin were 2.29 mg for men and 1.84 mg for women (Gregory *et al*. 1990). Up to 20% of this population (aged 16–64 years) had intakes below the RNI but very few below the LRNI (MAFF 1994).

Sources in the UK diet

The main contributors to dietary intake are (Gregory *et al*. 1990):

- milk and dairy products (27%)
- meat and meat products (>20%)
- cereal products (>20%)
- beverages (11%), with beer being a significant source for men (8%), but not for women.

Milk from cows fed on grass contains more riboflavin than that from those fed on dry rations or root crops, so levels tend to be lower in the winter months; the riboflavin content of milk is also reduced on exposure to light.

Concentrated sources of riboflavin are:

- yeast and yeast extracts
- liver and offal meats
- green leafy vegetables.

Deficiency

Deficiency symptoms are characterized by cracks and sores in the skin around the mouth and nose (cheilosis; angular stomatitis). Severe deficiency is unlikely in the UK population, but poor status and subclinical deficiency may be widespread in older people (Finch *et al*. 1998).

Toxicity

This is low, owing to the rapid elimination from the body of any surplus.

Niacin

The term describes both nicotinic acid and nicotinamide; the term 'vitamin B_3' is occasionally used. Both forms are found in foods although in the body, niacin occurs as nicotinamide. Humans are not entirely dependent on dietary niacin as it can also be synthesized from the amino acid tryptophan (60 mg tryptophan is required to produce 1 mg niacin). The contribution of niacin and tryptophan together is described as 'niacin equivalents'.

Function

Niacin is an essential constituent of the coenzymes NAD and NADP, which are required for oxidation–reduction reactions in metabolic pathways.

Requirement and intake

Because niacin is involved in energy metabolism, there is a direct association between requirements and energy intakes: the RNI is calculated to provide 6.6 mg niacin/ 1000 kcal. The RNI (as niacin equivalents) for children is 8–12 mg/day, for adult men 17 mg/day and for adult women 13 mg/day. During lactation there is an additional requirement of 2 mg/day (DH 1991).

The Survey of British Adults showed that average intakes of niacin equivalents were far above these levels: 40.9 mg for men and 30.3 mg for women (Gregory *et al*. 1990). Intakes from food were significantly lower in women under the age of 35 years, compared with older women. However mean consumption by the lowest 2.5th percentile of the population was still above the RNI (21.6 mg and 13.9 mg for men and women, respectively).

Sources in the UK diet

The major dietary contributors of niacin equivalents in the UK diet (Gregory *et al*. 1990) are:

- meat and meat products (33%)
- cereal products, including bread (14%) and breakfast cereals (8%)
- vegetables (about 10%)
- milk and dairy products (about 10%)
- beverages (about 10%).

Concentrated food sources of niacin equivalents are:

- meat and fish
- wholegrain and fortified cereals
- yeast extracts
- coffee.

Some of the nicotinic acid in foods is held in a bound unabsorbable form; this is of particular significance with low-protein, maize-based diets. Nicotinic acid becomes available in an alkaline medium, and in communities where maize is a staple food it can be prepared with lime water to release the nicotinic acid.

Deficiency

Severe niacin deficiency causes pellagra, characterized by lesions in areas of skin which are exposed to sunlight, but this is usually only seen in deprived populations whose staple food is maize. Deficiency is unlikely in the UK population; in general, protein intakes are more than adequate to maintain niacin status.

Toxicity

Nicotinic acid in excess of 200 mg/day causes vasodilatation and this effect has been used therapeutically in some circulatory disorders. Very high intakes of nicotinic acid (3–6 g/day) can affect liver function, carbohydrate tolerance and uric acid metabolism, although these appear to be reversible once supplementation ceases (DH 1991).

Vitamin B$_6$

Function

Vitamin B$_6$ (often called pyridoxine) covers the group of metabolically interchangeable compounds pyridoxal, pyridoxine and pyridoxamine; any of these can be converted into the coenzyme pyridoxal-5-phosphate, which is essential for many of the steps in the metabolism of protein. Pyridoxine-dependent enzymes are also involved in the metabolism of glycogen and lipids, in the synthesis of haem, and in the conversion of tryptophan to niacin.

Requirement and intake

Requirements for vitamin B$_6$ are related to protein intake, at 15 μg/g of dietary protein; from this, the following RNIs are derived (DH 1991):

- children: 0.7–1.0 mg/day
- adult men: 1.4 mg/day
- adult women 1.2 mg/day.

The Survey of British Adults showed that average intakes of vitamin B$_6$ were 2.68 mg for men and 2.84 mg for women (Gregory *et al.* 1990). The higher figure for women reflects the large contribution to total average intakes from supplemental sources of the vitamin: the average intake for women from food sources alone was 1.57 mg/day. About 20% of adult women, but only 6% of adult men, had intakes below the RNI (MAFF 1994).

Sources in the UK diet

Main dietary contributors (Gregory *et al.* 1990) are:

- cereal products (about 20%)
- meat and meat products (about 20%)
- beverages (about 20%)
- potatoes (15%)
- milk and dairy products (12%).

The significant contribution of beverages relates principally to beer, which contributes to 19% of vitamin B$_6$ intake in men (providing 0.47 mg/day), but only 3% of intake in women.

Vitamin B$_6$ is widely distributed in foods; rich sources are:

- meat
- wholegrain and fortified cereal products
- bananas
- nuts
- pulses.

Deficiency

Clinical deficiency is rare but has been associated with metabolic abnormalities in infants maintained on inappropriate synthetic diets, in severe alcoholics and as a consequence of drug–nutrient reactions. To some degree, vitamin B$_6$ status is affected by protein intakes: poor status is more likely to develop on a high-protein diet than on one low in protein.

Toxicity

Vitamin B$_6$ supplements are commonly taken by women suffering from premenstrual syndrome (PMS), although the benefits of this remain equivocal (Bussell 1998). The dosages taken to alleviate symptoms can sometimes be high (e.g. 200–800 mg/day; Abraham 1984) and this level of intake can cause severe symptoms of sensory neuropathy such as numbness, weakness and paraesthesia. In 1997, a review of the evidence by the Committee on Toxicity of Chemicals in Food, Consumer Products and the Environment (COT) concluded that neuropathic toxic effects can occur at intakes above 50 mg/day. As a result of this, and in order for there to be a sufficient margin of safety, the Department of Health recommended that the maximum daily intake of B$_6$ should be 10 mg/day (DH 1997). Following criticism that this figure is unrealistically low, and publication of a report by the US National Academy of Sciences recommending an upper limit of 100 mg/day (NAS 1998), the evidence was re-evaluated by COT, but the conclusion of the Committee, and hence Department of Health advice, remained unaltered (DH 1998).

Vitamin B12

Function

There are several related structures with vitamin B$_{12}$ activity, described as the cobalamins; all consist of a corrin nucleus surrounding a cobalt atom. These compounds are synthesized by micro-organisms and are not found in plants. Vitamin B$_{12}$ is required for the production of enzymes involved in isomerization reactions, in recycling of folate coenzymes and in the synthesis of methionine from homocysteine.

Requirement and intake

The RNI for children is 0.5–1.0 μg/day and for adults 1.5 μg/day. During lactation an additional increment of 0.5 μg/day is recommended (DH 1991).

The Survey of British Adults showed that average intakes of vitamin B$_{12}$ were 7.3 μg for men and 5.4 μg for women (Gregory *et al.* 1990). Intakes increased with age and were highest in the older age groups. The lower 2.5 percentile intake level was 2.4 μg and 1.3 μg for men and women respectively; 4% of 16–18 year olds (but fewer than 1% of adults over 18 years) had intakes below the LRNI (MAFF 1994).

Sources in the UK diet

Vitamin B$_{12}$ is only found naturally in animal food sources, principally being derived from (Gregory *et al.* 1990):

- meat and meat products (about 50%)
- milk and dairy products (18%)
- fish and fish dishes (13%)
- eggs (8%).

Small amounts of vitamin B$_{12}$ in the diet come from fortified foods such as breakfast cereals.

The most concentrated sources of vitamin B_{12} in the diet are meat, especially liver. Analysis of some fermented and seaweed products indicates that they contain vitamin B_{12} but it is probable that these are analogues with no vitamin activity in humans and so should not be considered dietary sources (Herbert 1988).

Deficiency

Prolonged B_{12} deficiency causes pernicious anaemia, resulting in potentially irreversible neurological damage and, since B_{12} affects folate metabolism, a megaloblastic anaemia similar to that resulting from folate deficiency. However, unlike most water-soluble vitamins, vitamin B_{12} can be stored in the liver, so even long periods of low intake may not affect B_{12} status. Deficiency due to inadequate dietary intake is very rarely observed, and isolated cases relate to young children on vegan or macrobiotic diets that also exclude fortified foods. Low vitamin B_{12} status is widely reported in older people (Stabler *et al.* 1997; Finch *et al.* 1998), but this is usually due to physiological changes resulting in reduced absorption of the vitamin (absence of gastric intrinsic factor and/or reduced pepsin activity and gastric acid secretion).

Treatment on diagnosis, or on the assessment of risk, is by oral supplementation if malabsorption only affects the protein-bound forms of vitamin B_{12}, or by injection where malabsorption is complete owing to lack of intrinsic factor.

Toxicity

No toxic effects have been reported in humans.

Pantothenic acid

Function

Pantothenic acid is widely distributed in plant and animal tissues, and is the precursor of coenzyme A which has a central role in energy metabolism.

Requirement and intake

No RNI has been defined for this vitamin. Current average intake levels of 3–7 mg/day are assumed to be adequate (DH 1991).

The Survey of British Adults showed that average intakes of pantothenic acid were 6.6mg for men and 5.1 mg for women (Gregory *et al.* 1990). The lower 2.5 percentile intake level was 2.9 mg and 2.1 mg for men and women, respectively.

Sources in the UK diet

Pantothenic acid is widely distributed in plant and animal foods. Particularly rich sources of pantothenic acid are:

- yeast
- offal
- peanuts
- meat

- eggs
- green vegetables.

Deficiency

No specific deficiency syndrome related to inadequate intakes has been identified in humans. Experimental deficiency has been reported to produce symptoms such as fatigue, dizziness, muscular weakness and gastrointestinal disturbances (DH 1991).

Toxicity

Large loads (10 g/day) of calcium pantothenate may cause diarrhoea and other gastrointestinal disturbances but no specific toxic effects.

Biotin

Function

There are eight stereoisomers of biotin but only one, D-biotin, has biological activity. Biotin is made by yeasts and bacteria, and is widely distributed in all plant and animal tissues. In addition to diet, biotin is also available from endogenous colonic bacterial synthesis. Biotin is a cofactor for several enzyme systems involved in the synthesis of fatty acids and in gluconeogenesis.

Requirement and intake

No RNI has been defined for this vitamin. Intakes of 10–200 μg/day are believed to be safe and adequate (DH 1991).

The Survey of British Adults showed that average intakes of biotin were 39.1 μg for men and 28.7 μg for women (Gregory *et al.* 1990). Intakes tended to increase with age. The lower 2.5 percentile intake level was 15.1 μg and 9.9 μg for men and women, respectively.

Sources in the UK diet

The main sources of biotin in the UK diet (Gregory *et al.* 1990) are:

- cereal products (23%)
- beverages (21%): beer provides about 12% of total intake for men (but only 1% for women), while coffee provides 9% of total intakes for men (and 12% for women)
- milk and dairy products (16%)
- eggs (15%)
- meat (11%).

Concentrated food sources of biotin are:

- liver and kidney
- yeast
- nuts
- pulses
- wholegrain cereals
- eggs.

Deficiency

Unlike most other water-soluble vitamins, biotin is stored in the liver and deficiency is unlikely to occur. Raw egg white contains the protein avidin which binds with biotin and prevents its absorption; however, no such effects occur when egg has been heated.

Folate

Folates occur naturally as a variety of polyglutamates (tetrahydrofolates), with different biological activity. Folic acid (pteroylglutamic acid) is the parent molecule; it does not occur naturally, but has a high degree of biological activity, is very stable, and is used for the fortification of foods and manufacture of supplements. Dietary folate equivalency has been proposed at:

1 μg food folate = 0.6 μg folic acid consumed with food
= 0.5 μg folic acid from supplements consumed without food (Yates 1998).

Function

Folate is essential for many of the methylation reactions involved in the synthesis of DNA and RNA, and hence plays a crucial role in cell division.

Requirement and intake

The RNI for children is 70–150 μg/day; for adults 200 μg/day (DH 1991). During pregnancy the RNI is increased by 100 μg and during lactation by 60 μg. Women who may or intend to become pregnant are advised to consume an additional 400 μg of folic acid/day, i.e. 600 μg/day in total, to reduce the risk of any pregnancy being affected by a neural tube defect (NTD). This level of intake is difficult to achieve from food sources alone and supplemental folate is advisable prior to, and for the first 12 weeks of, pregnancy. Women with a previous pregnancy affected by NTD are advised to take a daily supplement providing 5000 μg (5 mg) folic acid (see Section, 3.1 Pregnancy).

The Survey of British Adults showed that average intakes of folate were 312 μg for men and 219 μg for women (Gregory *et al.* 1990). The lower 2.5 percentile intake level was 145 μg and 95 μg for men and women respectively; 4% of women of child-bearing age (16–50 years) had a folate intake below the LRNI (MAFF 1994).

Sources in the UK diet

The main sources of folate in the average diet are:

- cereal products (21%)
- vegetables (16%)
- milk and dairy products (<10%)
- meat products (<10%).

In the average diet, fruits and fruit juices do not make a significant contribution to folate intake, typically providing about 5% of intake.

In men, but not women, beer can be a major source of folate, contributing 16% (49 μg) of average intake.

Concentrated sources of folate in the diet are:

- liver
- yeast extract
- green leafy vegetables
- pulses
- oranges.

Foods fortified with folic acid, particularly breakfast cereals, are now widely available, and can significantly increase total intake.

Deficiency

Deficiency of folate results in megaloblastic anaemia. It is most likely to occur as a result of:

- malabsorption
- the use of certain drugs which interfere with folic acid metabolism (e.g. anticonvulsants used to treat epilepsy)
- disease states which increase cell proliferation (e.g. leukaemia).

In early pregnancy, folate insufficiency can cause impaired neural tube development (see Section 3.1, Pregnancy).

It has recently been suggested that poor folate status may increase the risk of cardiovascular disease (CVD) (DH 2000). Folate intake is inversely related to blood homocysteine level, and elevated homocysteine levels are a known risk marker for CVD. However, as yet no intervention trials have been carried out to show that reducing blood homocysteine level by folate supplementation, or by any other means, is cardioprotective (DH 2000).

Toxicity

No adverse effects from high folate intakes have been reported, other than the risk of exacerbating a megaloblastic anaemia caused by undiagnosed B_{12} deficiency.

Vitamin C

Function

Most plant and animal tissues can synthesize vitamin C from glucose; however humans, primates, guinea-pigs and some birds lack this ability, so dietary intake of the pre-formed vitamin is essential to prevent deficiency resulting in scurvy. Vitamin C (ascorbic acid) is a powerful reducing agent and electron donor and affects many oxidation–reduction reactions. Its ability to convert the ferric (Fe^{3+}) ion to the more soluble ferrous (Fe^{2+} form) means that it assists the absorption of non-haem iron. Since it is water soluble, it functions as an antioxidant in the aqueous components of tissues, often in conjunction with vitamin E, which has an antioxidant role in lipid structures. Vitamin C is essential for the structure and maintenance of blood vessels, cartilage, muscle and bone.

Requirement and intake

The RNI for children is 30 mg/day and for adults 40 mg/day (DH 1991). During pregnancy the RNI is increased by 10 mg/day and during lactation by 30 mg/day. Regular cigarette smokers have an increased turnover of vitamin C, and their intakes need to be double, i.e. 80 mg/day, to achieve similar serum levels to those found in non-smokers.

The Survey of British Adults showed that average daily intakes of vitamin C were 74.6 mg for men and 73.1 mg for women (Gregory *et al.* 1990). The lower 2.5 percentile intake levels were 19.1 mg and 14.4 mg for men and women respectively.

Sources in the UK diet

In the average UK diet, the main contributors to vitamin C intake are:

- vegetables (46%): potatoes alone provide 16% of total vitamin C intake
- beverages, mainly fruit juice (22%)
- fruits (17%).

The most concentrated sources of vitamin C are:

- berries and currants
- guava
- strawberries
- citrus fruits

Vegetables such as green peppers, broccoli, cabbage, kale and spring greens are rich sources of vitamin C, but major losses of the vitamin can occur during food storage, preparation and cooking.

Deficiency

Frank deficiency in the form of scurvy is rarely seen in the UK; however, poor status affecting many aspects of health may affect people with:

- poor diets devoid of fresh fruit and vegetables
- higher requirements, e.g. cigarette smokers and post-operative patients.

Toxicity

High-dose supplemental intakes of vitamin C are commonly taken, often in the belief that they help to protect against colds. A recent Cochrane review (Douglas *et al.* 2000) concluded that there is no evidence that supplemental vitamin C prevents colds, although it may reduce the duration of cold symptoms to some extent. Higher doses appeared to produce greater benefits than lower ones.

However, intakes of vitamin C in excess of 1 g/day may result in diarrhoea and increase the risk of oxalate stone formation (DH 1991). Prolonged high intakes also increase the rate of vitamin C turnover and sudden cessation of high-dose supplementation can result in rebound scurvy (DH 1991). People who choose to take vitamin C supplements which significantly exceed requirement (e.g. 500 mg–1 g/day) should be advised not to take them for prolonged periods (e.g. not more than a few weeks), and then diminish the level of intake gradually. Intakes of more than 1 g/day may not be advisable.

2.6.4 Vitamin supplements

The use of vitamin and mineral supplements to prevent deficiency, or to treat particular symptoms or conditions, is a long-established practice; however, there was a large increase in the prevalence of use and in the variety and quantity of products consumed during the 1990s, with predictions for future increases in use in the UK population (Mintel 1997).

The reasons that people report for supplement usage vary. In general, people choose to take combination products (containing a variety of vitamins) for reasons of 'overall' health and well-being, and the prevention of future ill health. Supplements of single nutrients tend to be chosen for more specific reasons and to prevent or treat a particular condition or symptom (Neuhouser *et al.* 1999) (and see Vitamin B_6 and Vitamin C, above).

There have been many surveys investigating patterns of vitamin supplement usage in the UK; most indicate higher levels of usage in women, in older people, and in those with higher levels of education and income (Gregory *et al.* 1990; Scottish Office 1997). People with some knowledge of, and interest in health, are also more likely to choose to take supplements. Surveys of usage suggest that people who take supplements are often those least likely to be in need of them; intakes of micronutrients from food sources are higher in regular supplement users than in those not taking supplements (Gregory *et al.* 1990; Kirk *et al.* 1998).

Vitamin and mineral supplements are useful adjuncts to the diet on a temporary or long-term basis in situations where the intake or selection of foods is limited, or where physiological requirements for particular micronutrients are elevated. Particular recommendations for the general use of vitamin supplements can be made for several population subgroups in the UK (Table 2.11). In addition, there are often clear indications for vitamin supplementation in specific medical conditions where micronutrient intake, absorption or metabolism is affected. These are discussed further in the relevant sections of the manual.

The use of supplements cannot be assumed to be without risk, and specific concerns relate to intakes that are manifold overestimates of requirements, especially of the fat-soluble vitamins. Based on current knowledge, guidance on safe upper limits of vitamin and mineral supplementation has been produced by the US Council for Responsible Nutrition (Hathcock 1997a, b), although it is

Table 2.11 Indications for the possible use of vitamin supplements

Group	Vitamins
Infants (breast-fed)	A, D
Young children (1–5 years)	A, D
Women, pre-pregnancy	Folic acid
Pregnant women	Folic acid (1st trimester), D
Lactating women	D
Older people	B_{12}, D
Vegans	B_{12}, D
Smokers	C
Those not exposed to sun	D
Those on restricted diets	Multivitamins
Those at risk of osteoporosis	D

acknowledged that many uncertainties remain. Some data from epidemiological studies indicate associations between higher intakes of particular nutrients from supplements and health benefits, but evidence of cause-and-effect relationships can only be proven through intervention studies, and dietetic recommendations on the use of supplements should relate to such supportive evidence. If, in the absence of any medical or nutritional need for vitamin supplements, people still wish to take them, they should be guided towards multiple preparations providing no more than 100% of the recommended daily amount (RDA) as defined under EU legislation (BDA 1999). This can be ascertained from product packaging information, as it is a legal requirement that the vitamin content of supplements is stated as a percentage of these RDAs.

Text revised by: Ursula Arens and Briony Thomas

Further reading

Eastwood M. *Principles of Human Nutrition*. London: Chapman and Hall, 1997

Garrow JS, James WPT (Eds). *Human Nutrition and Dietetics*, 10th edn. Edinburgh: Churchill Livingstone, 1999.

References

Abraham GE. Nutrition and the premenstrual syndromes. *Journal of Applied Nutrition* 1984; **436**: 103–124.

Booth SL, Webb DR, Peters JC. Assessment of phylloquinone and dihydrophylloquinone dietary intakes among a nationally representative sample of US consumers using 14-day food diaries. *Journal of the American Dietetic Association* 1999; **99**: 1072–1076.

British Dietetic Association. Vitamin and mineral supplementation. Position paper. *Journal of Human Nutrition and Dietetics* 1999; **12**: 171–178.

Bussell G. Pre-menstrual syndrome and diet. *Journal of Nutritional and Environmental Medicine* 1998; **8**: 65–75.

Department of Health. Report of the Panel on Dietary Reference Values of the Committee on Medical Aspects of Food Policy (COMA). *Dietary Reference Values for Food Energy and Nutrients for the United Kingdom*. Report on Health and Social Subjects 41. London: HMSO, 1991.

Department of Health, Committee on Toxicity of Chemicals in Food, Consumer Products and the Environment (COT). *Statement on Vitamin B₆ (Pyridoxine) Toxicity*. London: DH, 1997.

Department of Health, Committee on Toxicity of Chemicals in Food, Consumer Products and the Environment (COT). *Statement on Preliminary Observations on the NAS Report on a*

Tolerable Upper Intake Level for Vitamin B₆. London: DH, 1998.

Department of Health, Committee on Medical Aspects of Food Policy (COMA). *Folic Acid and the Prevention of Disease*. Report on Health and Social Subjects 50. London: The Stationery Office, 2000.

Douglas RM, Chalker EB, Treacy B. Vitamin C for preventing and treating the common cold. (Cochrane Review). In *The Cochrane Library*, No. 4. Oxford: Update Software, 2000.

Finch S, Doyle W, Lowe C *et al*. *National Diet and Nutrition Survey: People Aged 65 Years and Older*. Vol. 1: *Report of the Diet and Nutrition Survey*. London: The Stationery Office, 1998.

Gregory J, Foster K, Tyler H, Wiseman M. *The Dietary and Nutritional Survey of British Adults*. London: HMSO, 1990.

Hathcock J. Vitamin and minerals: efficacy and safety. *American Journal of Clinical Nutrition* 1997a; **66**: 427–437.

Hathcock J. *Vitamin and Mineral Safety*. Washington DC: US Council for Responsible Nutrition, 1997b.

Herbert V. Vitamin B₁₂: plant sources, requirements, and assay. *American Journal of Clinical Nutrition* 1988; **48**: 852–858.

Kirk SFL, Cade JE, Connor MT, Barrett JH. Supplementary issues for women. *BNF Nutrition Bulletin* 1998; **85**: 197–202.

Ministry of Agriculture, Fisheries and Food. *The Dietary and Nutritional Survey of British Adults – Further Analysis*. London: HMSO, 1994.

Mintel. *Vitamin and Mineral Supplements*. London: Mintel International Group, 1997.

National Academy of Sciences, Food and Nutrition Board. *Dietary Reference Intakes for Thiamin, Riboflavin, Niacin, Vitamin B₆, Folate, Vitamin B₁₂, Pantothenic Acid, Biotin and Choline*. Washington, DC: National Academy Press, 1998.

Neuhouser ML, Patterson RE, Levy L. Motivations for using vitamin and mineral supplements. *Journal of the American Dietetic Association* 1999; **7**: 851–854.

Olson RE. Vitamin K . In Shils ME, Young VR (Eds) *Modern Nutrition in Health and Disease*, pp. 328–339. Philadelphia, PA: Lea & Febiger, 1988.

Scottish Office. *Scottish Health Survey 1995*. London: The Stationery Office, 1997.

Stabler SP, Lindenbaum, Allen RH. Vitamin B₁₂ deficiency in the elderly: current dilemmas. *American Journal of Clinical Nutrition* 1997; **66**: 741–749.

Trang HM, Cole DEC, Rubin LA *et al*. Evidence that vitamin D₃ increases serum 25-hydroxyvitamin D more efficiently than does vitamin D₂. *American Journal of Clinical Nutrition* 1998; **68**: 854–858.

Yates AA, Schlicker SA, Suitor CW. Dietary Reference Intakes: a new basis for recommendations for calcium and related nutrients, B vitamins, and choline. *Journal of the American Dietetic Association* 1998; **98**: 699–706.

2.7 Minerals and trace elements

Minerals and trace elements are, like vitamins, only required in small or even trace quantities but are nonetheless essential for normal body function. They have a variety of roles and may be necessary for:

- *Tissue structure*: Minerals such as calcium and phosphorus are important structural components of bone; iron is an essential constituent of haemoglobin in blood.
- *Enzyme systems*: Many minerals and trace elements are required as cofactors, coenzymes or metalloenzymes in metabolic pathways.
- *Fluid balance*: The concentration of elements such as sodium and potassium in body fluids, and their movement between extracellular and intracellular compartments, is part of the regulatory mechanism for fluid balance.
- *Cellular function*: Some are necessary for membrane stability and inter- and intracellular transport mechanisms.
- *Neurotransmission*: Some influence electrical activity and have an essential role in nerve function.

Minerals and elements known to be essential for humans are summarized in Table 2.12. Those required in milligram quantities (sometimes several hundred milligrams) tend to be referred to as minerals. Those required in smaller amounts (microgram quantities) are usually called trace elements. This is, however, an arbitrary distinction.

The precise role and requirements of some minerals and many trace elements remain to be established. As a result, there is some variability in the recommended levels of intake set by different countries or international advisory bodies, and UK dietary reference values (DRVs) are kept under review (see Section 1.3.2 in Dietary reference values).

Table 2.12 Minerals and trace elements known to be essential in humans

Minerals (required in milligram quantities)	Trace elements (required in microgram quantities)
Calcium	Copper
Phosphorus	Chromium
Magnesium	Manganese
Sodium	Molybdenum
Potassium	Selenium
Iron	Iodine
Zinc	
Fluorine[1]	

[1]Regarded as semi-essential. No physiological requirement can be shown to exist but it has known beneficial effects.

It can also be difficult to determine whether the estimated requirements for these micronutrients is being met, for the following reasons:

Difficulties in estimating the amount consumed: Their content in food, particularly in respect of trace elements, can vary according to factors such as the soil in which plants are grown, animal feedstuffs, the species, ripeness or age of the plant or animal, and food-processing techniques. There are also analytical difficulties in accurately measuring the content of elements present in only minute amounts. For these reasons, tables of food composition provide an indication of mineral and trace element content but cannot be regarded as infallible (see Section 1.4.2 in Food composition tables).

Difficulties in estimating the amount absorbed: The amount absorbed is variable. Not only are there differences between minerals and trace elements in terms of bioavailability (some are well absorbed, others much less so) but many other factors can further influence the absorption of a particular mineral or element, such as:

- Its dietary source: Calcium in milk is absorbed more effectively than calcium in cereal foods or vegetables.
- Its chemical form: Haem iron is absorbed by a different, and more efficient, mechanism than non-haem iron.
- The presence of other dietary components which inhibit absorption: Phytates, oxalates or some types of fibre can form unabsorbable complexes with minerals and elements and inhibit their absorption.
- The presence of other dietary components which enhance absorption: The absorption of non-haem iron is improved by the presence of vitamin C.
- The amount of other minerals consumed: Some minerals such as iron and zinc compete for the same absorption site; a high intake of one may therefore impair the absorption of the other.
- Its level of intake: Percentage absorption tends to decrease when dietary intake is high and increase when the level of intake is low.
- Physiological factors: The amount absorbed may increase in response to increased physiological need, e.g. pregnancy, lactation or conditions of depletion.
- Age: Absorption tends to decline with age.

DRVs for minerals and trace elements take some account of their bioavailability in an average mixed diet (although this is sometimes on the basis of limited data), and may also incorporate factors for age and physiological status.

Recommended intakes are usually therefore much higher than estimates of physiological requirement. (For this reason, mineral and trace element requirements for people fed parenterally are lower than for those fed orally because there is no loss of availability; see Section 1.15, Parenteral nutrition.) However, DRVs cannot take into account all of the variations in bioavailability between different foods, different diets or different people. These may be important considerations in people whose intakes are of marginal adequacy.

Difficulties in assessing mineral and trace element status: There are few simple or reliable biochemical ways of assessing this. Serum levels are often of limited value as indicators of nutritional inadequacy because either circulating levels are under tight homoeostatic control (e.g. calcium) or body stores must be severely depleted before circulating levels are affected (e.g. iron and zinc). Circulating and stored levels of micronutrients may also be altered by disease or the metabolic response to illness, infection or trauma.

In dietetic practice, micronutrient adequacy often has to be assessed on the basis of whether the type of diet habitually consumed by an individual contains the types and amounts of foods likely to be required to meet physiological needs. In general, people who consume small amounts of food in quantitative terms (due to a small appetite or impaired food intake) and/or who consume diets of limited variety are most likely to have an intake that is either inadequate or of only marginal adequacy. In such people, factors affecting bioavailability (in either a positive or negative direction) may make the difference between sufficiency and deficiency. Clinical factors that increase micronutrient requirements or enhance losses are also an important consideration (see Section 1.10.5 in Estimating nutritional requirements).

Detailed information about the structure and function of minerals and trace elements can be found in standard textbooks of nutrition. This section provides a summary of those aspects which are most relevant to dietetic practice.

2.7.1 Calcium

Function

The body requires considerable quantities of calcium in order to create and maintain its skeletal structures. Ninety-nine per cent of the body's calcium (about 1.0–1.5 kg in total) is deposited as calcium salts, principally hydroxyapatite [$Ca_{10}(PO_4)_6(OH)_2$], within the matrix of bones and teeth, providing structural rigidity. The remaining 1% is found within tissues and body fluids, where it plays a vital role at the cellular level, affecting membrane transport and stability, and influencing functions such as muscle contraction, nerve transmission and blood clotting.

About 45% of plasma calcium exists as free ions (ionized calcium), the remainder being complexed with citrate or bicarbonate. The level of ionized calcium in plasma is normally maintained within narrow limits (between 2.25 and 2.6 mmol/l) by means of hormonal influences on calcium absorption, excretion and mobilization of calcium from bone. Parathyroid hormone (PTH) raises plasma calcium by increasing renal tubule resorption of calcium and by stimulating the formation of 1,25-dihydroxycholecalciferol (the hormonal form of vitamin D), which increases calcium absorption from the gastrointestinal tract. The hormone calcitonin decreases plasma calcium levels by inhibiting the release of calcium from bone and by increasing urinary excretion.

Calcium is primarily absorbed by an active transport mechanism, which is enhanced by 1,25-hydroxyvitamin D. At higher levels of intake, calcium is also absorbed by passive diffusion. Calcium absorption decreases with age as vitamin D metabolism becomes less efficient and PTH production may also decline, although this is partially offset by a fall in calcium excretion due to a decrease in glomerular filtration rate.

Urinary calcium excretion primarily reflects calcium intake but can be increased by high intakes of sodium and protein, although to some extent the latter effect is offset by the high content of phosphorus in many protein-containing foods (Pannemans *et al*. 1997).

Requirement and intake

Requirements for calcium depend upon the rate at which calcium is incorporated into bone; they are therefore highest during periods of growth, especially during infancy and adolescence, and fall after peak bone mass is achieved at about 25 years of age. Individual requirements for calcium are, however, difficult to quantify because of variability in both the bioavailability of calcium from different foods and its rate of absorption. The reference nutrient intakes (RNIs) considered sufficient to meet the needs of the vast majority of the UK population (DH 1991) are:

- 1–3 years: 350 mg/day
- 4–6 years: 450 mg/day
- 7–10 years: 550 mg/day
- 11–18 year olds: 1000 mg/day for males and 800 mg/day for females.
- adults over 19 years: 700 mg/day.

Although the body's requirement for calcium increases considerably during pregnancy, this can be met by increased absorption of dietary calcium so no additional increment is made to the RNI for pregnant women. However, an additional 550 mg calcium/day is considered necessary to meet the needs of lactating women.

UK RNIs are lower than recommended calcium intakes in some other countries, especially for 11–14 year-old females (see Table 4.71. in Osteoporosis), and there has been debate as to whether they are sufficiently high to prevent osteoporosis (see Section 4.31). The UK recommendations have recently been reviewed by the COMA subgroup on bone health (DH 1998), who concluded that there was insufficient evidence to justify an increase in the RNIs. However, the subgroup emphasized the importance of older adults' meeting the RNI for vitamin D of 10 μg/ day (if necessary by supplementation) in order to offset the reduced efficiency in calcium absorption that occurs with age.

In the Dietary and Nutrition Survey of British Adults (Gregory *et al*. 1990; MAFF 1994) mean calcium intakes were 940 mg/day in men and 730 mg/day in women. In adults between the age of 19 and 50 years, 25% of men and 48% women had intakes below the RNI. This proportion was considerably higher in 16–18 years olds, among whom 64% of males and 71% of females failed to achieve the RNI for this age group (i.e. 1000 mg/day and 800 mg/day, respectively). A significant proportion of women (27% of 16–18 year olds and 10% of those aged 19–50 years) had a calcium intake which was below the lower reference nutrient intake (LRNI) for their age group.

These levels of intake suggest that many of the population, particularly teenage girls, are not consuming sufficient calcium to achieve maximum bone density and hence may be at increased risk of developing osteoporosis in later life.

Sources in the UK diet

In the average UK diet, calcium is derived from (MAFF 1999):

- milk and dairy products: 56% (milk 41%, yoghurt 3%, cheese 11%)
- cereal foods: 25% (white bread 5%, brown/wholemeal bread 2%, cakes and biscuits 4%, breakfast cereals 1.5%)
- vegetables: 6 % (fresh green vegetables 1.4%)
- meat and meat products: 3%
- fruit and fruit juices: 2.4%
- fish: 1.7%.

The bioavailability of calcium from different dietary sources is variable. Calcium in milk and dairy foods is absorbed much more readily than that in plant-based foods. Bioavailability may also be affected by dietary components which inhibit absorption, such as phytates (in many cereal foods), oxalates (in some green leafy vegetables) or supplemental intakes of minerals such as zinc. Percentage absorption can increase if habitual calcium intake is low or physiological need is high. It can decrease with age or in conditions of vitamin D insufficiency.

The dietary calcium:phosphorus ratio was formerly thought to be important in determining calcium absorption, but this is no longer thought to be the case in adults unless phosphate intake is excessive. However, it may be important in young infants, and infant formulae usually have a calcium:phosphorus ratio of about 2:1 which reflects that found in mature breast milk.

Concentrated dietary sources of calcium are:

- milk (whole milk, semi-skimmed or skimmed milk)
- dairy products (e.g. cheese, yoghurt, fromage frais)
- fish containing soft bones (e.g. canned pilchards and sardines)

- green leafy vegetables
- foods containing UK-produced white and brown flour (fortified with calcium)
- pulses (e.g. baked beans, dried lentils)
- tap water in hard-water areas.

Milk and dairy products are the best dietary sources of calcium as their calcium content and bioavailability are both high.

Quantities of foods providing approximately 200 mg calcium are shown in Table 2.13.

Deficiency

Lack of calcium can result in stunted growth and failure to achieve peak bone density in early adulthood, hence increasing the risk of osteoporosis in later life (see Section 4.31, Osteoporosis). The role of calcium supplementation in the prevention and management of osteoporosis is discussed in this section.

Failure to absorb sufficient calcium as a secondary consequence of vitamin D deficiency results in rickets in children and osteomalacia in adults, and may also be implicated in osteoporosis.

In healthy people, dietary deficiency of calcium does not affect the plasma calcium level because this is maintained under tight homoeostatic control. Hypocalcaemia resulting in symptoms such as tetany or cardiac arrythmias only occurs when other factors override the normal regulatory mechanisms, e.g. hypoparathyroidism, pancreatitis or severe malabsorption (see Section 1.10.4 in Estimating nutritional requirements). Only measurement of bone density provides an indicator of long-term calcium adequacy.

Toxicity

Supplemental intakes of calcium of even up to 2 g/day do not appear to have toxic effects. However, intakes at, or even below, this level may result in interactions between calcium and other minerals which could have a negative impact on health (Whiting and Wood 1997). High calcium intakes have been shown to reduce zinc absorption and balance in humans by as much as 50% (Wood and Ju Zheng 1997).

Table 2.13 Quantities of foods providing approximately 200 mg calcium

---

1/4 pint of milk (5–6 fl. oz)
A small piece cheddar cheese (28 g)
1 small carton of yoghurt (150 ml)
1 1/2 small cartons of cottage cheese or fromage frais (225 ml)
1/2 large can of creamed rice pudding (200 g)
A serving of canned sardines (56 g)
6 medium slices of white or brown bread (200 g)
10 medium slices of wholemeal bread (360 g)
2 scones (125 g)
2 servings of muesli (200 g)
5–6 servings of green leafy vegetables (500–600 g)
2 servings of baked beans in tomato sauce (400 g)
4 oranges (600 g)
Mixed nuts (200 g)

2.7.2 Phosphorus

Function

Phosphorus is present in all cells of the body and is closely linked to calcium and protein metabolism. The majority (85%) of the body's phosphorus is in bone in the form of hydroxyapatite. The remaining 15% is a constituent of substances such as phospholipids and nucleic acids, or is concerned with the release of oxygen and energy to the cells and the mediation of the intracellular effects of hormones. Phosphate excretion through the kidney is one of the mechanisms for regulating acid–base balance in the body.

Phosphorus shares similar homoeostatic mechanisms with calcium (see above). Phosphate balance is maintained largely by the renal tubules.

Requirement and intake

Phosphorus and calcium exist in the body in equimolar amounts and requirements for phosphorus parallel those of calcium. RNIs for phosphorus are therefore the same as those for calcium expressed in millimoles. When quantitatively expressed in milligrams, these represent an RNI for adults over the age of 19 years of 550 mg/day, with an additional 440 mg/day being required during lactation. For 11–18 year olds, the RNI is 775 mg/day for males and 625 mg/day for females (DH 1991).

Typical UK dietary intakes of phosphorus (Gregory *et al.* 1990; MAFF 1994) well exceed these levels, on average being 1452 mg/day in men and 1072 mg/day in women.

Sources in the UK diet

Phosphate is a major constituent of plant and animals and so is present in most foods. Inorganic phosphorus is added to processed foods, particularly baked goods and carbonated drinks, and these provide about 10% of total phosphorus intake.

The main sources of phosphorus in the UK diet (MAFF 1994) are:

- milk and milk products (25%)
- cereal products (25%)
- meat and meat products (20%)
- vegetables and potatoes (10%).

Milk and dairy products are the most concentrated sources of phosphorus in the UK, although meat, fish, egg, nuts, fruit, cereals and vegetables provide useful amounts.

Approximately 60% of dietary phosphorus is absorbed. Non-starch polysaccharide (NSP) decreases percentage phosphate absorption but, since high NSP diets also tend to be high in phosphate, quantitative absorption is not reduced. Phytic acid phosphorus from wholegrain cereals and pulses is not absorbed in the small intestine because mammals do not produce phytase; however, this enzyme is naturally present in some wholegrain cereals, making the phosphorus more available. In addition, some absorption may take place in the large bowel following bacterial fermentation.

Deficiency

In the healthy person, dietary phosphorus deficiency is unlikely to occur. However, phosphate depletion in blood and soft tissue may occur in any disorder where body pH is altered or where there is excessive loss of phosphate through urine or stools (e.g. diabetic ketoacidosis or malabsorption). Deficiencies have also been reported as a result of diuretic drug use in elderly people, excessive use of magnesium and aluminium antacids, and inappropriately formulated parenteral nutrition. Symptoms of hypophosphataemia include myopathy, respiratory and cardiac failure, neuropathy and tissue hypoxia.

Toxicity

The body can normally tolerate a wide range of phosphate intake, but intakes in excess of 70 mg/kg body weight per day (about 4.5 g/day for a 65 kg man) may result in hyperphosphataemia or other adverse effects. High phosphate intakes may be contraindicated in some forms of renal failure or chemotherapy treatment. The dietary calcium:phosphorus ratio is an important consideration in artificially fed infants (see Calcium, above).

2.7.3 Magnesium

Function

Magnesium functions in many enzyme systems, such as those involved in decarboxylation or phosphate group transfer and energy release. It plays a vital role in skeletal development, protein synthesis, muscle contraction and neurotransmission. Metabolically, it is closely linked with calcium. There appear to be no major hormonal factors controlling magnesium balance and homoeostasis is largely controlled by the kidney.

Requirement and intake

Requirements for magnesium have been difficult to establish (DH 1991). The RNI for adults over the age of 19 years has been set at 300 mg/day for men and 270 mg/day for women, with an additional increment of 50 mg/day during lactation.

The average UK dietary intake of people aged 16–64 years (Gregory *et al.* 1990; MAFF 1994) is 323 mg/day in men and 237 mg/day in women. About 73% of women have intakes below the RNI, and about 7% men and 13% women had intakes below the LRNI. Whether this is physiologically significant remains uncertain.

Sources in the UK diet

In the average UK diet (MAFF 1994) magnesium is derived from:

- bread and cereal products (30%)
- beverages, principally beer and coffee (20% in men; 14% in women)
- vegetables and potatoes (16%)
- milk and milk products (12%)
- meat and meat products (10%).

Magnesium is a component of chlorophyll, so green vegetables are a rich source. Meats, pulses and cereals (particularly wholegrain) also provide useful amounts. Hard drinking water may make a significant contribution to intake.

About 20–30% of dietary magnesium is absorbed, mainly from the small intestine, by both passive diffusion and an active process partly dependent on 1,25-dihydroxyvitamin D.

Deficiency

Since the body is efficient at conserving magnesium and the skeleton also acts as a magnesium store, dietary deficiency of magnesium is unlikely. However, hypomagnesaemia can result from high intestinal losses, increased renal excretion, or changes in tissue distribution of magnesium associated with disease or use of some types of drugs or other treatments (e.g. diuretic drugs, some bowel-cleansing solutions or plasmapheresis). Symptoms of hypomagnesaemia include muscle weakness and cramps, hypertension and cardiac arrhythmias.

Toxicity

Surplus magnesium is normally rapidly excreted by the kidneys and intakes in excess of about 2 g/day are not absorbed from the intestine. Hypermagnesaemia is however a risk in disease states such as renal failure or adrenal insufficiency, and can occur as a result of intravenous or enteral overadministration.

2.7.4 Sodium

Function

Sodium is the principal cation in extracellular fluid and plays a vital role in the regulation of fluid balance, blood pressure and transmembrane gradients.

Requirement and intake

The physiological requirement for sodium is small, in the region of 69–460 mg/day. In the UK, intake usually far exceeds these levels, typically ranging between 2 and 10 g/day. In the Dietary and Nutritional Survey of British Adults (Gregory *et al.* 1990), average sodium intakes, excluding discretionary sources added to food, were 3376 mg/day in men and 2351 mg/day in women. As a result of concerns over the possible adverse effects of a chronically high sodium intake on health, particularly in respect of blood pressure (see Section 4.24, Hypertension), the RNI for sodium has been set at a level which aims to reduce population intake of sodium from an total average intake of about 3.9 g/day to 1.6 g/day (70 mmol/day). The LRNI for adults is 575 mg/day (25 mmol/day). The Department of Health COMA report on Cardiovascular Disease (DH 1994) recommended that average intake of salt (i.e. sodium chloride) should decrease by at least one-third from its current average of 9 g salt/ day to 6 g/day; this is equivalent to a reduction in sodium consumption from 3.6 g/day to 2.4 g/day.

Sources in the UK diet

Many foods in their natural state contain small amounts of sodium but none contains large amounts. The sodium content can increase dramatically when foods are preserved or processed in some way, as a result of the addition of either salt or other sodium-containing additives such as sodium bicarbonate, sodium nitrite or monosodium glutamate. Salt is also often added directly to foods during cooking or at the table ('discretionary' salt). The proportions of sodium obtained from these sources are typically:

- 15–20% from sodium naturally present in food
- 15–20% from discretionary addition of salt to foods
- 60–70% from manufactured or processed foods.

In the average UK diet, non-discretionary sodium is primarily obtained from (MAFF 1994):

- bread and other cereals (35%)
- meat and meat products (27%)
- milk and milk products (9%)
- pickles and sauces (7%).

The remaining 22% is derived from a wide range of other foods.

Concentrated sources of sodium are fairly obvious because of their associated salty taste and include:

- ham
- bacon
- smoked fish (e.g. kippers or smoked mackerel)
- products canned in brine (e.g. frankfurters, fish)
- cheese
- butter (salted)
- salted foods (e.g. nuts, salted biscuits)
- yeast extract spreads, stock cubes, bottled sauces.

Less obvious but often significant sources of sodium include many meat and fish products, canned and packaged soups, 'instant' foods and ready meals. The majority of manufactured foods now provide nutrition labelling information in a format which includes a declaration of sodium content, and people should be encouraged to look for, and know how to interpret, this information.

Sodium restriction

As part of healthy eating guidance, people should be encouraged to reduce their sodium intake. Advising a reduction in the amount of salt added to food and limited consumption of salt-rich foods should be part of this. However, it should be borne in mind that to make a significant impact on habitual sodium intake, the average person's diet will need to contain fewer packaged and processed foods and more fresh and unprocessed foods, especially potassium-rich fruit and vegetables (see Section 1.2, Healthy eating).

Certain disease states may necessitate more severe sodium restriction to a level which may be classified as:

- *No Added Salt*: 80–100 mmol (1.8–2.3 g) sodium/day: Salt must not be added to food and only a minute amount is allowed in cooking. The level of consumption of some salt-rich foods is restricted (see Table 4.20 in Section 4.13, Liver and biliary disease).
- *Low salt*: 40 mmol (approx. 1 g) sodium/day: No salt must be added to foods either at the table or in cooking. Additional food restrictions apply (see Table 4.20 in Section 4.13, Liver and biliary disease).
- *Low sodium*: 22 mmol (0.5 g) sodium/day: This is now rarely used in clinical practice and necessitates extensive substitution with salt-free foods.

Diets that are therapeutically low in sodium lack palatability as a result of their bland flavour, and patients will require suggestions for alternative ways of flavouring foods, e.g. using lemon juice or permitted herbs and spices. Salt substitutes may also be helpful but, because of their high potassium content, are likely to be contraindicated in many of the disorders requiring therapeutic sodium restriction.

Deficiency

High sodium losses necessitating short-term salt repletion can occur as a result of excessive sweating in extreme conditions of heat or physical exertion. In elderly people, the combination of reduced tubular reabsorption of sodium and low sodium intake can result in a sodium depletion state characterized by anorexia and mental confusion.

Many clinical conditions also increase sodium losses and increase requirements; these are discussed in the relevant sections of the Manual.

Toxicity

Excessive oral loads of sodium have the potential to be fatal, but their powerful emetic effect also reduces the likelihood of this happening in normal circumstances. However, high sodium intakes administered artificially, or to someone with impaired renal, hepatic or cardiac function, can have rapid and severe detrimental consequences.

2.7.5 Potassium

Potassium is predominantly an intracellular cation and plays a fundamental role in acid–base regulation, fluid balance, muscle contraction and nerve conduction. Since 95% of the body's potassium is found within cells, body potassium content is directly related to (and can be used to estimate) lean muscle mass.

Requirement and intake

Although metabolically closely linked, the body's requirement for potassium is higher than that for sodium because there is an obligatory loss of potassium in the urine and stools which amounts to about 590 mg (15 mmol)/day.

Precise requirements are difficult to establish, but the RNI for adults over 19 years old has been set at 3500 mg/day (90 mmol/day).

The average daily potassium intake in the UK diet (Gregory *et al*. 1990) was found to be 3187 mg in men and 2434 mg in women. Approximately 67% of men and 93% of women have a potassium intake below the RNI (MAFF 1994). Since potassium has a reciprocal relationship with sodium and may have an important protective role in the development of hypertension (see Section 4.24, Hypertension), these intakes may be inappropriate for long-term health.

Sources in the UK diet

In the average UK diet (MAFF 1994), potassium is derived from:

- vegetables and potatoes (28%)
- beverages, particularly coffee (16%)
- milk and milk products (14%)
- cereal products (14%)
- meat and meat products (13%)
- fruit (5%).

Potassium is present in nearly all foods, but the most concentrated dietary sources are:

- fruit: especially bananas, apricots, rhubarb, blackcurrants, citrus fruits, dried and crystallized fruit, fruit juices
- vegetables: especially potatoes and potato snacks, mushrooms, beetroot, pulses including baked beans, tomato juice
- chocolate, cocoa and chocolate-flavoured products
- coffee and coffee-flavoured products
- malted milk drinks
- yeast extracts and spreads, stock cubes, bottled sauces and ketchups
- chutneys and pickles
- tinned and packet soups, packets of instant desserts
- wine, sherry, beer and cider
- cream of tartar, curry powder, chilli, ginger, salt substitutes.

Meat, fish, eggs, milk and dairy products and wholegrain cereals also provide significant amounts of potassium and intake may need to be regulated on potassium-restricted regimens (see Section 4.14, Renal disease). In some clinical circumstances, dietary potassium intake may need to be controlled by means of a system of potassium exchanges (see Appendix 6.2).

General population guidance to increase potassium intake should focus on the importance of, and many other health benefits from, increasing the dietary intake of fruit and vegetables.

Deficiency

Potassium depletion results in skeletal muscular weakness and may also affect heart muscle (causing cardiac arrhythmias and possibly cardiac arrest) or the muscles of the gastrointestinal tract (causing reduced motility or ileus). Mental impairment or confusion may also occur. However, these effects are unlikely to result from dietary deficiency per se, but as a secondary consequence of abnormal renal potassium losses, usually due to the use of potassium-losing diuretics.

Toxicity

The body's ability to excrete surplus potassium via renal tubular excretion is considerable and, provided that renal function is normal, it is almost impossible to induce potassium overload by dietary means. However, potassium retention is a high risk in some forms of renal disease and can cause fatal cardiac arrest (see Section 4.14, Renal disease).

2.7.6 Iron

The major role of iron is as an oxygen carrier in haemoglobin in blood and myoglobin in muscle. In addition, iron is required for many metabolic processes. It is part of the cytochrome system involved in electron transfer and hence has a central role in energy metabolism in all cells. Enzymes such as catalase and peroxidases (peroxide and superoxide metabolism) contain haem as part of their structure; other iron-containing proteins include flavoproteins and prolyl hyroxylase involved in nucleotide and collagen synthesis. Iron also acts as a cofactor for enzymes in the citric acid cycle and amino acid metabolism.

In its free state, iron is toxic and also has pro-oxidant effects. The transport and storage of iron is therefore closely regulated. Once absorbed, iron is transported in blood by the protein transferrin to receptors on cell membranes and to developing red blood cells in bone marrow. Iron surplus to requirements is stored mainly in the liver, spleen or bone marrow as ferritin, a labile and readily accessible source of iron, and haemosiderin, an insoluble form.

The adult human body contains 3–5 g iron, about two-thirds of which is in haemoglobin.

Requirements and intake

About 1 mg of iron per day is lost from the body via urine, faeces, sweat and desquamated cells. In women of reproductive age, menstruation accounts for an additional loss of, on average, about 20 mg iron/month, although this varies considerably and may be significantly more in women with menorrhagia. Additional iron will also be required to meet the expansion in blood volume that occurs during growth, particularly the rapid growth that occurs during adolescence and pregnancy.

The minimum requirement for absorbed iron is therefore about 1 mg/day in an adult male, and about 2–3 mg/day in menstruating women and adolescents. DRVs (DH 1991) take account of these differing needs and the fact that only about 5–10% of dietary iron consumed is absorbed.

The UK RNIs for iron for older children and adults are:

- males, 11–18 years: 11.3 mg/day
- males, >19 years: 8.7 mg/day
- females, 11–50 years: 14.8 mg/day
- females, >50 years: 8.7 mg/day.

Below the age of 11 years, the RNIs of boys and girls are assumed to be the same and increase incrementally with age:

- 0–3 months: 1.7 mg/day
- 4–6 months: 4.3 mg/day
- 7–12 months: 7.8 mg/day
- 1–3 years: 6.9 mg/day
- 4–6 years: 6.1 mg/day
- 7–10 years: 8.7 mg/day.

The body has the capacity to increase its iron absorption in the face of increased physiological demand such as during pregnancy, lactation or growth spurts, and in conditions of iron insufficiency or following acute blood loss. However, if in these circumstances habitual iron intake or iron stores are low, additional amounts of dietary iron will be required.

In the Dietary and Nutritional Survey of British Adults aged 16–64 years (Gregory et al. 1990) mean iron intake was 14.0 mg/day in men and 12.3 mg/day in women. The latter figure is below the RNI for those aged below 50 years. Very few men had an iron intake below the LRNI but in women, 33% of 16–18 year olds and 26% of those aged 19–50 years had intakes below the LRNI (MAFF 1994).

Sources in the UK diet

Dietary iron exists in two forms, haem and non-haem. Haem iron, which is contained in the haemoglobin and myoglobin of animal foods, is relatively available and its absorption is relatively unaffected by other food items or by the iron status of an individual. The absorbability of non-haem iron present in plant foods is much more variable. Non-haem iron can interact with dietary constituents such as tannins, phytates, some forms of protein and dietary fibre, and with other inorganic elements, making it less readily solubilized and available than haem iron (FAO 1988). Tea and eggs are notable inhibitors of non-haem iron absorption (Hurrell 1997). However, the absorption of this form of iron can also be enhanced by substances such as ascorbic acid (vitamin C) which reduce ferric ions to their more readily absorbed ferrous form. It is therefore particularly important that people whose iron intake is predominantly from non-haem iron sources also consume sufficient amounts of vitamin C (e.g. by consuming fruit or fruit juice with meals.)

In the average UK diet (MAFF 1994), iron is principally derived from:

- cereal products (42%)
- meat and meat products (23%)
- vegetables (15%).

The most concentrated sources of haem iron are:

- red meat
- liver and offal meats.

Smaller amounts of haem iron are present in animal foods such as poultry meat and fish.

Good sources of non-haem iron are:

- bread and cereal foods made from UK fortified white flour
- fortified breakfast cereals
- green leafy vegetables
- pulses
- dried fruit
- nuts and seeds.

Deficiency

Iron deprivation results in a reduced ability to transport oxygen around the body, with many detrimental effects, particularly in terms of cardiovascular, respiratory, brain and muscular function. In children, iron-deficiency anaemia can delay, or possibly permanently impair, mental and motor development.

Several haematological parameters are used to assess iron depletion. Early stages of deficiency may be indicated by the serum ferritin level, which reflects iron stores and falls prior to any change in blood haemoglobin. However, since serum ferritin levels may be increased by infection or some pathological states, and vary during pregnancy, they may not always reveal underlying deficiency. Accompanying indicators of iron depletion such as low serum transferrin, low transferrin saturation and increased total iron-binding capacity (TIBC) may be necessary to identify low iron status. As iron deficiency becomes more prolonged and haemoglobin production falls, a microcytic hypochromic anaemia develops, resulting in symptoms such as pallor, breathlessness and fatigue. Clinical anaemia is usually defined as a blood haemoglobin level below 110.0 g/l (although the cut-off point will vary according to age, gender and local reference ranges) in conjunction with reduced levels of haematological parameters such as the haematocrit, mean corpuscular volume (MCV), mean corpuscular haemoglobin concentration (MCHC) and mean corpuscular haemoglobin (MCH).

Iron deficiency is the most common nutritional deficiency in the world and the prevalence in the UK is also considerable. Sectors of the population most at risk are:

- Infants over the age of 6 months and toddlers, particularly those from deprived backgrounds and certain ethnic groups. This largely results from inadequate intake of iron as a result of inappropriate or delayed weaning (see Sections 3.3, Infants, and 3.4, Preschool Children).
- Menstruating women, especially female adolescents whose demands for iron are high but whose dietary intake is often low (see Section 3.6, Adolescents).
- Pregnant women: Although the demand for iron during pregnancy is high, the prevalence of anaemia is not considered to be as high as was once thought because the fall in haemoglobin which tends to occur largely reflects the expansion in blood volume (i.e. is a haemo-dilution effect). In addition, iron absorption increases considerably in response to the demand for iron. Nevertheless, anaemia is a risk in women who commence

pregnancy with low iron stores (see Section 3.1, Pregnancy).

- Unbalanced vegetarian diets. Strict or unbalanced vegetarian diets may increase the risk of anaemia, particularly if haem iron intake ceases abruptly, if insufficient non-haem iron is consumed and if vitamin C intake is poor.

Toxicity

Iron absorption is strictly regulated and iron overload is not normally a risk from dietary sources (Hulten *et al.* 1995). High intakes of iron in the form of supplements may, however, override normal homoeostatic controls and result in iron overload. High intakes of supplemental iron can also interfere with the absorption of other elements, especially zinc, inadvertently creating other micronutrient imbalances and deficiencies (Fairweather-Tait 1995; Fairweather-Tait and Hurrell 1996). Overdosage with iron supplements, especially by children, can be fatal.

2.7.7 Zinc

Zinc has a wide range of biological functions and is a component of more than 70 mammalian enzymes. It participates in carbohydrate, lipid, protein and nucleic acid synthesis and degradation. Zinc also plays a structural role in non-enzymic proteins such as insulin and growth hormone and helps to maintain the configuration of some gene-transcription proteins.

The human body contains about 2 g zinc, of which about 60% is present in muscle tissue, 30% in bone and 5% in skin.

Requirement and intake

Over the age of 15 years, the RNI for males is 9.5 mg/day and for females 7.0 mg/day. Considerable increments (6 mg/day for the first 4 months and 2.5 mg thereafter) are considered necessary during lactation.

In the Dietary and Nutritional Survey of British Adults (Gregory *et al.* 1990), mean zinc intake was 11.4 mg/day in men and 8.4 mg/day in women. About 30% of both groups had intakes below the RNI, but few were below the LRNI.

Sources in the UK diet

In the average UK diet (Gregory *et al.* 1990; MAFF 1994) zinc is primarily derived from:

- meat and meat products (40%)
- cereal foods (22%)
- milk and milk products (16%)
- vegetables and potatoes (9%).

Zinc bioavailability is, however, variable, being much higher from animal foods than from phytate-containing cereal foods (Sandstrom 1997). Zinc absorption therefore depends of the proportion of these sources of zinc in the diet. In the UK, where consumption of animal foods is generally high, dietary zinc bioavailability is probably in the region of 50–55%. However, the bioavailability of some vegetarian, and especially vegan, diets may be much lower (30–35%) (WHO 1996).

Rich sources of zinc with high bioavailability are:

- red meat
- fish and shellfish
- milk and milk products
- poultry and eggs.

Other good sources of zinc but with lower bioavailability include:

- bread and cereal products
- green leafy vegetables
- pulses.

Deficiency

Because of its importance in protein, enzyme and nucleotide synthesis, the effects of zinc deficiency are most apparent in tissues with a rapid turnover, such as those of the mouth, skin and intestinal mucosa. Reduced taste acuity due to loss of taste buds is a common symptom. Immune function and wound healing may also be impaired.

Overt zinc deficiency is rare, but subclinical deficiency may be relatively common, particularly in circumstances when requirements are high as a result of tissue injury, surgery or infection, but dietary intake is low due to poor appetite, or eating and swallowing difficulties.

Deficiency is also a risk on diets devoid of meat and animal products if the associated consumption of phytate-containing cereals is high and zinc intake from other foods is low.

Toxicity

Intake of zinc in excess of 2 g/day can cause nausea and vomiting. Long-term ingestion of high intakes of zinc may interfere with the absorption of other essential elements, especially iron, copper and manganese.

2.7.8 Copper

Copper is a component of a number of oxidative enzymes; cytochrome C oxidase is active at the terminal end of the mitochondrial electron transport chain, uricase is involved in the renal and hepatic metabolism of uric acid, and amine oxidases contribute to the elasticity and tensile strength of elastin and collagen, particularly in blood vessels.

Copper is also a component of caeruloplasmin, a glycoprotein, which appears to be important not only for copper transport but also for the enzyme (ferroxidase) in the control of free radicals, in defences against infection and in the intracellular oxidation of Fe^{2+} to Fe^{3+}.

Requirements and intake

There are very few data available on human requirements, and the COMA Panel on Dietary Reference Values was unable to derive estimated average requirements (EARs) or LRNIs (DH 1991). For both men and women over the age of 18 years, an RNI of 1.2 mg/day was set. An additional 0.3 mg/day is estimated to be required during lactation. In children, RNIs are:

- <1 year: 0.3 mg/day
- 1–3 years: 0.4 mg/day
- 4–6 years: 0.6 years
- 7–10 years: 0.7 mg/day
- 11–14 years: 0.8 mg/day.

The average UK dietary intake of adults aged 16–64 years (Gregory *et al.* 1990) is 1.63 mg/day in men and 1.23 mg/day in women.

Homoeostasis for copper is mainly achieved by adjustment of biliary excretion, and requirements may be increased in the presence of a jejunostomy or with other loss of bile such as chronic diarrhoea. Care should be taken when administering copper to intravenously fed patients with impaired biliary excretion, since copper overload is likely to occur if intake is high (Greene *et al.* 1988).

Sources in the UK diet

In the UK diet (MAFF 1994) copper is principally derived from:

- meat and meat products (27%)
- cereal products (27%)
- vegetables and potatoes (17%)
- beverages (mainly tea and coffee) (6%).

Concentrated sources of dietary copper are shellfish, liver, nuts and cocoa. Most foods provide some copper but milk and dairy products are generally poor sources. The copper content of drinking water can be high if copper plumbing is used.

About 35–70% of dietary copper is absorbed, its bioavailability being reduced by large amounts of phytate and some types of fibre. Owing to competition for binding sites, copper absorption is also inhibited by high intakes of zinc, iron, calcium and phosphorus. Absorption also tends to decrease with age and may be low in elderly people (Bunker *et al.* 1984).

Deficiency

Overt copper deficiency is rare and usually results from genetic disorders affecting copper transport or deposition. It can also occur as a result of malnutrition or chronic malabsorptive states and marginal copper deficiency may be more prevalent than has hitherto been appreciated (WHO 1996).

Copper deficiency may result in anaemia, neutropenia and pathological changes in bone similar to those of osteoporosis. Hair changes, especially pigment formation, may also occur. There is increasing speculation that an optimal level of copper may be important to maintain antioxidant defences and help to prevent disorders such as cardiovascular disease.

Toxicity

High intakes of copper are toxic but have only been reported in unusual circumstances such as contamination of drinking water.

As result of recent interest in the possible importance of copper to long-term health, supplemental use of copper by the general population is likely to increase. Since at upper ranges of intake, copper may have more of a pro-oxidant than antioxidant effect (Strain 1994), such a measure should be regarded with caution.

2.7.9 Chromium

Chromium may have a number of important influences on metabolism. It forms an organic complex with nicotinic acid, glutathione and other amino acids which appears to potentiate the action of insulin in cellular glucose uptake. This complex is often referred to as the 'glucose tolerance factor', although much remains to be learnt about its nature and effects (WHO 1996). Chromium may also play a role in lipid and amino acid metabolism, in maintaining the structure of nucleic acids and in gene expression. Chromium does not appear to form part of any enzyme system.

Requirements and intake

Human requirements remain uncertain and no UK RNIs have been set. A safe and adequate intake is estimated to be above 25 μg/day for adults and between 0.1–1.0 μg/kg per day for children and adolescents (DH 1991). More recently, the WHO Expert Group (1996) has suggested that the minimum chromium intake of adults should be 33 μg/day.

Observed intakes in adults range between 13 and 49 μg/day (DH 1991). Requirements may be affected by nutritional or physiological stress which alter glucose metabolism.

Sources in the UK diet

Chromium is usually present in food as trivalent chromium (Cr^{3+} or Cr III) and the absorption of this is 0.5–2% of intake. Hexavalent chromium (Cr VI) is less biologically active and is also more toxic.

There are few recent data on the chromium content of foods and many previously published values are likely to be unreliable and falsely high (DH 1991).

Rich sources of chromium are thought to include:

- brewers' yeast
- meat
- wholegrains
- legumes
- nuts.

Refined foods are generally low in chromium.

Deficiency

Overt chromium deficiency has only been documented in people on long-term parenteral nutrition. There is spec-

ulation that lesser degrees of deficiency may have adverse metabolic effects, particularly in terms of insulin resistance and glucose tolerance, but this remains to be established.

Toxicity

Trivalent chromium has low toxicity. High intakes of the hexavalent form (1–2 g/day) have resulted in renal and hepatic necrosis.

2.7.10 Manganese

Many enzymes require manganese as part of their structure or as a cofactor, including glycosyl transferases (glycoprotein synthesis), pyruvate carboxylase (carbohydrate synthesis) and superoxide dismutase (protection from free radical damage). Manganese is also a component of bone and cartilage.

Requirement, intake and sources in the UK diet

There are limited data on manganese turnover and metabolism. For this reason the UK COMA Panel on Dietary Reference Values (DH 1991) was unable to make precise recommendations. Safe intakes were estimated to be above 1.4 mg/day for adults and above 16 μg/kg per day for infants and children.

Because of analytical difficulties, few studies of intakes have been carried out. UK adult intakes of manganese have been estimated to be about 4.6 mg/day, about half of which is derived from tea (Wenlock *et al.* 1979).

Deficiency

Since deficiencies have never been described in free-living populations, current ranges of intake are presumed to meet requirements.

Toxicity

Manganese is one of the least toxic elements. The rate of absorption is low and any surplus is efficiently excreted via bile and the kidneys.

2.7.11 Molybdenum

Molybdenum is a cofactor in the enzyme involved in the metabolism of DNA and sulphites, especially xanthine oxidase, aldehyde oxidase and sulphite oxidase.

There have been few studies of molybdenum requirements and intakes (food levels are markedly affected by local soil concentration), and deficiency in free-living humans has never been clearly documented. The COMA Panel (DH 1991) was unable to set RNIs; safe intakes for adults are believed to lie between 50 and 400 μg/day. Current intakes of molybdenum are believed to be sufficient for normal health and development (WHO 1996).

2.7.12 Selenium

Selenium has aroused great interest as a result of its antioxidant effects and hence possible protective role against cardiovascular disease (CVD) and cancer. Selenium is an essential constituent of the enzyme glutathione peroxidase, which protects tissues from oxidative breakdown. It also appears to be a constituent of other enzymes or proteins and may affect the metabolism of lipids, carbohydrate, thyroid hormone and certain drugs (Arthur and Beckett 1994).

Requirement and intake

Based on limited data, the RNIs for selenium for adults over 19 years were set at 75 μg/day for men and 60 μg/day for women (DH 1991). An additional 15 μg/day was estimated to be necessary during lactation. The LRNI was set at 40 μg/day for adults since no evidence of deficiency has been observed in populations with this level of intake.

Typical intake in the UK is about 62 μg/day (Butcher *et al.* 1995).

Sources in the UK diet

Selenium is widely distributed in the environment but the selenium content of foods is greatly affected by the soil on which crops are grown or animals are grazed. In the UK, the selenium level in soil, and hence in the food chain, tends to be low (Holland *et al.* 1991).

In the UK diet, selenium is mainly derived from meats, fats, vegetables and cereals (Butcher *et al.* 1995). Fish is a particularly concentrated source but does not make a large contribution to average dietary intake. Absorption from food is thought to range between 55 and 65% (DH 1991).

Deficiency

Severe deficiency of selenium (resulting from intakes of less than 12 μg/day) can cause Keshan disease, a selenium-responsive cardiomyopathy which predominantly occurs in China. Selenium deficiency has also been associated with disturbances in lipid and carbohydrate metabolism and impaired immune function.

There is considerable interaction between selenium and vitamin E in the body and the effects of selenium deficiency may be decreased by high doses of vitamin E.

Any benefits from selenium supplementation in terms of preventing CVD or certain types of cancers remain to be established.

Toxicity

The margin between selenium requirements and toxicity is narrower than for many trace elements and over-supplementation may be hazardous. Disturbed selenium homoeostasis has been observed at intakes of 750 μg/day and it is recommended that intake from all sources should not exceed 450 μg/day (DH 1991). Since the kidney is the major route of excretion, additional caution may be warranted in people with renal insufficiency.

2.7.13 Fluorine

Fluorine is deposited in bones and teeth. Its incorporation into tooth enamel markedly increases the latter's hardness and resistance to decay (see Section 4.1.1, Dental caries).

Requirement and intake

There is little evidence that there is any physiological requirement for fluorine and therefore no RNIs have been set (DH 1991). However, the COMA Panel on Dietary Reference Values endorsed the recommendation that, where necessary, water should be fluoridated to a level of 1 ppm as a public health measure against dental caries (DH 1991).

Sources in the UK diet

The major source of fluoride in most diets is water (principally in the form of tea), with foods providing only about 25% of total intake. The mean daily fluoride intake of adults has been estimated to be about 1.82 mg fluoride/day, but may be significantly higher (up to 12 mg/day) if large quantities of drinks derived from fluoridated water are consumed (DH 1991). Young children may also ingest a certain amount of fluoride from toothpaste, a practice which should be discouraged as much as possible because of the risk of fluorosis.

Fluoride is rapidly and efficiently absorbed from the gut; unbound fluoride in water is more bioavailable than protein-bound forms, such as in milk. Excretion of fluoride is mainly by the kidney.

Deficiency

A deficiency of fluorine has never been demonstrated in humans, hence it is not considered to be an essential element. However, low levels of fluoride in drinking water significantly increase the risk of dental caries (McDonagh *et al.* 2000) (see Section 4.1.1).

Toxicity

Excessive intake of fluoride causes fluorosis, early signs of which are mottling and discoloration of the teeth. Pronounced changes in tooth enamel have been seen in children consuming 0.1 mg fluoride/kg body weight per day. To minimize this risk, an upper safe level of intake by infants and young children of 0.05 mg/kg per day has been set (DH 1991). The WHO Expert Group recommended that total intakes at the ages of 1, 2 and 3 years should not exceed 0.5, 1.0 and 1.5 mg/day, respectively (WHO 1996).

Fluoride increases osteoblast and osteoclast activity and has been used in the treatment of osteoporosis. However, large doses impair bone mineralization and lead to osteomalacia; fluoride therefore needs to be given with a calcium supplement to prevent this. A large-scale multicentre prospective trial has recently established that long-term exposure to fluoridated drinking water does not increase the risk of osteoporotic fracture (Phipps *et al.* 2000).

Intakes of fluoride in excess of 500 mg/day can be fatal.

2.7.14 Iodine

Iodine functions as part of the thyroid hormones thyroxine (T_4) and triiodothyronine (T_3). These are necessary for the maintenance of metabolic processes, thermoregulation, protein synthesis and the integrity of connective tissue. In the fetus and neonate, protein synthesis in the brain and central nervous system is dependent on iodine or an iodine-containing compound.

Requirement and intake

There are few data on iodine requirements in populations and the COMA Panel was unable to derive an EAR (DH 1991). Since, in adults, 70 μg/day appears to be sufficient to prevent goitre, the LRNI was set at this level. In order to provide a suitable margin of safety, the RNI was set at 140 μg/day.

In the Dietary and Nutritional Survey of British Adults (Gregory *et al.* 1990), mean iodine intakes were estimated to be 243 μg/day in men and 176 μg/day in women.

In Western countries, milk is the major source of iodine, and the iodine content of milk has risen in recent years as a result of the use of iodine-supplemented animal feedstuffs and contamination from iodine-containing sterilizing compounds. Seafoods and dried seaweeds are concentrated sources.

Iodine is normally well absorbed, but can be inhibited by goitrogens such as thiocyanates and cyanoglucosides found in foods such as turnips, cabbage, cassava, millet, maize, bamboo shoots, lima beans and sweet potato. Calcium, magnesium, manganese and fluoride may also impair absorption, but these influences are likely to be insignificant in the UK diet unless iodine intake is abnormally low.

Deficiency

Deficiency in adults causes a fall in the blood level of T_4, which in turn stimulates thyroid-stimulating hormone (TSH). TSH causes hyperplasia of the thyroid gland and the development, of a goitre. In pregnant women, iodine deficiency is associated with increased rates of stillbirths, spontaneous abortions, perinatal deaths and congenital abnormalities. In infants and young children, lack of iodine impairs brain development, resulting in cretinism, characterized by mental retardation, hypothyroidism and dwarfism. Iodine deficiency disorders continue to be a public health problem in many parts of the world, but are rare in Europe.

Toxicity

Persistently high iodine intakes can cause hyperthyroidism and may be linked to thyroid cancer. In the UK the recommended maximum safe upper limit has been set at 17 μg/kg per day, or nor more than 1000 μg/day in total (DH 1991).

Table 2.14 Non-essential elements

Essential for some species but not humans	No known physiological function in any species
Arsenic	Aluminium
Boron	Antimony
Bromine	Caesium
Cadmium	Germanium
Lead	Mercury
Lithium	Silver
Nickel	Strontium
Silicon	Titanium
Tin	
Vanadium	

2.7.15 Cobalt

The only known function of cobalt in humans is as a constituent of vitamin B_{12} and there is no dietary requirement for it other than in this form.

2.7.16 Other trace elements and contaminants

Some elements are present in body tissues but there is no evidence that there is a dietary requirement for them in humans (see Table 2.14). Others have no known role in any species. Many of these elements are highly toxic at relatively low levels of intake and hence the primary concern is to avoid their presence in food as much as possible. Levels of these elements in the UK diet are therefore closely monitored by Government agencies. Published food surveillance reports can be accessed via the Food Standards Agency website.

Text revised by: Briony Thomas

Useful address

Food Standards Agency
Website: www.foodstandards.gov.uk

Further reading

British Nutrition Foundation. *Calcium*. Briefing Paper 24. London: BNF, 1991.

British Nutrition Foundation. *Salt in the Diet*. Briefing Paper. London: BNF, 1994.

British Nutrition Foundation. *Iron. Nutritional and Physiological Significance*. London: Chapman and Hall, 1995.

Holland B, Welch AA, Unwin ID *et al. McCance and Widdowson's The Composition of Foods*, 5th edn. Cambridge: Royal Society of Chemistry/MAFF, 1991.

Linder MC, Hazegh-Azan M. Copper biochemistry and molecular biology. *American Journal of Clinical Nutrition* 1996; **63** (Suppl): 1347S–1356S.

Mertz W. Chromium in human nutrition: a review. *Journal of Nutrition* 1993; **123**: 626–633.

National Academy of Sciences, Food and Nutrition Board. *Dietary Reference Intakes for Calcium, Phosphorus, Magnesium,*

Vitamin D and Fluoride. Washington, DC: National Academy Press, 1997.

Swinkels JWGM *et al*. Biology of zinc and biological value of dietary organic zinc complexes and chelates. *Nutrition Research Reviews* 1994; **7**: 129–149.

World Health Organization. *Trace Elements in Human Nutrition and Health*. A Report of a Joint FAO/WHO/IAEA Expert Consultation. Geneva: WHO, 1996.

References

Arthur JR, Beckett GJ. New metabolic roles for selenium. *Proceedings of the Nutrition Society* 1994; **53**: 615–524.

Bunker VW, Lawson MS, Delves HT, Clayton BE. The uptake and excretion of chromium by the elderly. *American Journal of Clinical Nutrition* 1984; **39**: 797–802.

Butcher MA *et al*. Current selenium content of foods and an estimation of average intake in the United Kingdom. *Proceedings of the Nutrition Society* 1995; **54**: 131A.

Department of Health. Report of the Panel on Dietary Reference Values of the Committee on Medical Aspects of Food Policy (COMA). *Dietary Reference Values for Food Energy and Nutrients for the United Kingdom*. Report on Health and Social Subjects 41. London: HMSO, 1991.

Department of Health. Report of the Cardiovascular Review Group of the Committee on Medical Aspects of Food Policy (COMA). *Nutritional Aspects of Cardiovascular Disease*. Report on Health and Social Subjects 46. London: HMSO, 1994.

Department of Health. *Nutrition and Bone Health*. Report on Health and Social Subjects 49. London: The Stationery Office, 1998.

Fairweather-Tait S. Iron–zinc and calcium–iron interactions in relation to zinc and iron absorption. *Proceedings of the Nutrition Society* 1995; **54**: 465–473.

Fairweather-Tait S, Hurrell RF. Bioavailability of minerals and trace elements. *Nutrition Research Reviews* 1996; **9**: 295–324.

Food and Agriculture Organization. *Requirements of Vitamin A, Iron, Folate and Vitamin B₁₂*. Report of a Joint FAO/WHO Expert Consultation. Food and Nutrition Series 23. Rome: FAO, 1988.

Greene HL, Hambidge KM, Schanier R, Tsang RC. Guidelines for the use of vitamins, trace elements, calcium, magnesium, and phosphorus in infants and children receiving total parenteral nutrition. *American Journal of Clinical Nutrition* 1988; **48**: 1324–1342.

Gregory J, Foster K, Tyler H, Wiseman M. *The Dietary and Nutritional Survey of British Adults*. London: HMSO, 1990.

Holland B, Welch AA, Unwin ID *et al*. *McCance and Widdowson's The Composition of Foods*, 5th edn. Cambridge: Royal Society of Chemistry/MAFF, 1991.

Hulten L, Gramatkovski E, Leerup A, Hallberg L. Iron absorption from the whole diet. Relation to meal composition, iron requirements and iron stores. *European Journal of Clinical Nutrition* 1995; **49**: 794–808.

Hurrell RF. Bioavailability of iron. *European Journal of Clinical Nutrition* 1997; **51** (Suppl 1): S4–S8.

McDonagh MS, Whiting PF, Wilson PM *et al*. Systematic review of water fluoridation. *British Medical Journal* 2000; **321**: 855–859.

Ministry of Agriculture, Fisheries and Food. *The Dietary and Nutritional Survey of British Adults – Further Analysis*. London: HMSO, 1994.

Ministry of Agriculture, Fisheries and Food. *National Food Survey 1998. Annual Report on Food Expenditure, Consumption and Nutrient Intakes*. London: The Stationery Office, 1999.

Pannemans DLE, Schaafsma G, Westerterp RR. Calcium excretion, apparent absorption and calcium balance in young and elderly subjects: influence of protein intake. *British Journal of Nutrition* 1997; **77**: 721–729.

Phipps KR, Orwell ES, Mason JD, Cauley JA. Community water fluoridation, bone mineral density and fractures: prospective study of effects in older women. *British Medical Journal* 2000; **321**: 860–864.

Sandstrom B. Bioavailability of zinc. *European Journal of Clinical Nutrition* 1997; **51** (Suppl 1): S17–S19.

Strain JJ. Newer aspects of micronutrients in chronic copper disease. *Proceedings of the Nutrition Society* 1994; **53**: 583–598.

Wenlock RW, Buss DH, Dixon EJ. Trace elements. 2. Manganese in British foods. *British Journal of Nutrition* 1979; **41**: 253–261.

Whiting SJ, Wood RJ. Adverse effects of high-calcium in humans. *Nutrition Reviews* 1997; **55**: 1–9.

Wood RJ, Ju Zheng J. High dietary calcium intakes reduce zinc absorption and balance in humans. *American Journal of Clinical Nutrition* 1997; **65**: 1803.

World Health Organization. *Trace Elements in Human Nutrition and Health*. A Report of a Joint FAO/WHO/IAEA Expert Consultation. Geneva: WHO, 1996.

2.8 Fluid

Fluid is essential to life and, while humans can survive for a period of weeks without food, they cannot withstand deprivation of fluid for more than a few days, or even hours. Fluid has many vital functions in the body and is needed:

- to act as a solvent for ions and molecules
- to act as a transport medium, especially for the excretion of osmotically active solutes such as urea and salts
- as a lubricant
- to regulate body temperature.

In adults water comprises 50–70% of total body weight. The percentage varies according to age (being higher in infants than in adults) and gender (women have larger stores of adipose tissue and therefore less body water than men).

Body water is primarily divided between the intracellular and extracellular compartments, the latter being composed of the interstitial fluid and the plasma volume (Table 2.15). These compartments are separated by semi-permeable barriers which permit the free passage of salt and water but only limited movement of other solutes such as proteins. All three compartments are interdependent and movement of fluid between them is regulated largely by pressure gradients and osmosis. Since it is difficult to gain access to the intracellular fluid compartment, extracellular fluid volume is the most important consideration when providing clinical care for a patient, particularly in the acute stages of an illness.

2.8.1 Regulation of fluid balance

Regulation of the body fluid is under tight homoeostatic control. Normally, the total fluid volume fluctuates by less than 1% per day, despite variations in intake. Changes of as little as 1–2% can lead to illness and sometimes death.

Factors affecting fluid movement

Movement of water between the three compartments is controlled by a variety of sensitive and highly complex mechanisms which include osmosis and the effect of hydrostatic pressure gradients. Particles within the body fluid are electrically charged; the main extracellular cation is sodium and the main intracellular cation is potassium (Table 2.15). In normal circumstances, the osmolalities of the plasma and interstitial fluid are equal. Plasma osmolality usually reflects the serum sodium which, in turn, reflects the total extracellular volume. Provided water is distributed normally between the three compartments, a high serum sodium level may indicate dehydration while a low level could point to over-hydration.

Plasma osmolality

This is a key factor in the determination of fluid movement and slight alterations in plasma osmolality are usually corrected by the movement of fluid between the interstitial compartment and the plasma. This may be accompanied by variations in oral intake.

If the plasma osmolality increases then the hypothalamus is stimulated by a sensation of thirst and increased amounts of antidiuretic hormone (ADH) are released. This leads to the reabsorption of water from the distal renal tubules and correction of the plasma osmolality.

Decreased plasma volume can also lead to a raised osmolality; aldosterone is then released which results in increased sodium and water retention.

Renal function is therefore an important factor in the regulation of fluid balance and any impairment is often characterized by oedema.

'Pitting oedema' is the most common clinical symptom of an expanded interstitial volume. Fluid balance is normally maintained within the extracellular compartment but can be upset for a number of reasons. It is important to

Table 2.15 Body fluids: location, percentage and composition

Compartment	Location	% Body weight	Principal cation	Principal anion
Extracellular Interstitial	Fluid surrounding the cells	16%	Na^+	Cl^-
Vascular	Fluids within blood vessels (6.5% solids, mainly protein)	4%	Na^+	Cl^-
Intracellular	Fluids within the cells (protein content higher than plasma)	30–40%	K^+	PO_4^- (+ protein)

The only common feature between these three compartments is the osmolality, which is 290 mosmol/kg water.

remember that the location of pitting oedema is affected by gravity and that a bedridden patient may show signs of sacral oedema in the absence of ankle oedema. Correction of oedema should never be attempted without a precise knowledge of its cause. It is also important to remember that severe cases of disturbed osmolality or volume depletion can lead to the movement of water between the intracellular and extracellular compartments; this is more difficult to diagnose and can have fatal consequences if not treated promptly.

Hydrostatic pressure

Plasma volume is also maintained by the effects of hydrostatic pressure. Essentially, a higher pressure is exerted within the arterial end of the capillary. At the same time there is the lesser effect of osmotic pressure exerted by the plasma proteins (oncotic pressure), resulting in the movement of fluid into the interstitial space. The process is reversed at the venous end of the capillary with a consequent movement of fluid back into the plasma (Starling's hypothesis, summarized in Fig. 2.6). The plasma proteins therefore play an important role in the movement of fluid between the vascular and interstitial compartments.

2.8.2 Clinical aspects of fluid balance

Factors affecting fluid balance

Fluid intake

Fluid intake is normally controlled by the sensation of thirst, which is regulated by the hypothalamus. Fluid is derived from food as well as beverages. Small quantities of water are also produced by the metabolic processes of the body.

Fluid output

Fluid output is primarily controlled by the kidneys, but insensible losses also occur via the skin, lungs and gastrointestinal tract. The level of these losses depends on factors such as climate, activity, state of health and dietary intake.

Respiratory losses Respiratory function can affect the maintenance of fluid volume. Normally, a constant amount of water (approximately 400 ml) is lost daily from the lungs. This loss can increase dramatically in hyperventilation, whatever the cause.

Skin losses Fluid is lost by evaporation from the skin. Losses by this route amount to approximately 500–750 ml/day but will increase as a result of a hot climate, fever, burns or any other situation that increases the metabolic rate. Pyrexia increases fluid requirements by approximately 500 ml/day per 1°C rise in temperature.

Gastrointestinal losses These mainly result from losses incurred during bouts of diarrhoea and/or vomiting. Normally, the large quantities of digestive juices that are secreted into the gastrointestinal tract are reabsorbed. If abnormal gastrointestinal function results in excessive fluid loss, this is replaced by extracellular fluid, which crosses the mucosa into the gut. Losses may be particularly high in conditions such as short bowel syndrome following ileal resection (see Section 4.12.1 in Intestinal Resection). The average composition of various intestinal fluids is shown in Table 2.16.

Fluid requirements

Individual requirements for additional fluids vary considerably. The minimum intake should be sufficient to

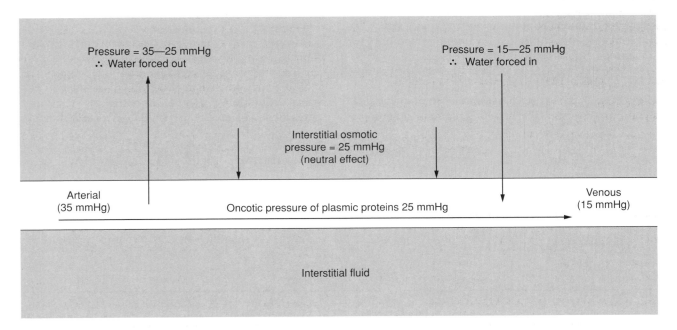

Fig. 2.6 Starling's hypothesis.

Table 2.16 Typical volume and composition of gastrointestinal secretions and sweat

Fluid	Average adult volume (ml/24 hours)	Electrolyte concentration (mEq/l)			
		Na^+	K^+	Cl^-	HCO_3^-
Gastric juice	2500	31–90	4.4–12.0	52–124	0
Bile	700–1000	134–156	3.9–6.3	83–110	38
Pancreatic juice	700–1000	113–153	2.6–7.4	54–95	110
Small bowel	3000	72–120	3.5–6.8	69–127	30
Faeces	100	<10	<10	<15	<15
Sweat	500–750	30–70	0–5	30–70	0

replace losses from all sources and provide adequate dilution for the excretion of solutes via the kidney. The maximum intake from oral liquids (or enteral or parenteral fluids) should be that which the kidney can excrete. In normal circumstances this is approximately 30–35 ml/kg body weight or 1 ml/kcal in adults and 1.5 ml/kcal in children (Kleiner 1999).

Renal solute load

It is essential to ensure that enough fluid is available for the excretion of solutes such as electrolytes and nitrogenous materials. This is a particularly important consideration in infants (because renal function is still relatively inefficient) or in patients with renal failure or any condition necessitating fluid restriction. In these circumstances the renal solute load of a feed or diet may need to be calculated. This is done by:

- calculating the dietary or feed content of protein, sodium, potassium, chloride and any other attendant anions. Dietary fats and carbohydrates do not affect the renal solute load because they are usually completely metabolized to carbon dioxide and water;
- assuming that each mmol of sodium, potassium, chloride or other anion will contribute 1 mmol to the renal solute load. If details of the attendant anion intake are not available, the content contributed by sodium and potassium should be doubled;
- assuming that each gram of protein will contribute 4 mmol to the renal solute load;
- adding the above figures together and then dividing by the urine osmolality. The resulting figure is the number

of litres of water needed to excrete the renal solute load generated by the diet or feed.

An additional allowance will need to be made for insensible losses from the lungs and skin (approximately 1000 ml in total/day); and additional losses as a result of pyrexia or abnormal gastrointestinal losses.

Estimation of fluid requirements is discussed further in Section 1.10.3 in Estimating nutritional requirements.

Monitoring fluid balance

Fluid balance is an important consideration in the management of any patient and the risk of fluid imbalance should always be assessed. The fluid status of some patients may need to be closely monitored by the meticulous completion of daily fluid balance charts recording fluid intake and output (Table 2.17), together with monitoring and evaluation of blood and urine results, with particular emphasis on sodium and osmolality.

2.8.3 People at risk of fluid imbalance

Severe fluid imbalance is usually only a risk in people who are critically ill or given inappropriate nutritional or hydration support.

However, mild to moderate fluid depletion is a high risk in many clinical circumstances (Table 2.18) and hydration status is an important consideration in the management of all patients. Acute dehydration is most likely in pathological conditions or clinical situations resulting in increased fluid losses. Rapid fluid depletion in infants and

Table 2.17 Fluid balance

Fluid input/24 hours		Fluid output/24 hours	
Source	Typical volume (ml)	Source	Typical volume (ml)
Oral liquids	1500	Urine	1500
Water contained in food[1]	1000	Faeces	150
Metabolism[2]	300	Lungs	400
		Skin	750
Total	2800	Total	2800

[1]The water content of food can be ascertained by looking up the appropriate item in McCance and Widdowson's *The Composition of Foods* (Holland *et al.* 1991). It may not always be necessary to calculate this figure accurately, but an estimate of the fluid derived from food should be included in the daily input. If the patient is not eating, the fluid usually derived from food should be replaced by another source.
[2]Metabolic yields: 1 g starch yields 0.6 g water; 1 g protein yields 0.4 g water; 1 g fat yields 1.1 g water.

Table 2.18 People at risk of dehydration

Principal reason	Examples
Increased fluid losses	Patients with tracheostomies or on ventilators Diarrhoea and/or vomiting Stomal losses Wound or burn exudates Pyrexia Diabetes insipidus Undiagnosed or uncontrolled diabetes mellitus Prolonged use of diuretic drugs Patients receiving high-protein/high-osmolar diets
Lack of awareness of, or inability to express, the need for fluid	Patients who are unable to communicate, e.g. those who are unconscious or who have suffered a stroke
Low fluid intake	Generally poor food intake due to anorexia, depression, apathy, chronic illness, physical immobility, etc. Eating difficulties, e.g. sore or painful mouth, fractured jaw Swallowing difficulties, e.g. post-stroke dysphagia Deliberate fluid restriction to reduce frequency of micturition or incontinence 'Nil-by-mouth' regimens

young children (e.g. due to gastroenteritis) can be life-threatening. Chronic dehydration is more likely to be caused by low fluid intake, and is particularly likely in people with generally poor food intake such as those who are elderly or unwell. The effects of chronic dehydration should not be underestimated as it can result in constipation, headaches, lethargy and mental confusion, and increases the risk of urinary tract infections and renal stones. Most healthy adults should drink at least 1.5–2 litres (3–4 pints) of liquid every day, and more in hot weather or if physically very active.

Fluid overload usually only occurs in people with impairment in cardiac, hepatic or renal function. Fluid restriction may therefore be an integral part of the management of these disorders (see relevant sections of the manual).

Text revised by: Briony Thomas

Further reading

Lipp J, Lord LM, Scholer LH. Fluid management in enteral nutrition. *Nutrition in Clinical Practice* 1999; **14**: 232–237.

Preston RA. *Acid–Base, Fluids and Electrolytes Made Ridiculously Simple*. USA: Medmaster, 1997.

Reference

Holland B, Welch AA, Unwin ID *et al. McCance and Widdowson's The Composition of Foods*, 5th edn. Cambridge: Royal Society of Chemistry/MAFF, 1991.

Kleiner SM. Water: an essential but overlooked nutrient. *Journal of the American Dietetic Association* 1999; **99**: 200–206.

2.9 Biologically active dietary constituents

Food contains many hundreds of chemical components, most of which are of no biological significance. Some have no nutritive function but nevertheless have physiological or pharmacological effects which may impact on nutrition or body function. The term 'phytochemicals' is increasingly being used to refer to biologically active substances present in the diet. Many have protective effects but some may be toxicants, or may become toxic if consumed to excess. Some of those which may be relevant to dietetic practice are discussed below.

2.9.1 Antioxidant and anticarcinogenic phytochemicals

In recent years there has been particular interest in phytochemicals which may have antioxidant or anticarcinogenic effects. It has become increasingly apparent from epidemiological studies that many plant foods, especially fruit and vegetables, have a protective role in terms of cardiovascular disease and some types of cancer, which cannot be explained solely by their content of antioxidant nutrients such as vitamin C, vitamin E and beta-carotene (DH 1994, 1998). It seems likely that these foods contain other naturally occurring biologically active compounds which confer additional protection against free radical damage, low-density lipoprotein (LDL) oxidation or DNA mutation, or inhibit abnormal cell proliferation.

Some of the phytochemicals which are currently the focus of such research and speculation are described below. To date, the nature and effects of many of these substances have only been investigated in experimental animal models or *in vitro* cellular studies, and their bioavailability, role and importance to humans remain to be established. It also seems likely that many other important biologically active compounds have yet to be identified. For these reasons, the best current dietary advice for cardiovascular or carcinogenic protection is to increase consumption of foods such as fruit and vegetables. Only these can provide all of the phytochemicals that may be relevant to health, and at safe levels of intake. Even if specific phytochemicals can be shown to be protective, abnormally high intakes of them may be unwise. The long-term safety of isolated supplements of antioxidant nutrients is questionable (Rapola *et al.* 1997) and the same may well apply to other substances with similar effects.

Carotenoids

These consist of about 100 naturally occurring plant pigments which provide the yellow/red colour of some vegetables and fruits. Some carotenoids can be metabolized in the intestinal mucosa to retinol (vitamin A). The most important of these is beta-carotene as its structure most closely resembles that of retinol; $6\,\mu g$ of beta-carotene is equivalent to $1\,\mu g$ retinol. Other provitamin A carotenoids are less potent, and $12\,\mu g$ is taken as being equivalent to $1\,\mu g$ preformed retinol. Other carotenoids such as xanthophyll (a yellow pigment) and lycopene (the red pigment of tomatoes) do not have provitamin A activity. However, many, or possibly all, carotenoids have an important role as dietary antioxidants because they can react with the unpaired electrons of free radicals, rendering them more stable and less reactive.

Lycopene has been of particular interest. Its ability to quench singlet oxygen makes it a powerful antioxidant and there is some experimental evidence that it may have inhibitory effects on cancer cell proliferation (Gerster 1997). Epidemiological studies have suggested that habitually high consumption of lycopene from tomato-based foods is associated with reduced risk of coronary heart disease (CHD)(Kohlmeier *et al.* 1997) and of cancer of the prostate, stomach, colon and rectum (Francheschi *et al.* 1994; Giovanucci *et al.* 1995). However, its comparative benefits in humans in relation to other dietary sources of antioxidants remain to be established.

About 85% of dietary lycopene is derived from tomatoes. Its bioavailability may be significantly improved by cooking or other processing that disrupts plant cells, and hence may be highest from tomato products such as ketchup, passatta, chopped tomatoes and tomato soup. Lycopene is also present in pink grapefruit, watermelon and guava, but these only make a small contribution to the lycopene content of most diets.

Polyphenols

Phenolic compounds are a common constituent of plants as part of their defence system against insects, humans and other animals. Many foods and beverages contain polyphenols, some of which have antioxidant effects, or potentiate the effect of other antioxidants. Polyphenols of particular current interest are flavonoids and phytoestrogens.

Flavonoids

Flavonoids are known to be very powerful antioxidants and there is some epidemiological evidence that high flavonoid consumption is inversely associated with CHD incidence and mortality (Hertog *et al.* 1993, 1995). They may also act as blocking agents in the expression of modified genes (i.e. have an anticarcinogenic effect) although, as yet, epidemiological studies have failed to find evidence that high intakes of flavonoids are protective against cancer (DH 1998). Flavonoids have also been suggested to have a variety of other biological effects, including antibacterial, antiviral, anti-inflammatory, antiallergic and vasodilatory actions (Formica and Regelson 1995; Cook and Sammen 1996).

Over 4000 types of flavonoid compound have been identified (Cook and Sammen 1996). They occur naturally in fruit, vegetables, nuts and seeds, and high concentrations are found in tea, onions and apples. However, many flavonoids are poorly absorbed from the gut and are subject to degradation by gut microflora. They may therefore not always be sufficiently available to have the *in vivo* effects demonstrated in the laboratory setting (Formica and Regelson 1995). It should also be borne in mind that, given the types of food in which they are found, some of their apparent cardioprotection may reflect the fact that a high flavonoid intake is also a marker of a healthy diet.

Flavonoids include compounds such as quercetin and catechins.

Quercetin This is the major component of a subclass of flavonoids called flavonols. Quercetin has been used in some epidemiological studies as an indicator of flavonoid intake and has been suggested to be protective against cardiovascular disease (Knekt *et al.* 1996). However, since quercetin is found in found in foods such as onions, apples, red wine and tea, it is difficult to distinguish its effects from those of other dietary flavonoids. Its biological availability also remains questionable (Formica and Regelson 1995).

Catechins About half of the flavonoids in tea are in the form of catechins, principally epigallocatechin gallate (EGCG), which is oxidized to other flavonoids such as theaflavins and thearubigens during the brewing process. The catechins, particularly EGCG, have a strong ability to scavenge free radicals (Wiseman *et al.* 1997) and *in vitro* studies have shown tea to have greater antioxidant activity than other sources such as fruits, vegetables (Cao *et al.* 1996), and isolated forms of vitamins C and E and the carotenoids (Vinson *et al.* 1995; Balentine *et al.* 1997). There is some evidence that these benefits may also apply *in vivo* (Tijburg *et al.* 1997; Leenen *et al.* 1999). The addition of milk to tea does not appear to impair its antioxidant capacity or the absorption of flavonoids across the gut (Balentine *et al.* 1997; Hollman *et al.* 1997; van het Hof *et al.* 1998; Leenen *et al.* 1999).

Catechins are also found in red wine, grapes and apple skins, but at a lower concentration than in tea.

Tannins

These phenolic compounds, which contribute to the flavour and colour of beverages such as tea and red wine, also have antioxidant activity. Tannins, particularly those in tea, have the less desirable effect of binding with iron and inhibiting its absorption (Brune *et al.* 1989; Disler *et al.* 1975). For this reason, people at risk of iron deficiency should be advised to avoid drinking large quantities of tea, or tea with meals. Other phenolic compounds, particularly those containing galloyl groups, found in the leaves of plants such as spinach, have a similar effect.

Phytoestrogens

Phytoestrogens are structurally similar to mammalian oestradiol. They compete for oestradiol receptors, and can modulate the effects of oestrogen (enhancing some effects and reducing others).

The most closely studied class of phytoestrogens comprises the isoflavones, found almost exclusively in soya and soya products. Other phytoestrogens such as lignans and coumestans are more widely distributed in foods such as oats, barley, wheatgerm, potatoes, apples, cherries, plums and vegetable oils derived from cotton seed, sunflower, corn, linseed, olive and coconut, but their effects have been less well documented.

Isoflavones

Isoflavones are diphenolic compounds present in soya beans and soya products. Types of isoflavones found in soya include genistein, daidzein and their glycosides. Daidzein is converted by gut microflora to equol, which may have particularly potent oestrogenic and antioxidant activity, although this conversion may not occur in everyone.

Soya isoflavones are known to influence hormonal function. A diet containing 60 g soy protein per day (46 g isoflavones) has been shown to be capable of affecting the menstrual cycle and levels of luteinizing hormone and follicle-stimulating hormone in adult premenopausal women (Cassidy *et al.* 1994), although the effects on ovarian function are variable and may be influenced by factors such as ethnicity, type of soya, level of phytoestrogen consumption and dietary composition (Wu *et al.* 2000; Lu *et al.* 2000). Soya phytoestrogens may help to alleviate menopausal symptoms, conserve bone density and reduce postmenopausal bone loss (Anderson and Garner 1998; Messina and Messina 2000), and be protective against the development of hormone-dependent cancers such as those of the breast and prostate (DH 1998; Lissin and Cooke 2000).

Soya isoflavones may also have beneficial non-hormonal effects. *In vitro* studies have shown that genistein and daidzein have the ability to inhibit the proliferation of some types of neoplastic tissue (Peterson and Barnes 1991, 1993; Lamartiniere 2000). The lipid lowering and cardioprotective effects of soya may also be partly, although not wholly, attributable to its content of isoflavones (Anderson *et al.* 1999; Sirtori 2000).

However, a recent review concluded that the effects of soya isoflavones are complex, and not necessarily uniform in everyone, or even beneficial in all target organs (Anderson *et al.* 1999). Different levels of intake can have different effects; excessive intakes may even have some cancer-enhancing properties (Anderson *et al.* 1999). For these reasons, some have cautioned against the use of isolated supplements of isoflavones until their effects have been explored more fully (Ginsberg and Prelevic 2000; Sirtori 2000).

There have also been concerns over the long-term safety of high intakes of isoflavones by infants and young children. Infants fed soya-based formulae have been found to have an isoflavone intake which is six to 11 times greater on a body weight basis than the amount that produces hormonal effects in adults. Circulating concentrations of isoflavones in soya-fed infants also greatly exceed plasma oestradiol levels in early life and may be sufficient to exert biological effects (Setchell *et al.* 1997). These could potentially impair sexual development and subsequent fertility and reproductive function (Irvine *et al.* 1998), although this remains to be established (Editorial 1996). An investigation by the Committee on Toxicity of Chemicals in Food, Consumer Products and the Environment (COT) found no evidence that the use of soya infant formula had any adverse effects (CMO 1996; MAFF 1998a). However, they also recommended that further research into the long-term effects of phytoestrogen consumption by infants should be carried out.

Sulphur-containing compounds

In animal studies, derivatives of sulphur-containing compounds present in foods of the *Allium* species, such as onions, garlic and leeks, have been found to have the ability to block or suppress carcinogenic mechanisms (DH 1998). Some may also modify the formation, activation or metabolism of carcinogenic substances such as *N*-nitroso compounds. There is some epidemiological evidence that diets containing a high proportion of *Allium* foods may reduce the risk of gastric cancer and colorectal cancers (DH 1998; Fleischauer *et al.* 2000), although this requires further substantiation.

Glucosinolates

Glucosinolates and their derivatives comprise about 120 different compounds found almost exclusively in brassica vegetables such as broccoli, Brussels sprouts, kale, cabbage and cauliflower. Experimental studies have shown that the breakdown products of these compounds, such as thiocyanates and indole-3-carbonol, have anticarcinogenic activity, being capable of inhibiting the induction of cancer via both blocking and suppressing mechanisms. However, these benefits may only apply at modest levels of intake. Human studies have suggested that high brassica intakes (e.g. 5 portions/day) may even increase phase 1 enzyme production and increase the risk of carcinogenesis (DH 1998). More research into their effects in humans is required.

2.9.2 Caffeine and methylxanthines

Caffeine, theophylline and theobromine are part of a group of chemicals called methylxanthines. These occur naturally in a number of plant-derived foodstuffs, in particular coffee, tea, cola drinks and cocoa products. Caffeine may also be added to specially formulated 'energy' drinks or to pharmaceutical products such as cold and flu remedies.

At intake levels of 150–250 mg/day (equivalent to about 4–6 cups of tea or 2–3 cups of instant coffee), caffeine is a mild stimulant and can increase mental alertness. However, individual sensitivity to its physiological effect varies greatly. Psychological factors may also affect the response to caffeine; some people may feel better after a cup of coffee because it provides a rest from other activities, or simply because they expect it to have a beneficial effect (Flaten and Blumenthal 1999).

Caffeine induces mild dependency and if regular caffeine consumption ceases abruptly, symptoms such as headache, irritability, fatigue, reduced alertness and mental performance occur. These are rapidly reversed by consumption of caffeine, and it has been suggested that the beneficial effects of coffee first thing in the morning reflect a reversal of negative effects of caffeine deprivation rather than a genuinely beneficial effect (Rogers and Dernoncourt 1998). Adverse symptoms of caffeine withdrawal disappear spontaneously after a few days.

In the short and medium term, drinking caffeinated coffee increases blood pressure (Nurminen *et al.* 1999; Jee *et al.* 1999) but there is little evidence to suggest that caffeine is a significant long-term contributor to hypertension; most people appear to develop tolerance to the cardiovascular responses (Nurminen *et al.* 1999). However, it cannot be ruled out that people susceptible to hypertension may be more sensitive to any adverse effects on blood pressure.

There is some experimental evidence that coffee can have an adverse effect on CHD risk factors such as blood cholesterol and homocysteine levels (Nygard *et al.* 1997; Grubben *et al.* 2000), but epidemiological prospective studies have failed to find an association between coffee consumption and CHD risk (Willett *et al.* 1996; Woodward and Tunstall-Pedoe 1999).

Caffeine crosses the placenta and women who consume more than 300 mg caffeine/day have been found to produce slightly lower birthweight infants (Hinds 1996), although this observation may be partly attributable to the confounding effect of smoking. Limitation of caffeine intake in pregnancy to below 300 mg/day may be advisable. Since caffeine also passes into breast milk, the same may apply to lactating women.

For the vast majority of the adult population, there is no evidence that current average levels of caffeine intake (about 300 mg/day) cause any harm. However, in children, the high levels of intake that can result from consumption of caffeine-supplemented soft drinks could produce transient behavioural changes such as increased irritability, nervousness or anxiety (MAFF 1999). At present, the EC Scientific Committee for Food advises a maximum content of 125 mg/l caffeine in soft drinks. However, there are no statutory controls in the UK other than the general provisions of the Food Safety Act 1990 (see Section 2.10, Food law).

Table 2.19 Caffeine content of foods and drinks (Figures based on those of MAFF 1998b)

Beverages

Type of product		Range of caffeine content (mg/l)	Average caffeine content per 200 ml serving
Tea	All types	204	40
	From tea bags	245–430	65
	From loose tea	95–105	20
	Instant	175–197	37
	Decaffeinated	5–20	<4
Coffee	Average	405	80
	Instant	210–340	58
	Filter/percolated	304–623[1]	104[1]
	Decaffeinated	10–11	2
Chocolate drinks[2]	All types	5.5–41	1–8
Cola drinks	Standard and sugar free	33–213	7–43
'Energy' drinks	All types	0.5–349 (Most contained >110 mg/l)	58[3]

Foods

Type of product		Range of caffeine content (mg/kg)	Average caffeine content per serving
Chocolate products[2]	Chocolate bar	110–430	5.5–21 (per 50 g bar)
	Chocolate mousse	21–50	2–5 (per 100 g)

[1] Estimated figures based on the average amount of ground coffee used by consumers.
[2] The main stimulant is theobromine.
[3] Based on the median content.

The content of caffeine and methylxanthines in a range of coffees, teas, chocolate products, 'energy' drinks and other soft drinks on sale in the UK has been surveyed by MAFF (1997, 1998b, 1999) and found to vary considerably. The amount of caffeine in a cup of tea depends on the brewing time, leaf size, water to leaf ratio, degree of agitation and water temperature. Different brews of percolated coffee can vary by more than three-fold in caffeine content. Cola drinks (both standard and sugar-free types) tended to fall into one of three bands of caffeine content: about 35 mg/l, 75 mg/l or >100 mg/l. Most 'energy' drinks had much higher caffeine levels than cola drinks, with all but one of 26 samples containing over 110 mg/l, and some containing as much as 350 ml/l.

Theobromine levels were low other than in chocolate products, while theophylline levels were so low as to be largely undetectable. Chocolate products with a high cocoa content (70% cocoa beans) had higher levels of caffeine and theobromine than average brands.

Decaffeinated tea and coffee are not completely caffeine free but usually contain about <5 mg/cup. They contain similar amounts of theobromine and theophylline to the standard products.

Guidance figures on the caffeine content of drinks are summarized in Table 2.19.

2.9.3 Vasoactive amines

Vasoactive amines such as histamine, tyramine, tryptamine and serotonin are present in many foods. Normally they are rapidly deactivated by the body, but high levels of intake or an impaired ability to metabolize them can result in their having significant vasoconstrictive effects. Monoamines can trigger migraine in susceptible individuals (see Section 4.34.4 in Food allergy and intolerance) and cause dangerous hypertensive side-effects in patients taking monoamine oxidase inhibitor type A drugs (see Section 2.12, Drug–nutrient interactions).

Text revised by: Briony Thomas

Further reading

Gutteridge J, Halliwell B. *Antioxidants in Nutrition, Health and Disease*. Oxford: Oxford University Press, 1996.
Halliwell B. Antioxidants and human disease: a general introduction. *Nutrition Reviews* 1997; **55**: 544–552.
Kumpulainen JT, Salonen JT (Eds). *Natural Antioxidants and Food Quality in Atherosclerosis and Cancer Prevention*. Cambridge: Royal Society of Chemistry, 1996.

References

Anderson JJ, Garner SC. Phytoestrogens and bone. *Baillieres Clinical Endocrinology and Metabolism* 1998; **12**: 543–557.
Anderson JJ, Anthony MS, Cline JM *et al*. Health potential of soy isoflavones for menopausal women. *Public Health Nutrition* 1999; **2**: 489–504.
Balentine DA, Wiseman SA, Vouwens LCM *et al*. The chemistry of tea flavonoids. *Critical Reviews in Food Science and Nutrition* 1997; **37**: 693–704.
Brune M, Rossander L, Hallberg L. Iron absorption and phenolic compounds: importance of different phenolic structures. *European Journal of Clinical Nutrition* 1989; **43**: 547–557.
Cao F, Sofic E, Prior RL. Antioxidant capacity of tea and common vegetables. *Journal of Agricultural and Food Chemistry* 1996; **44**: 3426–3431.
Cassidy A, Bingham S, Setchell KDR. Biologic effects of a diet of soy protein rich in isoflavones on the menstrual cycle of pre-

menopausal women. *American Journal of Clinical Nutrition* 1994; **60**: 333–340.

Chief Medical Officer. *Phytoestrogens in Soya Infant Formula Milk*. London: Department of Health, 1996.

Cook NC, Sammen S. Flavonoids – chemistry, metabolism, cardioprotective effects and dietary sources. *Nutrition and Biochemistry* 1996; **7**: 66–76.

Department of Health. Report of the Cardiovascular Review Group of the Committee on Medical Aspects of Food Policy (COMA). *Nutritional Aspects of Cardiovascular Disease*. Report on Health and Social Subjects 46. London: HMSO, 1994.

Department of Health. Report of the Working Group on Diet and Cancer of the Committee on Medical Aspects of Food and Nutrition Policy (COMA). *Nutritional Aspects of the Development of Cancer*. Report on Health and Social Subjects 48. London: The Stationery Office, 1998.

Disler PB, Lynch SR, Charlton RW *et al*. The effect of tea on iron absorption. *Gut* 1975; **16**: 193–200.

Editorial. Phytoestrogens and soy based infant formula. *British Medical Journal* 1996; **313**: 507–508.

Flaten MA, Blumenthal TD. Caffeine-associated stimuli elicit conditioned responses: an experimental model of the placebo effect. *Psychopharmacology* 1999; **145**: 105–112.

Fleischauer AT, Poole C, Arab L. Garlic consumption and cancer prevention: meta-analyses of colorectal and stomach cancers. *American Journal of Clinical Nutrition* 2000; **72**: 1047–1052.

Formica JV, Regelson W. Review of the biology of quercetin and related bioflavonoids. *Food and Chemical Toxicology* 1995; **33**: 1061–1080.

Francheschi S, Bidoli E, La veccia C *et al*. Tomatoes and risk of digestive-tract cancers. *International Journal of Cancer* 1994; **59**: 181–184.

Gerster H. The potential role of lycopene for human health. *Journal of the American College of Nutrition* 1997; **16**: 109–126.

Ginsberg J, Prelevic GM. Lack of significant hormonal effects and controlled trials of phytoestrogens. *Lancet* 2000; **355**: 163.

Giovannucci E, Ascherio A, Rimm EB *et al*. Intake of carotenoids and retinol in relation to risk of prostate cancer. *Journal of the National Cancer Institute* 1995; **87**: 1767–1776.

Grubben MJ, Boers GH, Blom HJ *et al*. Unfiltered coffee increases plasma homocysteine concentrations in healthy volunteers: a randomized trial. *American Journal of Clinical Nutrition* 2000; **71**: 480–484.

Hertog MGL, Feskens EJ, Hollman PC *et al*. Dietary antioxidant flavonoids and risk of coronary heart disease: the Zutphen Elderly Study. *Lancet* 1993; **342**: 1007–1011.

Hertog MGL, Kromhout D, Aravanis C *et al*. Flavonoid intake and long-term risk of coronary heart disease and cancer in the Seven Countries Study. *Archives of Internal Medicine* 1995; **155**: 381–386.

Hinds TS, West WL, Knight EM, Harland BF. The effect of caffeine on pregnancy outcome variables. *Nutrition Reviews* 1996; **54**: 203–207.

Hollman P, Tijburg LBM, Yang CS. Bioavailability of flavonoids in tea. *Critical Reviews in Food Science and Nutrition* 1997; **37**: 719–738.

Irvine CH, Fitzpatrick MG, Alexander SL. Phytoestrogens in soy-based infant foods: concentrations, daily intake and possible biological effects. *Proceedings of the Society for Experimental Biology and Medicine* 1998; **217**: 386–392.

Jee SH, He J, Whelton PK *et al*. The effect of chronic coffee drinking on blood pressure: a meta-analysis of controlled clinical trials. *Hypertension* 1999; **33**: 647–652.

Knekt P, Jarvinen R, Reunanen A, Maatela J. Flavonoid intake and coronary mortality in Finland: a cohort study. *British Medical Journal* 1996; **312**: 478–481.

Kohlmeier L, Kark JD, Gomez-Gracia E *et al*. Lycopene and myocardial infarction risk in the EURAMIC study. *American Journal of Epidemiology* 1997; **146**: 618–626.

Lamartiniere CA. Protection against breast cancer with genistein: a component of soy. *American Journal of Clinical Nutrition* 2000; **71** (6 Suppl): 1705S–1707S.

Leenen R, Roodenburg AJ, Tijburg LB *et al*. A single dose of tea with or without milk increases plasma antioxidant activity in humans. *European Journal of Clinical Nutrition* 1999; **53**: 1–6.

Lissin LW, Cooke JP. Phytoestrogens and cardiovascular health. *Journal of the American College of Cardiologists* 2000; **35**: 1403–1410.

Lu LJ, Anderson KE, Grady JJ *et al*. Decreased ovarian hormones during a soya diet: implications for breast cancer prevention. *Cancer Research* 2000; **60**: 4112–4121.

MAFF Food Safety Directorate. Survey of caffeine and other methylxanthines in energy drinks and other caffeine-containing products. *Food Surveillance Information Sheet* 103, March 1997.

MAFF. Soya infant formulae. *Food Safety Information Bulletin* 1998a; 102 (November): 10.

MAFF Food Safety Directorate. Survey of caffeine and other methylxanthines in energy drinks and other caffeine-containing products (Updated information). *Food Surveillance Information Sheet* 144, March 1998b.

MAFF. Caffeine in soft drinks. *Food Safety Information Bulletin* 1999; 109 (June): 13.

Messina M, Messina V. Soyfoods, soybean isoflavones and bone health: a brief overview. *Journal of Renal Nutrition* 2000; **10**: 63–68.

Nurminen ML, Niittynen L, Korpela R, Vapaatalo H. Coffee, caffeine and blood pressure: a critical review. *European Journal of Clinical Nutrition* 1999; **53**: 831–839.

Nygard O, Refsum H, Ueland PM *et al*. Coffee consumption and plasma total homocysteine: the Hordaland Homocysteine Study. *American Journal of Clinical Nutrition* 1997; **65**: 136–143.

Peterson TG, Barnes S. Genistein inhibition of the growth of human breast cancer cells: independence from oestrogen receptors and the multi-drug resistance gene. *Biochemistry and Biophysics Research Communications* 1991; **179**: 661–667.

Peterson TG, Barnes S. Genistein and biochanin A inhibit the growth of human prostate cancer cells but not as epidermal growth factor receptor tyrosine autophosphorylation. *Prostate* 1993; **22**: 335–345.

Rapola JM, Virtamo J, Ripatti S *et al*. Randomised trial of alpha-tocopherol and B-carotene supplements on incidence of major coronary events in men with previous myocardial infarction. *Lancet* 1997; **349**: 1715–1720.

Rogers PJ, Dernoncourt C. Regular caffeine consumption: a balance of adverse and beneficial effects for mood and psychomotor performance. *Pharmacology, Biochemistry and Behavior* 1998; **59**: 1039–1045.

Setchell KDR, Nechemias LZ, Cai J, Heubi J. Exposure of infants to phyto-oestrogens from soy-based infant formula. *Lancet* 1997; **350**: 23–27.

Sirtori CR. Dubious benefits and potential risk of soy phytoestrogens. *Lancet* 2000; **355**: 849.

Tijburg LBM, Mattern T, Folts JD *et al*. Tea flavonoids and cardiovascular disease: a review. *Critical Reviews in Food Science and Nutrition* 1997; **37**: 771–785.

van het Hof KH, Kivits GAA, Westrate JA, Tijburg LBM. Bioavailability of catechins from tea: the effect of milk. *European Journal of Clinical Nutrition* 1998; **52**: 356–359.

Vinson J *et al*. Plant flavonoids, especially tea flavonoids, are powerful antioxidants using an *in vitro* oxidation model for heart disease. *Journal of Agricultural and Food Chemistry* 1995; **43**: 2800–2802.

Willett WC, Stampfer MJ, Manson JE *et al*. Coffee consumption and coronary heart disease in women. A ten-year follow-up. *Journal of the American Medical Association* 1996; **275**: 458–462.

Wiseman SA, Balentine DA, Frei B. Antioxidants in tea. *Critical Reviews in Food Science and Nutrition* 1997; **37**: 719–738.

Woodward M, Tunstall-Pedoe H. Coffee and tea consumption in the Scottish Heart Health Study follow-up: conflicting relations with coronary risk factors, coronary disease and all-cause mortality. *Journal of Epidemiology and Community Health* 1999; **53**: 481–487.

Wu AH, Stanczyk FZ, Hendrich S *et al*. Effects of soy foods on ovarian function in premenopausal women. *British Journal of Cancer* 2000; **82**: 1879–1886.

2.10 Food law

2.10.1 History of food legislation in the UK

The earliest record of food legislation in this country was an act passed in 1266 which protected the purchaser against sale of unsound meat and short weight in bread. Whilst apparently far sighted, the enforcement of the act left a lot to be desired and was largely ineffective. However, guilds, which played a very important role at that time, helped to ensure that the commodities were as pure as possible. This meant checking a commodity such as pepper to ensure that there was no added gravel, leaves or twigs, checking coffee to ensure that there was no added grass, acorns or lard, and checking bread to ensure that no mashed potato, sand or ashes had been added.

As the population grew, the industrial revolution caused a massive shift from country to town; more people needed to be fed and a larger proportion of them were no longer able to grow their own food and became dependent on others for its supply. By the middle of the nineteenth century the abuses were appalling. Increased publicity to the problem of food adulteration was now being given in both the scientific journals and popular press of the day and as a result public pressure led to the establishment of a Select Committee on Food Adulteration. After much dissatisfaction concerning its effectiveness, another committee was set up, the result of which was the 1875 Sale of Food and Drugs Act. This Act is the basis of present UK law and includes the statement fundamental to current practice:

> No person shall sell to the prejudice of the purchaser any article of food or any food thing which is not of the nature, substance or quality demanded by such purchasers.

By the end of the nineteenth century, significant improvements had been made to the purity of basic commodities, in that bread, flour and coffee were no longer adulterated. The 1875 act remained in force until 1928, when it was replaced by the consolidated Food and Drugs (Adulteration) Act. It was at this time that regulations pertaining to food composition and labelling were first introduced.

In 1943 the Food and Drugs Act combined all previous legislation concerning the retailing of foodstuffs. This act was the basis of government control during the war years. In 1955 the Food and Drug Act came into being and was to remain the basis of food legislation until general legislation covering the composition, labelling, hygiene and safety of food in the UK was introduced in 1984 by the

Food Act. (The 'drug' aspect was superseded by the Medicines Act in 1968, and since 1974 has no longer been included in this schedule.)

In view of the considerable changes that had occurred in both food production and eating habits in the previous 50 years, food legislation became increasingly criticized for being out of date. As a result, food legislation underwent the first major review since the 1940s, culminating in the Food Safety Act 1990.

2.10.2 Current UK food legislation

Legislation relating to food can be primary or secondary. Primary legislation comes under an act (e.g. the Food Safety Act 1990 or Weights and Measures Act 1985). Regulations and orders made under an act (e.g. The Food Labelling Regulations 1996) are termed secondary legislation.

The Food Safety Act

The Food Safety Act 1990 is the primary UK legislation on food safety and consumer protection in Great Britain. A separate but similar law applies in Northern Ireland. The act provides the framework for UK food law and does not, in itself, contain the specific rules governing matters such as the safety, quality, description or labelling of food. These details are set out in regulations and orders (secondary legislation) made under the act. Codes of practice can also be issued under Section 40 of the Food Safety Act 1990. These are documents issued by ministers for the guidance of food authorities, the provisions for which can be enforced by direction and court order.

The aims of the Food Safety Act are to:

- ensure that all food produced for sale is safe to eat, meets quality expectations and is not misleadingly presented
- provide legal powers and penalties
- enable the UK to fulfil its responsibilities in the European Union (EU)
- keep pace with technological change.

The Food Safety Act 1990 is in four main parts.

Part I: Preliminary

This sets out the full scope of the act and the responsibilities for those involved in enforcing it. The scope of the Food Act 1990 is much more extensive than previous legislation. It covers the whole of Great Britain and its definitions of food and premises are wider, with the former now including slimming aids and dietary supplements as well as tap water, and the latter including most Crown properties as well as ships and aircraft. It provides provision for regulations covering all aspects of food production, processing and selling, from the farm to the retailer.

The act also sets out the principle that local authorities are responsible for enforcing most aspects of food law.

Part II: Main provisions

The main provisions of the act, namely food safety, consumer protection, regulation-making powers and defences, are covered in this part of the act.

Offences The main offences under the Food Safety Act are:

- selling, or possessing for sale, food which does not comply with food safety requirements
- rendering food injurious to health
- selling, to the purchaser's prejudice, food which is not of the nature or substance or quality demanded
- falsely or misleadingly describing or presenting food.

'Food safety requirements' apply to food throughout the food chain, not just that for retail sale. Food is 'injurious to health' if it could harm part of the population in either the short term (e.g. cause food poisoning) or long term (e.g. is contaminated with lead). 'Not of the nature or substance demanded' means that it is illegal to sell cod described as haddock, or cola instead of diet cola. A 'purchaser' can range from a customer at a shop to one supplier buying from another. 'Falsely or misleadingly described or presented' applies to written statements or pictorial representations which are untrue. (Additional constraints are also laid down in the Food Labelling Regulations 1995.)

Defences A new aspect of food legislation introduced under this act was that 'due diligence' is grounds for defence. Thus, for example, a retailer who unwittingly sold a contaminated food would not be guilty if it can be shown that the contamination occurred at an earlier stage in the supply chain and that the retailer could not have known that the product was unfit for sale. In practice, this means that the onus is on the food industry and food importers to supply safe food, and is considered to be a far-reaching and important aspect of the act.

Novel foods The act also contains powers to make regulations covering the sale of novel foods, i.e. those which are new or which have only been rarely eaten in this country. There is a system of prior approval for the marketing of foods resulting from genetic modification.

Part III: Administration and enforcement

This lays down procedures for the sampling and analysis of products, powers of entry, obstruction and enforcement. It also deals with legal aspects of prosecution and appeal procedures.

Part IV: Miscellaneous and supplemental

This covers the issuing of codes of practice to food authorities on the execution and enforcement of legislation, and directions on specific steps to be taken to comply with a code. Other details pertain to areas of coverage of the act and other aspects of its implementation.

Other food-related UK legislation

Several other Acts of Parliament, and their subsidiary regulations, also impact in various ways on the provision, sale or safety of food, and the main ones are listed below.

European Communities Act 1972

Because the UK is a member of the EU, its regulations and directives also have to be implemented. European regulations are effective in all member states as soon as they are adopted. European directives, in contrast, do not become effective until they are written into a country's own legislation in the form of regulations. Section 2(2) of the European Communities Act makes provision for any designated minister or department to make regulations in order to implement the UK's European obligations.

The Trade Descriptions Act 1968

This makes it an offence to make false or misleading statements about goods, services, accommodation or facilities.

The Prices Act 1974

Regulations made under this act require prices to be displayed on any premises where food or drink is offered for sale.

The Weights and Measures Act 1985

This makes short weight an offence. Most pre-packed food is required to carry an indication of net content and non-pre-packaged food has to be sold by either quantity or number. Trading standards officers enforce the provisions of this act.

The Consumer Protection Act 1987

Part I imposes civil liability for damage caused by defective products (including food). Part II provides for secondary legislation relating to consumer safety (e.g. governing the use of food contact materials). Part III makes it an offence for a consumer to be given a misleading indication of the price at which goods are available.

International Carriage of Perishable Food Stuffs Act 1976

Regulations made under this act govern the standards for the transport of perishable foodstuffs.

The Animal Health Act 1981

This provides powers to control diseases in animals which could pose a risk to human health, e.g. brucellosis, salmonella and bovine spongiform encephalopathy (BSE).

The Medicines Act 1968

This controls the manufacture and marketing of medicinal products for humans and animals.

Public Health (Control of Disease) Act 1984

Regulations made under Part II enable local authorities to impose controls to prevent the spread of food poisoning and food-borne infections in persons involved in the food trade.

Public Health (Scotland) Acts 1982 to 1907

Sections 58 and 59 prohibit infected persons engaging in any occupation connected with food unless proper precautions have been taken against spreading disease or infection.

The Agriculture Act 1970 (as amended)

This covers the use of fertilizers and animal feedstuffs.

The Food and Environment Protection Act 1985

This governs the control of pesticides and maximum permitted residue levels in food, crops and feeding stuffs.

Environmental Protection Act 1990

Part VI aims to prevent or minimize damage to the environment caused by the release of genetically modified organisms, and imposes restrictions on the importation, acquisition, release or marketing of such organisms.

Regulations

Most of the key provisions in food law are contained in regulations which set out the specific details governing matters such as:

- food labelling
- food hygiene
- animal, meat and meat products (e.g. those concerned with the examination for residues and maximum residue limits)
- registration of food premises
- regulations on milk and dairies
- food composition
- use of food additives
- use of food packaging materials.

Regulations may also be introduced in order to implement European directives (e.g. the Food Labelling Regulations 1996 which implement EC Food Labelling Directive 79/112/EC on nutrition labelling for foodstuffs).

New regulations introduced under the Food Safety Act 1990 include those concerned with:

- *Registration*: Premises used for food business now have to be registered with their local authority. These include premises, vehicles and market stalls used by charities, or at events where catering is provided over several consecutive days (e.g. at conference or sports events).
- *Training for food handlers*: The act requires that all those handling food should be trained to an appropri-

ate level in hygiene, and be shown to be competent in such practices through independent assessment.

Regulations are kept under review and subject to change (in the form of amendments), either as a result of that review or in order to harmonize food law within the EU.

Some important regulations pertaining to food are listed in Table 2.20.

2.10.3 Law enforcement

Most of the responsibility for enforcing the Food Safety Act lies with local authorities. However, central government is responsible for overseeing the work of the local authorities and advising them on enforcement via statutory codes of practice (e.g. relating to the timing and frequency of inspections). Central government also enforces some regulations such as those relating to licences for irradiated foods, and has the scope to become involved in certain emergency situations or where a local authority fails to discharge its duty under the act. The State Veterinary Service and Meat Hygiene Service may be involved in enforcement action on farms and at slaughterhouses, respectively.

Local authorities are responsible for enforcing the law in two main areas:

- Trading standards officers deal with the labelling of food, its composition and most cases of chemical contamination.
- Environmental health officers deal with hygiene, with cases of microbiological contamination of foods and with food which for any reason, including chemical contamination, is unfit for human consumption.

Under the Food Safety Act, local authority officers may, by right:

- enter any food premises to investigate possible offences
- take away samples for investigation
- detain suspect food or ask for it to be destroyed through local court procedures
- require food hygiene to be improved or, in an extreme case, close down premises if they are considered to be a public health risk.

In the non-metropolitan areas of England, trading standards work is carried out by county councils and environmental health work by district councils. London boroughs and metropolitan authorities carry out both functions, as do the unitary authorities in Wales. In Scotland, most food law enforcement is carried out by environmental health departments of district and island councils. In Northern Ireland, the work is carried out by environmental health departments of district councils.

Throughout the UK, public analysts are responsible for carrying out chemical analysis of food, and food examiners are responsible for microbiological examination of food. They both form an integral part of the enforcement team.

Table 2.20 Some important regulations relating to food

Regulation	Purpose
The Food Labelling Regulations 1996	Regulate the labelling, presentation and advertising of food for sale to the consumer (except for provisions relating to net quantity and certain additives) Implement EC directives relating to the use of claims for foods, nutrition labelling and labelling of alcoholic strength
The Food Labelling (Amendment) Regulations 1998	Introduced Quantitative Ingredients Declaration (QUID) and the requirement for origin of starch and modified starch to be declared on ingredients lists
The Sweeteners in Foods Regulations 1995 (and 1997 amendments)	Implement EC directives laying down specific criteria governing the use of sweeteners in foodstuffs
The Colours in Food Regulations 1995	Implement EC directives laying down specific criteria governing the use of colours in foodstuffs.
The Flavourings in Food Regulations 1992 (and 1994 amendments)	Implement EC directives on the use of flavourings in foods
The Miscellaneous Food Additives Regulations 1995 (and later amendments)	Implement EC directives on food additives, other than colours and sweeteners, together with various directives governing purity criteria
Lot Marking Regulations 1996	Implement an EC directive establishing a common batch-identification system to facilitate product recall along the whole of the food chain when a product constitutes a health risk to consumers
The Foods Intended for Use in Energy Restricted Diets for Weight Reduction Regulations 1997	Implement an EC directive on foods intended for use in energy-restricted diets for weight reduction
The Materials and Articles in Contact with Food Regulations 1987 (and later amendments)	Control the use of food-contact materials with the aim of ensuring that they do not transfer their constituents to food in quantities which could endanger human health or make food otherwise unacceptable to consumers
The Plastic Materials and Articles in Contact with Food Regulations 1998	Control the use of plastic packaging materials
The Cooking Utensils (Safety) Regulations 1972	Control the composition of coatings on kitchen utensils
The Ceramic Ware (Safety) Regulations 1988	Implement an EC directive setting limits for the migration of lead and cadmium from ceramic articles
The Mineral Hydrocarbons in Food Regulations 1996	Prohibit the use of hydrocarbons in the composition or preparation of food, apart from in some lubricants, chewing compounds and cheese rind
The Tryptophan in Food Regulations 1990	Prohibit the addition of tryptophan (an amino acid) to food intended for human consumption
The Lead in Food Regulations 1979 (and later amendments)	Lay down a general permitted limit of 1 mg/kg for lead in food
The Tin in Food Regulations 1992	Prohibit for sale or import any food containing a level of tin exceeding 200 mg/kg
The Pesticide (Maximum Residue Levels in Crops, Food and Feeding Stuffs) Regulations 1994 (and later amendments)	Set maximum residue levels (MRLs) for fruit, vegetables, cereals and animal products
The Animal and Animal Products (Examination for Residues and Maximum Residue Limit) Regulations 1997	Made under the European Communities Act 1972, these continue the ban on the use of hormonal growth promoters in food-producing animals within the EC and extend it to beta-agonists in some circumstances Harmonize, improve and extend the controls on the surveillance of veterinary medicinal residues in meat
The Food (Control of Irradiation) Regulations 1990	Implement the control system governing the production and safety of irradiated food
The Novel Foods and Novel Food Ingredients Regulations 1997	Introduced a Community-wide premarket approval system for all novel foods (including genetically modified foods)
EC Council Regulation EC No. 1139/98 concerning the compulsory indication of the labelling of certain foodstuffs produced from genetically modified organisms	Requires the presence of genetically modified protein or DNA in a food to be declared
The Food Safety (General Food Hygiene) Regulations 1995	Implement an EC directive requiring food business proprietors to ensure that their activities are carried out in a hygienic way
The Food Safety (Temperature Control) Regulations 1995	Require food business proprietors to observe temperature controls on the holding of food, where otherwise there would be a risk to health
The Organic Products Regulations 1992	Implement EC directives relating to the production and sale of organic foods

(Continued overleaf)

Table 2.20 Some important regulations relating to food (continued)

Additional specific regulations apply to the composition of foods such as:
  Bread and flour
  Cocoa and chocolate products
  Drinking milk, condensed and dried milk honey
  Spreadable fats
  Categories of foods such as infant formula and follow-on formula, and weaning foods

Specific hygiene regulations relate to the production of:
  Milk and milk products
  Ice-Cream
  Fishery products and live shellfish
  Meat
  Meat products
  Minced meat and meat preparations
  Animal byproducts

More details of these regulations and amendments can be found in *Food Law* (see Further reading at the end of this section).

At the extreme end of such control, when for example shutting down a food premises is insufficient to limit further contaminated food reaching the consumer, the Food Safety Act gives the government power to make emergency control orders.

2.10.4 International food legislation

Since food is both imported into and exported from the UK, legislation on standards of composition and labelling has to be compatible with, and in some instances, comply with, international standards.

European Union

Membership of the EU means that the UK is required to implement European regulations and directives and, as described above, this is now a major influence on UK food legislation.

The Codex Alimentarius Commission

Usually known as 'Codex', this sets worldwide food standards. It is the joint body of two United Nations organizations: the Food and Agriculture Organization (FAO) and the World Health Organization (WHO). Codex sets out to establish procedures and principles that are acceptable to member countries in relation to meeting agreed standards for food in international trade and to help to lower trade barriers. Codex recommendations have no statutory force but, where possible, are incorporated into European, and hence UK, legislation.

2.10.5 Monitoring food quality and safety

In the UK, the Food Standards Agency (FSA) provides advice to government on matters relating to the quality and safety of food (a responsibility formerly shared between the Department of Health and the Ministry of Agriculture,

Fisheries and Food). The FSA does this on the basis of expert guidance from a number of independent advisory scientific committees.

The principal advisory committee is the Food Advisory Committee (FAC), which provides guidance on any issue which impacts on the labelling, composition and safety of food. In order to do this, the FAC works closely with, and often seeks advice from, other scientific committees, in particular:

- The Committee on Toxicity of Chemicals in Food, Consumer Products and the Environment (COT): COT assesses and advises on the toxic risk to humans of a wide range of substances affecting everyday life. This may include evaluation of data on substances used or proposed for use as food additives, or substances which might contaminate food either naturally or during the food production process.
- The Advisory Committee on the Microbiological Safety of Food (ACMSF): This assesses the risk to humans of micro-organisms which are used or occur in food, and on matters relating to the microbiological safety of food.
- The Advisory Committee on Novel Foods and Processes (ACNFP): This provides advice on any matters relating to novel foods and processes, including food irradiation.

Other scientific committees which may provide advice to the FAC include:

- The Advisory Committee on Animal Feedingstuffs
- Committee on Mutagenicity of Chemicals in Food, Consumer Products and the Environment (CoM)
- Committee on Carcinogenicity of Chemicals in Food, Consumer Products and the Environment (CoC)
- Spongiform Encephalopathy Advisory Committee (SEAC)
- Expert group on Vitamins and Minerals (EVM).

Guidance can also be sought from the food working parties on:

- Chemical Contaminants in Food
- Chemical Contaminants from Food Contact Materials and Articles
- Dietary Surveys
- Food Additives
- Food Authenticity
- Nutrients in Food
- Radionuclides in Food.

Another key committee to the work of the FSA is the Scientific Advisory Committee on Nutrition (SACN), which has replaced the Committee on Medical Aspects of Food Policy (COMA). The role of the SACN is to advise the Chief Medical Officer, FSA or government on scientific aspects of nutrition and health, with particular reference to:

- the nutrient content of individual foods and advice on diet as a whole, including the definition of a balanced diet and the nutritional status of people
- monitoring and surveillance of the above
- wider public health policy issues where nutritional status is one of a number of risk factors, e.g. cardiovascular disease, cancer, osteoporosis and obesity
- vulnerable groups, e.g. infants, elderly people or disadvantaged people
- research requirements.

The FSA also oversees the UK's food surveillance programme, which monitors the microbiological, radiological and chemical safety of food.

More details of the role and responsibilities of the FSA and reports of the work of the advisory committees can be obtained from the FSA website (see Useful addresses at the end of this section).

Text revised by: Briony Thomas

Useful addresses

Department of Health
Richmond House, 79 Whitehall, London SW1A 2NL
Tel: 020 7210 4850
E-mail: dhmail@doh.gsi.gov.uk
Website: www.doh.gov.uk

Food Standards Agency
Room 6/21, Hannibal House, PO Box 30080, London SE1 6YA
Fax: 020 7238 6330
E-mail: helpline@foodstandards.gsi.gov.uk
Website: www.foodstandards.gov.uk

Food Standards Agency (Scotland),
St Magnus House, 6th Floor, 25 Guild Street, Aberdeen AB11 6NJ
Fax: 01224 28516

Food Standards Agency (Wales),
1st Floor, Southgate House, Wood Street, Cardiff CF10 1EW
Fax: 029 2067 8918/9

Food Standards Agency (Northern Ireland),
10B and 10C Clarendon Quay, Clarendon Dock, Clarendon Road, Belfast BT1 3BW
Fax: 028 9041 7726

Ministry of Agriculture, Fisheries and Food (MAFF)
3–8 Whitehall Place, London SW1A 2HH
Helpline: 0645 335577   Fax: 020 7270 8419
E-mail: helpline@maff.gsi.gov.uk
Website: www.maff.gov.uk

MAFF Publications
Admail 6000, London SW1A 2XX
Telephone orders (for free publications): 08459 556000

The Stationery Office
Details of their bookshops and online ordering can be found on their website at: www.tsonline.co.uk

Further reading

Food Standards Agency. *Food Law* (a freely available document containing guidance information on UK food legislation. Can be consulted or downloaded from the FSA website at: www.foodstandards.gov.uk/regulations/foodlaw.htm).
MAFF Food Sense booklets (available free from MAFF Publications (see Useful Addresses, above):
The Food Safety Act and You – A Guide (PB 2507).
The Food Safety Act 1990 and You: A Guide for the Food Industry (PB2507).
The Food Safety Act 1990 and You: A Guide for Caterers and their Employees (PB0370).
The Food Safety Act 1990 and You: A Guide for Farmers and Growers (PB0371).

2.11 Food and nutrition labelling

Food labelling is principally controlled by the Food Labelling Regulations 1996 (and later amendments) made under the Food Safety Act 1990 (see Section 2.10, Food law).

These Regulations set out the general requirements for the labelling, presentation and advertising of food for sale to the consumer (except for those relating to certain additives which are covered by other regulations). They also:

- make special provision for the labelling of
  - food which is not pre-packed and certain similar foods
  - fancy confectionery products
  - food which is packed in small packages and indelibly marked bottles
  - certain foods sold at catering establishments
  - seasonal selection packs
- specify additional labelling requirements for food sold from vending machines and for alcoholic drinks
- require warnings to be given with raw milk (health warning) and products consisting of skimmed milk together with non-milk fat (unsuitable for babies)
- specify an additional labelling requirement for food packaged in a gas to extend its durability
- specify additional labelling requirements for food containing sweeteners, added sugar and sweeteners, aspartame or more than 10% polyols
- specify requirements as to the manner of marking or labelling of food
- prohibit a claim in the labelling or advertising of a food that it has tonic or medicinal properties, and impose conditions for the making of claims relating to foods for particular uses and for claims relating to low energy value, protein, vitamins, minerals, cholesterol or nutrition content
- specify labelling requirements for nutrition information, whether or not a nutrition claim is also being made
- impose certain restrictions on the use of certain words and description in the labelling or advertising of food
- permit the use of the word 'wine' in composite names for drinks other than wine or table wine.

2.11.1 Food labelling

The Food Labelling Regulations require that all food supplied to either the consumer or a catering establishment (subject to certain exceptions) be marked or labelled with:

- the name of the food
- a list of ingredients
- an indication of its durability, either a 'best before' a 'use by' date
- any special storage conditions or conditions of use
- the name and an address of the of the manufacturer or packer, or of a seller established within the European Union (EC).

In certain circumstances it may be necessary to provide:

- particulars of the place of origin of the food, if failure to give such particulars might mislead
- instructions for use if it would be difficult to make appropriate use of the food in the absence of such instructions.

There are less onerous rules for foods which are non-pre-packed or pre-packed on the premises of sale.

Product name

This is required to be a clear description of the product, e.g. 'pilchards in tomato sauce'. If the product has a non-descriptive brand name (e.g. 'Marmite') some indication of its nature must be given (e.g. 'yeast extract'). The name must also indicate whether the form has undergone any form of processing, e.g. 'UHT milk' or 'smoked mackerel'. Descriptions must also not be misleading: if a product is described as 'raspberry yoghurt' then it must contain raspberries, not just raspberry flavouring. Some foods have 'customary names', e.g. 'cream crackers' do not contain cream but the name is considered to be sufficiently familiar not to be misleading. Other foods have 'prescribed' names with strict rules governing their use, e.g. 'margarine' has to contain 80% fat; if it contains less than this it must be called something else such as a 'spread'.

Ingredients

These are given in descending order of content so, for example, if water is the first item listed, then water is the largest ingredient. Until recently, food ingredients lists only provided a limited guide to food quality (e.g. whether a hamburger contains cereal filler as well as meat). Since 2000, this ability has been strengthened by the EC requirement for Quantitative Ingredients Declaration (QUID). Most food products now have to state the quantity of any ingredients which:

- appear in the name of a food or which are usually associated with that name by consumers
- are emphasized on the label in either words, pictures or graphics

- are essential to characterize the food and to distinguish it from products with which it might be confused because of its name or appearance.

Declarations must appear in, or next to, the name of the food, or in the ingredients list, and must be shown as a percentage (based on the amount of the ingredient used at the manufacturing stage). The aim is to help the consumer to compare the quality of similar foods by being able to see how much ham and mushroom is in a 'ham and mushroom pizza' or pork in 'pork sausages'.

For the purposes of food exclusion, ingredients lists can be useful to confirm that a food component such as wheat or gluten is *present* in a food. They do not, however, necessarily confirm that something is *absent*, because not all ingredients will necessarily be declared. Those which are part of a compound ingredient comprising less than 25% of the finished product do not have to be itemized separately. A compound ingredient (such as 'sponge cake' in a fruit trifle) may therefore be a source of hidden ingredients (such as milk, wheat and eggs). The ingredients of certain foods regarded as being of standard composition (such as butter and vinegar) also do not need to be declared. However, in order to make it easier for people to avoid gluten, it is now a requirement that the origin of starch or modified starch in an ingredients list is stated (i.e. whether it is derived from wheat, maize or other cereal; see Section 4.9, Coeliac disease).

Any additives that form part of compound ingredients usually have to be declared. However, residual amounts of additives remaining from a previous processing stage will not always be listed. For example, sulphite is often added to fruit to preserve it, and if the fruit is made into jam, some sulphite may remain in the finished product. If however, the amount carried over is too small to have any preservative effect on the jam, it need not be declared. The other exemption which may be important to dietitians is bread and bread flour. Flour is considered to be a single-ingredient food and, provided only the additives stipulated in the Bread and Flour Regulations are used, they need not appear on the label. Additives used solely as processing aids (e.g. tin-greasing agents), solvents or carriers of flavours also do not have to be listed.

As well as guidance on the use and limitations of food ingredients lists, consumers who need to avoid specific dietary components often also need guidance on the ways in which foods may be described on ingredients lists, e.g. 'milk' could be present in the form of whey, casein or lactoglobulin, or in many other guises (see Section 4.35, Food exclusion in the management of food allergy and intolerance).

Durability

This must be indicated by either a 'use by' or 'best before' date, and there is an important difference between the two. Highly perishable fresh foods (e.g. dairy products) must have a 'use by' date and after this time it should be assumed that the food is no longer safe to eat. To mini-

mize the risk of food poisoning, 'use by' dates should be strictly observed.

The 'best before' date applies to foods with a shelf life of weeks, months or even years (e.g. breakfast cereals or canned foods). After this date there may be some deterioration in the quality of the texture and flavour of the product, but the food will not necessarily be unsafe to eat.

In all cases, if any special storage conditions such as refrigeration are necessary, these must be shown close to the 'use by' or 'best before' date.

Quantity

Under separate Weights and Measures legislation, most foods are required to state the amount provided, either in terms of quantity (e.g. 200 g or 500 ml) or by number if the product is sold in units (e.g. 6 jam tarts). Net weight or volume of the contents may be indicated by the 'e' symbol, which means that the amount is an average figure; the contents of each product may vary slightly within strictly defined limits.

2.11.2 Claims

Types of claims which may be made in relation to foods are:

- *nutrition claims*, that the food is a source of a particular nutrient, or contains less or more of a nutrient than a standard product
- *health claims*, that the food is in some way beneficial to health (medicinal claims, i.e. that a food can prevent, treat or cure a human disease or a symptom of a disease, are not permitted unless a food is licensed as a medicine)
- *claims for particular nutritional uses*, that the food is suitable for particular nutritional purposes.

Nutrition claims

Nutrition claims can be a useful way of conveying information to consumers and helping them to choose foods with particular nutritional features. However, they need to be able to do so without being misled. Currently, the Food Labelling Regulations 1996 cover some nutrition claims but by no means all. Statutory requirements are only attached to claims that a food is:

- reduced or low in energy
- a source, or rich source, of protein
- a source, or rich source, of vitamins or minerals
- cholesterol free.

Because of the limited scope of this legislation, voluntary guidelines on claims made for other nutrients such as fat, saturates, sugars, sodium and fibre were drawn up by MAFF in consultation with the food industry (MAFF 1993, revised 1999). These cannot be legally enforced but most food manufacturers comply with the defined criteria. The voluntary guidelines on nutrition claims (which also incorporate the statutory requirements) are summarized in Table 2.21.

At the time of writing (2000), all nutrition claims legislation is under review by the EU, which is considering adopting the International Standards for Nutrition Claims set by FAO/WHO Codex Alimentarius Commission (FAO 1998). These set criteria for claims relating to energy, fat, saturated fat, cholesterol, sugars and sodium and are broadly similar to (although slightly more stringent than) those devised by MAFF.

Health claims

At present, existing law prohibits the claim that a particular food can prevent, treat or cure disease. It is permissible to state or imply that a food may in some way benefit health by mentioning a disease risk factor (e.g. 'can help to reduce blood cholesterol'), a nutrient's physiological function ('calcium can help to build strong bones') or general lifestyle (e.g. 'breakfast is a good start to your day'), as long as the information is true and does not mislead the consumer. However, the current legal framework is felt to be far from satisfactory, being too lax in some respects but too restrictive in others, and with too many areas of uncertainty open to subjective interpretation and dispute. Health claims legislation is therefore under review in order to provide greater clarity for food producers and more meaningful information for consumers.

Claims for particular nutritional uses

Commonly known as PARNUTS legislation, this governs the use of foods for special dietary purposes. This legislation is also undergoing major review by the EU and is likely to change in the near future.

2.11.3 Nutrition labelling

The Food Labelling Regulations 1996 lay down a prescribed format for the nutritional labelling of foods in accordance with the 1990 EC directive. Nutrition labelling is only compulsory when a nutrition claim is made, but most pre-packaged foods now voluntarily provide it.

If nutrition information is given, it must comply with strict rules governing its format. The minimum amount of nutrition information which must be given is the group 1 ('big 4') format, which comprises:

- energy (expressed as kJ and kcal per 100 g or 100 ml)
- protein (g/100 g or 100 ml)
- carbohydrate (g/100 g or 100 ml)
- fat (g/100 g or 100 ml)

The quantity of any nutrient for which a claim is made must also be declared.

Values per quantified serving may be given as well as, but not instead of, values per 100 g or 100 ml.

Alternatively, more detailed information can be provided in the group 2 ('big 8') format:

- energy (kJ and kcal/100 g or 100 ml)
- protein (g/100 g or 100 ml)
- carbohydrate (g/100 g or 100 ml)
- – of which sugars (g/100 g or 100 ml)
- fat (g/100 g or 100 ml)

Table 2.21 Statutory and voluntary guidelines for nutrition claims (MAFF 1993, 1999)

Claim	Criteria	
'Reduced'	Contains 25% less than comparable standard product	
	Applies to reduced energy[1], fat, sugar, and sodium	
'Low'	Contains less than a specified amount of the nutrient per 100 g and, sometimes, per serving of the food:	
	Energy[1]	<40 kcal per 100 g /100 ml and <40 kcal per serving[1]
		There is separate provision for 'low calorie' soft drinks which may not contain >10 kcal per 100 ml
	Fat[2]	<3 g per 100 g/100 ml
	Sugar(s)	<5 g per 100 g/100 ml
	Saturated fat	<1.5 g per 100 g/100 ml and less than 10% total energy of the product
	Sodium	<40 mg per 100 g/100 ml
'Free'	Contains virtually none per 100 g of the food:	
	Fat	<0.15 g per 100 g/100 ml
	Saturated fat	<0.1 g per 100 g/100 ml
	Cholesterol[1]	<0.005% (i.e. 5 mg per 100 g)[1]
	Sugars	<0.2 g per 100 g/100 ml
	Sodium	<5 mg per 100 ml/100 ml
'Source'	Contains more than a specified amount of the nutrient per 100 g and per serving of the food:	
	Protein[1]	The food contains >12% energy from protein and provides >12 g per day
	Vitamins/minerals[1]	Typical daily intake of the food will provide 17% (about one-sixth) RDA[3]
	Fibre	>3 g fibre/100 g food or 3 g in the reasonable expected daily intake of that food
'High/rich'	Contains more than a specified amount of the nutrient per 100 g and, sometimes, per serving of the food:	
	Protein[1]	Contains >20% energy from protein and typical daily intake will provide >12 g per day
	Vitamins/minerals[1]	Typical daily intake of the food will provide 50% RDA[3]
	Fibre	>6 g fibre/100 g food or 6 g in the reasonable expected daily intake of that food

[1] As specified by Food Labelling Regulations 1996. All other criteria are voluntary and not currently governed by legislation.
[2] Specific EU Regulations apply to spreadable fats and MAFF guidelines do not apply to these products.
[3] RDAs are as defined by EU legislation.

- – of which saturates (g/100 g or 100 ml)
- fibre (g/100 g or 100 ml)
- sodium (g/100 g or 100 ml).

This information may also optionally be provided per serving as well as that per 100 g/100 ml. With this format, the amounts of starch, polyols, monounsaturates, polyunsaturates and cholesterol can also be listed if desired.

The rules governing the labelling of vitamins and minerals are more complex. The content of these nutrients can only be declared if a food will provide a significant proportion (about one-sixth) of the recommended daily amount (RDA) for each vitamin and mineral as defined by European legislation.

Problems with nutrition labelling

The following aspects of nutrition labelling information should be noted.

Energy

For nutrition labelling purposes, energy content is derived using a conversion factor of 4 kcal/g for carbohydrate and sugars, rather than 3.75 kcal/g used by standard UK food tables. The energy content declared on food labels will therefore be slightly higher than food table values.

Fibre

The EC Directive on Nutrition Labelling provided no agreed definition of dietary fibre for nutrition labelling purposes and as a result, a variety of methods has been used to measure its content in food. Scientific opinion in the UK is that the Englyst method, which specifically measures non-starch polysaccharide (NSP), should be the preferred method. However, much of the UK food industry and most other countries have favoured the American Organization of Analytical Chemists (AOAC) method, which measures a wider range of dietary fibre constituents, including resistant starch, and results in a higher estimate of fibre content. It now seems likely that the AOAC method will become the Europe-wide standard method of analysis, and this will necessitate revision of the UK definition of 'high-fibre' foods and of the UK DRVs for fibre, both of which are set in terms of NSP (see Section 2.5, Dietary fibre).

Sodium

Some consumers are not aware that sodium figures are an indication of salt content. Others incorrectly assume that sodium content is the same as salt content. Those trying to reduce their salt intake to the UK target of 6 g/day should be aware that this is equivalent to 2.4 g sodium.

Accuracy

Nutrition information on food labels is not necessarily obtained by laboratory analysis. This is an expensive option for food manufacturers and they are permitted to estimate nutritional content on the basis of published data on food composition. There will therefore be some variability between stated and actual nutrient content. An acceptable margin for error is not specified by law, but trading standards officers usually regard ± 10% as being sufficiently accurate. A survey by the Consumers Association (1997) found that nearly half of the nutrients they measured analytically differed from the stated content by more than 10%.

Format

The requirement to give information per 100 g/100 ml, rather than per portion, is not always helpful to the consumer because foods are not always eaten or supplied in amounts of 100 g. While per 100 g information may be useful to compare brands of the same product, most people find it difficult to do the mental arithmetic to judge whether one beefburger will provide less fat than a portion of chicken pie. Fortunately, many manufactured foods provide the optional per serving information, but this often depends on packaging space; on small items such as chocolate bars this information is often lacking.

Terminology

Many consumers have poor understanding of terms such as saturates, polyunsaturates or kJ (kilojoules).

2.11.4 Guideline daily amounts

In a survey by MAFF (1995), 50% of a sample of 1079 people said they made use of nutrition labelling information when buying food and that they found it useful. However, the same survey also found that only two-thirds could correctly extract information from the label, and less than half if a simple calculation was required.

It was also clear that most consumers had little ability to interpret nutrition information. While most were aware of health messages such as 'eat less fat', few people had any idea of whether the amount of fat present in a food was 'a little' or 'a lot'. As a result, MAFF (1998) produced 'yardstick' guidance for the consumer on how this might be assessed (Table 2.22).

A further initiative by the Institute of Grocery Distribution (IGD) in conjunction with MAFF, the Department of Health, consumer groups, academic nutritionists and the food industry led to the development of *Voluntary Nutrition Labelling Guidelines to Benefit the Consumer* (IGD 1998). Based on a 3-year consumer research programme to determine what information could be added to food labels to help people to understand nutrition information, they advocate the use of a standardized set of benchmark guideline daily amounts (GDAs) on product packaging. These should be listed in conjunction with 'per serving' information so that a comparison between the two can easily be made. GDAs are derived from adult DRVs but, because people vary in terms of weight and activity level, are not intended to be individual 'target' or 'recommended' intakes, merely guidelines to help to interpret nutrition information. GDAs are not applicable to children.

Table 2.22 Guidance for consumers on interpreting nutrition information (MAFF Food Safety Directorate 1998)

Guidance on what is 'a little' or 'a lot'
Compared with either the per serving figure for a whole meal, or the per 100 g for a snack

	'A lot' is	'A little' is
Total fat	More than 20 g	Less than 3 g
Saturates	More than 5 g	Less than 1.0 g
Fibre	More than 3 g	Less than 0.5 g
Sodium	More than 0.5 g	Less than 0.1 g

Daily guidelines[1] for an average adult of normal weight

	Men	Women
Energy	2500 kcal	2000 kcal
Fat	95 g	70 g
Saturates	30 g	20 g
Sugar	70 g	50 g
Fibre	20 g	16 g
Sodium	2.5 g	2 g

[1]The figures for energy (as 'calories'), fat and saturates are now government-endorsed guideline daily amounts (GDAs) (IGD 1998, and see Table 2.23).

GDAs on product packaging are currently confined to fats and calories, as consumer research suggested that these would be the most helpful. The term 'calories' is used instead of 'kcal' as this was found to be much more readily understood. GDAs have been approved for saturates, but their use on food labels is not recommended until there is better consumer understanding of this term, and of the concept of GDAs in general.

To avoid any conflict with the legal constraints on nutrition labelling, GDA figures must be kept distinct from nutrition information. Ideally, the GDAs and per serving figures should be presented in a separate box (Table 2.23). Where there is inadequate space, the calories and fat per serving figures in the nutrition information panel can be highlighted.

GDA information is increasingly appearing on product labels and it is permissible for them to be accompanied by the statement 'Official Government figures for average adults'.

2.11.5 Food additives

The use of food additives is mainly governed by:

- The Sweeteners in Foods Regulations 1995
- The Colours in Food Regulations 1995

Table 2.23 Guideline daily amounts used on food labels (Official government figures for an average adult; IGD 1998)

Each day	Women	Men
Calories	2000	2500
Fat	70 g	95 g

- The Flavourings in Food Regulations 1992
- The Miscellaneous Food Additives Regulations 1995.

Many of these have later amendments.

These regulations implement EC directives governing which additives are permitted in foods, the purposes for which they may be used, and any conditions attached to their use in terms of content, purity or type of food.

The Food Labelling Regulations 1996 influence the way in which additives present in foods are declared on food labels. Those used as ingredients in pre-packaged foods must be listed in an ingredients list by:

- the appropriate category name of the function (e.g. preservative), which must be followed by
- their specific name (e.g. sulphur dioxide) or E number (e.g. E220).

If an additive has more than one function (e.g. emulsifier and thickener) the category name which describes its principal function should be used.

Flavourings are slightly different because there are so many of them and they are harder to categorize. They may therefore be declared either by the term 'flavourings' or by a more specific name.

Foods containing artificial sweeteners require a declaration that the food contains sweeteners, or sweeteners and sugar (any added monosaccharide or disaccharide or any other foods used for sweetening purposes).

There are additional labelling requirements for foods containing aspartame (stating that it is a source of phenylalanine) and polyols (that excessive consumption may have a laxative effect).

Non-pre-packed or foods packaged on the premises where they are sold only have to declare the presence of the following categories of additives: antioxidants, artificial sweeteners, colours, flavour enhancers or preservatives. This information can either be given on a label or displayed on a nearby notice.

Consumer attitude to additives

Many consumers view the presence of additives in foods with great suspicion, believing them to be undesirable in principle, synthetic in nature and a common cause of 'allergies'. Many of these anxieties are misplaced. In general, food additives fulfil a useful purpose in retarding microbial spoilage, prolonging shelf-life, and improving taste, colour and texture. Many food additives are natural or nature-identical substances, or even nutrients such as beta-carotene (used as a food colour) or vitamin C (used as an antioxidant). Although some people can react to certain additives, this type of food intolerance is relatively rare (see Section 4.34, Food allergy and intolerance).

In recent years, the food industry has responded to consumer concerns by reducing the level of usage of additives as much as possible, particularly the use of azo food dyes in soft drinks and sweets, and substituting synthetic compounds with more natural alternatives. These are welcome measures, although the reduced use of preservatives is arguably less desirable as this has significantly reduced the shelf-life of many perishable foods and could increase the risk of food poisoning if people are tempted to ignore 'use by' dates so that food is not wasted.

It is perhaps ironic that the E number classification system, originally intended as a way of providing assurance that an additive's safety had been evaluated, came to be regarded by the general public as a symbol of undesirable food. As a result of the bad image associated with E numbers, food manufacturers are increasingly declaring additives in ingredients lists by their chemical name rather than their E serial number (a permitted option under Food Labelling legislation). From a dietetic viewpoint, this can make it more difficult for clients who need to avoid particular additives as they now have to memorize complex chemical names rather than simple numbers.

The E number classification system for food additives is summarized in Appendix 6.2.

2.11.6 Enforcement

Enforcement of the law in relation to food labelling is primarily the responsibility of local authorities. Issues relating to the labelling of food, its composition and most cases of chemical contamination are enforced by trading standards officers. Those relating to the hygiene, cases of microbiological contamination of foods and food which is unfit for human consumption are the remit of environmental health officers (see Section 2.10.3 in Food law).

Text revised by: Briony Thomas

Useful addresses

British Nutrition Foundation
High Holborn House, 52–54 High Holborn, London WC1V 6RQ
Tel: 020 7404 6504
Website: www.nutrition.org.uk

Food Standards Agency
Website: www.foodstandards.gov.uk

Institute of Grocery Distribution (IGD)
Grange Lane, Letchmore Heath, Watford, Herts WD2 8DQ
Tel: 01923 857141

MAFF Publications
Admail 6000, London SW1A 2XX
Tel: 0645 556000

Further reading

British Nutrition Foundation. *Nutrition Claims*. Briefing Paper. London: BNF, 1996.
Food Standards Agency. Food Law (a freely available document containing guidance information on UK food legislation. Can be downloaded from the FSA website at: www.foodstandards.gov.uk/regulations/foodlaw.htm)
MAFF. *Use your Label. Making Sense of Nutrition Information* (a guide from the Food Safety Directorate Foodsense booklet PB 2362, 1998; available free from MAFF Publications).
MAFF *Understanding Food Labels*. Foodsense Booklet PB 0553, 1998 (available free from MAFF Publications).

References

Consumers Association. Don't believe all you read. *Which?* 1997; June: 16–19.
FAO/WHO Codex Alimentarius Commission. *Guidelines for Nutrition Claims*, 22nd Codex Alimentarius Commission (ALINORM 97/37). Rome: FAO, 1998.
Institute of Grocery Distribution. *Voluntary Nutrition Labelling Guidelines to Benefit the Consumer*. Watford: IGD, 1998.
MAFF Consumer Protection Division. *Guidelines for the Use of Certain Nutrient Claims on Food Labelling and Advertising*. London: MAFF, 1993 (Revised 1999).
MAFF. *Nutrition Labelling Study Report* (Research Services Ltd). London: MAFF, 1995 (RSL, Research Services House, Elmgrove Road, Harrow Middlesex HA1 2QG).
MAFF Food Safety Directorate. *Use your Label. Making Sense of Nutrition*. Foodsense Booklet PB 2362, 1998.

2.12 Drug–nutrient interactions

There are many interactions between drugs and nutrition. Drugs and nutrients are absorbed from similar sites and metabolized and excreted in similar ways so, just as one drug can interfere with the action of another drug, some drugs may interfere with the action of a nutrient or vice versa. Side-effects of drugs can increase, decrease or alter food intake. Use of medications is therefore an important part of a patient's clinical history (see Section 1.8, Assessment of nutritional status).

Prescribed drugs are likely to have the greatest nutritional impact since they are the most powerful or high-dose forms of medication. However, it should not be overlooked that people often self-administer other types of preparations with pharmacological effects and nutritional implications. These include:

- over-the-counter drugs, e.g. analgesics, indigestion remedies, laxatives; these can sometimes be an indicator of poor eating habits, as well as having nutritional implications by themselves
- herbal remedies, particularly Chinese herbal remedies
- nutritional supplements, e.g. fish oil capsules, megadoses of vitamins; multivitamins may be used as a substitute for healthy eating
- alcohol, which affects drug-metabolizing enzymes
- tobacco, which increases free radical production and the body's requirement for antioxidants
- illegal substances: drug abuse can cause many nutritional problems, both directly from the effects of the drug itself and indirectly from the poor dietary habits and living conditions often associated with abuse.

Drug–nutrient interactions can be broadly categorized into two aspects:

- effect of nutrition on drugs: the influence of nutritional factors on drug absorption, action and effectiveness
- effect of drugs on nutrition: the influence of drugs on nutritional intake, metabolism, excretion and requirements.

2.12.1 Effects of nutrition on drugs

The metabolism of a drug usually involves the following stages, any of which can be influenced by nutrition:

1 Absorption from the gastrointestinal tract (if the drug is orally administered).
2 Transport in the blood, usually bound to plasma proteins.
3 Deactivation by a two-stage metabolic process:

- oxidation by microsomal enzyme systems involving reduced nicotinamide adenine dinucleotide (NADPH) and cytochrome P450, predominantly in the liver but also in the lung and small intestine
- conjugation with glucuronic acid, sulphate or glycine.

4 Excretion of the conjugate in urine or bile.

Effect of nutrition on drug absorption

The pharmacological effect of an orally administered drug depends on the rate and extent to which it is absorbed from the gastrointestinal tract. This can be either delayed or enhanced by the presence or absence of food.

The presence of food in the stomach and proximal intestine may reduce drug absorption as result of:

- delayed gastric emptying
- altered gastrointestinal pH
- competition for binding sites with nutrients
- chelation of drugs by food cations (e.g. tetracyclines chelate with calcium ions present in milk)
- dietary fats impeding the absorption of hydrophilic drugs.

Some drugs must therefore be taken on an empty stomach in order to maximize their rate of absorption and therapeutic effect. Conversely, others must be taken with food to achieve a slower, more sustained rate of absorption, or to minimize side-effects.

Effect of nutrition on drug transport

Many drugs are transported in blood bound to plasma proteins. Severe malnutrition, or diseases affecting the synthesis of plasma proteins (such as liver disease) may reduce the body's ability to transport drugs and hence impair their effectiveness.

Effect of nutrition on drug metabolism

Factors which affect the deactivation or conjugation of a drug can alter its pharmacological or toxic effects.

Periods of short-term starvation or prolonged periods of nutritional inadequacy can influence the effectiveness or safety of drugs. The amount of a drug required to produce a certain pharmacological effect is determined by body weight. Sudden reduction in weight or dehydration may therefore result in overdosage. Undernutrition also reduces the activity of microsomal drug-metabolizing enzymes, and this can either diminish a drug's effectiveness (by reducing the rate of synthesis of an active metabolite) or enhance its toxicity (by reducing the rate of its excretion) (Dickerson 1988). These are additional reasons for ensuring nutritional adequacy during illness, particularly since this is when pharmacological drug use is most likely to be needed.

Alcohol, which is also a drug in its own right, often affects microsomal enzyme activity and can potentiate the action of some hypoglycaemic drugs (such as tolbutamide or insulin) or central nervous system depressants (such as barbiturates). The action of other drugs such as propanolol may be reduced by alcohol.

Certain nutrients can also have a direct influence on drug metabolism. Vitamin K reduces the anticoagulant effect of warfarin and the dosage has to be sufficient to counteract the effects of habitual vitamin K intake. Any significant alteration in vitamin K intake (e.g. the consumption of large quantities of vegetables or the commencement of enteral feeding) may necessitate adjustment in warfarin dosage.

Sodium intake inversely affects serum levels of the mood stabilizer lithium carbonate and, since this drug has a narrow range of therapeutic effectiveness, dietary sodium intake must be kept at a constant level in patients receiving this treatment (see Section 4.30.1 in Mental illness).

Effect of nutrition on drug excretion

Urinary acidity affects drug reabsorption from the renal tubules. Supplemental intakes of nutrients which increase urinary acidity (e.g. large amounts of vitamin C) can decrease the excretion of salicylate drugs such as aspirin.

2.12.2 Effects of drugs on nutrition

Drugs may affect food intake or the absorption, metabolism or excretion of nutrients. This may have implications in terms of food choice or nutritional requirements.

Effects of drugs on food intake

Food intake may be reduced as a result of drugs which:

- *Have an anorexic effect*, either as a direct effect of the drug on appetite (e.g. some antibiotics and many cytotoxic drugs) or as a result of side-effects such as drowsiness or lethargy (e.g. tranquillizers).
- *Cause nausea and vomiting*: this is a common side-effect of many drugs.
- *Affect the gastrointestinal tract*: non-steroidal anti-inflammatory drugs (NSAIDs) such as aspirin or ibuprofen often cause indigestion, heartburn or gastritis. Other drugs may produce gastrointestinal side-effects such as bloating or early satiety. Chronic abdominal pain or diarrhoea may reduce the inclination to eat.
- *Cause taste changes*: Several drugs (particularly cytotoxic and psychiatric drugs) result in either loss of taste (making food seem dull and bland) or change in taste perception (making some foods taste unpleasant). These effects can alter both the amount and type of food eaten.
- *Cause dry mouth*: Lack of saliva makes it difficult to masticate and swallow foods, especially those of a dry or fibrous consistency.
- *Cause sore or painful mouth*: This is a common side-effect of chemotherapy and can significantly impair food intake.
- *Confusion*: Drugs which impair memory or cause confusion can result in people forgetting to eat.

Drugs may also increase food intake if they:

- *Stimulate appetite*: This is a common side-effect of corticosteroids, insulin and psychotropic drugs.
- *Induce cravings for particular types of foods, particularly carbohydrates*: Some psychotropic drugs have this effect (see Section 4.30.3 in Mental illness).

Effects of drugs on nutrient absorption

Absorption can be impaired as a result of:

- *Formation of insoluble complexes*: Many drugs can chelate with minerals and trace elements, e.g. penicillamine (used occasionally in the treatment of rheumatoid arthritis) chelates zinc; cholestyramine binds with iron; antacids may bind with phosphorus.
- *Competition for binding sites*, e.g. salicylate drugs such as aspirin compete with vitamin C; sulphasalazine impairs folate absorption.
- *Damage to the absorptive surface of the intestinal mucosa*: Drugs used in chemotherapy can cause villous atrophy, resulting in malabsorption.
- *Lack of bile acids*: The absorption of fat-soluble vitamins, especially A, D and K, will be impaired by bile salt binding-drugs such as cholestyramine.
- *Increased intestinal motility*: Drugs which cause diarrhoea (e.g. some antibiotics) or stimulate peristaltic activity (e.g. laxatives such as senna or phenolphthalein) may result in nutrient losses.

Effects of drugs on nutrient metabolism

Carbohydrate metabolism

Hypoglycaemic drugs such as insulin and sulphonylureas are prescribed because of their ability to increase carbohydrate utilization, and their action has to be balanced with carbohydrate intake in order to maintain glycaemic control. Other drugs such as oral contraceptives or corticosteroids have adverse effects on carbohydrate metabolism and worsen glucose intolerance.

Lipid metabolism

Some drugs are used to correct lipid metabolism, whilst others such as chlorpromazine and phenobarbitone can induce hyperlipidaemia.

Vitamin and mineral metabolism

Micronutrients are required cofactors or coenzymes in many metabolic pathways, including those by which drugs are metabolized. Increased activity of these pathways as a result of drug metabolism may therefore increase micronutrient requirements.

Drugs can also compete with, or inhibit, the metabolic conversion of some micronutrients to their active metabolites, particularly folate. Methotrexate (used in the treatment of some cancers) directly antagonizes folic acid metabolism by inhibiting the activity of the enzyme dehydrofolate reductase. Anticonvulsants (such as phenytoin, phenobarbitone and primidone) impair vitamin D metabolism, probably by inhibiting the hydroxylation to its active form, with consequent disturbances in calcium metabolism and adverse effects on bone.

Drugs may also affect the metabolism of dietary components. Type A monoamine oxidase inhibitors (MAOI-A) exert their antidepressant effects by inhibiting the breakdown of endogenously produced amine neurotransmitters. However, they also inhibit the breakdown of dietary amines such as tyramine which, if allowed to accumulate, can produce a dangerous rise in blood pressure. Patients on these drugs therefore have to avoid dietary sources of tyramine and other vasoactive amines (see Section 4.34.4 in Food allergy and intolerance). More recently, reversible inhibitors of monoamine oxidase A (known as RIMA) such as moclobemide have been introduced and these drugs appear to cause less potentiation of the pressor effects of tyramine. Dietary precautions may not therefore need to be as strict as with other MAOI-A drugs, although high intakes of foods such as cheese, yeast extracts and fermented bean products should still be avoided. It should be noted that monoamine oxidase B inhibitors, such as selegiline used in the management of Parkinson's disease, do not have hypertensive effects or dietary implications in terms of amines (Merriman 1999).

Effects of drugs on nutrient excretion

As well as their intended increase in sodium excretion, diuretic drugs can also result in enhanced losses of other elements such as potassium, calcium, magnesium and zinc. Tetracycline increases the urinary excretion of vitamin C.

2.12.3 Clinical significance of drug–nutrient interactions

It should always be borne in mind that that poor nutritional status can impair drug metabolism, and that drug treatment can have a detrimental effect on nutritional status.

Not all drug–nutrient interactions are clinically significant. In many instances, any losses in nutrient availability or drug action will be small in scale and may be of short duration. Drugs which are most likely to have dietetic implications are those which:

- have a narrow range between therapeutic effect and toxicity (e.g. lithium, anticoagulants)
- need to be taken for a prolonged period
- have implications in terms of the timing of food intake (habitual meal pattern may need to be adjusted)
- necessitate dietary restrictions or regulation (food choice may need to be altered)
- have side-effects which impact on appetite or gastrointestinal function (e.g. cytotoxic drugs)
- compete directly with a nutrient (e.g. vitamin K and warfarin; anticonvulsants and folate)

People who are most at risk from drug–nutrient interactions are those:

- whose gastrointestinal, liver and/or renal function is inefficient or failing
- who are in a nutritionally compromised state, as a result of poor diet, alcoholism or disease
- who have had recent weight loss
- who are dehydrated
- who are on multiple drug therapy
- who are on prolonged drug therapy.

Many of these factors are likely to coexist in elderly people (Roe 1984). In addition, the physiological changes that occur with age, such as a decrease in lean body mass and body water, fall in plasma protein concentration, and general decline in renal and liver function, mean that the risk of adverse drug reactions is much higher (Hamilton Smith 1995). For this reason, it is now a requirement that drug data sheets provide details of suitable dosages for elderly people.

Elderly people are also more likely to be given the types of drugs with powerful effects and which are most likely to impact on nutrition, e.g. cytotoxic drugs, anti-Parkinson's drugs and antidiabetic drugs. Diminished salivation may make it more difficult to swallow tablets, and oesophageal motility disorders may lead to bulky drugs sticking in the oesophageal mucosa. Other problems such as failing memory, poor hearing and vision, and difficulty with opening containers may mean that drug regimens are not followed correctly, particularly if they are complex.

Drug usage is therefore an important aspect of the dietary assessment of elderly people. Drugs which may have particular nutritional implications in elderly people include:

- *Tolbutamide*: This can have a profound hypoglycaemic effect in older people owing to the decline in plasma albumin level with age and consequently more tolbutamide remaining free, rather than bound, in plasma. Liver mass, and hence the rate at which this drug is metabolized, may also be reduced. An alternative hypoglycaemic agent with a shorter half-life such as glipizide is preferable for older people with diabetes. If tolbutamide is used, it should be given with, or immediately after, food to lessen the risk of hypoglycaemia (see Section 4.16, Diabetes mellitus).
- *Levodopa*: The level of levodopa in the plasma is criti-

Table 2.24 Classes of drugs which are most likely to have nutritional implications

Class of drug	Common effects
Amphetamines	Increase appetite
Analgesics	Anti-inflammatory analgesics (NSAIDs) cause gastric irritation
Antacids	Can bind with minerals such as phosphorus, iron and zinc and reduce their absorption
Antibiotics	Anorexia
	Altered gut flora and diarrhoea
	Tetracycline forms complexes with calcium (in foods or mineral supplements), reducing the absorption of both
Anticoagulants	Warfarin action is affected by vitamin K
Anticonvulsants	Interfere with folate metabolism
	Interfere with vitamin D metabolism
Antidepressants	Anorexia
	MAOI type A usage necessitates avoidance of tyramine
Antihyperlipidaemics	Clofibrate and cholestyramine can result in malabsorption, especially of minerals and fat-soluble vitamins
Antipsychotics	Some types markedly increase appetite (see Section 4.30)
Corticosteroids	Anabolic effects and weight gain
	Glucose intolerance
Cytotoxic (anticancer) drugs	Anorexia
	Taste changes
	Nausea, vomiting and diarrhoea
	Damage to intestinal villi
	Interfere with folate metabolism
	Reduce thiamin status
Diuretics	Thiazide and loop diuretics can cause excessive urinary loss of potassium, calcium and zinc and water-soluble vitamins
	Dehydration
Hypoglycaemics	Action has to be balanced against carbohydrate intake
	Alcohol can potentiate their action
	Chlorpropamide can react with alcohol and cause facial flushing
Laxatives	Reduced absorption of nutrients (liquid paraffin)
Mood stabilizers	Lithium action is affected by dietary sodium
Oral contraceptives	Affect glucose and lipid metabolism
	Can cause weight gain

NSAID: non-steroidal anti-inflammatory drug; MAOI: monoamine oxidase inhibitor.

cal for clinical status in the later stages of Parkinson's disease (see Section 4.26.1 in Neurodegenerative disorders). All factors which delay gastric emptying of levodopa (the precursor of dopamine), including food and drugs such as anti-cholinergics, result in delayed and reduced peak plasma concentration. This, is turn, reduces conversion to dopamine and the drug's effectiveness. Since severe Parkinson's disease, with tremor and reduced swallowing ability, can markedly reduce food intake, the risk of undernutrition is high. This, is turn, may impact on the effect of other drugs as well as general health.

Classes of drugs which are most likely to have nutritional implications are summarized in Table 2.24. Drug–nutrient interactions associated with the management of some clinical disorders are also discussed in the other sections of the Manual (e.g. the effects of drugs used to treat psychiatric illness are discussed in Section 4.23). Specific details of the effects of particular drugs can be found in the *British National Formulary* (BNF) or the *Monthly Index of Medical Specialities* (MIMS) (see Further reading, below). The effects of drug therapy on vitamins and minerals have been reviewed by White and Ashworth (2000).

Text revised by: Briony Thomas

Acknowledgements: The British Dietetic Association's Nutrition Advisory Group for Elderly People (NAGE); Sheila Merriman.

Useful address

The United Kingdom Drug Information Pharmacists Group (UKDIPG)
Website: www.ukdipg.org.uk

Further reading

British National Formulary (BNF). A joint publication of the British Medical Association and the Royal Pharmaceutical Society of Great Britain. Revised at 6-monthly intervals. Available from bookshops.

Monthly Index of Medical Specialities (MIMS). A monthly publication available free to medical practitioners and available on subscription to other health professionals.

Thomas JA. Drug – nutrient interactions. *Nutrition Reviews* 1995; **53**: 271–282.

References

Dickerson JWT. The interrelationships of nutrition and drugs. In Dickerson JWT, Lee HA (Eds) *Nutrition and the Clinical Management of Disease*, 2nd edn, pp. 392–421. London: Edward Arnold, 1988.

Hamilton Smith C. Drug–food/food–drug interactions. In Morley JE, Glick Z, Rubinstein LZ (Eds) *Geriatric Nutrition: A Comprehensive Review*. New York: Raven Press, 1995.

Merriman SH. Monoamine oxidase drugs and diet. *Journal of Human Nutrition and Dietetics* 1999; **12**: 21–28.

Roe DA (Ed.). *Drugs and Nutrition in the Geriatric Patient*. Edinburgh: Churchill Livingstone, 1984.

White R, Ashworth A. How drug therapy can affect, threaten and compromise nutritional status. *Journal of Human Nutrition and Dietetics* 2000; **13**: 119–129.

SECTION 3
Nutritional needs of population subgroups

3.1 Pregnancy

3.1.1 Preconceptional and periconceptional nutrition

Preconceptional nutrition in men

The preconceptional (before the time of conception) and periconceptional (around the time of conception) effects of diet in men are poorly researched. Most studies have been carried out on animals and the relevance to humans is unclear.

Male reproductive function has recently attracted attention due to reports of a time-related decline in semen quality. However, the aetiology of male infertility remains largely unknown. Various physical and chemical agents have been shown to affect male reproductive function in animals but human data are often conflicting (Tas *et al*. 1996). It is often difficult to identify the role of a single agent because exposure conditions are often complex and various confounding factors related to lifestyle, such as smoking, alcohol and diet, and socioeconomic status may affect sperm quality, fertility or pregnancy outcomes. Data indicate that sperm counts may have declined in some parts of the world but there seem to be regional differences, both in the quality of semen and in this secular trend (Giwercman and Bonde 1998). It has been postulated that the decline in semen quality, together with an increase in the incidence of congenital malformations of the male reproductive tract and the incidence of testicular cancer, may be due to perinatal environmental and dietary exposure to phytoestrogens (Sharp and Shakkeback 1993). However, there is, as yet, no evidence that these agents are having an influence on male fertility.

Preconceptional nutritional advice for men

Although it is known that gross dietary inadequacies or excesses in men can affect both the likelihood of and the outcome of conception (Calloway 1983), the effects of lesser degrees of dietary imbalance are unknown. The most prudent preconceptional nutritional advice for men at the present time is therefore to:

- consume a balanced and varied diet
- moderate alcohol intake
- correct grossly abnormal body weight.

It is advisable that dietary changes should be made at least 2–3 months before the intended time of conception.

Preconceptional nutrition in women

Body fat content has an important influence on female fertility. The average body fat content of postpubertal women is 28% of body weight, and fat must comprise at least 22% of body weight for the maintenance of ovulatory cycles (Frisch and McArthur 1974). It has been established that it is the fat content of the body rather than absolute body weight that is critical because trained athletes of average or above average body weight who have a very low body fat content may be oligomenorrhoeic or amenorrhoeic.

Other causes of secondary amenorrhoea leading to subfertility include psychological stress, thyrotoxicosis and various malabsorption syndromes, as well as eating disorders such as anorexia nervosa and bulimia nervosa.

Conception can occur in women who are well below average or ideal weight (for height) and has been reported in women with a body mass index (BMI) as low as 14.9 (Treasure and Russell 1988). However, the infants of women who are thin at the time of conception are more likely to be of low birthweight and/or premature and to have significantly increased morbidity (Edwards *et al*. 1979). The likelihood of producing healthy offspring is increased if the diet of such mothers is adequate throughout pregnancy and weight is gained appropriately (Rosso 1985).

Obesity can affect ovulation and also the response to fertility treatment. In a prospective study, Clark *et al*. (1998) showed that adherence to a weight loss and exercise programme by anovulatory overweight women brought about spontaneous ovulation, conception and a successful pregnancy outcome in the majority of subjects. However, consumption of an energy-deficient diet immediately prior to conception or during pregnancy can disadvantage the fetus if it results in nutrient deficiencies.

A recent study showed that a woman's alcohol intake is associated with decreased fertility, even among women with a weekly alcohol intake corresponding to five or fewer units (Jensen *et al*. 1998), but this finding needs further corroboration. The effects of alcohol consumption during the preconceptional period on the outcome of pregnancy are unknown.

Nutrition and early fetal development

The fetus is most susceptible to nutritional imbalance during the first trimester of pregnancy, when rapid cell differentiation and the establishment of embryonic systems and organs are taking place. The time of greatest nutritional vulnerability is possibly before a woman even suspects she is pregnant and certainly before the first antenatal appointment. The effects of the Dutch 'Hunger Winter' of

October 1944 to May 1945 on the outcome of pregnancy in women who were or became pregnant during that time clearly showed that the stage of pregnancy at which the mother experiences food shortage determines which parameters are most affected. In the presence of adequate preconceptional nutrition, fetal growth is protected until maternal deprivation becomes extreme (Stein *et al.* 1995). However, among babies conceived towards the end of the food shortage there was greater perinatal mortality, as well as low birth weight (Wynn and Wynn 1981). There were also significantly increased rates of infertility (and malformations in those babies who were conceived) in the 4 months immediately *after* the end of the food shortage.

Although overt food shortage is rare in the UK, undernutrition due to other factors is not uncommon in a number of population subgroups. Among anorexia nervosa patients it can be particularly severe and, although pregnancy is unlikely to occur during the anorexic state itself, fertility can return during the recovery phase and the patient should be made aware of the possible risks to the fetus if conception occurs at this time. In other people, extremely poor eating habits resulting from ignorance or a low income may also lead to an inadequate nutrient intake, as may the deliberate restriction of food intake in an attempt to reduce body weight. Large numbers of young women spend periods of time following weight-reducing 'diets' of dubious nutritional quality which may result in very low energy intakes. In addition, overweight women trying to start a family are often encouraged to lose weight, not only to facilitate conception but because of the increased risk of late pregnancy complications and perinatal mortality in overweight mothers (Naeye 1979; Edwards *et al.* 1979).

Vitamin intake and congenital malformations

Folate There is now considerable evidence that folic acid is of crucial importance in early pregnancy to help protect against neural tube defects (NTD) (Smithells *et al.* 1980; MRC 1991; Czeizel and Dudas 1992). The Department of Health's Expert Advisory Group on Folic Acid and Neural Tube Defects (DH 1992) has recommended that:

(a) *To prevent the first occurrence of neural tube defects*, all women who are planning a pregnancy should:

- supplement their diet with 0.4 mg (400 μg) folic acid until the 12th week of pregnancy. (This is available on prescription but, except for those on a low income and exempt from prescription charges, it is cheaper to buy it than to pay the standard prescription charge);
- choose foods such as bread and breakfast cereals which are fortified with folic acid;
- consume more folate-rich foods, which should not be overcooked.

Women who have not been supplementing their diet with folic acid and become pregnant should immediately start supplementation and continue until the 12th week of pregnancy.

(b) *To prevent recurrence of neural tube defects* in the offspring of women or men with a history of a previous child with NTD, women who wish to become pregnant, or are at risk of becoming pregnant, should take a daily supplement of 5 mg (5000 μg) folic acid (available on prescription only) and supplementation should continue until the 12th week of pregnancy.

Despite government campaigns to raise the awareness of the importance of preconceptional and periconceptional folate, this advice has only had limited effect (DH 2000). Since as many as half of all pregnancies in some areas of the UK are unplanned, many women do not take additional folate until it is too late, if at all (McGovern *et al.* 1997). A report by the government's COMA committee (DH 2000) estimated that of the 107 NTD-affected births reported in 1988, many could have been prevented had folate intake been sufficient. COMA confirmed that current recommended supplementary measures and awareness campaigns should continue, but they also suggested that better protection could be offered to the entire childbearing population by fortifying flour used in food production with folic acid. They estimated that fortification at a level of 240 μg per 100 g would reduce the risk of NTD by 41%, without resulting in unacceptably high intakes in any group of the population (DH 2000).

Although it has been suggested that periconceptional intake of other vitamins may also be relevant to some types of structural malformation (Czeizel 1993), at present the evidence is that the influence of folate is of paramount importance. Women are therefore encouraged to take specific folate supplements rather than combinations of multivitamins and folate, because some of the latter preparations may not contain sufficient folate to be protective.

Vitamin A Although vitamin A requirements during pregnancy do increase, it has been known for many years that in animals a high intake of vitamin A in the form of retinol is teratogenic in the periconceptional period. In humans, one case-report described an infant with congenital renal abnormalities associated with maternal retinol intakes 10 times above the recommended dietary allowance (RDA) (Bernhardt and Dorsey 1974). Isotretinoin, an analogue of retinol, used for the treatment of acne, has been associated with miscarriage and congenital malformations (Benke 1984). Because isotretinoin is mainly prescribed to teenagers and pregnancies are more likely to be unplanned at this age, the risk of giving birth to offspring with congenital malformations may be increased.

In recent years, there has been significant concern over the dramatic rise in the vitamin A content of animal liver. Analytical data revealed that a typical portion could contain between 13 000 and 40 000 μg vitamin A/100 g. These excessively high levels were thought to result from the retinol being added to animal foodstuffs as a growth promoter. The maternal retinol dose threshold for increased risk of birth defects remains unknown (Hathcock *et al.* 1990). However, as a cautionary measure, in 1990 the

Department of Health and Social Security advised all women of child-bearing age to avoid excessive intake of retinol, either in the form of supplements or as liver products such as paté or liver sausage (DHSS 1990).

Preconceptional nutritional advice for women

Dietary advice for women planning a pregnancy should highlight the following:

- Make dietary changes (including any desired weight loss) at least 3–4 months before attempting conception.
- Follow the periconceptional folic acid recommendations (see above).
- Eat a diet with adequate energy.
- Eat a varied diet to ensure adequate intake of all nutrients and include at least 5 portions of fruit and vegetables daily.
- Restrict, or exclude, alcohol.
- Seek advice from a doctor before taking any over-the-counter medications or supplements and discuss any prescribed medication with the general practitioner (GP).

Much of the information relating to pre-pregnancy care (including nutrition) should form part of health education which should be started in schools and continued into the pre-pregnancy phase of life. Pre-pregnancy counselling should be available for both underweight and overweight women in order to modify pre-pregnancy BMI and reduce the risk of other adverse lifestyle factors. Ideally, weight loss should occur well in advance of conception to lessen the likelihood of the woman consuming a nutritionally deficient diet at a time which is critical to fetal development.

3.1.2 Nutritional considerations during pregnancy

The extra nutritional requirements imposed by pregnancy must be met by dietary intake and body stores. Fetal growth depends on the health and nutritional status of the mother before conception, the degree of energy demands placed on her during pregnancy, and the growth, energy and nutrient demands of the products of conception at different stages of gestation, but it is worth remembering that there is a number of ways in which the nutrient supply to the fetus may be regulated. These include:

- changes in maternal food choice and dietary intake
- maternal metabolic adaptation
- altered maternal absorption
- fetal uptake (i.e. maternal loss)
- varying placental transfer.

Nevertheless, there will be some pregnant women in whom nutritional needs will not be met and although results of studies to determine how nutrient intake of mothers during early and late pregnancy influences placental and fetal growth have been inconclusive (Doyle *et al.* 1990; Godfrey *et al.* 1996; Rogers *et al.* 1998; Mathews *et al.* 1999) there is some evidence that it will be detrimental to the fetus throughout life (see below).

Fetal origins of adult disease

Observational studies have been published suggesting that the long-term effects of fetal undernutrition depend on the trimester in which it occurs (Barker 1992, 1994, 1995) and that:

- First trimester undernutrition may lead to down-regulation of growth with reduced birthweight and a proportionately small infant who continues to grow poorly and still has a low weight at 1 year. In adult life such infants may be prone to hypertension and death from haemorrhagic stroke.
- Second trimester undernutrition occurring as a result of a disturbed fetoplacental relationship tends to lead to reduced birth weight but normal weight at 1 year and, in later life, may increase risk of hypertension, type II diabetes and excessive mortality from coronary heart disease.
- In the third trimester, undernutrition is most likely to cause growth retardation which is asymmetric, with brain growth spared at the expense of truncal growth, leading to a normal birthweight but short length, and low infant weight at 1 year. Increased blood pressure, low-density lipoprotein (LDL) cholesterol and fibrinogen may be a consequence in adult life, together with an increased risk of coronary heart disease and thrombotic stroke.

Barker (1994) suggested that these studies showed that disease prevention in the next generation can be achieved by directing attention to the nutrition of mothers and their babies (The Barker hypothesis). However, reanalysis of the data based on corrections for socioeconomic status in adult life has since suggested that postnatal environmental factors may play a more major role than originally suggested (Ben-Shlomo and Smith 1991). Other criticisms of the Barker hypothesis include the fact that extrapolations were made from results obtained on very small cohorts and selection bias could be operating (Paneth and Susser 1995).

The controlled study performed in the USA on low-income women whose diets were supplemented with specific foodstuffs in the government programme 'Women, Infant and Children' (WIC) showed a reduction in perinatal mortality and an increased head circumference but without any significant effect on birthweight (Rush *et al.* 1988), and whether the Barker hypothesis proves to be correct in the long term remains to be seen. In the meantime, health professionals should be aware that various aspects of the Barker hypothesis have been brought to the attention of the general public in a simplistic format and should be sufficiently informed themselves to allay any unnecessary concerns of those who are pregnant.

Nutritional requirements during pregnancy

Energy

There are wide variations between individuals and their energy requirements during pregnancy. This is because of the variation in amount of fat laid down and because some women have a reduction in basal metabolic rate during the early months of pregnancy whilst others show an increase, almost from the time of conception (Hytten 1991). Some of the energy costs of pregnancy are also assumed to be met by the reduction in energy expenditure due to reduced physical activity.

Weight gain during pregnancy   The Institute of Medicine (IOM 1990) has recommended a total weight gain during pregnancy for women based on the pre-pregnancy BMI:

- BMI in the normal range (19.8–26): a weight gain of 11.5–16 kg is advised
- BMI below 19.8, a weight gain of 1–2 kg more than this is encouraged
- BMI above 26: the weight gain should be below the minimum suggested for women with a BMI in the normal range.

However, Feig and Naylor (1998) have summarized data showing little evidence to advocate such liberal weight gain during gestation in well-fed Western societies. They suggest that the minimum threshold for maternal weight gain should be 6.8 kg and that the IOM recommendations are unnecessarily high. Much of their concern about excessive weight gain during pregnancy relates to the long-term risks of obesity for the mother. Studies have shown that weight gained at an excessive rate by women with a normal pre-pregnancy BMI does not enhance fetal growth but does contribute to postpartum maternal obesity (Scholl *et al*. 1995). A relationship has also been shown between high maternal weight gain and short-term adverse outcomes such as infant macrosomia and operative delivery (Shepard *et al*. 1986; Johnson *et al*. 1992).

An additional 200 kcal/day in the third trimester of pregnancy has been recommended (DH 1991) but the best practical advice for women during pregnancy is to eat according to appetite and monitor weight gain. Women with a pre-pregnancy BMI within the normal range should aim for a pregnancy weight gain of between 6.8 and 11.4 kg (Feig and Naylor 1998).

The optimal weight gain for pregnant adolescents who are themselves still growing is uncertain. A study by Rees *et al*. (1992) suggested that adolescents with a weight gain of about 0.6 kg/week in the second and third trimester were more likely to give birth to an infant with a weight within the normal range (3–4 kg) than those who gained less, and thus a greater and earlier increase in energy intake may be required.

Protein

The optimal protein requirements for pregnancy are unknown. The current UK dietary reference value (DRV) of an additional 6 g/day throughout pregnancy, making the reference nutrient intake (RNI) approximately 51 g/day, is based on calculations to allow for protein retention in the products of conception and in the maternal tissues associated with the birth of a 3.3 kg infant (DH 1991). However, most women consume more protein than this (Gregory *et al*. 1990) and it is unlikely that the majority of women need to increase their usual intake during pregnancy.

Iron

During pregnancy, iron is needed for the manufacture of haemoglobin in both maternal and fetal red blood cells. The fetus accumulates most of its iron during the last trimester and, at term, a normal-weight infant has about 246 mg iron in blood and body stores. Maintenance of erythropoiesis is one of the few instances during pregnancy when the fetus acts as a true parasite by ensuring its own production of haemoglobin, drawing iron from its mother. Maternal iron deficiency does not usually result in an infant that is anaemic at birth. The most common cause of iron deficiency anaemia in infants is prematurity, as an infant that has a short gestation simply does not have enough time to accumulate sufficient iron during the last trimester.

Maternal iron needs   The current DRV (DH 1991) for iron in adult women is 14.8 mg/day, with no recommended increase during pregnancy. In theory, the increased demand for iron in pregnancy is met through the combined actions of:

- mobilization of maternal iron stores
- increased dietary absorption
- savings made in basal iron losses due to cessation of menstruation.

In women who begin pregnancy with adequate iron reserves these adaptations allow the additional iron requirements to be met without the necessity for an increased dietary iron intake (DH 1991). The ideal level of storage iron at the beginning of pregnancy is not known, but studies in the UK (Gregory *et al*. 1990) have demonstrated low iron stores (ferritin) in considerable numbers of women of child-bearing age. In a recent study (Robinson *et al*. 1998), low iron stores in early pregnancy were strongly associated with multiparity, low socioeconomic grouping and low BMI.

Iron absorption from the gastrointestinal tract is increased during pregnancy by as much as 50% compared with the usual 10–20% in non-pregnant women. However, the bioavailability of dietary iron is of greater importance than the actual amount of iron in the diet (Hallberg 1994). Haem iron from the haemoglobin and myoglobin of animals is absorbed more efficiently than non-haem iron because the entire porphyrin ring containing the iron is taken up by mucosal cells, and thus the iron is protected from factors that inhibit its absorption. Non-haem iron is found in vegetables, cereals and eggs, and its bioavailability is affected by the balance of dietary factors enhancing and inhibiting iron absorption. Vitamin C increases bioavailability, and calcium and iron-binding polyphenols such as tannins from tea decrease it (Robinson *et al.* 1998).

Maternal iron status during pregnancy As pregnancy advances most women show haematological changes suggesting iron deficiency, but this simply reflects haemodilution which in itself is of no physiological significance. Haemoglobin and serum iron concentrations fall and the total iron binding capacity rises. The mean corpuscular haemoglobin concentration may remain constant or may fall. Haemodilution also makes the interpretation of serum ferritin levels (which correlate very well with the level of iron stores in non-pregnant individuals) more difficult during pregnancy itself (Whittaker *et al.* 1996).

In the UK, routine iron supplementation in pregnancy is a common practice but is probably unnecessary in many cases and may be disadvantageous in some if it results in side-effects such as constipation or nausea. It is probably only necessary in women with a history of anaemia, who are likely to have low iron stores at the commencement of pregnancy, or who develop clear haematological or clinical signs of anaemia during pregnancy. For most women, the advice to include some lean red meat in the diet every day is probably sufficient. In non-meat eaters, care should be taken to ensure that the diet is high in vitamin C to improve the absorption of inorganic iron.

Calcium

A baby at birth contains 25–30 g calcium, most of which is laid down in the last 10 weeks of pregnancy. There is a consensus (Misra and Anderson 1990), that the concentration of maternal free (biologically active) 1,25-dihydroxyvitamin D_3 is raised during pregnancy, increasing net calcium absorption. Thus, the increased requirement for calcium during pregnancy may be met entirely from increased absorption. No additional increment is therefore made to the current RNIs for calcium for adult women (i.e. 700 mg/day for women aged 19–50 years and 800 mg/day for those aged 15–18 years) (DH 1991).

The average UK calcium intake of 0.8–1.0 g/day will meet these needs. However, there are some subgroups who are at risk of calcium inadequacy:

- women who consume little or no milk or dairy products
- teenage mothers whose own calcium requirements are high as they have not yet achieved peak bone mass
- Asian women who, as well as having low vitamin D status (see below), may consume a high-fibre diet which additionally compromises calcium absorption.

It is important that such women are offered appropriate dietary guidance which improves either the consumption or absorption of calcium.

Zinc

Animal studies have shown that deficiency of zinc is associated with abnormalities in pregnancy, but this has not been clearly demonstrated in humans. There is no evidence that extra zinc is required during pregnancy and the UK RNI for zinc is 7 mg/day with no increment during pregnancy (DH 1991). Zinc intakes tend to parallel protein intake and rich sources of zinc include meat, fish, pulses and wholegrain cereals.

Folate

In addition to the preconceptional need for folic acid supplementation, the requirement for folate is increased during pregnancy. In order to prevent megaloblastic anaemia, the DRV for folate during pregnancy is increased by an additional 100 µg/day, i.e. raising it from 200 µg/day for non-pregnant women to 300 µg/day (DH 1991). This level of increase can be achieved by a well-balanced diet containing folate-rich foods such as green leafy vegetables and folate-fortified foods such as breakfast cereals.

Vitamin C

Vitamin C aids the absorption of non-haem sources of iron, and the recommended vitamin C intake is increased by 10 mg during the third trimester of pregnancy to 50 mg/day (DH 1991). Women should be encouraged to include some source of vitamin C at each meal, particularly from fruit and vegetables. If consumption of these foods tends to be low, fruit juice or vitamin C-enriched fruit squash should be encouraged. Vitamin C intakes have been found to be lower amongst women who smoke during pregnancy (Haste *et al.* 1990) and particular attention should be paid to intake in these women.

Vitamin D

Vitamin D is essential to sustain the heightened calcium absorption and utilization during pregnancy. Normally, the body's requirements for vitamin D are supplied through exposure to sunlight, but whether the increased needs during pregnancy can be met via this route is unclear. The current recommendation (DH 1991) is that pregnant women should receive supplementary vitamin D to achieve an intake of 10 µg/day. For most women, diets which regularly contain vitamin D-enriched margarine, cheese, fatty fish and eggs will probably supply sufficient vitamin D. However, supplements may be important for at-risk individuals, especially Asian women who are particularly likely to have compromised vitamin D status as a result of low sunlight exposure and reduced metabolic synthesis of the active forms of the vitamin.

Vitamin A

In Western countries, intakes of retinol and its precursors are usually adequate to meet the additional requirements of pregnancy, but an increment of 100 µg/day throughout pregnancy has been recommended to enhance maternal stores and allow for the rapid fetal growth of late pregnancy (DH 1991). However, because of the known teratogenic effects of high retinol intakes, the American College of Obstetrics and Gynaecology (Committee on Obstetrics 1993) recommended that pregnant women do not consume more than 5000 IU (1500 µg) per day as a supplement.

Other nutrition-related aspects of pregnancy

Smoking

How smoking relates to nutrition is complex and incompletely understood, but it is known that it raises metabolic rate, alters taste perception and affects the metabolism of a range of nutrients. It has long been known that smoking is associated with a decrease in birthweight of around 175–200 g (Lumley and Astbury 1989) and that smokers tend to weigh less and gain less weight during pregnancy than non-smokers. This may be linked more closely to social class than dietary intake, but Haste *et al.* (1990) reported that women who smoked had a poorer quality of diet (other than energy intake) than did non-smokers and this was independent of social background. Non-smokers were found to have persistently higher mean intakes of all nutrients (except for energy) analysed in all social class groups. More recent studies (Rogers *et al.* 1998) have found that women who smoke and those with more financial difficulties consumed less folate, iron and vitamin C than non-smokers and those with fewer financial difficulties.

Alcohol

The term fetal alcohol syndrome (FAS) is used to describe the congenital malformations associated with excessive maternal alcohol intake. These include growth retardation, abnormal craniofacial features, and developmental problems (Beattie 1992). FAS is likely to occur in the offspring of mothers regularly drinking more than 80 g pure alcohol per day. Some women drinking at this level produce children with full FAS; other infants may exhibit only partial FAS features and are considered to have fetal alcohol effect (FAE). The incidence of FAS is around 1–2 per 1000 live births, with 3–5 cases of FAE per 1000 in the general population (Spohr *et al.* 1993). However, the incidence varies from region to region and, in the UK, cases have mainly been seen in the west of Scotland, Liverpool and Belfast (Beattie 1992).

Although there is general agreement that women should not drink alcohol excessively during pregnancy there is no consensus opinion as to what is a safe amount to drink during pregnancy. Department of Health (1995) guidance is that women who are pregnant or planning a pregnancy should not consume more than 1–2 units once or twice a week, and should avoid intoxication. A recent review of the evidence by the Royal College of Obstetricians and Gynaecologists (1999) concluded that alcohol consumption in excess of three drinks per week during the first trimester of pregnancy increases the risk of spontaneous abortion, and social alcohol consumption above 15 units (120 g alcohol)/week can have a small negative effect on birthweight. They found no conclusive evidence of adverse effects on either fetal growth or IQ at levels of alcohol consumption below 120 g (15 units) per week. Nevertheless, their recommendation is that women should be cautious about alcohol consumption in pregnancy and limit this to no more than one standard drink per day.

Foodborne illness and food safety

Some types of foodborne infection pose a particular threat to pregnant women as they have the potential to cause death of, or damage to, the fetus.

Listeriosis Listeriosis is a rare form of food poisoning caused by the bacterium *Listeria monocytogenes*. Infection of the fetus can lead to abortion, stillbirth or delivery of an acutely ill infant (DH 1996). Pregnant women are therefore advised to avoid foods which could contain significant amounts of the organism. These are:

- soft ripened cheeses such as Camembert, Brie, goats' and sheep's milk cheeses. Care must also be taken with mould-ripened cheeses which have a higher pH and permit growth of *L. monocytogenes*. Hard cheeses, yoghurt and butter can be regarded as safe because of a low pH and lack of moisture. Processed cheese spread and cottage cheese are also likely to be free from contamination;
- unpasteurized milk (from the cow, sheep or goat) and any products made from it;
- precooked or ready-prepared cold foods which will not be reheated, e.g. purchased salads, paté, quiches, cold meat pies.

The organism is destroyed by heat, so properly cooked foods pose no risk. It is important that precooked ready meals are cooked according to manufacturers' instructions and that the product is piping hot throughout before being consumed. Leftover cooked food should be discarded.

Salmonellosis Salmonella is a major cause of food poisoning in the UK and, if severe, its effects can trigger miscarriage or premature labour. The most likely sources of salmonella are raw eggs, consumed either in home-made mayonnaise or desserts such as cold soufflés, undercooked poultry and cross-contamination from raw poultry. Pregnant women should take particular care regarding the handling and consumption of these foods.

Toxoplasmosis This is caused by the organism *Toxoplasma gondii*, commonly found in raw meat, unpasteurized milk and cat faeces. In pregnancy it can cause flu-like symptoms in the woman and a range of severe fetal abnormalities including mental retardation and blindness. In addition to general safe food hygiene measures, pregnant women should be advised to:

- wear disposable gloves when gardening
- wear disposable gloves whilst handling cat litter trays
- be particularly vigilant about hygiene practices if cats are allowed into the kitchen.

Campylobacter Campylobacter pathogens are a frequent cause of food poisoning, the most common sources of infection being poultry, milk, untreated surface water, domestic pets and soil. Campylobacter infections during pregnancy have been associated with prematurity, spontaneous abortion and stillbirth. As with other causes of food poisoning, risk is reduced by observing good hygiene practices.

Guidance on food safety during pregnancy The risk of contracting all types of foodborne illness can be greatly diminished by following simple but important rules regarding kitchen hygiene and the storage, preparation and cooking of food. Detailed guidance for pregnant women is given in the booklet *While you are Pregnant: Safe Eating and How to Avoid Infection from Food and Animals*, issued by the Department of Health (1996) in a variety of languages. The key points of guidance can be summarized as:

- Always wash your hands before and after preparing food.
- Keep kitchen surfaces, cooking utensils, tea-towels, etc., scrupulously clean.
- Do not let uncooked food (e.g. raw meat or fish) contaminate cooked or ready-to eat food (e.g. via chopping boards or by letting raw juices drip on to other foods in the fridge).
- Wash fruit, vegetables and salad before consumption.
- Never eat food after the 'use by' date.
- Cook food thoroughly and according to manufacturers' instructions.
- Cool leftover food quickly and use within 24 hours. Do not reheat.
- Make sure your fridge and freezer are operating at the right temperatures.
- Keep pets away from kitchen surfaces.
- Always wear rubber gloves when handling cat litter trays or gardening.

Peanut/nut allergy

The incidence of nut and peanut allergy in children is increasing and, because of its severity, is of considerable concern. The risk of peanut allergy is greatly increased in children from atopic families and there is some evidence that intrauterine exposure to peanut allergens may increase the risk of subsequent allergy in such children. The Department of Health (1998) has therefore suggested that pregnant women with a diagnosed allergic disorder, or if the father or another child in the family has such a disorder, may wish to avoid nuts and peanuts during pregnancy. There is no evidence that women from non-atopic families would benefit from doing so. Since peanut and nut products are widely used in food manufacture, their exclusion is far from simple and women will require expert dietetic guidance in order to be able to do so effectively (see Section 4.35.3 in Food exclusion).

3.1.3 Dietary guidance in pregnancy

Pregnant women are, in general, receptive to nutrition education and willing to adopt a healthier style of eating. Antenatal care thus provides a unique opportunity to influence the eating habits of large numbers of women, with the additional potential to influence the health of the next generation.

General dietary guidance for pregnant women should encompass the importance of:

- Eating regular meals and snacks.
- Sensible food choice based on healthy eating principles. Foods which should be encouraged include:
  - bread, rice, pasta, chappattis, breakfast cereals and potatoes
  - fruit and vegetables
  - milk, yoghurt and pasteurized cheeses
  - meat, fish, eggs (well cooked), beans or lentils.
- Eating according to appetite but also taking care that the consumption of fat-rich and sugar-rich food choices is not so excessive that they displace more nutrient-dense foods from the diet or lead to excessive weight gain.
- Being cautious over alcohol intake (suggested, although unconfirmed, guidance is a maximum of 1 unit per day) or avoiding it altogether.
- Avoiding potentially hazardous foods, i.e.
  - unpasteurized milk, cheeses made from unpasteurized milk or mould-ripened soft cheese
  - liver and foods made from it
  - raw or undercooked eggs
  - nuts and peanuts if the mother or her partner has a diagnosed history of atopic disease.
- Observing food-safety procedures.

However, within this framework, some women will require more targeted advice in order to counter individual nutritional problems or inadequacies, either at the onset of or during pregnancy. Ideally, a simple nutritional screening assessment should be an integral part of initial antenatal care so that any problems are identified at an early stage. In practice, this may not happen, particularly if dietetic input into local antenatal care services is minimal. In these circumstances, dietitians have an important role as educators of midwives and other health professionals to ensure that pregnant women with nutritional problems receive the dietary advice and follow-up that they need.

Women who are particularly likely to be nutritionally at risk during pregnancy are those who:

- are teenagers, especially those still in their young teens
- are more than 20% above or 10% below ideal body weight
- are from an ethnic minority group, especially recent immigrants or those with English language difficulties
- are from a low-income group
- are vegans or vegetarians who follow an inadequate diet (Drake *et al.* 1997)
- are restricting their food intake for reasons such as slimming or self-diagnosed food 'allergies'
- have, or have a recent history of, an eating disorder such as anorexia nervosa or bulimia nervosa
- have alcohol, smoking or drug problems
- have a pre-existing medical complication such as diabetes mellitus or gastrointestinal disease
- have a poor obstetric history including low birthweight babies (less than 2500 g), spontaneous abortion, prolonged labour and abruptio placenta
- have closely spaced pregnancies.

Nutritional assessment and monitoring is particularly important in women from such groups and expert dietetic guidance will often be warranted. However, nutritional considerations should remain an integral part of the monitoring process of all women throughout pregnancy, particularly in respect of weight gain. Those gaining weight too rapidly should be given guidance on how to lower their dietary energy density by reducing consumption of fat-rich and sugar-rich foods and snacks, while still maintaining a diet of high nutrient density via food choices such as fruit and vegetables, low-fat dairy products and cereal foods. Conversely, poor weight gain requires investigation for potential dietary origins and the need for appropriate measures to improve dietary nutrient and energy density.

3.1.4 Nutrition-related problems in pregnancy

Nausea and vomiting

Nausea and vomiting, especially 'morning sickness', are common occurrences during pregnancy, particularly in the first trimester. Nausea may be exacerbated by long journeys and smells (particularly those of cigarettes, coffee and toothpaste). It is a common experience that small, carbohydrate-rich snacks given at frequent (e.g. 2–3 hourly) intervals provide some relief from nausea, although the reason for this is not clear. Women should be reassured that more frequent consumption of small, well-balanced snacks (e.g. sandwiches, fruit, milk drinks) will be just as nourishing as occasional full meals and need not result in excessive weight gain.

General measures to help to alleviate nausea are described in Section 1.12.2 in Oral nutrition support, but advice which may be particularly helpful for pregnant women is to:

- eat some dry bread, biscuits or cereal before getting up in the morning. Get out of bed slowly, avoiding sudden movements
- drink liquids between, rather than with, meals to avoid abdominal distension which can trigger vomiting
- avoid large meals and greasy and highly spiced foods
- suck something sour, such as a slice of lemon
- relax and rest and get into the fresh air as much as possible. Keep rooms well ventilated and odour free
- slowly sip a fizzy drink when feeling nauseated
- try foods and drinks containing ginger as these sometimes relieve nausea (Erick 1995).

Alternative therapies such as acupuncture have been reported to help relieve nausea and vomiting in some mothers (Dundee 1988), and acupressure wrist bands used for the relief of travel sickness may be effective for some. Caution should be advised with other alternative remedies since their effects in pregnancy are largely unknown and, in the hands of untrained practitioners, could be hazardous (e.g. some aromatherapy oils are contraindicated in pregnancy).

Hyperemesis gravidarum

Hyperemesis gravidarum is the term used to describe the vomiting which occurs in pregnancy before the 20th week of gestation and may be of such severity as to require hospital admission. The aetiology is unknown, although factors such as multiple pregnancy, parity, race and social circumstances may contribute.

Early intervention is important in hyperemesis gravidarum to avoid severe dehydration and associated problems. Once hospitalized, initial attention must focus on intravenous rehydration, correction of electrolyte imbalance and energy provision. Vitamins, minerals and trace elements should also be supplied as these may be severely depleted. Total parenteral nutrition is rarely necessary. Once enteral feeding can commence, small frequent feeds of clear fluids should be offered and once these are well tolerated, small quantities of a complete food supplement should be given at frequent intervals. As tolerance improves the amount can be increased gradually until intake approaches the daily requirement. Even when three meals a day can be tolerated, supplemental drinks should still be given between meals and phased out gradually as the meals increase in size.

Body weight, electrolytes, urinary ketones, fluid balance and food consumption should be monitored throughout. Discharge can be planned once the oral regimen is tolerated and weight gain is occurring.

Cravings, aversions and pica

Food aversions and cravings have long been recognized as a common occurrence in pregnancy. Food aversions have been defined as 'a definite revulsion against food and drink not previously disliked' (Dickens and Trethalum 1971), with the most common aversions being to tea and coffee, alcohol, fried food and eggs in early pregnancy, and to sweet foods in later pregnancy.

Food cravings have been defined (Dickens and Trethalum 1971) as 'a compulsive urge for a food for which there was no previous excessive desire'. There is no pattern to the type of foods that have been identified and there is no evidence that such cravings adversely affect the nutritional intake of women during pregnancy.

Pica is the craving for and ingestion of substances usually considered inedible for human consumption. A wide variety of items has been described, including laundry starch, ice, rocks, matchboxes and clay. There is no convincing evidence that pica has any physiological significance or indicates any mineral deficiency.

Heartburn

Gastro-oesophageal reflux, the basis of heartburn in pregnancy, is very common and can start as early as the third month but is generally worst in the third trimester. It is the result of increased abdominal pressure, combined with altered gastrointestinal motility. The discomfort can be severe and sustained, and often exacerbated by lying down and by certain foods, particular those which are spicy, fatty, fizzy or acidic. Small, frequent meals or snacks are usually tolerated better than infrequent, large ones. Milk and yoghurt may help to relieve the symptoms in some people but antacids are widely used. General measures for the alleviation of reflux are given in Section 4.5.3 in Disorders of the stomach and duodenum.

Constipation

In the UK, many women suffer from constipation some time during pregnancy. Its aetiology is complex and probably a combination of physiological effects of pregnancy on gastrointestinal function, decreased physical activity and dietary changes.

Measures which may alleviate it include dietary modification, use of faecal bulking agents and changes in the type of any iron supplement used. Standard dietary guidance to increase consumption of fluids and cereal-fibre containing foods is appropriate (see Section 4.11.1 in Disorders of the colon). It should be borne in mind that lack of fluid may be a significant contributory cause of constipation in pregnant women because many deliberately restrict fluid intake to overcome the problem of frequency of micturition.

Pre-eclampsia

Pre-eclampsia is the presence of hypertension (diastolic pressure of 90 mmHg or more) together with significant proteinuria (above 0.2 g/l) in the absence of other causes of these symptoms such as renal disease, urinary tract infection and essential hypertension. There is no conclusive evidence that dietary restriction or supplementation can prevent pre-eclampsia.

Text revised by: Jacki Bishop, Fiona Ford and Briony Thomas

Useful addresses

National Childbirth Trust
Alexandra House, Oldham Terrace, London W3 6NH
Tel: 020 8992 8637

La Leche League
PO Box BM 3424, London WC1N 3XX
Website: www.lalecheleague.org

Maternity Alliance
5th Floor, 45 Beech Street, London EC2P 2LX
Tel: 020 7588 8583/020 7588 8582

References

Barker DJ. *Fetal and Infant Origins of Adult Disease*. London: BMJ Publishing, 1992.

Barker DJP. *Mothers, Babies and Diseases in Later Life*. London: BMJ Publishing, 1994.

Barker DJP. Fetal origins of coronary heart disease. *British Medical Journal* 1995; **311**: 171–174.

Beattie JO. Alcohol exposure and the fetus. *European Journal of Clinical Nutrition* 1992; **46** (Suppl 1): S7–S17.

Benke PI. The isotretinoin teratogen syndrome. *Journal of the American Medical Association* 1984; **251**: 3267–3269.

Ben-Shlomo Y, Smith GD. Deprivation in infancy or adult life: which is the more important for mortality risk? *Lancet* 1991; **337**: 1386–1387.

Bernhardt JR, Dorsey DJ. Hypervitaminosis A and congenital renal anomalies in human infants. *Obstetrics and Gynaecology* 1974; **43**: 750–755.

Calloway DH. Nutrition and reproductive function of men. *Nutrition Abstracts and Reviews* 1983; **53**: 361–377.

Clark AM, Thornley B, Tomlinson L *et al.* Weight loss in infertile women results in improvement in reproductive outcome for all forms of fertility treatment. *Human Reproduction* 1998; **13**: 1502–1505.

Committee on Obstetrics; Maternal and Fetal Medicine. Vitamin A supplementation during pregnancy. ACOG Committee Opinion. *International Journal of Gynecology and Obstetrics* 1993; **40**: 175.

Czeizel AE. Prevention of congenital anomalies by periconceptional multivitamin supplementation. *British Medical Journal* 1993; **306**: 1645–1648.

Czeizel AE, Dudas I. Prevention of the first occurrence of neural tube defects by periconceptional vitamin supplementation. *New England Journal of Medicine* 1992; **327**: 1832–1835.

Department of Health. *Dietary Reference Values for Food Energy and Nutrients in the UK*. Report on Health and Social Subjects 41. London: HMSO, 1991.

Department of Health. *Folic Acid and the Prevention of Neural Tube Defects*. Report from the Expert Advisory Group for Health Professionals. London: Department of Health, 1992.

Department of Health. *Sensible Drinking*. The report of an interdepartmental working group. London: DH, 1995.

Department of Health. *While you are Pregnant: Safe Eating and how to Avoid Infection from Food and Animals*. London: Department of Health, 1996.

Department of Health: Committee on Toxicity of Chemicals in Food, Consumer Products and the Environment. *Peanut Allergy*. London: DH 1998.

Department of Health. *Folic Acid and the Prevention of Disease*. Report on Health and Social Subjects 50. London: The Stationery Office, 2000.

Department of Health and Social Security. *Vitamin A and Pregnancy*. PL/CMO (90) 11, PL/CNO (90). London: HMSO, 1990.

Dickens G, Trethalum WH. Cravings and aversions during pregnancy. *Journal of Psychosomatic Research* 1971; **15**: 259–268.

Doyle W, Crawford MA, Wynn AHA, Wynn SW. The association between maternal diet and birth dimensions. *Journal of Nutritional Medicine* 1990; **1**: 9–17.

Drake *et al.* Are vegetarians receiving adequate dietary advice for pregnancy? *British Journal of Midwifery* 1997; **6**: 28–32.

Dundee JW. P6 acupuncture reduces morning sickness. *Journal of the Royal Society of Medicine* 1988; **81**: 456–457.

Edwards LE, Alton IR, Barrada MI, Hakanson EY. Pregnancy in the underweight woman. *American Journal of Obstetrics and Gynecology* 1979; **135**: 297–302.

Erick M. Vitamin B6 and ginger in morning sickness. *Journal of the American Dietetic Association* 1995; **95**: 416.

Feig DS, Naylor CD. Eating for two: are guidelines for weight gain during pregnancy too liberal? *Lancet* 1998; **351**: 1054–1055.

Frisch RE, McArthur JW. Menstrual cycles: fatness as a determinant of minimum weight for height necessary for their maintenance and onset. *Science* 1974; **185**: 949–951.

Giwercman A, Bonde JP. Declining male fertility and environmental factors. *Endocrinology and Metabolism Clinics of North America* 1998; **27**: 807–830.

Godfrey K, Robinson S, Barker DJP *et al*. Maternal nutrition in early and late pregnancy in relation to placental and fetal growth. *British Medical Journal* 1996; **312**: 410–414.

Gregory J, Foster K, Tyler H, Wiseman M. *The Dietary and Nutritional Survey of British Adults*. London: HMSO, 1990.

Hallberg L. Prevention of iron deficiency. *Baillieres Clinical Haematology* 1994; **7**: 805–814.

Haste FM, Brooke OG, Anderson HR *et al*. Nutrient intakes during pregnancy: observations on the influence of smoking and social class. *American Journal of Clinical Nutrition* 1990; **51**: 29–36.

Hathcock JN, Hattan DG, Jenkins MY *et al*. Evaluation of Vitamin A toxicity. *American Journal of Clinical Nutrition* 1990; **52**: 183–202.

Hytten FE. Weight gain in pregnancy. In Hytten FE, Chamberlain G (Eds) *Clinical Pathology in Obstetrics*, 2nd edn. pp. 173–203. Oxford: Blackwell Science, 1991.

Institute of Medicine (IOM). *Nutrition During Pregnancy*. Washington, DC: National Academic Press, 1990.

Jensen T, Hjollund NHI, Henriksen TB *et al*. Does moderate alcohol consumption affect fertility? Follow up study among couples planning first pregnancy. *British Medical Journal* 1998; **317**: 505–510.

Johnson JWC, Longmate JA, Frentzen B. Excessive maternal weight and pregnancy outcome. *American Journal of Obstetrics and Gynecology* 1992; **167**: 353–372.

Lumley J, Astbury J. Advice for pregnancy. In Chalmers I, Enkin M (Eds) *Effective Care in Pregnancy and Childbirth*.Oxford: Oxford University Press, 1989.

Mathews F, Yudkin P, Neil A. Influence of maternal nutrition on outcome of pregnancy: prospective cohort study. *British Medical Journal* 1999; **319**: 339–343.

McGovern E, Moss H, Grewal G *et al*. Factors affecting the use of folic acid supplements in pregnant women in Glasgow. *British Journal of General Practice* 1997; **47**: 635–637.

Medical Research Council Vitamin Study Group. Prevention of neural tube defects: results of the MRC Vitamin Study. *Lancet* 1991; **238**:131–137.

Misra R, Anderson DC. Providing the fetus with calcium. *British Medical Journal* 1990; **30**: 1220–1221.

Naeye RL. Maternal body weight and pregnancy outcome. *American Journal of Clinical Nutrition* 1979; **52**: 273–279.

Paneth N, Susser M. Early origins of coronary heart disease (the Barker Hypothesis). *British Medical Journal* 1995; **310**: 411–412.

Rees JM, Englebert-Fenton KA, Gong EJ *et al*. Weight gain in adolescents during pregnancy: rate related to birth-weight outcome. *American Journal of Clinical Nutrition* 1992; **56**: 868–873.

Robinson S, Godfrey K, Denne J, Cox V. The determinants of iron status in early pregnancy. *British Journal of Nutrition* 1998; **79**: 249–255.

Rogers I, Emmett P, Barker D, Golding J and the ALSPAC Study Team. Financial difficulties, smoking habits, composition of the diet and birthweight in a population of pregnant women in the South West of England. *European Journal of Clinical Nutrition* 1998; **52**: 251–260.

Rosso P. A new chart to monitor weight gain during pregnancy. *American Journal of Obstetrics and Gynecology* 1985; **41**: 644–652.

Royal College of Obstetricians and Gynaecologists. *Alcohol Consumption in Pregnancy*. London: RCOG, 1999.

Rush D, Sloon NL, Leighton J. The National WIC Evaluation V Longitudinal study of pregnant women. *American Journal of Clinical Nutrition* 1988; (Suppl): 439–483.

Scholl TO, Hediger ML, Schall JI *et al*. Gestational weight gain, pregnancy and postpartum weight retention. *Obstetrics and Gynecology* 1995; **86**: 423–427.

Sharp RM, Shakkebaek NE. Are oestrogens involved in falling sperm counts and disorders of the male reproductive tract? *Lancet* 1993; **341**: 1392–1395.

Shepard MJ, Hellenbrand KG, Bracken MB. Proportional weight gain and complications of pregnancy, labor and delivery in healthy women of normal pre-pregnant stature. *American Journal of Obstetrics* 1986; **155**: 947–954.

Smithells RW, Sheppard S, Schorah LJ *et al*. Possible prevention of neural tube defects by periconceptional vitamin supplementation. *Lancet* 1980; **ii**: 339–340.

Spohr HL, Willms J, Steinhausen HC. Prenatal alcohol exposure and long term developmental consequences. *Lancet* 1993; **i**: 907–910.

Stein AD, Ravelli ACJ, Lumley LH. Famine, third trimester pregnancy weight gain and intrauterine growth: the Dutch famine birth cohort study. *Human Biology* 1995; **67**: 135–150.

Tas S, Lauwerys R, Lison D. Occupational hazards for the male reproductive system. *Critical Reviews in Toxicology* 1996; **26**: 261–307.

Treasure JL, Russell GFM. Intrauterine growth and neonatal weight gain in babies of women with anorexia nervosa. *British Medical Journal* 1988; **296**: 1038.

Whittaker PG, Macphail S, Lind T. Serial hematologic changes and pregnancy outcome. *Obstetrics and Gynecology* 1996; **88**: 33–39.

Wynn M, Wynn A. *The Prevention of Handicap of Early Pregnancy Origin*. London: Foundation for Education and Research in Childbearing, 1981.

3.2 Preterm infants

3.2.1 Definitions

- A *preterm infant* is one born before 36 weeks' completed gestation.
- A *low birthweight* (LBW) infant is one born weighing <2500 g regardless of the length of gestation.
- Infants <1500 g are *very low birthweight* (VLBW).
- Those <1000 g are *extremely low birthweight* (ELBW).

Infants born smaller than expected may also be categorized as *small for gestational age* (SGA) and *intrauterine growth retarded* (IUGR).

Preterm infants in particular are prone to problems with all organ systems owing to immaturity, particularly compromised respiratory function, and many did not survive before the advent of mechanical ventilation. They have poor tolerance of both enteral and parenteral nutrition.

3.2.2 Nutritional requirements

Preterm infants have limited stores of many nutrients as accretion occurs predominantly in the last trimester (Friss-Hanson 1971). Thus, they are poorly equipped to withstand inadequate nutrition; theoretically, endogenous reserves in a 1000 g infant are only sufficient for 4 days (Heird *et al.* 1972). It is generally accepted that most infants < 1500 g will need some parenteral nutrition while enteral feeds are gradually increased. The following is a brief discussion of the requirements for the major nutrients, via the enteral route unless otherwise specified. The most recent set of recommendations is covered comprehensively by Tsang *et al.* (1993) and summarized in Table 3.1.

Energy

As a rough guide Tsang *et al.* (1993) suggest aiming for 80–90 non-protein kcal/kg parenterally and 110–120 kcal/kg enterally; occasionally infants with chronic cardiac or respiratory problems will require more. Intakes above requirements will lead to higher weight gains but this will usually be due to fat deposition in excess of uterine accretion rates (Tsang *et al.* 1993) and lead to higher metabolic rates (Brooke, 1980). There are no advantages for lean body mass or skeletal growth even when protein is also increased (see Protein, below).

Table 3.1 Recommended composition of preterm infant formulae (Tsang *et al.* 1993)

Nutrient	Recommended content per 100 ml or 80 kcal (unless otherwise stated)
Energy	80 kcal
Protein	
Infants < 1000 g	3.6–3.8 g/kg
Infants > 1000 g	3.0–3.6 g/kg
Fat	3.5–4.8 g (tentative)
Long-chain polyunsaturates	Conditionally essential
Linoleic acid	0.35–1.36 g
Linolenic acid	0.09–0.35 g
Carbohydrate	Not specified
Minerals	
Sodium	30–46 mg
Potassium	52–80 mg
Chloride	47–71 mg
Calcium	80–154 mg
Phosphorus	40–94 mg
Ca:P ratio	Not specified
Magnesium	5–10 mg
Iron	2.0 mg/kg
Zinc	0.7 mg
Copper	80–100 μg
Iodine	20–40 μg
Manganese	5 μg
Selenium	0.9 μg
Vitamins	
Vitamin A	Chronic lung disease (CLD): 450–840 μg/kg No CLD: 210–450 μg/kg
Vitamin D	2.4–6.4 μg (Min. 10 IU/day)
Vitamin E (TE)	2.7–5.4 mg (Max. 25 IU/day)
Vitamin K	5.3–6.7 μg
Thiamin B$_1$	0.12–0.16 mg
Riboflavin B$_2$	0.16–0.24 mg
Niacin	2.4–3.2 mg
Panthothenic acid	0.8–1.2 mg
Pyridoxine B$_6$	0.1–0.14 mg
Folic acid	17–34 μg
Vitamin B$_{12}$	0.2 μg
Biotin	2.4–4.0 μg
Vitamin C	12–16 mg
Choline	Not specified
Taurine	2.25–6.0 mg
Inositol	16–54 mg
Carnitine	Not specified
Nucleotides	Not specified
Beta-carotene (μg)	Not specified
Osmolality	Not specified
Estimated renal solute load (mOsmol/l)	Not specified

Protein

Tsang *et al.* (1993) suggest protein intakes stratified according to birthweight as *in utero* accretion rates decline with advancing gestation (<1000 g 3.6–3.8 g/kg per day; >1000 g 3.0–3.6 g/kg per day). Between 27 and 35 weeks' gestation, daily accretion is around 2 g/kg; this can be achieved postnatally as long as the above protein intakes are accompanied by recommended energy intakes. Protein gain increases in a linear fashion up to an intake of around 4 g/kg per day, after which it is static. Hepatic immaturity leads to the need for exogenous supplies of cysteine, glycine and taurine, normally considered non-essential in older individuals.

Fat

Absorption will be variable but the more immature the infant, the higher the risk for malabsorption due to smaller bile salt pools (Signer *et al.* 1974) and less pancreatic lipase (Hamosh 1987).

Controversy exists on the provision of the longer-chain derivatives of linoleic and linolenic acids, namely arachidonic (AA) and docosahexaenoic (DHA) acids. Although Tsang *et al.* (1993) felt that definite recommendations could not be made, other experts have suggested that both should be added to preterm formula (ESPGAN 1991). There seem to be advantages with respect to visual and neurodevelopmental outcome for preterm infants (Carlson *et al.* 1994; Gibson and Makrides 1998).

Theoretically, enteral medium-chain triglycerides should lead to improved fat absorption; however, no consistent advantage with respect to fat (Hamosh et al. 1991) or nitrogen balance (Sulkers *et al.* 1992) has been found.

Carbohydrate

Lactase levels are low in preterm infants, but feeding a lactose-containing milk will assist precocious development of lactase activity, thus aiding tolerance (Shulman *et al.* 1998).

Folic acid

Requirements for folic acid have been established (Ek *et al.* 1984) and preterm formulae are all fortified appropriately (Tsang *et al.* 1993). However, many neonatal units still give a folic acid supplement; although this is not regarded as toxic, the appearance of unmetabolized folic acid in the serum may be undesirable, particularly in those given a large weekly dose (Kelly *et al.* 1997).

Vitamin A

Many preterm infants are born with poor vitamin A stores (Mupanemunda *et al.* 1994) and there is some evidence that high-dose enteral supplementation (5000 IU/day) is needed to normalize serum levels (Landman *et al.* 1992). There is renewed interest in appropriate vitamin A supplementation as it may help to reduce the risk of chronic lung disease (CLD) (Kennedy *et al.* 1997).

Vitamin D

A daily intake of 400 IU/day to a maximum of 800 IU/day enterally is recommended, with a lower dose parenterally as the gut barrier is bypassed (Tsang *et al.* 1993). Higher enteral intakes had previously been thought necessary, but these have not been shown to improve outcome (Evans *et al.* 1989). A recent study demonstrated that even a population from northerly latitudes, likely to have the lower range of vitamin D status at birth, progressed well on 400 IU/day (Backstrom *et al.* 1999).

Vitamin E

At least 1.0 IU vitamin E/g linoleic acid and 0.7 IU vitamin E/100 kcal up to a maximum of 25 IU/day should be provided (Tsang *et al.* 1993).

Calcium, phosphorus and magnesium

The fetus acquires 80% of the normal term content of calcium during the last trimester (Ziegler *et al.* 1976) and thus preterm infants have high requirements for calcium and other minerals needed for bone formulation. Although a calcium:phosphorus ratio is not specified (Tsang *et al.* 1993), all current preterm formulae fall between 1.7: 1 and 2: 1, complying with previous guidelines (ESPGAN 1987).

Iron

Iron stores are low in preterm infants and without supplementation will become depleted by 8 weeks (Olivares *et al.* 1992). Current recommendations are that supplements should start any time between birth and 8 weeks as either a supplemented formula or medicinal iron at a level of 2 mg/kg per day to a maximum of 15 mg/kg per day (Tsang *et al.* 1993). Owing to the interactions of iron, copper and zinc during absorption, excessive amounts of each individually should be avoided.

Zinc

Zinc may be an important growth regulator during infancy. Tsang *et al.* (1993) suggest 0.7 mg/80 kcal; others have suggested that more is necessary (Friel and Andrews 1994). Renal losses may be exacerbated by repeated acute-phase responses and diuretic therapy (Askari *et al.* 1979; Wester 1980).

Conditionally essential nutrients

Nucleotides

Nucleotides may be conditionally essential for the gut and immune system during times of stress (Rudolph 1994). Despite the high levels in human milk, Tsang et al. (1993) felt that there were insufficient data at the time of publication to support formula supplementation. Since then, encouraging studies have been published suggesting that nucleotide supplementation can reduce diarrhoea in term infants (Brunser et al. 1994) and improve growth in SGA infants (Cosgrove et al. 1996).

Glutamine

Glutamine is an important fuel for the small intestine and immune system, possible becoming rate limiting during increased demand (Powell-Tuck 1993). Although at the time Tsang et al. (1993) could not recommend supplementation, glutamine has since been associated with improved outcome in both parenterally (Lacey et al. 1996) and enterally fed preterm infants (Neu et al. 1997). This may become an important supplement in the future.

3.2.3 Parenteral nutrition

With increased survival, preterm infants have become a major recipient of parenteral nutrition, usually in association with minimal enteral feeds (Berseth 1990). Early initiation of parenteral nutrition has been shown to be well tolerated (Gilbertson et al. 1991; Murdock et al. 1995; Van-Goudoever et al. 1995; see King 1998a for a comprehensive review).

3.2.4 Enteral nutrition

The advantages of early and minimal enteral feeding have been shown in many studies (Dunn et al. 1988; Meetze et al. 1992; Ehrenkranz et al. 1996; Schanler et al. 1999).

The milk of choice is undoubtedly the mother's own freshly expressed breast milk, which has the following advantages:

- improved feed tolerance (Lucas 1987; Uraizee and Gross 1989)
- reduced risk of sepsis (Uraizee and Gross 1989; Hylander et al. 1998; Schanler et al. 1999).
- long-term neurodevelopmental benefits (Lucas et al. 1992a, 1994).
- reduced risk of necrotizing enterocolitis (NEC), a serious gut disease with a high mortality rate found almost exclusively in preterm infants (Lucas and Cole 1990; Schanler et al. 1999).

Pasteurized banked donor breast milk retains some immunological advantages (Lucas and Cole 1990); however, heat-labile vitamins, bile salt stimulated lipase and live cells are reduced or destroyed, so it is recommend for initiation of feeds only in the absence of mother's own milk.

Note that the pasteurization process and maternal screening prevent any risk of human immunodeficiency virus (HIV) transmission from banked donor milk.

Human milk may be nutritionally adequate in many respects for infants >1500 g when fed in sufficient volumes, i.e. up to 220 ml/kg in well infants, although an iron supplement will be needed by 2 months. However, in infants below 1500 g, some nutrients may be limiting, particularly protein and some minerals and vitamins. Serum phosphate should be kept above 1.5 mmol/l, but below calcium levels. When serum phosphate is <1.5 mmol/l a supplement is required; 0.5 mmol twice daily has been given successfully (Holland et al. 1990), but should be titrated according to serum biochemistry. Milk produced during the first 2–3 weeks of lactation may have higher protein levels, although this is not a consistent finding and wide variations have been reported (Velona et al. 1999).

An indirect measure of protein intake may be the serum urea level. This was found to drop below 1.6 mmol/l in most cases when human milk protein intake fell below 3 g/kg per day (Polberger et al. 1990). Protein fortification can be considered once serum urea reaches 2 mmol/l after a consistent fall. A commercially produced human milk fortifier has many advantages over supplementing with formula, as this will allow the use of full volumes of mother's milk (Lucas et al. 1996).

See King (1999) for further details on all practical aspects of enteral nutrition.

Method of enteral feeding

As a result of an immature suck – swallow – breathe pattern, preterm infants require tube feeding until around 35–37 weeks of gestation, and sometimes longer.

There are advantages and disadvantages to both bolus and continuous gastric tube feeding. Boluses have been associated with less feed intolerance (Schanler et al. 1999) but they may lead to a deterioration in respiratory function compared with continuous feeds (Macagno and Demarini 1994). Continuous feeding of human milk can lead to excessive fat loss (Narayanan et al. 1984) and risk of sedimentation of added minerals. An alternative method is 2-hour slow infusion every 3 hours, which has been shown to improve feed tolerance (de Ville et al. 1998).

There is much evidence that rapid advancement of enteral feeds is associated with an increased risk of NEC (Uauy et al. 1991; McKeown et al. 1992). Limiting the increase to 20 ml/kg per day has been suggested, particularly in those considered to be at high risk of NEC.

For some infants, particularly those who have been very unwell, the transition to nipple feeding is very difficult. Liaison with an experienced speech and language therapist is invaluable in these circumstances. Some mother–infant pairs benefit from specialist advice on establishing breast feeding and, with support, infants born at as young as 24 weeks can leave neonatal units being totally breastfed.

3.2.5 Post-discharge nutrition

All mothers should be encouraged to breast feed their infants on demand wherever possible post-discharge; however, for those who cannot, alternatives to term formulae have been developed. Preterm infants have been observed to consume up to 300 ml/kg of term formula post-discharge (Lucas *et al.* 1992b). In response to this, nutrient-enriched post-discharge formulae (NEPDF) have been developed so that the nutrition required to maintain a rapid growth rate can be delivered in smaller volumes of feed. Although limited, there are data suggesting that enriched formulae may improve growth, bone mineralization and possibly neurodevelopment (Lucas *et al.* 1992c; Bishop *et al.* 1993; Carlson *et al.* 1994). Some also have the advantage of negating the need for separate iron and vitamin supplements post-discharge.

3.2.6 Weaning

Solids should not be introduced before 16 weeks post-delivery unless there are exceptional circumstances. A suggested upper limit is 7 months post-delivery.

Concern has been voiced about the safety of introducing a preterm infant to solids before 16 weeks post due date (i.e. 40 weeks' gestation). However, the introduction of milk feeds leads to a precocious development of the gastrointestinal tract with respect to digestion (Shulman *et al.* 1998) and motility (Berseth 1992). There is no evidence for increased risk of allergy (David and Ewing 1988) or of obesity, the latter theoretically as a result of passive overfeeding. However, preterm infants seem to have a higher prevalence of behavioural feeding problems (Douglas and Bryon 1996; Martin and Shaw 1997). This may be due to solids (particularly lumps) having been delayed beyond a critical period for their acceptance (Illingworth and Lister 1964).

Once weaning has started it should proceed according to COMA guidelines (DH 1994). See King 1998b) for further details on weaning preterm infants.

Text revised by: Caroline King

Further reading

Shaw V, Lawson M (Eds). *Clinical Paediatric Dietetics*, 3rd edn. Oxford: Blackwells, 2001.

References

Askari A, Long CL, Blakemore WS. Urinary zinc, copper, nitrogen, and potassium losses in response to trauma. *Journal of Parenteral and Enteral Nutrition* 1979; **3**: 151–156.

Backstrom MC, Maki R, Kuusela AL *et al.* Randomised controlled trial of vitamin D supplementation on bone density and biochemical indices in preterm infants. *Archives of Disease in Childhood* 1999; **80**: F161–F166.

Berseth CL. Neonatal small intestinal motility: motor responses to feeding in term and preterm infants. *Journal of Paediatrics* 1990; **117**: 777–782.

Berseth CL. Effect of early feeding on maturation of the preterm infants small intestine. *Journal of Paediatrics* 1992; **120**: 947.

Bishop NJ, King FJ, Lucas A. Increased bone mineral content of preterm infants fed a nutrient enriched formula after discharge from hospital. *Archives of Disease in Childhood* 1993; **68**: 573–578.

Brooke OG. Energy balance and metabolic rate in preterm infants fed with standard and high-energy formulas. *British Journal of Nutrition* 1980; **44**: 13–23.

Brunser O, Espinoza J, Araya M *et al.* Effect of dietary nucleotide supplementation on diarrhoeal disease in infants. *Acta Paediatrica* 1994; **83**: 188–191.

Carlson SE, Werkman SH, Peeples JM, Wilson WM. Long-chain fatty acids and early visual and cognitive development of preterm infants. *European Journal of Clinical Nutrition* 1994; **48**: 527–530.

Cosgrove M, Davies DP, Jenkins HR. Nucleotide supplementation and the growth of term small for gestational age infants. *Archives of Disease in Childhood* (Fetal and Neonatal Edition) 1996; **74**: F122–F125.

David TJ, Ewing CI. Atopic eczema and preterm birth. *Archives of Disease in Childhood* 1988; **63**: 435–436.

de Ville K, Knapp E, Al Tawil Y, Berseth CL. Slow infusion feedings enhance duodenal motor responses and gastric emptying in preterm infants. *American Journal of Clinical Nutrition* 1998; **68**: 103–108.

Department of Health, Committee on Medical Aspects of Food Policy *Weaning and the Weaning Diet*. Report on Health and Social Subjects 45. London: HMSO, 1994.

Douglas JE, Bryon M. Interview data on severe behavioural eating difficulties in young children. *Archives of Disease in Childhood* 1996; **75**: 304–308.

Dunn L, Hulman S, Weiner J, Kliegman R. Beneficial effects of early hypocaloric enteral feeding on neonatal gastrointestinal function: preliminary report of a randomized trial. *Journal of Paediatrics* 1988; **112**: 622–629.

Ehrenkranz RA, Younes N, Fanaroff AA *et al.* Effect of nutritional practices on daily weight gain in VLBW infants. *Pediatric Research* 1996; **39**: 308A.

Ek J, Behncke L, Halvorsen KS, Magnus E. Plasma and red cell folate values and folate requirements in formula fed premature infants. *European Journal of Paediatrics* 1984; **142**: 78–82.

ESPGAN. Nutrition and feeding of preterm infants. *Acta Paediatrica Scandinavica* 1987; Suppl 336.

ESPGAN. Comment on the content and composition of lipids in infant formula. *Acta Paediatrica Scandinavica* 1991; **80**: 887–896.

Evans JR, Allen AC, Stinson DA *et al.* Effect of high-dose vitamin D supplementation on radiographically detectable bone disease of very low birth weight infants. *Journal of Paediatrics* 1989; **115**: 779–786.

Friel JK, Andrews WL. Zinc requirement of premature infants. *Nutrition* 1994; **10**: 63–65.

Friss-Hanson B. Body composition during growth: *in-vivo* measurements and biochemical data correlated to differential anatomical growth. *Pediatrics* 1971; **47**: 264–274.

Gibson RA, Makrides M. The role of long chain polyunsaturated fatty acids (LCPUFA) in neonatal nutrition. *Acta Paediatrica* 1998; **87**: 1017–1022.

Gilbertson N, Kovar IZ, Cox DJ *et al.* Introduction of intravenous lipid administration on the first day of life in the very low birth weight neonate. *Journal of Paediatrics* 1991; **119**: 615–623.

Hamosh M. Lipid metabolism in premature infants. *Biology of the Neonate* 1987; **52** (Suppl 1): 50–64.

Hamosh M, Mehta NR, Fink CS *et al.* Fat absorption in premature infants: medium-chain triglycerides and long-chain triglycerides are absorbed from formula at similar rates. *Journal of Pediatric Gastroenterology and Nutrition* 1991; **13**: 143–149.

Heird WC, Driscoll JM, Jr, Schullinger JN *et al*. Intravenous alimentation in pediatric patients. *Journal of Paediatrics* 1972; **80**: 351–372.

Holland P, Wilkinson A, Diez J, Lindsell D. Prenatal deficiency of phosphate, phosphate supplementation and rickets in very low birth weight infants. *Lancet* 1990; **335**: 697–701.

Hylander MA, Strobino DM, Dhanireddy R. Human milk feedings and infection among very low birth weight infants. *Pediatrics* 1998; **102**: E38.

Illingworth RS, Lister J. The critical or sensitive period with special reference to certain feeding problems in infants and children. *Journal of Paediatrics* 1964; **65**: 839–849.

Kelly P, McPartland J, Goggins M *et al*. Unmetabolized folic acid in serum: acute studies in subjects consuming fortified food and supplements. *American Journal of Clinical Nutrition* 1997; **65**: 1790–1795.

Kennedy KA, Stoll BJ, Ehrenkranz RA *et al*. Vitamin A to prevent bronchopulmonary dysplasia in very-low-birth-weight infants: has the dose been too low? The NICHD Neonatal Research Network. *Early Human Development* 1997; **49**: 19–31.

King CL. *Neonatal Unit Parenteral Nutrition Policy*. London: Dietetics Department, Hammersmith Hospital, 1998a.

King CL. *Neonatal Unit Weaning Policy*. London: Nutrition and Dietetic Department, Hammersmith Hospital, 1998b.

King CL. *Neonatal Unit Enteral Feeding Policy*. London: Nutrition and Dietetic Department Hammersmith Hospital, 1999.

Lacey JM, Crouch JB, Benfell K *et al*. The effects of glutamine-supplemented parenteral nutrition in premature infants. *Journal of Parenteral and Enteral Nutrition* 1996; **20**: 74–80.

Landman J, Sive A, De V *et al*. Comparison of enteral and intramuscular vitamin A supplementation in preterm infants. *Early Human Development* 1992; **30**: 163–170.

Lucas A. Aids and milk bank closures. *Lancet* 1987; **i**: 1092–1093.

Lucas A, Cole TJ. Breast milk and neonatal necrotising enterocolitis. *Lancet* 1990; **336**: 1519–1523.

Lucas A, Morley R, Cole TJ. Breast milk and subsequent intelligence quotient in children born preterm. *Lancet* 1992a; **339**: 261–264.

Lucas A, King F, Bishop NB. Post discharge formula consumption in infants born preterm. *Archives of Disease in Childhood* 1992b; **67**: 691–692.

Lucas A, Bishop NJ, King FJ, Cole TJ. Randomised trial of nutrition for preterm infants after discharge. *Archives of Disease in Childhood* 1992c; **67**: 322–327.

Lucas A, Morley R, Cole TJ, Gore SM. A randomised multicentred study of human milk vs formula and later development in preterm infants. *Archives of Disease in Childhood* 1994; **70**: F141–F146.

Lucas A, Fewtrell MS, Morley R. Randomised outcome trial of human milk fortification and developmental outcome in preterm infants. *American Journal of Clinical Nutrition* 1996; **64**: 142–151.

Macagno F, Demarini S. Techniques of enteral feeding in the newborn. *Acta Paediatrica*. 1994; **402** (Suppl): 11–13.

Martin M, Shaw NJ. Feeding problems in infants and young children with chronic lung disease. *Journal of Human Nutrition* 1997; **10**: 271–275.

McKeown RE, Marsh D, Amarnath U. Role of delayed feeding and of feeding increments in necrotising enterocolitis. *Journal of Paediatrics* 1992; **121**: 764–770.

Meetze WH, Valentine C, McGuigan JE. Gastrointestinal priming prior to full enteral nutrition in very low birth weight infants. *Journal of Pediatric Gastroenterology and Nutrition* 1992; **15**: 163–170.

Mupanemunda RH, Lee DS, Fraher LJ *et al*. Postnatal changes in serum retinol status in very low birth weight infants. *Early Human Development* 1994; **38**: 45–54.

Murdock N, Crighton A, Nelson LM, Forsyth JS. Low birthweight infants and total parenteral nutrition immediately after birth. II. Randomised study of biochemical tolerance of intravenous glucose, amino acids, and lipid. *Archives of Disease in Childhood* (Fetal and Neonatal Edition) 1995; **73**: F8–F12.

Narayanan I, Singh B, Harvey D. Fat loss during feeding of human milk. *Archives of Disease in Childhood* 1984; **59**: 475–477.

Neu J, Roig JC, Meetze WH *et al*. Enteral glutamine supplementation for very low birth weight infants decreases morbidity. *Journal of Paediatrics* 1997; **131**: 691–699.

Olivares M, Llaguno S, Marin V *et al*. Iron status in low-birth-weight infants, small and appropriate for gestational age. A follow-up study. *Acta Paediatrica* 1992; **81**: 824–828.

Polberger SKT, Axelsson IE, Raitia NCR. Urinary and serum urea as indicators of protein metabolism in very low birth weight infants fed varying human milk protein intakes. *Acta Paediatrica Scandinavica* 1990; **79**: 737–742.

Powell-Tuck J. Glutamine, parenteral feeding, and intestinal nutrition. *Lancet* 1993; **342**: 451–452.

Rudolph FB. Symposium: dietary nucleotides: a recently demonstrated requirement for cellular development and immune function. *Journal of Nutrition* 1994; **124**: 1431S–1432S.

Schanler RJ, Shulman RJ, Lau C *et al*. Feeding strategies for premature infants: randomized trial of gastrointestinal priming and tube-feeding method. *Pediatrics* 1999; **103**: 434–439.

Shulman RJ, Schanler RJ, Lau C *et al*. Early feeding, feeding tolerance, and lactase activity in preterm infants. *Journal of Paediatrics* 1998; **133**: 645–649.

Signer E, Murphy GM, Edkins S, Anderson CM. Role of bile salts in fat malabsorption of premature infants. *Archives of Disease in Childhood* 1974; **49**: 174–180.

Sulkers EJ, von Goudoever JB, Leunisse C *et al*. Comparison of two preterm formulas with or without addition of medium-chain triglycerides (MCTs). 1: Effects on nitrogen and fat balance and body composition changes. *Journal of Pediatric Gastroenterology and Nutrition* 1992; **15**: 34–41.

Tsang RC, Lucas A, Uauy R, Zlotkin S. *Nutritional Needs of the Preterm Infant: Scientific Basis and Practical Guidelines*. Baltimore, MD: Williams & Wilkins, 1993

Uauy RD, Fanaroff AA, Korones SB. Necrotising entercolitis in very low birth weight infants. Biodemographic and clinical correlates. *Journal of Paediatrics* 1991; **119**: 630–638.

Uraizee F, Gross SJ. Improved feeding tolerance and reduced incidence of sepsis in sick very low birth weight (VLBW) infants fed maternal milk. *Pediatric Research* 1989; **25**: 298A.

Van-Goudoever JB, Colen T, Wattimena JL *et al*. Immediate commencement of amino acid supplementation in preterm infants: effect on serum amino acid concentrations and protein kinetics on the first day of life. *Journal of Paediatrics* 1995; **127**: 458–465.

Velona T, Abbiati L, Beretta B *et al*. Protein profiles in breast milk from mothers delivering term and preterm babies. *Pediatric Research* 1999; **45**: 658–663.

Wester PO. Tissue zinc at autopsy – relation to medication with diuretics. *Acta Medica Scandinavica* 1980; **208**: 269–271.

Ziegler EE, O'Donnell AM, Nelson SE, Komon SJ. Body composition of the reference fetus growth. *Growth* 1976; **40**: 329–341.

The nutritional requirements of infants are high. This is a period of rapid growth and development and, in its first year of life, an infant will triple its birthweight and increase its length by 50%. Compared with adults, infants have a higher requirement per kilogram body weight for energy, protein, iron and calcium. In addition, many of the newborn infant's body systems are immature and it is therefore important that they receive food in a form that they can digest and metabolize. The consequences of inadequate or unbalanced nutritional intake may not only affect growth and development during the early years but may also influence disease in later life (Barker 1992).

Parents may receive information about infant feeding from a variety of sources. Advice before and after the birth should be based on careful observation and scientific facts in order that parents can make informed choices about the way they feed their child. In the UK, mothers can exercise considerable choice over how to feed their infants; however, many are ill informed about the implications and practicalities of the feeding method chosen.

3.3.1 Breast feeding

Breast milk provides the best source of nourishment for the early months of life. Mothers should be encouraged to and supported in breast feeding for at least four months (DH 1994).

To some mothers, breast feeding is a natural progression of pregnancy, but others find the idea less attractive. Despite the clear advantages of breast feeding, the number of women choosing to breast feed their babies is low. A 1995 survey (Foster *et al.* 1997) showed that:

- In England and Wales, about two-thirds (68%) of babies were breast fed from birth. In Scotland the figure was just over half (55%) of the infant population, while in Northern Ireland fewer than half (45%) of infants were initially breast fed.
- There was a sharp decline in breast-feeding rates within the first few weeks, particularly in Northern Ireland where only 56% of initially breast-fed infants were still receiving breast milk at 6 weeks compared with 65% of breast-fed infants in Scotland, England and Wales.
- Breast-feeding rates were higher amongst women of Asian origin, with 90% of Bangladeshi women, 82% Indian and 76% Pakistani women choosing to breast feed. However, Pakistani and Bangladeshi mothers stopped breast feeding at an earlier stage than either white or Indian mothers.
- The highest incidence of breast feeding was amongst first-time mothers. However, mothers who had successfully breast fed a previous child were most likely to continue feeding after the first few weeks.

Benefits of breast feeding

It is a complete food

Breast milk provides complete nutrition once feeding is successfully established, with no additional nutrients being required until about the age of 6 months. Furthermore, the bioavailability of the nutrients that it contains is high.

Fatty acid composition

Breast milk contains the long-chain polyunsaturated fatty acids (LCPs) arachidonic acid (AA) and docosahexaenoic acid (DHA). These LCPs play an important part in brain (Farquharson *et al.* 1995; Jamieson *et al.* 1999) and retinal development (Birch *et al.* 1998). Adults are able to synthesize LCPs but infants, in particular low birthweight infants, are unable to do so in the amounts that their bodies require. They therefore require an adequate supply which breast milk provides, although the content of LCPs in breast milk is variable and dependent on the mother's diet (Koletzko and Rodriguez-Palmero 1999). Lack of LCPs has been linked with impaired cognitive development in low birthweight and preterm infants (Carlson 1999; Willatts and Forsyth 2000), although whether deficiency has any long-term cognitive effects in infants of normal birthweight remains to be established.

Protection against infection

It is well documented that breast feeding offers protection for the baby against many types of bacterial and viral infection (Hanson 1999). Human milk contains macrophages (which produce lysozymes and lactoferrin), lymphocytes (which secrete interferon and secretary immunoglobulin A), bifidus factor (which enhances the growth of *Lactobacillus bifidus*) and antibodies (Yap *et al.* 1979; Brock 1980). Significantly less gastrointestinal disease is found in babies who are breast fed for at least 13 weeks, with the effect persisting beyond the period of breast feeding (Howie *et al.* 1990). Breast-fed infants also have less respiratory illness than those who are artificially fed (Howie *et al.* 1990; Burr *et al.* 1993), a trend which also may persist into childhood (Wilson *et al.* 1998).

Atopic disease

Exclusive breast feeding offers some protection against the development of atopic disorders and other allergies

(Halken *et al.* 1992; ESPGAN 1993; Saarinen and Kajosaari 1995) as it avoids exposure to large quantities of potential triggering antigens such as cow's milk or soya protein. The extent to which maternal antigen avoidance provides additional protection is less certain (Kramer 1988) (see also Section 4.34.3, Prevention of food allergy).

No risk of solute overload

Unlike powdered milks, breast milk cannot be reconstituted incorrectly.

Availability

Breast milk is immediately available at the correct temperature and no additional preparation is required.

Effect on mother–infant relationship

Suckling ensures frequent contact between mother and infant and assists bonding. A recent systematic review shows that early contact is associated with greater communication between mother and infant (Renfrew *et al.* 2000).

Maternal benefits

Breast feeding assists uterine involution and utilizes surplus body fat deposited in pregnancy, thus facilitating a return to normal body weight. Breast feeding also temporarily reduces fertility which, while this cannot be relied on as a method of contraception, may be advantageous in countries with poor family-planning facilities. In the long term, breast feeding may have a protective effect in respect of premenopausal cancer (Labbok 1999).

Cost

Breast feeding is cheaper than bottle feeding, even when the cost of the additional nutritional needs of the lactating mother is taken into account.

Issues to be challenged

Demands on the mother's time

The mother has to be available day and night to feed the baby, especially in the early weeks whilst breast feeding is being established. It is therefore important that the mother receives encouragement and as much rest as possible during the early stages of breast feeding. Family members can provide invaluable support at this time by helping with other children or taking over household duties.

Physical problems

Establishing a successful lactation is not always straightforward. Physical discomfort in the early days from engorged breasts and sore nipples discourages some mothers. It is important that mothers trying to breast feed are made aware that this is a normal, but short-lived, stage in establishing lactation and are encouraged to persevere.

Difficulty in measuring supply

Some mothers like the reassurance of knowing how much milk their infant has consumed and find it disconcerting that this is not possible with breast feeding. As a result, some worry that their milk supply may be inadequate. It is important that mothers are taught that the infant itself provides the best guide; a baby who is contented and is gaining weight is adequately fed. Mothers should also be encouraged to discuss any concerns about the adequacy of the child's feed or progress with a health professional before abandoning or supplementing breast feeding for this reason.

Embarrassment

Some mothers are embarrassed to breast feed even within the home, particularly those in lower socioeconomic groups (Foster *et al.* 1997). Many women find that the attitude of other people to breast feeding in public, coupled with the frequent lack of facilities to feed in private, make prolonged excursions outside the home very difficult. In addition, many mothers do not receive the support they need from health-service providers (Beeken and Waterston 1992). In an effort to change this, UNICEF has launched its Baby Friendly Initiative, which aims to improve breast-feeding support in maternity and community health services and encourage strategies to promote breast feeding (UNICEF 1999).

Breast feeding can create jealousy

Husbands, relatives and siblings may, in different ways, resent the exclusive role of the mother in breast feeding. Involving everyone in all other aspects of caring for the infant can help to alleviate this problem.

Incompatibility with work

Owing to the lack of suitable child-care facilities in most places of work, returning to work shortly after giving birth makes continuing with full breast feeding almost impossible. Baby-friendly initiatives in the work place would help to support breast-feeding mothers. However, partial breast feeding (e.g. in the mornings and evenings) is often possible and should be encouraged.

Contraindications to breast feeding

Usage of certain drugs

Since many drugs are passed into the breast milk, serious maternal illness necessitating the use of some types of medication may prevent breast feeding. However, in many clinical situations there are choices of drugs which are compatible with breast feeding. Maternal diabetes mellitus, epilepsy or caesarean section are not usually contraindications to breast feeding. Details of drugs which are contraindicated in lactation can be found in the *British National Formulary*.

Human immunodeficiency virus

Mothers in the UK who are HIV positive are at present advised against breast feeding their babies (DHSS 1988; WHO 1992). However, this remains controversial, particularly in developing countries, where formula feeding greatly increases the risk of mortality from gastrointestinal infections. Further research is necessary to establish the risks and benefits of this measure (Morrison 1999).

Medical problems in the infant

Physical problems such as cleft palate or illness in the infant may make breast feeding difficult or not practicable. Where possible, infants who have to be tube fed should be given expressed breast milk. Breast milk, possibly supplemented with human milk fortifiers, is also usually suitable for low birthweight infants who need to be tube fed (see Section 3.2.4 in Preterm infants). Breast feeding is contraindicated in a few rare inborn errors of metabolism such as galactosaemia or alactasia.

Promoting breast feeding

The promotion of breast feeding in the population is dependent on changing attitudes within society. This is a long-term process. However, much could be done to support those who choose to breast feed. It is recognized that professionals may not always provide the most appropriate support. For this reason the Department of Health in 1988 recommended that 'all professionals who are concerned with infant feeding should review their policy and practice to ensure that parents receive adequate advice to encourage the mother to breast feed her baby.' Support for staff should include training in breast-feeding management and improving the information given to mothers wishing to feed their babies.

Establishing and maintaining breast feeding

The decision to breast feed

Virtually all women decide before the birth how they intend to feed their infant. The most common reason given for breast feeding is that it is best for the baby. Convenience is also important to many mothers (Foster *et al.* 1997).

Breast feeding is most common amongst mothers:

- of first babies
- aged 25 years or more
- of higher social class
- educated beyond 18 years
- living in London and the south-east of England.

Initiation of breast feeding

Consistent and appropriate advice from midwives and other staff is essential for the optimal care of the breast-feeding mother and her baby. In practice, many new mothers receive conflicting advice and this is unhelpful and confusing. The provision of extra support by professionals with special skills in breast feeding results in more women exclusively breast feeding their babies and for longer periods (Sikorski and Renfrew 2000). A good understanding of the physiology of lactation is essential for all who are involved in the care of breast-feeding mothers. The

book *Successful Breast Feeding*, published by the Royal College of Midwives (see Further Reading), provides guidance on the management of breast feeding.

The composition of breast milk is not homogeneous. It alters between feeds, within feeds and during the course of lactation (Table 3.2). The first milk produced by the breast is colostrum and is only produced for the first few days after birth. Although colostrum is produced in a small volume its protein content is very high. Furthermore, much of this protein is present as immunoglobulins (mainly IgA), which are important in protecting against infection. Colostrum is lower in fat than mature milk and therefore lower in energy. It is, however, a rich source of minerals and vitamins A, D and B_{12}.

Breast-milk composition changes during the transition to mature milk (Table 3.2) and the calculated composition can only be based on average values (DHSS 1977) (Table 3.3). The hindmilk has a higher fat and thus greater energy content than the foremilk obtained at the beginning of a feed. Incomplete emptying of the breasts may lead to a baby receiving an inadequate energy intake (Woolridge and Fisher 1988).

Early contact between mother and baby increases breast-feeding success. Putting the baby to the breast immediately after birth assists in developing the suckling reflex, which is particularly strong for a short while after delivery (Righard and Alade 1990).

The supply of breast milk is determined largely by demand and is stimulated by frequent, rather than prolonged, suckling. Therefore, feeding 2–3 hourly or even more frequently, for a few minutes at each breast will help the milk supply to become established by the third or fourth day postpartum. Complementary feeds are not necessary and will hinder the establishment of breast feeding.

It takes 3–6 weeks for lactation to become fully established; it is during this period that feeding 'on demand' round the clock is most valuable. Once lactation is well established, feeds can be spaced further apart without diminishing the milk supply.

If the baby is unable to suckle at birth, the mother can use an electric or hand pump to simulate suckling and the baby can be fed expressed breast milk until normal breast feeding can commence. Milk supply can be reduced by

Table 3.2 Changes in breast-milk composition during lactation

Days postpartum	Type of milk	Description
1–3	Colostrum	Thick, yellowy milk, high in protein, antibodies and certain vitamins and minerals
3–7+	Transitional	Thinner, white appearance; composition approaching mature milk
7–10+	Mature	More watery appearance, almost blue in colour as the feed begins and becoming white by the end of a feed as the fat content increases

Table 3.3 Composition of mature breast milk and term infant formula milk

Nutrient	Average content per 100 ml mature breast milk[1] (DH and literature sources)	Recommended content per 100 ml term formula milk (EC Directive 1991)
Energy	65–75 kcal 270–315 kJ	60–75 kcal 250–315 kJ
Protein (g)	1.2–1.4	1.8–3.0 (modified cow's milk) 2.5–3.0 (unmodified cow's milk)
Casein:whey ratio	40:60	
Fat (g)	3.7–4.8	3.3–6.5
Essential fatty acid ratio linoleic acid (n-6): α-linolenic acid (n-3)	5:1	Not specified
Carbohydrate (g)	7.1–7.8	7–14
Calcium (mg)	32–36	50
Phosphorus (mg)	14–15	25–90
Calcium:phosphorus ratio	2.3:1	Not specified
Sodium (mg)	11–20	20–60
Potassium (mg)	57–62	60–145
Chloride (mg)	35–55	50–125
Magnesium (mg)	2.6–3.0	5–15
Iron	62–93 μg	0.5–1.5 mg
Zinc	260–330 μg	0.5–1.5 mg
Iodine (μg)	2–12 μg	5
Manganese (μg)	0.7–1.5 μg	Not specified
Copper (μg)	37–43 μg	20–80
Vitamin A (μg retinol equivalents)	40–76	60–180
Vitamin D_3 (cholecalciferol) (μg)		1.0–2.5
Vitamin E (α-tocopherol) (mg)	0.29–0.39	0.5
Vitamin K (phytomenadione) (μg)	–	4
Thiamin (μg)	13–21	40
Riboflavin (μg)	31	60
Vitamin B_6 (pyridoxine) (μg)	5.1–7.2	35
Vitamin B_{12} (cyanocobalamin) (μg)	0.01	0.1
Nicotinic acid (μg)	210–270	250
Pantothenic acid (μg)	220–330	300
Biotin (μg)	0.52–1.13	1.5
Folic acid (μg)	3.1–6.2	4.0
Vitamin C (mg)	3.1–4.5 mg	8.0
Potential renal solute load (mosmol/l)	86	Not specified

[1]Data compiled from DHSS (1977), DHSS (1980), DH (1991) and other literature sources.

tiredness and tension, so practical and emotional support is very important. Establishing lactation is more difficult to achieve in some babies than in others. Some infants seem to fight at the breast or may be irritable and scream or cry. This may be a result of the rapid initial flow of milk, which overwhelms and frustrates the baby. Expressing a little milk before the feed often resolves the problem. Mothers should be reminded that crying in a baby does not always signal a demand for food. It may be because the baby is uncomfortable, overtired, or just bored and lonely.

Maintaining lactation

Support for the lactating mother from family, friends, midwife, health visitor, National Childbirth Trust breast feeding counsellors or other national or local support organizations and groups is important if breast feeding is to continue. Foster *et al*. (1977) found that one-third of mothers stopped breast feeding within six weeks. The most common reason given for this was 'insufficient milk' but

few had been offered or received any guidance as to whether this was really the case.

Once the milk supply is established, the mother may wish to express breast milk to feed her baby. This expressed milk can be given to the baby via a spoon, cup or a bottle, although not all babies co-operate with an occasional feed in this way. Expressed breast milk can be stored in a refrigerator for up to 48 hour or it can be frozen for up to 6 months. Careful attention to hygiene is important; bottles, containers for storage and other utensils must be sterilized. Guidelines on the collection, storage and handling of expressed breast milk have been produced by the British Association of Perinatal Medicine (1997).

Complementary bottle feeds   Some mothers complement breast feeds with milk formula from a bottle. This may be for reasons of convenience, illness in the mother or an inadequate supply of breast milk. If done for the latter reason it is likely that the mother's own milk supply will diminish further, making a return to complete breast feeding impossible. Wherever possible, other measures to improve her lactation should be tried before starting complementary feeds (see below). If complementary feeds are used, they should be given after the breast feed.

Additional nutritional requirements of the breast-fed infant

Vitamins

Provided that the maternal diet is adequate, breast milk will meet the vitamin requirements of the baby until 6 months of age. After this time, additional supplements of 200 μg vitamin A, 20 mg vitamin C and 7 μg vitamin D are currently recommended for breast-fed infants until the age of 2 or preferably 5 years of age (DH 1994), and are available from infant welfare clinics. It should be noted that the composition of these supplements is under review and may change in the near future.

Fluid

Additional fluid is not necessary for exclusively breast-fed babies and should be discouraged in the early days of breast feeding as it may interfere with the establishment of lactation. A thirsty baby will demand more breast milk. Older infants may be offered cooled, boiled water from a feeding cup or by cup and spoon, as part of the weaning process.

Maternal nutritional considerations

Lactation imposes a heavy nutritional cost on the mother and requirements for energy, calcium and many other minerals and vitamins are increased (DH 1991; and see Appendix 6.2). However, much of the increased need for energy can be met from maternal adipose stores deposited during pregnancy, and this will also assist the restoration of normal body weight.

In well-nourished women, the influence of maternal diet on the volume of breast milk produced is minimal. Lactational capacity (the ability to produce milk) usually far exceeds milk production (the volume actually produced) and increased demand by the infant will be met by increased supply, irrespective of maternal energy intake. This may not be the case in poorly nourished women (Brown et al. 1986) or those who follow extreme weight-reducing diets (IOM 1991), although the body's ability to maintain lactation in conditions of energy shortage is considerable (Whitehead et al. 1980)

Maternal diet also has a relatively small impact on milk composition. Women can produce milk containing adequate protein, fat, carbohydrate and most micronutrients even when their own supplies are limited (National Academy of Sciences 1991; Rasmussen 1992). Only prolonged lactation in nutritionally depleted women is likely to impact on milk composition and, in these circumstances, its content of calcium, folate, and vitamins B_6, B_{12}, A and D may be reduced (National Academy of Sciences 1991).

The maternal diet may, however, affect the fatty acid composition of the milk, particularly that of LCPs (AA and DHA) (Koletzko and Rodriguez-Palmero 1999), which may be relevant to brain and retinal development (see Benefits of breast feeding, above).

In general, if the nutritional costs of lactation are not met, it is the mother who will be affected, not the infant. Milk quantity and quality will be maintained at the expense of the maternal stores. Women most at risk of depletion are those who have a poor nutritional intake during pregnancy followed by similarly inadequate intake during lactation. Any significant fall in nutritional status, particularly in respect of calcium, may have long-term consequences on health, especially bone health. It is estimated that the calcium loss during lactation is approximately 210 mg/day, although to some extent this may be offset by adaptation in calcium homoeostasis (Fairweather-Tait et al. 1995). Lactating women should ingest at least 1200 mg calcium/day in order to meet their needs (DH 1991). In lactating young women and adolescents who will not have achieved maximum bone density, it has been suggested that daily calcium intake should be 1500 mg/day (NIH Consensus Panel 1994).

Maternal fluid intake does not affect the volume of breast milk produced, but a lactating women needs to consume more fluid (about 2 l/day) to protect herself from dehydration (Dusdieker et al. 1990). A useful strategy is for the mother to drink a glass of water, milk or fruit juice every time the baby feeds, in addition to her usual fluid intake and extra drinks when thirsty.

Some aspects of the maternal diet can affect breast milk. Alcohol and caffeine both pass readily into breast milk and high intakes of either should be avoided during lactation. Highly spiced or strong tasting foods can alter the taste of breast milk and this may unsettle some infants. Infants who are highly sensitive to cow's milk protein or other allergens can react to the presence of these antigens in breast milk, or may be sensitized by them, although maternal dietary exclusion of such foods is rarely justified as a routine measure because of the risk of nutritional depletion in the mother (see Section 4.34.3 in Food allergy and intolerance).

Monitoring the progress of a breast-fed baby

General observation of the infant

A thriving breast-fed infant will:

- have a good skin colour
- be alert, responsive and mostly contented
- have frequent wet nappies
- produce bright yellow soft stools (frequency is unimportant).

Monitoring weight gain

Most breast-fed babies gain weight and thrive. Some weight loss usually occurs during the first few days of life but this usually ceases by days 4–7, with birth weight being regained within 7–10 days. Only loss of weight in excess of 10% of birth weight or failure to regain weight is a matter for concern.

Over the first 3 months, weight gain is approximately 200 g/week, which then reduces to about 150 g/week between the ages of 3 and 6 months. A healthy full-term baby of average birthweight doubles its weight by about 5 months and trebles it by the end of the first year of life. Typically, a successfully breast-fed infant gains weight more rapidly than a bottle-fed infant in the first 2–3 months but the rate of weight gain tends to slow from around 4 months and may be less than that of a bottle-fed infant between 6 and 12 months. However, weight gain is not always consistent and overfrequent weighing can cause unnecessary anxiety. A meaningful assessment of an infant's growth can only really be made by the regular use of centile growth charts (see Section 1.8.7 in Assessment of nutritional status).

Test weighing Test weighing the infant (recording weight before and after several feeds) is usually only recommended if there are problems with fluid balance in the baby, e.g. renal failure or heart failure. It should not be used as a method for recording milk intake as it is not a particularly meaningful figure. In addition, it is frequently traumatic for the mother and may even result in a reduced milk supply. The disadvantages of test weighing strongly outweigh any advantages.

Possible reasons for failure to thrive at the breast

Poor weight gain and growth and an unsettled or over-quiet, listless baby are clear indications of an inadequate milk intake. Reasons for this may include:

- *Inadequate milk supply*: Illness, tension or fatigue in the mother can interfere with her lactation. However, the most common cause is a lactation which has never been properly established.
- *Fixing difficulties*: Breast engorgement, inverted nipples or a poor suckling position can prevent the correct fixing or attachment of a baby to the nipple. This is essential if the baby is to obtain the complete volume and nutrient content of the feed.
- *Feeding frequency*: The baby may not be being fed frequently enough. Some babies need to be fed more frequently than others. Rigid feeding schedules should be discouraged; infants should be fed on demand and allowed to feed for an unrestricted length of time. More frequent feeding will increase the milk supply.

Mothers should be encouraged to seek advice on solving these or other problems from an experienced midwife, health visitor or breast-feeding support counsellor.

Problems associated with breast feeding

'Posseting' or vomiting

Many babies regurgitate small amounts of milk at the end of a feed. This is of no consequence. Projectile vomiting, vomiting both after and between feeds, the presence of blood or bile-stained vomit or other signs of illness require prompt medical attention. (Occasionally, traces of blood may originate from cracked and bleeding nipples.)

Irregular bowel habits

The baby's stools will normally be bright yellow and loose or soft. A breast-fed baby may pass several stools during one day and then several days may elapse before another one. Even after 4–5 days without a bowel movement, the breast-fed baby is not constipated if the stool, when passed, is soft.

Illness

Temporary nasal obstruction due to an upper respiratory tract infection commonly interferes with feeding. A prescribed short course of decongestant nose drops may be helpful.

It is unusual for a breast-fed baby to develop gastroenteritis but, if this does occur, breast feeding should continue, supplemented with an oral rehydration solution (Walker-Smith 1990).

Occasionally, serious illness (e.g. congenital heart disease) may present with feeding difficulties and failure to thrive.

3.3.2 Bottle feeding

At the age of 1 month the majority of babies in the UK are having some bottle feeds and at 6–10 weeks 62% are fully bottle fed (Foster *et al*. 1997).

Infant formulae

Modified cow's milk formulae

Most infant feeding formulae are based on cow's milk modified to mimic the nutrient profile of mature breast milk. Although nutritionally complete, none can provide the immunological and anti-infective properties of breast milk. Since 1995, the composition, labelling and marketing of formulae for term infants has had to comply with the *UK Infant Formula and Follow-on Formula Regulations* which implement the 1991 EC Directive.

As a result of concerns over requirements for LCPs (see under Advantages of breast feeding, above), infant milk manufacturers are now adding these to some of their term formulae. The European Society of Paediatric Gastroenterology and Nutrition (ESPGAN) committee on nutrition has recommended that term infant formulae should contain at least a similar concentration and same ratio of LCPs as that which occurs in breast milk, and suggested a ratio of linoleic to α-linoleic acid of between 5:1 and 15:1 (Aggett *et al*. 1991). While the addition of these to preterm formulae have shown positive effects on visual acuity and later intelligence quotient, the evidence for their efficacy in term formulae is inconclusive (Willatts *et al*. 1998; Lucas *et al*. 1999; Birch *et al*. 2000).

Modified cow's milks available in the UK can be divided into three groups: whey-dominant, casein-dominant and follow-on formulae (Table 3.4). Some 'Organic' infant formulae have also recently been introduced further details of which can be obtained from their manufacturers.

Whey-dominant formulae These are the most highly modified milks available. They have a ratio of whey to casein of about 60:40, similar to that found in breast milk.

Table 3.4 Nutritionally complete cow's milk-based infant formulae

Type of formula	Product name (Manufacturer)	Recommended age of use
Whey-dominant infant formulae	SMA Gold (SMA Nutrition)	Birth to 1 year
	Premium (Cow & Gate)	Birth to 1 year
	Farley's First Milk (Farley)	Birth to 1 year
	Aptamil First (Milupa)	Birth to 1 year
	Infant Formula 1 (Boots)	Birth to 1 year
	Hipp Organic Infant Milk (Hipp)	Birth to 1 year
	Omneocomfort 1 (Cow & Gate)	Birth to 1 year
Casein-dominant infant formulae	SMA White (SMA Nutrition)	Birth to 1 year
	Plus (Cow & Gate)	Birth to 1 year
	Farley's Second Milk (Farley)	Birth to 1 year
	Aptamil Extra (Milupa)	Birth to 1 year
	Milumil (Milupa)	Birth to 1 year
	Infant Formula 2 (Boots)	Birth to 1 year
Follow-on milks (all casein-dominant)	Progress (SMA Nutrition)	From 6 months to 2 years
	Step Up (Cow & Gate)	From 6 months to 2 years
	Forward (Milupa)	From 6 months to 2 years
	Follow on Milk (Boots)	From 6 months to 2 years
	Farley's Follow on Milk (Farley)	From 6 months to 2 years
	Hipp Organic Follow-on Milk (Hipp)	From 6 months to 2 years
	Omneocomfort 2 (Cow & Gate)	From 6 months to 2 years
	Next Steps (Cow & Gate)	From 6 months to 2 years

Information compiled September 2000. It should be noted that the range and availability of products may change and be different to that noted here. Compositional data can be obtained from the manufacturers.

Whey-dominant formulae are generally considered the most suitable for infants from birth onwards, and their use can continue throughout the first year of life and beyond.

Casein-dominant formulae These have a whey:casein ratio of about 20:80, similar to that found in cow's milk. There is a common belief that changing from a whey-based formula to a casein-based one will help to satisfy a hungry baby, but there is no scientific basis for this (Taitz and Scholey 1989).

Follow-on formulae Follow-on formulae have a higher iron content than infant formula milk and are an alternative to infant formulae for infants over 6 months (Table 3.4). They may play a part in preventing iron-deficiency anaemia in certain groups of infants, e.g. Asian children and those living in inner cities (Williams *et al.* 1999) if continued as an alternative to cow's milk after the age of 12 months.

Specialist infant formulae

Preterm formulae Milk formulae adapted to meet the special nutritional needs of low birth-weight infants are available (see Section 3.2, Preterm infants). Other nutrient-enriched post-discharge formulae which bridge the gap between preterm and term formulae are now available for use in the community but their role remains controversial (Buttriss 1995).

Soya-based formulae Infant formulae based on soya protein isolates should only be used for infants with clinically diagnosed lactose or cow's milk protein intolerance, and even then may not be suitable for all such cases (see Section 4.35.2 in Food exclusion in the management of allergy and intolerance). Nutritionally incomplete soya-based drinks, available from supermarkets and health-food shops, are not suitable for infants or children below the age of 2 years.

Soya formulae contain glucose polymers and hence may be more cariogenic than those containing lactose (DH 1994). If these formulae are used, good dental hygiene is essential and extended use of bottle feeding should be avoided.

Concern has been expressed over the phytoestrogen content of soya formula and the possible consequences of their weak oestrogenic effect on sexual development and fertility in later life (see Section 2.9.1 in Biologically active dietary constituents). This was investigated by the Department of Health's Committee on Toxicity of Chemicals in Food, Consumer Products and the Environment (COT), which found that the phytoestrogen content of normally reconstituted soya infant formula ranged between 18 and 41 mg/l, but no evidence that this level of consumption had adverse effects (MAFF 1998). They therefore advised that children fed on a soya formula under medical direction should continue to do so. However, they also recommended that further research into the long-term effects of phytoestrogen consumption by infants should be carried out.

Changing milk formulae

Foster *et al.* (1977) reported that 35% of mothers changed infant formula by 6–10 weeks of age (most commonly from a whey-dominant to casein-dominant formula). Three-quarters (76%) of mothers did so because they believed that their infants were 'hungry' or 'not satisfied' with their milk feed. Many mothers, and some health professionals, wrongly believe that casein-dominant milks contain more energy.

It seems likely that a variety of problems is wrongly attributed to the choice of milk feed. Frequent changes, particularly in an attempt to treat minor symptoms of wind, posseting or colic, should be discouraged.

International code of marketing of breast-milk substitutes

An international code of marketing of breast-milk substitutes was adopted as a resolution by the World Health Organization in 1981, its aim being to promote breast feeding and ensure the correct use of infant formulae (WHO 1981). Within the UK, a voluntary code of practice relating to the marketing of infant formulae was drawn up by the Food Manufacturers' Federation (FMF) in 1988. This can be summarized as follows:

- The advertising of infant formulae should be restricted to professional journals.
- Maternity hospitals should not use promotional material such as posters or cot tags.
- Breast-feeding mothers should not be given free samples of formula.
- All packaging should state that breast feeding is best for babies.

Since 1995, the marketing of infant formulae has to comply with the *UK Infant Formula and Follow-on Formula Regulations* implementing a 1991 EC Directive.

Establishing bottle feeding

Most maternity hospitals use 'ready to feed' sterilized bottles of infant formulae. Most offer a choice of product. A range of infant formulae is available and recipients of income support receive vouchers, which they can exchange for infant formula at local clinics, supermarkets or chemists. This does not, however, apply to follow-on milks, soya formulae or low birthweight formulae.

Bottle-feeding techniques

Infants usually readily accept feed from a bottle, and only refuse to do so if they have become accustomed to breast or tube feeding. Occasionally a baby will show frustration by crying, refusing the teat or feeding reluctantly, and this is usually due to an inappropriate flow rate of milk from the bottle. Changing to a larger or smaller-holed teat can alter this. A teat that resembles the human nipple in size and shape may be more successful than the traditional bottle teat. Some teats have an automatic vacuum release, which ensures a continuous flow of milk from the bottle. The use of 'soft spout' teats from the age of 4 months can facilitate the move towards feeding from a cup.

The correct feeding technique is important. The bottle should always be angled so that the teat is full of milk, thus minimizing the amount of air consumed. It is usual to 'wind' bottle-fed babies half way through a feed and after a feed.

Calculating the bottle feed

The average milk intake from 1 week of age until weaning is 150 ml/kg per day. Some babies will take more milk. A baby regularly taking significantly less is likely to be underfed.

As with breast feeding, mothers should be encouraged to feed on demand. However, most young babies will feed 3–4 hourly, for example, a 2-week-old, 4 kg baby might take 100 ml at six feeds every 4 hours. As the volume of feed taken increases, the interval between feeds increases and a typical 3-month-old baby weighing 6 kg might take 180 ml at five feeds every 4 hours (missing one feed overnight).

Hygiene

It is essential to encourage high standards of hygiene in feed preparation and storage. Bottles, teats and bottle caps must be rinsed after use, washed in hot water with detergent, rinsed and then sterilized for the recommended time with a commercial sterilizing solution. Dummies, spoons and other non-metallic items should also be sterilized in this way. Sterilizing solutions must be changed daily. Alternatively, equipment may be boiled for 3 minutes. Steam sterilizers are also available. Domestic microwave ovens do not sterilize infant feeding equipment sufficiently well for this to be considered a safe method.

Reconstitution of formula

Traditionally, powdered infant milks are reconstituted on the basis of one level scoop of milk powder to every 30 ml (or 1 fluid ounce) of cooled boiled water, but some manufacturers now provide milk powder in sachets to be added to a specified volume of water. If scoops are used, it is important to use the ones provided with the chosen formula because different products have different scoop sizes. Feeds are usually prepared in the feeding bottle, with the milk powder being added to the measured water. A water temperature of 70°C will ensure a final pasteurization in the bottle (DHSS 1988). Bottle feeds may be prepared in advance and stored in a refrigerator for up to 24 hours.

Feeds can be warmed by standing the bottle in hot water or using an electric bottle warmer. The temperature of the feed should be checked by shaking a few drops on to the inside of the wrist before it is given to the infant. Any milk remaining after a feed should be discarded. Care should be taken if milk is warmed in a microwave oven as the milk heats unevenly and resultant 'hot spots' can easily scald a baby's mouth. To avoid this, the bottle should be shaken thoroughly after heating, before checking the milk temperature as described above.

Use of bottled water

Some parents wish to use mineral or spring waters for their babies, as they perceive them to contain fewer chemicals and other contaminants. However, bottled waters are not sterile and must be boiled for infants under the age of 6 months (DH 1994). Only products that comply with EC guidelines on the mineral content of tap water should be used to make up infant feeds (DH 1994). The sodium content of the water is a particularly important consideration and should not exceed 200 mg/l. Some brands of spring water currently exceed this level, and parents should be aware of the need to check labelling information to ascertain that the product is suitable.

Use of filtered and softened waters

The use of a water filter to remove organic and inorganic constituents in tap water has become popular in recent years. However, water filters are breeding grounds for bacteria and filtered water used for infants under 6 months of age must be boiled. Freshly filtered water can be given to older infants.

Softened water produced by an ion-exchange system contains high levels of sodium and must not be used to prepare infant formulae (DH 1994).

Additional nutritional requirements of the bottle-fed infant

Vitamins and minerals

All infant milk formulae are supplemented with vitamins and minerals to meet EC guidelines (EC 1991). Additional supplements are not, therefore, required for infants under 6 months who consume at least 500 ml of formula per day.

Additional fluids

If formula-fed infants are given additional drinks, these should be confined to cooled boiled water. This advice is frequently ignored; by the age of 6 weeks, virtually all bottle-fed babies have been given drinks other than formula milk or water (Foster *et al.* 1997).

Any infant with fever, diarrhoea or vomiting will need additional fluids and possibly electrolytes to replace losses.

Monitoring the progress of a bottle-fed infant

The most important factors to consider in the bottle-fed infant are the growth rate (weight gain in relation to length) and the contentment of the baby.

Because the volume of feed consumed is known, it is easier to assess the nutrient intake of the bottle-fed than the breast-fed infant. However, this assumes that the feed is being made up correctly, and this factor must be borne in mind when either an inadequate or excessive weight gain is being investigated. Lucas *et al.* (1991) measured the energy content of infant formulae as made up by a group of bottle-feeding mothers and found that the energy content ranged from 41 to 91 kcal/100 ml, whereas the manufacturer's intended energy content was 68 kcal/100 ml. One-third of feeds contained less than 50 kcal/100 ml and around half the feeds over 80 kcal/100 ml.

Inadequate weight gain may be due to:

- feeds being either too few or too small
- feed being overdiluted
- underlying illness
- intolerance to a component of the feed.

Excessive weight gain may be due to:

- feeds being either too frequent or too large
- feeds being overconcentrated
- rusk or cereal being added to the bottle. Although this practice, once common, is discouraged by health professionals in the UK it still occurs, mainly because well-meaning relatives often recommend it. The practice is still advocated by health professionals in France and The Netherlands.

Problems associated with bottle-feeding

Wind, posseting and vomiting

Bottle-fed babies tend to take in more air with their feed than breast-fed infants and are therefore more likely to suffer discomfort. For the same reason, regurgitation during or after a feed is also more common. Both problems can be minimized by allowing the baby to rest from feeding at intervals in a vertical position so that the swallowed air can escape. Reducing the flow rate of the milk may also help.

If a considerable proportion of the feed is being persistently regurgitated, medical advice should be sought. A prescribable thickening agent can be added to the feed and this is usually very effective, although it necessitates the use of a large-holed or cross-cut teat. Alternatively, one of the recently introduced infant formulae which thicken in the acid conditions of the stomach can be used. Currently, such products are Omneocomfort 1 (for infants from birth) or Omneocomfort 2 (follow-on formula) produced by Cow & Gate and based on hydrolysed whey protein, or Efamil AR (Mead Johnson), which is derived from whole protein.

Stool appearance

Artificial feeding results in stools which are often greenish in colour and these are not always easily distinguished from the green stools which occur when a gastrointestinal infection is present. Loose stools may be normal for a particular baby but can occasionally indicate dietary intolerance. The sudden appearance of loose stools associated with vomiting or other signs of illness suggests the presence of infection necessitating medical advice.

Constipation

This is more likely to occur in bottle- than breast-fed infants and may reflect an inadequate fluid intake or overconcentrated feeds. Bottle-fed infants should be offered cooled boiled water at intervals, particularly in hot weather.

Hyperosmolar dehydration and hypernatraemia

As a result of immature renal function, a high solute load this can result in hyperosmolar dehydration and hypernatraemia. Fortunately, these conditions are much rarer than they used to be, owing to modifications in infant milk formulae. However, they can still arise from a combination of factors such as overconcentrated feeds, high extra-renal fluid losses (e.g. due to diarrhoea or excessive sweating), a reduced renal output and no additional fluid.

Hypercalcaemia and hyperphosphataemia

As with the above, modern milk formulae are less likely to cause these problems. The ratio of calcium to phosphorus in breast milk is 2.3:1 and artificial formulae now reflect this.

Milk intolerance

The diagnosis and management of the various types of allergy and intolerance to milk are discussed in Section 4.35.2 (Food Exclusion in the management of allergy and intolerance).

3.3.3 Weaning

Weaning is a time of nutritional vulnerability as the increasing requirement for many nutrients coincides with the gradual depletion of the infant's nutrient stores which were present at birth.

Infants are weaned for two main reasons:

- *Nutritional reasons*: Energy and nutrient needs become too large to be met by milk alone. Stores of iron, for example, are depleted by about 6 months of age and additional sources of iron need to be introduced.
- *Developmental reasons*: Feeding behaviour progresses from immature sucking and swallowing to biting and chewing. To encourage this phase of development it is important to introduce a variety of tastes and textures from 6–7 months. Pridham (1990) has reviewed the development of feeding behaviour at weaning.

In the UK, guidance on weaning is based on the COMA report *Weaning and the Weaning Diet* (DH 1994).

Commencement of weaning

It is recommended (DH 1994) that weaning should commence between the ages of 4 and 6 months. The introduction of solids is undesirable before 4 months of age because:

- The renal function of the infant may not be capable of dealing with the increased solute load.
- The production of digestive enzymes may not have fully developed, and the increased permeability of the immature gastrointestinal tract increases the risk of allergic reaction to food antigens.
- The neuromuscular co-ordination of baby may not be sufficiently developed to enable transfer of a food bolus from the front to the back of the mouth, or safe swallowing ability.

However, if an infant is not weaned by 6 months, its intake of energy, protein, minerals such as iron and zinc, and vitamins A and D may be inadequate. Late weaning may also delay development in eating behaviour and speech.

Indications that the child is ready for solid food are:

- if the infant seems hungry after a milk feed, even when the amount has been increased
- if the baby is demanding more feed

- if the baby begins to wake in the night having previously slept through.

It is clear that many mothers are misinformed or ignore guidance as to when weaning should commence. The 1995 survey of the diets of British infants (Foster *et al.* 1997) found that 55% of babies had received solids by 3 months of age. The reasons given for this early introduction of solids included a desire for the baby to sleep through the night, wanting the baby to move on to the next stage of feeding, the feeling that milk was not sufficient, and peer and family pressure. Other factors that influence the age at which weaning commences include:

- socioeconomic grouping (lower income groups are more likely to commence early weaning than higher income groups)
- cultural beliefs
- method of infant feeding (bottle-fed infants tend to be weaned earlier than breast-fed infants)
- professional advice
- growth rate
- medical conditions.

Nutritional aspects of weaning

The nutritional content of the weaning diet needs to be sufficient to make up the increasing shortfall between nutritional needs and nutritional provision from breast or formula milk. In the early stages of weaning the nutrient content provided by solid food will be almost negligible but, as the weaning process progresses, the infant becomes more reliant on solids to meet its nutritional requirements.

Energy

If an infant does not receive sufficient energy, growth will be impaired. Since, at this stage of life, energy requirements are relatively high but food can only be consumed in small quantities, energy much be provided in a concentrated form. Foods that are reduced in fat or high in fibre are not appropriate in this age group.

Sugars are an important source of energy at this stage but most will be derived from milk and those present in fruit and vegetables. Unnecessary addition of sugars to food should be avoided because of the risk, of dental caries, but this does not necessarily preclude the use of sugar altogether. In practice, many of the intrinsic forms of sugar (e.g. whole fruit) will be given to the infant in an extrinsic form (e.g. fruit is likely to be stewed or puréed), and improving the palatability of a fruit purée by adding a small amount of sugar is only giving it the composition of a purée made from riper, sweeter fruit. What is most important is that infants are not encouraged to develop a taste for sweetness by being offered sugar-rich foods or drinks, particularly between meals.

Minerals and vitamins

It is important that a wide variety of foods is included in the diet from an early age as this helps to ensure that all essential minerals, trace elements and vitamins will be provided. Particularly important considerations at this age are as follows.

Iron By 6 months of age, the iron stores present at birth will have diminished but the demand for iron to meet the needs of growth and development will be high. A dietary source of iron is therefore imperative. Iron-deficiency anaemia is common in this age group (Mills 1990) and may have consequences in terms of mental development (Walter 1996). Food rich in haem iron (meat) should be encouraged in preference to non-haem iron sources (cereals, pulses and vegetables) because the iron is better absorbed. Many weaning foods are fortified with iron and can make a significant contribution to the iron content of the diet. Infant formulae and follow-on milks are fortified with iron, and the latter are useful as a drink for infants over the age of 6 months (since cow's milk is contraindicated for this purpose until the age of 1 year).

Zinc Deficiency of zinc can impair growth. Since the main source of zinc in the diet is meat, intake may be inadequate if meat is excluded from the weaning diet.

Sodium Salt should not be added to weaning food owing to the inability of the infant to excrete sodium efficiently.

Vitamin D This vitamin is important in the diet of the infant because of its role in calcium metabolism. There is a risk of deficiency between 6 and 12 months of age owing to the rapid rate of bone growth but possibly low provision as a result of lack of exposure to sunlight and consequent minimal synthesis. Formula milk is fortified with vitamin D but breast-fed infants will require a supplement from the age of 6 months, such as Department of Health vitamin drops. Most commercial weaning foods are fortified with vitamin D.

Vitamin C High intakes of vitamin C will improve the absorption of non-haem iron from the diet. Vitamin C is included in the Department of Health infant drops, and many commercial weaning foods are also fortified.

Fluid and drinks

Before 6 months of age, no additional drinks are needed by breast-fed infants, and formula-fed infants only need additional water. Breast or formula milk should be continued until 1 year of age. From 6 months babies can be offered follow-on milks. Cow's milk should not be used as a drink until the child is 1 year old, although it may be used in cooking from the age of 6 months. The milk should be pasteurized and full-fat in composition; skimmed and semi-skimmed milks are insufficiently energy and nutrient dense for children below the age of 5 years and 2 years, respectively.

From the age of 6 months, fruit juices or baby drinks can be given as part of a meal. Because the high acidity and sugar content of these drinks may adversely affect dental health, it is suggested that they should be diluted, 1 part fruit juice to at least 4–5 parts water (HEA 1996).

Drinks between meals should be confined to water or breast/formula milk. By 6 months infants should be encouraged to drink from a cup and the use of a bottle should be discontinued after the age of 1 year. Infants should never be left with a bottle or feeding reservoir containing sugar-containing drinks as this can lead to rampant caries (see Section 4.1.1 in Dental disorders).

Soft drinks such as fruit squashes and carbonated beverages should not be included in the weaning diet because of their high cariogenic potential (Duggal and Curzon 1989). Colas and some other drinks also contain large amounts of caffeine which should be avoided. Drinks containing artificial sweeteners ('diet' drinks) are not recommended for use in infants, and may in any case be just as acidic and detrimental to teeth as sugar-containing alternatives (see Section 4.1.2 in Dental disorders).

Some bottled waters are unsuitable for infants as they have a high mineral content (see Use of bottled water, above). It will still be necessary to boil and cool bottled water before it is given to babies below the age of 6 months (DH 1994).

Goat's or sheep's milk should not be given to children under 1 year of age and should be boiled before use if it has not been pasteurized. Additional vitamins, particularly folate, may also be necessary.

Tea is not a suitable drink for young children as the tannin content interferes with iron absorption (DH 1994).

Practical aspects of weaning

Mothers lack confidence about weaning, feeling unsure when to start, what to give and whether they are doing it properly. Many find the advice offered by health professionals vague and theoretical. They may also worry unduly about some aspects of the diet, such as additives, not realizing that nutritional adequacy is more important.

Choice of foods

Cow's milk should not be added to foods such as breakfast cereals before 6 months and not given as a drink until 1 year of age. However, cow's milk products (such as yoghurt) can be used from the age of 4 months. Cow's milk can also be used as a food ingredient (e.g. in custard) from this age.

Foods most likely to provoke allergic reactions (wheat, gluten, egg, fish and citrus fruits) should not be given before the age of 6 months. If there is a family history of food allergy, it may be advisable for foods to be introduced one at a time.

To reduce the risk of peanut allergy, infants in a family with a history of atopy or allergic disease should not be given peanut-containing products until the age of 3 years (DH 1998). No child under the age of 5 years should be given whole peanuts, because of the risk of choking.

Infants below the age of 12 months should not be given set or spoonable liquid honey because of the very small risk of infant botulism from clostridial spores which are not removed in normal processing (Fenicia *et al.* 1993; Balslev *et al.* 1997). This restriction does not apply to honey which has been added to commercial baby foods.

As the intestine matures the spores are unable to germinate and by 12 months of age the risk is negligible.

Nutrient content This is relatively unimportant in the early stages of weaning owing to the small amounts offered. Commercially available foods such as baby rice are popular as first foods. The range of food offered should increase as the infant progresses.

Flavour Bland foods with a neutral or milky flavour are likely to be better accepted than strongly flavoured or spicy foods. No salt or sugar should be added to home-made or manufactured food. The food should suit the immature palate of the baby, not that of an adult.

Consistency Initially the food should be of a smooth, semi-liquid consistency. Manufactured weaning food can be reconstituted to the correct texture. Home-made weaning food will require sieving, mashing with a fork or liquidizing to achieve a suitable texture. Gradually, food can progress to being more textured (grated or minced) and then chopped. This should progress at the child's own pace.

From 6 months finger foods can be introduced. To reduce the risk of choking (see below) these should initially be foods which soften in the mouth, with harder foods such as pieces of apple or carrot only being offered when the child can chew well.

Home-made versus manufactured baby foods Mothers often ask whether they should use home-made or manufactured baby foods. Either type is suitable, it is simply a matter of personal preference and convenience.

Some mothers like to prepare all of their infant's food and have the satisfaction of knowing exactly what their baby is eating. Others find it frustrating to take time and trouble preparing a suitable purée only for it to be rejected after one spoonful. In theory, home-made baby foods are more economical than manufactured ones, although this is not always the case if they are prepared separately from the family meals (e.g. to avoid the use of excess salt or sugar), thus incurring extra fuel costs, or if the baby dislikes what has been produced. Home-made baby foods can also be nutritionally inadequate (Morgan and Stordy 1995; Stordy *et al.* 1995), whereas commercially prepared infant foods must adhere to strict compositional guidelines.

In the early stages, many mothers opt for the convenience of dried manufactured foods which can be made up in small quantities, and gradually supplement these with suitably modified items from the family meals. Home-made baby food can be prepared and frozen in sterilized ice-cube trays and later in small pots (e.g. empty yoghurt cartons). Ready-made baby foods are likely to be particularly useful when travelling or eating away from home.

From 6–7 months it is reasonable to offer the baby suitable food from family meals. Commercially prepared infant foods tend to be bland and their prolonged use can make some babies reluctant to enjoy the varied textures and tastes of family food.

For an older infant sharing family food, it is unrealistic to suggest that no salt be used in cooking. It is, however, a time when people can be made aware of their unnecessary use of salt. In particular, the practice of adding extra salt at the table is a habit that many children copy and one that can be beneficially avoided by the entire family.

Rate of progress of weaning

The main stages in weaning are outlined in Table 3.5. It is, however, important to realize that each child will be different and the time taken to reach each stage will vary.

Nutritional adequacy

Although a satisfactory growth rate is the most obvious sign of an adequate diet, the baby's general contentment, sleeping pattern and bowel habits are also valuable indicators. Some mothers worry over the apparent minute quantities eaten by their child. They should be discouraged from trying to force the child to eat more and be reassured that a healthy baby will not go hungry.

Additional vitamins Children should be given Department of Health vitamin drops (currently containing vitamins A, D and C) from the age of 6 months, unless they are receiving 500 ml of infant formula or follow-on milk per day. Supplementation should continue the age of at least 2 years, and preferably 5 years (DH 1994). The supplements are sold at low cost at infant clinics and are free to families on income support. The composition of these supplements is currently under review as a result of concerns over high vitamin A intakes and the need for folate in the infant diet.

Problems associated with weaning

Risk of choking

It is important that a baby is never left alone whilst feeding. Initially, finger foods should be those which soften easily in the mouth (e.g. rusk, bread or banana). Harder foods such as apple or carrot should only be given when the child has learnt to chew well. All parents and carers of children should be taught the emergency procedures that can save the life of a choking child.

Rejection of solids

It takes time for a baby to become accustomed to feeding from a spoon and to each new taste. There will inevitably be some rejections, but provided that weaning coincides with the infant's development, solids will be taken.

A reluctance to accept lumpy food is a common problem; this is often the result of smooth purées being offered for too long. Slow weaning progress can sometimes stem from parental desire to avoid the mess associated with independent feeding and infants being fed, rather than being allowed to attempt to self-feed, for too long. Other weaning problems are most likely to be associated with late weaning (e.g. after 9 months), developmental problems in the infant and prolonged periods of enteral or intravenous feeding in the early months of life.

Table 3.5 Timetable for weaning

	Stage 1 Initially	Stage 2 4–6 months	Stage 3 6–9 months	Stage 4 9–12 months
Aim	To get the infant used to the idea of the spoon rather than to provide nourishment	To introduce new tastes and provide some nourishment	To lessen the dependence on milk as a source of nourishment	To learn to chew and feed themselves
Frequency	Once a day, after (or during) one feed	After two, then after three feeds per day	Three to five times per day. Solids should be given before the milk feed.	A regular meal pattern.
Quantity	Initially 1, then 1–2 teaspoons	Dictated by appetite	More substantial servings	Dictated by appetite
Suitable foods	Baby rice. Puréed vegetables cooked without salt (e.g. potato, carrot) Puréed non-citrus fruit (e.g. apple, pear, banana)	Baby rice (or cereal) at one meal only Wider variety of puréed vegetables Wider variety of puréed non-citrus fruits Puréed meat, chicken, fish or liver Puréed pulses (e.g. split lentils) Custard, plain yoghurt.	Cow's milk for mixing cereals Cauliflower/macaroni cheese Rice pudding Wheat-containing cereals Dairy foods (yoghurt, fromage frais, cheese) Eggs (well cooked) Citrus fruits More family foods without added salt, sugar or spices	Normal family food, mashed or chopped as necessary
Texture	Smooth purée	Smooth purée	Can be less smooth, e.g. mashed, minced or scrambled and then chopped	Mashed or chopped
Introduce			Soft finger foods, e.g. bread, pitta bread, banana, orange segments Harder finger foods (carrot, apple) as competence improves	
Milk feeds	No change	Usual number	Being reduced	500 ml either as a drink or mixed with food

Infants should never be unduly coerced or forced to eat. Parents encountering persistent or severe feeding weaning problems should receive expert help and support, ideally from a team including a speech therapist experienced in assessing feeding development.

Poor weaning practices

Common causes include ignorance, child neglect, and economic and social problems. Some ethnic groups delay weaning and allow the child to remain almost exclusively on cow's milk until 2–3 years of age. This problem requires tactful handling.

Over-zealous application of healthy-eating guidelines to infants (especially high-fibre, low-fat diets) can cause a number of nutritional problems, as the resultant low intake of energy and minerals may be inadequate to meet the requirements for growth. Some mothers are reluctant to introduce foods other than fruit and vegetables into the weaning diet, unaware perhaps that inclusion of some foods with a higher energy density is essential.

Parental diagnosis of food allergy and consequent food restrictions or the use of goat's milk or nutritionally incomplete soya milk substitutes can also result in diets that are nutritionally unbalanced and inadequate, especially in nutrients such as calcium (see Section 4.34, Food allergy and intolerance). Restrictive diets may also be followed for religious, social or cultural reasons, and the nutritional implications of these may need to be addressed (see Sections 3.9, People from ethnic minority groups, and 3.10, Vegetarianism and veganism).

Failure to thrive

Poor weaning practices can, if prolonged, result in the infant failing to thrive. However, the possibility of a functional cause of poor growth such as coeliac disease or cystic fibrosis should not be overlooked.

Constipation

Some babies are more prone to constipation than others. Constipation can occur if the fluid or fibre intake is inadequate. Consumption of these should be increased, and high-fibre cereals and wholemeal bread can be introduced at around 6–9 months.

Diarrhoea

This can be due to:

- infection
- excessive fibre intake
- food intolerance
- excessive consumption of fructose or sucrose (e.g. via concentrated fruit juice).

Severe or persistent diarrhoea should always be medically investigated.

Inconsistent advice

The new mother is usually bombarded with advice from professionals, the mass media, baby-food manufacturers, lay groups, relatives and friends, much of which may be contradictory (Clark and Laing 1990). The implementation of a local child nutrition policy that endeavours to introduce some degree of uniformity to the advice given by health professionals within a particular area may help to reduce these problems. Dietitians should be available not only to give advice directly to mothers but also to train the advisers.

Text revised by: Diane Talbot
Acknowledgements: Judy More, Vanessa Shaw, Jackie Lewin and Karen Shukla.

Useful addresses

Association of Breastfeeding Mothers
26 Hearnshaw Close, London SE26 4T11

British Association of Perinatal Medicine
50 Hallam Street, London W1W 6DE
Tel: 020 7307 5640
Website: www.bapm-london.org

Joint Breastfeeding Initiative
Department of Health, Skipton House, 80 London Road, London SE1 6LW
Tel 020 7972 2000

La Leche League (Breastfeeding Help and Information)
PO Box BM 3424, London WC1N 3XX
Website: www.lalecheleague.org

National Childbirth Trust, Breastfeeding Promotion Group
Alexander House, Oldham Terrace, Acton, London W3 6NH
Tel: 020 8992 8637
Website: www.nct-online.org

Further reading

Department of Health. *Breastfeeding: Good Practice Guidance to the NHS*. London: DH, 1996.
La Leche League International. *The Art of Breastfeeding*. London: Angus and Robertson, 1990.
Royal College of Midwives. *Successful Breastfeeding*. Edinburgh: Churchill Livingstone, 1991.
Smale M. *The NCT Book of Breastfeeding*. London: Vermilion, 1992.
Stanway P, Stanway A. *Breast is Best*. London: Pan Books, 1983.

Thompson J. (Ed.). *Nutritional Requirements of Infants and Young Children: Practical Guidelines*. Oxford: Blackwell Science, 1998.
Wardley BL, Puntis JWL, Taitz LS. *Handbook of Child Nutrition*, 2nd edn. Oxford: Oxford University Press, 1997.

References

Aggett PJ, Hascheke F, Heine W, Hernell O. Comment on the content and composition of lipids in infant formula. ESPGAN Committee on Nutrition. *Acta Paediatrica Scandinavica* 1991; **80**: 887–896.
Balslev T, Ostergaard E, Marsden IK, Wandall DA. Infant botulism. The first culture-confirmed Danish case. *Neuropediatrics* 1997; **28**: 287–288.
Barker DJP (Ed.). *Foetal and Infant Origins of Adult Disease*. London: British Medical Journal, 1992.
Beeken S, Waterston T. Health service support of breast feeding – are we practising what we preach? *British Medical Journal* 1992; **305**: 285–287.
Birch EE, Hoffman DR, Uuay R *et al*. Visual acuity and the essentiality of docosahexaenoic acid and arachidonic acid in the diet of term infants. *Pediatric Research* 1998; **44**: 201–209.
Birch EE, Garfield S, Hoffman DR *et al*. A randomized controlled trial of early dietary supply of long-chain polyunsaturated fatty acids and mental development in term infants. *Developmental Medicine and Child Neurology* 2000; **42**: 174–181.
British Association of Perinatal Medicine. *Guidelines for the Collection, Storage and Handling of Mother's Breast Milk to be Fed to her Own Baby on a Neonatal Unit*. London: British Association of Perinatal Medicine, 1997.
Brock JH. Lactoferrin in human milk: its role in iron absorption and protection against enteric infection in the newborn infant. *Archives of Disease in Childhood* 1980; **55**: 417–422.
Brown RH, Akhtor NA, Robertson AD, Ahmed MG. Lactational capacity of marginally malnourished mothers: relationships between maternal nutritional status and quantity and proximate composition of milk. *Pediatrics* 1986; **78**: 909–916.
Burr ML, Limb ES, Maguire MJ *et al*. Infant feeding, wheezing and allergy: a prospective study. *Archives of Disease in Childhood* 1993; **68**: 724–728.
Buttriss J. (Ed.). *Nutrition in General Practice: Promoting Health and Preventing Disease*. London: Royal College of General Practitioners, 1995.
Carlson SE. Long chain polyunsaturated fatty acids and development of human infants. *Acta Paediatrica* 1999; **88** (Suppl): 72–73.
Clark BJ, Laing SC. Infant feeding: a review of weaning. *Journal of Human Nutrition and Dietetics* 1990; **3**: 11–18.
Department of Health. *Dietary Reference Values for Food Energy and Nutrients in the United Kingdom*. Report on Health and Social Subjects 41. London: HMSO, 1991.
Department of Health, Committee on Medical Aspects of Food Policy. *Weaning and the Weaning Diet*. Report on Health and Social Subjects 45. London: HMSO, 1994.
Department of Health: Committee on Toxicity of Chemicals in Food, Consumer Products and the Environment. *Peanut Allergy*. London: Department of Health, 1998.
Department of Health and Social Security. *The Composition of Mature Human Milk*. Report on Health and Social Subjects 12. London: HMSO, 1977.
Department of Health and Social Security. *Artificial Feeds for the Young Infant*. Report on Health and Social Subjects 18. London: HMSO, 1980.

Department of Health and Social Security. *Present Day Practice in Infant Feeding*. Report on Health and Social Subjects 32. London: HMSO, 1988.

Duggal MS, Curzon MEJ. An evaluation of the cariogenic potential of baby and infant fruit drinks. *British Dental Journal* 1989; **166**: 327–330.

Dusdieker LB, Stumbo PJ, Booth BM *et al*. Prolonged maternal fluid supplementation in breast-feeding. *Pediatrics* 1990; **86**: 737–740.

ESPGAN. Comment on antigen-reduced infant formulae. *Acta Paediatrica* 1993; **82**: 314–319.

European Commission. *Directive on Infant Feeding Formulae and Follow-on Formulae*. 91/321/EC, O.J.No.L. 175/35. 1991.

Fairweather-Tait S, Prentice A, Heumann KG *et al*. Effect of calcium supplements and stage of lactation on the calcium absorption efficiency of lactating women accustomed to low calcium intakes. *American Journal of Clinical Nutrition* 1995; **62**: 1188–1192.

Farquharson J, Jamieson EC, Abbasi KA *et al*. Effect of diet on the fatty acid composition of the major phospholipids of infant cerebral cortex. *Archives of Disease in Childhood* 1995; **72**: 198–203.

Fenicia L, Ferrini AM, Aureli P, Pocecco M. A case of infant botulism associated with honey feeding in Italy. *European Journal of Epidemiology* 1993; **9**: 671–673.

Foster K, Cheesbrough S, Lader D. *Infant Feeding 1995*. London: HMSO, 1997.

Halken S, Host A, Hansen LG, Osterballe O. Effect of an allergy prevention programme on incidence of atopic symptoms in infancy. A prospective study of 159 'high-risk' infants. *Allergy* 1992; **47**: 545–553.

Hanson LA. Human milk and host defence: immediate and long-term effects. *Acta Paediatrica* 1999; **88** (Suppl): 42–46.

Health Education Authority. *Feeding your Child From Birth to Three*. London: HEA, 1996.

Howie PW, Forsyth JS, Ogaton SA *et al*. Protective effect of breast-feeding against infection. *British Medical Journal* 1990; **300**: 11–16.

Institute of Medicine (IOM) Subcommittee on Nutrition during Lactation. *Nutrition during Lactation*. Washington DC: National Academy Press, 1991.

Jamieson EC, Farquharson J, Logan RW *et al*. Infant cerebellar gray and white matter fatty acids in relation to age and diet. *Lipids* 1999; **34**: 1065–1071.

Koletzko B, Rodriguez-Palmero M. Polyunsaturated fatty acids in human milk and their role in early human development. *Journal of Mammary Gland Biology and Neoplasia* 1999; **4**: 269–284.

Kramer MS. Does breast feeding help protect against atopic disease? *Journal of Paediatrics* 1988; **112**: 181–190.

Labbock MH. Health sequelae of breastfeeding for the mother. *Clinical Perinatology* 1999; **26**: 491–503.

Lucas A, Lockton S, Davies PSW. Milk for babies and children (Letter). *British Medical Journal* 1991; **302**: 350–351.

Lucas A, Stafford M, Morley R *et al*. Efficacy and safety of long-chain polyunsaturated fatty acid supplementation of infant-formula milk: a randomised trial. *Lancet* 1999; **354**: 1948–1954.

MAFF. Soya infant formulae. *Food Safety Information Bulletin* 1998; 102.

Mills AF. Surveillance patterns for anaemia: risk factors in patterns of milk intake. *Archives of Disease in Childhood* 1990; **65**: 428–431.

Morgan J, Stordy J. Infant feeding practices in the 1990s. *Health Visitor* 1995; **68**: 56–58.

Morrison P. HIV and infant feeding: to breast-feed or not breast feed: the dilemma of competing risks. *Breast Feeding Review* 1999; **7**: 5–13

National Academy of Sciences, Food and Nutrition Board. *Nutrition during Lactation*. Washington, DC: National Academy Press, 1991.

NIH Consensus Panel on Optimal Calcium Intake. NIH Consenses Conference. Optimal Calcium intake. *Journal of the American Medical Association* 1994; **272**: 1942–1948.

Pridham KF. Feeding behaviour of six to twelve month old infants. Assessment and sources of parental information. *Journal of Pediatrics* 1990; **117** (Suppl): S174–S190.

Rasmussen KM. The influence of maternal nutrition on lactation. *Annual Review of Nutrition* 1992; **12**: 103–119.

Renfrew MJ, Lang S, Woolridge MV. Early versus delayed initiation of breastfeeding (Cochrane Review). The *Cochrane Library*, Issue 4. Oxford: Update Software, 2000.

Righard L, Alade M. Effect of delivery room routines on success of first breast feed. *Lancet* 1990; **336**: 1105–1107.

Saarinen UM, Kajosaari M. Breastfeeding as prophylaxis against atopic disease: prospective follow-up study until 17 years old. *Lancet* 1995; **346**: 1065–1069.

Sikorski J, Renfrew MJ. Support for breastfeeding mothers. The *Cochrane Library*, Issue 2. Oxford: Update Software, 2000.

Stordy BJ, Redfern AM, Morgan JB. Healthy eating for infants – mothers' actions. *Acta Paediatrica* 1995; **4**: 733–741.

Taitz LS, Scholey E. Are babies more satisfied by casein based formulas? *Archives of Disease in Childhood* 1989; **64**: 619–621.

UNICEF. Baby Friendly Initiative website: www.unicef.org/bfhi/junebfhi99.

Walker-Smith JA. Management of infantile gastroenteritis. *Archives of Disease in Childhood* 1990; **65**: 917–918.

Walter T. Effect of iron deficiency anaemia on cognitive skills in infancy and childhood. In *Iron Nutrition in Health and Disease*. London: John Libbey, 1996.

Whitehead RG, Paul AA, Rowland MGM. Lactation in Cambridge and the Gambia. *British Medical Bulletin* 1980; **37**: 77–82.

Willatts P, Forsyth JS. The role of long chain polyunsaturated fatty acids in infant cognitive development. *Prostaglandins, Leukotrienes and Essential Fatty Acids* 2000; **63**: 95–100.

Willatts P, Forsyth JS, DiMondugno MK *et al*. Effect of long-chain polyunsaturated fatty acids in infant formula on problem solving at 10 months of age. *Lancet* 1998; **352**: 688–691

Williams J, Wolff A, Daly A *et al*. Iron supplemented formula milk related to reduction in psychomotor decline in infants from inner city areas: randomised study. *British Medical Journal* 1999; **318**: 693–698.

Wilson AC, Forsyth JS, Greene SA *et al*. Relation of infant diet to childhood health: seven year follow up of cohort of children in Dundee infant feeding study. *British Medical Journal* 1998; **316**: 21–25.

Woolridge MW, Fisher C. Colic, 'overfeeding', and symptoms of lactose malabsorption in the breast fed baby. A possible artefact of feed management. *Lancet* 1988; **ii**: 382–384.

World Health Organization. International Code of Marketing of Breast Milk Substitutes. Geneva: WHO, 1981.

World Health Organization. Global program on Aids. Consensus statement from WHO/UNICEF consultation on HIV transmission and breastfeeding. 30 April–1 May, 1992, Geneva. WHO GPAINF 92.1

Yap PL, Pryde A, Latham PJ, MeLelland DB. Serum IgA in the neonate. Concentration and effect of breast feeding. *Acta Paediatrica Scandinavica* 1979; **68**: 695–700.

3.4 Preschool children

Children aged between 1 and 5 years have:

- high energy and nutrient requirements relative to their size;
- a small stomach which prevents them consuming large quantities of food at one time;
- a variable appetite, related to fluctuations in growth rate and level of physical activity.

These factors must be taken into account if nutritional needs are to be met. A meal pattern of several small meals with snacks in between is the most appropriate to achieve these needs at this age. Much of the food offered should be of high nutrient density to meet micronutrient as well as energy requirements.

The developments that take place in a child between the ages of 1 and 5 years are numerous and, directly or indirectly, affect eating habits. At this age, children are almost totally dependent on others for their food, and parents and other carers should realize that their own eating habits, likes and dislikes will be the ones that the child imitates.

Early food experiences have an important effect on eating patterns in adult life. Attitudes to eating, including which types of foods are considered 'normal' and whether meals are regarded as social occasions or just something to be eaten whilst watching television, will develop during the early years. Meal times are also an important time to communicate and interact with young children. Good eating habits enhance communication skills and language development, and delayed speech and poor eating habits often coexist (Thomas 1996).

Food and eating are wonderful sources of learning for children (e.g. cooking, shopping, helping to lay the table and eating out). Food can also be a source of frustration and a cause of arguments between the food provider and child.

Increasing numbers of preschool children spend long periods being cared for outside their home environment and thus, for many, parents are not the only or indeed the main meal providers. This has been recognized, and an excellent report providing nutritional guidelines for food prepared in child-care settings has been published (Caroline Walker Trust 1998).

Because children at this age have high energy requirements but a limited capacity to consume food, healthy-eating guidelines designed for adults are not always appropriate. However, the food intake of young children cannot be considered in isolation from that of their families, and healthy-eating advice should be directed at the whole family, bearing in mind the special nutritional needs of the young child.

3.4.1 Dietary intake of preschool children

Energy

Many young children show chaotic eating patterns, consuming very little at one meal but making up later. Others have days of poor eating followed by a period of improved intake. Some children have one meal a day which they eat particularly well, commonly breakfast. Despite variability in eating patterns, a study of 2–5-year-old American children (Birch *et al.* 1991) found that, while food consumption from meal to meal was highly erratic, total daily energy intakes were relatively constant. Minor illness, which frequently occurs in this age group, is a common cause of short-term impaired food intake.

The 1992/93 National Diet and Nutrition Survey (NDNS) of 1859 children between the ages of $1\frac{1}{2}$ and $4\frac{1}{2}$ years provides the most recent comprehensive information about the dietary intake of this age group (Gregory *et al.* 1995). The survey found that, in terms of total energy intake, children of this age group were generally well nourished, being taller and heavier but not fatter than those of 25 years ago. Prynne *et al.* (1999) compared the data obtained for the $3\frac{1}{2}$–$4\frac{1}{2}$-year-old children in this survey with similar data derived from a 1950 survey on 4 year olds. They found that the mean energy intake of the 1950 cohort was 17% greater than that of the 1990s sample. In addition, the records for 1950 did not include energy derived from the sweet ration, which would have increased mean intake by about 80 kcal/day. Since children were shorter and thinner in 1950 (Gregory *et al.* 1990), the fact that they had a higher energy intake than today's 4 year olds suggests that they were also considerably more active. The importance of regular physical activity for optimal growth and development has long been recognized and it is recommended that, by the age of 5 years, children should be physically active, at a level of at least moderate intensity, for a minimum of half an hour, and preferably for 1 hour, every day (HEA 1998).

Carbohydrate

The mean carbohydrate intake of children in the NDNS sample provided approximately 51% of total energy intake, with starch accounting for 22% of this. About 65% starch came from cereals and cereal products and a further 25% from vegetables, potatoes and savoury snacks.

Although most children consumed adequate energy for their needs, approximately 20% was derived from non-milk extrinsic sugars (NMES) found in foods such as biscuits, confectionery, sugar added to cereals and drinks, as well as sugar-containing drinks. The latter provided one-third of the NMES intake. About 10% of the children surveyed were deriving more than one-third of their energy intake from NMES (Gregory *et al.* 1995). This has implications in terms of nutrient density; diets with a high proportion of NMES-containing foods tend to be low in micronutrients relative to their energy content. Frequent consumption of sugar-containing foods also increases the risk of dental caries (see Section 4.1, Dental disorders).

Non-starch polysaccharides (dietary fibre)

There is no official recommendation for fibre intake in children, but children should have a proportionally lower intake than the 18 g non-starch polysaccharide (NSP)/day recommended for adults (Caroline Walker Trust 1998). The NDNS found that children aged 1½ and 4½ years consumed approximately 6 g NSP/day, the majority of which was derived from potatoes and other vegetables (Gregory *et al.* 1995). This survey found a positive correlation between NSP intake and the number of daily bowel movements.

Dietary fibre intake of young children needs to be sufficient but not excessive. High-fibre diets are bulky and young children with small appetites may not be able to eat sufficient of them to meet their energy needs (Burkitt *et al.* 1980). An associated high intake of phytate may also adversely affect mineral absorption and trigger deficiencies in those with marginal intakes. This risk is increased for children following vegetarian diets (see Section 3.10.4 in Vegetarianism and veganism).

Some young children appear sensitive to a relatively modest amount of fibre in their diet. The result is symptoms of wind, colic and loose frequent stools (see Toddler's diarrhoea, below).

Fat

Eating less fat poses no nutritional problems for adults but, in the small child, fat restriction can result in a diet of insufficient energy content. It is physically difficult for those with small appetites to eat enough of a diet high in fibrous carbohydrate foods to meet their energy needs.

Nevertheless, in order to encourage the development of eating habits which help protect against atherosclerosis in later life, progress towards lower fat food choices as part of a healthy family lifestyle should be encouraged. Semi-skimmed milk can be introduced from the age of 2 years if the child is growing well, but skimmed milk is too low in energy and vitamins for the under-5s. It is recommended (Tarlow 1989) that, by the age of 5 years, dietary fat should comprise no more than 35% of energy intake. Since the percentage of energy from dietary fat already falls from about 50% in a breast- or formula-fed infant to about 36%

by the age of 4½ years (Gregory *et al.* 1995), this target would appear to be achievable.

Young children with familial hypercholesterolaemia are special cases who require early and intensive management to improve their prognosis (Tarlow *et al.* 1988).

Vitamins

The NDNS (Gregory *et al.* 1995) showed that the majority of children had adequate intakes of most vitamins, with the exception of vitamin A, for which half the children had a mean daily intake below the reference nutrient intake (RNI) value of 400 μg. The main food sources of vitamin A were milk and vegetables. Since only a limited number of foods are a rich source of this vitamin, and young children tend not to consume large quantities of vegetables, a supplementary source of vitamin A (from Department of Health vitamin drops) is advisable.

Vitamin C intake may be only marginally adequate in this age group. Only 1% of children had vitamin C intakes below the lower reference nutrient intake (LRNI) but, even taking into consideration the amount obtained from dietary supplements, 35% of the sample had a daily vitamin C intake below the RNI.

The Department of Health recommends that children up to 5 years of age are given supplements of vitamins A, C and D. These are available free to families receiving Income Support and certain other state benefits (Caroline Walker Trust 1998).

Minerals

Some foods and ingredients which are regularly consumed by children in this age group are fortified with iron (breakfast cereals) and iron and calcium (white flour), and therefore cereals and cereal products are a major source of these minerals for children in this age group (Gregory *et al.* 1995).

Between the ages of 1 and 3 years the RNI for iron is 6.9 mg/day, reflecting a high requirement during this period of rapid growth and development. The RNI is reduced to 6.1 mg/day in those aged 4–6 years. Gregory *et al.* (1995) found that 84% of this age group had intakes below the RNI, and almost 20% had very low intakes.

The main source of calcium in the diet of 1½ and 4½ year olds is milk and milk products, which provide approximately 65% of the mean intake, with milk alone providing 51%. However, the contribution of milk and milk products to calcium intake is highest in the youngest children in this age band, and decreases as children progress across it (Gregory *et al.* 1995). Cereal and cereal products are the other main source of dietary calcium and the proportion derived from these foods increases with age.

3.4.2 Healthy eating in preschool children

Ideally, children should look forward to meal times as social occasions as well as for provision of food. They should be encouraged, but not forced, to try a variety of foods and be able to use the adults present as role models for both the type of foods eaten and eating behaviours. At this age, children will need to eat little and often, but snacks should be treated as meals and children expected to sit and eat, rather than continuing their activities with a snack in their hand.

Their diet needs to an appropriate balance of foods from all four main food groups (see Section 1.2, Healthy eating):

- bread, cereals and potatoes
- fruit and vegetables
- milk and dairy foods
- meat, fish and alternatives.

Most of their food should be rich in essential nutrients, especially calcium and iron. Children, as well as adults, are advised to eat five portions of fruit or vegetables a day. Any of the following would be a suitable portion for a child under 5 years:

- 25 ml orange or apple juice diluted with water
- small banana or half an apple or pear, small bowl of tinned fruit (preferably tinned in its own juice)
- 40 g portion of broccoli, carrots, corn, green beans, peas or tomatoes.

Sugary or savoury snack foods such as crisps, biscuits, sweets and chocolate can be part of the diet but should be treats rather than daily items. Better choices of snack foods include:

- plain biscuits, breadsticks, melba toast, bread, toast, crumpets, currant buns or teacakes, pitta bread or sandwiches
- home-made plain popcorn or breakfast cereals which are not sugar coated
- dried or fresh fruit, carrot sticks
- yoghurt or fromage frais, preferably plain with added fruit.

Milk and water are the best drinks to serve between meals. Sweetened drinks, including diluted fruit juice, should only be consumed with, rather than between, meals to reduce the risk of dental caries. Consumption of sugar-free fizzy or fruit-based drinks should also be confined to meal times because the high acidity level of these drinks can cause dental erosion (see Section 4.1.2, in Dental disorders).

In order to reduce the risk of peanut allergy, peanut-containing foods should not be given to children below the age of 3 years if a parent or sibling has a diagnosed allergy or history of atopy (DH 1998; see Section 4.34.3 in Food allergy and intolerance). Whole nuts should not be given to any child below the age of 5 years because of the risk of choking.

3.4.3 Nutritional problems in preschool children

Dental caries

There was a dramatic fall in the incidence of dental caries in young children in the UK between 1973 and 1983, largely due to the introduction and widespread use of toothpaste with added fluoride. Since then the progress has slowed, and although 57% of preschool children had no evidence of caries in 1993, the average number of decayed and filled teeth in 5 year olds remained at 1.6 (O'Brien 1994). It has also become evident that young children from more deprived sectors of the population are particularly at risk from, and have an increased prevalence of, dental disease (see Section 4.1.1 in Dental disorders).

The NDNS Dental Survey (Hinds and Gregory 1995; Gibson and Williams 1999) provided evidence that the most important preventive measure in preschool children is brushing teeth twice a day with a fluoridated toothpaste. This procedure should be supervised as young children lack the dexterity to brush properly, and care should be taken to avoid swallowing toothpaste. The frequency of consumption of sugar-containing drinks and foods should be reduced and ideally kept to meal times only (Levine 1996). The NDNS Dental Survey highlighted the high prevalence of bedtime and nocturnal consumption of sugar-containing beverages (Hinds and Gregory 1995); an important caries-prevention measure in this age group is therefore the policy of 'only water after brushing at night'.

Iron-deficiency anaemia

Iron deficiency is common in preschool children, particularly in socially disadvantaged groups and in the immigrant population. Incidence figures for iron-deficiency anaemia of around 25% in the second year of life have been reported in studies from Birmingham and Nottingham (Aukert et al. 1986; James et al. 1989). Iron deficiency is associated with frequent infections, poor weight gain, developmental delay and behaviour disorders (Aukert et al. 1986) and is an important treatable condition in early childhood.

Iron deficiency in young children is usually of dietary origin. It is associated with late weaning, inappropriate weaning foods and the early introduction of cow's milk, which not only is a poor source of iron but may cause intestinal blood loss in some young children (Ziegler et al. 1990). Williams and Sahota (1990) suggested that the lack of manufactured halal meat-based weaning foods may be partly responsible for the low iron intakes commonly found in infants of Asian origin.

Prevention of iron deficiency

Dietary advice around the time of weaning is particularly important. Extended use of iron-fortified infant formulae or a follow-on milk should be encouraged.

Foods such as meat, fish, fruit and vegetables should be included on a daily basis. Liver is a good source of iron but also a very rich source of vitamin A, which can be harmful in large amounts. It has therefore been suggested that liver and liver-containing products should not be given to a child more than once a week (MAFF 1997). Haem iron is absorbed much more efficiently than non-haem iron but the absorption of iron from plant sources can be enhanced by the simultaneous consumption of foods and drinks rich in vitamin C, such as citrus fruits and juices or tomatoes. This is a particularly important measure in vegetarian children (see Section 3.10.4 in Vegetarianism and veganism).

Obesity

Because preschool children are totally dependent on other people for their food, obesity in this age group can be regarded as the fault of the parents (or carers) rather than the child. Very often it is a consequence of having allowed high-energy foods such as sweets, biscuits and crisps to figure to excess in the diet of a fussy eater. Management of childhood obesity is discussed in Section 4.17.11 in Obesity.

Poor eating

'My child hardly eats a thing' is a common reason for referral to a general practitioner, health visitor, paediatrician or dietitian. Food refusal by a toddler is a powerful weapon and causes much parental anxiety.

In the absence of underlying disease, if a child is growing normally it is unlikely that there is a significant problem. Height and weight centiles should be plotted together with previous measurements if available. Since there is considerable variability in the rate of growth, isolated centile measurements are only of concern if they fall below the 0.4th centile (Cole 1994). Deviation of growth from a centile line is more indicative of impaired growth, and a growth curve which crosses a centile line between two annual measurements (e.g. crossing from the 25th to the 9th centile) warrants further investigation. A growth curve which crosses a centile line over a period of 2 years (i.e. three annual assessments) is an indication for further assessment a year later and subsequent referral if necessary.

If the child appears healthy, management of the poor eater revolves around education and reassurance. Many parents have unrealistic expectations of their child's weight gain and requirements for food and are worrying unnecessarily. They should be reminded that from birth to 1 year a child gains about 6 kg (15 lb) but during the second, third and fourth years, the average weight gain is only 2 kg (5 lb). The rapid growth and constant increases in food intake of a baby do not continue.

It is important to discover what the child is actually eating. Taking a detailed dietary history or asking the parents to keep a 3-day food diary can be very revealing. Common findings include:

- *Frequent drinks of milk or juice*: Many young children prefer drinking to eating and readily fill themselves up with drinks. Useful advice is that drinks are avoided for 1 hour before meals and only offered at the end of a meal, not along with food. If a toddler still drinks from a bottle, a cup should be encouraged as this will help

to decrease fluid intake. Those responsible for children who consume a large volume of milk should be advised that 3 cups a day and the milk added to breakfast cereal is sufficient.
- *Frequent snacking*: Small children may need to eat between meals, but some end up eating most of their food between meals. Consumption of snack foods at frequent intervals throughout the morning will stop most toddlers eating lunch. Less frequent and more appropriate snacks (such as half a banana or one plain biscuit instead of a bag of crisps or several chocolate biscuits) should be suggested.

Some parents feel that they have to offer snacks if meals are uneaten. They should be reassured that no healthy child will starve if appropriate food is offered at meal times. A consistent approach is essential and all those involved in the care of the child, including relatives and childminders, must co-operate with any measures suggested.

There is never a place for threats, bribery or other measures to force a child to finish a meal. Battles over food will only make the situation worse. If food offered at meal times is rejected, it should be removed without comment but nothing substituted in its place or offered before the next meal. Other strategies such as picnics in the garden, eating at friends' homes and meals out can also be employed to help the fussy eater; food and meal times should, after all, be an enjoyable part of a child's day. Preschool children's eating habits often improve dramatically once they come into contact with other children and, once they start school, they tend to expend more energy and have less opportunity to eat between meals, and so be hungrier at meal times.

Toddler's diarrhoea

This is a common problem in children who are otherwise healthy. Frequent, loose stools containing recognizable food matter (e.g. peas, carrots, sweetcorn) may be passed up to eight or more times daily. The stools often become looser later in the day but are not passed at night. Typically, the first stool of the day is passed soon after the child first eats or drinks. The condition is thought to be due to a degree of immaturity of gut function and often improves spontaneously around the age of 3–4 years. Parents often present for advice when they hope to start toilet training or when the child is due to attend nursery school.

Toddler's diarrhoea is a harmless condition and careful explanation reassures many parents. Consumption of large quantities of fruit or fruit juice is a common cause as the immature gut is inefficient in absorbing fructose, which therefore remains in the gut and results in osmotic diarrhoea. Sucrose, which is metabolized to glucose and fructose, may have similar effects if consumed in large quantities.

Reducing fibre intake is particularly likely to help children whose families have adopted a high-fibre diet. This can be achieved by a short-term change to white bread and refined breakfast cereal, and reducing fruit and vegetable intake to one portion of each daily until tolerance to fibre has improved.

Constipation

Young children may become constipated, particularly following an anal fissure or after an intercurrent infection. There may also be a behavioural element to the problem. The child should be encouraged to consume foods with a higher fibre content, which are also enjoyed (e.g. wholegrain breakfast cereal, fruit, baked beans, high-fibre white bread). Nothing will be achieved by trying to make the child eat vegetables they do not like. Young children should not be given unprocessed bran as it can cause bloating and flatulence as well as having a detrimental effect on the absorption of micronutrients.

Constipation can also result from inadequate fluid consumption; some young children are 'poor drinkers' rather than 'poor eaters'. It should also be borne in mind that an increased dietary fibre intake will only be beneficial in terms of constipation if fluid intake is also increased.

Food and poverty

Families on low incomes can face major problems in feeding their children, and dietary problems and health risks are much more prevalent in children growing up in disadvantaged circumstances (NCH 1991). This subject is discussed in more detail in Section 3.8 (People in low-income groups).

Text revised by: Jacki Bishop

Useful addresses

Caroline Walker Trust (publications)
22 Kindersley Way, Abbots Langley, Herts WD5 0DQ
Tel: 01923 269902
Website: www.cwt.org.uk

Further reading

British Dietetic Association. *Children's Diets and Change*. Report of the Child Health and Nutrition Working Party. Birmingham: BDA, 1987.

Morse E. *My Child Won't Eat*. London: Penguin, 1988.

Baxter B, Rich H. *Healthy Eating for Little People: A Quick and Simple Guide for Busy Parents*. RB Publishing, 1994.

References

Aukert MA, Parks YS, Scott PH, Wharton BA. Treatment with iron increases weight gain and psychomotor development. *Archives of Disease in Childhood* 1986; **61**: 849–857.

Birch LL, Johnson SL, Andresen G, Peters JC. The variability of young children's energy intake. *New England Journal of Medicine* 1991; **324**: 232–235.

Burkitt D, Morley D, Walker A. Dietary fibre in under and over nutrition in children. *Archives of Disease in Childhood* 1980; **55**: 803–807.

Caroline Walker Trust. *Eating Well for Under 5s in Child Care: Practical and Nutritional Guidelines*. Report of an expert working group. London: Caroline Walker Trust, 1998.

Cole TJ. Do growth centile charts need a face-lift? *British Medical Journal* 1994; **308**: 641–642.

Department of Health. *Dietary Reference Values for Food Energy and Nutrients for the United Kingdom*. Report on Health and Social Subjects 41. London: HMSO, 1991.

Gibson S, Williams S. Dental caries in pre-school children: associations with social class, tooth-brushing habit and consumption of sugars and sugar-containing foods. Further analysis of data from the National Diet and Nutrition Survey of children aged 1.5–4.5 years. *Caries Research* 1999; **33**: 101–103.

Gregory JR, Foster K, Tyler H, Wiseman M. *The Dietary and Nutritional Survey of British Adults*. London: HMSO, 1990.

Gregory JR, Collins DL, Davies PSW et al. *National Diet and Nutrition Survey: Children Aged 1½ and 4½ Years*. Vol. 1. *Report of the Diet and Nutrition Survey*. London: HMSO, 1995.

Health Education Authority. *Young and Active Policy Framework for Young People and Health-Enhancing Physical Activity*. London: HEA, 1998.

Hinds K, Gregory JR. *National Diet and Nutrition Survey: Children Aged 1.5 to 4.5 Years*. Vol. 2. *Report of the Dental Survey*. London: HMSO, 1995.

James T, Lawson P, Male P, Oakhill A. Preventing iron deficiency in pre-school children by implementing an educational and screening programme in an inner city practice. *British Medical Journal* 1989; **299**: 838–840.

Levine R. *The Scientific Basis of Dental Health Education: A Policy Document*. London: HEA, 1996.

Ministry of Agriculture Fisheries and Food (MAFF), in association with the Department of Health and Health Education Authority. *Healthy Diets for Infants and Young Children*. A Foodsense booklet. London: MAFF, 1997.

National Children's Home. *NHC Poverty and Nutrition Survey 1991*. London: NCH, 1991.

O'Brien M. *Children's Dental Health in the United Kingdom 1993*. Office of Population Censuses and Surveys, Social Survey Division. London: HMSO, 1994.

Prynne CJ, Paul AA, Price GM et al. Food and nutrient intake of a national sample of 4 year old children in 1950: comparison with the 1990s. *Public Health Nutrition* 1999; **2**: 537–547.

Tarlow M, Green A, Worthington D, Buchanan E. The paediatric lipid clinic in Birmingham. *Journal of Inherited Metabolic Disease* 1988; **11** (Suppl 1): 91–93.

Tarlow MJ. Cholesterol and diet. *Archives of Disease in Childhood* 1989; **64**: 647–648.

Thomas BJ. *Nutrition in Primary Care*. Oxford: Blackwell Science, 1996.

Williams S, Sahota P. An enquiry into the attitudes of Muslim Asian mothers regarding infant feeding practices and dental health. *Journal of Human Nutrition and Dietetics* 1990; **3**: 393–402.

Ziegler EE, Fomon SJ, Nelson SE. Cow milk feeding in infancy: further observations on blood loss from the gastrointestinal tract. *Journal of Pediatrics* 1990; **116**: 11–18.

3.5 School-aged children

When children leave the comparative safety of the nursery or home to attend school for the first time, learning about food and coming into contact with new eating situations is part of the process. At home, children's food choices might be limited by the family; however, at school, there are school meals, breakfast clubs, tuck shops, the opportunity to share food with friends, lessons on nutrition and the nearby corner shop, all of which shape the development of eating behaviour.

Children may find it difficult to relate to this new plethora of choice and retreat into familiar habits or food fads, or they may embrace the challenge and enjoy the opportunity to broaden their tastes. This section will focus on the nutritional requirements and nutritional intake of school children, prior to puberty. Encouragement rather than restriction should be the watchword for dietitians working with this age group, unless there are compelling therapeutic reasons, such as inborn errors of metabolism or allergy, to indicate otherwise.

3.5.1 Nutritional requirements and dietary intake

There are three distinct periods in childhood when growth is rapid: during infancy, adolescence and between the ages of 6 and 8 years (often called the mid-growth spurt). The greatest changes occur in adolescence but it is still important in the years preceding puberty to meet the nutrient requirements that allow for growth. Boys are slightly taller and heavier than girls at this time and this is reflected in their greater energy requirements, although other nutrient requirements, such as for protein and micronutrients, are similar (DH 1991). There are few differences in body fat content between boys and girls aged 5–7 years but after this time, girls begin to gain body fat at a greater rate than boys, culminating in the rapid deposition of adipose tissue on the hips and thighs during adolescence in response to sex-hormone production.

Energy

Energy requirements expressed per kilogram of body weight are higher in prepubertal children than in adults (DH 1991) as would be expected for steady growth. The midgrowth spurt is shortlived but can impact on both requirements and appetite. Children have remarkably good coupling between energy needs and energy intake and tend to adjust their food consumption appropriately. This can be at odds with the desire of parents to see children finish what is on their plate.

The most recent Government Report on the diet and nutritional status of 4–18 year olds in the UK, the National Diet and Nutrition Survey (NDNS) (Gregory et al. 2000), found that the mean energy intake of all age groups was below the estimated average requirement. However, children were taller and heavier than those in the 1983 survey and it is therefore likely that the lower energy intakes are sufficient and reflect the reduced level of physical activity. Data collected on physical activity indicated that about one-third of boys aged 7 years and over, and more than half the girls of the same age, failed to meet the Health Education Authority recommendation for young people to participate in at least moderate intensity exercise for 1 hour/day (HEA 1998).

Protein

Protein is needed for the formation of bone tissue and lean body mass. Reference nutrient intake (RNI) values range from the region of 20 g/day for 4–6 year olds to almost 30 g/day for 7–10 year olds. In the UK, achieving an adequate protein intake is not usually a problem and it is more likely that intake will be too high, which can contribute to rapid deposition of weight and an enhanced risk of obesity (Rolland-Cachera et al. 1995).

The NDNS found that the most common types of meat eaten by children aged 4–10 years were chicken and turkey dishes, including coated products, sausages, bacon and ham (Gregory et al. 2000). Red meat and offal were less significant contributors to protein intake; this has important implications in relation to iron intake. The proportion of children eating fried or coated white fish, including fish fingers, decreased significantly with age.

Iron and vitamin C

Maintaining adequate iron status is important for growth, cognitive function and the immune system. However, some of the major sources of dietary iron, such as offal, red meat, pulses and green leafy vegetables, are not always popular food choices among young children. The more common sources of iron in the childhood diet are bread, chips, meat and meat products (Gregory et al. 2000). Fortified foods, such as breakfast cereal, also make an important contribution to iron intakes in children; however, the iron added to such foods may not always be of good bioavailability and the high fibre content of certain breakfast cereals can hamper iron absorption.

Vitamin C assists the absorption of non-haem iron as well as being important for growth, wound healing and immunocompetence. While the NDNS found that most children had adequate vitamin C intakes, these were most likely to be derived from fruit, fruit juice and fortified soft drinks; only about 40% of 7–10 year olds consumed green leafy vegetables (Gregory et al. 2000). Children living in the north of England and Scotland and/or in lower socio-economic groups are likely to have the lowest intakes of fruit and vegetables.

Calcium

Lack of calcium in childhood can result in poor bone density and an increased chance of developing osteoporosis in later life (see Section 4.31, Osteoporosis). The NDNS survey showed that, while most children consumed adequate dietary calcium, between 2 and 5% of children aged 4–10 years had intakes below the RNI.

3.5.2 Dietary patterns of school-aged children

Meals

The frequency of breakfast consumption is at its highest in the prepubertal years, tending to decline as adolescence approaches, especially in girls. Breakfast can be a major source of nutrients and contribute between 6 and 20% of daily energy intake and approximately 20% of daily carbohydrate intake in young children. The most commonly eaten foods at breakfast have been shown to be ready-to-eat cereals, followed in popularity by toast and jam (Gibson and O'Sullivan 1995). Breakfast cereals consumed with milk provide an important source of B vitamins, calcium, iron, zinc and folate, and children who consume breakfast cereals on a regular basis are more likely to meet recommendations for micronutrient intake than children who consume them rarely or not at all (Nicklas 1995).

In addition to the nutritional benefits, breakfast consumption may have other advantages in terms of improved concentration and cognitive performance later in the morning (see Section 1.2.2. in Healthy eating).

Snacking

As a result of relatively high activity levels and small appetites, it is difficult for many children to meet their nutritional requirements by consuming only three meals a day; snacking is therefore reasonable childhood behaviour. It also contributes to socialization in the playground since many snack foods are shared, swapped and bartered. Snacking should not be discouraged, but care should be taken that the foods eaten are varied and as dense in micronutrients as possible. The most common snack food eaten by young children is potato crisps, aver-

age intakes of which have been reported to be 170 g/week, and can be as high as 1040 g (42 regular-sized packets) (Ruxton et al. 1996b). Other popular snack foods are jelly/boiled sweets, biscuits, sandwiches, fruit and milk chocolate.

Snack foods contribute around 25% of daily energy intakes, and can be considerably higher than this in children from lower socioeconomic groups. Ruxton et al. (1996b) compared mean daily dietary intake and body composition of children deriving a high percentage of energy from snacks (>35%) to those with a low percentage of energy intake derived from snacks (<15%). No significant differences were found. It was concluded that children who ate more snacks had smaller meals, resulting in the overall intakes being similar. The diets of children who snacked on breakfast cereals were closer to recommendations with respect to fat, fibre and micronutrients. However, frequent consumption of sugar-rich snacks does have implications in terms of dental health (see Section 4.1, Dental disorders).

3.5.3 Dietary targets and healthy eating

Dietary compositional targets, such as a relatively low proportion of dietary energy from fat, apply to adults and are not always appropriate for young children. There is no dietary reference value (DRV) for fibre for young children and, given their small appetites, high fibre intakes can decrease energy density to such an extent that it becomes difficult to eat sufficient food to meet energy and nutrient needs.

Nevertheless, since the development of eating habits starts in childhood, there should be gradual encouragement of food choices that will help to achieve healthy eating in later life. In healthy children with adequate energy intakes, low-fat diets can be compatible with satisfactory growth (Boulton and Magarey 1995). However, the extent and pace at which this occurs should be dictated by considerations of appetite, the likelihood of energy and micronutrient intakes being met and rate of growth.

Most carbohydrate should be derived from starchy foods such as bread, potatoes, breakfast cereals, pasta and rice. Sources of intrinsic and milk sugars such as fruit and dairy products and fruit can be encouraged as these are valuable sources of other nutrients. It is reasonable for extrinsic sugars from sugar-containing snack and drinks (including fruit juice) to make some contribution to carbohydrate and energy intake, but consumption should not be excessive (preferably below 11% of dietary energy) and the frequency with which such foods are consumed should be low. Some sources of both insoluble fibre (from cereal foods) and soluble fibre (from fruit, vegetables, pulses and oat-based cereals) should be encouraged.

In the drive to promote better eating habits, it is important not to prohibit specific foods. Restricting access to foods that children enjoy will focus attention on those foods and exacerbate the desire to eat them. Using food as a reward, particularly for consuming foods which are not liked, is equally counterproductive as the reward food will gain a higher status than other foods. It is better to use non-food treats where possible.

3.5.4 The impact of school on diet and health

Nutritional standards and guidelines for school meals

Formal nutritional guidelines for school lunches in the UK were abolished in 1980. Since then the few studies that have evaluated school meals have found that they provided sufficient micronutrients and protein but were high in fat (Ruxton 1996a). Recent recommendations on the composition and provision of school meals include *Nutritional Guidelines for School Meals* (Caroline Walker Trust 1992) and the three-part Health of the Nation document *Eating Well at School* (DfEE 1997).

The UK government has announced its intention to return to formal nutritional standards for school lunches, and the consultation paper *Ingredients for Success* (DfEE 1998) set initial suggestions for standards. Following this, draft regulations and guidance for nutritional standards for school lunches were published (DfEE 1999a).

Food consumption during the school day

A national school-meals survey (Gardner Merchant 1998) found that 42% of children bought sweets on the way to school and a further 24% bought crisps and savoury snacks.

A comparison of packed lunches and school meals in 7–8-year-old children found that school lunches were higher in fat and lower in starch, sugars, fibre and iron than packed lunches (Ruxton 1996a). Home lunches had a nutrient composition that fell between the two. School lunches provided around 22% of daily energy and also 22% of fibre intakes, whereas packed lunches provided 33% of energy and 36% of fibre intakes. This may have implications for children in lower socioeconomic groups who often have free school meals (Ruxton *et al.* 1996a). The most popular school-meal choices have been found to be pizza, chips, roast dinner, burgers and sausages (Gardner Merchant 1998).

However, while packed lunches can make a valuable contribution to nutritional intake, direct observation of children eating packed lunches shows that their composition in terms of food choice often leaves much to be desired. Typically, a packed lunch is comprised of sandwiches, a chocolate bar, savoury snack and sweetened drink. Fresh fruit is often absent. Providing parents with suggestions for packed lunches which are equally appealing but healthier in composition is an important aspect of health promotion within schools.

Nutrition education

Within school, children learn about food and nutrition through the National Curriculum. At Key Stage 2 (7–11 years), children learn about themselves as growing and changing individuals. Most of this work is carried out under the personal and social health education (PSE) subject area, but crosses into other curriculum areas such as science and physical activity. Pupils are taught about nutrition with regard to their own health and the importance of variety in their diet. They are also taught about the importance of exercise on health and, since August 2000, the government has suggested that at least 2 hours of physical education should be included within the curriculum each week.

Further details about the nutrition content of the National Curriculum can be obtained from their website. The DfEE Standards and Effectiveness Unit also has a website which gives practical examples of how nutrition education can be incorporated into other subject areas such as mathematics. The website details for these can be found in Useful Addresses at the end of this section.

It is also important that the nutrition education derived from the curriculum is complemented and reinforced in other food-related areas of school life such as breakfast clubs, tuck shops, packed lunches, vending machines, school meals and cooking skills. In order to achieve this there is a need for a 'whole school approach' to food and nutrition, such as the establishment of School Nutrition Action Groups (see Section 3.6, Adolescents). This has recently been endorsed by the publication of the National Healthy School Standard (DfEE 1999b) which aims to encourage all schools to become part of a 'Healthy Schools Programme'.

3.5.5 Common dietary problems in school-aged children

Obesity

Between 5 and 15% of prepubertal children are classified as overweight and the proportion is increasing with each generation, primarily as a result of falling levels of physical activity (Gregory *et al.* 2000). Normal preschool children have a high level of adiposity which falls around the age of 4–5 years and increases again at 7 years. This is called the 'adiposity rebound'. Children who become obese in adolescence have been shown to experience adiposity rebounds before the age of 6 years. Risks for childhood obesity have been reported to be high protein intakes, high fat intakes, high parental body mass index (BMI) and inactivity. This is discussed in more detail in Section 4.17.11 in Obesity.

The Health Survey for England (Prescott-Clarke and Primatesta 1998) found that a high birthweight was related to later obesity. It also found that young children are already developing perceptions about their weight and acting on their concerns. Seven per cent of 8–9-year-old boys reported being too heavy and 12% reported trying to lose weight. The corresponding figures for girls were 9% and 13%. Between the ages of 10 and 12 years the findings were more worrying, with 10% of boys believing they were too heavy and 15% trying to diet, while the corresponding figures for girls were 10% and 23%. The actual incidence of obesity in this group was 7%.

Underweight

Many young children are naturally lean, particularly during the mini-growth spurt that occurs around the age of 7 years. However, children who persistently fall below the 10th centile of weight for height should be investigated (see Section 1.8.7 in Assessment of nutritional status). Failure to thrive is rare but may be due to an underlying medical condition, poor appetite, family problems, concern about body image or self-imposed dietary restriction. Eating disorders are not common amongst prepubertal children but are recognized to occur (Sands *et al.* 1997).

Dental caries

Children are more susceptible to dental caries than adults, although the incidence of caries in children in the UK has decreased substantially since the introduction of fluoride toothpaste in the 1970s. However, the type of food regularly consumed and eating frequency still play an important role in caries prevention (Kandelman 1997). These factors are discussed in detail in Section 4.1.1 in Dental disorders).

Anaemia

Although iron intake in prepubertal children has been found to be generally adequate (Gregory *et al.* 2000), iron-deficiency anaemia does occur in this age group, particularly in children who are vegetarian or from ethnic minorities. The NDNS found that 3% of boys and 8% of girls aged 4–6 years had haemoglobin levels below 11.0 g/dl (the defining cut-off point for anaemia) (Gregory *et al.* 2000).

Practical approaches to increasing iron intake include encouraging greater consumption of foods such as fortified breakfast cereals, dried fruit, baked beans, corned beef, red meat, pilchards and sardines. Mincing meat and adding pulses to meals may also be beneficial. Iron uptake can be maximized by offering fruit juice with meals and avoiding foods which tend to hamper absorption, such as tea or high-fibre cereals.

Allergy, intolerance and hyperactivity

Parents often believe their child to have 'allergies' or behavioural problems which are related to food. Many of these beliefs will be unfounded, but dietitians must consider all such parental concerns seriously and establish whether there is a basis for them by means of detailed dietary enquiry and diet – symptom records. Trial food-exclusion measures should only be considered when dietary investigations suggest that these are justified (see Section 4.34, Food allergy and intolerance).

Some parents may have already imposed dietary restrictions, and the nature and implications of these should be explored. Exclusion of foods which are major nutrient contributors such as milk and dairy products, or wheat, can seriously compromise nutritional status in this age group. Remedial dietetic advice may be necessary to correct or avert this.

Text revised by: Diane Talbot, Helen Storer and Carrie Ruxton

Useful addresses

Department for Education and Employment (DfEE)
DfEE Publications Centre: 0845 60 22260
Website: dfee.gov.uk

DfEE Standards and Effectiveness website: www.standards.dfee.gov.uk
National Curriculum website: www.nc.uk.net

Wired for Health (This is a website primarily designed for teachers covering health-related topics such as accidents, alcohol, healthy eating, mental health, smoking, substance misuse and sun safety)
Website: www.wiredforhealth.gov.uk.

References

Boulton TJC, Magarey AM. Effects of differences in dietary fat on growth, energy and nutrient intake from infancy to eight years of age. *Acta Paediatrica* 1995; **84**: 146–150.

Caroline Walker Trust. *Nutritional Guidelines for School Meals*. Report of an Expert Working Group. London: Caroline Walker Trust, 1992.

Department for Education and Employment (DfEE). *Eating Well at School: Dietary Guidance for School Food Providers*. Part 1: *Guidance for Governors and Head Teachers in Schools Which do not Manage their own School Meals Contract*. Part 2: *Guidance for Policy Makers in Local Education Authorities and Schools which Manage their own School Meals Contracts*. Part 3: *Guidance for Catering Contract Managers and Caterers in Schools*. London: DfEE, 1997.

Department for Education and Employment. *Ingredients for Success*. A Consultation Paper on Nutritional Standards for School Lunches. London: DfEE, 1998.

Department for Education and Employment. *Draft Regulations and Guidance for Nutritional Standards for School Lunches*. London: DfEE, 1999a.

Department for Education and Employment. *The National Healthy School Standard*. London: DfEE, 1999b.

Department of Health. *Dietary Reference Values for Food Energy and Nutrients for the United Kingdom*. Report on Health and Social Subjects 41. London: HMSO, 1991.

Gardner Merchant School Meals Survey. *What are Today's Children Eating?* Gardner Merchant, 1998.

Gibson SA, O'Sullivan KR. Breakfast cereal consumption patterns and nutrient intakes in British school children. *Journal of the Royal Society of Health* 1995; **115**: 336–370.

Gregory J et al. National Diet and Nutrition Survey: Young People Aged 4 to 18 Years. Vol. 1. *Report of the National Diet and Nutrition Survey*. London: The Stationery Office, 2000.

Health Education Authority. *Young and Active: Policy Framework for Young People and Health – Enhancing Physical Activity*. London: HEA, 1998.

Kandelman D. Sugar, alternative sweeteners and meal frequency in relation to caries prevention: new perspectives. *British Journal of Nutrition* 1997; **77** (Suppl 1): S121–S128.

Nicklas TA. Dietary studies of children: the Bogalusa Heart Study experience. *Journal of the American Dietetic Association* 1995; **95**: 1127–1133.

Prescott-Clarke P, Primatesta P. (Eds). *The Health of Young People 1995–1997*. London: The Stationery Office, 1998.

Rolland-Cachera MF, Deheeger M, Akrout M, Bellisle F. Influence of macronutrients on adiposity development: a follow up study of nutrition and growth from 10 months to 8 years of age. *International Journal of Obesity* 1995; **19**: 573–578.

Ruxton CHS, Kirk TR, Belton NR, Holmes MAM. The contribution of specific dietary patterns to energy and nutrient intakes in 7–8 year old Scottish schoolchildren. II. Weekday lunches. *Journal of Human Nutrition and Dietetics* 1996a; **9**: 15–22.

Ruxton CHS, Kirk TR, Belton NR, Holmes MAM. The contribution of specific dietary patterns to energy and nutrient intakes in 7-to-8-year old Scottish schoolchildren. III. Snacking habits. *Journal of Human Nutrition and Dietetics* 1996b; **9**: 23–31.

Sands R, Tricker J, Sherman C *et al*. Disordered eating patterns, body image, self-esteem, and physical activity in pre adolescent school children. *International Journal of Eating Disorders* 1997; **21**: 159–166.

3.6 Adolescents

Adolescence is a period of transition between childhood and adulthood. This applies not only to physical and emotional change but also to the development of dietary and other health-related behaviours. Whereas childhood is often characterized by resistance to new foods or experiences, the opposite is the case in adolescence where experimentation reigns. Young people will choose foods for many reasons other than their nutritional content. These can include slimming or weight control (whether justified or not), peer-group pressure to consume certain foods or brands, the development of personal ideology such as the use of vegetarian diets, following a specific diet to enhance sporting prowess or even just plain convenience. Understanding why adolescents eat the foods they do is the first step to discovering the challenges and pitfalls of health education in this group.

3.6.1 Nutritional implications of adolescence

Physical development

The main human growth spurt occurs in adolescence, although the exact time-point varies enormously and is influenced by genetics, gender, race and body weight. During childhood, growth rates are fairly similar between boys and girls, with boys being slightly larger and heavier than girls up to around the 9th year of life. Once the pubertal growth spurt commences, these gender differences are temporarily reversed. Girls begin their phase of rapid growth first, a process lasting up to $3\frac{1}{2}$ years, and reach their near adult height by the age of 14 years, whereas boys start their growth spurt 2 years later and will be shorter than girls for a period of time. The greatest gains in adolescent height occur in the year preceding menarche for girls and around 14 years for boys, while the greatest gains in weight occur at 13 years for girls and 14 years for boys. Growth may not cease completely at the end of adolescence; height increases of up to 2 cm can still occur between the ages of 17 and 28 years.

Adolescence is also the time when sexual development occurs. The onset of the sexual characteristics of puberty may be a better marker of the stage of adolescence (and thus nutritional requirements) than age *per se*. In girls, the onset of menarche varies widely. Adipose stores are a major factor and tall, heavy girls will tend to begin their periods earlier than their smaller, leaner classmates. Vigorous exercise, such as athletics, can delay menarche, due both to the physiological effects of training and to depletion of body fat.

Nutritional requirements

Requirements for energy and protein intakes are highest during the period of peak growth, particularly in boys who gain a greater amount of height and lean body mass than girls. Undernutrition at this time can inhibit bone development, resulting in a lower peak bone mass, and produce a low height velocity, leading to stunting. Severe undernutrition can also delay puberty or halt its progression.

Other major nutrients important for growth are iron, calcium, vitamin C and zinc. Calcium is particularly important during adolescence as the production of sex hormones results in rapid accretion of bone tissue. It is important to maximize bone density during this time because, once it peaks in the early twenties, little can be done to augment the calcium stored in the bone. Low bone density is related to increased osteoporosis risk in later life, especially in women and people with a history of anorexia nervosa (see Section 4.31, Osteoporosis).

Iron is another key nutrient during growth since it is a component of muscle and blood. Achieving adequate iron stores becomes important for girls as menstrual periods become more regular and heavier.

3.6.2 Dietary intake of adolescents

Nutritional intake of adolescents

There is a common belief that the adolescent diet is nutritionally inadequate. In terms of meeting the energy needs for growth, this is clearly not generally the case since the average height of teenagers has continued to increase in recent decades. Furthermore, the incidence of obesity in this age group is rising, suggesting that energy surplus (coupled with physical inactivity) is a more likely problem.

There are, however, some concerns in relation to micronutrient deficiency. The recent National Diet and Nutrition Survey (NDNS) (Gregory et al. 2000) found that the average intakes of zinc, potassium, magnesium and calcium in older boys and girls were below the reference nutrient intake (RNI), as was that of iron in girls. Significant proportions of these young people had intakes below the lower reference nutrient intake (LRNI), almost certainly insufficient to meet their needs. Almost 20% of older girls, and 12% of older boys, had intakes of vitamin A below the LRNI. About one-fifth of girls also had riboflavin intakes below the LRNI.

In terms of energy composition, the average teenage diet was not ideal, although the same can be said about the diet of much of the adult UK population (see Table 1.1 in Section 1.1, Diet, health and disease). While the percentage of dietary energy derived from fat was in the region of 35% energy (i.e. close to the recommended percentage), this was partly due to the relatively high proportion of energy derived from non-milk extrinsic sugars (about 16.5% of energy, compared with the recommended 11%). Total intake of carbohydrate was less than the recommended 50% of energy. Intake of saturated fat exceeded recommendations (14.2% of energy compared with the recommended 11%). Average intake of dietary fibre was well below adult recommendations. Salt intake, excluding any additions during cooking and at the table, was high.

Nutritional status of adolescents

Despite the low dietary intakes of a number of minerals and some vitamins by adolescents, there is little evidence of widespread biochemical deficiency. The NDNS did, however, highlight a number of concerns (Gregory *et al.* 2000). Low serum ferritin levels, indicative of low iron stores, were found in 13% of boys and 27% of girls. A significant proportion (13%) of 11–18 year olds had poor vitamin D status. Some individuals were found to have poor nutritional status in respect of vitamin C, folate, riboflavin and thiamin, particularly young people in Scotland and northern England. Therefore, subgroups of the adolescent population appear to have poor vitamin or mineral status and dietitians should be alert to this possibility.

Others may also have borderline deficiency, evidence of which is difficult to detect biochemically as homoeostatic mechanisms can mask the effects of nutrient deficiencies until an advanced stage of depletion (see Section 1.8.5 in Assessment of nutritional status). It is also conceivable that, in some adolescents, overt deficiency is offset by the use of multivitamin and mineral supplements; Gregory *et al.* (2000) found that 20% of this age group regularly took these products.

The risk of low folate status is an important consideration in this age group where unplanned pregnancies are increasingly common. Young women who do not consume fortified breakfast cereals, and have low intakes of other important dietary sources of folate such as green leafy vegetables, pulses and citrus fruits, are particularly at risk.

Other adverse parameters of nutritional status which impact on health were also apparent. In the NDNS, 8% of boys and 11.5% girls had a plasma cholesterol concentration above 5.2 mmol/l. In both boys and girls, use of salt at the table was associated with increased systolic blood pressure.

Food choices of adolescents

Food choice by teenagers explains many of the dietary imbalances found. Gregory *et al.* (2000) found that the most commonly consumed foods in this age group were white bread, savoury snacks, potato chips, biscuits, boiled, mashed and jacket potatoes, and chocolate confectionery.

Consumption of red meat and milk tended to be low, and that of fruit and vegetables was particularly low. Boys consumed, by weight, nearly four times as many biscuits as green vegetables; girls consumed four times the quantity of sweets and chocolate as green vegetables. Use of carbonated soft drinks was high, whereas only 12–15% of 15–18 year olds drank milk. Marked contrasts in health-related behaviour were also apparent; for example, 33% of 15–18-year-old girls smoked but only 20% ate citrus fruit.

This pattern of food intake inevitably increases the likelihood of higher than desirable intakes of fat and non-milk extrinsic sugars, and a diet of relatively low micronutrient density. As a result, fortified foods, particularly breakfast cereals, can be an important source of micronutrients in the teenage diet. Other foods, not normally regarded as significant sources of micronutrients, can also make a significant contribution to total intake; for example, up to 12% of daily iron intake may be derived from foods such as crisps and chocolate. However, it should also be borne in mind that the bioavailability of these and other non-haem sources of iron may not be high in adolescents who consume little fruit or fruit juice and hence have low intakes of vitamin C.

The main predictor of micronutrient adequacy in any diet is total energy intake: the more food that is eaten, the more likely it is that micronutrient needs will be met. The same applies to the diets of adolescents, even if they contain a high proportion of sugar-rich foods; dietary surveys show that total sugar intake is positively correlated with micronutrient intakes (Gibson 1993). The risk of micronutrient inadequacy on a diet containing a preponderance of high-fat, high-sugar, low-micronutrient density food choices therefore depends on total energy intake; if this is inadequate the likelihood of micronutrient insufficiency is also increased.

Dietary patterns in adolescents

Boys and girls appear to have different dietary patterns, although the findings from different surveys are not always consistent. In general, boys appear to prefer meat and dairy products, while girls are more likely to favour fruit, low-fat products and artificially sweetened drinks, perhaps through a desire to control body weight (Andersen *et al.* 1995).

As in adults, there are distinct regional differences in dietary intake, with young people living in Scotland consuming more high-fat foods and less fruit and vegetables than those in the south of England. This impacts nutritionally with lower intakes of fibre, retinol equivalents and riboflavin in Scottish children. Noticeable socioeconomic differences are also apparent, with adolescents from the least affluent groups having lower intakes of energy, fat, and most vitamins and minerals (Gregory *et al.* 2000).

Snacking or 'grazing' is a common pattern of eating in this age group, with most adolescents eating on at least six occasions during the day rather than the traditional three meals a day. This is not necessarily undesirable, since increasing eating frequency is acknowledged to be a useful way of meeting high energy needs. A 'grazing' pattern of eating has also been associated with leaner physiques and better blood lipid profiles (Drummond *et al.* 1996). However, much depends on the nature of the snacks which, among teenagers, are more likely to be comprised of crisps, biscuits, confectionery and carbonated drinks rather than fresh fruit, sandwiches or milk-based products (Gregory *et al.* 2000). Young people from lower socio-economic groups tend to derive a greater proportion of their daily energy intake from snacks than those from more advantaged groups, and this may have a nutritional impact if the snacks are of low nutrient density, particularly if breakfast is also omitted (Adamson *et al.* 1996).

Other surveys relating to the dietary intake and food habits of adolescents are summarized in Tables 3.6 and 3.7. When comparing and interpreting the results, it is important to bear in mind that selective under-reporting rather than dietary inadequacy can often be a reason for low reported intakes of energy and certain nutrients, particularly in girls or people who are overweight.

3.6.3 Promoting healthy eating in adolescents

Health is rarely top of the list when adolescents make food choices. Preference, taste, brand name, fashion and convenience are more likely to be the motivation factors unless there is a preoccupation with control of body weight. In an American survey, eating healthy food was the least valued option when compared with other health behaviours such as not using drugs or wearing seatbelts (Neumark-Sztainer *et al.* 1998).

This does not mean that health promotion is not worthwhile in adolescents. While a young person might not be concerned about their risk of disease in middle age, they are likely to want to have an acceptable body image and feel good about themselves. If these short-term gains can be addressed in the context of food, attention might be paid to attempts at nutrition education.

Another factor is control. Adolescents are at a stage where they are becoming empowered and taking more responsibility for themselves. Education which implies that adult authority figures 'know best', will not be well received. Education which involves the adolescent in a journey of discovery and justifies the dietary changes that are being recommended might be more successful.

Dietary adequacy

The UK dietary reference values (DRVs) (DH 1991) for adolescents are summarized in Appendix 6.2. For the active adolescent, a wide range of food intakes can be compatible with good health. The adolescent body is going through a period of rapid growth, and dietary energy sufficiency is a greater priority than dietary energy composition. Any concern about the ability of an adolescent's diet to meet micronutrient targets can be addressed by encouraging the consumption of a wide range of foods, particularly those which are fortified such as bread and breakfast cereals.

If the nutritional demands for growth in adolescence are accompanied by additional physiological demands as a result of pregnancy, lactation or intensive sports training, nutritional requirements can increase considerably. Intakes of iron, calcium, folate and zinc are major priorities in pregnancy, whereas strenuous sporting activity will require attention to energy, carbohydrate and iron intake. If these needs cannot (or will not) be met by dietary manipulations such as a greater consumption of nutrient-dense foods or a better balanced food choice, supplements should be considered.

Healthy eating messages

The purpose of modern dietary guidelines is not just to ensure adequate intakes of nutrients but to prevent chronic diseases that occur in later life such as cancer, coronary heart disease and stroke. For the population in general, reducing the intake of dietary fat, particularly saturated fat, is an important protective measure and, since raised blood lipids and pathological evidence of atherosclerosis are detectable in quite young children, it may be important that dietary protective measures commence sooner rather than later in life. However, it should not be overlooked that, in young people with high energy and nutrient needs, fat can be an important source of both

Table 3.6 Surveys of adolescent dietary behaviour

Authors	Date	Sample *n*	Age (years)	Method
Bull	1985	1015	15–18	14 day unweighed record
Department of Health	1989	1723	10–11	7 day weighed record
		974	14–15	
Irish Nutrition Survey	1990	207	12–14	Diet history
(Lee and Cunningham)		183	15–18	
McNeill *et al.*	1991	61	12	7 day weighed record
Adamson *et al.*	1992	379	11–12	6 day unweighed record
Crawley	1993	4760	16–17	4 day unweighed record
Southon *et al.*	1994	51	13–14	7 day weighed record
				7 day duplicate diet sample
Gregory *et al.*	2000	1700	4–18	7 day weighed record

Table 3.7 Average daily dietary intakes of adolescents in the UK and Ireland

Authors	Gender (age range, years)	Energy (MJ)	Protein (% energy)	CHO (% energy)	Fat (% energy)	Fe (mg)	Ca (mg)	B$_1$ (mg)	B$_2$ (mg)	B$_{12}$ (µg)	Niacin (mg)	Folate (µg)
Bull (1985)	M (15–25)	10.1	13	44	42	11.0	1000	1.16	1.91	5.98	34.3	153
	F (15–25)	7.8	13	43	43	8.5	885	0.9	1.51	4.63	26.1	125
Gregory et al. (2000)	M (10–11)	8.7	12	50	38	10.0	833	1.21	1.70		26.5	
	F (10–11)	7.7	12	50	38	8.6	702	1.03	1.40		23.1	
	M (14–15)	10.4	12	50	38	12.2	925	1.47	1.89		32.6	
	F (14–15)	7.8	12	49	39	9.3	692	1.04	1.32		24.0	
Irish Nutrition Survey (Lee and Cunningham 1990)	M (12–14)	11.3	13	50	37	14.7	1208	1.8	2.5	4.9	40.2	246
	F (12–14)	9.1	14	50	36	11.0	962	1.4	1.9	3.9	32.0	198
	M (15–18)	14.0	14	49[1]	36	19.3	1549	2.2	3.1	7.2	51.7	306
	F (15–18)	8.9	14	49	37	11.6	950	1.3	1.8	4.0	31.5	182
McNeill et al. (1991)	M	9.0	11	50	39	10.0	822	1.2	1.5	1.1	27	105
	F	8.1	11	49	40	10.0	767	1.0	1.4	1.0	24	90
Adamson et al. (1992): 1980	M (11–12)	8.9	12	49	39	10.0	850					
	F (11–12)	8.3	11	49	40	9.0	751					
1990	M (11–12)	8.6	12	49	39	12.0	786					
	F (11–12)	8.2	12	48	40	11.0	763					
Crawley (1993)	M (16–17)	11.4	12	47	41							
	F (16–17)	8.8	12	46	42							
Southon et al. (1994)	M	(9.5)[2]	13	52	35	(13.2)	899	(2.0)	(1.8)	4.0	32.4	(332)
	F	(7.4)	12	51	37	(9.8)	761	(1.5)	(1.2)	2.6	25.3	(252)

[1] Numbers do not add up to 100 owing to alcohol supplying 0.4% of energy.
[2] Numbers in parentheses denote a measured, rather than estimated, variable.

energy and essential fatty acids. While it is reasonable to discourage excessive reliance on concentrated sources of saturated fat, over-restriction of fat is not usually appropriate in this age group. Overzealous or restrictive dietary messages in respect of fat or sugar reduction may also inadvertently contribute to disordered eating patterns in some vulnerable individuals who already have concerns about their body image. It is more important to stress the importance of dietary variety and overall balance. *The Balance of Good Health* (HEA 1994) is a useful teaching model to show how individual preferences for particular foods can be fitted into a healthy diet, and to encourage greater consumption of starchy foods, milk and dairy products, and fruit and vegetables (see Section 1.2, Healthy eating).

It should also be borne in mind that healthy-eating messages are not the only, or necessarily the most important, way of promoting health in this age group. The rising prevalence of adverse health behaviours such as smoking and excessive consumption of alcohol by young people is a serious concern (Gregory *et al.* 2000) and it may be more important to tackle these issues. An American survey found that 60% teenagers were restricting their intake of fat and 57% were avoiding sugar, but suggested that a redirection of efforts towards reducing smoking and increasing physical activity might reap far greater health benefits (Neumark-Sztainer *et al.* 1998).

In the adolescent population, healthy-eating messages may have most benefit when targeted at those with adverse health behaviours. In a study of 16–17 year olds, those who smoked also consumed diets that were lower in thiamin, vitamin C and fibre than those of non-smokers (Crawley and While 1995). Eighteen-year-old male smokers have been found to consume diets relatively high in fat and low in iron (Andersen *et al.* 1995). Australian adolescents who smoked also had less satisfactory lipid profiles and took little physical activity (Milligan *et al.* 1997). It is in these groups that the lack of protective antioxidants from foods such as fruit and vegetables, and other dietary distortions resulting from inappropriate food choice, will have most impact on long-term health.

Influence of school on healthy eating

Although about 40% of all schoolchildren consume school lunches, teenagers increasingly opt for snack foods, packed lunches or, if allowed off the school site, to eat at cafés or obtain foods from sandwich bars or fast-food outlets. As a daily habit, this can result in diets of lower nutrient density, i.e. high in sugars but low in iron, calcium and vitamin C (Adamson *et al.* 1996).

While no control can be exercised over off-site food purchases, much can be done to improve the type and uptake of foods available on the school site. The provision of foods available in cash cafeterias (the most common form of food service in secondary schools) can often be improved in terms of the choice and price of food on offer. Much can also be done to encourage pupils to make appropriate food choices. School Nutrition Action Groups (SNAGs)

(Harvey and Passmore 1994), have been widely acknowledged as a way of developing school food policies and influencing the food choice of pupils. The aims of a SNAG are to:

- provide a health-promoting environment in the school
- involve the pupils
- establish, monitor and evaluate a school food policy
- help children and staff to make improved choices about food.

A SNAG will adopt a whole-day, whole-school approach to nutrition, covering aspects such as the provision of breakfast, tuckshops, school meals, packed lunches and vending machines. Dietitians may be invited to attend SNAG meetings along with senior teaching staff, pupils, parents, caterers and school nurses. The composition and mode of operation will depend on the local circumstances, but SNAGs should be owned and managed at school level.

3.6.4 Common dietary problems in teenagers and young adults

Obesity

Adipose stores increase rapidly in adolescence, so it is no surprise that this stage of life is one of the key points for the development of obesity. During puberty, girls deposit adipose tissue at a greater rate than boys, laying down stores in the breast and hip regions. Fat deposition in boys tends to be more central. This physiological accumulation of adipose tissue should not, in itself, result in obesity but, when combined with energy-dense diets and a lack of physical activity, the likelihood of obesity increases. Excessive body fat, particularly in the truncal region, markedly increases health risks in later life. Adolescent obesity can also predispose to gall stones, sleep apnoea and asthma but, most crucially for the teenager, social development can be hindered as a result of bullying, victimization and exclusion.

Physical inactivity tends to increase during adolescence as self-consciousness about body image, or a preference for television or video games, supplants the desire for sporting activities. A Norwegian study of adolescents found that only 34% of boys and 21% of girls exercised regularly (Andersen *et al.* 1995). In the UK, Gregory *et al.* (2000) found that 15–18-year-old girls were the least active of all the 4–18 year olds studied.

'At-risk' adolescents can be tracked using percentiles for body mass index (BMI) or skinfold thickness. BMI centile charts for use in boys and girls from birth to 20 years have been produced by the Child Growth Foundation (see Section 1.8.7 in Assessment of nutritional status). BMI above the 91st percentile is indicative of overweight requiring intervention. However, it should be borne in mind that full height may not have been reached and the overweight may not persist into adulthood. In older adolescents, waist circumference is a useful way of estimating truncal fat stores.

Inappropriate slimming

Research shows that the proportion of children who are concerned about their body image and adopting self-imposed slimming measures is rising and increases with age. This trend is far more marked in girls than in boys, the latter usually being more concerned that they are not muscular enough. The Minnesota Adolescent Health Survey of 30 000 teenagers revealed that 12% girls were dieting, 30% binge eating, 12% vomiting and 2% using laxatives or diuretics (Neumark-Sztainer *et al.* 1998). In the UK, 16% of 15–18-year-old girls (and 3% of the boys) said that they were dieting to lose weight (Gregory *et al.* 2000).

Unsupervised and unnecessary slimming can result in low micronutrient intakes as 'the diet' often involves missing meals, particularly breakfast. Body image can be improved by encouraging physical activity, but care must be taken when discussing diet with girls who are concerned about their weight in case an overfocus on food encourages a drift towards an eating disorder. Emphasis on variety and balance rather than restriction or 'good versus bad foods' is important.

Eating disorders

Sometimes a concern about body image does end up being more serious. Adolescence is the peak age of onset of eating disorders such as anorexia nervosa and bulimia nervosa, the former condition being the most common, affecting 3% of children. Bulimia is rare in children but may affect as many as 1% late adolescent and young adult women (Shaw and Lawson 1994). In many cases, the eating disorder is short lived or incomplete, e.g. use of obsessive exercise without the other signs. Peer pressure, academic concerns and emotional stresses are likely catalysts. More persistent cases require specialist psychiatric and dietetic management as the resulting long-term energy depletion can have lasting effects on growth, sexual development and peak bone mass (see Section 4.19, Eating disorders).

Vegetarianism

Adolescence is a period of experimentation with new ideas, and diet is no exception. Many young people try special diets such as vegetarian, vegan or macrobiotic regimens. In the NDNS, 10% of 15–18-year-old girls stated that they were either vegetarian or vegan (but only 1% boys of the same age) (Gregory *et al.* 2000). This is not a problem in itself but, if the diets are poorly planned and imbalanced, the result can be an inadequate intake of some micronutrients. Common pitfalls are failure to consume foods which sufficiently compensate for the loss of haem iron from the diet and, in the vegan diet, alternative sources of protein and vitamin B_{12} (see Section 3.10, Vegetarianism and veganism).

Alcohol

Most adolescents will try alcohol at some point. A 1995 survey by the Health Education Authority (Turtle *et al.* 1997) found that 74% of 11 year olds and 96% of 15 year olds had consumed alcohol. There is also evidence that both the prevalence and level of alcohol consumption have increased markedly in this age group. Between 1990 and 1996, the average alcohol consumption of 11–15 year olds had more than doubled, rising from 0.8 units to 1.8 units per week (ONS 1997).

High alcohol intakes are a cause for concern for both health and social reasons. Young people have less ability to metabolize alcohol than fully mature adults and are more susceptible to its adverse effects. As in adults, excessive alcohol consumption is associated with an increased risk of accidents and death (DH 1993). From a nutritional point of view, regular alcohol consumption can displace more nutrient-dense foods from the diet and, since alcohol has a high energy density but little impact on appetite, regular drinking can easily lead to overconsumption of energy.

Health advice on alcohol should not be too negative in tone or it will simply be ignored. It is more productive to ensure that young people are aware of safe drinking limits and know how to assess the alcoholic strength of products, particularly some of the recently marketed 'designer drinks' or special brews of lagers which may have a deceptively high alcohol content (see Section 1.2.4, Sensible use of alcohol).

Text revised by: Diane Talbot, Helen Storer, Carrie Ruxton and Briony Thomas

Further reading

British Paediatric Association/ Royal College of Physicians. *Alcohol and the Young.* London: BPA/RCP, 1995.

References

Adamson AJ, Rugg-Gunn AJ, Appleton DR *et al*. Dietary sources of energy, protein, unavailable carbohydrate and fat in 11–12-year-old English children in 1990 compared with results in 1980. *Journal of Human Nutrition and Dietetics* 1992; **5**: 371–385.

Adamson AJ, Rugg-Gunn AJ, Butler TJ, Appleton DR. The contribution of foods from outside the home to the nutrient intake of young adolescents. *Journal of Human Nutrition and Dietetics* 1996; **9**: 55–68.

Andersen LF, Nes M, Sandstad B *et al*. Dietary intake among Norwegian adolescents. *European Journal of Clinical Nutrition* 1995; **49**: 555–564.

Bull N. Dietary habits of 15–25 year olds. *Human Nutrition: Applied Nutrition* 1985; **39A** (Suppl 1): 1–68.

Crawley H. The energy, nutrient and food intakes of teenagers aged 16–17 years in Britain. *British Journal of Nutrition* 1993; **70**: 15–26.

Crawley H, While D. The diet and body weight of British teenage smokers at 16–17 years. *European Journal of Clinical Nutrition* 1995; **49**: 904–914.

Department of Health. *Diets of British Schoolchildren*. London: HMSO, 1989.

Department of Health. *Dietary Reference Values for Food Energy and Nutrients for the United Kingdom*. London: HMSO, 1991.

Department of Health. *Health of the Nation: Key Area Handbook*. London: DH, 1993.

Drummond S, Crombie N, Kirk T. A critique of the effects of snacking on body weight status. *European Journal of Clinical Nutrition* 1996; **50**: 779–783.

Gibson SA. Consumption and sources of sugars in the diets of British schoolchildren: are high-sugar diets inferior? *Journal of Human Nutrition and Dietetics* 1993; **6**: 355–371.

Gregory J et al. *National Diet and Nutrition Survey: Young People Aged 4–18 Years*. Vol. 1: *Findings*. London: The Stationery Office, 2000.

Harvey J, Passmore S. *School Nutrition Action Groups: A New Policy for Managing Food and Nutrition in Schools*. Birmingham: Health Education Unit, 1994.

Health Education Authority. *The Balance Of Good Health*. London: HEA, 1994.

Lee P, Cunningham K. *Irish National Nutrition Survey*. Irish Nutrition and Dietetic Institute, 1990.

McNeill G, Davidson L, Morrison DC, *et al*. Nutrient intake in schoolchildren: some practical considerations. *Proceedings of the Nutrition Society* 1991; **50**: 37–43.

Milligan RA, Burke V, Dunbar DL *et al*. Associations between lifestyle and cardiovascular risk factors in 18 year old Australians. *Journal of Adolescent Health* 1997; **21**: 186–195.

Neumark-Sztainer D, Story M, Resnick M, Blum R. Lessons learnt about adolescent nutrition from the Minnesota Adolescent Health Survey. *Journal of the American Dietetic Association* 1998; **98**: 1449–1456.

Office of National Statistics (ONS), Social Survey Division. *Young Teenagers and Alcohol in 1996*. Vol. 1: *England*. London: The Stationery Office, 1997.

Shaw V, Lawson M (Eds). *Clinical Paediatric Dietetics*. Oxford: Blackwell Science, 1994.

Southon S, Wright AJA, Finglas PM, *et al*. Dietary intake and macronutrient status of adolescents: effect of vitamin and trace element supplements on indices of status and performance in tests of verbal and non-verbal intelligence. *British Journal of Nutrition* 1994; **71**: 887–918.

Turtle J, Jones A, Hickman M. *Young People and Health. The Health Behaviour of School-aged children*. London: HEA, 1997.

3.7 Older adults

The greatest challenge in the twenty-first century will be to improve the quality of life as we all age. Health is the most important prerequisite for people to enjoy life, especially in their older years (Brundtland 1998).

3.7.1 Number and proportion of older people

Deciding when someone is old is arbitrary. The World Health Organization uses chronological age, classifying people aged 45–59 years as 'middle aged', 60–74 years as 'elderly', 75–89 years as 'old' and 90+ years as 'very old'. In the UK, the normal retirement age of 65 years is generally accepted when describing someone as 'elderly'. This may be further divided into age bands of 65–74 years, 75–85 years and over 85 years.

One of the main features of the world population in the twentieth century was the considerable increase in the absolute and relative number of older people in both developed and developing countries. This phenomenon is referred to as 'population ageing'. At present there are approximately 580 million elderly people (60 years and over) in the world, of whom 355 million live in developing countries. By 2020 this number will have increased to over 1000 million worldwide.

In Europe 20% of the population are elderly (over 60 years), but by 2020 this is expected to have risen to 25%.

In 1994, 16% of the UK population (representing 9 million people) were over the retirement age of 65 years. By 2031 this will have increased to 23% of the population. The greatest percentage increase will be in the over 85-year-old age group which will nearly double, meaning that over 10% of the total population will be aged over 75 years. It is estimated that by 2031 there will be 36 000 centenarians (people aged 100 years and over) compared with just 300 in 1951.

In recent years the number of older people living in nursing and residential care homes has increased in absolute terms but the percentage remains at about 5%. Most older people live in the community, in their own homes (either alone or with a partner) or with other family members, and either with or without formal paid support.

Implications of this demographic shift

This demographic shift has important implications for health planners and the general population. As the proportion of older people and, more significantly, the number of very old people increases, new demands will be made on health and welfare (social) services with economic and structural implications for the government and national policy. Several initiatives, including the Millennium Debate of the Age co-ordinated by Age Concern and the Royal Commission on the Long Term Care of Older People (1999), demonstrate that this matter is being acknowledged, although no obvious answers have yet materialized. The Royal Commission recommended, for example, that more care be given to people in their own homes, and that the costs of care for those individuals who need it should be split among living costs, housing costs and personal care. On funding they recommended that, as a first step, the government should ascertain precisely how much money, whether from National Health Service (NHS), local authority social services and housing budgets, or from social security budgets, goes to supporting older people in residential settings and in people's own homes.

Consideration also has to be given to meeting the health needs of an ageing population who are more likely to develop chronic debilitating diseases such as diabetes, heart disease, stroke and dementia. Other problems such as hearing loss and visual impairment also increase dramatically with age.

Services available in the community

A range of health and social services is available in the community for vulnerable older individuals to assist them to maintain their independence and live in their own home for as long as possible (Table 3.8). These may involve local government, statutory bodies, the private sector or voluntary organizations. Their availability varies considerably across the UK, both between and within counties and between rural and urban areas. General practitioners (GPs) or local social services are often the access route for many of these provisions. The vast majority of help and support is still provided by family and friends.

3.7.2 Nutritional aspects of ageing

Ageing is a normal process involving a range of biochemical and physiological changes in all parts of the body (Table 3.9). The rate of decay for a specific organ or tissue varies between individuals. Webb and Copeman (1996) identify four issues that are of particular importance to the general nutrition of older people:

- fluid balance and renal function
- skeletal changes

Table 3.8 Services available to support older people living in the community

Local community services	Luncheon clubs
	Community centres
	Day centres
	Cultural/religious activities
	Cookery classes
Services within the home	Community meals (meals on wheels)
	Cleaning
	Home care assistance with activities of daily living
	Bath nurse
	Laundry service
Shopping services	'Dial a ride' – for a free ride to the shops
	Access bus – meeting the needs of people with restricted mobility
	Telephone shopping
Local support groups	Alzheimer's Disease Society
	Carers Association
	CRUSE
	Stroke Association
After discharge from hospital	24 hour home-care packages
	'Hospital at home' Rapid response multidisciplinary team assessment and treatment in an emergency

Table 3.9 Changes in the body as part of the ageing process (Based on Copeman and Hyland 1999)

Part of body	Changes produced by ageing
Skin	Wrinkling
	Loss of hair
	Reduced function of sweat and sebaceous glands
Heart	Loss of heart muscle
	Increased fibrous tissue
	Decreased cardiac output
Renal function	20–30% decrease in weight and volume affecting nephrons and resulting in decreased filtration rate and increased glucose threshold
Bone	Increased resorption
Immune system	Impaired T-cell function and hence greater susceptibility to viral infections
Small and large intestine	Decreased motor function and muscle tone
	Impaired digestive capacity
	Diverticula
Muscle	Loss of tension
	Atrophy, especially in lower body
Hearing	Elevated sound threshold
	Loss of perception of high frequencies
Pain and touch	Touch and pain thresholds increase
Taste and smell	Decreased number of taste buds
	High taste threshold (loss of taste sensitivity)
	Reduced number of nasal sensory cells
Vision	Diminished colour fidelity
	Decreased visual acuity
Height	Reduced
Homoeostatic regulation	Reduced
Whole body composition	Proportion of fat increases
	Lean body mass decreases

- physical fitness and strength
- changes in the immune system.

Gariballa and Sinclair, in their review of nutrition, ageing and ill health, also highlight changes in the gastrointestinal tract (1998). These range from a decrease in the number of taste buds in the mouth to decreased motor function and muscle tone in the intestine. Some of these changes jointly act to cause 'anorexia of ageing', where a person's appetite and intake are reduced.

3.7.3 Food choice and food selection

Food plays many roles apart from the biological function to alleviate hunger. Social, psychological and economic influences can play a significant part in determining whether food is actually consumed.

Webb (1995) developed a framework for food selection to explain how different factors act in a hierarchical way to influence food choice and consumption:

1 The first requirement is for *food to be physically available*, thus the development of large supermarkets and the closure of small local shops will restrict food choice if someone does not have a car or is unable to travel by public transport with heavy shopping.
2 *Economic availability* is the next requirement. As many older people are on a limited budget, even if the food is physically available they may not be able to afford it. Larger supermarkets tend to cater for the family and buying for one or two people is more expensive per head. Larger bargain packs are not helpful if the food item deteriorates before it is eaten, or if the individual cannot afford the initial outlay.
3 The third stage is *cultural availability*. Some individuals will have restrictions related to religious belief but many other people have cultural habits that influence the acceptance of a particular food.
4 *The gatekeeper – the person who purchases and brings food into the house*, traditionally the woman, has a powerful impact on the food available. When people are living in residential care or need others to purchase food on their behalf, they lose this control.
5 The final part of the framework is *personal choice*, which can affect the availability of food that has overcome the earlier barriers in the hierarchy.

Some of the factors which influence food choice and eating patterns are listed in Table 3.10. Many are associated with previous experience, current living conditions or state of health. The actual dietary intake may be less if, for example, appetite is reduced.

3.7.4 Nutritional status and eating habits of older people

Between October 1994 and September 1995, a large survey was undertaken to determine the eating habits and nutrition of people aged 65 years and older in the UK (Finch *et al.* 1998; Steele *et al.* 1998). This was part of the

Table 3.10 Factors affecting food choice, eating patterns and dietary intake

Previous experience	Current living conditions	State of health
Budgeting skills	Availability of food	Confusion
Cultural traditions	Cooking ability	Constipation
Education	Cooking facilities	Depression
Habit	Cooking for self and/or others	Drug side-effects
Individual likes and dislikes	Cost of food items	Dysphagia
Nutrition knowledge	Eating alone or with others	Loss of taste, smell and thirst
Previous food experience	Living conditions	Physical illness
Religious belief	Time available	Poor dentition
Willingness to experiment		

MAFF/DH planned programme of National Diet and Nutrition Surveys (NDNS) covering representative samples of defined age groups.

Two nationally representative samples were drawn from adults aged 65 years and over, one sample comprised of free-living individuals and the other of individuals living in institutions. Detailed measurements of food and nutrient intakes, dental and oral health, heights, weights and blood pressure were obtained from nearly 1700 people. The main findings were:

- For people not in institutions, those with lower socio-economic status had significantly lower average intakes of energy, protein, carbohydrates, fibre, some vitamins, notably vitamin C and minerals.
- The better their oral health, including how many natural teeth they had, the better their diet and nutritional status.
- The oral health of older adults living in an institutional environment was poor compared with their free-living counterparts. Poor oral hygiene and root decay were particularly prevalent.
- The presence of root decay showed a strong relationship with the frequency of intake of foods containing high levels of sugar, independent of age, gender, social class and region of origin.
- People who were not in institutions were heavier than people of this age 30 years earlier, but their recorded food energy intakes were lower.
- Taken as a group, people met COMA (Committee on Medical Aspects of Food Policy) recommendations for total fat intakes as opposed to the national adult average, but ate too much saturated fat and non-milk extrinsic sugars, and too little fibre.
- For each of the vitamins and minerals, biochemical status as measured by blood levels was generally adequate for most participants.
- Vitamin D status was poor in some people, particularly those living in institutions and particularly in the winter months.
- Folate status was poor in a significant proportion of this age group, particularly among those who were older, i.e. over 85 years.
- In the context of security of household food stocks, 90% of people not in institutions had in their home seven or more items from a list of ten staple items.

- 86% of free-living individuals visited the shops to do their food shopping, although 55% said that their food shopping was sometimes done by someone else.
- Of those living in their own houses 53% had milk delivered.
- A traditional diet was common, especially in older people and those living in institutions. The foods and drinks most commonly consumed included tea, boiled, mashed or baked potatoes, white bread and biscuits.
- People living in institutions were more likely to consume sugar, preserves, buns, cakes and pastries, and cereal-based milk puddings.
- One in three free-living individuals reported that they took non-prescribed dietary supplements, the most common being cod liver oil (60% of supplement users).

3.7.5 General nutritional considerations

The Working Party on the Nutrition of Elderly People (DH 1992) recommended that the majority of people aged 65 years or more should adopt, where possible, similar patterns of eating and lifestyle to those advised for maintaining health in younger adults. The recommendations of the COMA Panel on Dietary Reference Values (DH 1991) are endorsed for well elderly people. However, an area of particular concern is the impact of acute or chronic illness and disability in this population group on nutritional status, which can be rapidly compromised as a result of low body weight and reduced nutrient intake. There needs to be greater awareness of the importance of good nutrition for maintaining the health of elderly people and its contribution to recovery from illness, and more use of appropriate practical guidance.

Elderly people can be considered to have an elevated risk of specific nutrient deficiencies but caution must be exercised because of the great diversity of this population group. The distribution of nutrient requirements is not necessarily symmetrical [as is assumed to be the case in the calculation of dietary reference values (DRVs)] and, in an elderly population, may well be skewed. A low intake will not always be a deficient one, owing to variations in individual requirements or adaptation. Conversely, some nutrient intakes may seem adequate compared with reference nutrient intakes (RNIs), but may be inadequate for those individuals with extra requirements due to short-term trauma, or as a result of long-term changes.

In order to maintain good nutritional status, it is recommended (DH 1992) that elderly people should:

- consume a diet containing a variety of nutrient-dense foods
- maintain an active lifestyle, with prompt resumption after episodes of intercurrent illness
- follow the same recommendations concerning dietary intake of non-milk extrinsic sugars as applied to the younger adult population
- have an intake of non-starch polysaccharide comparable to that recommended for the general population
- increase dietary intake of vitamin C; in those dependent on institutional catering, measures should be taken to ensure vitamin C intake is optimal
- be advised to eat more fresh vegetables, fruit and wholemeal cereals
- be encouraged to consume oily fish and fats fortified with vitamins A and D
- have doorstep milk deliveries if available (to encourage milk consumption)
- expose some skin to sunlight regularly during May to September (DH 1998)
- if exposure to sunlight is not possible, vitamin D supplementation should be considered, particularly during the winter and early spring (DH 1998)
- have nutritional status assessed as a routine aspect of history taking and clinical examination, when admitted to hospital.

Good nutrition contributes to the health of elderly people and to their ability to recover from illness. Focus on nutrition is becoming increasingly important. Ultimately, it may lessen the burden of health costs by enabling elderly people to remain independent for as long as possible, and improve the overall quality of life.

Nutritionally, it is important to consider elderly people according to biological and not chronological age. As their dependence increases, so the nutritional status of elderly people in the UK declines (Beales *et al.* 1998).

Energy

The consumption of sufficient energy to maintain satisfactory body weight is important. Recommendations for dietary energy intakes of elderly people should be generous, except for those who are obese. The decline in estimated average energy requirements with age is relatively small (Table 3.11).

Table 3.11 Changes in energy requirements with age (Based on DH 1991)

Age band (years)	Men (kcal/day)	Women (kcal/day)
51–59	2550	1900
60–64	2380	1900
65–74	2330	1900
≥75	2100	1810

Calcium and vitamin D

In older people, intake of calcium and vitamin D (together with sunlight exposure) is an important consideration in order to maintain bone health. Osteoporosis and the fractures resulting from it are a major cause of morbidity and mortality in elderly people. In people aged over 50 years, osteoporosis is a contributory factor in at least 85% of fractures at all sites, most of which occur in the wrist, spine or hip. Hip fractures dominate any assessment of mortality, disability and health-care costs, but there are real and significant consequences of all osteoporotic fractures. Dietary and lifestyle measures which help to prevent bone loss are therefore important (see Section 4.31, Osteoporosis).

The COMA report on *Nutrition and Bone Health* (DH 1998) recommends that the RNI for calcium for adults (including older adults) should continue to be 700 mg/day, which can be obtained by daily intake of milk and milk-based foods, white (fortified) flour products and vegetables.

For vitamin D, the COMA recommendation from the age of 65 years is an RNI of 10 μg/day. Older people are particularly susceptible to vitamin D deficiency because they have a reduced efficiency of vitamin synthesis in the skin and also tend to have less sunlight exposure than younger groups (as a result of rarely going out of doors or, when they do, being well covered up). In addition, dietary intake of vitamin D from sources such as oily fish may be poor, particularly in those living in institutions (Finch *et al.* 1998). Supplementation with vitamin D is therefore usually needed to achieve the recommended intake of 10 μg/day, particularly during the winter months.

The influence of factors such as body weight and physical activity should also not be overlooked. Being underweight increases osteoporotic risk, while being overweight can impair mobility and increase the risk of falls. Taking weight-bearing exercise is of major importance in helping to preserve bone mass. As people reach retirement age, they should be discouraged from a sedentary lifestyle and made aware of the many health benefits from regular physical activity. Those of more advanced years should be encouraged to remain as active as possible (see Physical activity, below).

Vitamin C

Although there is no evidence that the RNI of 40 mg vitamin C/day for adults needs to be higher for elderly populations, consumption of fruit and vegetables by this group may not be sufficient to achieve this level of intake, especially in those who are frail and institutionalized or who have poor appetites. Fortified drinks and vitamin C supplements may be necessary to ensure adequate intake.

Supplementation should not be at a level which greatly exceeds the RNI. Although the role of vitamin C in connective tissue growth and wound healing is well recognized, excessive doses are not associated with better healing of pressure sores and leg ulcers and may have some disadvantages (see Section 5.8, Wound healing and tissue viability).

Folate

Institutionalized elderly people, particularly those who are frail, disabled or have dementia, may be at risk of folate deficiency as a result of overcooked food and a poor dietary intake.

Vitamin B$_{12}$

Although Vitamin B$_{12}$ deficiency anaemia is usually caused by a failure of absorption, and less commonly due to a dietary deficiency, higher intakes may be beneficial for older people. The vitamin B$_{12}$ intakes of older people who are vegans or strict vegetarians, or with conditions such as gastric atrophy, hypochlorhydria/achlorhydria or Crohn's disease, or who have had a gastrectomy require particular consideration (Finch *et al*. 1998).

Iron

Although elderly people (especially women) may require less iron to maintain iron status than when they were younger, they also have a higher prevalence of disorders which interfere with efficient iron absorption, thus reducing dietary iron bioavailability. Iron losses may also be increased as a result of occult gastrointestinal blood loss (a common cause of anaemia in this age group). It is therefore important that a good dietary iron intake is maintained, together with sufficient vitamin C to promote non-haem iron absorption. If people cannot consume or, in institutions, are not offered adequate amounts of a sufficiently varied diet, iron requirements may not be met.

Zinc

Zinc is necessary for tissue repair and wound healing may be delayed in the presence of overt zinc deficiency. Decreased taste acuity in anorexic elderly subjects has also been associated with zinc deficiency (Goode *et al*. 1991).

Physical activity

At all ages, an active lifestyle has many health benefits. Weight-bearing exercise promotes bone health and all types of physical activity contribute to energy expenditure (which is generally desirable), promote cardiovascular health and mental well-being.

In older people, even modest amounts of daily physical activity such as walking at a normal pace may increase appetite (thus helping to prevent nutritional inadequacies), improve balance and muscle co-ordination (lessening the likelihood of falls and fractures) and increase lean body mass (Bassey 1985; Fiatanon *et al*. 1994). For those who can safely cope with greater levels of weight-bearing exercise such as walking briskly, stair climbing or recreational activities such as dancing, the benefits may be much greater.

Fluid and hydration

The risk of dehydration is much more common in older people for a number of reasons:

- With ageing the skin becomes thinner and therefore more water is lost via this route.
- The kidney is not able to concentrate urine to the same degree because both renal plasma flow and glomerular filtration rate decline with age.
- The thirst mechanism is not as sensitive, so older people may not feel thirsty.

Some common causes of dehydration in older people are summarized in Table 3.12.

The effects of dehydration on older people can include:

- loss of skin elasticity
- increased risk of pressure-sore development
- unpleasant taste in the mouth
- drowsiness
- confusion
- constipation
- urinary tract infection
- electrolyte imbalance
- altered cardiac function.

Effects of dehydration such as drowsiness or confusion may further impair thirst perception and so compound the problem. Severe dehydration is a particular risk in elderly people who are unable to procure or request fluids as a result of disability or mental impairment. A fluid loss of 20% can be fatal.

About 10% of older people admitted to community hospitals suffer from clinical dehydration, and as many as 25%

Table 3.12 Common causes of dehydration in older people (Based on Copeman and Hyland 1999)

Pathological causes	Effects of ageing	Iatrogenic causes
Pyrexia	Increased skin losses	Drugs such as diuretics
Renal failure	Reduced total body water	Institutionalization
Immobility	Reduced renal function	Fluid restriction
Confusion	Altered thirst perception	Urinary incontinence
Drowsiness		
Depression		

of immobile elderly patients suffer from mild chronic dehydration (Rolls and Phillips 1990). Restoration of normal hydration, even if it is achieved via a nasogastric tube regimen or peripheral/ subcutaneous fluids, will increase the sense of well-being and comfort.

In order to prevent chronic dehydration, the provision of adequate fluids must be made a priority in the care of older people and the most appropriate drinking vessel used. A daily intake of about 1500–2000 ml is necessary. A suggested fluid regimen of 1500 ml (6–8 cups/day) for an older person is outlined in Table 3.13. Additional fluid will normally also be obtained from food items such as gravy, custard, ice-cream and milk puddings.

3.7.6 Maintaining function in chronic illness

Although the types of disease which occur in older people are in many instances no different to those which occur at younger ages, the presentation of disease in older people is often more obscure and its management more complex. Older people may delay consulting a doctor because they dismiss symptoms as simply being due to 'old age', are reluctant to 'bother the doctor', may not appreciate the benefits to be gained from modern treatments or may think that doctors may be less willing to help older people.

Older people may present in an apparently non-specific manner which can be summarized by the acronym IF OLD:

- incontinence
- falls
- off Legs (immobility)
- delirium (acute confusional state).

However, among these factors underlying presentations may include:

- the presence of multiple impairments often requiring rehabilitation
- multiple medical problems
- polypharmacy

Table 3.13 A suggested 1500 ml fluid intake regimen for an older person

Time of day	Beverage	Volume (ml)
Early morning	Tea	150
Breakfast	Fruit juice	100
	Tea/coffee	150
Midmorning	Tea/coffee/milky drink	150–200
Midday meal	Soup/water	200
	Tea/coffee after meal	150
Afternoon	Tea	150–200
Evening meal	Tea/coffee with meal	150
Supper/evening drink[1]	Tea	150
Bedtime drink	Milky drink	150
	TOTAL	1500–1600 ml/day

[1]Often omitted to reduce night time micturition

- sensory or cognitive impairment leading to an inability to remember or recount an accurate history
- complications of disease.

Many chronic illnesses have nutritional implications either because food intake is changed (e.g. appetite is reduced) or because nutrient and energy requirements are altered. These problems can be caused by physical, physiological or emotional factors (Table 3.14).

Prompt identification of these factors and suggesting practical measures to offset their effect on food intake are important. Practical difficulties such as not being able to use a tin opener, lift a saucepan or grip ordinary cutlery may be overcome by specially adapted cutlery and other aids to assist in food preparation. Dietary measures to help

Table 3.14 Effects of chronic illness on the nutrition of older people (Based on Copeman and Hyland 1999)

Problem	Possible causes
No interest in food	Poor appetite
	Anorexia
	Nausea
	Depression
	Altered or impaired sense of taste and smell
	Side-effect of radiotherapy
	Side-effect of chemotherapy
	Cachexia
Inability to place food in mouth	Unable to use cutlery
	Unable to unwrap food
	Reduced manual dexterity
	Poor hand–mouth co-ordination
	Stroke, rheumatoid arthritis, Osteoarthritis
Oral problems	Sore mouth
	Dry mouth
	Mouth infection
	Ill-fitting dentures
	Inability to chew
	Inability to move food round mouth
	Lack of saliva
Swallowing difficulties	Delayed swallow
	Poor posture
	Oesophageal stricture
	Physical abnormality
	Parkinson's disease, stroke
Indigestion	Hiatus hernia
	Poor posture
	Gastric ulcer
	Rapid ingestion of food
	Achlorhydria
Malabsorption	Drug interaction
	Bacterial overgrowth
	Coeliac disease
	Pancreatic insufficiency
	Food intolerance
Constipation	Low fibre intake
	Reduced mobility
	Low fluid intake
	Reduced peristaltic action
Incontinence	Bladder dysfunction
	Infection

to alleviate problems such as dry or sore mouth, nausea, anorexia or other factors compromising food intake, often resulting from drug side-effects, can be suggested (see Section 1.12.2 in Oral nutritional support). People whose food intake is markedly affected by depression, anxiety and other psychological problems may need to be referred for expert help.

It should also be borne in mind that drug–nutrient interactions can affect vitamin and mineral status and are likely to have most impact in the nutritionally compromised elderly person (see Section 2.12, Drug–nutrient interactions).

3.7.7 Malnutrition

Types of malnutrition

Several types of malnutrition can be found in elderly people, and these can either be distinct entities or occur simultaneously. Davies (1988) has identified four which require diagnosis and appropriate intervention:

- *specific*: deficiency of a particular nutrient or a nutrition-related disease such as scurvy, pellagra or osteomalacia;
- *long-standing*: the clinical appearance of energy and nutrient deficiencies after a period of inadequate eating, often linked with general neglect;
- *sudden*: results from a sudden marked change in food intake, often following a significant disruptive life event such as a major fall or a bereavement;
- *recurrent*: typified by the older person with a barely adequate nutritional status who, following a period of illness, can enter a cycle of poor nutrition and repeated episodes of illness.

Consequences of malnutrition

The consequences of malnutrition can be profound. Weight loss with muscle wasting and loss of subcutaneous fat has many physical effects such as decreased muscle strength, mobility and immune function. Psychological effects such as depression, apathy, fatigue, weakness, anorexia and anxiety can also occur, even when their appearance is not significantly abnormal. These effects are discussed in detail in Section 1.11 (Undernutrition).

In older people, the effects of malnutrition can include:

- *increased liability to heart failure* as a result of muscle wasting occurring in the heart and hence compounding the decline in cardiac function which occurs as part of the ageing process;
- *increased risk of pneumonia and other respiratory tract infections* because the weakened muscles of the respiratory system mean that the ability to cough effectively is reduced;
- *increased risk of thromboembolism* as a result of immobility;
- *increased risk of pressure sores* due to loss of protective subcutaneous fat and increased immobility;

- *increased risk of infection* due to depressed cellular immunity, exacerbated by the normal decline in immune competence with age.

As a result, the malnourished older person is likely to have a greater risk of mortality, a reduced rate of healing, increased morbidity, a protracted rehabilitation and a longer stay in hospital.

Causes of malnutrition in institutions

Table 3.15 gives some examples of individual or institutional factors that may lead to malnutrition, but it is not an exhaustive list. It is important that the specific causes of malnutrition in a particular individual are identified and relevant action is taken.

3.7.8 Nutritional interventions

When considering the nutrition of vulnerable older people, it is essential to remember that an informal carer, a relative or friend will often give most of the practical care. An important role of the health-care professional is to provide appropriate information and support to carers so that they have both the knowledge and confidence to provide the correct type and level of care, and also know how, when and where to refer to 'the professional'.

Choosing the appropriate intervention

A systematic approach should be adopted when considering the appropriate action for someone who has been identified as nutritionally vulnerable. The NAGE publica-

Table 3.15 Some causes of malnutrition among older people in institutions

Individual factors	Institutional factors
Illness, disease process	Inadequate staff to assist patients with eating
Anorexia due to illness or treatment, or in response to hospitalization	Staff breaks coincide with meal times
Swallowing difficulty, ill-fitting dentures	Medical ward rounds over lunch time
Physical problems with eating, e.g. cannot hold fork due to arthritis or stroke	Poorly served food, poor nutritional content
Food is unfamiliar or unappetizing	Food served at wrong temperature, kept warm for long periods
Confused or forgetful	Lack of patient choice
Lack of mobility	Lack of facilities for able-bodied patients to make a drink or snack
Afraid to ask for assistance, or feel they may be bothering the busy staff	Lack of storage for patient's own food
	Medical investigations require fasting or absence at meal times
	Inappropriate meal times with long gaps when no food or fluid is offered
	Money dictates food provided

tion *Taking Steps to Tackle Eating Problems – A Handbook and Poster for those who Care for Older People* (1994) provides practical suggestions for tackling the key nutritional issues in older people (Fig. 3.1).

The factors affecting nutritional status of older people can be broadly categorized into three areas:

- *intrinsic factors*: naturally occurring ageing processes that affect nutritional status
- *pathological factors*: disease status that may directly or indirectly affect nutritional status
- *extrinsic factors*: environment, alcohol, dependency, social isolation and drugs.

Ideally, every older person should be considered individually to ensure that their nutrition is optimal and any relevant nutritional risk factor recognized and tackled.

Davies and Knutson (1991) have developed a grid system to help with the identification of elderly people at risk of poor nutritional intake (Fig. 3.2). Using the grid helps to identify known risk factors. These are factors or circumstances that are known to increase the risk of malnutrition and include living alone and not having regular cooked meals. In themselves they are not indicators of the presence of malnutrition, but when warning signals occur (*y*-axis on the grid), if the situation is left unchecked without early intervention, the client is likely to develop malnutrition. The warning signals are interrelated and cumulative, so that each one must be evaluated in relation to the others.

Screening is the process of identifying older people who are already malnourished, or at risk of becoming so. One example for use in day hospitals and community settings

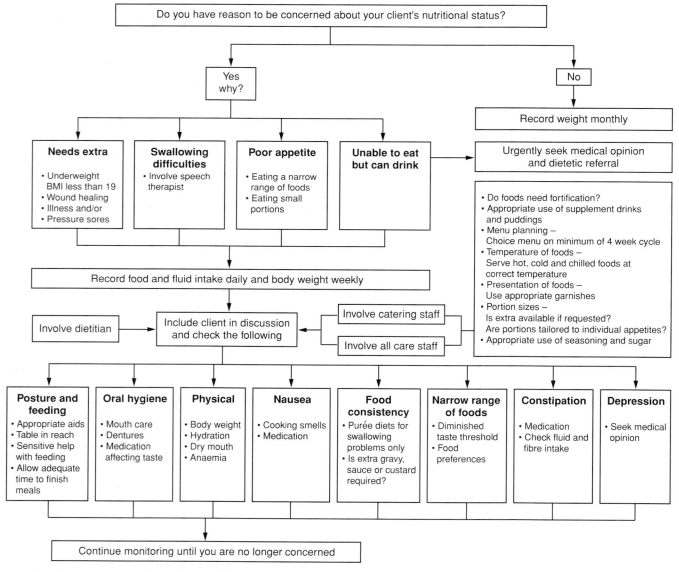

Fig. 3.1　Taking steps to tackle eating problems. Reproduced with permission from the British Dietetic Association's Nutrition Advisory Group for Elderly People (NAGE, 1994).

Relevant risk factors and observed warnings signals

Name _____

Address _____

Date _____

WARNING SIGNALS	Living alone	Housebound	No regular cooked meals	Low mental test score	Clinical diagnosis of depression	Chronic bronchitis/emphysema	Gastrectomy	Poor dentition and/or difficulty in swallowing
Recent unintended weight change + or – 3 kg (7 lb)	O	O	O	O	O	O	O	O
Physical disability affecting food shopping preparation or intake	O	O	O		O	O		
Lack of sunlight		O			O			
Bereavement and/or observed depression/loneliness	O	O	O	O	O	O		
Mental confusion affecting eating	O		O	O				
High alcohol consumption	O		O		O			
Polypharmacy/long-term medication	O		O	O	O			
Missed meals/snacks/fluids	O	O	O	O	O	O	O	O
Food wastage/rejection	O	O	O	O	O	O	O	O
Insufficient food stores at home	O	O	O	O	O	O		
Lack of fruit/juices/vegetables	O	O	O					O
Low budget for food	O		O					
Poor nutritional knowledge		O	O	O			O	O

Fig. 3.2 The Nutrition Assessment Grid. (adapted from Davies and Knutson 1991); reproduced with permission of Dr L. Davies.

is the Birmingham Heartlands Hospital and Sefton Health Authority Nutrition Risk Score (Hickson and Hill 1997). Nutritional Risk Assessment is discussed in more detail in Section 1.9.

Strategies for the community

Although the majority of the elderly UK population lives in the community, many of those who are more vulnerable are in need of nutritional support in order to prevent chronic or (acute) sudden malnutrition, and unnecessary institutionalization. To identify those in need of nutrition support, checks can be made by the GP or other members of the primary care team at the general screening of all patients over 75 years using a community nutrition risk-assessment tool.

However, the 10 main risk factors highlighted by Davies (1981) are still relevant today:

- fewer than eight main meals, hot or cold, eaten in a week
- very little milk consumed
- virtual abstention from fruits and vegetables
- wastage of food, even that supplied hot and ready to eat
- long periods in the day without food or beverages
- depression or loneliness
- unexpected weight change, either a significant gain or loss
- shopping difficulties
- poverty
- indication in medical records of disabilities, including alcoholism.

Elderly people living in residential homes

Research on nutrition and catering in old people's residential homes led to the identification of 26 risk factors, any of which may influence food intake and affect nutritional intake (Davies and Holdsworth 1979). These risk factors are listed in Table 3.16.

An expert working group (Caroline Walker Trust 1995) has published practical guidelines for meals in residential and nursing homes, and also suggested some nutritional

Table 3.16 An A–Z checklist of potential risk factors in residential homes (Based on Davies and Holdsworth 1979)

A. Weekly cyclic menu or monotony of menu
B. Difficulties with tea/supper meal menu (this highlights a lack of experience in menu planning and recipe ideas, and may affect costing)
C. Tea/supper meal at or before 5 pm (this frequently occurs in the UK mainly because of staffing difficulties: biscuits often have to be supplied later in the evening because some residents become hungry before bedtime)
D. Lack of rapport between head of home and cook, or the cook resists and resents suggestions
E. Residents' suggestions (e.g. for recipes) unheeded; Residents' need for special diets ignored. Inadequate contact between the residents and the home's decision-making committee or board
F. Residents not allowed choice of portion size, or poor portion control or no second helpings available
G. No heed taken of food wastage
H. Very little home-style cooking (residents frequently express a desire for familiar foods they have been used to eating, rather than institutional type catering)
I. No special provision for food treats from the local community or from the home, apart from Christmas
J. For active residents: poor or no facilities for independence in providing food and drink (e.g. tea making)
K. Hot meals served lukewarm or poorly flavoured
L. Poor presentation of food, including table setting and appearance of dining room
M. Unfriendly or undignified waitress service; meal too rushed
N. No observation of weight changes in the residents (significant changes in weight can be used as a diagnostic tool for illness, depression or other conditions which can affect nutritional status)
O. No help in feeding very frail residents; no measures taken to protect other residents from offensive eating habits
P. Head of home and cook lacking basic nutritional or catering knowledge; isolation from possible help
Q. Lengthy periods between preparation, cooking and serving; time lag between staff meals and resident meals
R. Lack of vitamin C-containing foods or risk of destruction of vitamin C due to poor cooking procedures
S. Few vitamin D-containing foods used, combined with lack of exposure of residents to sunlight
T. Low-fibre diet and complaints of constipation
U. Possible low intake of other nutrients, e.g. iron, folate and vitamin B_{12}
V. Preponderance of convenience foods of poor nutritional content
W. Disproportionate expenditure between animal protein/fruit and vegetables/high-energy foods may lead to a nutritionally imbalanced menu
X. Obvious food perks to staff to detriment of residents' meals. High proportion of food served to others
Y. Conditions conductive to food poisoning; lack of cleanliness
Z. Recommendations may not be implemented

standards for community meals. The working group recommended that there should be regular monitoring of the quality of meals in residential and nursing homes and that failure to meet nutritional standards should ultimately be grounds for rescinding of registration if advice on ways of improving standards proves ineffective.

Nutritional supplementation

The simplest way of providing nutritional support is to encourage the older person to eat more, but the provision of, or access to, small snacks and frequent meals is not always easy. Useful guidance includes:

- Eat little and often: try to have some food every 2–3 hours during the day.
- Have snacks between meals, such as milky drinks, biscuits or crackers. Make everything as nutritious as possible.
- Enrich an ordinary food with another energy- and/or nutrient-dense food that does not increase the volume of the meal, such as adding milk powder to ordinary milk which is then used for drinks, breakfast cereals, puddings or soups, or adding cream, grated cheese, butter or margarine to soup, vegetables, potatoes, etc. (see Section 1.12.3 in Oral nutritional support).

If dietary measures alone are insufficient, or if malnutrition is severe, proprietary energy/nutrient supplements may be helpful (see Section 1.12.4 in Oral nutritional support). However, the use of nutritional supplements needs to be monitored and subjected to regular review, particularly in terms of their impact on consumption of other foods and fluids. In the longer term, dietary methods of improving nutrient density and intake, if necessary in conjunction with multivitamin supplementation, are preferable.

Changes in the texture of food

The texture of food is very important to its palatability, and in general meals should consist of a variety of different textures. In some instances, the texture of food will need to be modified as a result of:

- problems in the mouth, e.g. ill-fitting dentures, candida, cancer of the mouth
- problems with the swallowing reflex, e.g. dysphagia
- physical obstruction, e.g. oesophageal stricture
- some psychiatric disorders
- neurological changes, e.g. following a stroke.

Various texture classifications of food have been devised by dietitians and speech and language therapists (see Section 4.3, Dysphagia) and one which may be particularly useful with older adults is given in Table 3.17.

An individual with progressively worsening levels of dysphagia might be offered a:

- *soft diet*, e.g. using minced meat, flaked fish, soft fruit, vegetables and mashed potato (with food enrichment

Table 3.17 A food texture classification appropriate for older adults (Based on Webb and Copeman 1996)

Texture classification	Example of food
Hard	Apple
Chewy	Cooked meat
Soft	Cake, bread/butter (no crust)
Liquid hard lump	Muesli
Liquid soft lump	Cornflakes and milk
Thickened soft lump	Plain yoghurt and banana
Thickened hard lump	Stew with chewy meat
Liquid	Milk, water, orange juice
Slides down easily	Butter, peanut butter, mousse

via added butter, margarine or milk powder if appropriate);

• *soft smooth diet*, where food is soft and mashed, e.g. puréed meat with gravy, fish in sauce, mashed soft vegetables, soft mashed potatoes, milk pudding or fruit yoghurts (with food enrichment);

• *puréed (homogenized) diet*, where food is puréed using a blender and additional fluid is added, e.g. puréed meat, potato, vegetables and fruit, smooth yoghurt, mousse or ground rice pudding.

As the degree of restriction increases so does the likelihood of an inadequate intake. Puréed food becomes more dilute with added fluid, and often has a watery taste and an unacceptable appearance. If a whole meal is liquidized together, the resulting mixture is often revolting, and bears little resemblance in appearance or taste to the original. This is not recommended, but commercial food moulds can be used to serve puréed vegetables separately from potatoes and meat or fish. Some puréed foods benefit from being prepared with a little thickening agent such as cornflour, potato flour or arrowroot. As the puréed diet is generally inadequate in energy, food usually needs to be fortified with milk powder, butter or margarine, glucose or glucose polymer, and vitamin C to prevent malnutrition.

Dysphagia is discussed in more detail in Section 4.3.

Making the meal service a good experience

Recent reports such as *Hungry in Hospital?* (Association of Community Health Councils 1997) and *Not Because They are Old* (Health Advisory Service 1998) provide clear evidence that many elderly patients in hospital are inadequately fed. The Counsel and Care Study (1997) showed that similar problems exist in residential care settings. The NDNS of people aged 65 years and over (Finch *et al.* 1998) also provided evidence that institutionalized individuals fare worse than free-living people with regard to nutrition.

In all of these studies, patients and relatives were concerned about the non-availability and poor quality of food and drink, and the inflexibility of hospital and some nursing care home routines. Relatives frequently reported a lack of help from staff in relation to feeding, and that staff did not always recognize or respond to the people who needed their help with reaching or eating their food. There was uncertainty about who was responsible for ensuring that older patients achieve adequate levels of nutrition, and lack of communication between staff and patients about treatment and care programmes; this is contrary to the good practice set out in *Eating Matters* (Bond 1997).

The Association of Community Health Councils of England and Wales (1997) recommended that:

1 The roles and responsibilities of staff at meal times must be clearly defined.
2 Staff training should be strengthened to emphasize the importance of nutrition in recovery from illness.
3 Existing guidance concerning hospital catering must be enforced. For example:
  • those patients needing assistance with eating and drinking must be helped while their meals are still hot and appetising;
  • all patients should have an initial assessment made of their food and fluid intake and eating and drinking patterns. Any significant changes in weight or eating and drinking patterns should be noted and acted upon;
  • patients at risk of malnutrition should be reviewed as agreed in their individual care plan;
  • local groups should be set up to implement the guidance and should include patient representatives.
4 The Department of Health should collect and disseminate examples of good practice at meal times to encourage hospitals to improve their services.

Further discussion of these aspects and their implementation can be found in *The NHS Plan* (DH 2000) and *The National Service Framework for Older People* to be published in 2001.

The Health of the Nation *Guidelines for Hospital Catering* (Nutrition Task Force 1994) reached similar conclusions to the Association of Community Health Councils and recommended that 'there must be a locally agreed policy for keeping written records of the proportion of a meal eaten by a patient, and a system of reporting this information to the nurse responsible for the patient's care'. The key areas addressed include:

• the timing of meals, which should be served at times which reflect the normal eating times of the majority which is, according to the Association of CHCs, a hot meal in the evening and a snack in the middle of the day
• positioning of the person in relation to food
• utensils
• physical problems
• medication
• eating environment
• roles and responsibilities identified and communicated.

Meal times and the service of meals

The physical and social environment in which meals are served is important as it affects the quantity of food and drink consumed, and food wastage (see Section 1.16, Food Service in hospitals and institutions). The dining room should be attractive, comfortable in temperature and clean, with easy access and suitable furniture. The type of meal service can also be influential; conventional cooking with bulk trolley service may be more acceptable than a plated cook–chill meal service which can offer less flexibility. Factors to consider in meal service are listed in Table 3.18.

When helping people with a poor appetite, small and attractive meals should be offered, together with snacks between main meals. As every mouthful must count in nutrient and energy terms, the food must be nutrient rich.

Copeman (1999) examined the possible nutrition-related outcomes of memory loss among older people with dementia and offered some practical suggestions to combat the weight loss that may occur. Other practical and organizational strategies are offered by an expert multi-disciplinary group (VOICES 1998). When working with this client group, it is important to remember that an individual's ability to feed him or herself will remain longer than good table manners (see Section 4.29, Dementias).

Teamwork

A comprehensive nutritional assessment will identify individuals who require nutritional support and referral to a multidisciplinary team. Effective multidisciplinary and interdisciplinary working can improve nutritional status. Interprofessional working has been spurred on by concerns with quality, both inside and outside the health-care system. Each profession has its own knowledge base, skills and expertise, which are not always recognized by other occupations. By working interprofessionally across occupational boundaries, both dietitians and non-dietitians gain a view of, and learn to listen to, what colleagues from another profession are doing and saying.

Fostering multidisciplinary working leads to improved communication, effective collaborative working, and improved quality of care for patients and clients. As the demand for health care continues to rise, the need to use available health and social care resources carefully and to maximum effect increases. This has resulted in a diversity of initiatives, particularly focused on the division of labour between professional groups so that, for example, in the community there is a shift from nurse to social worker in the care of long-term dehospitalized patient or resident living in local authority accommodation.

Successful multidisciplinary working requires a continuing acknowledgment of the contribution which others have to make, supported by effective communication. Team meetings help to facilitate teamwork and are an ideal forum for information sharing, problem solving and decision making, as well as discussing service quality, monitoring, audit, throughput of clients, activity assignments and updates on specific topics regarding clinical practice.

Multidisciplinary care in both primary (community) and secondary (hospital acute) sectors is comprised of teams of different composition which often overlap (Fig. 3.3). In the hospital setting, multidisciplinary team members who may be involved in nutritional aspects of care will usually include dietetic, nursing, medical, pharmacy and catering

Table 3.18 Factors to consider in meal service (Based on Webb and Copeman 1996)

Physical environment	Seating arrangement
	Chairs of appropriate height and type
	Appropriate cutlery
	Noise level
	Distractions
	Avoidance of offensive odours
Social environment	Sufficient time allocated for eating
	Compatibility of dining companions
	Personal preferences, e.g. resident who wishes to eat alone
	Pleasant and non-patronizing serving staff
	Appropriate and discreet assistance
The meal	Portion size
	Appearance
	Taste, smell, colour and texture
	Individual likes and dislikes
	Familiarity and cultural acceptability
	Temperature
	Second helping available
	Sufficient fluid (tea, coffee, fruit juice, water)

personnel, with additional input from a physiotherapist, occupational therapist, speech and language therapist, social worker, clinical psychologist, dentist, nutrition and infection-control nurse, health-care assistants and ward operative staff. In the community setting, the nutritional support team members may comprise a GP, specialist nurse, community nurse, dietitian, physiotherapist, occupational therapist, speech and language therapist, social worker, discharge co-ordinator and home carer.

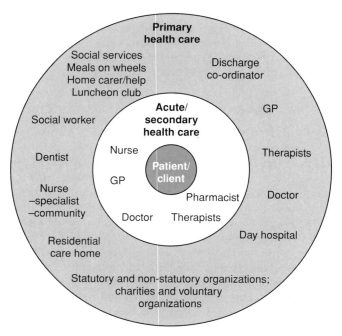

Fig. 3.3 Members of the multiprofessional team caring for older people (based on Copeman et al. 1999).

It is essential that the members of the numerous types of team involved in the care and support of older people are aware of the main determinants of health. These are:

- age, sex and constitutional factors
- individual lifestyle factors
- social and community networks
- general socioeconomic, cultural and environmental conditions (including education, living conditions, housing, access to health care and income).

The Acheson Report (1998) reiterated the importance of considering the complex nature of inequalities in health. Factors such as poverty, income, tax and benefits, education, employment, housing and environment, mobility, transport, pollution and nutrition all have a significant impact on inequalities in health. Many of these inequalities are experienced by a large number of older people, making them more vulnerable to malnutrition and illness. These factors must be taken into account when individual care plans for the older person are constructed.

Text revised by: June Copeman, Karen Hyland and other members of the British Dietetic Association's Nutrition Advisory Group for Elderly People (NAGE)

Useful addresses

Age Concern England
1268 London Road, London SW16 4ER

Alzheimer's Disease Society
Gordon House, 10 Greencoat Place, London SW1P 1PH
Tel: 020 7306 0606

British Geriatric Society
1 St Andrews Place, London NW1 4LB
Tel: 020 7935 4004

Carers National Association
20–25 Glasshouse Yard, London EC1A 4JS

Caroline Walker Trust (publications)
22 Kindersley Way, Abbots Langley, Herts WD5 ODQ
Tel: 01923 269902
Website: www.cwt.org.uk

Centre for Policy on Ageing
25–31 Ironmonger Row, London EC1V 3QP
Tel: 020 7253 1787

Cruse Bereavement Care
Cruse House, 126 Sheen Road, Richmond, Surrey TW9 1UR
Tel: 020 8940 4818

Disabled Living Foundation
380–384 Harrow Road, London W9 2HU
Tel: 020 7289 6111

Help the Aged
St James Walk, Clerkenwell Green, London EC1R 0BE
Tel: 020 7253 0253

Research into Ageing
Braid House, 15–17 St Cross St, London EC1N 8UN

Stroke Association
CHSA House, Whitecross Street, London EC1Y 8JJ
Tel 020 7490 7999. Fax: 020 7490 2686
(There are local support groups of this association in many areas)

VOICES (Voluntary Organisations Involved in Caring in the Elderly Sector)
c/o Association of Charity Officers, Beechwood House, Wyllyotts Close, Potters Bar, Herts EN6 2HN

Useful resources

The British Dietetic Association's Nutrition Advisory Group for Elderly People (NAGE) publishes a number of leaflets and resources for use with elderly clients. Details of current publications can be found on the British Dietetic Association website at www.bda.org.uk (or by contacting the Association directly).

References

Acheson D. *Independent Inquiry into Inequalities in Health*. London: The Stationery Office, 1998.

Association of Community Health Councils for England and Wales. *Hungry in Hospital*. London: Association of Community Health Councils for England and Wales, 1997.

Bassey J. Benefits of exercise in the elderly. In Issago B (Ed.) *Recent Advances in Geriatric Medicine*, 3rd edn. Edinburgh: Churchill Livingstone, 1985.

Beales D, Denham M, Tulloch A. *Community Care of Older People*. Abingdon: Radcliffe Medical Press, 1998.

Bond S (Ed.). *Eating Matters. A Resource for Improving Dietary Care in Hospital*. Newcastle upon Tyne: University of Newcastle, Centre for Health Service Research, 1997.

Brundtland GH (Director General of the World Health Organization). Speech to the fifty-first World Health Assembly. Geneva, 13 May 1998.

Caroline Walker Trust Expert Working Party. *Eating Well for Older People*. London: Caroline Walker Trust, 1995.

Copeman JP. *Nutritional Care for Older People: A Guide to Good Practice*. London: Age Concern, 1999.

Copeman JP, Hyland K. Nutrition issues in older people. In Corley G (Ed.) *Older People and Their Needs*. London: Whurr Publishers, 1999.

Copeman J, Hyland K, Oldfield G. Post registration education and training. The NAGE experience. *Journal of Human Nutrition and Dietetics* 1999; **12**: 395–402.

Counsel and Care. *Appetite for Life*. Birmingham: Counsel and Care, 1997.

Davies L. *Three Score years … and then?* London: Heinemann Medical Books, 1981.

Davies L. Practical nutrition for the elderly. *Nutrition Reviews* 1988; **46**: 83–87.

Davies L, Holdsworth D. A technique for assessing nutritional 'at risk' factors in residential homes for the elderly. *Journal of Human Nutrition* 1979; **33**: 165–169.

Davies L, Knutson KC. Warning signals for malnutrition in the elderly. *Journal of the American Dietetic Association 1991*; **91**: 1413–1417.

Department of Health. *Dietary Reference Values for Food Energy and Nutrients for the UK*. Report of the Working Group of the Committee on Medical Aspects of Food Policy. Report on Health and Social Subjects 41. London: HMSO, 1991.

Department of Health. *The Nutrition of Elderly People*. Report of the Working Group on the Nutrition of Elderly People of the Committee on Medical Aspects of Food Policy. Report on Health and Social Subjects 43. London: HMSO, 1992.

Department of Health. *Nutrition and Bone Health*. Report of the Working Group of the Committee on Medical Aspects of Food Policy. Report on Health and Social Subjects 49. London: The Stationery Office, 1998.

Department of Health. *The NHS Plan. A plan for investment. A plan for reform*. London: The Stationery Office, 2000.

Fiatanon MA, O'Neill EF, Ryan ND *et al.* Exercise training and nutritional supplementation for physical frailty in very elderly people. *New England Journal of Medicine* 1994; **330**: 1769–1775.

Finch S, Doyle W, Lowe C *et al. National Diet and Nutrition Survey: People Aged 65 Years and Over*. Vol. 1: *Report of the Diet and Nutrition Survey*. London: The Stationery Office, 1998.

Gariballa SE, Sinclair AJ. Nutrition, ageing and ill health. *British Journal of Nutrition* 1998; **80**: 7–23.

Goode H, Penn ND, Kelleher J, Walker BE. Evidence of cellular zinc depletion in hospitalized but not in healthy elderly subjects. *Age and Ageing* 1991; **20**: 345–348.

Health Advisory Service. *Not Because They are Old*. London: HAS, 1998.

Hickson M, Hill M. Implementing a nutritional assessment tool in the community: a report describing the process, audit and problems encountered. *Journal of Human Nutrition and Dietetics* 1997; **10**: 373–377.

NAGE. *Taking Steps to Tackle Eating Problems*. Birmingham: Nutrition Advisory Group for Elderly People (NAGE), 1994. (Available from NAGE, The British Dietetic Association, Unit 21 Goldthorpe Industrial Estate, Goldthorpe, Rotherham, South Yorkshire S63 9BL.)

Nutrition Task Force. *Nutrition Guidelines for Hospital Catering*. London: Department of Health, 1994.

Rolls BJ, Phillips PA. Aging and disturbances of thirst and fluid balance. *Nutrition Reviews* 1990; **48**: 137–144.

Royal Commission on Long Term Care. *With Respect to Old Age*. London: The Stationery Office, 1999.

Steele JG, Sheiham A, Marcenes W, Walls AWG. *National Diet and Nutrition Survey: People Aged 65 Years and Over*. Vol. 2: *Report of the Oral Health Survey*. London: The Stationery Office, 1998.

VOICES Expert Working Party. *Eating Well for Older People with Dementia*. Potters Bar: Voluntary Organisations involved in Caring in the Elderly Sector (VOICES), 1998. (Available from PO Box 5, Manchester M60 3GE.)

Webb G. *Nutrition: A Health Promotion Approach*. London: Edward Arnold, 1995.

Webb G, Copeman JP. *The Nutrition of Older Adults*. London: Edward Arnold, 1996.

3.8 People in low-income groups

The relevance of food as a factor in, and on occasions determinant of, health is beyond question. The epidemiological evidence on the contemporary diet has become increasingly clear. Food plays a role in inequalities in health and is implicated in the West's main causes of premature death: heart disease and some cancers (breast, colon) (World Health Organisation, 1990). There is near unanimity in the scientific literature about the connection between diet and health (Lang *et al*. 1999)

This section explores the links between diet and poor health. It considers why it is that those with the lowest incomes experience the poorest diets and examines some of the difficulties that people encounter when eating on a low income. It discusses the size and nature of the problem, the barriers to eating a healthy diet and some of the ways in which the problems that people experience may be overcome.

Dietitians cannot alleviate poverty directly but they can, by means of sensitive appropriate advice, help to minimize some of the nutritional consequences. In addition, dietitians have a responsibility to highlight the nutritional problems which can result from low income to policy makers and planners.

3.8.1 The links between diet and health

The evidence shows that there is a wide health divide between the richer and poorer sections of society (Low Income Project Team Report 1996; James *et al*. 1997). People in lower income groups have a higher prevalence of obesity, hypertension, high serum cholesterol and anaemia, and are more likely to suffer a premature death from coronary heart disease or cancer (Table 3.19). In addition to this, their children are more likely to have a low birthweight, birth abnormalities, poor growth or dental caries, or to die in the perinatal period.

While many factors contribute to the increased risk of certain diseases, it is now widely accepted that dietary factors are important. Put very simply: a poor diet can make you ill. Virtually every dietary survey shows the same pattern, that lower income groups consume a diet containing fewer essential nutrients but more fat and sugars than those in higher income groups (DH 1989; Gregory *et al*. 1990; MAFF 1993). Several studies have shown that poorer households have a less diverse diet and that they also have consistently lower nutritional outcomes than richer members of society (Dowler and Dobson 1997). The questions that arise are: who are the poor and how many people live in poverty?

3.8.2 The size and nature of the problem

Unlike most other European countries, the UK government does not have an official poverty line below which people are agreed to be poor. However, a range of measures is

Table 3.19 Observed prevalence of disease and risk factors within social class, in men and women of all ages (James *et al*. 1997)

	Social class					
	I	II	IIINM	IIIM	IV	V
Men						
Ischaemic heart disease	5.1	5.4	6	7.7	7	6.4
Stroke	1.3	1.6	1.7	2.3	2.7	2.1
Mean blood pressure (mmHg)	136/76	137/77	138/76	139/77	138/77	139/77
Cholesterol >6.5 mmol/l	26	28	27	27	27	26
Smoking >20 cigarettes/day	31	31	33	44	40	40
Obesity (BMI >30)	9.9	13.5	13.7	15	15	14
Physically inactive	14	14	15	20	21	21
Women						
Ischaemic heart disease	1.8	3.4	5.2	4.4	5.9	7.2
Stroke	0.5	0.9	2.3	1.5	2.0	2.5
Mean blood pressure	130/72	132/72	136/73	134/73	136/73	141/75
Cholesterol >6.5 mmol/l	26	29	35	33	33	36
Smoking >20 cigarettes/day	24	24	23	28	30	30
Obesity (BMI >30)	11.8	14.3	15	19.7	21.9	22.6
Physically inactive	15	15	17	24	22	22

The values are percentages of the population, with the exception of mean blood pressure which is in mmHg.
Reproduced with permission of the BMJ Publishing Group.

frequently used to identify those in society with insufficient resources. While each measure of poverty has advantages and disadvantages, it is important to note that each often produces different estimates and identifies different groups as poor.

> There is no right nor wrong answer, rather we need to be aware of the implications of accepting one definition of poverty and rejecting another, because the way in which we conceptualise poverty will in a very real sense determine our own, and indeed any political response to poverty (Dobson 1997).

It would be wrong to assume that poverty is a static phenomenon and that the poor are a homogeneous group. There have always been groups in societies who are vulnerable, such as people who are elderly, disabled or chronically ill, and those from ethnic minorities. Often these groups have fewer resources and many have struggled to make ends meet. Traditionally, the poor were thought to comprise individuals from these groups as well as some others who were responsible for their own misery (Hantrais 1995). However, there is a growing awareness of a 'new poverty', that is poverty experienced by the able-bodied of working age, some of whom are in the labour market (Cross 1993). Research suggests that individuals or households may enter the ranks of the new poor either because they are excluded from employment or because their wages are insufficient to provide their families with adequate resources. The evidence demonstrates that people move in and out of poverty and that some experience repeated spells in poverty. While some move out of poverty this escape is shortlived and they oscillate between being in and out of poverty. This movement affects the financial and other resources to which individuals have access, and in turn limits their opportunities for adopting a healthy diet.

There has been a rise in the number of poor people and a widening of the gap between the rich and the poor (Hills 1995). Since 1977 the proportion of the British population with less than half the average income has more than trebled, so that by 1994 63% of individuals had incomes less than the national average. In 1994, after housing costs, the national average income was £247 per week. However, 81% of families in which the head of house was unemployed had incomes of less than £150 per week (DSS 1996). In 1999 official government figures estimated that one in three children was living in poverty.

A several studies have investigated the effects of living in poverty. The 1991 National Children's Home Poverty and Nutrition survey (NCH 1991) found that:

- One in five parents and one in 10 children had gone hungry because they did not have enough money to buy food.
- Two-thirds of the children and over half of the parents had nutritionally poor diets.
- Nearly half of the parents had gone without food to ensure that their children had something to eat.

In the UK, social security benefit levels are sometimes used as an indicator of those living on a low income as,

in theory, they represent the 'safety net', that is the amount of income required to live on. In 1995 almost one-fifth of people lived in families that were reliant on means-tested benefits. However, the amount of income received by a family living on benefit is not generous. For example, in 1999/2000 a family of four (two adults and two children) would receive just less than £150 per week. This equates to roughly £5.30 per person per day and this money has to cover all household and family expenses such as food, utility and other bills, school costs, travel, household consumables such as washing powder as well as larger items such as furniture, birthdays and presents. A report produced by the Family Budget Unit (1998) estimated the cost of a modest but adequate diet to be £49.12 per week for a family. However, a study in Leicester (Dobson et al. 2000) found that low-income families are spending less than this a week. Its findings suggest that, after paying bills, a family of four is left with £30–35 per week for food. This is approximately £1.16 per person per day on food. Given the limited income of families in this study, it is not surprising that they were unable to afford to follow the healthy-eating guidelines. Their difficulty was compounded by the fact that healthier foods not only cost more than cheap filling foods (which are not always 'healthy') but also cost more in the shops near to where poorer people live (Dowler and Rushton 1994).

3.8.3 Nutritional consequences of low income

The UK National Food Survey (DSS 1994) showed that the intakes of many nutrients are less likely to be adequate in households receiving benefits, or in those with the lowest incomes. In particular, the intakes of vitamin C, folate, iron, zinc and magnesium are less likely to be adequate in households with more than three children or in those headed by a lone parent (Dowler and Calvert 1995).

The Diet and Nutrition Survey of British Adults (Gregory et al. 1990) showed than men and women who were unemployed or who lived in households in receipt of benefit had significantly lower intakes of many vitamins and minerals than adults not in these circumstances. This survey also found that adults from social classes IV and V had lower intakes of most vitamins and minerals than those in the higher social classes.

The National Diet and Nutrition Survey (NDNS) of Children (Gregory et al. 1995) found that young children from manual social classes, or who lived in households who were unemployed or in receipt of benefit, had lower intakes and/or blood levels of carotene, niacin, vitamin C, iron, calcium, phosphorus and potassium than those from non-manual or more advantaged households. There were no significant differences in energy intakes by any other social characteristic (Gregory et al. 1995). Similar findings are seen in other large-scale surveys (Braddon et al. 1988; Bolton-Smith et al. 1991; Moynihan et al. 1993).

The work of Dowler and Calvert (1995) on lone-parent households showed that those who had been in receipt of income support for some time had intakes of iron, folate, vitamin C and fibre which were approximately half those of people not living in similar circumstances. These parents were much less likely to reach 100% reference values, regardless of whether or not parents smoked.

3.8.4 Low-income issues and dietetic practice

When working with low-income households dietitians have to address a very complex situation in which access to food and shops, prices, budgeting strategies, patterns of food choice, and the need for social and cultural acceptability all interact. The challenge for dietitians is to find ways to maximize the opportunities available to people on a low income in order to incorporate a healthier diet into their daily lives. Dietitians must understand how these factors interact in order to ensure that the information and advice given is appropriate and that the particular individual or family has the resources to implement such guidance.

The difficulties experienced by families living on a low income are compounded by the problems of price and access to foods. Although poorer households spend less in absolute terms on food than richer households, they spend a much higher proportion of their income on food: 26% as opposed to 15% (Central Statistics Office 1992). Evidence from the National Food Survey (1995) showed that poorer households were the most efficient purchasers of nutrients per unit cost, and other studies call into question the image of the poor as 'inefficient'. The work of Kempson (1996) demonstrated that those living on low incomes were highly skilled at budgeting but their difficulty was that food was often the only flexible item of the budget. This was the item which was cut back on when bills had to be paid. Therefore, those advocating changing eating patterns which may involve added costs must be aware of how little room for manoeuvre people have.

The difficulties encountered by families living on a low income were explored in a report published by Dobson *et al.* (1994). This examined in detail the food choices of families and identified some of the difficulties and barriers faced when eating on a limited budget. The principal findings were:

- All families who participated in this study struggled to make ends meet. Their main concern was feeding their families and preventing children from being hungry. Families had a definite rationale for their food purchases. All had changed their food-buying habits in an attempt to economize and the cost of food took precedence over issues of taste, cultural acceptability and healthy eating.
- The responsibility for budgeting and feeding the family rested with the mothers. Many found themselves having to ration food to ensure that there would be enough to go round. They had to decide where and when to shop, and what to foods to buy, and most shopped alone to avoid confrontation with children who wanted other non-essential items. Shopping and cooking under such constraints were difficult and time-consuming. Not sur-

prisingly, the majority had lost interest in food and few derived any pleasure from eating.
- Families tended to shop little and often at local discount supermarkets as they could not commit income to buying in bulk or in advance from large supermarkets or food co-operatives.
- Families resisted radical changes and tried to maintain conventional eating patterns, often eating cheaper versions of familiar 'mainstream' meals. Families had worked out that it was cheaper to buy prepared foods from discount supermarkets than to buy raw ingredients. A limited income also discouraged experimentation with new foods in case children and partners did not like them and so refused to eat them. To reduce costs, many families ate together as they could not afford to prepare separate meals.
- Parents were concerned that their children should not seem different from their peers; having crisps or chocolate to take to school was not seen as a luxury but as a way of participating in conventional behaviour.
- Families were aware of the need to eat healthily but the difficulty for many was knowing how to achieve this given the constraints of a limited income.
- Advice on healthy eating was often not considered feasible or could only be partially carried through. The advice that many families received would have involved making substantial changes to their diets, which few could risk or afford. When considering what to buy, families tended to think in terms of meals rather than the nutritional value of individual foods. Dietary advice did not reflect this. Some of the advice given recommended using unfamiliar foods, most of which were not available locally or were too expensive.

This study did not include people who were homeless or those living in temporary accommodation such as hostels or bed and breakfasts. For these individuals and families, the difficulties are even more severe as many will not have access to cooking or storage facilities. Therefore, the advice given to these groups needs to reflect the realities of their everyday life.

In 1997 the National Food Alliance (now called Sustain) published a document that dispelled many of the myths about food and low income (Lobstein 1997). It challenged the widely held assumption that people in the UK can choose to eat a healthy diet if they want to. The evidence in this report refuted myths such as 'healthy food isn't expensive' and 'they [the poor] should learn to cook like everyone else', and is therefore useful reading for dietitians and others working on issues related to food and low income.

3.8.5 The policy response to low-income issues

The link between diet, poverty and health has been well documented, together with the overwhelming evidence that a poor diet increases the risk of certain diseases (Low Income Project Team 1996). While there have been national policies aimed at improving the diets of the poor, since the 1970s many of these have been eroded so that there is minimal dietary help available to those living on low incomes. For example, there has been a reduction in the provision of free school milk and school meals have been deregulated. Leather (1996) concluded that food poverty (i.e. less than optimal nutrition) exists in Britain and that those on low incomes struggle to afford a healthy diet.

It has only been within the last few years that the problems associated with a poor diet have again merited government attention. A number of reports such as *Saving Lives: Our Healthier Nation* (DH 1999a), the Nutrition Task Force's *Eat Well II* (DH 1996), *Inequalities in Health* (Acheson 1998) and *Bringing Britain Together* (Social Exclusion Unit 1998) acknowledge the link between diet and health and highlighted the difficulties of those living on a low income. This interest has resulted in a number of policies such as New Deal for Communities, SureStart, Single Regeneration Budget, Health Action Zones, Education Action Zones and Healthy Living Centres. Although many of these policies are not primarily aimed at improving nutrition *per se*, they call for co-ordinated and holistic approaches so as to tackle 'all the things which make people ill' (DH 1999b).

The aim of many of these policies is to reduce inequalities and improve health through developing coherent strategies for renewal that involve working with local people.

Increasingly, dietitians are becoming involved in many community initiatives, especially those stemming from Health Action Zones, Single Regeneration Projects and Healthy Living Centres. McGlone *et al.* (1999) examined a number of community food projects and identified certain factors that both facilitated and hindered the development and sustainability of local initiatives (Table 3.20). They concluded that although there were many different types of food project, none was found to be more sustainable than another. Two key factors influencing sustainability were secure funding and community involvement.

An important lesson from this research for all those involved in community food projects, is that initiatives must be seen to be meeting local needs as well as being of interest and practical use. When local people were asked why they used food projects, the majority of them cited social reasons as their prime motivation. Given this, those

involved in community food projects need to ensure that local people enjoy food initiatives.

Dietitians are increasingly looking for alternative ways of encouraging people to make changes to their diets since empirical research has shown that, for low-income groups, nutrition education has a limited role (Kennedy *et al.* 1999). The reasons for this are summarized in Table 3.21.

Some of the community projects involving dietitians are adopting a community development approach. Community development is an interactive and iterative process that should involve genuine partnership between local people, local workers and professionals. It is a process that has been described as 'working to stimulate and encourage communities to express their needs' and then to work with all those concerned to address these needs (Ewles and Simnett 1995).

Two examples of dietitians using a community development approach are the Bolton Community Nutrition Assistants Project (Kennedy *et al.* 1999) and the Saffron Food and Health Project (Dobson *et al.* 2000). While these projects differ in terms of their content they are similar in that dietitians have developed models of working *with* local people to bring about changes in eating behaviours. The needs and food concerns of local people have influenced how these projects developed and ensured that many of the initiatives brought theory and practice together in a format that was accessible to local people. Both projects used familiar foods that were available locally, and the dietitians worked with local people to identify dietary changes that they could achieve and afford, and which were acceptable to the whole family.

An interesting development in both of these food projects has been their use of community food workers who are members of the communities in which the projects are based. In the Bolton project they are called community nutrition assistants and in the Saffron Food and Health Project they are referred to as community food workers. In both instances these workers received training and support to enable them to go into communities and to work with

Table 3.20 Factors affecting the sustainability of food projects (McGlone *et al.* 1999)

Factors which facilitate	Factors which hinder
Reconciling different agendas	Opposing agendas
Secure funding	Instability of funding
Community support	Meeting limited needs
Professional support	Lack of support
Credibility	Changing agendas
Shared ownership	Exclusively owned
Dynamic worker	
Responsiveness	

Reproduced with permission of the Joseph Rowntree Foundation.

Table 3.21 Reasons why nutrition education has a limited role for low-income groups (After Kennedy *et al.* 1999)

- Traditional approaches to nutrition education have shown limited success in changing food consumption patterns of low-income households
- The main barrier to change is not ignorance of nutrition but the sum effect of social, cultural and economic factors
- The unidimensional model of knowledge, attitudes and behaviour is too simplistic
- The combination and interrelationship of factors has a more powerful effect on the individual's ability to exercise informed choice
- Nutrition education is clearly only part of the solution
- Even using more contemporary methods of nutrition education, people with limited resources are less likely to adopt recommended dietary changes unless other factors are also dealt with
- More comprehensive approaches are needed
- Evaluation of the effectiveness of nutrition prevention and health-promotion work at the community level is urgently required

Table 3.22 Key characteristics of community development and possible organizational constraints

Characteristics of community development projects	Possible organizational constraints encountered by professionals
Area or community based	Work with individuals, or groups and locality based
Encourages community participation	Patients or clients referred to a service
Meets local needs and has an open agenda	Must achieve specified targets
Enhances community capacity	Often task driven
Open-ended in terms of time and outcomes	Time limited, outcomes specified and work on a sessional basis
The boundaries extend beyond single issues such as eating behaviour	Funding and professional boundaries restrict workers to single issues
Involves local residents, workers and professionals	Difficulties associated with cross-disciplinary and multiagency working

local people to address their food concerns. Their involvement has included running a number of different sessions including 'cook and eat' and food tasting, as well as providing healthy-eating advice and supporting food-related community activities.

The use of community food workers represents an important development in dietetic practice and one that requires further investigation. The conclusion of both of these projects is that, given adequate training, support and resources, community food workers can make an effective contribution to improve eating behaviours. However:

> ... [A] firm policy on what the CNA [community nutrition assistant] should not attempt is necessary. Clear guidelines are needed on when CNAs should refer clients or seek support (Kennedy *et al.* 1999).

Finally, there are certain practical difficulties that dietitians may encounter as they attempt to incorporate community development into current working practices, as this approach requires different working practices, resources and organizational infrastructure to traditional therapeutic working. Table 3.22 highlights the key characteristics of community development as well as the possible constraints that health professionals may experience. Although community development offers dietitians an innovative way in which to work with local people to change eating behaviour, it also presents them with a number of challenges that must be addressed if this approach is to prove effective.

Text revised by: Barbara Dobson and Diane Talbot

References

Acheson D. *Inequalities in Health: An Independent Inquiry*. London: The Stationery Office, 1998.

Bolton-Smith C, Smith W, Woodward M, Tunstall-Pedoe H. Nutrient intakes in different social classes: results from the Scottish health study. *British Journal of Nutrition* 1991; **65**: 321–325.

Braddon F, Wadsworth M, Davies J, Cripps H. Social and regional differences in food and alcohol consumption and their measurement in a national birth cohort. *Journal of Epidemiology and Community Health* 1988; **42**: 341–349.

Central Statistics Office. *Family Spending: A Report on the 1991 Family Expenditure Survey*. London: HMSO, 1992.

Cross, M. Generating the new poverty: a European comparison. In Simpson R, Walker R (Eds) *For Richer for Poorer*. London: Child Poverty Action Group, 1993.

Department of Health. *Eat Well II: A Progress Report from the Nutrition Task Force on the Action Plan to Achieve the Health of the Nation Targets on Diet and Nutrition*. London, DH, 1996.

Department of Health. *Saving Lives: Our Healthier Nation*. London: The Stationery Office, 1999a.

Department of Health. *Reducing Health Inequalities: An Action Report*. London: DH, 1999b.

Department of Health, Committee on Medical Aspects of Food Policy (COMA). *The Diets of British School Children*. Report on Health and Social Subjects 36. London: HMSO, 1989.

Department of Social Security. *Income Support Statistics: Annual Inquiry, May 1993*. London: Department of Social Security, 1994.

Department of Social Security. *Households Below Average Income: A Statistical Analysis 1979–1993/94*. London: HMSO, 1996.

Dobson B. The paradox of want amidst plenty. In Kohler BN, Feichtinger E, Barlosius E, Dowler E. (Eds) *From Food Poverty to Social Exclusion in Poverty and Food in Welfare Societies*, pp. 33–46. Berlin: Sigma, 1997.

Dobson B, Beardsworth A, Keil T, Walker R. *Diet, Choice and Poverty: Social, Cultural and Nutritional Aspects of Food Consumption among Low Income Families*, p. 36. London: Family Policy Studies Unit, 1994.

Dobson B, Kellard K, Talbot D. *A Recipe for Success: An Evaluation of a Community Food Project*. Loughborough: Centre for Research in Social Policy, 2000.

Dowler E, Dobson B. Nutrition and poverty in Europe: an overview. *Proceedings of the Nutrition Society* 1997; **56** (1A): 51–62.

Dowler E, Calvert C. *Nutrition and Diet in Lone Parent Families in London*. London: Family Policies Studies Centre, 1995.

Dowler E, Rushton C. *Diet and Poverty in the UK: Contemporary Research Methods and Current Experience: A Review Working Paper for the Committee on Medical Aspects of Food Policy (COMA) and the Nutrition Task Force*. Department of Health, Department of Public Health and Policy Publication Number 11. London: London School of Hygiene and Tropical Medicine, 1994.

Ewles L, Simnett I. *Promoting Health: A Practical Guide*. London: Scutari Press, 1995.

Family Budget Unit. *Low Cost But Acceptable. A Minimum Income Standard for the UK: Families with Young Children*. Parker H (Ed.). Bristol: Policy Press, 1998.

Gregory J, Foster K, Tyler H, Wiseman M. *The Diet and Nutrition Survey of British Adults*. London: HMSO, 1990.

Gregory J, Collins D, Davies P *et al*. *National Diet and Nutrition Survey: Children aged 1 1/2 to 4 1/2 Years*. London: HMSO, 1995.

Hantrais L. *Social Policy in the European Community*. Basingstoke: Macmillan, 1995.

Hills J. *Inquiry into Income and Wealth*. York: Joseph Rowntree Foundation, 1995.

James W, Nelson M, Ralph A, Leather S. The contribution of nutrition to inequalities in health. *British Medical Journal* 1997; **314**: 1545–1549.

Kempson E. *Life on Low Income*. York: Joseph Rowntree, 1996.

Kennedy L, Ubido J, Elhassan S *et al*. Dietetic helpers in the community: the Bolton Community Nutrition Assistants project. *Journal of Human Nutrition and Dietetics* 1999; **12**: 501–512.

Lang T, Caraher M, Dixon P, Carr-Hill R. *Cooking Skills and Health*. London: Health Education Authority, 1999.

Leather S. *The Making of Modern Malnutrition: An Overview of Food Poverty in the UK*. London: Caroline Walker Trust, 1996.

Lobstein T. *Myths about Food and Low Income*. London: National Food Alliance, 1997.

Low Income Project Team. *Low Income, Food, Nutrition and Health: Strategies for Improvement*. London: Department of Health, 1996.

MAFF. *The National Food Survey, 1992*. London: HMSO, 1993.

McGlone P, Dobson B, Dowler E, Nelson M. *Food Projects and How they Work*. York: Joseph Rowntree Foundation, 1999.

Moynihan P, Adamson A, Skinner R *et al*. The intake of nutrients by Northumbrian adolescents from one parent families and from unemployed families. *Journal of Human Nutrition and Dietetics* 1993; **6**: 433–441.

National Children's Home. *Action for Children's Poverty and Nutrition Survey*. London: NCH, 1991.

Social Exclusion Unit, Cabinet Office. *Bringing Britain Together*. London: The Stationery Office, 1998.

Britain is a multicultural society. The 1991 census showed that just over 3 million people (5.5% of the population) are of minority ethnic origin (Balarajan and Raleigh 1993; Raleigh and Balarajan 1994). About half of these are people of South Asian origin (2.7% of the UK population). The second largest group is comprised of people of African-Caribbean origin (0.9% of the population). Their geographical distribution is uneven, with most living in greater London, the West Midlands and other metropolitan counties.

It is now acknowledged that people from black and ethnic minorities are a disadvantaged group of the population in terms of health (DH, 1992; Balarajan and Raleigh 1995). Overall, the prevalence of disorders such as heart disease, diabetes, hypertension, stroke and mental illness tends to be high but, despite these increased health needs, uptake of health-care services tends to be low. Health problems are often compounded by factors such as poverty, unemployment, poor housing, communication difficulties and social isolation, particularly of women. Many of these problems have nutritional implications.

There is enormous diversity in culture, traditions and food habits both between and within different ethnic groups, and even within a single family, and it is vital that dietitians understand and are familiar with these factors when offering dietary guidance. About half of those of minority ethnic origin in the UK were born in this country, a proportion which will steadily increase with time, and as a result, Western influences on diet have affected traditional eating patterns to a considerable extent. Some people consume a diet which is no different to that of their indigenous peers; others, particularly older people or those who have recently immigrated, retain their traditional eating practices. Dietitians should never make assumptions about an individual's food habits simply on the basis of ethnic origin.

3.9.1 South Asian people

Although used generally (and also for brevity in this section) the description 'Asian' should more correctly be denoted as 'South Asian' since it refers to people whose ancestors originated from the Indian subcontinent, i.e. from countries such as India, Pakistan, Sri Lanka and Bangladesh (Fig. 3.4). The group also includes Indian people who subsequently migrated to other areas such as East Africa (Fig. 3.5). In terms of dietary customs, they are a very heterogeneous group and there is enormous cultural diversity both between and within them.

In the UK, older South Asian people are more likely to be first-generation immigrants and to follow traditional customs, although this is the less the case than it used to be. Some may not read or speak English. In contrast, the younger population may have adopted many aspects of the Westernized way of life, including dietary habits.

The extended family is the centre of all Asian cultures. Family members often live near each other and get together for an evening meal several times a week. Senior members of the family are held in great respect and their views (including those on dietary matters) may have considerable influence.

Traditional dietary practices of South Asian people

Religious influences on diet and lifestyle

Religion is an integral part of life. The three main religions of Asians living in the UK are Hinduism, Islam (Muslims) and Sikhism. Each has its specific dietary restrictions but there are some points in common (Table 3.23).

Hindus Hinduism is founded on reverence for life, non-violence and a belief in reincarnation. As a result, many Hindus are lactovegetarians.

Geographical origin: Many Hindus in the UK will have come from Gujarat on the north-west coast of India, and Gujarati is likely to be their first language. A significant proportion will have originated from the Punjab and speak Punjabi and/or Hindi. Some will be from East Africa.

Food restrictions:

- Hindus rarely eat beef and most will not eat meat or fish of any kind. Less strict Hindus (particularly men) may eat lamb, chicken or white fish.
- Very strict Hindus do not eat eggs since they are potentially a source of life.
- Animal-derived fats such as dripping or lard are not acceptable. Ghee (clarified butter) and vegetable oil are used in cooking.
- Strict Hindus will be unwilling to eat food unless they are certain that the utensils used in preparation and service have not been in contact with meat or fish.
- Alcohol is not forbidden but may not be consumed, especially by women.

Festivals and fasting: Three festivals in the Hindu calendar are observed as fast days:

- *Mahashivratri*: the birthday of Lord Shiva (March)

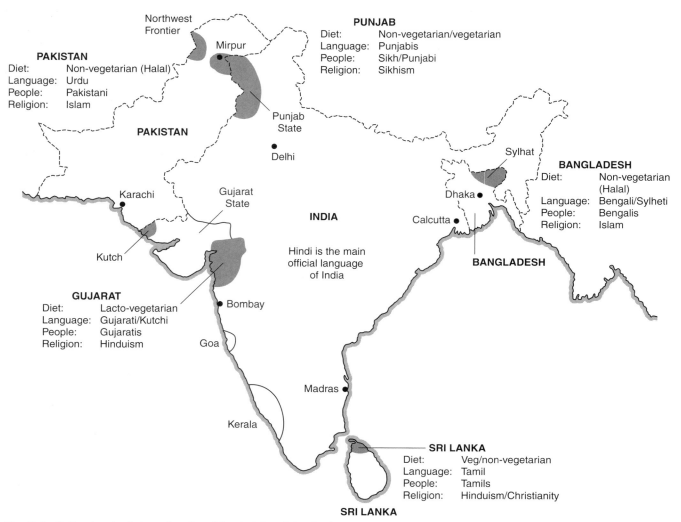

Fig. 3.4 Cultural and religious diversity of South Asians living in the UK. Copyright: Aruna Thaker, South West London Community NHS Trust.

- *Ram Navmi*: the birthday of Lord Rama (April)
- *Janmastami*: the birthday of Lord Krishna (late August).

Some devout Hindus will fast quite regularly during the week and on religious days. The fast is observed from dawn to sunset and so some may have one cooked meal a day, or only eat 'pure' foods such as yoghurt and fruit, whilst others forego all food and may take fluids only. It is mostly a matter of individual preference.

Two important festivals where an abundance of rich food is available are Holi (in March), Raksha Bandhan (August) and Diwali (October/November).

Note that all of the above dates are only approximate as they are based on the lunar calendar.

Muslims The religion of Muslims is Islam. The word Islam is an Arabic word meaning 'submission'. All Muslims acknowledge the obligation to signify their submission in terms of 'the five pillars of Islam'. These are:

1 Belief in one God and that Mohammed is his true messenger;
2 Prayer: five times a day;

3 Zakat: give 2.5% of their wealth to the poor and needy;
4 Fasting: complete abstention from food and drink from dawn to sunset in the month of Ramadan;
5 Pilgrimage: once in a lifetime, Muslims should make a pilgrimage to Mecca if they can afford it.

Geographical origin: The Asian Muslim community in Britain comes mainly from Pakistan, Bangladesh and East Africa. However, some UK Muslims will have originated from the Middle East, Malaysia, Indonesia, Sri Lanka and Africa.

Language: Many Muslims of Asian origin will speak Punjabi, Mirpuri or Bengali; Urdu and Gujarati may also be commonly used. Those of Middle Eastern origin will speak Arabic.

Food restrictions: In Islam, all wholesome things may be used for food and the general rule is that every food is lawful (*Halal*) unless it is declared unlawful (*Haram*). Unlawful foods (Haram) are:

- foods and food products from the pig
- all other meat which has not been ritually slaughtered (Kosher meat may be acceptable)

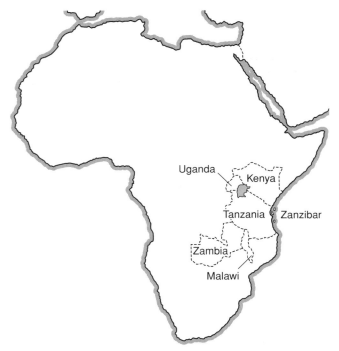

Fig. 3.5 Map of Africa showing countries from where the South Asians have come to Britain. Copyright: Aruna Thaker, South West London Community NHS Trust.

- foods containing ingredients or additives derived from the pig, or from any animal which not been ritually slaughtered, or from any Haram source. In practice, this means that a wide range of manufactured foods containing gelatine, animal fats or emulsifiers derived from animal sources will be avoided
- shellfish or seafood without fins and scales
- alcohol, including that used in cooking or for medicinal purposes.

It should be noted that a Muslim may refuse a food if he cannot be sure that it does not contain an unlawful ingredient. Similarly, a devout Muslim will be concerned that the dishes used for cooking have not been in contact with unlawful foods.

The Muslim Food Board (UK) produces a regularly updated *Halaal Food Directory* listing UK manufactured foods which are Halal.

Festivals and fasting: There are two major festivals in the Muslim calendar:

- *Eid-al Fitr* (festival breaking the Fast), 'little Eid', marks the end of the month of Ramadan, and celebrations are held both in the community and at home.
- *Eid-al Adha* ('big Eid') commemorates the pilgrimage to Mecca and is celebrated, by those who can afford it,

Table 3.23 Traditional diet of the South Asian Communities (compiled by Aruna Thaker, Community Dietitian, South West London Community NHS Trust)

	Indian Punjab		Gujarat		Pakistan	Bangladesh	Sri Lanka
	Sikhs	Hindus	Hindus	Muslims	Muslims	Muslims	Tamil
Main staple cereal	Chapatis made from wheat flour	Chapatis made from wheat flour	Chapatis made from wheat flour Rice	Chapatis made from wheat flour Rice	Chapatis made from wheat flour	Rice	Brown rice Brown rice flour
Vegetables and fruit	Vegetables cooked with spices Salad Fresh fruit	Vegetables cooked with spices Salad Fresh fruit	Vegetables cooked with spices Salad Fresh fruit	Vegetables cooked with spices Salad Fresh fruit	Vegetables cooked with spices Salad Fresh fruit	Vegetables cooked with spices Salad Fresh fruit	Vegetables cooked with spices Salad Fresh fruit
Meat	No beef Eat mainly chicken or mutton	No beef Mostly lacto-vegetarians	No beef Mostly lacto-vegetarians	No beef Halal meat only Chicken Mutton Lamb	Beef Halal meat only Chicken Mutton Lamb	Beef Halal meat only Chicken Mutton Lamb	No beef Chicken Mutton Lamb
Fish	–	–	–	Little if any fish	Little fish	A lot of fresh or dried fish	Fish
Eggs	Not a major part of the diet	Not eaten by strict vegetarians	Not eaten by strict lacto vegetarians	Usually hard boiled, fried or omelette	Usually hard boiled, fried or omelette	Few: usually hard boiled, fried or omelette	Hard boiled or omelette
Pulses and dals	Major source of protein	Major source of protein	Major source of protein	Important	Important	Important	Major source of protein
Dairy products	Full-fat milk, yoghurt, paneer	Full-fat milk, yoghurt, paneer	Full-fat milk, yoghurt and cheese	Full-fat milk, yoghurt	Full-fat milk, yoghurt	Full-fat milk yoghurt,	Full-fat milk, yoghurt
Fats/oils	Ghee Butter	Ghee Butter	Groundnut/ mustard oil Ghee Butter	Groundnut/ mustard oil Ghee Butter	Ghee or groundnut oil Butter	Groundnut/ mustard oil A little ghee Butter	Coconut oil Vegetable oil Sesame oil Butter

Asian families in East Africa ate a diet largely based on the area of the subcontinent from which they emigrated.

by the sacrifice of a lamb, sheep, cow or goat and sharing the meat amongst family, friends and the poor (only one-third may be consumed by the family).

Both of the Eids are marked with additional prayers to regular daily prayers, celebratory meals and, especially for children, the giving of presents and wearing of new clothes.

Muslims are required to fast from dawn to sunset during the month of Ramadan, which is the ninth month of the Muslim (lunar) calendar. Fasting involves abstinence from all food and drink. Feelings of weakness and lethargy can occur as a result of this abstinence and, to help overcome this, most Muslims rise early and eat a substantial high-carbohydrate, high-fat meal before dawn. Another heavy meal is taken after sunset. Elderly people and children under 12 years old are exempt from fasting. Women who are pregnant, breast feeding or menstruating, and people who are ill or travelling during Ramadan are exempt from fasting, but are expected to compensate by fasting at some other time. Chronically ill people such as those with diabetes, for whom fasting would be physically harmful, are exempt. Devout Muslims may fast once or twice a week in addition to Ramadan.

Sikhs Sikhism, which began 300 years ago as an offshoot of Hinduism and Islam, has developed into a religion in its own right. Sikhs believe in one personal God, with whom each Sikh must make his own relationship and through that lead a virtuous, useful life in the community. The five signs of a Sikh man are uncut hair, a special comb, a steel bangle, a dagger and a particular type of underwear. Orthodox Sikh men will wear turbans and grow a beard. Unorthodox younger men may be clean shaven. The Sikh 'Gurdwara' traditionally serves three meals daily and most people will partake in one of these meals at least once a week. In the UK, meals are usually cooked at weekends and on religious days by women who give voluntary service.

Geographical origin: Most Sikhs in Britain originate from the Punjab in India, but some come from East Africa. Their first language is Punjabi but many speak English, Hindi or Urdu.

Food restrictions: For Sikhs this is a matter for each individual's conscience. As a group they are less strict than Hindus and Muslims, but for each Sikh their own self-imposed restrictions are binding. Some Sikhs (especially women) are lactovegetarian, but many eat chicken, lamb and fish. They are unlikely to eat pork, and beef is forbidden. Alcohol is also forbidden, but in practice its consumption (and sometimes excessive consumption, particularly of spirits) is becoming increasingly common amongst men.

Festivals and fasting: There are three main festivals in the Sikh calendar:

- *Baisakhi*: the Sikh New Year's Day (April)
- *Diwali*: the Festival of Light (October/November)
- *Birth of Guru Nanak*: the founder of Sikhism (November).

Fasting is not a religious requirement but some devout Sikhs may fast in the same way as the Hindus.

Food choices of South Asian people

The traditional Asian diet has many healthy features, its main components being wheat, rice, pulses, dairy products, vegetables and fruit. The forms in which these foods are consumed or cooked are described below. Data on the nutritional composition of foods commonly consumed by South Asians in the UK have recently been published (Judd *et al.* 2000).

Cereal foods

Chapattis (*Roti or Rotli*), the main type of Indian bread, are generally in the UK made from 85% extraction wheat flour. They are unleavened and may contain oil and/or salt in the dough. Oil or butter is often spread on the surface of chapattis, particularly if they are prepared in advance of the meal. The thickness and size vary according to the region of origin. Gujarati chapattis are normally thin and small, the dough usually contains some oil, and oil or butter is often spread on the surface. Punjabi chapattis (both Sikh and Pakistani) are usually larger and thicker, the dough is usually prepared with just water and some salt, and fat is not normally spread on the surface. Tandori roti are a traditional Pakistani type of chapatti made from the same dough, but bigger and thicker in size and cooked in a tandoor (clay oven).

Parathas are comprised of the same dough used to make chapattis. Parathas are prepared by layering the ghee/butter (rather like puff pastry) and are shallow fried on a cast-iron griddle (called a Tava).

Poories/puries are deep-fried types of Indian bread made from a dough comprised of refined white flour, oil or ghee, and water. They are normally very thin and small, and eaten at weekends or on special occasions.

Batura are made with self-raising flour, yoghurt and water, and deep fried. They are similar to poories but much thicker and bigger.

Nans/naans are traditionally a Pakistani bread but now used by all groups. The dough (comprised of flour, water and salt) is leavened with yeast. A special (rogani) nan dough may additionally contain yoghurt and eggs, and be leavened with either flour-raising agent or yeast. Nans are usually cooked in a clay oven.

Rice is usually boiled, although fried varieties (pilau) may be eaten at weekends and on special occasions. The consumption of brown rice is minimal, despite the fact that brown basmati rice is now widely available. Brown rice and brown flour are mainly used by the Tamil community.

Vegetables and fruit

Vegetables are usually cooked in fat or oil, or as a component of dishes such as curries. Only very rarely will vegetables be cooked in water in typical British style. Common vegetables used include aubergines, bitter gourds (karela), valor (beans), okra, courgettes, dodi, spinach and cauliflower. People from southern India and Sri Lanka may use coconut (cream, milk or milk powder) in cooking.

Side salads, especially of raw onion, cucumber and tomato and sometimes incorporating a yoghurt, vinegar or lemon-based dressing, are frequently eaten at main meals.

Fruits: Traditional fruits include mango, papaya, sack fruit, passion fruit, melon and custard pears but, since many of these are expensive in the UK, commonly available fruits such as apples, bananas and oranges are more likely to be consumed.

Milk and dairy foods
Milk: Most Asian people use full-fat rather than reduced-fat milk because it is considered to be superior and unadulterated.

Yoghurt is often served as an accompaniment to main meals (when it is known as raita). This usually contains added fruits or vegetables, and may be spiced with salt, cumin powder, mustard powder, green chillis or fresh coriander leaves. The yoghurt may be home-made (usually from full-fat milk) or bought.

Home-made curd cheese (paneer) is quite unlike cheddar-type cheese; the nearest equivalent is cottage cheese, but since paneer is normally made from full-fat milk it is not a low-fat product. It is also often fried prior to consumption, which further adds to its fat content. Paneer is usually home-made by adding lemon juice or vinegar to full-fat milk and the resultant curds are separated from the whey using a muslin cloth. In Punjab, paneer is traditionally used for cooking savoury dishes; in Bangladesh it is used in sweet dishes.

Meat, fish, eggs, pulses and meat alternatives
Considerable use is made of pulses, seeds and nuts, especially by Sikhs and Hindus.

Pulses (dals) such as moong, urad, toor, masur, channa, chick peas, black-eyed beans and kidney beans are a common component of traditional South Asian cuisine. They can be cooked to varying consistencies, ranging from a watery soup to a thick purée, or even a whole bean/lentil curry eaten with either rice or chapattis.

Meat and fish: The extent to which these are consumed will depend on the constraints imposed by religious beliefs (Table 3.23). Some Asian people will be strict vegetarians; others, particularly younger age groups, may eat a totally Westernized diet. If meat is eaten, it is most likely to be lamb or chicken, and least likely to be pork or beef. Fish, even if permitted, is not usually a major dietary feature, although it is more popular among Bangladeshi people. Oily fish is rarely eaten.

Eggs, when consumed, are usually eaten hard boiled, curried, fried as an omelette, or a constituent of cakes and manufactured products.

Fat-rich foods
Fat in the form of oil, butter or ghee is an integral part of Indian cooking. Many foods are fried or are coated with fat prior to cooking. Spices and onions are usually fried in fat before the main ingredients are added when making curries or dahl. Fried snacks such as samosa, chevda, ganthia, sev, pakora and bhajia are also commonly eaten.

The use of ghee (a clarified butter, made by boiling butter for at least an hour to reduce its moisture content) is becoming less common and polyunsaturated oils are increasingly used instead (often in liberal quantities). Monounsaturated oils are less popular, although rapeseed oil may be used if its benefits are known. Olive oil is disliked because of its distinctive flavour which impairs the flavour of traditional Asian dishes, and also because of its cost implications.

As a result, the total dietary fat content of many Asian people in the UK tends to be high and may also have an undesirably high ratio of $n6:n3$ fatty acids.

Sugar-rich foods
Sweetmeats: Indian sweetmeats (collectively known as methai) such as burfi, halwa, jalebi, ladoo and gulab juman are widely consumed during festivities, which are held frequently to celebrate births, marriages and other special occasions. Sweetmeats are prepared using a combination of sugar, ghee, full-cream milk powder, nuts, chick-pea flour and sweetened condensed milk, and are highly energy dense.

Asian puddings include kheer (a rice pudding which contains nuts and green sultanas) and seviaan (sweet vermicelli).

Sugar-rich drinks such as cola, fruit squash or glucose drinks are popular, and sugar may be routinely added to Indian-style tea and coffee (usually made with a 50:50 mixture of milk and water).

Accompaniments and flavourings
Home-made pickles and chutneys often accompany main-course dishes. These are often very oily, salty or sweet to help the preservation process.

Spices are used individually (e.g. turmeric/haldi, cumin, cinnamon, peppercorns) or in specific combinations (e.g. garam masala). 'Curry powder' as used in Britain is not comparable. Freshly ground garlic, ginger and green chillies are commonly used.

'Hot' and 'cold' foods
This classification bears no relationship to the temperature or spiciness of a food or the temperature at which it is served, but is regarded as an inherent property of the food itself and one which affects the body's 'balance' and state of health.

'Hot' foods are thought to increase body temperature, excite the emotions and increase activity. 'Cold' foods are considered to reduce body temperature and impart strength and cheerfulness. Normally, a diet containing a mixture of hot and cold foods would be consumed. However, hot foods may be restricted during 'hot' conditions (e.g. mangoes are restricted during pregnancy). The intake of cold foods is controlled during 'cold' conditions (e.g. potatoes are consumed only in small amounts during lactation). This belief can have nutritional implications if important sources of nutrients are restricted in vulnerable people. For example, consumption of dairy products may be reduced in people who have arthritis and the consequent lower calcium intake may be significant in those who are elderly.

Dietary manipulations based on 'hotness' and 'coldness' tend to have less influence on the diets of people originating from the Indian subcontinent than on those from Far East Asian countries such as China (see Chinese people, below). There is also much more variation among different South Asian groups as to which foods are considered 'hot' and 'cold', and the younger generation may not follow these practices at all.

Meal patterns of South Asian people

Traditional South Asian meal patterns

These may comprise the following.

Breakfast: Rice or chapattis, *or* leftover curry and chapattis from the previous evening meal, *or* Indian snacks, *or* egg with bread, *or* Cereal with full-fat milk; tea with hot milk and sugar. Poories/puries (deep-fried Indian bread) and parathas may be consumed with yoghurt at weekends. This traditional form of breakfast is becoming less common in the UK and it is more likely that foods such as breakfast cereals and toast will be eaten.

Main meals: Rice or chapattis, meat dish if acceptable (fish dishes are rare), several vegetable or pulse dishes, pickles, side salad and yoghurt, and desserts: kheer, trifle, fresh fruit (usually those commonly available in Britain). Variations occur within this pattern and food choices increasingly include Western foods.

Snacks: Traditional deep-fried snacks such as samosas, pakoras (e.g. onion bhaji) and chevda (similar to Bombay mix) are popular. The consumption of Western-style biscuits, crisps and chocolate is also becoming increasing common, particularly by young people.

Customs associated with meals

- Hands are always washed before and after meals.
- Food is generally consumed with the right hand.
- Many people like to rinse their mouths with water after a meal.
- Strict vegetarians will not wish to use china or utensils which may have been in contact with meat or fish.

Nutritional implications of South Asian diets

Because of the heterogeneity of diets consumed by South Asians, it is impossible to generalize about the nutritional implications. These will vary from person to person depending on the nature of the diet and the extent to which it meets individual nutritional needs and provides overall dietary balance. The younger generation is increasingly moving away from traditional dietary practices in favour of Western food habits.

The traditional 'Asian' diet, rich in starchy cereal foods, pulses and vegetables, is in principle a very healthy one, being high in complex carbohydrate and fibre and low in fat. In practice, a number of factors associated with living in the UK may erode this dietary pattern:

- The best aspects of the Asian diet may be supplanted by less desirable components of the Western diet, e.g.

pulse and vegetable consumption may be replaced by chips.
- Liberal use of oil, butter or ghee in cooking may result in a high intake of fat and energy.
- Traditional vegetables and pulses may not be easily obtainable, or at an affordable price (although this is less of a problem nowadays).
- Poor cooking facilities may make traditional methods of cooking difficult, resulting in greater reliance on fried and convenience foods.
- Women are more likely to work and have less time for traditional methods of food preparation which are very time-consuming.
- Western dietary attitudes (e.g. to infant feeding) may be regarded as superior to traditional practices.
- Physical activity levels may be reduced to the level of inactivity typical of most of the UK population.

As a result, there may be a number of nutritional problems with the diets of South Asian people in the UK. At one end of the spectrum are people with an inadequate intake of energy and micronutrients as a result of inappropriate food choice, ignorance or the problems associated with low income. At the opposite end, and becoming increasingly common, are people, especially young people, whose consumption of high-fat convenience and snack foods in preference to fruit, vegetables and starchy cereal foods results in a diet which is energy dense and nutritionally imbalanced. The range of nutritionally related health problems within the Asian community is similarly wide, extending from problems such as undernutrition, anaemia and rickets to those of obesity, diabetes and heart disease.

Common health problems in South Asian people

Diabetes

South Asians in the UK are more likely to develop diabetes than their white counterparts. Up to 20% of Asians aged 40–69 years have type II diabetes, compared with about 5% of white people. The difference in prevalence may be even greater than this since it is likely that many Asian diabetics remain undiagnosed (Simmons *et al.* 1989; UK Prospective Diabetes Study Group 1994). Since the disease also tends to develop at a younger age than in white people, and duration of diabetes is one of the strongest risk factors for development of complications, problems such as diabetic nephropathy and end-stage renal failure are significantly more common in Asian diabetics (Burden *et al.* 1992). Mortality from diabetes among people born in the Indian subcontinent is about 3.5 times the national rate for England and Wales (Raleigh 1997).

Cardiovascular disease

South Asian men and women living in the UK have a greatly increased risk of coronary heart disease (CHD). CHD mortality is 36% higher in Asian men (20–69 years) and 46% higher in Asian women than in the general population (Balarajan 1991). The prevalence of hypertension and risk of stroke are also higher than in the white population, although not as high as in the African–Caribbean population (Balarajan 1991; Raleigh 1997).

Obesity

The rising prevalence of obesity, particularly central obesity, and low levels of physical activity among Asian people are likely to be significant contributory factors to the development of insulin resistance and type II diabetes in this group (McKeigue and Sevak 1994; HEA 1995).

Rickets

Although the prevalence of rickets associated with vitamin D deficiency has declined since the 1960s, cases still occur among some Asian groups in the UK, particularly among Hindu vegetarians, and may be severe (Iqbal *et al*. 1994).

Anaemia in young children

Although the prevalence of breast feeding is higher among Asian mothers than white mothers, weaning is more likely to be delayed and, by the age of 9 months, cow's milk is more likely to be used as a main drink than continuation of formula milk (Thomas and Avery 1997). As a result, the risk of anaemia in Asian children is much higher. Lawson *et al*. (1998) found that 29% of Pakistani, 25% of Bangladeshi and 20% of Indian children had haemoglobin levels below 110 g/l, compared with about 12% of 2-year-old children in the general UK population (Gregory *et al*. 1995).

Providing dietary guidance to South Asian people

In this client group, compliance with dietary guidance is often poor, and this often stems from inappropriate guidance being given in the first place. Without proper understanding of an individual's customs, food habits, level of understanding of any health problems and the reasons for suggested changes, advice is bound to be ineffective. Communication difficulties may also hamper partnership between the client and the health professional (see Communicating with non-English speaking clients, below).

Before offering dietary guidance the health professional must ascertain:

- *dietary food patterns and customs*: ascertain the extent to which traditional customs are followed within the household and the form that these take;
- *hierarchy within the family*: establish who decides what is eaten, who does the shopping and who does the cooking;
- *Social pressures within the home*: identify factors which may be a barrier to dietary change. For example, a young daughter-in-law living within an orthodox extended family may not be able to modify her diet and cooking methods if her mother-in-law governs what is bought and how it is cooked. Similarly, a woman may not have a desire to lose weight if her husband finds rounded women more attractive;

- *socioeconomic factors*: income constraints and social factors such as poor housing and unemployment may need to be considered, although it should also be remembered that many Asians will not be living in deprived circumstances.

As with any client, dietary guidance must be tailored to these individual needs and circumstances. *The Balance of Good Health* can be usefully adapted for both healthy eating and many types of therapeutic dietary advice in order to encourage better balanced food choice (see below). Specific guidance on the modification of traditional recipes (particularly in terms of the use of oil), cooking methods and meal pattern may also be advisable.

Guidance in pictorial form (e.g. photographs or drawings of foods which should be eaten more or less often) is particularly valuable because, even if the client is fluent in English, other members of the family (who may be the ones who do the shopping or cooking) may not be. Other innovative methods such as cookery demonstrations can also be effective.

Information in different Asian languages (Urdu, Bengali, Punjabi, Hindi and Gujarati) can be useful, although it should be borne in mind that some people, especially older women, may be illiterate in their own language. In contrast, younger Asian people often prefer to be given written information in English. Rather than make assumptions, it is usually better to ask the client (if necessary via an interpreter) which written language would be most helpful. Dietitians will also need an English text of the translated version to refer to.

Guidance on healthy eating

The general framework of the *Balance of Good Health* can be used as a basis for guidance, with appropriate modifications in terms of food choice.

Starchy foods

These should be a main part of every meal.

Good choices: bread, chapattis/rotis, pitta bread, nan, rice, unsweetened breakfast cereals, rolls, pasta and potatoes.

Main dietary message to get across: the importance of using less fat in the preparation, cooking and serving of these foods.

Encourage:

- medium brown to wholemeal choices of breads and flours
- wholegrain breakfast cereals not coated with sugar or honey
- use of flours made from millet (bhajira), maize (cornmeal) and gram flour (besan), as well as wheat flour (e.g. to make rotis)
- incorporating puffed rice or flaked rice into dishes.

Discourage:

- adding fat to chapatti dough (chapattis can be kept soft by covering with a cloth as made)
- addition of oil or ghee/butter to the surface of chapattis or other breads

- pooris/puries (deep-fried chapattis) and parathas; their use should be kept to special occasions
- pilau rice or biryani: these are high in fat and only suitable for occasional use. Rice which is either boiled or prepared by a low-fat cooking method should be recommended instead.

Fruit and vegetables:
At least five servings should be eaten per day.

Good choices: all types of fresh and frozen vegetables, fresh fruit, fruit canned in natural juice, dried fruit and fruit juice.

Main dietary message to get across: using as little fat or oil as possible in the cooking of vegetables and dishes containing them.

Encourage:

- fresh or dried fruit as snacks instead of fat-rich or sugar-rich snacks
- adding fruit instead of sugar to breakfast cereals and desserts
- storing vegetables in a cool, dark place and using them while still fresh
- cooking vegetables for the shortest time possible and serving immediately
- plenty of salad vegetables with meals
- chutneys made with tomatoes, mangoes, onions, chillis, etc. (without added oil)
- pickle made with lemon juice or vinegar.

Discourage:

- tinned fruit in syrup
- sweetened fruit juice
- adding fat to vegetables during cooking
- reheating cooked vegetables (as this destroys their vitamin content)
- oily pickles (as these have a high fat and salt content).

Milk and dairy foods:
Two to three servings should be eaten every day

Good choices: reduced-fat milk, yoghurt and cheeses (full-fat varieties for children under 2 years old).

Main dietary message to get across: the benefit from switching to reduced-fat milk because it contains the same nutrients but less fat. This measure tends to be resisted by Asian people because they dislike the 'thinner' taste.

Encourage:

- semi-skimmed or skimmed milk rather than full-fat milk
- making home-made yoghurt with semi-skimmed milk
- curd cheese, low-fat soft cheese or low-fat cheese spread in preference to full-fat cheeses.

Discourage:

- frying paneer: small amounts can be chopped or cubed and added to curries unfried
- gold-top milk
- adding gram-flour balls (boondi) to yoghurt
- condensed milk.

Meat, fish, pulses, dals and alternative protein sources
Two servings should be eaten every day.

Good choices: lean meat, poultry, fish, eggs, beans (e.g. moong, kidney beans, black-eyed beans, blackgram), dals (e.g. redgram, chick peas, lentils), nuts (e.g. almonds, cashews, pistachios).

Main dietary message to get across: the need to watch the amount of fat used during cooking

Encourage:

- eating pulses and dals more often
- sprouting pulses (which have an increased nutritional value)
- removing fat and skin from meat and poultry skin before it is cooked
- draining off surplus fat from cooked dishes
- using as little ghee or oil as possible (and in measured amounts) when cooking.

Discourage: Frying or coating foods in oil or ghee.

Fat-rich foods
Minimum amounts should be eaten.

Examples: ghee, butter, margarines, cooking oils, fried foods, parathas, pies, pastry, crisps, Indian snacks.

Main dietary message to get across: the importance of consuming less of these dietary components

Encourage:

- using as little oil or ghee as possible when cooking
- measuring the amount that is used
- using minimum amounts of spreading fats such as ghee, butter, margarines or other spreads
- eating fewer deep-fried foods such as samosa, pakoras, bhajias and chips
- choosing dry-roasted snacks such as chick peas, peanuts and popcorn rather than high-fat ones such as chevda, ganthiya, sev or crisps
- using low-fat cooking methods such as baking, grilling, steaming or microwaving rather than frying or roasting
- substituting some monounsaturated oil for polyunsaturated oil.

Sugar-rich foods
Minimum amounts

Examples: cakes, biscuits, Pakistani rusks, chocolate, sweetmeats, jam, sweetened fizzy drinks, glucose drinks, sweetened fruit juice, sugar, gurr, honey.

Main dietary message to get across: too many of these foods may lead to dental and weight problems.

Encourage:

- sugar-free drinks or unsweetened fruit juice
- reducing the amount of sugar added to tea or coffee or replacing it with an artificial sweetener
- choosing fresh or dried fruit as a snack instead of cakes, biscuits, sweets and chocolate
- keeping sweetmeats and sugar-rich desserts for special occasions.

Other aspects of lifestyle advice covering aspects such as alcohol consumption or physical activity may also be necessary. As with any type of dietary advice, follow-up is essential.

Therapeutic dietary guidance

These general principles of healthy eating are relevant in a wide variety of therapeutic applications. Aspects which may need to be considered or emphasized in the management of specific disorders are outlined below.

Obesity The general difficulties in achieving permanent weight loss apply to all groups, but there may be additional cultural barriers among Asian people. In South Asian societies, a rounded body shape may be regarded as being more attractive and possibly even a sign of affluence and good health. Thus, there may be little desire or social pressure for losing weight. The benefits of weight loss for health reasons, particularly in terms of reducing the risk from diabetes and heart disease, may need to be stressed.

Weight-reducing advice should be based on the above healthy-eating guidelines, but with particularly strong emphasis on the need to reduce fat intake via changes in food choice and cooking practices (either Asian or Western).

Like many other people in the UK, South Asians often mistakenly believe that starchy foods are 'fattening' and need to assured that these foods can, and should, be a major part of each meal. Wholegrain and wholemeal food choices should be promoted to help to maintain dietary satiety.

It is important to stress that increased physical activity is a vital component of a weight-management programme. With Asian clients, it is necessary to ensure that suggested forms of exercise are culturally acceptable.

Diabetes The management of Asian people with diabetes is often inadequate and ineffective (Cruickshank 1989). Patients often lack knowledge about the disease, its complications and the importance of self-management, problems which stem from poor communication, provision of inadequate or culturally inappropriate information, and non-availability of educational material in minority languages (Goodwin et al. 1987; Hawthorne 1990; Close et al. 1995).

The Balance of Good Health model adapted for the South Asian community is appropriate for those with diabetes (Govindji 1991). Particular emphasis may need to be placed on:

- the timing of meals, particularly for those on insulin or oral hypoglycaemic drugs. It is sometimes also necessary to remind patients of the importance of these medications being taken at the specified times (and in the specified amounts)
- the need for an even and relatively constant distribution of starchy cereal foods throughout the day, and which is appropriate for any hypoglycaemic therapy given

- the need to avoid rich sources of sugars, particularly sweetmeats and sugar-containing fizzy drinks which are often consumed in large quantities
- the need to reduce fat consumption (principally by using less during cooking)
- the importance of weight loss for those who are overweight (via restriction of energy intake, primarily from fat, and increased physical activity).

It should be noted that herbal medicines such as karela (bitter gourd) capsules tend to be popular among Asian people with diabetes and these types of products are sometimes promoted on Asian TV and radio channels. Although such remedies may have some hypoglycaemic effects, there is little clinical evidence regarding their effects on long-term safety, particularly at the high doses taken by many people (Bailey and Day 1989; Gray and Flatt 1997). They may also lead to the attitude that, as long as the capsules are taken, diet does not matter and that, for example, sweetmeats can be eaten with impunity.

Health promotion in South Asian people

There is evidence that UK health services are not reaching South Asian communities effectively (Balarajan and Raleigh 1995). Attendance rates at outpatient clinics are notoriously low and compliance with treatment and advice can be similarly poor. These result not from feelings of indifference to health among Asian people but more from a sense of vulnerability (Hawthorne 1990). They may be reluctant to approach health professionals because they feel that their ignorance will be exposed, their personal lifestyle scrutinized and possibly ridiculed, and their culture neither understood nor respected.

In order to overcome these barriers, it is necessary for health professionals to develop multicultural competencies and go to the community rather than expecting the community to come to them. Local community initiatives, where links are built with respected leaders of the community and health-promotion work is conducted within the community, are essential. It is often more productive and hence time- and cost-effective to run specific 'healthy-eating' sessions, cookery classes, group sessions in a local centre or even someone's home. It is also important that health education is focused on specific ethnic groups rather than just being targeted at 'Asians'.

Communicating with non-English-speaking clients

A skilled interpreter or linkworker is an essential part of a health-care team which has clients with little command of English. One-to-one teaching between the professional and the patient via the interpreter is ideal, although may not be time- or cost-effective. When using interpreters on a one-to-one basis, the following points should be borne in mind:

- An interpreter needs to be chosen with sensitivity. The patient may not feel comfortable relating to an interpreter if personal lifestyle and habits are being exposed. A hospital porter or domestic worker may not be a good choice as time may be limited, there may be a lack of interest and commitment and there may be unacceptable class differences. Similarly, using a member of the family may not always be appropriate. This is particularly the case when a young child is used as an interpreter, or when a man is used to interpret to a female patient. It is important to try to choose someone considered to be an equal and, even then, confidentiality and sensitivity may be a problem.

- The interpreter may not understand what the dietitian is saying, and therefore language needs to be appropriate to the interpreter as well as the patient. It is important that dietitians use non-jargonistic, plain English.
- The interpreter may not be able to translate accurately since some words may not have an equivalent in the Asian language.
- It is not unlikely that the interpreter will give some of his or her own advice, and may neglect to pass on some of the more important advice. Some prior basic training on nutrition and health for the interpreter can help to avoid this.

Interpreters may also be invaluable for group teaching sessions, for example introducing a video presentation, especially if the group uses a common language. If the group is varied, Hindi is usually the most appropriate language to use, since Indian films are produced in Hindi and these are generally widely understood.

In health-promotion work, educational sessions which use a respected and well-known elder within the community as an interpreter are likely to be particularly well received by a particular community. However, it must not be forgotten that some people within the group may not be prepared to reveal information of a personal nature in a public setting.

3.9.2 African–Caribbean people

The name African–Caribbean collectively refers to people of African descent who come from the many Caribbean islands. The majority of people from the Caribbean moved to the UK during the 1950s and 1960s, notably from Jamaica (HEA 1993).

As with people of Asian origin, it is important to remember that the dietary customs of people from the Caribbean are not uniform. The dietary traditions of each island have been influenced by different historical, political, social and geographical factors; the development of the sugar colonies, for example, brought many different cultures to the Caribbean (HEA 1993). As a result, dietary practices can vary considerably and dishes with similar or the same names can contain different ingredients. Alternatively, the same dish may have several names, e.g. journey cakes are also called Jonny cakes (Douglas 1987). There will also be variation in the degree to which individuals follow traditional eating habits; some people will consume a diet indistinguishable from the typical UK diet.

Traditional dietary practices of African–Caribbean people

Food choices

Starchy foods These generally form the main part of the diet and primarily consist of rice, corn and cornmeal, oats and wheat-based foods such as pasta, cakes and bread (often West Indian bread, which is known as hard dough bread).

Starchy fruits, roots and tubers are also an important part of a meal. Starchy fruit may include green banana, plantain and breadfruit. Starchy roots and tubers (sometimes referred to as provisions) include cassava, yam, sweet potato, dasheen and coco yam.

Fruits and vegetables Dark-green leafy and yellow vegetables are commonly used in soups, stews and one-pot meals, often with meat and fish. Examples include callaloo (spinach), kale, peppers, karela and carrots. Other vegetables commonly eaten include sweetcorn, okra, cabbage, tomato, aubergine, pumpkin and cho cho (christophene).

A wide variety of fruit is eaten, popular choices being pawpaw, guava, banana and pineapple.

Milk and dairy foods A variety of milk and dairy products may be used but, traditionally, condensed and evaporated milks are used in preference to fresh milk.

Meat, fish, eggs, peas, beans, nuts and seeds Particularly popular varieties of fish include snapper, red bream, red mullet, mackerel, and tinned fish such as sardines and pilchards.

A wide variety of pulses in the form of peas and beans is included in the diet via stews and one-pot meals, and as an accompaniment to meals (e.g. as a mixture of rice and peas).

Cashew nuts, almonds and coconut are often eaten as a snack. Watermelon, pumpkin and sesame seeds may be consumed by some Rastafarians.

Fat-rich foods Butter, margarine and different types of oils are used. Coconut cream may be used for flavour.

Sugar-rich foods Sweetened foods and beverages are popular with this community. Many of the preferred flavours of fizzy drinks and cordials/syrups such as sarsparilla or kola 'champagne' are not available in low-sugar varieties. However, low-calorie varieties of ginger beer, another popular drink, are more easily obtained. Other major sources of sugar include added table sugar, honey, sugary (and fatty) snacks, cakes, biscuits and chocolate.

Meal pattern

The meal pattern varies with the individual or family. Traditional dishes may take a long time to prepare, and are more likely to be eaten at weekends and evenings. At weekends there is a tendency towards eating two meals each day, omitting lunch.

Popular cooking methods include stewing, braising, steaming, frying and roasting, and very often involve the use of added fat. Food is highly seasoned.

Desserts are traditionally only eaten on special occasions, although this trend appears to be changing. Foods such fruit, fruit salads and ice-cream may be eaten quite commonly, and other items such as apple pie and gateaux are being increasingly consumed.

Within the African–Caribbean community, beliefs about diet and health may influence dietary practices, e.g. the use of herbal (bush) teas as a cure for disease (Springer and Thomas 1983).

Influence of religious beliefs

Religious beliefs influence food choice, preparation and cooking methods. Although African–Caribbean people are generally Christian (Cruickshank and Beevers 1989), there are many faiths in the Caribbean. Two main religions which affect dietary practice are Seventh Day Adventism and Rastafarianism.

Seventh Day Adventists   Followers are often vegetarian. If meat and fish are eaten, pork is avoided, as are fish without fins and scales. Alcohol and other stimulants (e.g. coffee and tea) are not consumed.

Rastafarians   The degree of dietary restriction depends upon the individual. Many are vegetarian or vegan. The majority of followers will only eat ital foods, which are foods considered to be in a whole and natural state. Processed or preserved foods are excluded. Specific foods not consumed are pork, fish without fins and scales, vine fruit and stimulants such as alcohol, coffee and tea.

Nutritional implications of African–Caribbean diets

Most of the traditional dietary practices of African–Caribbean people are compatible with guidelines for healthy eating. Dietary imbalance tends to occur when traditional food habits are eroded or supplanted by some of the less desirable aspects of the European diet. Most people eat a combination of African–Caribbean foods and European foods. Typically, traditional foods such as corn-meal, coconut, green banana, plantain, okra and yam feature alongside foods such as breakfast cereals, cakes, biscuits, crisps, burgers and chips. As a result, many African–Caribbean people living in the UK consume a diet which tends to be high in fat, sugar and salt (Sharma *et al.* 1996).

A high fat intake can result from:

- the frequent consumption of convenience, snack and fast foods
- foods being fried before another method of cooking, such as steaming, is used
- the consumption of large amounts of coconut cream which may be used in dishes such as rice and peas

- the use of cheaper cuts of meat (e.g. trotters, tails) which have a high fat content.

Sugar intake may be high because of the popularity of:

- homemade beverages based on condensed milk with added sugar or honey)
- glucose energy drinks, squashes, milk-based energy or malt drinks (e.g. Nutriment, Nourishment, Supermalt)
- sweet snack foods such as cakes (both Caribbean and European), biscuits, sweets and chocolate.

Salt intake may be high if there is frequent consumption of:

- salted fish
- salted meat
- convenience and snack foods
- salt-rich seasonings.

Alcohol consumption may also be high, particularly in men (HEA 1993).

Common health problems in African–Caribbean people

Hypertension

The prevalence of hypertension in people of African descent is high throughout the world. Hypertension is the most common chronic disease in the Caribbean and a major contributor to mortality, particular from hypertensive renal failure (Grell 1989). In the UK, 25–35% of African–Caribbeans are hypertensive compared with 10–20% of white people (Beevers and Beevers 1993). Mortality from hypertension among African–Caribbean-born people is 3.5 times greater than the national rate, and possibly as much as six times higher in Caribbean-born women (Raleigh 1997).

Because hypertension is often asymptomatic, it often remains undiagnosed and untreated. This is particularly likely to be the case in the African–Caribbean sector of the population who tend to be a socioeconomically deprived group and whose access to and use of health-care services tends to be below the national norm. Poor communication between African–Caribbean patients and their general practitioners (GPs) may also lead to poor compliance with anti-hypertensive therapy and thus poorly controlled blood pressure (Morgan 1995).

The reason for the high prevalence of hypertension among African–Caribbean people is not entirely clear, but is likely to be exacerbated by factors such as obesity, high salt intake, stress and a sedentary lifestyle. Their typically high salt intake may also play a part and there is also some evidence to suggest that African–Caribbean people may be more sensitive to the hypertensive effects of salt than white people (Beevers and Beevers 1993; Kaplan 1994).

Cardiovascular disease

The risk of stroke in significantly higher in the African–Caribbean sector of the population (Stewart *et al.* 1999), and is closely associated with hypertension.

In contrast, it appears that African–Caribbeans have a lower rate of CHD than the indigenous European population, possibly because rates of smoking tend to be low and lipid profiles are relatively favourable (Chaturvedi *et al*. 1993). Nevertheless, CHD is a still major cause of death in African–Caribbeans in Britain (Balarajan 1995) and health-intervention measures to reduce the risk are still a priority, although the primary focus should be on the need to control blood pressure, particularly via control of body weight and increased physical activity.

Diabetes

As with the South Asian community, the prevalence of diabetes is significantly higher among African–Caribbeans living in the UK than their white counterparts. About 13% of men and 18% of women aged 40–64 years have type II diabetes, i.e. about two to four times the rate found in the white population (Chaturvedi *et al*. 1994). Mortality from diabetes, particularly as a result of diabetic nephropathy and end-stage renal failure, is also significantly higher (Cruickshank 1989; Roderick *et al*. 1996). Obesity is an important contributory factor in the development and progression of type II diabetes.

African–Caribbean people with diabetes appear to be less susceptible to CHD than white diabetic people, but because diabetes is more prevalent in African–Caribbeans the net effect is still one of a high overall risk of mortality from CHD in this group. African–Caribbeans are as susceptible to microvascular complications as other groups of diabetic people.

Obesity

As with the general UK population, the rising prevalence of obesity is of concern and, in this population, a major factor in the development of hypertension and type II diabetes (see above).

Providing dietary guidance to African–Caribbean people

With some adaptations to preferences for ethnic foods, *The Balance of Good Health* is a good teaching model to encourage healthy eating in this population, with particular emphasis on the need to eat more starchy foods, fruit and vegetables and beans, and fewer fatty, sugary and salt-rich foods.

Starchy cereal foods

These should be a main part of every meal.

Good choices: bread (including hard dough bread), rice, plantain, yam, cassava, sweet potato, cornmeal, green banana, dumplings, dasheen, breadfruit, coco yam, pasta.

Encourage:

- high-fibre choices such as cassava, yam, brown rice and wholemeal bread, particularly for those who are overweight
- more use of bread, toast, crispbreads or plain crackers as an alternative to fatty snacks

- plain high-fibre or wholegrain breakfast cereals rather than sugar- or honey-coated ones

Discourage: frying foods or adding unnecessary amounts of fat.

Fruit and vegetables

At least five servings should be eaten every day.

Good choices: pumpkin, tomato, sweetcorn, eggplant, spinach, callaloo, cho-cho, cabbage, okra, pineapple, guava, banana, pawpaw, mango, melon, strawberries, lime, apple, pear, orange.

Encourage:

- steaming or boiling vegetables for the minimum amount of time
- use of fresh or dried fruit as snacks and desserts
- tinned fruit in natural juice.

Discourage:

- frying vegetables or coating them with fat
- adding condensed or evaporated milk to fruit.

Milk and dairy foods

Two to three serving should be eaten every day.

Good choices: reduced-or low-fat varieties of milk, cheese, yoghurt, fromage frais.

Encourage: use of reduced fat (and reduced sugar) varieties of milk and dairy products.

Discourage: use of condensed milk (occasional use only). Evaporated milk can be used on a more regular basis if a person is not overweight or does not have raised lipid levels.

Meat, fish and alternatives

Two servings should be eaten every day.

Good choices: peas (e.g. gungo), beans (e.g. black-eyed and kidney beans), lentils, fish, egg, skin-free chicken, lean meat.

Encourage:

- removing visible fat or skin from meat and poultry before cooking
- using the least possible amounts of oil when cooking
- use of peas and beans such as black-eyed beans, kidney beans, gungo peas and baked beans as a partial substitute for meat
- soaking salt-rich foods such as salt fish, salted mackerel, salted beef and salted pig's tail before cooking
- using herbs and spices rather than salt-rich seasonings.

Discourage: frying foods or meal components.

Fat-rich foods

Minimum amounts should be eaten.

Examples: butter, margarine, spreads, oils, coconut cream, pies, patties, fried dumplings, tails and trotters, fried foods.

Encourage:

- grilling, boiling, baking, steaming or microwaving foods rather than frying (e.g. dumplings can be boiled rather than fried)

- only using cooking oil in small and measured amounts
- using small amounts of a low-fat spread instead of butter, margarine or other spreads.

Sugar-rich foods
These should only be eaten in small amounts.
Examples: sugar, honey, molasses, sarsparilla, cordials, fruit punch, carrot juice, sugar-containing fizzy drinks, glucose drinks, malted milk drinks, cakes, buns, biscuits, sweets, chocolate.

Encourage:

- adding less sugar (either white or brown) to drinks or cereals
- choosing sugar-free or 'diet' drinks
- use of fruit as an alternative to sugary snacks such as buns, cakes and biscuits.

General aspects
Other diet and lifestyle changes which offer additional protection against hypertension and obesity and their associated health problems should also be encouraged, in particular regarding salt consumption and physical activity.

Reducing salt consumption
Encourage:

- less use of salt in cooking and at the table
- less consumption of salted meat and fish and other high-salt foods such as bacon, ham, cheese, corned beef, crisps and packet soups
- more use of herbs and spices as an alternative to salt-rich seasonings such as chicken and meat seasoning, monosodium glutamate, garlic salt, soya sauce and stock cubes.

Increasing physical activity
Encourage: 20 minutes of moderate-level activity (e.g. walking) every day.

3.9.3 West African people

The majority of West Africans in the UK originate from Nigeria and Ghana and have settled in major cities.

Traditional dietary practices of West African people

The diet consumed by West Africans is in general similar to those consumed by African–Caribbean people, but there are some differences in both food choice and cooking methods.

Starchy foods   Cassava (usually boiled) is more frequently used, sometimes in a pounded form (*eba*). Green bananas, yam and plantain (called *fufu* when pounded) are common starchy vegetables. Other starchy foods include ground rice, cornmeal, gari and kenkey.

Fruits and vegetables   Ugu, green leaf and okazi are common choices

Meat, fish and alternatives   Meat and fish such as egusi, khobi and stockfish are popular. Among Nigerians, black-eyed beans (*akara*) may be cooked as a stew.

Cooking methods
Palm oil is commonly used to give flavour and colour to dishes.

Meal pattern
Typical food combinations may be meat/fish with a starchy food such as cassava, yam or plantain (possibly pounded) plus a vegetable stew or soup. Desserts are not usually served. Nuts and seeds (often in the form of products such as peanut butter) are more likely to form part of a meal than to be used as snack foods.

Common health problems and dietary guidance

The incidence of diabetes, hypertension and obesity is high in the West African community. General weight-reducing dietary advice is often necessary and areas which need to be highlighted are:

- reducing the amount of oil used in stews: palm oil and palm nut oil are commonly used but are rich in saturated fats; if possible a limited amount of sunflower, corn or groundnut oil should be used instead
- reducing the amount of peanut butter used in soups
- reducing the amount of fried foods such as fried fish or meat. Fish, for example snappers, may be stewed or baked instead of being fried
- the portion size of green bananas, yam, ground rice and other starchy foods is often quite substantial and may need to be reduced
- the frequent use of glucose drinks such as Lucozade and other sugar-rich drinks should be discouraged.

3.9.4 East African people

Some dietary characteristics of this group are summarized in Table 3.24.

3.9.5 Chinese people

Food has a prominent position in Chinese culture and is used as a major way of marking family, religious and social events. The dietary pattern is believed to be an important determinant of the body's 'balance' and state of health, and manipulations of this pattern to restore equilibrium lost as a result of disease or changes in physiological status may have considerable influence on food habits.

Table 3.24 Typical East African meal structure (compiled by the BDA's DHIVA Group)

Food group	Examples	Notes
Carbohydrates (staples)	Starchy fruits: matooke/cooking banana	Usually steamed or boiled
	Roots: cassava, sweet potato, yam, 'Irish' potato	Large portions usually eaten at a meal
	Grains: maize, millet, sorghum, rice	Maize meal/millet sometimes made into a porridge with water for breakfast or made into more solid 'food' to eat at main meals.
Protein	Fish (tilapia) Chicken, beef, goat Legumes Groundnuts	Usually cooked as a sauce or soup with a base of onions, tomatoes and seasoning Groundnuts made into a sauce and often served with dried fish
Fruit and vegetables	Green leafy vegetables, e.g. spinach Wide variety of fruit Freshly squeezed juice	Added to sauces above Fruit eaten as a snack
Desserts rarely eaten		

Traditional dietary practices

Regional variations

China is a vast country and not surprisingly there is considerable variation in food choice and cuisine within its regions as a result of the different climatic and geographical influences on crop production and the availability of non-locally produced foods. In broad terms, dietary customs can be divided into those of the rice-growing areas in the southern and central parts of the country, and those of the wheat- and mixed grain-producing regions in the north. Within this division, four distinctive cuisines can be identified (usually named after the large cities which have been the focus of their development), although many other minor variants exist.

Northern China (Peking/Beijing)   Northern China is the main wheat-growing area, and wheat-based foods are major dietary components. Wheat-flour dumplings are a particularly common dietary feature; these may be steamed or perhaps stuffed with a sweet or savoury filling and boiled or shallow fried. Other wheat-containing items such as noodles and bread are also common features. A sandwich may be created by filling pockets of wheat-flour bread (similar to pitta) with thinly sliced and flavoured barbecued meat.

Peking cuisine developed around the royal court, and hence emphasis is placed on the presentation of dishes and the exquisiteness of recipes. Liberal use is made of strongly flavoured ingredients such as peppers, garlic, ginger, leek and coriander. Oil is used lavishly in cooking and dishes tend to be more energy dense than those of other regions.

Southern China (Canton)   As in much of South-East Asia, rice is a major dietary component in this region: a meal without rice is not considered a meal at all. As well as being consumed boiled, rice is also made into flour, noodles, cakes, confectionery and many fermented products (e.g. vinegars).

Wheat is also imported from northern China, and bread and other baked products have become increasingly popular in areas exposed to Western influence, such as Hong Kong.

To many non-Chinese, Cantonese cooking is typified by dishes such as chop suey and sweet and sour pork. In fact, these are Western modifications of Chinese dishes which bear little resemblance to the authentic style of cooking. True Cantonese food contains little sugar, and sweet and sour dishes are rare. Instead, Cantonese cuisine is known for its fresh and delicate flavours. Typically, freshly bought ingredients are prepared the same day and cooked just before serving, using little oil or spicy seasonings. Much more characteristic of Cantonese cooking are stir-fried dishes, often flavoured with black beans. Commonly used foods are meat and seafood (often together in the same dish), cured meats (sausage, pork and duck), fried rice, fried noodles and a variety of finely cut vegetables.

Cantonese are famous for their 'small eats' (dim sum). These are simple snacks which can now either be purchased in Britain ready-made and chilled, or eaten in a restaurant. The snacks consist of chopped meat, seafood and vegetables wrapped up in a wafer-thin coating of pastries or dough and then either steamed, braised, fried or boiled. Dim sum differs from other kinds of Chinese eating since a variety of small savoury and sweet items is consumed throughout the meal. In southern China and Hong Kong, dim sum is traditionally eaten at breakfast and mid-afternoon. Among immigrant Chinese populations in the UK, its consumption tends to be confined to weekends, often with family and friends in restaurants.

Hakka cuisine is also characteristic of this region, typified by the style of cooking which usually involves using every part of an animal.

Western China (Szechuan-Hunan and Yunnan)   In the west of China, Szechuan cooking is distinguished by:

- intensive use of hot spices such as fugara (brown pepper), chillies, garlic and pepper oil
- extensive use of dairy products such as yoghurt, cheese and fried milk curd (unlike most other regions of China)
- wide use of nuts, poultry and pork
- use of mountain products such as game or fungi
- noodles and steamed bread being eaten in preference to rice
- common use of salting, drying, smoking and pickling as a means of food preservation.

Characteristic dishes include hot and sour soup, camphor and tea smoked duck, beef with dried tangerine peels and an oily walnut paste and sugar dessert.

Eastern China (Shanghai)   Shanghai, a port in eastern China, does not have a traditional cuisine of its own but comprises a variety of cuisines from the surrounding provinces. Particular features of the diet are:

- Dishes are usually cooked for longer and contain much more oil (usually vegetable) than dishes of other regions.
- There is great emphasis on soups, stews and rich meaty stocks and all sorts of congee (rice porridge). Soup bases are commonly made from fishballs, turtle meat, fungi or small clams.
- A wide variety of seawater and freshwater products is used.
- Pork, coagulated pig and poultry blood, cabbage and soya beans are commonly used.
- Noodles are more common than rice and often mixed with soups and other dishes.

Food choices

Cereal foods   Rice, wheat and maize (corn) are all staple components of Chinese diets, with rice predominating in southern areas and wheat-containing foods in the north.

Rice, as well as being boiled, is made into flour, noodles, cakes and fermented products such as vinegar.

Wheat flour is used to make dumplings, noodles and bread. Wheat gluten (separated from the starch) is widely used to make imitation meats in vegetarian cookery.

Maize may be used to make foods such as noodles or cornmeal cakes and is also used in the production of alcohol.

Pulses, legumes and nuts

Soybeans are widely used, being used either to make beancurd or in the production of fermented products such as soy sauce.

Mung beans are also used to make beancurd and the resulting beanstarch is used to make fine transparent noodles. Beansprouts are usually also derived from mung beans.

Red beans such as adzuki, kidney and rice are boiled and used as constituents in soups.

Fresh green beans, often long ones, are commonly sliced into sections and used in stir-fries.

Nuts only play a minor role in most types of cuisine, the most commonly used varieties being walnuts, chestnuts, hazelnuts, pine nuts and ginkgo nuts.

Vegetables and fruits

Most vegetables are of the green leafy or gourd variety (e.g. Chinese broccoli, flowering cabbage and water melon). All parts of China rely on vegetables from the cabbage and onion family, but other fruits and vegetables differ between the north and south. The north is the land of peaches, jujubes, apricots, apples and turnips, while the southern rice region uses citrus, lychees, banana, taro and lotus.

Green leafy vegetables of the cabbage (brassica) family such as Chinese cabbage, paak choi and mustard greens are the most commonly eaten vegetables.

Spinach may also be used in clear soups.

Lettuce and watercress may also be components of soups but are never eaten on their own (as in a European salad).

Spring onion is used as a garnish or meal component.

Seaweeds may be used as a vegetable and in soups.

Fungi: many types of Chinese mushroom (e.g. shitake and straw mushrooms) are commonly eaten and various types of dried bracket fungi used as ingredients in dishes.

Aubergine, tomato and chilli peppers are used.

Fruits may be used as vegetables, such as various types of melon (squash, pumpkin and cucumber) and gourds. Particular varieties of melon seeds may also be consumed.

Fruit is usually eaten green, or salted and pickled. Such fruits include peach, apricot, apple, Chinese pears, Chinese cherry, loquat, jujube (Chinese date) and carambola (star fruit).

Citrus fruits such as orange, mandarins, tangerines, pomero and kumquat are also popular.

Animal foods

Most animal products are eaten, depending mainly on their availability.

Fish: many types of fish and seafood are eaten. Fresh lobsters, crabs and shrimps are regarded as particular delicacies. Some types of seafood such as sea cucumbers or shark's fin are dried and then stewed, acting like a sponge absorbing the flavours of other foods cooked with them. Marine white fish, either steamed or made into fishballs, are also popular. Salted fish (used as a traditional means of preservation) is also commonly eaten.

Meat: Pork and chicken are the most commonly eaten types of meat, particularly in the south. Mutton is a more important meat in the north. Beef is eaten but not widely available. Meat derived from other animals and birds, such as water buffalo, dog, rabbit, duck, guinea fowl and pigeon is eaten in some areas depending on custom and availability.

Milk and dairy products   These do not feature in the diets of most Chinese people and are only common among the nomadic people in the west.

Fats and oils   Vegetable oil is usually used in Chinese cooking, derived from either rapeseed or, increasingly, peanut oil. Lard is occasionally used.

Herbs, spices and flavourings

Chinese food uses less herbal and spice flavouring than in other parts of Asia. Those which are most commonly used are:

- *spices*: ginger, and lesser use of star anise, brown pepper, cassia bark
- *herbs*: coriander leaves and chives
- *Flavourings*: mainly derived from fermented beans or their products such as soy sauce, soyabean pastes or pickled bean curd.

Festival food includes moon cakes, eaten to mark the August Moon Festival, which coincides with the end of the harvest year. These are sweetened, mashed lotus nuts which are encased in a thin, sweet pastry which sometimes contains duck egg. Glutinous rice (sweet or savoury and sometimes stuffed with meat) is eaten at the time of the Dragon Boat Festival. It is served wrapped in lotus leaves and then steamed.

The diet of immigrant Chinese children and young Chinese adults is normally very Westernized. Popular foods are white bread, beefburgers, pork chops, ham, bacon, peas, butter, crisps, chips and those from fast-food outlets. Lamb and frozen vegetables are less commonly eaten. Elderly people still consume the more traditional diet but often incorporate Western foods such as white bread and cornflakes for convenience at breakfast (Chan 1991).

Food preparation

Most of the staple foods in the Chinese diet (e.g. rice or wheat dumplings) are cooked by being boiled. Other prominent dietary components such as soups and stews will also be boiled.

More delicately flavoured items such as aquatic foods and dim sum are more likely to be steamed (usually by placing them on slatted wooden or bamboo trays over boiling water).

Roasting is used as a cooking method for items such as pork, chicken and duck.

Baking has become more common in areas exposed to Western influence, with items such as cakes, tartlets and buns being produced in this way. However, in northern China, where wheat consumption has always been common, buns made from wheat flour and sesame seeds have traditionally been baked by sticking them to the sides of a large pot or pot-shaped oven.

Fried foods are stir fried. Oil is heated until it smokes, than meat and vegetables sliced into small pieces are tossed into it and rapidly stirred around the searingly hot pan so that the food cooks without being burnt. This usually only takes a few seconds. Larger pieces of fish, poultry and egg may be cooked for longer with more oil and less stirring.

It is also a common practice to cook a food item by sequential methods. For example, a food may be smoked, then boiled and finally stir-fried. Alternatively, it may be partly boiled, then set aside until needed and the cooking processed completed by further additional boiling as part of another dish, or by another cooking method.

Meal pattern

This depends on the degree of Westernization. Most children and young adults will consume a Western-style breakfast and lunch, and only the evening meal is likely to be typically Chinese. Older adults are more likely to maintain traditional customs.

The Chinese style of eating, particularly in the evening, is usually a communal affair where everyone helps themselves to dishes placed in the centre of the table. The bite-sized pieces are easily picked up by chopsticks and often dipped into various complementary sauces to enhance their flavour. For example, steamed chicken may be dipped into minced ginger, scallion and oil; roast chicken may be dipped into peppercorn-flavoured salt or Worcestershire sauce. Soy sauce and chilli sauce are also popular. The Chinese like hot foods to be served very hot (in temperature).

Breakfast Traditionally, this consists of congee (a type of porridge), steamed buns, rice or noodles. The congee may contain soya bean sticks and nuts or chicken or fish. However, this is time-consuming to prepare and most people, even older adults, eat a Western-style breakfast such as egg and ham with toast, breakfast cereals with milk, or a combination of Chinese and Western foods (such as cheese with Chinese bread). Some drink tea with milk.

Main meals The midday or evening meal consists of the staple such as rice or wheat noodles or dumplings with several main dishes, usually containing meat, poultry or fish. Bean curd or tofu may be used as an alternative to meat. A clear soup (made from meat or poultry stock with added herbs or vegetables) and at least one vegetable dish are also likely to be served. Fried rice is eaten usually only at the end of a special meal.

Desserts Traditionally, desserts are not usually eaten, but fresh fruits, especially oranges, are often consumed after a meal.

Snacks Fruit is also eaten as a snack between meals, as are cakes, nuts and biscuits.

Beverages The most popular drinks are hot water and tea. Coffee is not commonly consumed. Sweet liquid drinks, *tong sui*, may be taken as an afternoon snack and may be included at the end of the evening meal on special occasions. These are comprised of an unrefined cane sugar base to which a variety of ingredients is added such as:

- sweet potato chunks and a little root ginger
- red mung beans and dried citrus peel
- soya bean shoots and nuts
- beans, ground roasted peanuts and dried citrus peel
- sago or tapioca soup with coconut cream.

Alcoholic drinks tend to be used either for medicinal purposes or during celebrations such as birthdays and weddings. The most popular types of alcohol are spirits such as brandy or whisky, and fortified wines such as sherry or port. Herbs steeped in brandy or whisky are popular among older people.

Yin and yang

According to traditional Chinese medicine, good health depends on a balance of two opposite elements (in the body), yin and yang. In illness, the balance is disturbed and the body becomes too 'hot' (an excess of yang) or too 'cold' (an excess of yin). Each individual has a body base or equilibrium point. This is not a fixed point but varies according to the person's age and also during pregnancy and lactation. In general, infants and young children are thought to be on the 'hot' side of the hot–cold equilibrium, whereas women and older people lie on the 'cold' side. A person is seen as being healthy when his or her equilibrium is maintained.

A person's base can be shifted through diet, drugs, tonics, herbs and the weather. The healthy state is maintained (when the body is not invaded by an outside agent such as a virus) by readjusting the base to equilibrium.

Diet is believed to play an important role in maintaining the individual's normal healthy balance and in correcting imbalances. Different foods have different properties: some are 'heating', some 'cooling' and some 'neutral'. Different cooking methods have different properties. A person whose body equilibrium was on the 'cold' side of the scale would avoid 'cold' foods. It is important to take these considerations into account when giving dietary advice. Some general guidelines on Chinese 'hot' and 'cold' foods are given in Table 3.25, although it must be borne in mind that there may be variations in this classification, and in the extent to which it is followed.

The concept of yin and yang is particularly relevant in illness and pregnancy. Pregnancy is thought of as a 'hot' condition and a pregnant woman may cut down on red meat and some types of fish. A traditional stew, *keung chow*, made from pigs' trotters and boiled eggs soaked in vinegar and ginger, is given to a woman after childbirth to help recovery and in celebration of the birth of a child. Childbirth is often followed by the practice known as 'doing the month', where the lactating woman is 'confined' to the house for a month after birth to avoid disease in the future (e.g. to avoid catching 'wind' which might manifest as arthritis in later years, Pillsbury 1978). During this time a woman will avoid raw and 'cold' foods and will be encouraged to consumed 'hot' ones in order to regain strength.

Other influences of yin and yang in physiological and disease states include:

- Infant formula milk is seen as very 'hot', so a Chinese mother may want to give her bottle-fed baby 'cooling' drinks such as boiled water or barley water.
- A lactating mother may want to eat 'cooling' foods because they may impart 'cool' properties to the breast milk.
- Foods used during convalescence include steamed white fish, finely minced meat, congee and chicken essence.
- Elderly people tend to avoid 'cold' foods.

Table 3.25 General guidelines on the Chinese classification of foods

	'Cold' foods	'Neutral' foods	'Hot' foods
Food	Most fruit Vegetables Barley water Some herbal teas	White fish Rice, bread Papaya Orange Beancurd	Oily fish, meat Alcoholic drinks Ginger, spices Some fruit, e.g. mango, pineapple Fried foods
Cooking method	Boiling	Deep frying Steaming	Roasting Stir-frying 'warm')

In addition to yin and yang, people may hold other traditional beliefs in the therapeutic qualities of certain foods and dishes; for example, that snakemeat combats rheumatism and female frogs are an antidote for asthma.

Nutritional implications of Chinese diets

The high sodium intake of some Chinese people as a result of the widespread use of monosodium glutamate (MSG) used to be of some concern, but MSG is now used less often in domestic cooking.

Lack of calcium is likely to be a more significant problem, due to the typically low level of consumption of milk and dairy products, particularly among older Chinese immigrants. Bean curd is an important source of calcium in Chinese diets and if neither milk nor bean curd is regularly consumed, calcium intake is likely to be inadequate.

Fibre intake (particularly of cereal fibre) may be low as Chinese people eat few wholegrain cereals. Fruit and vegetable consumption, however, tends to be high.

Common health problems in Chinese people

Thalassaemia
Alpha-zero-thalassaemia is an important genetic risk for people originating from Hong Kong, Singapore, Vietnam, Thailand, the Philippines and south China.

Hepatitis B infection
There is estimated to be between 10 and 20% carriage of hepatitis B virus among South-East Asian Chinese (House of Commons Report, 1985).

Cancer
Cancers of the nasopharynx, oesophagus and liver are particularly common among Chinese people and may be linked with the traditionally high consumption of salted, smoked and pickled foods. There is some evidence that the prevalence of these cancers is lower in Chinese migrants born in Western countries such as the USA, but the prevalence of other cancers such as those of the colon, lung and breast is higher (Cruickshank and Beevers 1989). Cigarette smoking (common among Chinese men) is a strong predictor of cancer risk and mortality.

Cardiovascular disease
The prevalence of stroke and coronary artery disease has also increased in Chinese people, along with increasing industrialization and adoption of more Westernized lifestyles. Cigarette smoking in men and hypertension are particularly prevalent risk factors.

Dental caries
The prevalence of caries among Chinese children is much higher than in other ethnic minority groups and indigenous white children, largely because of the lack of routine dental care (teeth may only be wiped with a cloth or cotton buds, or not at all) and the lack of use of dental services.

Providing dietary guidance to Chinese people

In addition to the distinctive but variable dietary customs of this population group, problems with communication may add to the difficulties in providing dietary guidance. Many first-generation Chinese speak little English and some cannot read Chinese. Western medical treatment (including dietary treatment) may also be supplemented by traditional Chinese strategies and herbal remedies, especially by the older generation.

Several organizations have produced, or are developing, resource material for use in this client group and details of these can be found at the end of this section (see Useful Resources).

3.9.6 Vietnamese people

Vietnamese civilization has its origins in China but has gradually developed its own distinctive traditions. France, as a colonial power, has also exerted some influence on Vietnamese culture. Many of the Vietnamese community in Britain are ethnic Chinese and speak Cantonese. Some also speak Vietnamese or French and many now speak English.

Traditional dietary practices of Vietnamese people

Given the strong southern Chinese influence, many Cantonese dishes are familiar to the Vietnamese. Some, such as Vietnamese spring rolls, have been adapted. Chopsticks and bowls are used.

The Chinese concept of yin and yang also plays a part in Vietnamese life. There are, however, major differences between the Chinese and Vietnamese cuisine and these lie in the seasonings used, the cooking methods employed and the differing emphasis on basic ingredients.

Regional variations

Vietnam can be divided into three regions, each with its own cuisine.

In the north, food tends to have the smallest variety of ingredients and spices, and is somewhat lighter and less spicy. Black pepper is widely used as a condiment. Although seafood, particularly crab, is popular, fish constitutes a surprisingly minor part of the diet. Stir-fried dishes appear more frequently, perhaps due to the greater Chinese influence.

In the central area of Vietnam, the cuisine is famous for its highly decorative presentation of foods. Meals consist of small portions of many dishes. Foods are very spicy and there is frequent use of hot chilli peppers and shrimp sauce.

In the south, the diet includes a great variety of vegetables, fruits, meat and game. A French influence is apparent by the use in the fondues, and there is more frequent use of vegetables such as white potatoes and asparagus. Sugar and sugar cane are used widely.

Although each region has its own style, the lines of distinction between them are blurred (Ngo and Zimmerman 1986). People from the north eat dishes typical of the south and vice versa.

Food choices

Starchy foods   Rice is the main cereal staple and is served either boiled or fried at main meals. Rice grown in Vietnam is a useful source of iron and calcium.

Starchy vegetables such as cassava, sliced green bananas, coconut, maize, peanut, soya beans, sugar cane and sweet potatoes may also be served.

Vegetables   Fresh, uncooked vegetables and salads are an integral part of many Vietnamese meals, and lettuce, cucumber, coriander and mint (of which there are many varieties) are almost always included. Shallots are used in great abundance, as are fresh herbs such as lemon grass. Vegetables are cooked only lightly, if at all, and bear little resemblance to British cooked vegetables.

Milk and dairy foods   Fresh milk is not available in Vietnam and so tends not to be used much in the diet, but some use is made of evaporated and sweetened condensed milk. Cheese is only eaten in small amounts and is usually of a processed type.

Fats and oils   Vegetable oils or lard are used in stir-fry cooking. Butter and margarine are used sparingly.

Snacks   Roast nuts, sweet potato, rice or noodle soup, rice with shreds of meat, spring rolls and fresh fruit are popular snacks between meals.

Seasonings   A commonly used Vietnamese seasoning is *nuoc mam,* a fermented salted fish sauce. Nuoc mam is combined with garlic, chilli peppers, fresh lime and sugar to give a sauce which takes the place of salt at the table. In Britain, when this is not available, dark soy sauce is used instead. Other popular flavourings are vinegar, chilli sauce and MSG.

Beverages   Tea, coffee and fruit juice are the usual drinks. Alcohol tends to be used for celebrations.

Unpopular foods   These include lamb, ox liver and tinned or cooked fruit.

Cooking methods   Barbecuing is an important cooking method in Vietnam and some dishes must be barbecued at the table. Simmering, long, slow cooking in a covered pan, with liquid, over charcoal is also popular.

Festivals   The Vietnamese calendar includes a number of festivals with associated traditional foods and meals. The main festival of New Year, in late January/early February, is celebrated over 7 days. Rice cakes, soya-bean soup, fruit and seeds are enjoyed, and the end of the celebrations is marked with a special feast.

Within the family, special ritual meals are associated with births, weddings, anniversaries and funerals.

Nutritional and health implications of Vietnamese diets

With its emphasis on rice as a staple part of the diet and minimal use of fat in cooking, the Vietnamese diet tends to be low in fat. Possible dietary problems as are follows.

Low calcium intake

Calcium intake may be low in the diet of Vietnamese people in Britain because:

- rice grown in Vietnam contains much more calcium than the rice imported into Britain
- fruit and vegetables in the UK contain less calcium than some tropical varieties
- milk and cheese are only consumed in small amounts, if at all.

Vitamin D deficiency

Low vitamin D intake has been identified in some Vietnamese children. In Vietnam the principal source of this nutrient in sunlight, and oral supplements may be necessary for those living in Britain.

3.9.7 Jewish people

Judaism is an ancient religion. Many Jewish people in Britain were born here, sometimes to families who have been resident in the UK for several generations. Most originate from Europe and some from the Middle East. For the majority, English is their native language. Some traditional dietary practices of Jewish people are summmarized below.

Jewish dietary laws

The Jewish people, like all other peoples, have food customs traditionally associated with their daily lives, their holidays and festivals. In addition to these, regulations are prescribed in a code of dietary laws (Kashrut), from the slaughter of animals used for food, to the kinds of dishes prepared for special holidays, festivals and the Sabbath. These food traditions have accumulated through the long, historical experience of the Jewish people. Maintenance of health and food hygiene underlie these laws, which are:

- The flesh of animals which may be used for food are quadrupeds that chew the cud and have cloven hoofs such as sheep, goats, deer and cattle. Pork and all products of the pig are forbidden.
- Permitted birds are chicken, duck, goose and turkey. Birds of prey, which are more prone to disease than herbivorous birds, are forbidden.
- Fish with scales and fins are allowed. Shellfish are not allowed as they are considered to be a source of disease. Fish does not have to be killed or koshered in any way.
- Meats must not be cooked with milk or milk derivatives, or be served at the same meal. Utensils, crockery, china pots and pans used for milk and meat must be stored, washed and dried separately.
- Animals and birds must be slaughtered by the Jewish method; this procedure, which must be carried out by a trained and authorized person, entails a rapid cut with a sharp knife to sever the jugular vein and carotid artery. The meat is then salted and soaked in water to remove the blood and render it kosher (permitted).

Festivals and fasting (the main holy days)

The seventh day of the week is the Sabbath, a day of prayer at synagogue and complete freedom from work. Sabbath begins at sundown on Friday and ends when the first star becomes visible on Saturday evening. On Friday night the Sabbath meal is served. No preparation of food is done on the Sabbath, but food prepared in advance is eaten.

The Jewish year is based on lunar calculations. The beginning of the Hebrew calendar is marked by the holiday called Rosh Hashanah (September). On the New Year it is customary to serve apple slices dipped in a bowl of honey, signifying the heart-felt yearning for a sweet and happy year.

Ten days after Rosh Hashanah is the Day of Atonement (Yom Kippur). This is the holiest day of the Jewish calendar and one of prayer and repentance. It is also a fast day; no food or drink is permitted for 25 hours (from sundown to sunset).

Passover, which commemorates the exodus of Jews from Egypt, is celebrated for 8 days in April. No foods made with wheat, barley, oats or rye may be eaten. Unleavened bread (matzo) is eaten in place of normal bread, and cakes and biscuits are made from matzo meal.

Text revised by: Briony Thomas

Acknowledgements: Aruna Thaker, Nuzhat Ali, Verona Bryant, Wynnie Chan, KaYee Chan, Usha Chappiti, Sarah Jean-Marie, Ruth Kander, Surinder Ghatoray, Azmina Govindji, Farhat Hamid, Avni Vyas, Sunita Wallia and other members of the British Dietetic Association's Multi-Cultural Nutrition Group.

Useful addresses

British Dietetic Association's Multi-Cultural Nutrition Group
c/o The British Dietetic Association, 5th Floor Charles House, 148–9 Great Charles Street, Birmingham B3 3HT
Tel: 0121 200 8080

Diabetes UK (formerly the British Diabetic Association)
10 Queen Anne Street, London W1M 0BD
Tel: 020 7323 1531

British Nutrition Foundation
High Holborn House, 52–54 High Holborn, London WC1V 6RQ
Tel: 020 7404 6504

Health Development Agency (formerly the Health Education Authority)
Trevelyan House, 30 Great Peter Street, London SW1 2HW
Tel: 020 7222 5300
Website: www.hda-online.org.uk

London Beth Din (for Kosher food enquiries)
735 High Road, London N12 0US
Tel: 020 8343 6259
Website: www.kosher.org.uk

The Muslim Food Board (UK)
PO Box 1786, Leicester LE5 5ZE
Tel: 0116 273 8228
Website: www.halaal.org

Useful resources

Many excellent dietetic resources have produced for use with South Asian, African-Caribbean, Chinese and other ethnic minority clients. Materials available range from health promotional materials such as adaptations of *The Balance of Good Health* to dietary guidance for conditions such as obesity and diabetes, often written in a variety of languages. For details of resources currently available and how they may be obtained, contact the British Dietetic Association's Multi-Cultural Nutrition Group (for address see above).

Local community and religious leaders may be able to help with general information, translation of leaflets and the establishment of contacts with relevant individuals or groups. Local temples and religious establishments or local council offices may be a useful starting point of contact.

Local health-promotion units may have produced resource material relevant to local minority groups.

Local voluntary organizations who cater for relevant communities may be a useful source of support when producing resources.

Further reading

Ethnicity in the 1991 Census
Volume 1: *Demographic Characteristics of Ethnic Minority Populations*. Coleman D, Salt J (Eds.). London: HMSO, 1996.
Volume 2: *The Ethnic Minority Populations of Great Britain*. Peach C (Eds.). London: HMSO, 1996.
Volume 3: *Social Geography and Ethnicity in Britain: Geographical Spread, Spatial Concentration and Internal Migration*. Ratcliffe P (Ed). London: HMSO, 1996.
Volume 4: *Employment, Education and Housing Among the Ethnic Minority Populations of Britain*. Karn V (Ed). London: Stationery Office, 1997.
Health Education Authority. *Nutrition in Minority Ethnic groups*. Asians and Afro-Caribbeans in the United Kingdom. Briefing Paper. HEA: London, 1993.
Health Education Authority. *Health-related Resources for Black and Minority Ethnic Groups*. London: HEA, 1994.
Judd PA, Kassam-Khamis T, Thomas JE. *The Composition and Nutrient Content of Foods Commonly Consumed by South Asians in the UK*. London: The Aga Khan Health Board for the United Kingdom, 2000.
Tan SP, Wenlock RW, Buss DH. *Second Supplement to McCance and Widdowson's The Composition of Foods*, 4th edn: *Immigrant Foods*. London: HMSO; Cambridge: Royal Society of Chemistry, 1985.

References

Bailey C, Day C. Traditional plant medicines as treatment for diabetes. *Diabetes Care* 1989; **12**: 553–561.

Balarajan R. Ethnic differences in mortality from ischaemic heart disease and cerebrovascular disease in England and Wales. *British Medical Journal* 1991; **302**: 560–564.

Balarajan R. Ethnicity and variations in the nation's health. *Health Trends* 1995; **27**: 114–119.

Balarajan R, Raleigh VS. The ethnic populations of England and Wales: the 1991 Census. *Health Trends* 1993; **24**: 113–116.

Balarajan R, Raleigh VS. *Ethnicity and Health in England*. London: HMSO, 1995.

Beevers G, Beevers M. Hypertension: impact upon black and ethnic minority people. In: Hopkins A, Bahl V (Eds). *Access to Health Care for People from Black and Ethnic Minorities*. London: Royal College of Physicians, 1993.

Burden AC, McNally PG, Feehally J, Walls J. Increased incidence of end-stage renal failure secondary to diabetes mellitus in Asian ethnic groups in the United Kingdom. *Diabetic Medicine* 1992; **9**: 641–645.

Chan W. *Concept of illness, dietary beliefs and food related health practices*. PhD Thesis, University of London, 1991.

Chaturvedi N, McKeigue PM, Marmot MG. Resting and ambulatory blood pressure differences in Afro-Caribbeans and Europeans. *Hypertension* 1993; **22**: 90–96.

Chaturvedi N, McKeigue PM, Marmot M. Relationship of glucose tolerance to coronary risk in Afro-Caribbeans compared with Europeans. *Diabetologia* 1994; **37**: 765–772.

Close CF, Lewis PG, Holder R *et al.* Diabetes care in South asian and white European patients with type 2 diabetes. *Diabetic Medicine* 1995; **12**: 619–621.

Cruickshank JK. Diabetes: contrasts between peoples of black (West African), Indian and white European origin. In Cruickshank JK, Beevers DG (Eds). *Ethnic Factors in Health and Disease*. London: Wright, 1989.

Cruickshank JK, Beevers DG (Eds). *Ethnic Factors in Health and Disease*. London: Wright, 1989.

Department of Health. *Health of the Nation: A Strategy for Health in England*. London: HMSO, 1992.

Douglas J. *Caribbean Food and Diet, Food and Diet in a Multiracial Society*. Cambridge: National Extension College, 1987.

Goodwin AM, Keen H, Mather HM. Ethnic minorities in British Diabetic clinics: a questionnaire survey. *Diabetic Medicine* 1987; **4**: 266–269.

Govindi A. Dietary advice for the Asian diabetic. *Practical Diabetes* 1991; **8**: 202–203.

Gray A, Flatt P. Nature's own pharmacy: the diabetes perspective. *Proceedings of the Nutrition Society* 1997; **56**: 506–517.

Gregory JR, Collins DL, Davies PSW *et al. National Diet and Nutrition Survey of Children Aged $1\frac{1}{2}$–$4\frac{1}{2}$ Years*. London: HMSO, 1995.

Grell GAC. Management of hypertension in the Caribbean: the Jamaican perspective. In Cruickshank JK, Beevers DG (Eds). *Ethnic Factors in Health and Disease*. London: Wright, 1989.

Hawthorne K. Asian diabetics attending a British hospital clinic: a pilot study to evaluate their care. *British Journal of General Practice* 1990; **40**: 243–247.

Health Education Authority. *Nutrition in Minority Ethnic groups*. Asians and Afro-Caribbeans in the United Kingdom. Briefing Paper. London: HEA; 1993.

Health Education Authority. *Health and Lifestyles: Black and Minority Ethnic Groups in England*. London: Hea, 1995.

House of Commons Home Affairs Report Committee 1984–1985. *The Chinese Community in Britain*. Vols I and II. London: HMSO, 1985.

Iqbal SJ, Kaddam I, Wassif W *et al*. Continuing clinical severe vitamin D deficiency in Asians in the UK (Leicester). *Postgraduate Medical Journal* 1994; **70**: 708–714.

Judd PA, Kassam-Khamis T, Thomas JE. *The Composition and Nutrient Content of Foods Commonly Consumed by South Asians in the UK*. London: Aga Khan Health Board for the United Kingdom, 2000.

Kaplan NM. Ethnic aspects of hypertension. *Lancet* 1994; **344**: 450–451.

Lawson MS, Thomas M, Hardiman A. Iron status of Asian children aged 2 years living in England. *Archives of Disease in Childhood* 1998; **78**: 420–426.

McKeigue P, Sevak L. *Coronary Heart Disease in South Asian Communities: A Manual for Health Promotion*. London: Health Education Authority, 1994.

Morgan M. The significance of ethnicity for health promotion: patients' use of anti-hypertensive drugs in inner London. *International Journal of Epidemiology* 1995; **24** (Suppl 1): S79–S84.

Ngo B, Zimmerman G. *The Classic Cuisine of Vietnam*. Ontario: Penguin Books, 1986.

Pillsbury B. Doing the month: confinement and convalescence of Chinese women after childbirth. *Social Science and Medicine* 1978; **11**: 22.

Raleigh VS. Diabetes and hypertension in Britain's ethnic minorities: implications for the future of renal services. *British Medical Journal* 1997; **314**: 209– 213.

Raleigh VS, Balarajan R. Public health and the 1991 census. *British Medical Journal* 1994; **309**: 287–288.

Roderick PJ, Raleigh VS, Hallam L, Mallick NP. The need and demand for renal replacement therapy among ethnic minorities in England. *Journal of Epidemiology and Community Health* 1996; **50**: 334–339.

Sharma S, Cade J, Jackson M *et al*. Development of food frequency questionnaires in three population samples of African origin from Cameroon, Jamaica and Caribbean migrants to the UK. *European Journal of Clinical Nutrition* 1996; **50**: 479–486.

Simmons D, Williams DDR, Powell MJ. Prevalence of diabetes in a predominantly Asian community: preliminary findings of the Coventry diabetes study. *British Medical Journal* 1989; **298**: 18–21.

Springer L, Thomas J. Rastafarians in Britain. A preliminary study of their food habits and beliefs. *Human Nutrition: Applied Nutrition* 1983; **37a**: 120–127.

Stewart JA, Dundas R, Howard RS *et al*. Ethnic differences in incidence of stroke: prospective study with a stroke register. *British Medical Journal* 1999; **318**: 967–971.

Thomas M, Avery V. *Infant Feeding in Asian Families: Early Feeding Practices and Growth*. London: The Stationery Office, 1997.

UK Prospective Diabetes Study Group. UK Prospective Diabetes Study XII: differences between Asian, Afro-Caribbean and white Caucasian type 2 diabetic patients at diagnosis of diabetes. *Diabetic Medicine* 1994; **11**: 670–677.

3.10 Vegetarianism and veganism

Increasing numbers of people are choosing to follow a vegetarian diet. In 1997, 5.4% of the British adult population claimed to be vegetarian and an additional 8.9% avoided red meat (Realeat 1997), compared with 2.1% and 2.6%, respectively, in 1984 (Realeat 1984). Vegetarianism is more common amongst women (6.5% compared with 4.1% of the male population); and approximately 23% of women aged 16–34 years eat no red meat. There are more vegetarians amongst social classes AB and C1 (6.1% and 6.7%) than C2 and DE (3.9% and 4.6%). Vegetarianism is least popular in Scotland (3.3%). There are approximately 250 000 vegans in Britain (Realeat 1997).

3.10.1 Type of vegetarian diets

People adopt vegetarian diets for a variety of reasons, including religion and culture (see Section 3.9, People from ethnic minority groups); moral and ethical beliefs (animal welfare); health; environmental, ecological and economic concerns. As a result, vegetarianism often involves not just an eating pattern but a philosophy which affects the whole lifestyle. There is wide variation in vegetarian dietary practices, so it is essential that health professionals do not assume what an individual's diet may involve, but investigate the extent and variety of food exclusions, and any associated food and health beliefs. Even lacto-ovovegetarians can differ in their level of exclusion (Table 3.26). For example, some may just avoid obvious sources of meat, poultry and fish, while those following current guidelines from The Vegetarian Society will avoid:

- eggs unless they are free range
- manufactured foods containing genetically modified (GM) ingredients (except for cheese containing GM chymosin)

- milk derivatives such as whey and skimmed milk powder
- cheese produced using animal rennet
- food additives derived from animal sources, e.g. edible bone phosphate (E542), cochineal (E120), emulsifiers E471 and E471a (these latter two also have non-animal sources)
- wine 'fined' with isinglass, chitin, gelatine or egg albumin (if non-free range).

The most common types of vegetarian diets are outlined in Table 3.26. In this section, the term 'vegetarian' will refer to lacto-ovovegetarians.

3.10.2 Health implications of vegetarian diets

The vegetarian population is very heterogeneous and there can be both benefits and drawbacks to vegetarian and vegan diets. Their 'healthiness' will depend on how nutritionally well balanced the particular vegetarian diet is, relative to individual needs. Overall, vegetarians appear to have a lower mortality from some chronic diseases and a lower incidence of chronic disease risk factors (Thorogood 1994). However, it is important to remember that people who choose to exclude meat from their diet are also more likely to modify other aspects of their diet and lifestyle, e.g. to eat more fruit, vegetables and wholegrains, not smoke, drink less alcohol and be more active. To what degree the apparent health benefits are distinct from lifestyle effects, and due to the vegetarian diet and/or not eating meat *per se*, continues to be investigated. However, current evidence suggests that all of these factors play contributory roles (Willett 1999).

Table 3.26 Common types of vegetarian diets

Type of vegetarian	Characteristics
Demivegetarian or Semivegetarian	Excludes red meat, but usually eats fish and/or poultry
Piscatarian	Eats fish but excludes red meat and poultry
Lacto-ovovegetarian	Excludes all meat, poultry, fish, shellfish and ingredients derived from them e.g. gelatine, rennet. Eats dairy products and eggs (although possibly only of free-range origin)
Vegan	Excludes all animal flesh and products, derived ingredients and additives
Fruitarian	A type of vegan diet which consists mainly of raw fruit, vegetables, nuts, seeds, sprouted pulses and grains
Macrobiotic	Based on the Chinese philosophy of yin and yang. Aims to balance foods which contain qualities of these two opposing but complementary forces of nature. Has seven levels which become increasingly restrictive. Lower levels are most varied and contain fish but still exclude all meat, poultry, eggs and dairy products. The highest level consists only of brown rice.

Benefits

Vegetarian diets tend to be lower in saturated fat, and higher in starchy carbohydrates, dietary fibre, fruit and vegetables than omnivorous diets (Bull and Barber 1984; Mann *et al*. 1997; Hoffman *et al*. 1999; Key *et al*. 1999). Vegan diets are generally lower in fat, at 30–35% of energy, with saturated fat intakes comprising 5–7% of energy (Roshanai and Sanders 1984; Thorogood and Mann 1990; Haddad *et al*. 1999a). Thus, vegetarian diets more closely approach key UK dietary recommendations (DH 1991, 1994a, 1998a) than omnivorous diets.

Vegetarians tend to have a lower body mass index (Appleby *et al*. 1998) but this has not been shown in all studies (Harman and Parnell 1998). Vegetarians also tend to have lower blood lipid levels (Dwyer 1988, 1991; Melby *et al*. 1994; Thorogood 1995), and lower rates of hypertension (Thorogood 1995) and heart disease (Thorogood *et al*. 1994; Key *et al*. 1999) than non-vegetarians. Nagyova *et al*. (1998) found that vegetarians had significantly increased plasma total antioxidant status compared with non-vegetarians, which indicates a more effective protection against lipoprotein oxidation.

Past studies have indicated that vegetarians have lower mortality rates from all cancers and all causes than non-vegetarians (Thorogood *et al*. 1994). When data from five prospective studies was combined to compare the death rates from common diseases of vegetarians with those of non-vegetarians with similar lifestyles, a 24% reduction in mortality from ischaemic heart disease was found; however, there were no significant differences in mortality from cerebrovascular disease; stomach, colorectal, lung, breast and prostate cancer, or all other causes combined (Key *et al*. 1999).

A review by Dwyer (1988) highlighted evidence for lower risks of type II diabetes and gall stones. There is also evidence of benefit from a vegetarian diet for some people with rheumatoid arthritis (Kjeldsen-Kragh 1999) and for slowing the progression of chronic renal failure (Soroka *et al*. 1998). Dwyer (1991) noted that the health benefits of vegetarian diets seem to be related to both the lifestyle and diet of vegetarians, so could be achieved without totally eliminating meat from the diet.

Risks

For some individuals, adoption of a vegetarian diet is an attempt to mask their dieting behaviour from others (Martins *et al*. 1999). However, the main risk associated with vegetarian diets is nutritional deficiency, particularly amongst vegans and population subgroups with increased needs, e.g. infants, children, and pregnant or lactating women.

3.10.3 Nutritional implications of vegetarian diets

Vegetarian diets in developed countries can be nutritionally adequate if sensibly selected; problems only arise if the variety and quantity of foods is quite restricted (Sanders 1999a).

Energy

Vegetarians tend to have similar energy intakes to non-vegetarian diets (Thorogood and Mann 1990; Draper *et al*. 1993; Nathan *et al*. 1996) but intakes can be lower amongst vegans (Abdulla *et al*. 1981), especially in men (Draper *et al*. 1993). Vegan and vegetarians diets can be bulky, which is a potential problem for infants, young children and people with small appetites. It is important to ensure sufficient energy intake for growth, and to prevent the catabolism of dietary protein by including more of the energy-dense vegan foods such as nuts, nut spreads, pulses, dried fruit, soya cheese, vegetable oils and margarines, suitable cakes and biscuits (lacto-ovovegetarians can also include milk and milk products).

Protein-energy malnutrition, growth retardation and delayed psychomotor development have been reported among infants and children fed on very restrictive macrobiotic and Rastafarian diets (Truesdell and Acosta 1985; Dagnelie *et al*. 1989b). Weaning foods with a low energy density and extended unsupplemented breast feeding account for most of the cases (Jacobs and Dwyer 1988). Lower rates of growth in the first few years of life have been reported in some vegan children. They do catch up and achieve normal height and development but overall vegan children tend to be lighter in weight and leaner than omnivores (O'Connell *et al*. 1989; Sanders and Manning 1992). Lacto-ovovegetarian children have similar energy intakes and growth patterns to omnivores (Sabate *et al*. 1991; Nathan *et al*. 1996, 1997).

Protein

Historically, there have been nutritional concerns about plant foods being lower in total protein and protein quality compared with animal foods. While the percentage of energy from protein is slightly lower amongst vegetarians and vegans, intakes meet recommended levels (Draper *et al*. 1993). Vegetarians receive all of their essential amino acids from milk or eggs. For vegans, combinations of different plant sources of protein (protein complementation) also provide adequate amounts of essential amino acids, as long as energy needs are met (to prevent protein catabolism). Pulses (including peanuts) with grains, or pulses with nuts and seeds are effective combinations. Research suggests that complementary proteins do not need to be eaten at the same time and a varied intake of different amino acid sources over the day should ensure adequate nitrogen use and retention (Young and Pellett 1994). Interestingly, soya protein has a similar protein quality to animal protein when assessed using the FAO/WHO/UNU approved scoring method PDCAAS (protein digestibility corrected amino acid score) (Young 1991).

Fat

While vegetarians generally eat diets lower in saturated fat, their total fat intake is often similar to the national average due to compensatory intake of fat from other foods, e.g. cheese, nuts, vegetable fats, cakes, chocolate and processed foods (Bull and Barber 1984; Draper *et al*. 1993; Nathan *et al*. 1997).

Concern has been expressed about the balance of essential fatty acids in vegetarian diets (Sanders 1999b; British Nutrition Foundation 1999) and vegan diets (Sanders and Manning 1992), which can be especially high in linoleic acid. A high ratio of linoleic acid (18:2*n*6) to alpha-linolenic acid (18:3*n*3) fatty acids may inhibit endogenous production of the long-chain polyunsaturated fatty acids eicosapentaenoic acid (EPA) and docosahexaenoic acid (DHA), which are virtually absent from vegetarian and vegan diets (as fish and red meat are not eaten). Functions of long-chain polyunsaturates include development of new tissue, especially brain and retinal tissue, and production of eicosanoids. A poor ratio between *n*6 and *n*3 families of fatty acids may also influence the types and potency of eicosanoids formed (British Nutrition Foundation 1999). While research continues, it is recommended that vegans and vegetarians use soya, rapeseed (or olive oil) and their margarines rather than sunflower, safflower or corn oil, in order to reduce the linoleic to alpha-linolenic ratio of the diet. Including other food sources of alpha-linolenic acid, e.g. linseeds, walnuts and walnut oil, sweet potatoes, soya beans, pumpkin seeds and green leafy vegetables, is also advisable.

Carbohydrate

Vegetarian diets can be higher in carbohydrate than those of non-vegetarians (Bull and Barber 1984; Roshanai and Sanders 1984). Vegans have the highest carbohydrate intakes, providing 50–55% of total energy intake (Thorogood and Mann 1990; Draper *et al*. 1993). Total sugar intakes are similar (Draper *et al*. 1993), although the intake of sugars from fruit may be quite high. One study found that vegan children were consuming 15% of their energy as sugar, mostly in the form of fruit juice (Sanders and Manning 1992).

Dietary fibre

Vegetarians generally have fibre intakes that meet or exceed the population average dietary reference value (DRV) of 18 g/day non-starch polysaccharides, while vegans have very high fibre intakes as a result of their preference for wholegrains (Thorogood and Mann 1990; Sanders and Manning 1992; Draper *et al*. 1993). While high intakes of fibre are generally recommended, an excessive level of fibre is not advised for infants, young children and the frail elderly as it adds bulk to the diet. Replacement of some high-fibre foods with more refined cereal products and/or including more energy-dense foods is recommended.

In vitro studies highlight that plant food components such as phytic and oxalic acids complex with minerals in food and reduce their bioavailability. However, populations who regularly eat balanced high-fibre diets do not appear to have a compromised mineral status (DH 1991). Phytates are found in appreciable amounts in wholegrain cereals, pulses (especially soya beans), nuts and seeds. While refining these foods removes some of the inhibitors of absorption it also removes some of the minerals, but there is less net zinc absorption from white bread than from wholemeal bread (Turnlund 1982).

Most vegetarians and vegans have adequate mineral status (see below). However, if mineral intakes are borderline, excessive intake of foods which are fibrous, oxalate rich (spinach, nuts, peanuts, chocolate, parsley, rhubarb) or phytate rich (e.g. concentrated isolates of fibre and phytates such as wheat bran) should be avoided.

Vitamins

Vitamin intakes of vegetarians are generally adequate, but vegans can have lower than recommended intakes of vitamin B_{12}, riboflavin and vitamin D (Draper *et al*. 1993). Sources of these three vitamins are shown in Table 3.27. Vegetarians and vegans will have relatively low intakes of preformed retinol, but the typically high intakes of carotenoid-rich fruit and vegetables by these groups is considered to provide sufficient compensation.

Vitamin D

Dietary sources of vitamin D are limited to animal foods (egg yolk, oily fish, liver) and fortified foods such as margarine, soya milk and breakfast cereals. For most British people the main source is from the action of sunlight on the skin, and blood levels in winter depend on exposure during the rest of the year. Vitamin D status in adults who spend sufficient time outdoors is usually adequate, but people with darker skin appear to have less ability to meet their requirements in this way (Clemens *et al*. 1982). There have been several reports of rickets in children on Rastafarian and macrobiotic diets and some among Asian children (Jacobs and Dwyer 1988; Dagnelie *et al*. 1990). The COMA report on Diet and Bone Health (DH 1998b) recommended that the following groups should take vitamin D supplements:

- people who rarely go out of doors or wear clothes that fully conceal them
- babies, young children and pregnant women from Asian communities
- young African–Caribbean children on strict vegan diets
- older people who eat no meat or fish, or who live in residential care, or who are housebound.

Vegetarian Asians appear to have a blunted response to increases in serum vitamin D levels after exposure to summer sunshine, compared with Caucasians and non-vegetarian Asians (Finch et al. 1992), so may also benefit from supplementation.

Cholecalciferol (vitamin D_3) is obtained from fish oil or lanolin. Ergocalciferol (vitamin D_2) is the non-animal form acceptable to vegans, and is found in some fortified vegan margarines, soya milks and soya cheeses.

Table 3.27 Sources of vitamins D, B_{12} and riboflavin for vegans

Vitamin	Sources	Comments
Vitamin D	Exposure to 'gentle' sunlight	30 minutes per day, April to October
	Fortified soya milk	
	Fortified breakfast cereals	⎫ Amount varies according to brand
	Fortified soya cheeses and soya yoghurts	⎬
	Fortified vegan margarines	e.g. Vitaquell, Tomor, Granose
	Vitamin supplements	
Vitamin B_{12}	Fortified yeast extract/vegetable stock	
	Fortified soya milk	⎫
	Fortified textured soya protein	⎬ Amount varies according to brand
	Fortified breakfast cereals	⎭
	Vitamin supplements	
Riboflavin	Yeast extract	Amount varies according to brand
	Wheat germ	0.7 mg/100 g
	Fortified breakfast cereals	Amount varies according to brand
	Almonds	0.8 mg/100 g
	Soya beans	0.3 mg/100 g
	Tempeh	0.5 mg/100 g
	Fortified soya milk	Amount varies according to brand
	Pumpkin, sunflower, sesame seeds, tahini	0.2 mg/100 g
	Mushrooms	0.3 mg/100 g
	Seaweeds:	
	kombu	0.3 mg/100 g
	nori	1.3 mg/100 g
	Avocado	0.2 mg/100 g
	Dried apricots, prunes	Both 0.2 mg/100 g
	Carob flour	0.5 mg/100 g

Vitamin B_{12}

Cobalamins are synthesized only by bacteria, fungi and some algae, and accumulate from microbial action in animals. Plant foods contain no appreciable amounts unless they are contaminated by bacteria or insects. Much of the B_{12} present in spirulina, nori, tempeh and miso has been shown to be the inactive B_{12} analogue rather than the active vitamin, and may even compete with the active form for uptake (Herbert 1988; Dagnelie *et al.* 1991).

Vitamin B_{12} deficiency has been reported, but the prevalence in the UK vegetarian population is uncertain (Sanders 1999a). Vegans and vegetarians have good intakes of folic acid which mask the megaloblastic anaemia of B_{12} deficiency, so sufferers tend to present with neurological symptoms. There have also been isolated reports of low blood levels of vitamin B_{12} with associated neurological symptoms in exclusively breast-fed infants of vegan mothers (Langley 1988) and in people of all ages on macrobiotic or Rastafarian diets (Campbell *et al.* 1982; Dagnelie *et al.* 1989a). Others have reported low serum levels in the breast-milk of vegan mothers (Specker *et al.* 1990) and adult vegans and vegetarians (Helman and Darnton-Hill 1987; Reddy and Sanders 1990; Haddad *et al.* 1999a; Hokin and Butler 1999). All vegans, as well as vegetarians who limit dairy foods or eggs, should regularly include a reliable source of vitamin B_{12} in their diet or take a B_{12} supplement. Good sources of B_{12} are shown in Table 3.27. The Vegan Society (address at end of this section) can advise on newer fortified products and suitable supplements.

Riboflavin

Dairy products and meat are the major sources of riboflavin. Vegan women have been shown to have intakes lower than the reference nutrient intake (RNI) but greater than the estimated average requirement (EAR) (Draper *et al.* 1993). Some vegan children also have intakes less than the RNI, but still greater than the lower reference nutrient intake (LRNI) (Sanders and Manning 1992). However, other studies have shown satisfactory serum levels amongst women (Helman and Darnton-Hill 1987). It remains prudent for all vegans, and especially children and pregnant and lactating women, to ensure an adequate riboflavin intake.

Minerals and trace elements

Vegans and vegetarian have similar or greater intakes of most minerals. Exceptions are iodine, calcium (vegans only) and possibly selenium. Extra care must be taken with iron and zinc because of their low bioavailability from plant-based diets. Good sources of some of these minerals for those on vegetarian diets are shown in Table 3.28.

Iron

The iron intake of adult vegetarians and vegans equal or exceeds that of omnivores (Reddy and Sanders 1990; Draper *et al.* 1993), but most of it will be in the less well-absorbed non-haem form. Vegetarians, especially women of child-bearing age, tend to have lower serum ferritin (iron

Table 3.28 Sources of iron, calcium and zinc for vegans and vegetarians

	Calcium (Amount[1] providing approximately 100 mg calcium)	Iron (Amount[1] providing approximately 2 mg iron)	Zinc (Amount[1] providing approximately 1 mg zinc)
Soya products	Tofu made with calcium chloride or sulphate (25 g) Soya cheese (25 g) Fortified soya milk (70–120 ml)	Soya flour (30 g) Tempeh (70 g)	Soya flour, miso (30 g) Soya cheese, tempeh (55 g)
Pulses	Soya, kidney, haricot beans (120–150 g)	Soya, haricot, pinto, kidney beans, lentils, chickpeas (70–100 g) Peas, split peas (120–130 g)	Chickpeas, split peas, lentils (70–85 g) Haricot, pinto, soya beans, peas (100 g)
Nuts, peanuts and seeds	Almonds (40 g) Brazil nuts (60 g) Hazelnuts (70 g)	Peanuts, pecans, Brazil nuts, peanut butter (80–100 g) Almonds, hazelnuts (60 g) Pine nuts, cashews (35 g) Sunflower seeds (35 g) Pumpkin seeds (20 g)	Almonds, peanuts (30 g) Walnuts (40 g) Cashews (20 g) Pumpkin, sunflower seeds (20 g)
Cereal products	White/brown bread (100 g) Wholemeal bread (185 g)	Wholemeal bread (75 g) Brown bread (90 g) White bread (125 g) Wheatgerm (25 g) Fortified breakfast cereals (10–50 g)	Wheat germ (5 g) Wholemeal bread (55 g) Brown rice (140 g) Fortified breakfast cereals (50 g)
Dried fruit	Dried figs (40 g)	Dried figs, dried apricots, raisins (50 g) Prunes (70 g)	
Green leafy vegetables	Spinach[2], watercress, kale (70 g) Spring greens (130 g)	Watercress, kale (90–105 g) Spinach– (125 g)	Watercress (140 g)
Seaweeds	Kombu, wakame, nori (15–25 g)	Kombu, wakame, nori (15 g)	Kombu (15 g)
Miscellaneous	Black treacle (20 g)	Black treacle (20 g)	Cocoa powder (15 g)
Additionally suitable for vegetarians Milk and dairy foods	Milk (75–90ml) Hard cheeses (20 g) Yogurt (50–70 g)		Hard cheeses (30–50 g)
Other		Eggs[2] (100 g)	Eggs (75 g)

Mineral bioavailability from plant foods tends to be lower than from animal sources.
[1] Cooked/edible weights.
[2] Particularly low bioavailability.

storage) levels (Helman and Darnton-Hill 1987; Reddy and Sanders 1990; Craig 1994), but the clinical importance of this is unclear as there is generally no significant difference in the incidence of iron deficiency anaemia amongst these groups (Anderson *et al.* 1981; Craig 1994; Ball and Bartlett 1999). Iron deficiency may carry a greater risk of the development of iron deficiency anaemia if iron needs are increased (infancy, pregnancy, blood loss). There is also evidence that iron deficiency can impair the immune response and compromise physical performance (Nelson *et al.* 1994; British Nutrition Foundation 1995).

The more restricted the diet the greater the risk of iron-deficiency anaemia. Fifteen per cent of children following a macrobiotic diet showed low blood levels of haemoglobin and ferritin in the study by Dagnelie *et al.* (1989a), while Nelson *et al.* (1994) postulated that being a 'new' vegetarian, and having a less balanced diet, increased the likelihood of iron-deficiency anaemia amongst teenage girls.

The absorption of non-haem iron in plant foods (and eggs) is enhanced by vitamin C, meat, fish, citric acid and ethanol, and inhibited by phytates, oxalates, tannins and other polyphenols in the diet (British Nutrition Foundation 1995). Hunt and Roughead (1999), showed there is 70% lower non-haem iron absorption from a vegetarian diet than from a non-vegetarian diet, but after an 8 week period there is an associated decrease in faecal ferritin, suggesting some physical adaptation to increase the efficiency of iron absorption. Vegans and vegetarians should be advised to include plant sources of iron daily, e.g. pulses, fortified cereals, wholegrain breads and cereals, to include vitamin C-rich foods with meals, and to minimize absorption inhibitors such as tannins.

Calcium

Vegetarians have similarly adequate calcium intakes to omnivores (Bull and Barber 1984; Draper *et al.* 1993). However, because of the exclusion of milk and dairy products, adult vegans tend to have average calcium intakes lower than the RNI (Draper *et al.* 1993). Sanders and Manning (1992) also found suboptimal intakes amongst vegan children.

Studies have found equal or greater bone densities amongst vegetarians compared with matched omnivores (Marsh *et al.* 1988; Hunt *et al.* 1989; Johnston 1999). However, Johnston (1999) also found that premenopausal vegan women had significantly lower spinal bone mineral density than matched vegetarians and omnivores. More research is needed concerning vegetarian and vegan diets and osteoporosis, as the lower protein and higher alkalinity of vegan diets improve conservation of calcium intake compared with omnivorous diets (Remer and Manz 1994). The body also adapts to lower intakes of calcium by increasing the rate of intestinal absorption, provided vitamin D status is adequate (DH 1998b). In addition, there is some evidence that diets rich in the phytoestrogens isoflavones (mainly found in soya beans) may have a positive effect on the bone health of postmenopausal women (Anderson *et al.* 1999).

A good calcium intake is needed as part of balanced diet throughout life to reduce the risk of osteoporosis (DH 1998b). Particular care should be taken to include good food sources of calcium and/or supplements in the diets of vegan children, teenagers and adults, especially breast-feeding women. Vegetarian and vegan women should also be encouraged to avoid being underweight (Barr *et al.* 1998).

Iodine

Both vegetarians and vegans have lower iodine intakes than omnivores (Draper *et al.* 1993; Remer *et al.* 1999). Vegans are at greater risk of low intakes as milk is a major source of iodine in the British diet. Compromised iodine status increases blood levels of thyroid-stimulating hormone (TSH), and mean TSH levels have been found to be 47% higher in a group of British male vegans compared with male omnivores (Key *et al.* 1992). Vegans should be encouraged to use iodine supplements, iodized salt or kelp fortified yeast extracts regularly.

Selenium

Concern has been expressed about the general decrease in selenium intakes in Britain, which is largely due to the change in the late 1970s to a bread-making flour with a lower selenium content (Rayman 1997). Vegetarians and vegans may be at most risk from low selenium intakes because of their reliance on cereals (omnivores now receive proportionally more of their selenium from meat). Significantly lower toenail selenium concentrations have been found amongst vegetarians and vegans compared with omnivores (Judd *et al.* 1997). Brazil nuts, other nuts, seeds, soya beans, mushrooms, grains and bananas are all vegan sources of selenium, but actual content will vary according to the selenium content of the soil in which these foods were grown.

Zinc

Vegetarians and vegans of all ages generally have dietary intakes of zinc equal to or higher than omnivores (Freeland-Graves 1988; Sanders and Manning 1992;

Draper *et al.* 1993). Most also have adequate blood levels, although lower than those of matched omnivores, and inadequate plasma levels have been found in a minority (Anderson *et al.* 1981; Sanders 1983). Zinc is similar to iron in that its richest sources are animal foods and it has a low bioavailability from plant foods (phytates are particularly strong inhibitors of zinc absorption). Vegetarians, and particularly vegans, should ensure intakes which meet or exceed the RNI.

3.10.4 Practical dietary advice for vegetarians

General considerations

The beliefs, attitudes and lifestyle of people following vegan and vegetarian diets should be taken into consideration when providing dietary guidance. A well-balanced vegetarian diet can be in line with healthy-eating targets, e.g. rich in fruit, vegetables, pulses and wholegrains, and low in saturated fat and salt. However, some vegetarians, especially young people, may rely too much on cheese as a meat substitute, as well as vegetarian convenience meals, burgers, pies, pizzas and chips. Many of these are low in iron and high in fat and sodium.

New vegetarians or vegans, parents of vegan or vegetarian children, and pregnant or breast-feeding vegetarian women are the groups most likely to benefit from dietary advice. They should be encouraged to experiment with a variety of cereals, grains, pulses, nuts, seeds, soya products, fruit and vegetables. Parents should be aware of the relatively high energy and nutrient needs of infants and young children.

There is an ever-increasing range of vegetarian and vegan ingredients from around the world as well as ready-prepared meals (of variable nutritional quality). Many vegetarian and vegan cookbooks are also available from the relevant societies (see the end of this section), book shops and local public libraries.

Meal planning for vegetarian diets

National guidelines for healthy eating can be adapted to suit the dietary preferences of vegetarians. A subcommittee of the Third International Congress on Vegetarian Nutrition 1999 developed a specific vegetarian food pyramid with supporting documentation (Haddad *et al.* 1999b). In the UK, dietary guidance can be based on *The Balance of Good Health* (see Section 1.2.2 in Healthy eating).

Bread, other cereals and potatoes These foods should form the basis of meals and snacks. Some should be wholemeal or wholegrain, but these should not be used exclusively for children with small appetites. A variety of different cereals and grains can be used. If calcium intake is low, white and brown bread may be a better choice than wholemeal (which is made with unfortified flour in the UK).

Fruit and vegetables At least five portions of a variety of fruit and vegetables should be consumed each day. Young children should have a similar variety but in smaller portions. The vitamin C content of fruit and vegetables is important for boosting non-haem iron absorption.

Milk and dairy foods Lactovegetarians of all ages should have two to three servings daily. For non-dairy consumers, calcium-fortified soya milk and orange juice will provide similar amounts of calcium per serving. Other good sources of calcium include: brown or white bread, tofu, green vegetables (except for spinach), pulses, nuts, sesame seeds and dried figs. Vegans should ensure an adequate riboflavin intake from other sources. Infants and young children not consuming milk and dairy products will need appropriate infant formulae or fortified soya milks (see below).

Alternatives to meat group Two to three servings are required daily to provide alternative sources of iron, zinc, B vitamins (including B_{12}), protein and selenium. Vegans must complement proteins over the day. Walnuts, pumpkin seeds and soya beans are also useful sources of alpha-linolenic acid. Good food choices are:

- peas: green, split peas, chick peas
- beans: mung, kidney, soya, black-eyed, etc.
- lentils
- tofu, textured vegetable/soya protein, soya protein isolate, Quorn (contains non-free-range eggs) and convenience foods made from them
- nuts and nut butters
- seeds and seed pastes, e.g. tahini.

Foods containing fat, and foods containing sugar As for the general population, these foods should be eaten sparingly. Oils which provide *n*3 fatty acids are a good choice, e.g. rapeseed oil, soya oil and walnut oil to help optimize the *n*6:*n*3 ratio (which should be somewhere between 4:1 and 10:1; Sanders 1999b). Olive oil is also a good choice as it rich in neither *n*3 nor n6 fatty acids so it does not further upset the ratio between these two families.

Other points

- Vegans and vegetarians should regularly include a reliable source of iodine, e.g. seaweed, iodized salt, Vecon or kelp-containing supplements.
- Vegans (and vegetarians who eat limited dairy products) should regularly include a source of vitamin B_{12}, and a source of vitamin D if sun exposure is limited.
- Fat should not be restricted in the diets of children under 5 years, and especially in those under 2 years.

Dietary considerations in particular population groups

Pregnant women

Well-planned vegetarian and vegan diets are adequate to maintain the health of both mother and child during pregnancy. General guidelines for planning diets in pregnan-

cy can be found in Section 3.1, Pregnancy. Birthweights of infants born to well-nourished vegetarian women are similar to those of infants of non-vegetarians (O'Connell *et al.* 1989). However, a UK study found early onset of labour and emergency caesarian section to be more common in Asian vegetarian women than in white omnivorous women. Gestation was on average 5–6 days shorter and birthweights were lower in the infants born to the Asian vegetarians (Reddy *et al.* 1994). Lower birthweights have also been reported in communities following macrobiotic diets and in vegans (O'Connell *et al.* 1989). The increased requirements of protein, vitamins A and C, thiamin, riboflavin and folate are not difficult to meet with varied vegetarian diets. Vegans must take more care with riboflavin. Adequate vitamin B_{12} intake is also vital. As for all women planning pregnancy and for the first 12 weeks of pregnancy, a daily 400 μg folic acid supplement is also advised.

The bulkiness of a vegetarian diet may be a problem, particularly if energy intake is reduced through appetite changes or morning sickness. A reduction in fibre intake and an increase in energy-dense and nutrient-dense foods may be necessary. Frequent, smaller meals may also help.

Pregnant women with limited exposure to sunlight and those with darker skins are recommended to ensure a dietary intake of 10 μg/day of vitamin D. This generally requires a vitamin supplement (DH 1991).

There is no recommendation for increased mineral intake in pregnancy as maternal stores and increased absorption balance higher needs (DH 1991). However, as mineral adequacy can be borderline in some vegetarian diets, adequate intakes must be ensured. If iron stores were low prior to pregnancy, supplementary iron is advisable.

Essential fatty acid requirements during pregnancy and lactation Long-chain polyunsaturated fatty acids (LCPs) derived from the parent fatty acids linolenic acid (18:2*n*6) and alpha-linolenic acid (18:3*n*3) are needed for the normal development of the retina and central nervous system. As LCPs are generally absent from plant foods, and the extent to which they can be synthesized from their parent fatty acids is still debated, it is vital to ensure that vegetarian mothers women choose a diet that optimizes the potential for LCP production. The developing foetus obtains LCPs via its mother's plasma, LCPs are present in the breast milk of vegetarians and there is no evidence that the capacity to synthesize LCPs is limited in vegetarians (Sanders 1999b). However, lower concentrations of DHA (22:6*n*3) have been observed in blood and artery phospholipids of infants of vegetarians and it is currently unclear whether their brain lipids contain lower proportions of DHA than do those of infant omnivores. Experiments in primates have shown altered visual function with diets with a high ratio of linolenic to alpha-linolenic acid (which is typical of vegetarian and vegan diets), so it would be prudent to advise pregnant and breast-feeding women (and all vegetarians) to avoid excessive intakes of linolenic acid and preferentially use sources of alpha-linolenic acid (Sanders

1999b). See Nutritional implications of vegetarian diets, above, for practical information.

Lactating women

Principles for diet planning during lactation are discussed in Section 3.3.1 in Infants. The DRVs for energy, protein and most B vitamins (including B_{12}) during lactation are increased by at least 25% compared with those for non-pregnant women, with greater increases for riboflavin and vitamins A, C and D. These increased needs should be met with nutritious vegetarian foods and sufficient exposure to sunlight for vitamin D synthesis. Women with darker skin or limited exposure to sunlight need 10 μg/day of vitamin D through diet or supplementation. Vegans should take extra care to ensure sufficient riboflavin and B_{12} intake from supplements or reliable sources to prevent deficiency in the breast-fed infant.

Calcium and zinc RNIs are about 80% higher than for non-breastfeeding women, so vegetarians and vegans should include extra food sources of zinc and calcium (vegans may need supplements). Inhibitors of mineral absorption, e.g. phytates, oxalates and tannins, should also be moderated.

Infants

The nutritional status of exclusively breast-fed infants depends largely on the nutrient stores and intake of the mother. For those who choose to use infant formula, a soya-based brand acceptable to vegans is essential. Carton soya milk has not been suitably modified and fortified for infant use.

Vitamin D status in infants and young children can be maintained by 'safe' sunlight exposure (i.e. in the shade) of the lower arms, legs and face for 30 minutes daily in the summer months or by appropriate supplementation (DH 1994b, 1998b).

Weaning on to solid foods should follow the same principles as for omnivorous babies (see Section 3.3.3 in Infants). Very restrictive macrobiotic and Rastafarian diets carry a high risk of deficiencies and cannot be recommended (Jacobs and Dwyer 1988; DH 1994b). Ensuring adequate energy intakes is vital. Excessive intake of fibrous or watery foods, e.g. very dilute porridges, excess fruits, vegetables and wholegrains, should be avoided and energy-dense cereal products, pulses, vegetable oils, etc., included. (Avocados are also useful.)

Commonly used first weaning foods such as cereals, fruit and vegetables are suitable for vegans, although many packaged baby cereals are fortified with animal-derived vitamin D_3. Several manufactured baby foods are suitable for vegetarians, but fewer are completely free of animal products; these are listed in the Vegan Society's *Animal-free Shopper*. Later weaning foods, e.g. after 6 months, appropriate for vegan babies are bread, mashed beans and lentils, nut spreads such as peanut butter and tahini (not whole nuts), tofu, rice and pasta, soya formula, soya yoghurt and vegan margarine. Vegetarians can include vegetarian cheese, yoghurt and well-cooked eggs.

Vegan infants may have low vitamin B_{12} stores at birth and may receive low levels in breast milk (this is also true for riboflavin). The weaning diet (and the diet of breast-feeding vegan women) must contain foods fortified with vitamin B_{12} and riboflavin, such as fortified soya formula, margarines or cereals. Protein complementation at meals is also wise to ensure maximum utilization of essential amino acids at this time of rapid growth.

Children

Infants should be progressing toward a varied diet by the age of 9–12 months. Whole cow's milk can be introduced to vegetarian children after 12 months. Non-breast fed vegan children should be kept on a soya infant formula until at least 2 years of age, as carton soya milk is lower in energy and nutrients. Advice regarding dental health is required owing to the use of non-milk sugars in soya infant formula (DH 1994b). Low-fat, high-fibre diets are not appropriate for children under 2 years, and care should be taken to limit mineral absorption inhibitors, e.g. tannins and phytates (DH 1994b). Providing frequent, smaller meals and energy-dense snacks is helpful. The growth of young children, particularly vegans, should be monitored closely for early identification of any problems (Nutrition Standing Committee the BPA 1988).

Adequate iron intake is a problem for children in general and good sources of iron should be included regularly, accompanied by vitamin C-rich foods. For children with limited sunlight exposure, 7 μg/day of vitamin D, from the diet or supplementation, is recommended until the age of 2 years. Children on vegan or macrobiotic diets may benefit from supplements until 5 years of age (DH 1994b). Vegan children should have a reliable source of vitamin B_{12}. The Vegan Society maintains a 'Vegan families list' for the mutual support of parents raising children on a vegan diet and lifestyle.

Adolescents

The nutritional needs of adolescents are described in Section 3.6 (Adolescents). Vegetarians and vegans should take special care to meet the requirements of energy, protein, iron, calcium and vitamin B_{12} during the adolescent growth spurt. Teenage males have particularly high requirements for iron and calcium. Health advantages from vegetarian and vegan diets in adolescence include low serum lipid levels and less body fat compared with omnivores (Jacobs and Dwyer 1988; Hebbelinck *et al.* 1999).

Adolescence is a popular time for adopting a vegetarian diet, often for ethical and environmental reasons and within an omnivorous household. Young people, and their parents, may be in particular need of nutritional and practical advice about well-balanced vegetarian diets (Nelson *et al.* 1994). Families should be aware of suitable meat alternatives (and dairy alternatives for vegans), especially since many vegetarian convenience foods are not good sources of iron, and fizzy drinks are preferred to milk. The Vegetarian Society and the Vegan Society provide information for young people.

Elderly people

There has been little research concerning elderly vegetarians, but the basic diet principles for this group are the same as for omnivores (see Section 3.7, Older adults). Older vegetarians have more nutrient-dense diets than omnivores but they need to pay attention to intakes of vitamins D and B_{12}, iron and zinc (Brants *et al.* 1990). Elderly people frequently do not receive adequate exposure to sunlight to maintain adequate vitamin D status, so an intake of 10 μg of vitamin D daily, through diet or supplementation, is recommended for people over 65 years of age (DH 1991, 1998b).

Absorption of micronutrients, especially of vitamin B_{12}, decreases with age, and regular use of reliable B_{12} sources is important (British Dietetic Association 1999). Older vegetarians benefit from being leaner than omnivores (Dwyer 1991) and from improved bowel regularity due to a high-fibre diet. The Department of Health, however, cautions against excessive intakes of non-starch polysaccharide and phytate in all elderly people as their diets may have marginal mineral contents (DH 1991).

Sports people

There is no convincing evidence that vegetarian athletes cannot meet their requirements for protein, iron, zinc and other trace minerals. There has been some concern than vegetarian female athletes are at increased risk of amenorrhoea, but evidence suggests that their low energy intake relative to needs, not dietary quality, is the major cause. Well-planned vegetarian diets can meet the nutritional needs of both recreational and elite athletes (Nieman 1999).

Text revised by: Lyndel Costain

Useful addresses

Realeat Survey Office
Howard Way, Newport Pagnell, Bucks BK16 9PY
Tel: 01908 211311

The Vegan Society
7 Battle Road, St Leonards-on-Sea, East Sussex TN37 7AA
Tel: 01424 427 393

The Vegetarian Society
Parkdale, Denham Road, Altrincham, Cheshire WA14 4QG
Tel: 0161 928 0793

Further reading

Background information

American Dietetic Association. Position of the American Dietetic Association: vegetarian diets. *Journal of the American Dietetic Association* 1997; **97**: 1317.

American Society for Clinical Nutrition. Third International Congress on Vegetarian Nutition. *American Journal of Clinical Nutrition* 1999; **70**: 3. (Suppl).

British Dietetic Association. *Vegetarian Diets*. Position Paper. Birmingham: BDA, 1995.

British Nutrition Foundation. *Vegetarianism*. Briefing Paper. London: BNF, 1995.

Langley, G. *Vegan Nutrition*. 2nd edn: The Vegan Society, 1995.

Melina V, Davis D, Harrison V. *Becoming Vegetarian: The Complete Guide to Adopting a Healthy Vegetarian Diet*. Canada: Macmillan, 1994. (Also suitable for the general public.)

Practical information

Wakeman A, Baskerville G. *The Vegan Cookbook*. Faber and Faber.

Elliot R. *Learning to Cook Vegetarian*. Phoenix.

The Animal-free Shopper. The Vegan Society.

Timperley C. *Baby and Child Vegetarian Recipes*. Ebury Press.

Vegetarian Issues: A Resource Pack for Secondary Schools. The Vegetarian Society

Additional resources (information about good sources of nutrition, recipe books, magazines, etc.) and details of local contacts are available from The Vegetarian Society and The Vegan Society (addresses above).

References

Abdulla NI, Andersson I, Asp N *et al*. Nutrient intake and health status of vegans. Chemical analyses of diets using the duplicate portion sampling technique. *American Journal of Clinical Nutrition* 1981; **34**: 2464–2477.

Anderson BM, Gibson RS, Sabry JH. The iron and zinc status of long-term vegetarian women. *American Journal of Clinical Nutrition* 1981; **34**: 1042–1048.

Anderson JB, Anthony M, Messina M, Garner SC. Effects of phytoestrogens on tissues. *Nutrition Research Reviews* 1999; **12**: 75–116.

Appleby P, Thorogood M, Mann JI, Key TJ. Low body mass index in non meat eaters: the possible roles of animal fat, dietary fibre and alcohol. *International Journal of Obesity* 1998; **22**: 454–460.

Ball B, Bartlett MA. Dietary intake and iron status of Australian vegetarian women. *American Journal of Clinical Nutrition* 1999, **70**: 353–358.

Barr SI, Prior JC, Janelle KC, Lentle BC. Spinal bone mineral density in premenopausal vegetarian and nonvegetarian women: cross-sectional and prospective comparisons. *Journal of the American Dietetic Association* 1998; **98**: 760–765.

Brants HA, Lowik MR, Westenbrink S *et al*. Adequacy of a vegetarian diet in old age. *Journal of the American College of Nutrition* 1990; **9**: 292–302.

British Dietetic Association. Vitamin and mineral supplementation. Position Paper. *Journal of Human Nutrition and Dietetics* 1999; **12**: 171–178.

British Nutrition Foundation. *Iron*. Task Force Report. London: British Nutrition Foundation, 1995.

British Nutrition Foundation. *n-3 Fatty Acids and Health*. Briefing Paper. London: British Nutrition Foundation, 1999.

Bull NL, Barber SA. Food and nutrient intakes of vegetarians in Britain. *Human Nutrition: Applied Nutrition* 1984; **38A**: 288–293.

Campbell M, Lofters WS, Gibbs WN. Rastafarianism and the vegans' syndrome. *British Medical Journal* 1982; **285**: 1617–1618.

Clemens TI., Henderson SL, Adams JS, Hollick MF. Increased skin pigment reduces capacity of skin to synthesize vitamin D_3. *Lancet* 1982; **i**: 74–76.

Craig WJ. Iron status of vegetarians. *American Journal of Clinical Nutrition* 1994; **59**: 1233S–1237S.

Dagnelie PC, van Staveren WA, Vergote FJVRA *et al*. Increased risk of vitamin B-12 and iron deficiency in infants on macrobiotic diets. *American Journal of Clinical Nutrition* 1989a; **50**: 818–824.

Dagnelie PC, van Staveren WA, Vergote FJVRA *et al*. Nutritional status of infants aged 4–18 months on macrobiotic diets and matched omnivorous control infants: a population-based mixed longitudinal study. II. Growth and psychomotor development. *European Journal of Clinical Nutrition* 1989b; **43**: 325–338.

Dagnelie PC, Vergote FJVRA, van Staveren WA *et al*. High prevalence of rickets in infants on macrobiotic diets. *American Journal of Clinical Nutrition* 1990; **51**: 202–208.

Dagnelie PC, van Staveren WA, van den Berg H. Vitamin B-12 from algae appears not to be bioavailable. *American Journal of Clinical Nutrition* 1991; **53**: 695–697.

Department of Health. *Dietary Reference Values for Food Energy and Nutrients in the United Kingdom*. Report on Health and Social Subjects 41. London: HMSO, 1991.

Department of Health. *Nutritional Aspects of Cardiovascular Disease*. Report on Health and Social Subjects 46. London: HMSO, 1994a.

Department of Health. *Weaning and the Weaning Diet*. Report on Health and Social Subjects 45. London: HMSO, 1994b.

Department of Health. *Nutritional Aspects of the Development of Cancer*. Report on Health and Social Subjects 48. London: HMSO, 1998a.

Department of Health. *Nutrition and Bone Health*. Report on Health and Social Subjects 49. London: HMSO, 1998b.

Draper A, Malhotra W, Wheeler E. The energy and nutrient intakes of different types of vegetarians: a case for supplements? *British Journal of Nutrition* 1993; **69**: 3–19.

Dwyer JT. Health aspects of vegetarian diets. *American Journal of Clinical Nutrition* 1988; **48**: 712–738.

Dwyer JT. Nutritional consequences of vegetarianism. *Annual Review of Nutrition* 1991; **11**: 61–91.

Finch P, Ang L, Colston KW *et al*. Blunted seasonal variation in serum 25-hydroxyvitamin D and increased risk of osteomalacia in vegetarian London Asians. *European Journal of Clinical Nutrition* 1992; **46**: 509–515.

Freeland-Graves J. Mineral adequacy of vegetarian diets. *American Journal of Clinical Nutrition* 1988; **48**: 859–862.

Haddad EH, Berk LS, Kettering JD *et al*. Dietary intake and biochemical, hematologic and immune status of vegans compared with non vegetarians. *American Journal of Clinical Nutrition* 1999a; **70**: 586S–593S.

Haddad EH, Sabate J, Whitten CG. Vegetarian food guide pyramid: a conceptual framework. *American Journal of Clinical Nutrition* 1999b; **70**: 615S–619S.

Harman SK, Parnell WR. The nutritional health of New Zealand vegetarian and non vegetarian Seventh Day Adventists: selected vitamin, mineral and lipid levels. *New Zealand Medical Journal* 1998; **111**: 91–94.

Hebbelinck M, Clarys P, De Malsche A. Growth, development and physical fitness of Flemish vegetarian children, adolescents and young adults. *American Journal of Clinical Nutrition* 1999; **70**: 579S–585S.

Helman AD, Darnton-Hill I. Vitamin and iron status in new vegetarians. *American Journal of Clinical Nutrition* 1987; **45**: 785–789.

Herbert V. Vitamin B-12: plant sources, requirements and assay. *American Journal of Clinical Nutrition* 1988; **48**: 852–858.

Hoffman I, Groenweld MJ, Leitzmann C. Nutrient intake and nutritional status of vegetarians and low meat eaters consuming a diet meeting preventive recommendations. *American Journal of Clinical Nutrition* 1999; **70**: 626S–629S.

Hokin BD, Butler T. Cyanocobalamin (vitamin B_{12}) status in Seven-day Adventists ministers in Australia. *American Journal of Clinical Nutrition* 1999; **70**: 576S–578S.

Hunt JR, Roughead ZK. Non-heme absorption, faecal ferritin excretion, and blood indexes of iron status in women consuming controlled lacto-ovo vegetarian diets for 8 weeks. *American Journal of Clinical Nutrition* 1999; **69**: 944–952.

Hunt IF, Murphy NJ, Henderson C *et al*. Bone mineral content in postmenopausal women: comparison of omnivores and vegetarians. *American Journal of Clinical Nutrition* 1989; **50**: 517–523.

Jacobs C, Dwyer JT. Vegetarian children: appropriate and inappropriate diets. *American Journal of Clinical Nutrition* 1988; **48**: 811–818.

Johnston PK. Bone mineral status in vegan, lacto-ovovegerarian, and omnivorous women premenopausal women. *American Journal of Clinical Nutrition* 1999; **70**: 626S–629S.

Judd PA, Long A, Butcher M *et al*. Vegetarians and vegans may be most at risk from low selenium intakes (Letter). *British Medical Journal* 1997; **314**: 1834.

Key TJ, Thorogood M, Keenan J, Long A. Raised thyroid stimulatory hormone associated with kelp intake in British men. *Journal of Human Nutrition and Dietetics* 1992; **5**: 323–326.

Key TJ, Davey GK, Appleby MN. Health benefits of a vegetarian diet. *Proceedings of the Nutrition Society* 1999; **58**: 271–275.

Kjeldsen-Kragh J. Rheumatoid arthritis treated with vegetarian diets. *American Journal of Clinical Nutrition* 1999; **70**: 594S–600S.

Langley G. *Vegan Nutrition: A Survey of Research*. The Vegan Society, 1988.

Mann JI, Appleby PN, Key TJ, Thorogood M. Diet determinants of ischaemic heart disease in health conscious individuals. *Heart* 1997; **78**: 450–455.

Marsh AG, Sanchez TV, Michelsen O *et al*. Vegetarian lifestyle and bone mineral density. *American Journal of Clinical Nutrition* 1988; **48**: 837–841.

Martins Y, Pliner P, O'Connor R. Restrained eating among vegetarians: does a vegetarian eating style mask concerns about weight? *Appetite* 1999; **32**: 145–154.

Melby CL, Toohey ML, Cebrick J. Blood pressure and blood lipids among vegetarian, semi vegetarian and non vegetarian African Americans. *American Journal of Clinical Nutrition* 1994; **59**: 103–109.

Nagyova A, Kudiackova M, Grancicova E, Magalova T. LDL oxidizability and antioxiative status of plasma in vegetarians. *Annals of Nutrition Metabolism* 1998, 42; **6**: 328–323.

Nathan I, Hackett AF, Kirby S. The dietary intake of a group of vegetarian children aged 7–11 years compared with matched omnivores. *British Journal of Nutrition* 1996; **75**: 533–544.

Nathan I, Hackett AF, Kirby S. A longitudinal study of the growth of matched pairs of vegetarian and omnivorous children aged 7–11 years, in the north-west of England. *European Journal of Clinical Nutrition* 1997; **51**: 20–25.

Nelson M, Bakaliou F, Trivedi A. Iron-deficiency anaemia and physical performance in adolescent girls from different ethnic backgrounds. *British Journal of Nutrition* 1994; **72**: 427–433.

Niemen DC. Physical fitness and vegetarian diets: is there a relation? *American Journal of Clinical Nutrition* 1999, 70; **3**: 570S–575S.

Nutrition Standing Committee of the British Paediatric Association. Vegetarian weaning. *Archives of the Diseases of Childhood* 1988; **63**: 1286–1292.

O'Connell JM, Dibley MJ, Sierra J *et al*. Growth of vegetarian children: the Farm Study. *Pediatrics* 1989; **84**: 475–481.

Rayman M. Dietary selenium: time to act. *British Medical Journal* 1997; **314**: 387–388.

Realeat Foods Ltd. *The Realeat Survey 1984; 1997*. London: Realeat Foods Ltd, 1984, 1997.

Reddy S, Sanders TAB. Haematological studies on premenopausal Indian and Caucasian vegetarians compared with Caucasian omnivores. *British Journal of Nutrition* 1990; **64**: 331–338.

Reddy S, Sanders TAB, Obeid O. The influence of maternal vegetarian diet on essential fatty acid status of the newborn. *European Journal of Clinical Nutrition* 1994; **48**: 358–368.

Remer T, Manz F. Estimation of the renal net excretion by adults consuming diets containing variable amounts of protein. *American Journal of Clinical Nutrition* 1994; **59**: 1356–1361.

Remer T, Neubert A, Manz F. Increased risk of iodine deficiency with vegetarian nutrition. *British Journal of Nutrition* 1999; **81**: 45–49.

Roshanai F, Sanders TAB. Assessment of fatty acid intakes in vegans and omnivores. *Human Nutrition: Applied Nutrition* 1984; **38A**: 345–354.

Sabate J, Lindsted KD, Harris RD, Sanchez A. Attained height of lacto-ovo vegetarian children and adolescents. *European Journal of Clinical Nutrition* 1991; **45**: 51–58.

Sanders TAB. Vegetarianism: dietetic and medical aspects. *Journal of Plant Foods* 1983; **5**: 3–14.

Sanders TAB. The nutritional adequacy of plant-based diets. *Proceedings of the Nutrition Society* 1999a; **58**: 265–269.

Sanders TAB. Essential fatty acid requirements of vegetarians in pregnancy, lactation, and infancy. *American Journal of Clinical Nutrition* 1999b; **70**: 555S–559S.

Sanders TAB, Manning J. The growth and development of vegan children. *Journal of Human Nutrition and Dietetics* 1992; **5**: 11–21.

Soroka N, Sliverberg DS, Greemland M *et al*. Comparison of vegetable-based (soya) and an animal-based low protein diet in predialysis chronic renal failure patients. *Nephron* 1998; **78**: 173–180.

Specker BL, Black A, Allen L, Morrow F. Vitamin B_{12}: low milk concentrations are related to low serum concentrations in vegetarian women and to methylmalonic aciduria in their infants. *American Journal of Clinical Nutrition* 1990; **52**: 1073–1076.

Thorogood M. Epidemiology of vegetarianism and health. *Nutrition Research Reviews* 1995; **8**: 179–192.

Thorogood M, Mann JI. Diet and plasma lipids in a group of vegetarians and omnivores. *Proceedings of the Nutrition Society* 1990; **49**: 59A–61A.

Thorogood M, Mann J, Appleby P, McPherson K. Risk of cancer and ischaemic heart disease in meat and non-meat eaters. *British Medical Journal* 1994; **308**: 1667–1670.

Truesdell DD, Acosta PB. Feeding the vegan infant and child. *Journal of the American Dietetic Association* 1985; **85**: 837–840.

Turnlund JR. Bioavailability of selected minerals in cereal products. *Cereal Foods World* 1982; **27**:152–157.

Willett W. Convergence of philosophy and science: the Third International Congress on Vegetarian Nutrition. *American Journal of Clinical Nutrition* 1999, **70**: 434S–438S.

Young VR. Soya protein in relation to human protein and amino acid nutrition. *Journal of the American Dietetic Association* 1991; **91**: 828–835.

Young VR, Pellett PL. Plant proteins in relation to human protein and amino acid nutrition. *American Journal of Clinical Nutrition* 1994; **59**: 1203S–1213S.

3.11 People with physical or learning disabilities

3.11.1 Physical disabilities

Physical disabilities may be present at birth as a result of congenital disease or malformation (e.g. cerebral palsy or spina bifida), or acquired later in life as a result of trauma or disease (e.g. head injury, stroke, multiple sclerosis or arthritis). The disability may impair physical movement and/or sensory function such as vision or hearing. Some people who are physically disabled may also have a learning disability (see Section 3.11.2).

The 1995 Health Survey for England (DH 1997) found that 18% of the adults surveyed had a physical disability, and about one-quarter of these were classified as 'serious disability'. Ten per cent of men and 12% of women had a locomotor disability, most commonly as a result of disease of the musculoskeletal system. Marked regional and social class differences were found to exist, with the prevalence of disability being highest in the north west and the more disadvantaged socioeconomic groups.

Physical disabilities in children

Physical disabilities which are present in infancy or early childhood can have profound consequences on both the ability to feed and the development of feeding skills, speech and normal eating habits. They may also create considerable problems for parents and carers since the feeding process may be difficult and protracted, sometimes resulting in parent–child conflict and behavioural disturbances (Jones 1989).

Congenital disabilities can result in impaired sucking and swallowing ability at birth, and may necessitate enteral feeding. The process of weaning is likely to be problematical and may take years to complete. Dysphagia may make it difficult for new tastes and textures to be introduced without choking and aspiration, while spoon feeding may be difficult in a child with a tonic bite reflex. The nutritional implications and management of children with disorders such as cerebral palsy, muscular dystrophy and cleft palate comprise a specialist dietetic area and readers are referred to paediatric textbooks for further guidance.

Physical disabilities in adults

The presence of a physical disability may affect food choice and nutrient intake as a result of difficulties with procuring and preparing food, and problems with eating or swallowing food. The extent to which these impair nutritional status or social functioning depends on the nature and severity of the disability and also on the level of care support available to the individual. People with less serious disabilities, particularly if they live alone, may be at greater nutritional risk than those whose disability necessitates a high level of care provision, because emerging nutritional problems are less likely to be identified and rectified at an early stage (Markson 1997; Stuck et al. 1999).

People with a physical disability can be regarded as being at 'nutritional risk', but their needs and difficulties will vary and must be assessed and managed on an individual basis. Problems which are most likely to require dietetic intervention are outlined below.

Difficulty with self-feeding

Following the sudden acquisition of a disability which impairs the ability to self-feed (such as head injury or stroke), it is important to try to overcome feeding problems as quickly as possible in order to help the person to regain self-confidence and self-respect (see Section 4.28, Neurorehabilitation). If the onset of the disability is more insidious (e.g. as a result of arthritis or neurodegenerative disease), emerging difficulties with self-feeding can easily be overlooked until their impact on nutritional intake is considerable.

In many instances, quite simple measures can do much to assist the feeding process.

Positioning People with poor head and trunk control should be well supported during feeding and a physiotherapist will be able to provide guidance on the best feeding position. Patients who have to lie flat (e.g. those with spinal injuries under traction) will have considerable difficulty in swallowing and may only be able to tolerate semi-solid food.

Feeding aids The inability to self-feed without spillage or dribbling is frustrating and demeaning, especially for adults, and many feeding aids are available to help to overcome these difficulties. Non-slip mats can be helpful for people who only have the use of one arm (such as those with stroke or arthritis). Modified dishes which are less easily tipped up, or which have a higher wall on one side so that food can be pushed up against it may be useful. Adapted cutlery with large handles may help people with weak or stiff hand grips who find ordinary conventional cutlery too thin and slippery. Alternatively, ordinary cutlery can be adapted by enlarging the diameter of the handle with sponge or rubber tubing. Specially shaped cutlery is available for those with little wrist movement (Fig. 3.6).

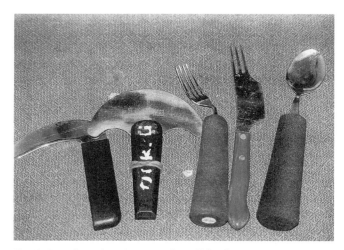

Fig. 3.6 Adapted cutlery to assist self-feeding.

Occupational therapists can assess individual needs and provide advice on suitable aids.

Drinking aids Flexistraws are useful for people unable to hold a cup. A plastic container with an airtight lid with a hole for the straw will prevent any spills if the container is knocked over. Special beakers with cutaway stems which can be lifted with the palm of the hand as well as the fingers are useful for those people with poor grip. Disabled children often find mugs with two handles easier to hold, and these also encourage the maintenance of a stable and symmetrical position whilst drinking.

Underweight

The presence of a physical disability can increase the risk of undernutrition because:

- The inability to shop, prepare and cook food, or the physical difficulties associated with eating it (e.g. causing increased food spillage) can result in a limited and inadequate food intake.
- Chewing and swallowing difficulties can lead to avoidance of whole groups of foods such as fruit and vegetables, or meat, and result in limited food choice and nutritional imbalance. There may also be reliance on inappropriate liquidized diets of low nutrient density.
- Psychological factors such as depression resulting from an acquired disability, or as a side-effect of drugs used to treat an underlying disorder, can impair appetite and interest in food.
- Those who are dependent on carers may have a poor intake as a result of lack of time available for feeding, or the food offered being of an inappropriate consistency or nutritional composition (e.g. soft or puréed diets of low nutrient density). Other factors such as poor positioning during feeding, lack of variety or unattractive meals may also compound the problem.

The way in which these problems are tackled depends on the individual circumstances. For those with limited mobility living in the community, guidance on food choice which is both nutritious and easy to prepare and cook may be helpful. Use should also be made of available community support services to assist with shopping, the provision of meals or feeding aids. For those with overt nutritional depletion, oral support measures may be indicated (see Section 1.12, Oral Nutritional support). For those dependent on others for food, education needs to be targeted at carers.

Inadequate hydration

People with reduced mobility often have a low fluid intake. Those with communication difficulties (e.g. following stroke or head injury) may be unable to indicate that they are thirsty. Others may be reluctant to drink much for fear of incontinence, or because of the physical effort involved in reaching the lavatory. Some may have increased fluid losses through excess saliva production and dribbling. In the care setting, the importance of providing fluids and monitoring fluid status may be overlooked. As a result, chronic dehydration is a common problem, increasing the risk of urinary infections and exacerbating problems such as constipation and renal stones.

Obesity

Immobility results in a decreased requirement for energy. In addition, lack of mobility may result in food choice being heavily dependent on easy-to-eat snack foods and confectionery. Others, perhaps confined to a wheelchair, may consume considerable quantities of confectionery, either as a source of comfort or because they are frequently given them by friends and relatives. All of these factors increase the risk of obesity.

The principles of dietary management of obesity are the same as for any other group of the population but progress may be slower owing to the inability to increase physical activity. A major problem is often monitoring the rate of weight loss, since it may be difficult to weigh people, particularly in the domestic setting. Alternative means of assessing and monitoring adiposity may be necessary (see Section 1.8, Assessment of nutritional status).

Constipation

This is commonly associated with immobility, particularly when injury or disease also has the effect of reducing gut motility (e.g. as a consequence of spinal injuries or multiple sclerosis). It may also be a side-effect of some drugs, particularly those used to relieve pain. In many people the problem will be exacerbated by a low fibre intake (particularly if a diet of a semi-solid consistency is consumed) and low fluid intake Pain or discomfort associated with defecation or episodes of incontinence may also make patients reluctant to increase fibre and fluid intake.

However, the combination of a modest increase in consumption of higher fibre food choices together with a greater fluid consumption may be sufficient to alleviate symptoms and reduce the need for laxatives. In people who require a soft or semi-solid diet, this can be achieved by use of high-fibre breakfast cereals soaked in milk, adding wholemeal breadcrumbs or well-cooked soft pulses to main meals, and the use of puréed fruit and vegetables or prune juice.

Communicating with people with visual or aural disabilities

Visual disability

In the UK, the most common causes of visual impairment are diabetes, cataracts and glaucoma. About 1 million people are registered as blind in the UK, and 600 000 people are registered as partially sighted. Many of these people are also elderly, and those who have a combination of both sight and mobility problems are a particularly nutritionally vulnerable group. However, most visually impaired adults cope with their disability remarkably well and are not at any particular nutritional risk. Nevertheless, they may, like the rest of the population, at times require therapeutic guidance for unrelated clinical disorders. Dietitians therefore need to be aware of how best to communicate with this client group.

Basic rules when communicating with someone who is totally blind are:

- Make sure that the person is aware of your presence before you start talking to them. Gain their attention by using their name and gently touching the person on the shoulder. Say who you are.
- Do not raise your voice while talking to them.
- Before you leave, make sure that the person knows you are going.

If supportive information is required for the patient, it can be transcribed into Braille or other readable form, or on to audiotape. Only a minority of blind people read Braille, since people who lose their sight in later years find it particularly hard to learn. The Royal National Institute for the Blind (RNIB) can advise on written or audio transcription services and also produces some general resources on nutrition and cookery. Local transcription services for visually impaired people may also be available.

People who are partially sighted may be able to cope with written material produced in large-print format. However, it is important to realize that the size of the print is not the only criterion affecting readability; other aspects which need to be considered include:

- *Contrast:* Black on a white background with high density print is best. Poorly photocopied material is often hard to read.
- *Spacing:* Letters should be spaced so that the area between them is similar; the width of a '0' should be left between words; and at least half the height of a letter should be left between lines.
- *Case:* Words produced in lower case can be recognized by their shape more readily than those in upper case.
- *Style of print:* There needs to be sufficient contrasting background within the letters.

Aural disability

Deafness poses a considerable barrier to communication. Listening through a hearing aid is rather like listening over a very bad telephone line; the sounds are distorted and there may be a lot of background noise. For this reason, many people with a hearing aid also try to lip-read what is being said, a process which requires a great deal of concentration.

When talking to someone who is deaf or hard of hearing, the following measures may help the person understand what is being said:

- Try to ensure the absence of distracting voices and sounds.
- Face the deaf person directly. Make sure that your face is clearly visible.
- Speak clearly and slowly, raising your voice slightly. Never shout.
- Do not overexaggerate lip movements
- Make sure that your mouth is not hidden by your hand (or anything else)
- Use gestures to make your meaning clear.
- Do not expect a deaf person to listen to you and look at a diet sheet or something else at the same time.

The assistance of a speech and language therapist familiar with Makaton sign language may be helpful for consultations with people with profound hearing problems.

3.11.2 Learning disabilities

The term 'learning disability' (which has replaced the term 'mental handicap') describes permanent intellectual impairment to an extent which hampers an individual's ability to lead a fully independent life. The effects may range from mild behavioural and educational difficulties to being totally dependent on others for care.

General aspects

Learning disabilities may be acquired for a number of reasons and at any stage of life:

- *prenatally*: inherited chromosome abnormalities (e.g. Down's syndrome), exposure to harmful agents *in utero* (e.g. rubella or maternal drug abuse), intrauterine growth retardation;
- *perinatally*: oxygen starvation during birth, premature birth;
- *postnatally*: infections affecting the brain (e.g. encephalitis, meningitis), exposure to toxins (e.g. carbon monoxide), physical injury to the brain, expression of undiagnosed inherited metabolic disorder (e.g. phenylketonuria), impaired brain development of physical or psychological origin (e.g. starvation; neglect)

Some people require specialist multidisciplinary health care. People whose disabilities are inherited or stem from early life are usually under the remit of a learning disabilities team, while those with learning disabilities acquired later in life as a result of accident or brain injury are more likely to be the responsibility of a neurorehabilitation team or other specialist unit. The needs of people with less severe disabilities will be overseen by the primary health care team. People with learning disabilities are disadvantaged in many respects and the aim of all those professionally involved in their care is to help them to lead a life that is as normal and independent as possible.

The principles of normalization

'Normalization' is a theoretical framework that underpins the movement of services for people with learning disabilities from long-stay hospitals and institutions into the community. Dietitians need to be familiar with its concepts as these influence how advice is given and the type of advice offered.

Normalization is not a single principle but a family of ideas with a common ancestry which has been evolving and developing since the early 1970s. It has been described as the 'utilisation of means which are culturally normative as possible, in order to establish and/or maintain personal behaviours and characteristics which are as culturally normative as possible' (Wolfensburger 1972) and 'the creation and support and defence of valued social roles for people who are at risk of devaluation' (Wolfensburger 1983).

O'Brien and Tyne (1981) set out the implications of normalization in terms of what services should achieve, for example, service user participation in community life and support in making choices. This has implications for dietitians, who will need to ensure that advice given is compatible with these principles, such as recognizing the importance of meals out, and ensuring clients that are fully involved in choosing and preparing their meals. Dietitians also need to know how to help clients to make valued and informed choices about health issues. Readers are referred to Brown and Smith (1992) for more detailed discussion of this subject.

Nutritional implications of learning disabilities

The nutritional implications of learning disabilities vary according to the level of disability and the quality of support that people receive, but many people with learning disabilities are nutritionally vulnerable for a variety of reasons:

- *Problems with communication:* People may find it difficult to express their thoughts and wishes in a way which others can understand.
- *Impaired cognitive skills:* People may find it difficult to understand what is said to them, or to comprehend written or verbal advice given for weight control or managing diabetes, for example. Problems with decision making, planning and sequencing may make tasks such as preparing a meal very difficult.
- *Poor social skills:* A lack of social skills may make it

difficult to form friendships, resulting in isolation, loneliness and depression.
- *Behavioural problems:* Problems such as food refusal may directly affect nutritional intake; other behavioural problems may lead to rejection by others and exacerbate social isolation.
- *Altered activity levels:* Some people may be hyperactive and others relatively inactive.
- *Coexisting mental health problems,* e.g. manic depression.
- *Coexisting physical disabilities:* These may make it difficult or impossible to shop, cook or self-feed.
- *Side-effects of medication:* These may affect appetite or mood.

Among those who are dependent on others for food, particularly those in residential care, nutritional inadequacies may result from:

- being given inappropriate, unappetizing or insufficient food
- lack of dietary variety or different food textures
- lack of account taken of individual likes and dislikes
- inflexible meal times: food may not be available when an individual is hungry
- insufficient time to consume food: a half-finished meal may be taken away because it is 'time to clear up'
- insufficient help with feeding if this is required
- being fed too quickly
- lack of attention paid to any swallowing difficulties
- overuse of medication such as laxatives to correct problems such as constipation.

Those who have made the transition from institutionalized to community care may, without adequate care and support, develop a number of nutritional problems (see Section 4.30, Mental illness). Some people will find the process of learning to cope for themselves very stressful and, as a result, eat very little. Alternatively, freely available food may cause a person to eat excessively or make inappropriate food choices and gain weight. Those who have spent years in residential care may have little concept of food preparation, e.g. that a raw potato can be turned into mashed potato. Others may find the choice of foods available in the modern supermarket so bewildering and daunting that making any choice becomes impossible.

For those who live independently, there may also be problems associated with low income, since many people with learning disabilities are unemployed. These problems may be compounded by difficulties in budgeting and managing money: all available income may be spent on other things before it is realized that none is left for food.

Nutritional problems of people with learning disabilities

Relatively few studies have investigated the nutritional status of learning disabled people, particularly those living in the community. The high risk of malnutrition among people in institutional care has long been recognized (Macdonald *et al.* 1989) but there has been little evaluation of the nutritional impact of recent community-care policies. One recent study (Bryan *et al.* 2000) suggested that unintentional weight change remained a significant problem in people who had moved from large institutions to smaller community homes.

However, the high prevalence of health problems, many of them nutritionally related, in this population group is well recognized (DH 1995). Furthermore, many of these problems are often unidentified and untreated (Wilson and Haire 1990) as people with learning disabilities are less likely to seek health care. They may be less aware of the need to visit the general practitioner (GP), or find making the arrangements to do so a daunting task. Once there, they may find it difficult to explain their concerns or to understand the advice that they are given. Problems may not be recognized as clinical symptoms but attributed to the person's learning disability. As a result, chronic disorders such as coeliac disease or diabetes are less likely to be diagnosed or properly managed (DH 1995). Kerr *et al.* (1996) highlighted the need for proactive health surveillance in this vulnerable group.

Some of the nutritional problems include the following:

Underweight or overweight

Adults with learning disabilities have a polarized weight distribution with a higher prevalence of both underweight and overweight than in the general population (Simila and Nishanen 1991; Wood 1994; Lea 1999).

Undernutrition is a high risk among those who:

- have difficulties in procuring food (e.g. shopping, cooking)
- have difficulties with eating food. Nutritional intake may be inadequate if people are not offered sufficient food or given sufficient time to self-feed. Food may be lost as a result of poor hand to mouth co-ordination, or dribbled from the mouth
- have swallowing difficulties, particularly those which have not been professionally assessed, and result in people consuming or being given inadequate amounts of a small range of foods
- suffer from anorexia, perhaps as a result of depression, isolation or medication
- have behavioural problems which result in food refusal
- have literacy problems which make it difficult to read instructions for cooking food
- have repeated episodes of vomiting and regurgitation. This may result from physical problems or because food is eaten too quickly or swallowed in large lumps.

Undernutrition is often not identified because body weight is not monitored. In the past this has been a particular problem in the institutional setting where underweight is often not perceived to be a problem; a history of chronic low body weight may simply be assumed to be a person's 'normal' weight. In addition, carers tend to prefer a lighter body weight which is easier to lift and carry.

Overweight may be associated with:

- disorders such as Down's syndrome, which is often associated with hypothyroidism (Kinnell *et al.* 1987; Dinani and Carpenter 1990)
- hyperphagia or compulsive eating resulting from an underlying disorder (e.g. Prader–Willi syndrome) or sometimes as a side-effect of medication
- lack of physical activity, sometimes because of a lack of opportunity or an inability to exercise
- excessive energy intake in the form of fat-rich and sugar-rich snack foods and confectionery, often given as a sign of affection by well-meaning relatives, and used by carers to pacify challenging behaviour or reward progress.

The management of underweight and overweight is, in principle, the same as for the rest of the population, but in practice will depend on the individual needs, problems and circumstances. Dietary guidance to those who are underweight, or their carers, should aim to achieve more frequent consumption of meals and snacks, with particular emphasis on the inclusion of foods of high nutrient density. Additional supplementary measures may be necessary if nutritional depletion is severe (see Section 1.12, Oral nutritional support).

Guidance to those, or the carers of those, who are overweight should focus on devising a healthy-eating plan which achieves a balance between individual food preferences and the need to reduce dietary energy intake. Issues such as a high consumption of confectionery (or large amounts of pocket money being spent on such items) may need to be addressed. The management of obesity associated with behavioural problems or eating disorders will require specialist help. In all cases, a planned programme of follow-up in order to monitor weight change and encourage progress is essential.

In some instances, relatives or carers may be resistant to the idea of correction of overweight. Restricting food choice may be seen as unwarranted denial of one of life's major pleasures and may also be regarded as problematical if food is used as a means of calming or rewarding people with challenging behaviour. There may also be ethical concerns over altering the food intake of those unable to give informed consent. Dietitians may need to spend time explaining that the reasons for proposed dietary changes are to benefit the health of the individual (and can therefore be considered to be a part of duty of care) and are not being imposed merely for the sake of achieving some norm.

Some carers may also feel guilty when people in their care are identified as being underweight or overweight, feeling that their care has been deficient in some way; others may even be resentful at such an implication. These feelings need to be defused by acknowledging that the efforts involved in caring for vulnerable people are considerable, and ensuring that any guidance given is positive and supportive rather than negative and judgemental.

Eating and swallowing difficulties

Neurological problems or drug-treatment side-effects may cause problems with mastication and swallowing, and people with learning disabilities people have an increased risk of avoidable death from choking (Dupont and Mortensen 1988). These problems often receive little professional attention and, as a result, fear of choking may make people afraid or unable to eat, or chronic aspiration may lead to recurrent chest infections. Alternatively, people may be given sloppy or liquidized diets which are inappropriate and unappetizing, and of low nutrient density. All people with swallowing difficulties should receive expert speech and language therapy assessment, and appropriate dietary guidance should be given to individuals and/or their carers (see Section 4.3, Dysphagia).

Constipation

This is a common problem, particularly in people in residential care. Although it can result as a side-effect of medication (particularly tranquillizers), the problem is nearly always dietary in origin, resulting from a lack of fluid and fibre together with a lack of physical exercise. It is often compounded by the overuse of laxatives, which may be administered routinely and for prolonged periods, resulting in the colon being unable to function normally (Moriaty and Silk 1988). Standard remedial dietary measures are usually appropriate (see Section 4.11.1), but the education of carers and health professionals is often essential if they are to be effective.

Faecal incontinence

This may be exacerbated by poor bowel control, constipation, medication or behavioural problems. Undiagnosed food intolerance may also be a contributory factor in some people.

Dental caries

The combination of a high consumption of sugar-rich snack foods and drinks, poor dental hygiene and a lack of professional dental care increases the risk of dental caries and periodontal disease (see Section 4.1, Dental disorders).

Dietary management of people with learning disabilities

Nutritional assessment

In order to help people with learning disabilities, it is essential that individual needs and problems are accurately identified. Nutritional assessment therefore needs to consider not only dietary intake but also the factors which impact upon it and are likely to affect nutritional status.

Communication difficulties may make the assessment process difficult. Some people will find it extremely hard to express themselves verbally and need to be given sufficient time to do so. Others may overcome these difficulties by gestural or other means of communication. Dietitians therefore need to adopt a patient, receptive attitude and develop keen observational skills so that they can identify and respond to the signals being conveyed. It should also be borne in mind that some people may have sight or hearing impairment.

Assessing nutritional requirements In general, the nutritional requirements of people with learning disabilities will be the same as for the rest of the population. However, some people may have increased energy requirements as a result of challenging behaviours manifesting as hyperactivity, pacing or restless agitated behaviour. Others may have energy requirements at the lower end of the normal range if they are markedly inactive as a result of withdrawal, lethargy or severe depression. Some types of medication may also have nutritional implications (see Table 4.66 in Mental illness and Section 2.12, Drug-nutrient interactions).

Assessing nutritional status Body mass index (BMI) is one of the most practical and useful indicators of nutritional status in people with learning difficulties (Wood 1994) as this will highlight severe cases of undernutrition or obesity. Changes in body weight over a period of time are also indicative of emerging problems and the weight of anyone identified as being at risk of undernutrition or overnutrition should be regularly monitored. As with the rest of the population, the aim should be to maintain BMI within the normal range of 20–25. If the measurement of height and weight is difficult as a result of accompanying physical disabilities, alternative parameters of adiposity can be used (see Section 1.8.4 in Assessment of nutritional status).

Assessing nutritional risk Because of the scarce availability of dietetic expertise, the technique of nutritional risk assessment is increasingly being recognized as a valuable means of identifying people most in need of dietetic referral and support. The development of nutritional screening tools is still in its infancy; most are targeted at the general population and few have been well validated (see Section 1.9, Assessment of nutritional risk). However, Bryan *et al.* (1998) have devised and validated a nutrition screening tool specifically for people with learning disabilities. This assesses three areas of nutritional risk:

- nutritional adequacy of the diet
- body weight
- nutrition-related problems such as swallowing difficulties or constipation.

The assessment form is quickly and easily completed by nursing staff from their knowledge of the client, nursing and medical records, and weight and medication charts. For each of the three areas the client is allocated as being 'at risk' or 'not at risk'. Any identified risks are referred to the client's doctor and/or care team and if necessary a nutrition care plan is formulated to address the needs. The care plan is then monitored, reviewed and amended as necessary.

This strategy has many advantages as it:

- enables nutritional problems to be identified and corrected at an early stage

- raises awareness of nutritional needs among carers and health professionals
- provides the basis for a planned programme of nutritional care
- promotes nutritional health and hence general health, thus reducing the risk of problems requiring health care.

Further developments in this approach are likely.

Providing dietary guidance

The overall objective is to encourage the consumption of a well-balanced varied diet, along the lines of the *Balance of Good Health*. However, other considerations may impact on the type of advice offered and the way in which this is conveyed to clients. Close collaboration with other members of the care team is essential to ensure that dietary objectives are compatible with other aspects of care and that everyone conveys the same dietary messages.

Individual care plans should be implemented for those identified as being at nutritional risk. These may, for instance, provide guidelines for when to contact the dietitian, e.g. when body weight falls below a certain level, thus enabling people to become responsible for their own or their client's care.

Dietary guidance to the client usually needs to comprise a few simple messages, i.e. two or three key dietary measures which are the most important for that individual. These messages should be reinforced on every possible occasion and also by other members of the care team.

The dietary messages may need to be supported with practical suggestions for meals and snacks, e.g. baked beans on toast, pizza and salad, or items to look for in the supermarket. Information in pictorial or model form may be useful, although the use of real food, meals, and visits to supermarkets and shops may be cognitively less confusing for those people who have difficulty with abstract concepts.

Many clients are able to learn about and manage their own diets if given appropriate guidance and support, a fact which is sometimes overlooked by professionals (Cole 1990). Group support may be appropriate and simple dietary guidance on meal planning, shopping list suggestions, easy-to-prepare recipes and solutions for common nutritional problems can often be built into teaching programmes devised to assist independent living.

Dietary management of specific learning disabilities

Autism

Autism is a disability which affects a person's ability to interpret and make sense of the world around them. As a result, the ability to communicate and interact with other people is severely impaired. The condition is a spectrum of disorders ranging widely in symptoms and severity, but the effects of which may include profound psychological disturbance such as:

- obsessional or compulsive behaviour
- repetitive behaviour and/or speech
- fixation on one object; fascination with lights
- hyperactivity, e.g. jumping up and down; arm flapping when excited; sleep problems
- fear or anxiety resulting in withdrawal and misery
- giggling and/or screaming for no reason
- pica (eating inedible substances such as earth, sand, paper or soap)
- difficulties with verbal and/or non-verbal communication
- general learning disability.

Autism is thought to affect between 10 and 15 people per 1000 in the UK and is about four times as common in boys as in girls, but the rate of diagnosis is rapidly rising as awareness of the condition increases. The symptoms usually become apparent during the first 3 years of life. Autism also includes the condition of Asperger syndrome, which describes children who have characteristics of autism but are of average or above average intelligence and have good communication skills.

The causes are not yet fully understood, although they may be associated with factors affecting brain development either before, during or after birth, such as maternal rubella, lack of oxygen at birth, and complications of whooping cough and measles. Genetic traits may also be relevant. There is no cure but specialized education and structured support can help to maximize a child's skills and minimize behaviour problems.

Nutritional implications of autism

Because of the unique communication difficulties posed by autism, it is important that dietitians working directly with autistic people receive expert training to help them to understand the needs and problems of this client group. The following two aspects of autism are particularly relevant to dietetic practice.

Dietetic problems associated with autism: because of the profound behavioural disturbance which can occur, disturbed and erratic eating habits are common. Clients may be very obsessional about food, only eating a narrow range of foods presented in set ways. Pica (consuming items normally considered inedible) may also be a significant problem. Assessing the extent and impact of these problems often depends on information supplied by parents or carers since the autistic sufferer is usually unable to respond to questions from outsiders. The way in which such problems are managed is a specialist area requiring expert psychiatric help alongside dietetic input, and is beyond the scope of this book. Readers are referred to an excellent review of the subject by Cornish (1998).

Possible links between diet and autism: it has been suggested that some, but by no means all, cases of autism may be triggered by intolerance to foods and/or chemicals. Some parents have observed that autistic behavioural symptoms such as continual screaming and violence appear to be aggravated by certain foods such as cheese, chocolate, bananas, oranges, tomatoes, yeast extract, pickled fish or those with artificial food colourings. This has led to speculation that impaired breakdown of amines, salicylates or phenolic compounds, possibly as a result of metabolic enzyme deficiencies, could result in alterations in mood-altering chemicals in the brain (Alberti *et al.* 1999). Other dietary components such as gluten, wheat or casein have also been linked with autistic symptoms (Ashkenazi *et al.* 1980; Lucarelli *et al.* 1995). While these findings are of interest, at present they remain to be substantiated and their clinical significance determined. They have, however, already resulted in many parents of autistic children imposing various types of exclusion diets in an attempt to reduce behavioural problems. While this is understandable, such regimens are likely to be imposed without any dietetic guidance and the dangers of nutritional imbalance if foods such as wheat and milk are removed from the diets of children are obvious. It is therefore important that dietitians who work with autistic clients are aware of this possibility and that the implications of such diets are discussed with parents and carers.

Text revised by: Briony Thomas

Acknowledgements: Fran Bryan, Hilary Bradshaw, Rosemary Hoskins, Karen Lake and the British Dietetic Association's Mental Health Group.

Useful resources

The British Dietetic Association's Mental Health Group can advise on resources currently available for those working with learning-disabled clients and can be contacted c/o the British Dietetic Association.

Useful addresses

Action for Blind People
14–16 Verney Road, London SE16 3DZ
Tel: 020 7732 8771

Association for Spina Bifida and Hydrocephalus (ASBAH)
ASBAH House, 42 Park Road, Peterborough, Cambridgeshire PE1 2UQ
Tel: 01733 555988

Cleft Lip and Palate Association (CLAPA)
235–237 Finchley Road, London NW3 6LS
Tel: 020 7431 0033
Website: www.clapa.cwc.net

Deafblind UK
100 Bridge Street, Peterborough, Cambridgeshire PE1 1DY
Tel: 01733 358100
Helpline: 0800 132 320

Disabled Living Foundation
380–384 Harrow Road, London W9 2HU
Helpline: 0870 603 9177
Website: www.dlf.org.uk

Down's Syndrome Association
15–155 Mitcham Road, London SW17 9PG
Tel: 020 8682 4001

MENCAP (Royal Society for Mentally Handicapped Children and Adults)
117–123 Golden Lane, London EC1Y 0RT
Tel: 020 7454 0454

Muscular Dystrophy Group
7–11 Prescott Place, Clapham, London SW4 6BS
Tel 020 7720 8055

National Autistic Society (NAS)
393 City Road, London EC1V 1NE
Tel: 020 7833 2299
NAS Information Service: 020 7903 3599

Royal Association for Disability and Rehabilitation (RADAR)
12 City Forum, 250 City Road, London EC1V 8AF
Tel: 020 7250 3222

Royal National Institute for the Blind (RNIB)
224 Great Portland Street, London W1N 6AA
Tel: 020 7388 1266
Helpline: 0845 766 9999

Royal National Institute for Deaf People (RNID),
19–23 Featherstone Street, London EC1Y 8SL
Tel: 020 7296 8000
Helpline: 0808 808 0123/0808 808 9000

Scottish Down's Association
158–160 Balgreen Road, Edinburgh EH11 3AU
Tel: 0131 313 4225

Further reading

Holmes A, Parrish A. Health of the nation for people with learning disabilities. *British Journal of Nursing* 1996; **5**: 1184–1188.
Home Farm Trust. *Nutritional Guidelines for People with Learning Disabilities*. Leamington Spa: Home Farm Trust, 1993.

References

Alberti A, Pirrone P, Elia M *et al.* Sulphation deficit in 'low functioning' autistic children: a pilot study. *Biological Psychiatry* 1999; **46**: 420–424.
Ashkenazi A, Levin S, Krasilowsy D. Gluten and autism. *Lancet* 1980; **i**: 157.
Brown H, Smith H (Eds). *Normalisation. A Reader for the Nineties*. London: Routledge, 1992.
Bryan F, Jones JM, Russell L. Reliability and validity of a nutrition screening tool to be used with clients with learning difficulties. *Journal of Human Nutrition and Dietetics* 1998; **11**: 41–50.
Bryan F, Allan T, Russell L. The move from long-stay learning disabilities hospital to community homes: a comparison of clients' nutritional status. *Journal of Human Nutrition and Dietetics* 2000; **13**: 265–270.
Cole A. Teaching people how to manage their own 'special' diets: some lessons from practice. *Mental Handicap* 1990; **18**: 156–159.

Cornish E. A balanced approach towards healthy eating in autism. *Journal of Human Nutrition and Dietetics* 1998; **11**: 501–509.

Department of Health. *The Health of the Nation: A Strategy for People with Learning Disabilities*. London: DH, 1995.

Department of Health. *Health Survey for England: 1995*. London: The Stationery Office, 1997.

Dinani S, Carpenter S. Downs syndrome and thyroid disorder. *Journal of Mental Deficiency Research* 1990; **34**: 387–392.

Dupont A, Mortensen NPB. Avoidable death in a cohort of mentally retarded. In Fraser I (Ed.) *Key Issues in Mental Retardation Research*. London: Routledge, 1988.

Jones PM. Feeding disorders in children with multiple handicaps. *Developmental Medicine and Child Neurology* 1989; **31**: 404–406.

Kerr M, Fraser W, Felie D. Primary health care for people with a learning disability. *British Journal of Learning Disabilities* 1996; **24**: 2–8.

Kinnell HG, Gibbs N, Teale JD, Smith J. Thyroid dysfunction in institutionalised Downs syndrome adults. *Psychological Medicine* 1987; **17**: 387–392.

Lea A. Assessment of body mass index for the residents of a long-stay institution for people with learning disability. *Journal of Human Nutrition and Dietetics* 1999; **12**: 141–149.

Lucarelli S, Frediani T, Zingoni AM *et al*. Food allergy and infantile autism. *Panminerva Medica* 1995; **37**: 137–141.

Macdonald NJ, McConnell KN, Stephen MR, Dunnigan MG. Hypernatraemic dehydration in patients in a large hospital for the mentally handicapped. *British Medical Journal* 1989; **299**: 1426–1429.

Markson EW. Functional, social and psychological disability as causes of loss of weight and independence in older community-living people. *Clinical Geriatric Medicine* 1997; **13**: 639–652.

Moriaty KJ, Silk DA. Laxative abuse. *Digestive Diseases* 1988; **6**: 15–29.

O'Brien J, Tyne A. *The Principle of Normalisation: A Foundation for Effective Services*. London: The Campaign for Mentally Handicapped People, 1981.

Simila S, Nishanen P. Underweight and overweight cases among the mentally handicapped. *Journal of Mental Deficiency Research* 1991; **35**: 160–164.

Stuck AE, Walthert JM, Nikolaus T *et al*. Risk factors for functional status decline in community-living elderly people: a systematic literature review. *Social Science Medicine* 1999; **48**: 445–469.

Wilson DN, Haire A. Health care screening for people with mental handicap living in the community. *British Medical Journal* 1990; **301**: 1379–1381.

Wolfensburger W. *The Principle of Normalisation in Human Services*. Toronto: National Institute on Mental Retardation, 1972.

Wolfensburger W. Social role valorisation. A proposed new term for the principle of normalisation. *Mental Retardation* 1983; **21**: 234–239.

Wood T. Weight status of a group of adults with learning disabilities. *British Journal of Learning Disabilities* 1994; **22**: 97–99.

3.12 Nutrition for exercise and sport

3.12.1 Exercise versus sport

Exercise

The role of nutrition in sport has become well accepted. Those who undertake regular training, either for pleasure or in order to compete in their chosen discipline, might consider themselves to be taking part in sport. However, there are increasing numbers of individuals who take part in physical activity at a different level, usually with the aim of maintaining health or assisting in the loss of weight. With the establishment of rehabilitation programmes in clinical areas such as coronary heart disease and diabetes we have also seen the advent of 'exercise on prescription'. These individuals may not consider themselves athletes in the true sense of the word. Each clinical area involving exercise as part of treatment or rehabilitation has its own dietary considerations, which are outlined elsewhere in this book, but the major basic principles underlying their diets are those of healthy eating (see Section 1.2). In the world of sport, the main dietary principles are also based on healthy eating; however, there are some aspects that need more specific recommendations. The more in-depth recommendations for sport may be unnecessary for individuals who take part in exercise as opposed to those who train regularly. However, there are a number of issues important to sport, to which every active individual should pay particular attention in order to gain the maximum benefit from their exercise:

- *Carbohydrate*: An adequate carbohydrate intake is important, and active people should ensure an intake of carbohydrate which at least matches the recommendations for health.
- *Timing*: Excessively long gaps between eating and exercising should be avoided and snacks used if necessary. After more strenuous exercise some participants may find it useful to include a small, high-carbohydrate snack immediately after exercise, e.g. fruit or bread-based snacks.
- *Fluid*: An adequate intake of fluid is important to all active individuals and the section of this chapter on fluid for sport should be noted when considering any type of exercise or sport.

Sport

In the world of sport, coaches and athletes appreciate the role played by nutrition in improving both health and sports performance. Diet directly affects an athlete's ability to train and recover from training, to compete and keep on competing. 'An adequate diet, in terms of quantity and quality, before, during and after training and competition, will maximize performance. In the optimum diet for most sports, carbohydrate is likely to contribute about 60–70% of total energy intake and protein about 12%, with the remainder coming from fat' (Consensus Statement 1991).

Owing to the wide diversity of different sporting activities and the vastly differing demands placed on the individual by their particular sport, level of performance and commitment, it is clearly beyond the scope of this chapter to provide detailed guidelines for every sport. However, two specific nutritional principles are applicable to most sports irrespective of the standard of the participant:

- the intake of sufficient dietary carbohydrate to maintain muscle glycogen levels during training and competition
- the intake of sufficient fluids to maintain normal thermoregulatory function during exercise.

3.12.2 Energy metabolism during exercise

In order to appreciate the relationship between diet and performance, it is helpful to summarize the effects of exercise on energy metabolism.

Energy is largely stored in the body as glycogen and fat. The body stores an average of 375–475g of glycogen, up to a maximum of approximately 600 g in muscle and a further 100 g in the liver. This is sufficient to run around 32 km (20 miles). The bodily reserves of fat are, for all practical purposes, unlimited even in the leanest of athletes. The third fuel is phosphocreatine, but only very small amounts of this are stored in the muscle, sufficient to run for 5 or 6 seconds.

During exercise the working muscles convert this stored energy into kinetic energy, to fuel movement and heat. The energy needs of the muscles are covered by accelerating the rate of adenosine triphosphate (ATP) resynthesis to match the rate at which ATP is being utilized. ATP is produced when muscle cells metabolize carbohydrate and fatty acids in the presence of oxygen. This process is called aerobic metabolism. ATP can also be produced without the presence of oxygen, but during this anaerobic metabolism only carbohydrate can be utilized. Thus, the two main fuels for muscle metabolism are carbohydrate and fat. Fatigue often coincides with depletion of the carbohydrate reserves.

As exercise intensity increases there is increased reliance on carbohydrate, but as exercise duration increases there is a declining contribution from carbohydrates. This is partly due to progressively depleted muscle glycogen and glucose as exercise continues, but also to the increased availability of free fatty acids. Training enables the working muscles to take up more oxygen from the blood supply and produce more energy aerobically, i.e. utilizing more free fatty acids and therefore sparing the limited glycogen stores.

3.12.3 The role of carbohydrate in sport

It is important to appreciate that whatever exercise is performed, some carbohydrate will always be used; the longer or harder the exercise, the greater the demands placed upon the carbohydrate stores of the body to maintain the desired rate of ATP resynthesis. Consequently, without adequate muscle glycogen reserves, the ability to perform high levels of work is markedly impaired. This important principle was established as long ago as 1967 when scientists such as Bergstrom *et al.* (1967) carried out their 'classic' studies. Many researchers have studied this area in more recent times and the *International Journal of Sports Nutrition* is a good source of recent work in this and other areas of sports science relating to nutrition.

This requirement for carbohydrate and the importance of carbohydrate as a fuel for exercise have consequences not only in competition but more importantly in training. It is only through training that performance can improve, and this can only be achieved if each training session is started with muscles well stocked with glycogen.

The role of carbohydrates in training

Every time an athlete trains, the amount of glycogen within the working muscles will fall. As these stores are limited, they must be restocked adequately before the next training session, or it will be started with lower than normal glycogen reserves. If the reserves are lower than normal, the point at which glycogen could become limiting may be attained more rapidly, impairing both the quality and quantity of training which can be accomplished within the training session. If the process of incomplete refuelling is repeated over successive days of training it will result in:

- a progressive depletion of glycogen stores within the working muscles
- difficulty in completing even the lightest exercise
- the feeling of continual lethargy and heavy, tired muscles
- incomplete recovery between training sessions.

The latter point may contribute to an overtraining syndrome, which may be related to trying to train with insufficient restocking of muscle glycogen.

In view of the importance of carbohydrates in exercise, replacing the glycogen reserves (particularly muscle glycogen following exercise) is a critical metabolic process in the recovery period. Exercise activates glycogen synthase in muscle, but full restoration of muscle glycogen during recovery is dependent on an adequate intake of dietary carbohydrate (Hargreaves 1991).

Factors influencing the rate of glycogen repletion

The main factors influencing the rate of muscle glycogen synthesis are the type and amount of carbohydrate ingested and the timing of ingestion. Muscle glycogen becomes totally depleted after 2–3 hours of continuous exercise at intensities of 60–80% VO_2max (Table 3.29).

Muscle glycogen can also be severely depleted after only 15–30 minutes of exercise at intensities of 90–130% VO_2max when the exercise takes the form of intervals of 1–5 minutes of exercise followed by rest, followed by exercise, rest, etc. (Coyle 1991). This type of short, intermittent, high-intensity exercise is a pattern found typically in many individual and team sports such as soccer, hockey and tennis. Increasing the carbohydrate intake of those taking part in intermittent activity can improve their exercise capacity (Nicholas *et al.* 1997). This stresses the importance of carbohydrate as a fuel for all types of sport and not just the endurance sports. Many athletes who train daily need to increase their carbohydrate consumption if they are to avoid residual fatigue, poor performance and the overtraining syndrome.

Glycogen is restored to the muscles at a rate of about 5% per hour and after exhaustive exercise up to 20 hours are needed fully to replenish muscle glycogen stores. During the first 2 hours after exercise, muscle glycogen resynthesis proceeds at the rate of 7% per hour. It is therefore essential that athletes consume sufficient carbohydrate during this time. It is generally recommended that athletes should aim to eat 50 g carbohydrate during the first 2 hour period after exercise (for 70 kg body weight adjustments should be made for actual body weight, using 0.7 g of carbohydrate/kg).

Dietary carbohydrate recommendations for training

Recommended dietary carbohydrate intakes are often described in different ways:

- Diets providing up to 70% of daily energy needs supplied by carbohydrate are better able to maintain the glycogen stores of athletes.
- In quantitative terms an intake of 500–600 g is often quoted as the recommended amount for the replenishment of muscle glycogen stores on a daily basis.

Table 3.29 Definition of VO_2max

As an individual moves from rest to running the oxygen uptake increases in an almost linear fashion until the individual reaches a point where there is no further increase in O_2 consumption. This is the maximum O_2 uptake or VO_2max for the individual

When the exercise intensity is expressed as a percentage VO_2max it is called the relative exercise intensity and it reflects the physiological and psychological demands on the individual

- Expressing carbohydrate requirements in terms of body weights can be used for males or females and is the most useful method of estimation. Athletes involved in regular training usually require a daily intake of 6–10 g/kg body weight depending on the type, length and intensity of training.

These principles represent similar, although more specific, guidelines to those recommended for the general population. Indeed, an interest in sport may present the opportunity to introduce healthy eating to an otherwise non-compliant population, particularly the young adolescent.

Starchy and sugary carbohydrates appear to be equally effective in glycogen refuelling. Athletes with high energy requirements will be eating large amounts of carbohydrate, and if they limit themselves to starchy foods the diet will become excessively bulky. The use of more sugary sources of carbohydrate may therefore become a necessity to athletes with high-energy requirements. As this varies from the usual healthy-eating message, parents of younger athletes may need an explanation of the reasons for this. In guiding athletes to include sugary sources of carbohydrate, care must be taken that fat intake is not greatly increased and that a healthy balance is achieved between the contribution of carbohydrate from these sources and the starchy sources.

Many athletes find solid food immediately after exercise unacceptable and, in order to achieve the required intake of carbohydrate during the first 2 hour period, drinks containing glucose, sucrose, maltodextrin or fructose in concentrations of 6 g/100 ml or higher may be more acceptable. There are many such commercial drinks available, more details of which are provided below. After the initial 2 hour period, 50 g (or the body weight equivalent) of carbohydrate should continue to be consumed every 2 hours. However, as such frequent meals are not usually practical, subsequent meals should take this into account. Meals should thus contain sufficient carbohydrate to cover the time interval before the next meal (i.e. 150 g for a 6 hour interval, 250 g for a 10 hour interval, etc.); see Coyle (1991) for more details of this issue. Foods with a high glycaemic index are generally thought to be beneficial during this post-exercise period. However, there still remains some debate concerning the use of the glycaemic index of foods eaten before, during and after sport (Burke *et al.* 1998). The issue is complicated by other attributes of carbohydrate sources such as palatability, cost, gastric comfort and portability.

The practical constraints placed on athletes by their lifestyle can make it difficult for them to achieve a balanced, healthy diet high in carbohydrates. These constraints are specific to each individual athlete and should be taken into account when giving advice. A single standardized set of dietary guidelines will result in poor compliance.

For example, one of the greatest difficulties facing the athlete is fitting in the purchase, preparation and consumption of relatively large amounts of food with training, travel, competition and employment or education. Many athletes rely heavily on the use of confectionery and convenience foods to satisfy their appetite. If athletes remove such foods from their usual diet in order to improve the overall quality of the diet, alternative sources of carbohydrate of comparable density must be included or total carbohydrate intake will fall considerably. Ease and speed of preparation of meals are important considerations.

General recommendations for carbohydrate during preparation for competition

The most important nutritional consideration is ensuring that the athlete arrives at the competition fully recovered from training with at least normal glycogen stores. Therefore, the best approach would be for athletes to consume a high carbohydrate diet at all times and then simply taper their training in preparation for competition.

The traditional 'carbohydrate loading' method popular during the late 1960s and 1970s is no longer used, having been replaced by a tapering of training and an increase in carbohydrate over the 3–5 days prior to competition.

Such increases in glycogen stores not only benefit the endurance athlete such as the marathon runner, triathlete or distance cyclist, but may be of help in tournament situations where competition lasts for several days. Starting the competition with high glycogen stores may help to offset the progressive depletion of muscle glycogen stores with each bout of competition. One possible disadvantage of increasing glycogen stores is the commensurate increase in body weight through the associated storage of water with glycogen. This may be an important consideration where an athlete competes in a weight-category sport such as judo or boxing.

Increasing the carbohydrate intake of those taking part in intermittent activity can improve their exercise capacity (Nicholas *et al.* 1997) and supercompensating muscle glycogen stores may also improve performance during maximal exercise of short duration (Maughan 1990).

Pre-exercise

The precompetition meal should:

- be carbohydrate-based
- be low in fat
- contain some but not excessive protein
- avoid excess fibre
- be readily digested.

It is generally recommended that approximately 200–300 g of carbohydrate be ingested during the 4 hours before competition. The use of carbohydrate feeding immediately before exercise can be considered. The effect of carbohydrate taken as a special feed during the last hour before exercise begins has been reported in a number of studies. The concern that sugar feedings can cause insulin-induced hypoglycaemia seem less well founded (for review see Coyle 1991) and there is now little support for the idea that such feedings before exercise impair peformance.

During competition

The consumption of carbohydrate during competitions of long duration or between bouts of intermittent competition will enhance performance (Walberg-Rankin 1995). Whilst increasing consumption of carbohydrate during exercise can be difficult, athletes:

- should remain well hydrated
- may use fluid as a vehicle for extra carbohydrate, which should be ingested at regular intervals throughout exercise (where the sport permits) rather than waiting until signs of fatigue appear.
- may eat solid food during certain long events: this should be carbohydrate based and low in fat.

Appropriate volumes and concentrations should be used depending on the circumstances, preferences and need for fluid replacement.

After exercise

- Refuelling should begin as soon as possible.
- Fifty grams (or body weight equivalent) of carbohydrate should be taken within the first 30 minutes to 2 hours.
- This should be repeated every 2 hours.
- Fluids may have to be used initially.

3.12.4 Fluid balance

Thermoregulation during exercise

During exercise, when the rate of energy utilization increases, the rate of heat production will also increase. In order to prevent an excessive rise in body temperature (hyperthermia) the body must lose this additional heat. It can do this by several mechanisms, the most important of which is through the evaporation of sweat on the surface of the skin. Where sweat losses greatly exceed replacement, the circulatory system is unable to cope and skin blood flow falls. With this comes a reduction in sweating and a reduction in the ability to lose heat, thus body temperature will rise with potentially fatal consequences. Although sweating is a very effective way of losing heat, care must be taken to ensure that this process is not impaired through dehydration. Sweat is simply a dilute version of blood. Thus, when sweating is prolonged or pronounced, the body loses both water and electrolytes.

The addition of sodium to sports drinks aids the absorption of water and thus the process of rehydration. Further, this sodium prevents the drop in plasma sodium concentration and plasma osmolality that would occur during exercise with the ingestion of large amounts of plain water. The drop in plasma sodium concentration and plasma osmolality would result in diuresis (Maughan and Leiper 1995), and would also result in a lowered desire to drink, resulting in a lower fluid consumption.

Considerable care should be taken to ensure adequate hydration before, during and after exercise so as to avoid thermal distress. These principles apply equally to training and competition, as progressive depletion of the body water can occur over several days of insufficient fluid intake in the same way as the progressive depletion of glycogen.

It should also be remembered that these points apply equally to all sportsmen and women, not just marathon runners, and especially to those exercising indoors. The rate of sweating depends on a number of factors – work rate, environmental temperature, humidity, body surface area, hydration status, training status, acclimatization and clothing (Brouns 1991) – and these should be taken into account when considering the volume and concentration of fluids to be ingested.

Dietetic advice concerning fluid balance

The fluid used during sport should be palatable to the athlete. Ideally, it should contain sodium, and most sports drinks contain levels of 10–25 mmol/l. The addition of carbohydrate to a drink also provides an additional source of fuel for the working muscles.

There are now several commercial preparations available that athletes can use for rehydration (e.g. Gatorade, Isostar, Lucozade Sport). Athletes can also make their own drinks by dissolving 4–8 g glucose or glucose polymer in 100 ml water (warm or hot water helps the glucose to dissolve, but the drink should be cooled for palatability) and adding one-fifth of a teaspoon of salt to every litre. Any flavouring should be 'sugar free', such as sugar-free squash. Where rehydration is a priority, the carbohydrate content should be low; where provision of additional fuel is paramount a higher concentration of glucose can be used (Table 3.30).

Before exercise

The athlete should be fully hydrated prior to taking any exercise training or competition. Sporting activities should never be started in a dehydrated state. This can be achieved by:

- constantly being aware of fluid status and maintaining a good fluid intake (a useful check is to ensure that the urine is the colour of pale straw)
- having a high intake of fluid in the days running up to competition or heavy training
- continuing to drink on the day of competition or heavy training
- drinking 400–600 ml of fluid during the last 10–30 minutes before competition. Drinking earlier than this can cause problems because of the need to urinate once the event has started.
- avoiding large amounts of alcohol the night before.

During exercise

- The use of a sports bottle is to be encouraged.
- Drinking should be encouraged at an early stage and *before* thirst has developed.
- Frequent ingestion of small amounts of fluids keeps up the rate of gastric emptying.
- Athletes are often encouraged to consume up to 150 ml fluid every 15 minutes. In reality this will be affected by palatability and tolerance to fluid in the stomach (Brouns 1991)
- Athletes should use training sessions to grow used to drinking during exercise.

Table 3.30 Sports drinks

- Sports drinks labelled *isotonic* usually contain carbohydrate at a level of 4–8 g/l. This is sufficient to provide a small amount of carbohydrate as energy during sport, but not sufficient for the carbohydrate to hinder fluid absorption. This makes them useful before, during and after sport.
- *Hypertonic* solutions containing >10 g carbohydrate/l will inhibit the absorption of fluid and these are therefore not generally to be recommended during sport.
- *Hypotonic* solutions containing <4 g carbohydrate/l will assist fluid replacement, especially if sodium is added, but will not make any major contribution to energy intake.

The addition of sugar in its various forms is necessary in a sports drink. However, the dietitian should bear in mind that advice should be given to encourage adequate oral hygiene.

Cold drinks were believed to be better than warm because they left the stomach more quickly, but research has cast doubts on the importance of temperature (Maughan 1991). The athlete's own preference is the best guide: a larger volume is more likely to be consumed if the athlete finds the drink palatable, and cooled drinks tend to be more palatable.

Sporting activities in warm climates require careful preparation and sufficient time for acclimatization before competition.

After exercise

- Athletes should carry their own supply of fluid in their kit bag and not rely on fluids always being available at events.
- Rehydration should start immediately, particularly when repeated bouts of exercise have to be performed.
- Drinks should contain some sodium.
- Drinks containing some carbohydrate will also help to replace energy needs.

The volume of fluid consumed needs to replace that lost as sweat, but also needs to take account of the ongoing losses during recovery. Therefore, fluid intake should exceed losses by as much as 50% i.e. for every litre lost 1.5 litres should be drunk (Shirreffs *et al.* 1996). The amount of fluid lost can be measured by weighing dry and without clothes before and after exercise: 1 kg of lost weight equates to 1 litre of lost fluid.

3.12.5 Other considerations

Energy

The energy expenditure due to physical activity can account for 25–35% of the daily energy turnover and up to 75% during intense training of long duration. Energy intakes can therefore vary from 1500 kcal/day for young female gymnasts to 6000–7000 kcal/day for Tour de France cyclists. In sports where a specific body image is required (e.g. female gymnastics, bodybuilding, dancing) or where a sport requires the athlete to compete in a weight category (e.g. judo, wrestling, boxing, lightweight rowing), athletes will often restrict energy intake to lose weight or maintain a particular body composition.

Athletes who repeatedly restrict energy intake for competition, then regain weight afterwards (weight cycling) may find it increasingly harder to lose weight, although regaining weight becomes easier. Female athletes who follow intensive training programmes while restricting energy intake may experience other related problems such as menstrual dysfunction (including amenorrhoea), decreased bone density and iron-deficiency anaemia (Westerterp and Saris 1991). Lower energy intakes may also be associated with low intakes of vitamins. There is also the potential risk that elite female athletes, and to a lesser degree male athletes, competing in weight-category sports or sports where weight or body composition is relevant for performance may present with eating disorders.

Rapid weight loss in days before competition to 'make weight' is also achieved in some sports by increasing rather than tapering training, fasting or vomiting, restricting fluids and by the use of saunas, sweat suits, laxatives and diuretics. Such practices will lead to diminished body reserves which more than offset any advantages of competing in a lower weight category. Long-term planned weight-reduction programmes are essential if athletes are to maintain training and not impair their performance.

Where high energy intakes are required, it is still important to provide a high proportion of carbohydrate for maximal power output and not to rely on increasing the intake of more energy-dense, fatty foods. The lifestyle of athletes often limits the amount of time available to eat, and for those athletes requiring a high energy intake it is not practical to recommend that the carbohydrate is provided solely by starchy, unrefined foods such as wholegrain cereals, potatoes and pulses. In such cases the diet will need to be supplemented with sources of simple carbohydrate in solid or liquid form.

Weight control

The aim of a weight-loss diet for an athlete is to decrease the body's fat store without affecting the glycogen, water or lean body-mass content. It is essential that the diet contains sufficient carbohydrate to restock the glycogen stores between each training session. The diet must therefore be very low in fat and provide all the essential nutrients in a total energy intake that will achieve the desired weight loss. Rapid weight loss by dietary or non-dietary methods should be discouraged if loss of performance due to dehydration and glycogen depletion is to be avoided (for review see Smith 1984).

In gaining weight, an athlete will want to increase lean body mass rather than body fat content. Muscle mass is determined by the training effect, and the best dietary advice for an athlete desiring to gain weight is to ensure an adequate diet with a high proportion of carbohydrate to support training. A conscious effort should be made to keep up food intake, meals should not be missed and high-carbohydrate snacks should be included between meals whenever possible.

Protein

Many athletes believe that they must eat large amounts of protein to build muscles and increase strength, yet most expert committees on nutrition throughout the world have not provided additional allowances of protein for active individuals when recommending dietary protein intakes. Experimental evidence seems to indicate that regular exercise increases protein needs. Several factors, including the composition of the diet, total energy intake, the type, intensity and duration of exercise, ambient temperature, gender and maybe even age, can influence protein requirements.

The recommendations for protein requirements for athletes are still a matter for research and discussion, but current evidence suggests that endurance athletes require 1.2–1.4 g protein/kg body weight per day, whilst strength or speed athletes may need as much as 1.7 g protein/kg body weight per day (Lemon 1998). Unless total energy intake is insufficient to meet requirements, such quantities of protein can usually be met by a diet providing 12–15% energy from protein. The high energy intakes typical of most athletes makes these recommendations easy to attain without any dietary manipulation. Athletes at the lower end of the energy intake range may require dietary manipulation to achieve their protein requirements. Vegetarian athletes may also need some guidance to ensure adequate protein intake, particularly those also consuming low-energy diets.

Fat

Unlike glycogen, which can only be stored in limited amounts, fat is not a limiting factor for exercise. Even the leanest of competitors (male and female endurance athletes have only about 7–10% of their body weight as fat) has a large reserve of fat for energy. There is no need to supplement the normal diet with additional fat, indeed intakes of more than 30% energy from fat are likely to indicate an inadequate intake of carbohydrate. Athletes therefore should aim to avoid excessive amounts of fat in the diet, and would normally be encouraged to look to lower-fat versions of foods where appropriate.

Vitamins

Vitamin supplements do not enhance the performance of athletes who are already consuming an adequate diet. However, there may be situations where intakes should be increased by altering the diet or recommending the use of supplementation, e.g. poor eating habits giving rise to limited intakes, or restriction of food intake to maintain low body weight. Athletes who need to consume high energy intakes may be including foods of low nutrient density in order to achieve their energy intake without too much bulk. In both extremes of energy intake it may be necessary to recommend the use of a vitamin supplement, but without megadosing (van der Beek 1991).

Whilst the antioxidant nutrients (carotenes, and vitamins A and E) do not appear directly to affect exercise performance, theories are emerging from studies to propose that supplemental dietary antioxidants may reduce the oxidative stress and skeletal muscle damage associated with strenuous exercise (Applegate 1999).

Minerals

Particular attention should be paid to iron and calcium intakes. Some athletes are predisposed to poor iron status due to low intakes of iron because of restricted food intakes or because dietary iron is predominantly in the form of non-haem iron. Such at-risk groups of athletes should be detected as early as possible and monitored for iron depletion. Treatment may include iron supplementation as well as dietary modification to maximize iron absorption.

Female athletes with amenorrhoea or dysmenorrhoea have an increased risk of developing osteoporosis because of the reduced levels of bone-protecting oestrogen. Improved calcium intakes are particularly important in athletes with low bone density, menstrual irregularities and low calcium intakes since stress fractures are particularly common in this group of athletes (Clarkson 1991).

Ergogenic aids

Ergogenic aids are substances that supposedly raise athletic performance above what would normally be expected, i.e. that will give the athlete that competitive edge. Substances that are claimed to be ergogenic aids include branched-chain amino acids, caffeine, coenzyme Q10, creatine, ginseng, glutamate, guarana, and many, many more. By the very nature of these substances the list is forever changing.

There is a definite lack of any scientific evidence to support the performance-enhancing claims for most of these substances. Taking such substances is unlikely to have any effect on performance except as a result of a placebo effect. However, research into the use of such substances continues and claims for their effectiveness continue to be made. Creatine has been the subject of much research in recent years (Greenhaff 1995). There would appear to be benefits to athletes in longer-sprint and possibly multi-sprint events in using creatine. However, research has not been carried out for sufficient time to determine the absence of side-effects from long-term use. Caffeine has increasingly been studied as an ergogenic aid and some studies have shown a positive effect on performance during prolonged endurance exercise and intense exercise of short duration (Spriet 1995). Ergogenic aids can be expensive but, more importantly, little is known about the possible side-effects or toxic levels of these substances. Commercially produced preparations can contain impurities which may be harmful or illegal (banned substances). Dietitians discussing ergogenic aids with athletes need to keep up to date with current research on the topic to enable them to give a full picture to athletes. The athlete is the one who will then make the decision whether to use any ergogenic aids. Athletes should be encouraged to accept training programmes, technique, good diet, good equipment, adequate rest and sleep, and the right mental approach as the effective ways to aid performance.

Text revised by: Jeanette Crosland

Acknowledgement: Helen Brown.

Useful addresses

Sports Nutrition Interest Group of the British Dietetic Association
Contact via the BDA Office, Birmingham.

National Coaching Foundation
114 Cardigan Road, Headingley, Leeds LS6 3BJ
Tel: 0113 274 4802

Further reading

Practical advice

Bean A. *The Complete Guide to Sports Nutrition*, 2nd edn. London: A&C Black, 1996.

Entry-level text

Crosland J. *Fuelling Performers*. Leeds: National Coaching Foundation, 1999.

Advanced text

Burke L, Deakin V (Eds). *Clinical Sports Nutrition*. Sydney: McGraw & Hill, 1994.
Proceedings of the Nutrition Society 1998; **57**: 1–103 (A summary of a meeting held in Dublin, 16–18 June 1997).

Physiology text

McArdle WD , Katch FI, Katch VL. *Exercise Physiology*, 4th edn. Philadelphia, PA: Williams and Wilkins, 1996.

Ergogenic aids

Williams MH. *The Ergogenics Edge*. Leeds: Human Kinetics, 1998.

Journal

International Journal of Sports Nutrition, published by Human Kinetics
UK contact: Human Kinetics, PO Box 1W14, Leeds LS16 6TR
Tel: 0113 278 1708

References

Applegate E. Effective nutritional ergogenic aids. *International Journal of Sports Nutrition* 1999; **9**: 229–239.

Bergstrom J, Hermansen L, Hultman E, Saltin B. Diet, muscle glycogen and physical performance. *Acta Physiologica Scandinavica* 1967; **71**: 140–150.

Brouns F. Dehydration–rehydration: a praxis oriented approach. *Journal of Sports Science* 1991; **9**: 143–152.

Burke LM, Collier GR, Hargreaves M. Glycemic index – a new tool in sport nutrition? *International Journal of Sports Nutrition* 1998; **8**: 401–415.

Clarkson PM. Minerals: exercise performance and supplementation in athletes. *Journal of Sports Science* 1991; **9**: 91–116.

Consensus Statement from the Conference on Foods, Nutrition and Sports Performance. *Journal of Sports Science* 1991; **9**: iii.

Coyle EF. Timing and method of increased carbohydrate intake to cope with heavy training, competition and recovery. *Journal of Sports Science* 1991; **9**: 29–52.

Greenhaff PL. Creatine and its application as an ergogenic aid. *International Journal of Sports Nutrition* 1995; **5**: S100–S110.

Hargreaves M. Carbohydrates and exercise. *Journal of Sports Science* 1991; **9**: 17–28.

Lemon PWR. Effects of exercise on dietary protein requirements. *International Journal of Sports Nutrition* 1998; **8**: 426–447.

Maughan RJ. Effects of diet composition on the performance of high density exercises. In Monod H (Ed.) *Nutrition et Sport*, pp. 200–211. Paris: Masson, 1990.

Maughan RJ. Fluid and electrolyte loss and replacement in exercise. *Journal of Sports Science* 1991; **9**: 117–142.

Maughan RJ, Leiper JB. Sodium intake and post-exercise rehydration in man. *European Journal of Applied Physiology* 1995; **71**: 311–319

Nicholas C, Green P, Hawkins R, Williams C. Carbohydrate intake and recovery of intermittent running capacity. *International Journal of Sports Nutrition* 1997; **7**: 251–260.

Shirreffs SM, Taylor AJ, Leiper JB, Maughan RJ. Post exercise rehydration in man: effects of volume consumed and sodium content of ingested fluids. *Medicine and Science in Sports and Exercise* 1996; **28**: 1260–1271.

Smith NA. Weight control in the athlete. In Hecker AL (Ed.) *Nutritional Aspects of Exercise. Clinics in Sports Medicine*, pp. 693–704. Philadelphia, PA: WB Saunders, 1984.

Spriet LL. Caffeine and performance. *International Journal of Sports Nutrition* 1995; **5**: S84–S99.

van der Beek EJ. Vitamin supplementation and physical exercise performance. *Journal of Sports Science* 1991; **9**: 77–89.

Walberg-Rankin J. Dietary carbohydrate as an ergogenic aid for prolonged and brief competitions in sport. *International Journal of Sports Science* 1995; **12**: S13–S28.

Westerterp KR, Saris WHM. Limits of energy turnover in relation to physical performance, achievement of energy balance on a daily basis. *Journal of Sports Science* 1991; **9**: 1–15.

SECTION 4
Dietetic management of disease

4.1 Dental disorders

At any age, dental disease can result in acute pain, increased sensitivity and disfigurement, and increases the risk of tooth loss. The chronic effects of dental disease can also have a significant impact on food intake, nutritional status and general health, particularly in older people. The National Diet and Nutrition Survey of people 65 years and over (Steele *et al*. 1998) found clear evidence that the better the oral health of people aged 65 years and over, including how many natural teeth they have, the better their diets and nutritional status. Consideration of a patient's ability to eat is an important aspect of both dietary assessment and guidance.

Damage to, or loss of, teeth may result from:

- dental caries
- acid erosion
- periodontal disease.

Both dental caries and dental erosion result from the corrosive effects of acid on tooth structure. Caries is caused by bacterial acid production in tooth plaque which, if it remains in close proximity to an area of tooth for prolonged periods, can result in deep localized lesions. Erosion results from acid derived from foods and drinks, or regurgitated from the stomach, repeatedly washing over the tooth surface, and tends to result in shallower but more widespread lesions. There has been little awareness until recently of the contribution of acid erosion to dental damage.

Periodontal disease results from inflammation of the gum (gingivitis) which gradually causes destruction of the bone supporting the teeth. Periodontal disease is the main cause of tooth loss associated with ageing.

4.1.1 Dental caries

Prevalence

The prevalence of dental decay in children in the UK has fallen significantly since the 1970s, largely as a result of the introduction of fluoridized toothpaste and fluoridization of water supplies (O'Brien 1994). In 1968, 40% of preschool children had evidence of dental decay; by 1995, the prevalence had decreased to 17% (Hinds and Gregory 1995). More than one-third of 15 year olds were found to be caries free in 1993 compared with fewer than 10% a decade previously (O'Brien 1994).

Nevertheless, dental caries remains a significant problem. O'Brien (1994) found that almost half of all 5-year-old children had some tooth decay, 60% of 9-year-old children had decayed, missing or filled teeth, and the average 12-year-old child had four diseased permanent teeth.

There is also evidence that the overall fall in prevalence has not occurred throughout the whole population and that some subgroups, particularly children from deprived backgrounds, still have very high levels of the disease (Winter 1990). Caries may also be more prevalent in some ethnic minority groups. A study in Camden found that 18% of Asian children had rampant caries compared with 6% of a similar Caucasian population and 3% of African and African–Caribbean children (Holt *et al*. 1996). In all age groups, the prevalence of caries is higher in northern areas of the UK and in people from lower socioeconomic groups (O'Brien 1994).

It should also not be overlooked that dental caries can be a problem in later life. The National Diet and Nutrition Survey of older adults found a strong relationship between the presence of root decay and the frequency of intake of foods containing high levels of sugars, independent of age, gender, social class and region of origin (Steele *et al*. 1998). Among free-living older people with natural teeth, 13% reported that the condition of their mouths adversely affected their day-to-day life on a regular basis. Since older people tend to have fewer teeth than younger people, the consequences of caries may have a greater effect on food intake, particularly if it results in further tooth loss or the necessity for dentures.

Causation

The development of dental caries is a complex process which can be influenced by a number of factors. It originates in dental plaque, a microbial biofilm which occurs naturally on teeth in order to prevent colonization by pathogenic organisms (Marsh 1999). The composition of this microbial population varies but is principally comprised of acidogenic bacteria such as *Streptococcus mutans* and lactobacilli. These bacteria ferment carbohydrate (sugars and starches), resulting in the production of acid (mainly lactic and acetic acids), a process which begins within minutes of exposure of the bacteria to a suitable substrate. Once the mouth pH falls below about 5.7, tooth enamel begins to be demineralized and become more porous.

At this stage, surface damage to tooth enamel can be repaired. Tooth enamel is not a static structure but constantly dissolving (demineralization) and reforming (remineralization). Acid produced by bacterial action will dissipate after about half an hour and, once the pH rises above 5.7, enamel can be remineralized with calcium and phosphate released from saliva. However, this process requires that the pH remains at or above this level for a period of time. As soon as more fermentable carbohydrate is consumed, more acid will be generated, the pH will fall, remineralization will cease and further demineralization will occur. If this process is continually repeated, gradual loss of mineral from the enamel will lead to its eventual breakdown. In time, the damage may progress into the dentine beneath the enamel, resulting in a cavity and gradual destruction of the tooth.

Children's teeth are particularly vulnerable to this process during the first 6 years of life when tooth enamel is still being developed and is relatively soft. Caries can also attack the roots of teeth if they become exposed as a result of gum recession; this is a common problem in older adults.

Diet and cariogenesis

Any fermentable carbohydrate substrate can cause dental caries, but sugars such as sucrose, glucose and fructose are most likely to do so because they are a readily available substrate for oral bacteria. Dietary sucrose may also be able to promote *S. mutans* selection and development in the oral cavity, thus increasing the risk of dental caries (Petti and Pezzi 1996). Sugars such as lactose or galactose have a lower cariogenic potential; furthermore, foods that contain them (milk and dairy products) tend to be high in protein, calcium and phosphates which help to neutralize acid production. Starch can also contribute to caries because saliva contains amylase which breaks it down to glucose and maltose in the mouth. However, the extent to which this occurs varies with the type of starch and the cooking and processing techniques applied to it (Moynihan 1995). Sugar alcohols (xylitol, mannitol and sorbitol) do not depress plaque pH and these sweeteners can therefore be considered non-cariogenic.

However, the type of carbohydrate consumed is not the sole determinant of caries risk. Other dietary and non-dietary factors influence the impact of carbohydrate on cariogenesis.

Frequency of exposure to substrate The association between intake of rapidly fermented carbohydrate such as sugars and caries prevalence is much more closely associated with the frequency of consumption than with the total amount (Holt 1991; Sahoo *et al*. 1992). Small amounts of sugar consumed at frequent intervals will cause far more damage than the same quantity of sugar consumed on a single occasion because acid conditions in the mouth are perpetuated, preventing remineralization and permitting further demineralization to occur.

Food texture Sticky or 'chewy' foods remain in the mouth longer and small particles of them may be left wedged between the teeth where bacterial acid production can continue. For this reason, foods such as dried fruit (e.g. dates, raisins) have a much greater cariogenic potential than fresh fruit (Mundorff *et al*. 1990). Sugars present in soft or liquid form will leave the mouth more quickly and more completely.

Oral hygiene Failure to clean teeth regularly results in the build-up of tooth plaque and the accumulation of food debris in teeth crevices, thus providing both the means and substrate for continuous bacterial acid production.

Salivary flow Saliva helps to protect against dental caries in several ways:

- It helps to remove food particles from the teeth; literally 'washing the mouth'.
- It contains bicarbonate which has a buffering action and helps to neutralize acid production.
- It delivers minerals such as calcium, phosphate and fluoride to the tooth surface, thus enabling remineralization to take place.

Reduced saliva production is thought to be an important factor in the development of root caries in older adults (Faine *et al*. 1992). Measures that stimulate salivary flow (such as chewing sugar-free gum) can therefore be protective.

The resistance of the teeth to decay There is considerable individual variability in the resistance of tooth enamel to decay. Some of this is due to the influence of genetic factors on tooth production (e.g. affecting enamel hardness or causing crowded teeth which are more susceptible to decay). Age is also relevant; both the young (with immature enamel) and the elderly (with worn enamel) are at greater risk. Nutritional factors also affect tooth structure. Fluoride markedly increases enamel resistance since it results in the formation of fluorhydroxyapatite crystals in the tooth matrix which are more resistant to acid erosion than unfluoridated hydroxyapatite. The maximum benefit from fluoride is obtained if it is available during the period of tooth formation, i.e. before the tooth erupts through the gum. Once the tooth has emerged, further protection can be obtained from topical or dietary fluoride. Deficiency of vitamin D causes defective calcification of the dentine of the teeth and may increase susceptibility to dental caries. Eruption of the teeth may be delayed in children with rickets.

The relationship between diet and caries development therefore depends on a complex interplay of factors. There seems little doubt that the frequent consumption of fermentable carbohydrates, particularly those with low oral clearance rates, increases the risk of enamel caries and may be even more damaging to root surfaces (Kandelman 1997; Jensen 1999). The risk of caries can also be compounded by the effect of acid erosion (see below). Foods such as milk and cheese contain phosphate and other components which help to neutralize acid and may be protective when consumed at the end of a meal (Jensen 1999).

However, while the frequency of sugar consumption is an important contributor to dental caries, oral hygiene may be of greater significance. Further analysis from the National Diet and Nutrition Survey of 1450 preschool children suggests that toothbrushing frequency is a more significant predictor of caries risk than sugar consumption frequency (Gibson and Williams 1999). An association between caries and consumption of sugar confectionery (both in amount and frequency) was only present in children whose teeth were brushed less than twice a day. Beighton *et al.* (1996) found that poor oral hygiene in children had a greater impact on the salivary levels of caries-associated micro-organisms than the frequency or amount of sugar consumed. Lack of oral hygiene measures and general lack of dental care are likely to account for a significant proportion of the excessive caries prevalence in deprived groups.

It is also clear that the relative importance of the aetiological role of sugar has changed in recent decades (Harel-Raviv *et al.* 1996; Kandelman 1997). On a population basis, sugar consumption does not affect caries prevalence as much as it used to because factors such as the caries-resistance effect of fluoride, better oral hygiene (e.g. use of flossing procedures and bactericidal mouthwashes) and other preventive dental measures (such as tooth coating and plaque removal) have reduced the impact of sugar on teeth. The overall fall in caries prevalence since the late 1970s has occurred despite little change in sugar consumption.

The significance of sugar consumption is that, in the absence of these protective measures, its frequent consumption can have a devastating impact on teeth. Infants who continually suck a bottle containing a sugar-containing drink develop a typical pattern of dental destruction known as nursing bottle caries. In young children, the combination of poor oral hygiene, limited exposure to fluoride and frequent exposure to sugary snacks and drinks results in rampant or early childhood caries (Ismail 1998). It is to these high risk groups that guidance about sugar consumption needs to be targeted. For the rest of the population, sugar consumption frequency remains an important aspect of dental health promotion but its contribution to caries development will be less as long as other protective measures are in place.

4.1.2 Acid erosion

A certain amount of attrition, abrasion and erosion is a normal part of tooth wear associated with ageing. However, the damage to teeth from acid erosion is now thought to be a significant contributor to dental disease (British Nutrition Foundation 1999). In the 1993 Children's Dental Health Survey, about half of a sample of children aged between 4 and 6 years had evidence of dental erosion, and in 20% of them, the enamel of their front teeth had been sufficiently worn to expose the dentine beneath (O'Brien 1994). The dramatic increase in consumption of acidic soft drinks in recent decades is thought to be a major reason for this.

Susceptibility to dental erosion is partly determined by factors such as the buffering capacity of saliva or solubility of the tooth structure. As with caries, young children are particularly susceptible to erosion because the tooth enamel is more easily damaged. Furthermore, it is this age group whose consumption of potentially damaging soft drinks tends to be high.

The erosive capacity of acidic food and drink depends on the following factors:

- *Titratable acidity*: The pH value provides some guide to acidity. However, some fruit juices (particularly apple, orange and grapefruit juice) have been found to have greater erosive potential than other soft drinks with a lower pH (such as cola and other carbonated drinks). This is thought to reflect the high content of free acids in some fruit juices and hence titratable acidity is a more useful indicator of erosive potential (BNF 1999).
- *Frequency of consumption*: There needs to be sufficient time between exposure to acidic foods and drinks for remineralization to occur. Repeated acid exposure causes repeated damage and also prevents remineralization occurring.
- *Timing of consumption*: Acid drinks consumed at bedtime cause the most damage. If acidic food or drink is consumed immediately before going to sleep, the low level of saliva production during the night enables the acid to continue demineralizing the teeth for several hours.
- *Consumption in relation to tooth brushing*: It may be particularly important that consumption of acidic foods or drinks is *not* immediately followed by toothbrushing. Contact between teeth and acid results in an immediate decalcification of a layer of tooth. Much of this can be reversed if sufficient time elapses for saliva to be produced and remineralization to occur. If people brush their teeth immediately after a demineralizing challenge, a layer of enamel or dentine may be removed. The traditional advice to clean teeth immediately after meals may therefore not be helpful in respect of dental erosion (BNF 1999).
- *Method of consumption*: Liquids sucked through a straw have less contact with the teeth and are therefore less damaging than those consumed from a glass.

Endogenous acids reaching the mouth as a result of gastro-oesophageal reflux or persistent vomiting (particularly the self-induced vomiting associated with bulimia) can also be significant causes of dental erosion.

4.1.3 Periodontal disease

The initial stage of periodontal disease is gingivitis (inflammation of the gums) usually resulting from infection from debris which accumulate in crevices at the base of the teeth. If gingivitis persists, periodontal disease may gradually develop beneath the gum surface, leading to bone loss around the teeth. As a result, the teeth become more mobile and may eventually fall out.

The main significance of periodontal disease and resultant tooth loss is that it impairs the ability to chew and can restrict food choice (Sheiham *et al.* 1999). This may be of considerable nutritional significance in older adults. The National Diet and Nutrition Survey of adults over 65 years found that those with natural teeth are more likely to consume foods which require an effort to chew such as fresh fruit and vegetables and as a result had both higher intakes and blood levels of vitamins A, C and E (Steele *et al.* 1998).

Although extraction as a result of caries still accounts for most tooth loss, there appears to be an increasing trend for tooth loss in adulthood resulting from periodontal disease (Ong 1998). The Adult Dental Survey (OPCS 1991) found that about 95% of the UK population had some signs of gum disease. Gingivitis and periodontal disease can be minimized by good plaque control, i.e. regular brushing and flossing of teeth, dental scaling (the removal of calculus or tartar, calcified plaque on teeth) and general good oral hygiene.

There is a strong correlation between smoking and the severity of periodontal disease (Ong 1998) which may account for the observed association found in a number of studies between periodontal disease and cardiovascular disease (Joshipura *et al.* 1998).

4.1.4 Prevention of dental disease

Dental disease is not an inevitable consequence of ageing and much can be done to prevent it. Dental health promotion is therefore relevant to the whole population but particularly important for those in high-risk groups such as:

- infants, especially at the time of weaning
- children and adults living in deprived circumstances
- elderly people (in whom the level of mouth care is often poor).

General protective measures against dental disease

These require a combination of the following measures.

Good oral hygiene practices

Proper cleaning of the teeth and gums by means of brushing and flossing is essential to remove plaque build-up and accumulation of debris at the base of the teeth. However, teeth should not be brushed immediately after consumption of acidic food or drink as this may hinder remineralization (see Acid erosion above).

The importance of mouth care in those who are infirm or unwell and possibly unable to do this themselves should not be overlooked. Patients undergoing radiotherapy to the head and neck or chemotherapy may be more susceptible to dental caries and good oral hygiene is essential throughout their treatment.

Regular dental check-ups are important in all age groups.

Fluoride protection

Fluoride is incorporated into tooth enamel in the form of fluorhydroxyapatite making it harder and more resistant to acid attack. Regular use of a fluoride-containing toothpaste has contributed to much of the fall in caries prevalence in children. (Other antimicrobial agents added to

toothpastes such as triclosan and zinc citrate provide additional caries protection.)

The fluoride content of drinking water is also an important factor, and caries prevalence is lower where water is naturally or artificially high in fluoride than in low fluoride areas (McDonagh *et al.* 2000). Water fluoridation to a level of 1 ppm is a safe and effective way of significantly reducing caries prevalence (Beal 1998), systematic review suggesting its only long-term drawback to be an increased prevalence of fluorosis (brown mottling of tooth enamel) (McDonagh *et al.* 2000). It is also the most effective public health strategy for caries prevention since it protects all children including those from deprived backgrounds where take-up of other preventive measures is likely to be poor (HEA 1996).

If local water fluoride content is significantly below 1 ppm, children may benefit from supplementary fluoride in the form of drops or tablets or by topical application by a dentist. Fluoride mouth rinses can be useful for adults. Supplements should not be used in areas with a higher water fluoride content because of the risk of tooth discoloration. Very high doses can be toxic. Community dental health officers can advise on appropriate levels of supplementation in a local area.

Dietary measures

These should emphasize the importance of:

- reducing the frequency of consumption of sugar-containing foods, particularly those of a sticky or chewable nature
- avoiding sugar-containing foods or drinks between meals
- only consuming acidic drinks (fruit-based or carbonated beverages) at meal times. Between meals, drinks should be non-acidic, e.g. water, milk or tea. To avoid causing further damage to teeth, acidic food or drink teeth should not be consumed immediately before brushing the teeth, or after doing so at night
- leaving a gap of 1–2 hours between 'eating occasions' (i.e. consumption of any food or drink). Since most foods and drinks contain some fermentable carbohydrates, this interval is necessary to allow saliva to neutralize mouth acids and allow remineralization to occur
- ending a meal with milk or cheese rather than fruit or fruit juice.

People at risk of damage from extrinsic acids (e.g. as a result of chronic gastro-oesophageal reflux or eating disorders associated with self-induced vomiting) should be identified and be given appropriate treatment.

Specific guidance for particular population subgroups

Infants

Prolonged bottle feeding, particularly with high sugar drinks and with soya formulae which contain sugars, should be discouraged (British Dietetic Association 1994). From the age of 6 months, infants should be encouraged to drink from a beaker and the use of a bottle should be discontinued after 1 year. Infants and young children should never be given a bottle or beaker as a comforter.

Weaning practices can have a major influence on both immediate and future dental health (Holt and Moynihan 1996). Weaning foods should be low in non-milk extrinsic sugars and acid content. Drinks other than milk or water should constitute a minority of total drinks and be given only at main meal times. They should not be given in bottles or at bedtime. Fruit juices and concentrates should only be consumed at meal times.

It is particularly important that this advice is targeted at mothers in high risk, socially deprived groups, along with other dental health promotion measures.

Children

Parents can make an enormous contribution to their child's dental health by:

- minimizing the frequency of consumption of sugar-containing and acidic drinks
- not giving children sugary or acidic drinks at bedtime or during the night
- supervising teeth cleaning with a fluoride toothpaste. Parents should clean the teeth of children under 6 years themselves
- ensuring that children have regular dental check-ups.

Elderly people

Aspects which are particularly relevant in this age group are:

- the importance of good mouth care, especially in those unable to do this themselves
- avoiding overfrequent consumption of sugar-rich foods while still maintaining the enjoyment of food
- ensuring that teeth or dentures are properly cleaned every day
- having regular dental checks to identify problems and ensure that dentures fit properly.

Text written by: Briony Thomas

Further reading

British Nutrition Foundation. *Oral Health: Diet and Other Factors*. London: BNF, 1999.
Health Education Authority. *The Scientific Basis of Dental Health Education – A Policy Document*, 4th edn. London: HEA, 1996.
National Dairy Council. *Diet and Dental Health*. Topical Update 5. London: National Dairy Council, 1996.
Rugg-Gunn AJ. *Nutrition and Dental Health*. Oxford: Oxford Medical Publications, 1993.

References

Beal JF. Water fluoridation is safe and effective. *British Medical Journal* 1998; **316**: 1830.
Beighton D, Adamson A, Rugg-Gunn A. Associations between dietary intake, dental caries experience and salivary bacterial

levels in 12 year old English schoolchildren. *Archives of Oral Biology* 1996; **41**: 271–280.
British Dietetic Association. *Soya Infant Formulae and Tooth Decay*. Birmingham: BDA, 1994.
British Nutrition Foundation. *Oral Health: Diet and Other Factors*. London: BNF, 1999.
Faine MP, Allender D, Baab D *et al.* Dietary and salivary factors associated with root caries. *Special Care in Dentistry* 1992; **12**: 177–182.
Gibson S, Williams S. Dental caries in pre-school children: associations with social class, toothbrushing habit and consumption of sugars and sugar-containing foods. Further analysis of data from the National Diet and Nutrition Survey of children aged 1.5–4.5 years. *Caries Research* 1999; **33**: 101–113.
Harel-Raviv M, Laskaris M, Chu KS. Dental caries and sugar consumption into the 21st century. *American Journal of Dentistry* 1996; **9**: 184–190.
Health Education Authority. *The Scientific Basis of Dental Health Education – A Policy Document*, 4th edn. London: HEA, 1996.
Hinds K, Gregory JR. *National Diet and Nutrition Survey: Children aged $1^1/_2$ to $4^1/_2$ years*. Vol. 2: *Report of the Dental Survey*. London: HMSO, 1995.
Holt RD. Foods and drinks at 4 daily intervals in a group of young children. *British Dental Journal* 1991; **170**: 137–143.
Holt RD, Moynihan PJ. The weaning diet and dental health. *British Dental Journal* 1996; **181**: 254–259
Holt RD, Winter GB, Downer MC *et al.* Caries in pre-school children in Camden in 1993/4. *British Dental Journal* 1996; **181**: 405–410.
Ismail AI. Prevention of early childhood caries. *Community Dentistry and Oral Epidemiology* 1998; **26** (1 Suppl): 49–61.
Jensen ME. Diet and dental caries. *Dental Clinics of North America* 1999; **43**: 615–633.
Joshipura KJ, Douglass CW, Willett WC. Possible explanations for the tooth loss and cardiovascular disease relationship. *Annals of Periodontology* 1998; **3**: 175–183.
Kandelman D. Sugar, alternative sweeteners and meal frequency in relation to caries prevention: new perspectives. *British Journal of Nutrition* 1997; **77** (Suppl 1): S121–S128.
Marsh PD. Microbiologic aspects of dental plaque and dental caries. *Dental Clinics of North America* 1999; **43**: 599–614.
McDonagh MS, Whiting PF, Wilson PM *et al.* Systematic review of water fluoridation. *British Medical Journal* 2000; **321**: 855–859.
Moynihan PJ. The relationship between diet, nutrition and dental health: an overview and update for the 1990s. *Nutrition Research Reviews* 1995; **8**: 193–224.
Mundorff SA, Featherstone JDB, Bibby BG *et al.* Cariogenicity of foods in the rat model. *Caries Research* 1990; **24**: 344–355.
O'Brien M. *Children's Dental Health in the United Kingdom 1993*. Office of Population Censuses and Surveys, Social Survey Division. London: HMSO, 1994.
Office of Population, Censuses and Surveys (OPCS). *Adult Dental Health 1988*. London: HMSO, 1991.
Ong G. Periodontal disease and tooth loss. *International Dental Journal* 1998; **48** (3 Suppl 1): 233–238.
Petti S, Pezzi R. Effect of sucrose consumption on the level of *Streptococcus mutans* in saliva. *New Microbiologica* 1996; **19**: 133–140.
Sahoo PK, Tewari A, Chawla HS, Sachdev V. Interrelationship between sugar and dental caries – a study in a child popula-

tion of Orissa. *Journal of the Indian Society of Pedodontics and Preventive Dentistry* 1992; **10**: 37–44.

Sheiham A, Steele JG, Marcenes W *et al.* The impact of oral health on stated ability to eat certain foods: findings from the National Diet and Nutrition Survey of Older People in Great Britain. *Gerodontology* 1999; **16**: 11–20.

Steele JG, Sheiham A, Marcenes W, Walls AWG. *National Diet and Nutrition Survey: People Aged 65 Years and Over.* Vol. 2: *Report of the Oral Health Survey.* London: The Stationery Office, 1998.

Winter GB. Epidemiology of dental caries. *Archives of Oral Biology* 1990; **35** (Suppl): 1S–7S.

4.2 Disorders of the mouth and throat

Damage and disease in the oral area always have the potential to compromise nutritional intake because they can affect the amount and type of food consumed. Even quite minor disorders can have a major impact on nutritional status, particularly if they are persistent and occur in people whose nutritional status is already poor. Food choice and consumption can be profoundly affected by symptoms such as:

- *Pain*: Oral ulceration or infection, dental disease, anaemia, trauma or surgery to the mouth or radiotherapy can have a pronounced anorexic effect as a result of the pain associated with eating.
- *Loss or alteration of taste sensation*: Food may taste insipid, unacceptably sweet or bitter, and some previously well-liked foods may taste unpleasant. A number of foods may be avoided and general appetite impaired.
- *Dry mouth*: Reduced salivary production as a result of radiotherapy or as a side-effect of anticholinergic drugs (such as antispasmodics, tricyclic antidepressants or some antipsychotics) causes difficulties with bolus production, mastication and swallowing. Dry mouth also increases the risk of dental caries or periodontal disease and oral infections such as candidiasis.
- *Difficulties with chewing*: Lack of teeth, ill-fitting dentures and physical problems with jaw movement can markedly affect food choice in favour of a limited range of soft or liquid foods.
- *Difficulties with swallowing*: Fear of choking can result in reluctance to eat and consumption of a diet restricted in variety, texture and nutritional content.

The possible presence of these factors and their likely impact on food and nutrient intake should always be explored as part of a dietary assessment.

The presence of minor oral disorders can also alert a dietitian to underlying micronutrient deficiency and poor nutritional status. Both iron-deficiency anaemia and pernicious anaemia (caused by lack of vitamin B_{12}) can result in the tongue becoming very red, sore and smooth. Deficiencies of practically all the vitamins of the B group can have an effect on the soft tissues of the mouth and cause symptoms such as angular stomatitis (an infection of the skin at the corners of the mouth, often associated with riboflavin deficiency) and cheilosis (a zone of red denuded epithelium at the line of closure of the lips, which often coexists with angular stomatitis). Although cheilosis is a classic symptom of pellagra (deficiency of niacin), in the UK it is more likely to be a sign of generalized vitamin B deficiency and undernutrition.

Vitamin A deficiency can affect the mucous membranes of the mouth and, in children, can result in hypoplasia in tooth enamel and dentine, increasing the susceptibility to caries.

Remedial measures for problems associated with mouth disorders are described in Section 1.12 (Oral nutritional support) along with general measures which may be necessary to restore or improve nutrient consumption and poor oral intake.

4.2.1 Disorders of the salivary glands

Inflammation of the parotid glands, due to either the mumps virus or bacterial infection, may make chewing and swallowing painful and difficult. The condition is usually temporary, and energy and nutrient needs should be met by encouraging consumption of nutrient-dense beverages (e.g. milk-based or glucose drinks) and soft or semi-liquid foods (e.g. as yoghurt, stewed fruit or milk puddings).

Salivary calculi cause pain and difficulty on eating. A soft or semi-fluid diet should be consumed and liquid energy supplements may be advisable if the condition becomes prolonged. Removal of the stones is usually by surgical excision and the diet is gradually regraded to normal as the mouth heals.

4.2.2 Fractured jaw and oral surgery

Jaw wiring is likely to be necessary in patients with fractured jaws and in some cases of oral surgery.

A liquid diet will be necessary and, since the jaws may remain wired for 6–8 weeks, the use of nutritionally complete liquid feeds is advisable to ensure that energy and nutrient needs are met. Most patients can sip these through a straw. In order to prevent taste fatigue, and hence reduced intake, variety is important and both savoury and sweet flavoured products should be used. Liquidized meals can also be consumed if the patient wishes and is willing to do so.

If patients are unable to suck for sufficient periods, or unwilling to take adequate amounts, feeding via the nasogastric route may be necessary.

As the wires are relaxed and ultimately removed, the diet should be regraded from a liquid to a soft or semi-solid diet, with protein and energy supplements if indicated, until a normal diet can be taken.

Careful attention should be given to oral hygiene as protein and energy-containing fluids are an ideal medium for bacterial growth.

4.2.3 Oral Crohn's disease

Crohn's disease is primarily an inflammatory disorder of the small bowel (see Section 4.10, Inflammatory bowel disease) but lesions can occur anywhere along the gastro-intestinal tract and can appear in the mouth.

Crohn's disease of the mouth may result in multiple lesions in the oral mucosa and on the lips, either as part of a generalized condition or without other gut involvement (Tyldesley 1979). The mouth becomes sore, making eating painful and difficult. During an acute attack, an energy-dense soft or fluid diet should be advised and hot, salty and spicy foods should be avoided (see Section 1.12, Oral nutritional support). Additional nutritional support measures may be necessary if the patient is already nutritionally compromised as a result of the prolonged effects of the condition.

4.2.4 Head and neck cancers

Cancers of the upper aerodigestive tract (Fig. 4.1), collectively known as head and neck cancers, constitute only a small percentage of all cancers, but when they occur their potential impact on the individual's nutritional intake and status can be devastating. Nutrition plays a vital role in the care of the individual with head and neck cancer, from the point of diagnosis onwards.

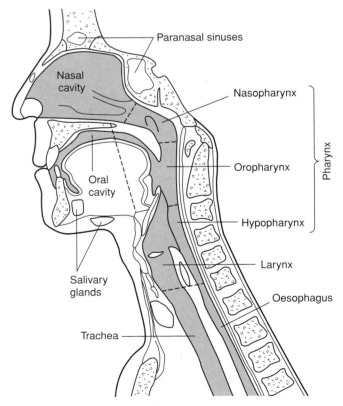

Fig. 4.1 Main sites of head and neck cancers. Adapted from Vokes *et al.* (1993).

Patients with head and neck cancer are at high risk of developing undernutrition both before diagnosis and during the course of treatment (van Bokhurst-de van der Schueren *et al.* 1999). Prior to diagnosis, many patients will have poor dietary habits and some will additionally have chronic histories of excessive alcohol intake and heavy tobacco use (DH 1998). Both before and after diagnosis, tumours of the oral cavity may result in problems such as pain on eating, ulcerated mouth, dysphagia or poorly fitting dentures, all of which can markedly impair food intake. Following diagnosis, treatments such as surgery, radiation therapy or chemotherapy are likely to create further nutritional problems and increase the risk of nutritional depletion (see Section 4.37, Cancer).

Pre-operative weight loss and post-operative complications have been shown to have a marked negative effect on the survival of patients with head and neck cancers (van Bokhurst-de van der Schueren *et al.* 1999).

Nutritional effects of treatment

Multimodality therapy significantly increases the likelihood of undernutrition, immunosuppression and morbidity (Daly *et al.* 1995), with more than 80% of head and neck cancer patients losing a significant amount of weight (Chencharick and Mossman 1983). Supplementary enteral feeding can significantly improve many of these parameters (Daly *et al.* 1995). It is important that nutritional assessment and monitoring is incorporated into each stage of the cancer treatment process to ensure that dietetic intervention is optimized.

Surgery

Nutritional problems related to surgery can be both complex and extensive. Van Bokhorst-de van der Schueren *et al.* (1997) studied 64 patients undergoing major surgery for advanced cancer and found that patients with a weight loss of more than 10% during the 6 months before surgery had a greater risk of post-operative complications such as wound infections, anastomotic leakage and septicaemia. Early nutritional assessment is therefore essential to identify those in need of pre-operative nutritional support. In some cases, aggressive nutritional support measures will be required (Flynn and Leighty 1987).

The post-surgical risk of undernutrition is high and prolonged enteral feeding may be necessary (Gardine *et al.* 1988). Surgical resection of tumours of the head and neck area is highly likely to affect or even prevent oral intake. In addition, post-operative complications such as infection, development of fistulae or sepsis, will increase nutritional requirements (Elia 1990). Early initiation of post-operative enteral nutrition has been shown to improve peripheral protein kinetics (Harrison *et al.* 1997) and result in a more rapid recovery of nutritional and immunological status (Braga *et al.* 1996).

Treatment strategies influence the type and level of artificial nutritional support provided. If it is anticipated that short-term support is required, enteral feeding via a nasogastric tube is often the most appropriate choice. Gastrostomy feeding may be more appropriate if long-term support is indicated (Shike *et al.* 1989). When assessing the likely duration of artificial support measures, the patient's pre-operative oral intake and nutritional status should be taken into account as well as the potential post-surgical feeding problems and delays in rehabilitation.

Chemotherapy

Chemotherapy, although not used widely for head and neck cancer patients, can compromise nutritional status and intake. The process is particularly likely to affect the rapidly dividing cells of the buccal and gastrointestinal mucosa, causing damage to the mucosal lining of the mouth. The resulting pain and ulceration can markedly impair the intake and enjoyment of food.

Nausea and vomiting may be additional side-effects and, if not well controlled with antiemetics, can lead to dehydration, weight loss and lethargy. Anticipatory nausea and vomiting, often triggered by factors such as taste, smell and anxiety, can also be a problem (Love *et al.* 1982).

Radiotherapy

Radiotherapy of the head and neck affects the normal tissues in and around the oral cavity and symptoms such as reduced or abnormal taste sensations, dry mouth, mucositis, loss of appetite and dysphagia commonly develop or worsen (Chencharick and Mossman 1983).

Xerostomia (dry mouth) can be temporary or permanent. Alongside good oral hygiene, modifications to food texture and consistency and increasing fluid intake can help (see Section 1.12, Oral nutritional support). The use of artificial saliva immediately prior to meals may benefit some patients, as may sugar-free pastilles or chewing gum. The reduction in salivary function during radiotherapy can cause loss of palatal seal in denture patients and general difficulty in chewing.

Chencharick and Mossman (1983) found that taste problems were a common consequence of radiotherapy. In their study, aversion to meat was common, as was a decreased taste threshold for sweetness, resulting in a noticeably high sugar consumption. In contrast, salt tended to be avoided because of its irritative effect on the oral cavity and because patients reported that their saliva already tasted salty.

The sore oral mucosa may also be irritated by items such as alcohol, smoking, extremes of temperature and spicy food. Patients tend to discover their own individual food sensitivities by trial and error. General remedial measures for a sore or painful mouth can be found in Section 1.12 (Oral nutritional support).

Dysphagia can occur during radiotherapy treatment necessitating changes in food texture and/or consistency (see Section 4.3, Dysphagia). Additional supplementary or oral nutritional support measures may also be necessary.

Artificial nutritional support, either as an adjunct to oral feeding or as a sole means of support, will be indicated if nutritional requirements are not being met by oral foods and fluids alone. If, in the planning stage of radiotherapy, an individual is identified as being at high risk of nutritional inadequacy, early instigation of partial or total artificial support should be considered.

A useful screening tool to assess nutritional need in patients undergoing head and neck therapy has been described by Macqueen and Frost (1998).

Text revised by: Briony Thomas and Julie Ashton

Acknowledgement: Hayley Wordsworth.

Further reading

Bruera E. ABC of palliative care: anorexia, cachexia and nutrition. *British Medical Journal* 1997; **315**: 1219–1222.

Daly JM, Hoffman K, Lieberman M *et al.* Nutritional support in the cancer patient. *Journal of Parenteral and Enteral Nutrition* 1990; **14** (6, Suppl): 2445–2485.

Dunlop RJ, Ellershaw JE, Baines MJ *et al.* On withholding nutrition and hydration in the terminally ill: has palliative medicine gone too far? A reply. *Journal of Medical Ethics* 1995; **21**: 141–143.

Grindel CG, Whitmer K, Barsevice A. Quality of life and nutritional support in patients with cancer. *Cancer Practice* 1996; **4**: 81–87.

Kouba J. Nutritional care of the individual with cancer. *Nutrition in Clinical Practice* 1988; **3**: 175–182.

References

Braga M, Vignali A, Gianotti L *et al.* Immune and nutritional effects of early enteral nutrition after major abdominal operations. *European Journal of Surgery* 1996; **162**: 105–112.

Chencharick J, Mossman KL. Nutritional consequences of the radiotherapy of head and neck cancers. *Cancer* 1983; **51**: 811–815.

Daly JM, Weintraub FN, Shou J *et al.* Enteral nutrition during multimodality therapy in upper gastrointestinal cancer patients. *Annals of Surgery* 1995; **221**: 327–338.

Department of Health, Committee on Medical Aspects of Food Policy (COMA). *Nutritional Aspects of the Development of Cancer*. Report on Health and Social Subjects 48. London: DH, 1998.

Elia M. Artificial nutritional support. *Medicine International* 1990; **82**: 3392–3396.

Flynn MB, Leighty FF. Pre-operative outpatient nutritional support of patients with squamous cancer of the upper aerodigestive tract. *American Journal of Surgery* 1987; **154**: 359–362.

Gardine RL, Kokal WA, Beatty D, Riitimati du Wagman LD. Predicting the need for prolonged enteral supplementation in the patient with head and neck cancer. *American Journal of Surgery* 1988; **156**: 63–65.

Harrison LE, Hochwald SN, Heslin MJ *et al.* Early postoperative enteral nutrition improves peripheral protein kinetics in upper gastrointestinal cancer patients undergoing complete resection: a randomised trial. *Journal of Parenteral and Enteral Nutrition* 1997; **21**: 202–207.

Love CR, Nerenz DR, Levanthal H. The development of anticipatory nausea and vomiting during cancer chemotherapy. *Proceedings of the American Society of Clinical Oncologists* 1982; **23**: 47.

Macqueen CE, Frost G. Visual analogue scales: a screening tool for assessing nutritional need in head and neck radiotherapy patients. *Journal of Human Nutrition and Dietetics* 1998; **11**: 115–124.

Shike M, Berner Y, Gerdes H *et al*. Percutaneous endoscopic gastrostomy and jejunostomy for long-term feeding in patients with cancer of the head and neck. *Otolaryngology – Head and Neck Surgery* 1989; **101**: 549–554.

Tyldesley WR. Oral Crohn's disease and related conditions. *British Journal of Oral Surgery* 1979; **17**: 1–9.

van Bokhorst-de van der Schueren MA, van Leeuwen PA, Sauerwein HP *et al*. Assessment of malnutrition parameters in head and neck cancer and their relation to post-operative complications. *Head and Neck* 1997; **19**: 419–425.

van Bokhorst-de van der Schueren MA, van Leeuwen PA, Kuik DJ *et al*. The impact of nutritional status on the prognoses of patients with advanced head and neck cancer. *Cancer* 1999; **86**: 519–527.

Vokes EE, Weichselbaum RR, Lipman SM, Hong WK. Head and neck cancer. *New England Journal of Medicine* 1993; **328**: 184–194.

4.3 Dysphagia

Swallowing is a highly complex process requiring appropriate posture of the head and neck, good lip and tongue movement and the presence of the swallow reflex. Many factors can impair the ability to swallow and the physical and nutritional consequences of this can be profound, even life threatening.

Dysphagia is a common consequence of many different types of illness or injury resulting in mechanical or neurological impairment of the swallowing process (Table 4.1). Dysphagia is most likely to be encountered in patients with stroke, progressive neurological disorders (e.g. Parkinson's disease, motor neurone disease and multiple sclerosis), anoxic brain injury, and other conditions or injury affecting the head and neck.

This section refers to dysphagic people over the age of 5 years. The normal swallow does not mature fully until this age, and details of the management of dysphagia in infants and young children should therefore be sought in paediatric textbooks.

4.3.1 The normal swallow

The normal swallow can be divided into four main stages and impairment in any one of these can result in dysphagia:

1 *Preparatory stage*: This stage is mainly under voluntary control, comprising the transfer of food (or liquid) into the mouth. As food or liquid approaches the mouth, the head moves forward, the tongue protrudes and the lips and jaws open in preparation. Food or drink is placed in the mouth and the lips and jaw close to seal the mouth. Saliva production will have been stimulated by the sight, smell and taste of the food.

2 *Oral stage*: This stage where food is prepared for passage from the mouth into the pharynx is also mainly under voluntary control. The tongue moves the food and positions it between the teeth. Chewing (mastication) is achieved by upward, downward and rotary movements of the jaw in order to grind the food and mix it with saliva. The tongue forms a central groove to collect the food, with its tip sealed against the hard palate. The resulting bolus is propelled backwards by the posterior movement of the tongue.

3 *Pharyngeal stage*: This is an involuntary stage where the food bolus passes from the mouth through the pharynx and into the oesophagus. At the same time, the airway is temporarily sealed off to prevent the entry of food or fluid into the lungs. The process is initiated when sensation of the bolus at the anterior faucal arch

Table 4.1 Common causes of dysphagia

Mechanical
  Oesophageal stricture
  Oesophageal spasm
  Cancers in the head, neck and oesophageal areas
  Pharyngeal pouch
  Goitre
  Injury or surgery to the tongue, lips, mouth or jaw
  Severe infections of the mouth or throat
Neurological
  Brain injury
  Stroke
  Spinal injury or deformity
  Motor neurone disease
  Parkinson's disease
  Multiple sclerosis
  Cerebral palsy
  Huntington's disease
  Guillain–Barré syndrome
  Drug-induced (psychotropic drugs)
Psychological
  Globus hystericus

(towards the back of the mouth) stimulates the swallowing centre in the brainstem. The swallow reflex is then triggered:

- the soft palate elevates to seal off the nasopharynx
- the larynx elevates and so forces the epiglottis down to cover the larynx
- the vocal cords (within the larynx) close
- respiration stops momentarily.

Food passes through the pharynx mainly by peristalsis, i.e. the muscles of the pharynx contract and move the bolus through, although gravity has some effect. The cricopharyngeal sphincter relaxes, and is opened by the upward pull of the larynx; the food bolus then passes into the oesophagus.

4. *Oesophageal stage*: This stage is also involuntary. The food bolus passes down the oesophagus into the stomach by peristalsis and gravity, the cardiac sphincter relaxes and food enters the stomach.

4.3.2 Consequences of dysphagia

Dysphagia is potentially fatal. Attempting to swallow foods or liquids without the ability to do so carries a high risk of aspiration (foods or liquids entering the lungs) which if extensive can cause acute asphyxiation and in lesser degrees is a major contributor to chest infections, lung abscesses and aspiration pneumonia (Gordon *et al.* 1987; Smithard 1995). Aspiration may also be 'silent', causing no outward signs of distress but still capable of causing pulmonary complications (Teasell *et al.* 1996).

An impaired ability to swallow has many nutritional implications. The physical effects of dysphagia make the process of feeding slow, difficult and tiring, and as a result food intake is often inadequate in terms of both quantity (sometimes further compromised by food leakages from the mouth) and variety of food consumed. Fear of choking (especially if there has been an unpleasant experience of aspiration) may cause food aversions or panic attacks at meal times. Other psychological factors such as depression or anxiety (stemming from the patient's reaction to the illness and its effects) may further depress appetite. Physiologically, inadequate intake of food and fluid will lead to undernutrition, weight loss, compromised immune function and a high risk of dehydration. These may in turn lead to deterioration of the patient's physical or mental condition and delay recovery or hasten death (Lennard-Jones 1992).

4.3.3 The dysphagia care team

Effective treatment of dysphagia, whether in primary or secondary care, requires multidisciplinary care from a team which should include:

- *clinicians*: who will have overall responsibility for diagnosis and treatment. In the hospital setting, this will be a consultant; in the community setting, responsibility may be passed to the patient's general practitioner (GP);
- *nursing staff*: to provide assistance with feeding and oral care, monitor the effectiveness of the measures recommended and act as a link with other health professionals in terms of need for further assessment and advice. In the community, nurses have an important supportive and advisory role to both patients and carers;
- *speech and language therapists (SLT)*: to assess the nature and extent of dysphagia and provide guidance on the safest position for eating and drinking, the appropriate texture and consistency of food and when oral feeding can safely be resumed in a patient maintained on artificial nutritional support;
- *dietitians*: to ensure that nutritional needs are met by assessing and monitoring nutritional status, estimating nutritional requirements, providing guidance on food consumption of appropriate texture and consistency and recommending additional nutritional support measures when indicated;
- *physiotherapists*: to implement remedial measures to reduce the risk of chest infection and improve posture and mobility;
- *occupational therapists*: to advise on feeding aids and equipment;
- *pharmacists*: to provide prescribed products such as commercial thickeners or nutritional supplements, and advise on the availability of medication in different forms and the possible effects of drugs on the swallowing mechanism;

- *the patient and/or carers*: who should be closely involved in the construction of any care plan.

Other personnel may need to be involved. In the hospital setting, these may include radiologists, psychologists and diet cooks. In the community, liaison with social workers and support personnel such as home helps or meals-on-wheels providers may be essential.

Multidisciplinary care will only work effectively if an effective system of communication is established and the procedure concerning cross-referral and feedback of information is clear.

4.3.4 Management of dysphagia

Dysphagia requires prompt and skilled remedial action in order to reduce the risk of aspiration and minimize nutritional deterioration, particularly if the onset has been acute (Odderson *et al.* 1995; Finestone *et al.* 1995). Nearly half of all stroke patients admitted to hospital will have swallowing difficulties (Gordon *et al.* 1987).

The primary aims of management are to:

- assess the nature of the swallowing problem
- determine a safe and adequate feeding route
- determine the appropriate texture and consistency of orally consumed food and fluids
- ensure that nutritional needs are met
- ensure that fluid needs are met
- educate the patient, carers and other members of the care team
- monitor progress
- ensure continuity of care.

Assessing the nature of the swallowing problem

Suspected dysphagia should always be expertly assessed so that it can be managed most effectively. Following a stroke, it is now recommended that all patients are given a simple bedside assessment of swallowing ability using a validated protocol administered by trained personnel (RCP 2000). Patients with suspected difficulties should be referred to a SLT. If a bedside assessment is inconclusive (difficulties at the pharyngeal stage can be particularly difficult to ascertain) videofluoroscopy (radiological examination of the swallowing process) may be carried out.

In primary care, a dysphagic patient identified by a GP or district nurse should be referred to a hospital for specialist assessment if this cannot be done within the community setting. Dysphagia is a significant contributory factor to undernutrition in elderly people living in the community or care homes (Finch *et al.* 1998) but its presence is often regarded as being of little significance and its management confined to liquidizing the patient's food.

It should be noted that the presence or absence of a gag reflex is not in itself an indication of the ability to swallow; many fit elderly people do not have a gag reflex (Davies *et al.* 1995) and the absence of a gag reflex after a stroke does not indicate either inability to swallow or the presence of aspiration (Smithard *et al.* 1994).

The first three stages of the normal swallow (preparatory, oral and pharyngeal) are most likely to be disrupted when there is neuromuscular dysfunction resulting in weakness, paralysis and/or sensory loss in the muscles associated with swallowing (e.g. as a result of stroke, motor neurone disease or anoxic brain injury). The oesophageal stage is more likely to be affected by mechanical problems such as stricture (e.g. oesophageal carcinoma). The types of problem that can result are summarized in Table 4.2.

Determining a safe and adequate feeding route

The first priority is to decide whether feeding via the oral route is safe. If it is not, alternative routes have to be considered, e.g. nasogastric, surgical gastrostomy, percutaneous endoscopic gastrostomy (PEG) and parenteral nutrition (see Section 1.13, Artificial nutritional support).

Determining the appropriate texture and consistency of orally consumed food and fluids

After establishing that the patient can safely manage an oral intake, the SLT will provide guidance on appropriate dietary consistency to ensure safe bolus transport and minimize the risk of aspiration. This may range from a diet in liquid form to one comprised of normal foods which are least likely to cause choking.

Liquid or puréed diets may be appropriate for patients with dysphagia of mechanical origin who are unable to chew (e.g. those with a fractured jaw). However, in patients with oropharyngeal disorders, diets comprised of thinned and fluid foods increase the risk of aspiration because:

- they cannot be controlled in the mouth
- the disordered swallowing mechanism cannot respond in time with sufficient control to protect the airway
- they lack the taste, temperature and pressure requirements to elicit an adequate swallow/protective reflex.

Foods and liquids therefore need to be modified to a consistency which provides the patient with best control over the rate at which foods and liquids pass through the pharynx (Curran and Groher 1990; O'Sullivan 1990).

The principle of texture modification in dysphagia management has been recognized for many years but the way in which it is implemented has never been standardized. A comprehensive review by Penman and Thomson (1998) revealed wide variation in practice. The most widely used system is a series of graded alterations in food consistency, typically ranging from:

- thin purée: homogenous consistency which does not hold its shape
- thick purée: thickened cohesive consistency which does hold its shape
- soft/finely minced: soft, cohesive and consistent textures requiring some chewing
- minced/normal: normal foods of varied textures, avoiding foods which pose a particular choking hazard.

However, many other classifications are in use.

Penman and Thomson suggested that collaboration between the SLT and dietetic professions was urgently needed to produce national guidelines on the use of textured diets in the management of dysphagia. As a first step, texture classification tables have been produced by the British Dietetic Association (Table 4.3a, 3b). Their aim is to help to ensure the safe management of patients with dysphagia and to assist in the provision of appropriately textured foods. The tables are intended as a resource that can be adapted to local needs.

The guidelines provide separate classifications for foods and fluids. This is because:

- fluid needs must be considered in addition to nutrient needs;
- patients often have different abilities to swallow liquids and solids; it is not unusual for a dysphagic patient to be able to manage a normal diet but be unable to swallow thin liquids (Pardoe 1993). Liquids may therefore be avoided, thus increasing the risk of dehydration.

Commercial thickening agents derived from food starch are ACBS prescribable for dysphagia and can be added to foods or liquids to provide the desired consistency and thickness (Table 4.4).

Table 4.2 Disruption of the normal swallowing process

Stage of the normal swallow	Affected by	Consequences
Preparatory stage	Reduced range of movement of facial muscles, lips, tongue and jaw Loss of sight, smell and/or taste	Difficulty in getting food/liquid into the mouth Difficulty in sealing the mouth Reduced saliva production
Oral stage	Reduced range of movement of facial muscles, lips, tongue and jaw and lack of saliva	Difficulty in mastication Difficulty in forming a food bolus Difficulty in controlling a food bolus
Pharyngeal stage	Absence of swallow reflex	Inability to swallow safely
Oesphageal phase	Impaired peristalsis or obstruction	Food fails to move into the stomach Aspiration after the swallow

Table 4.3a Texture classification of liquids
British Dietetic Association, Post Registration Course in the Nutritional Management of Dysphagia (1997)

Texture	Description of liquid texture	Consistency to aim for
1	A thickener must be added A straw will stand on its own in this liquid Cannot be sipped from a cup; requires a spoon	Thick custard
2	A thickener may be added A straw will move slowly through the liquid Can be sipped from a cup but not through a drinking straw	Double cream (before whipping)
3	A thickener may be added A straw will move easily through the liquid Can be sipped from a cup or through a straw	Single cream
4	A thickener is not required A straw falls freely through the liquid Can be drunk or sipped from a cup and easily taken through a drinking straw	Water Tea Coffee Milk Most fruit juices

Table 4.3b Texture classification of solids
British Dietetic Association, Post Registration Course in the Nutritional Management of Dysphagia (1997)

Texture	Description of solid texture	Consistency to aim for
A	Food that has been puréed and sieved to remove fine particles A smooth, uniform consistency A thickener may be added to maintain stability of texture Sauce-like; it drips rather than pours off a spoon Can only be eaten with a spoon	Tomato ketchup Salad cream Tinned custard
B	Food that has been puréed and sieved to remove fine particles A thickened, smooth, uniform consistency A thickener must be added to maintain stability of texture Must not separate into liquid and solid components during swallow It should be moist, not sticky Will hold its own shape on a plate and can be moulded, layered and piped	Mousse Smooth fromage frais Whipped cream
C	Food that is soft, moist and has not been puréed and sieved Consists of food pieces which are easily mashed with a fork and break into pieces not more than 0.5 cm (¼ inch) in size These foods should be served or coated with a thick gravy or sauce	Flaked tuna in a sauce Mashed cauliflower cheese Mashed banana

D	Dishes consisting of soft, moist, bite-sized pieces
	Suitable foods can be broken into 1.5 cm (¾ inch) pieces with the flat edge of a fork
	Avoid foods which pose a choking hazard, e.g.
	  Dry and crisp: muesli, crisps, battered or breaded foods, toffee
	  Sticky: white bread/rolls, peanut butter
	  Stringy: gristle, fruit skins and shells of peas, beans, sweetcorn
		Moist pasta in a sauce
		Crustless egg mayonnaise sandwiches

E	Dishes made up of solids and liquids together are allowed Suitable foods which can be broken into 1.5 cm (¾ inch) pieces with the flat edge of a fork Avoid foods which pose a choking hazard, as for D above	Mince Casserole of tender meat Weetabix crushed into milk
F	No modification of texture is necessary Free choice of foods available	

Foods suitable or unsuitable for inclusion in an individual diet depend on the grade of consistency required. As a general guideline, single texture foods such as well-mashed potato, semolina, custard, Greek yoghurt, instant desserts and sieved soup are more appropriate than combination foods such as stews or risotto. However, foods that are dry, sticky (e.g. peanut butter) or in the form of discrete particles such as nuts, corn or rice are usually contraindicated. Foods that change consistency from solid to liquid in the mouth (e.g. ice-cream, sorbets) may also be unsuitable for patients dysphagic to liquids.

In addition to appropriate texture modification, the SLT may suggest other measures that may assist those with oropharyngeal disorders; for example, the use of cold or stimulating foods in those with delayed triggering of the pharyngeal swallow, or alternate mouthfuls of hot and cold foods for those with reduced oral awareness (Penman and Thomson 1998). Other members of the care team may

Table 4.4 Commercial proprietary thickeners

The following products, available in the form of powders comprised of modified food starch, are ACBS prescribable to thicken foods and liquids in the management of dysphagia:
Nutilis (Nutricia Clinical Care)
Thick & Easy (Fresenius Kabi)
Thixo-D (Sutherland Health)
Vitaquik (Vitaflo)
Resource Thicken Up (Novartis Consumer Health)

A number of pre-thickened fruit drinks have been given ACBS approval and it is likely that others will be prescribable in the near future.

Note: None of the above products is normally suitable for infants and young children. Thickeners based on carob seed flour such as Instant Carobel (Cow & Gate) and Nestargel (Nestlé) are used to thicken infant feeds for the treatment of recurrent vomiting. They are not suitable for the management of dysphagia.

Data compiled January 2001.
Full compositional details of these products and prescribing indications can be found in the British National Formulary or the Monthly Index of Medical Specialties (MIMS) or obtained directly from the manufacturers (for addresses see Appendix 6.9).

provide guidance on the best posture or sitting position for eating, or the most appropriate eating utensils and drinking vessels. It is also important that patients and their carers are provided with specific guidance on dietary modification measures and compensatory swallowing techniques to help to minimize problems such as aspiration (DePippo *et al.* 1994).

Ensuring that nutritional needs are met

As well as being of the appropriate consistency, the diet has to be capable of meeting the individual's nutritional needs. When dysphagia is managed without dietetic input, this aspect is often overlooked.

People with dysphagia often consume a very limited variety of foods, either because of the constraints imposed by the need for texture modification, or because patients themselves limit their intake to a few foods which they know they can tolerate. Retextured food can also look unappetizing. Foods such as bread, fresh fruit, meat, pulses and nuts are often absent from the diet and, as a result, intake of dietary fibre and micronutrients such as water-soluble vitamins and iron may be inadequate. In addition, because dysphagia inevitably makes the process of eating difficult and a physical effort, the total quantity of food consumed may be insufficient to meet total energy needs.

It is therefore important that in any dysphagic patient, recent dietary intake and nutritional status are taken into account and their implications incorporated into an assessment of likely nutritional needs. Dietary guidance must ensure that these needs will be met, and not focus solely on texture modification. Patients (or their carers) require guidance on appropriate food choices from all of the *Balance of Good Health* food groups. If, as is often the case, total food intake is poor, guidance on food fortification measures to increase the nutrient density of the diet may be helpful (see Section 1.12.3 in Oral nutritional support). If intake remains inadequate, additional energy and nutrient supplementation may need to be considered (see Section 1.12.4). Sip feed supplements may, if necessary, be thickened to an appropriate texture with commercial thickeners, or one of the more semi-solid fortified dessert supplements may be used.

The adequacy of these measures should be continuously reviewed, along with the progress of the dysphagia itself (see Monitoring Progress, below).

Ensuring that fluid needs are met

Dehydration is a high risk in the dysphagic patient, so steps need to be taken to ensure that fluid intake is adequate. SLT guidance on the appropriate degree of thickening should be followed. It should be borne in mind that the consistency of unthickened drinks may change with time and temperature. Some liquids become thicker as they cool (e.g. gravy, home-made custard, sauces), whereas others become more watery (e.g. manufactured custard from cartons or cans).

Most liquids, both hot and cold, can if necessary be thickened with one of the commercial thickeners available (Table 4.4). It is important that appropriate guidance is given to ward staff and carers concerning the degree of thickness required (Table 4.3a). The SLT can also give guidance on head position to promote safer swallowing (e.g. it is usually unsafe to use a feeder cup that requires the head to tip back).

Educating the patient, carers and other members of the care team

People with dysphagia often need to be encouraged to eat. Factors such as anxiety or depression (often as a consequence of the underlying illness), confusion (perhaps as a result of stroke or dementia), fear (of choking) plus the sheer physical effort of consuming food all tend to act as barriers to eating. Appropriate education on food placement, maintaining the temperature of food, serving favourite foods and feeding at a comfortable pace can all increase food consumption. It is important that patients and/or carers understand that good nutrition is just as important as any other dietary measures being recommended such as texture modification. All members of the care team, not just dietitians, should reinforce this message.

Patients or carers should be given clear practical guidance on:

- overall dietary balance
- daily fluid intake
- food choice (suitable and unsuitable)
- appropriate texture, and how this can be achieved (e.g. by use of thickeners)
- other measures needed to help boost nutrient intake (e.g. food fortification strategies or use of supplements)
- who to contact in the event of queries.

Other members of the care team should also be informed of the dietary measures implemented.

Monitoring progress

In some patients, dysphagia may be regarded as 'stable' (i.e. the level of dysphagia remains unchanged for a considerable period) but in most instances this is not the case. Following stroke or acute brain injury, there is nearly always some improvement or even complete resolution of dysphagia. Conversely, in progressive neurological disorders or terminal illness, dysphagia may gradually (or suddenly) worsen. Management of dysphagia should therefore be regarded as a dynamic process which is likely to change with time, rather than as a static solution to a clinical problem. For this reason, frequent monitoring is essential to assess whether current measures are appropriate for the level of dysphagia and to identify when they need to be modified. This monitoring process requires close collaboration between all members of the care team, from carers or nursing staff who may be the first to notice feeding problems or improvements, to SLTs, dietitians and medical staff who can assess the situation and modify the care plan.

If dysphagia is resolving, patients may gradually progress towards a more normal diet in a stepwise process as outlined in the guidelines given in Table 4.3a and b. If dysphagia is worsening, or there are signs of aspiration such as choking or recurrent chest infection, a different grade of texture modification may be required. In some cases, it may be necessary to change to an alternative feeding route such as enteral feeding, sometimes only as a temporary measure until a certain amount of recovery or remission has occurred.

Ensuring continuity of care

Measures need to be in place to ensure that the dysphagic patient in hospital receives continuing assessment and support following discharge back into the community. Many areas now have a liaison nurse who acts as a link between the primary and secondary care sectors, liaising with ward staff to ascertain a patient's needs and ensuring that district nursing services are aware of and able to meet these needs.

Community dietetic provision is variable. In some areas, community dietetic services are an integral part of primary care support teams; in others, liaison with hospital-based dietetic departments will be required. When responsibility for dietetic care is transferred from secondary to primary care, it is vital that this accompanied by the provision of relevant information. The community dietitian will require details of:

- the patient, including relevant medical and contact details
- the discharge date
- the discharge location
- details of the patient's GP
- details of the patient's carer and home circumstances
- details of the initial and most recent nutrition assessment
- details of dietary measures implemented (together with their acceptability and effectiveness)
- the type of follow-up required.

The patient's GP will require:

- a summary of the dietetic management of the patient to date
- details of any proprietary thickeners or supplements prescribed and predicted usage
- an indication of likely future dietetic needs.

The patient (or carer) will require:

- the name and contact details of the dietitian responsible for their care
- written details of any dietary guidance that they have been given.

Text written by: Briony Thomas

Acknowledgements: Sheila Merriman, Helen Molyneux and the British Dietetic Association's NAGE and DINT Groups.

Further reading

Langley J. *Working with Swallowing Disorders*. Winslow Press, 1993.

Logerman JA. Factors affecting ability to resume oral nutrition in the oropharyngeal dysphagic individual. *Dysphagia* 1990; **4**: 202–208.

O'Gara JA. Dietary adjustments and nutritional therapy during treatment for oropharyngeal dysphagia. *Dysphagia* 1990; **4**: 209–212.

References

British Dietetic Association, Post Registration Course in the Nutritional Management of Dysphagia. *Texture Classification of Liquids and Solids*. Birmingham: BDA, 1997.

Curran J, Groher ME. Development and dissemination of an aspiration risk reduction diet. *Dysphagia* 1990; **5**: 6–12.

Davies AE, Kidd D, Stone SP, MacMahon J. Pharyngeal sensation and gag reflex in health subjects. *Lancet* 1995; **345**: 487–488.

DePippo KL, Holas MA, Reding MJ *et al*. Dysphagia therapy following stroke: a controlled trial. *Neurology* 1994; **44**: 1655–1660.

Finch S, Doyle W, Lowe C *et al*. *National Diet and Nutrition Survey: People Aged 65 Years and Over*. Vol. 1: *Report of the Diet and Nutrition Survey*. London: The Stationery Office, 1998.

Finestone HM, Greene-Finestone LS, Wilson ES, Teasell RW. Malnutrition in stroke patients on the rehabilitation service and at follow-up: prevalence and predictors. *Archives of Physical Medicine and Rehabilitation* 1995; **76**: 310–316.

Gordon C, Langton Hewer R, Wade DT. Dysphagia in acute stroke. *British Medical Journal* 1987; **295**: 411–414.

Lennard-Jones JE. A *Positive Approach to Nutrition as a Treatment*. London: King's Fund Centre, 1992.

Odderson IR, Keaton JC, McKenna BS. Swallow management in patients on an acute stroke pathway: quality is cost effective. *Archives of Physical Medicine and Rehabilitation* 1995; **76**: 1130–1133.

O'Sullivan N. Nutritional considerations. In O'Sullivan N (Ed.) *Dysphagia Care: Team Approach with Acute and Long-term Patients*. Los Angeles: Cottage Square, 1990.

Pardoe EM. Development of a multistage diet for dysphagia. *Journal of the American Dietetic Association* 1993; **93**: 568–571.

Penman JP, Thomson M. A review of the textured diets developed for the management of dysphagia. *Journal of Human Nutrition and Dietetics* 1998; **11**: 51–60.

Royal College of Physicians, The Intercollegiate Working Party for Stroke. *National Clinical Guidelines for Stroke*. London: RCP, 2000.

Smithard DG. Dysphagia assessment after acute stroke. *Hospital Update* 1995; December: 555–561.

Smithard DG, England R, Renwick DS *et al*. Aspiration following acute stroke: incidence and diagnosis. In Proceedings of the 2nd International Stroke Conference, Geneva, 1993. *Cerebrovascular Diseases* 1994; **4** (Suppl): 52.

Teasell RW, McRae M, Marchuk Y, Finestone HM. Pneumonia associated with aspiration following stroke. *Archives of Physical Medicine and Rehabilitation* 1996; **77**: 707–709.

4.4 Disorders of the oesophagus

The oesophagus is a muscular tube about 25 cm in length with an upper oesophageal sphincter below the pharynx and a lower oesophageal sphincter at the gastro-oesophageal junction. The function of the oesophagus is relatively simple, i.e. the transport of food from the mouth to the stomach.

Disease or stricture of the oesophagus is likely to result in pain, discomfort or difficulty in swallowing. The management of dysphagia (which may result from a number of oropharyngeal and neurological problems as well as those of the oesophagus) is discussed in Section 4.3.

4.4.1 Oesophagitis

This is inflammation of the mucosa lining the oesophagus and is usually a consequence of gastro-oesophageal reflux (see Section 4.5.2). Symptoms develop if reflux becomes frequent and the mucosa of the oesophagus becomes sensitive to the acidic reflux material. Dietary management is as for gastro-oesophageal reflux, with the patient being advised to consume soft, bland and non-irritant foods and liquids while the symptoms are acute.

4.4.2 Achalasia

Achalasia is characterized by weak peristalsis of the oesophagus and the inability of the lower oesophageal sphincter to relax after a swallow. It is relatively uncommon. Food collects in the oesophagus, causing discomfort, and eventually may pass through the sphincter by the action of gravity and the weight of food consumed. Regurgitation of food is common but lacks the bitter taste of acid or bile which is typical of reflux. Aspiration of food from the oesophagus may lead to pneumonia. Repeated collection of food in the oesophagus can irritate the mucosa, resulting in secondary oesophagitis and pain.

Loss of weight is uncommon unless the patient becomes afraid to eat. Relief may be obtained by advising the patient to:

- consume small, frequent meals
- avoid fried foods or any other foods which aggravate dyspepsia
- avoid very hot or cold foods (these tend to increase the intake of air into the stomach)
- avoid strong tea or coffee or large amounts of alcohol.

The patient may also find that standing up during a meal, drinking a glass of water and exhaling hard may help to force food into the stomach.

If dietary measures are ineffective, surgical myotomy or mechanical dilatation may be necessary.

4.4.3 Oesophageal perforation

If the oesophagus perforates spontaneously or is perforated as a result of dilatation, oesophagoscopy or caustic burns, any food or liquid consumed would enter the thoracic cavity with potentially fatal consequences.

The perforation may be allowed to heal naturally or may need surgical repair. Patients should be 'nil by mouth' and an alternative means of nutritional support instituted, usually via nasogastric or jejunostomy feeding; parenteral feeding may be necessary.

4.4.4 Benign oesophageal stricture

Benign stricture usually results from mucosal injury, as a consequence of either chronic gastro-oesophageal reflux or damage following intubation with wide-bore gastric tubes. Stricture may initially be due to muscular spasm or it may result from physical scarring and thickening of the oesophageal wall.

The first symptom is usually difficulty in swallowing solid foods or foods 'sticking', particularly items such as bread and meat which tend to remain in a bolus as they pass down the oesophagus. Dysphagia with solid foods may soon progress to dysphagia with semi-solids and liquids. Appetite is usually reduced and severe weight loss may be reported. Patients may suffer these difficulties for some time before seeking help, and may be dehydrated and malnourished on presentation. Some patients who are very depleted may need intravenous rehydration and nutritional support prior to treatment, which is usually by oesophageal dilatation.

Following dilatation, swallowing should be improved, although most patients still need to choose their foods carefully (see Section 4.3, Dysphagia). Some patients may require repeated dilatations and should be observed closely for possible oesophageal perforation.

If gastro-oesophageal reflux has been a contributory factor, it is important that this is corrected to prevent recurrence of the stricture (see Section 4.5.2).

4.4.5 Malignant oesophageal stricture (Oesophageal carcinoma)

Carcinoma of the oesophagus is more common in elderly people and is seen more frequently in men than in women. The lower third of the oesophagus is the most likely area to be affected. Patients may present with loss of body weight, dysphagia and retrosternal pain on eating. The extent of weight loss tends to be related to the degree and duration of the dysphagia.

The diagnosis of cancer of the oesophagus is by barium swallow, endoscopy, biopsy and brush cytology. By the time patients present with symptoms, the disease is often advanced and deterioration may occur rapidly. Treatment may involve surgery, radiotherapy, chemotherapy, endoscopic techniques such as dilatation, the insertion of a prosthetic tube, or a combination of these measures. If the cancer is very advanced, palliative care may be all that can be offered.

Oesophageal resection

Surgical treatment of carcinoma of the oesophagus may be by partial or total oesophagectomy or oesophagogastrectomy, depending on the site and extent of the cancer. Since many of these patients will be severely nutritionally debilitated, pre-operative nutritional support, if practicable, is highly advisable to help them to withstand the effects of surgery.

Early post-operative nutritional support is essential. Enteral feeding by a route that bypasses the oesophagus and stomach is usually appropriate (e.g. jejunostomy feeding). In severely malnourished patients undergoing chemotherapy, there may be some benefits from parenteral nutrition (De Cicco *et al.* 1993).

Before oral feeding is resumed, the integrity of the anastomosis must be confirmed. Once this has been done, oral fluids followed by graded introduction of solid foods (see Section 4.3.4) should be phased in as enteral nutrition or parenteral nutrition is phased out. Regular dietetic advice and supervision are essential, both during hospitalization and following discharge.

Persistent post-operative nutritional problems can include:

- poor appetite
- early satiety
- fear of eating, particularly foods that were difficult to eat pre-operatively
- difficulty in regaining or maintaining body weight
- nausea
- reflux.

Dietary management should aim to prevent further nutritional deterioration and weight loss, and attempt to restore good nutritional status, which may have been severely compromised prior to surgery.

Practical guidance should focus on:

- eating small, frequent meals
- chewing foods well
- drinking fluids separately from meals
- good choices of nutrient- and energy-dense foods and useful food enrichment strategies (see Section 1.12, Oral nutritional support)
- good choices of nutrient-rich beverages
- avoiding foods that cause discomfort or gastrointestinal symptoms
- measures to reduce the likelihood of reflux (e.g. not eating late at night, not lying down soon after eating, avoiding strong tea, coffee and alcohol).

Additional support measures such as sip feed supplementation may be indicated if nutritional needs cannot be met by these measures alone.

Radiotherapy

Radiation therapy, i.e. external beam radiation therapy (EBRT) or intraluminal radiation (brachytherapy), may be used to treat oesophageal carcinoma. This may be the sole treatment or used in combination with chemotherapy or following surgery. During a course of radiotherapy, the tissues will become oedematous, inflamed and swollen, and it is therefore likely that dysphagia will worsen before it improves. These effects are usually temporary but, as these patients are often already severely malnourished and have suffered marked weight loss, it may be important for the dietitian to raise the issue with the medical team as to whether enteral feeding is indicated prior to or during treatment. Nutritional support via gastrostomy or jejunostomy (depending on the site of the tumour) at this stage may prevent further deterioration of already poor nutritional status. If such support is implemented, it is important to explain to the patient why such intervention is advisable at this stage, and that this is to avert possible problems and not a sign that their condition has worsened.

During radiotherapy treatment, patients may find that bland foods (avoiding strong flavours, artificial or natural acidity or spices) are tolerated best. Foods will also need to have a smooth consistency (e.g. liquidized meals, strained thickened soups, custard, milk pudding) or a crumbly texture (e.g. water biscuits or crispbread).

Reintroduction of a normal diet should be gradual. Meals will need to be well moistened and accompanied by frequent sips of drinks to assist the passage of food past the inflamed area. Sip feed supplements may be necessary to maintain adequate energy and nutrient intake. Most patients will continue with a soft diet for some time as some difficulties with swallowing often persist. Some will also be afraid to try foods with which they associate problems, particularly meat, poultry and bread. Patients may find that such foods can be well tolerated if consumed with plenty of sauce or gravy.

Chemotherapy

Side-effects such as nausea, vomiting and taste changes commonly associated with this form of therapy may have an additional impact on oral intake. General remedial measures to help to alleviate these effects are discussed in Sections 1.12 (Oral nutritional support) and 4.37 (Cancer).

Other treatment strategies

When radical surgery is contraindicated because of surgical risk due to medical history, metastatic spread or because the patient is too weak to withstand its effects, endoscopic techniques such as dilatation, laser therapy or the insertion of either a prosthetic tube or, increasingly, a stent is used as a palliative procedure to relieve dysphagia.

Intubation with a prosthetic tube (e.g. a celestin tube) is carried out under general anaesthesia. The procedure has a high rate of complications such as perforation or haemorrhage and an increased risk of mortality. Since the diameter of the lumen is relatively small (10–12 mm) there is a also a high risk of blockage from food. However, insertion of the device does usually bring about an immediate improvement in dysphagia and, with appropriate guidance, many patients are able to resume eating a diet comprised of soft normal foods.

Self-expanding metal stents are increasingly being used in preference to prosthetic tubes. Although these devices are more costly, they are easier to insert, so can be carried out under sedation and, since the lumen size is greater (16–25mm) and more flexible, there is much less risk of food blockage as well as other complications (Siersema *et al.* 1998). The main complication is that of stent migration, which can cause nausea and vomiting. It is likely that future changes in stent design will minimize this problem.

Guidelines for the dietary management of patients who have been intubated with either a prosthetic tube or a stent vary according to the type of device inserted and local policy. However, general guidelines are:

- The position of a stent must be confirmed (usually by barium swallow) before oral intake is resumed.
- Initially, oral intake is confined to clear fluids.
- When foods are introduced, they should be soft or semi-soft and consumed with plenty of moisture.
- Food must be chewed well.
- Hard, lumpy or fibrous foods which are difficult to chew into a soft mass before swallowing must be avoided; this is vital in people with prosthetic tubes (Table 4.5).
- Powdered food supplements should be mixed thoroughly as lumps of dry powder can block the tube.
- Meals should be small and frequent.
- People should eat slowly and never hurry meals in order to keep up with others.
- After eating a meal, a fizzy drink (such as soda water or lemonade) should be consumed to help clear the tube of any food particles.

If swallowing problems suddenly recur or the patient suddenly experiences the sensation of food 'sticking', it is likely that the tube has become blocked. If this happens, the patient should be advised not to panic but to take sips of fizzy drinks, walk around, jump up and down and take more fizzy drinks. If the blockage persists for more than 3 hours, medical advice should be sought. Patients should be reassured that if their tube does block, they will come to no harm.

As is common with upper gastrointestinal tract malignancies, many of these patients will be nutritionally compromised and should be encouraged to consume a nutrient dense diet via appropriate food choice, food

Table 4.5 Guidance on food consistency for people with prosthetic tubes

	Suitable consistency	Unsuitable consistency
Meat	Meat which is very tender, minced, finely chopped or liquidized	Meat in large lumps or which is tough and difficult to chew
Fish	Flaked or mashed. Ensure all bones are removed	Fish with bones
Cheese	Grated or in a sauce. Cottage or curd cheese	Cubes of hard cheese
Eggs	Scrambled, boiled, poached or made into an omelette	Hard-boiled eggs, unless well mashed. Fried egg white. Raw or undercooked egg (risk of food poisoning)
Bread	Day-old bread	New bread (has a tendency to 'stick'). Crusty bread (e.g. French sticks). Toast
Breakfast cereals	Porridge-type cereals or those which readily soften in milk	High-fibre cereals containing nuts or dried fruit, or of a fibrous consistency (e.g. muesli)
Vegetables	Well cooked or mashed	Raw or stringy vegetables. Salad vegetables. Hard chips
Fruit	Well cooked, puréed or liquidized. Fruit juice	Raw apple, unless peeled and chewed thoroughly. Orange or grapefruit segments or pith. Fruit skins, in jam and stewed fruit
Desserts	Any of a soft, fairly uniform consistency, e.g. milk puddings, individual cream desserts, creamy yoghurt, fromage frais, egg custard, crème caramel	Yogurts containing chunks of fruit

enrichment strategies and, if necessary, use of proprietary supplements (see Section 1.12, Oral nutritional support).

Guidance on texture modification may be helpful in some cases (see Section 4.3, Dysphagia). However, tolerance to different foods varies between patients, and may even vary on a day-to-day basis in the same patient; it is therefore difficult to give precise guidance as to which foods will or will not cause problems. Many patients establish a diet of suitable texture by a process of trial and error.

Occasionally the tube or stent may need to be replaced if the tumour has grown and obstructed its entrance or the exit. This procedure carries a high risk of mortality, particularly in those with prosthetic tubes.

Text revised by: Briony Thomas

Acknowledgement: Hayley Wordsworth.

Useful address

Oesophageal Patients Association
16 Whitefields Crescent, Solihull, West Midlands B91 3NU
Tel: 0121 704 9860

References

De Cicco M, Panarello G, Fantin D *et al*. Parenteral nutrition in cancer patients receiving chemotherapy: effects on toxicity and nutritional status. *Journal of Parenteral and Enteral Nutrition* 1993; **17**(6): 513–518.

Siersema PD, Dees J, Van Blankenstein M. Palliation of malignant dysphagia from oesophageal cancer. Rotterdam Oesophageal Tumor Study Group. *Scandinavian Journal of Gastroenterology Supplement* 1998; **225**: 75–84.

4.5 Disorders of the stomach and duodenum

4.5.1 Nausea and vomiting

Nausea and vomiting are symptoms rather than 'disorders'. They can be the pathological consequences of disease or its treatment, but can also be physiological (e.g. early morning sickness in pregnancy) or psychological (e.g. bulimia nervosa) in origin.

Severe and/or persistent vomiting can cause severe dehydration, particularly in those who are very young, very old or very ill, or if accompanied by diarrhoea. Chronic nausea can have a profound impact on food intake and is a significant risk factor for undernutrition.

Acute nausea and vomiting

In normally healthy adults and children, nausea and vomiting caused by infection or food poisoning will usually resolve spontaneously, possibly without the need for medical advice. Food should be stopped until acute symptoms have diminished and replaced with frequent consumption of small quantities of glucose drinks, sugar-containing soft drinks or oral rehydration solutions.

Medical advice should always be sought for severe or persistent vomiting in infants, young children or elderly people since fluid and electrolyte replacement therapy, possibly intravenously, may be required.

Chronic nausea and vomiting

These are potentially serious dietetic problems because, if persistent, they may seriously compromise intake of both foods and fluids, and may exacerbate an already poor nutritional status resulting from underlying disease.

Dietetic management depends on the nature of the underlying problem, but measures that may help to alleviate symptoms and other strategies to improve oral nutritional intake are described in Section 1.12 (Oral nutritional support).

4.5.2 Indigestion

Frequent feelings of discomfort or unusual fullness after eating may, if persistent, be a sign of inappropriate eating habits or a symptom of underlying, possibly serious, disease. It is important to establish which is the case.

Contributory dietary factors are likely to be:

- erratic eating habits, particularly long periods without food followed by a large meal
- hurried meals
- frequent consumption of heavy, fat-rich meals
- eating late at night
- excessive consumption of tea, coffee or alcohol, or heavy use of tobacco
- a 'stressed' lifestyle.

Simple indigestion can nearly always be alleviated by diet and lifestyle changes which result in a regular meal pattern and healthier balance of foods.

4.5.3 Gastro-oesophageal reflux (Heartburn)

This is a common accompaniment to indigestion and characterized by a sharp, burning pain either just below the breast-bone or between the shoulder blades. Sometimes the chest pain may be so severe that it may be mistaken for angina. Typically, the symptoms occur after meals or during the night, and may be aggravated by bending, lying flat, lifting or straining.

It is caused by the reflux of the contents of the stomach (containing acid and enzymes) back into the oesophagus, some of which may reach the mouth or be sensed in the back of the throat (Fig. 4.2). The presence of acid and enzymes irritates the mucosa, causing pain, and repeated

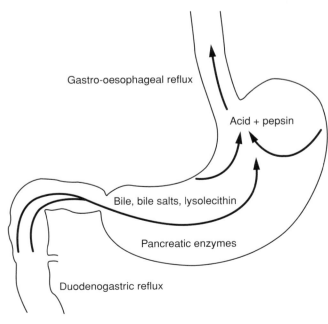

Fig. 4.2 Constituents of gastro-oesophageal reflux.

attacks may cause mucosal damage and inflammation (oesophagitis). This in turn increases the risk of adeno-carcinoma (Kahrilas 1996).

Reflux may occur as a result of:

- weakness of the sphincter at the junction of the oesophagus and stomach
- high pressure within the stomach (e.g. due to the consumption of a large quantity of food or liquid)
- high pressure from the abdominal area (e.g. obesity, pregnancy)
- hiatus hernia (see below).

These influences are illustrated in Fig. 4.3. Symptomatic reflux may also occur after operations in the gastro-oesophageal region (e.g. truncal vagotomy and proximal partial gastrectomy).

Diet and lifestyle modifications are the mainstay of treatment (Kitchin and Castell 1991), although it is acknowledged that the effectiveness of commonly advised measures such as weight loss, reduction of intake of fatty foods or smoking cessation in relieving gastro-oesophageal reflux *per se* has not been conclusively established by well-controlled trials. However, since such measures are of general benefit to health and may result in symptom relief in some patients, it is considered reasonable to encourage them on the grounds of health promotion (Galmiche *et al*. 1998).

Measures which are generally accepted as being helpful to people with gastro-oesophageal reflux are:

- eating smaller meals at regular intervals
- avoiding eating late at night
- avoiding bending, lifting or lying down after meals
- reducing weight if obese
- avoiding excessive consumption of tea, coffee or alcohol
- avoiding highly spiced or irritant foods or particular foods known to exacerbate symptoms
- sleeping in a semi-upright position or with the head of the bed raised a few inches to help to prevent nocturnal symptoms of reflux.

Additional symptom relief is obtained by the use of antacids and short courses of drugs which suppress gastric acid production such as H_2-receptor antagonists (e.g. cimetidine, ranitidine), proton pump inhibitors (e.g. omeprazole) or prokinetics (e.g. metoclopramide, domperidone), which improve functioning of the gastro-oesophageal sphincter.

4.5.4 Hiatus hernia

The diaphragm has several openings through which the abdominal viscera can enter the thorax. The opening for the oesophagus, the hiatus, is loosely attached to the oesophagus. In middle age this attachment weakens and abdominal pressure may cause the hiatus to herniate (tear). This is particularly likely to happen as a result of becoming overweight but may also occur as a consequence of pregnancy, chronic coughing or chronic constipation (from straining when the bowels are opened).

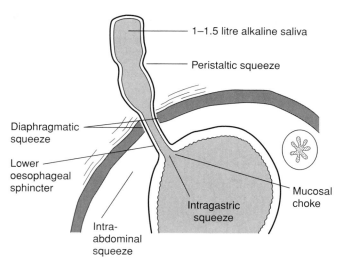

Fig. 4.3 Factors preventing the reflux and regurgitation of food from the stomach.

The major symptoms of hiatus hernia are pain and discomfort as a result of reflux and oesophagitis. Patients may also complain of the sensation of foods such as bread and salad components 'sticking' in the gullet.

In many patients, the priority is weight loss, which will help to reduce abdominal pressure and may also be advisable if surgical repair is necessary.

Most patients will benefit from healthy eating guidance along *The Balance of Good Health* guidelines. The importance of a sensible meal pattern comprised of small meals at regular intervals should be stressed. Symptom relief from gastro-oesophageal reflux can be obtained by following the preventive measures listed above. If particular foods cause dysphagic symptoms, they should be avoided. People with chronic constipation should be encouraged to choose high-fibre cereal foods and increase their fluid intake.

4.5.5 Gastritis

Gastritis is an inflammatory lesion of the gastric mucosa and may be an acute, erosive gastritis or a chronic, atrophic gastritis. Acute gastritis may be triggered by alcohol, non-steroidal anti-inflammatory drugs (NSAIDs) such as aspirin, other chemical irritants and exposure to certain pathogens. Chronic gastritis may follow repeated attacks of acute gastritis and is closely associated with infection by *Helicobacter pylori*. It tends to be more common in patients who smoke and drink alcohol heavily.

Iron-deficiency anaemia may result from repeated bleeding, and pernicious anaemia may result from reduced production of intrinsic factor and consequent reduced absorption of vitamin B_{12}. Untreated chronic gastritis also increases the risk of gastric carcinoma.

Acute gastritis

Acute gastritis usually causes pain, nausea and vomiting. Dietary treatment comprises:

- resting the stomach by avoiding solid food

- preventing dehydration by the frequent consumption of soft, glucose or sugar-containing drinks
- restoring electrolyte balance, if necessary by oral rehydration fluids.

Regeneration of healthy mucosa should occur in 2–5 days.

Chronic gastritis

Chronic gastritis is treated by:

- resting the inflamed gastric mucosa for 1-2 days by a fluid or very bland diet
- identifying and attempting to correct dietary and non-dietary factors which are contributing to the condition (e.g. alcohol, smoking, drugs, poor eating habits)
- encouraging patients to consume a well-balanced diet based on healthy eating principles together with a sensible meal pattern
- correcting any deficiencies (e.g. iron, vitamin B_{12}) which have occurred.

Medical treatment comprises the use of drugs which suppress gastric acid production, together with a course of antibiotics to eliminate Helicobacter infection.

4.5.6 Peptic ulcer

Peptic ulcer is an erosion in the mucosal lining of the stomach or duodenal areas. Ulcers may be single or multiple, acute or chronic, large or small. Gastric ulcers are less common than duodenal ulcers. The majority of duodenal ulcers occur in the duodenal cap and duodenitis is invariably present. Ulceration may also occur in the pyloric antrum and the resultant scar tissue may cause pyloric stenosis causing delayed gastric emptying and the accumulation of fermenting food debris in the stomach, causing discomfort, nausea and bad breath. If untreated, ulcers can eventually result in perforation of the gastric or duodenal wall, a potentially fatal complication.

For many years it was thought that peptic ulcer resulted primarily from hypersecretion of gastric acid or inadequate buffering of acid stomach contents in the duodenum, these being exacerbated by factors such as a stressed lifestyle, irregular meals, eating quickly and inadequate mastication. These factors may affect the healing process but it is now clear that the primary cause of peptic ulcer is the bacterium *Helicobacter pylori*. Other cases may also be a direct consequence of NSAID use.

Treatment of peptic ulcer has been transformed by the use of antibiotic treatment to eradicate Helicobacter. To promote healing, this is usually accompanied by a 4–8 week course with an H_2-receptor antagonist or proton pump inhibitor to reduce gastric acid production. Most patients will benefit from healthy diet and lifestyle advice to minimize the risk of recurrence.

4.5.7 Gastric carcinoma

Development of gastric cancer is now known to be closely associated with the carcinogenic consequences of infection with *H. pylori*, which leads to chronic atrophic gastritis and eventual gastric neoplasia (IARC 1994). This helps to explain why gastric cancer is more prevalent in deprived populations where infection with this bacterium occurs at an early age, and the socioeconomic gradient associated with the disease (OPCS 1986). Gastric carcinoma is more common in men than women and the risk of its development increased by smoking (DH 1998).

The disease is often diagnosed late because its early symptoms may be dismissed as indigestion or heartburn. By the time patients present with anorexia, nausea, vomiting, pain on eating and severe weight loss, the disease may be well advanced, possibly with metastatic spread.

If the condition is operable, partial or total gastrectomy is performed (see below). If gastrectomy is contraindicated, a gastroenterostomy may relieve symptoms and allow the patient to eat such foods as can be tolerated. The additional use of supplements or other support measures is usually necessary to make up the shortfall in energy and nutrient intake.

Gastric resection and reconstruction

The type of procedure performed may have a considerable impact on subsequent food intake, weight recovery and quality of life. Gastric replacement with various enteric reservoirs has been used to improve the postprandial symptoms and nutrition of patients after total gastrectomy, and Pouch and Roux-en-Y reconstructions have been shown to be the most useful of the commonly performed procedures for improving the post-operative quality of life (Nakane *et al.* 1995).

As a result of the combination of cancer-related cachexia and chronic symptoms such as nausea, vomiting or discomfort on eating, gastric carcinoma patients often present in a highly malnourished state and nutritional support measures should be instituted as soon as possible, preferably before surgery or as soon as possible afterwards, and via the enteral rather than parenteral route (see Section 5.6, Surgery).

During surgery a jejunostomy catheter may be positioned as a route for post-operative nutritional support. Jejunostomy feeding may also be required for certain patients receiving palliative treatment for gastric outlet obstruction.

Disturbances in gastrointestinal function often occur following gastric resection and reconstruction (Table 4.6) and these may affect nutritional intake and nutritional status. Some of these problems occur soon after eating and are described as early or postcibal syndromes; others result from the long-term consequences of disturbed gastric function.

Early symptoms

Small stomach syndrome The majority of patients experience early satiety and may feel distended and uncomfortable during or after eating. This is particularly likely after total and partial gastrectomy but may also occur

Table 4.6 Gastrointestinal consequences of gastric resection and reconstruction

Rapid emptying of the stomach remnant
Reduced secretion of intrinsic factor
Reduced secretion of pancreatic enzymes
Inadequate mixing of food with enzymes and bile
Reduced absorption of certain food substances, especially protein and fat
Rapid absorption of glucose
Abolition of the normal pH gradient in the small intestine
Increased intestinal motility

after vagotomy and pyloroplasty. Small, frequent meals should be eaten and fluids should be consumed separately from solid food (see Section 1.12, Oral nutritional support).

'Dumping syndrome'

Early dumping occurs soon after eating, causing symptoms such as sweating, dizziness, faintness, rapid weak pulse and hypotension as a response to the rapid and early delivery of a hyperosmolar meal into the jejunum. The symptoms usually recede 2–3 months after surgery, but in the meantime may be relieved by consuming small meals, limiting the consumption of rapidly absorbed carbohydrate and not consuming liquids with meals.

Late dumping: some patients may also experience symptoms similar to hypoglycaemia about 2 hours after a meal as a result of overproduction of insulin in response to the rapid absorption of glucose. Patients typically feel weak, faint, cold and sweaty and the symptoms can be relieved by consumption of a small amount of carbohydrate. Preventive measures are as described for early dumping.

Diarrhoea Diarrhoea frequently occurs following vagotomy or total gastrectomy. The problem may be alleviated by codeine phosphate or loperamide, and should disappear within 1–2 months of surgery.

Bile vomiting Pancreatic and biliary secretions may accumulate in the afferent loop and, after a meal has left the stomach, can enter the gastric remnant causing nausea and vomiting. Surgical correction may be needed.

Long-term consequences

Weight loss and undernutrition Weight loss and nutritional inadequacy are common occurrences after gastric surgery, and nearly always reflect poor food intake. Problems such as early satiety or dumping syndrome tend to make people reluctant to eat, and side-effects of treatments such as radiotherapy or chemotherapy may further affect appetite and food consumption. Dietary guidance should aim to improve meal frequency and nutrient density via appropriate food choice and enrichment measures (see Section 1.12, Oral nutritional support). Additional supplementation may also be indicated.

Patients should be monitored regularly so that progress can be assessed and nutritional support measures adjusted as necessary.

Malabsorption Malabsorption, particularly of fat, may result from a number of alterations in gastrointestinal function following gastrectomy (Table 4.6). If this occurs, it is important to ensure that energy intake is increased to compensate for faecal energy losses and that micronutrient intake does not become compromised, particularly that of calcium, iron and fat-soluble vitamins. Steatorrhoea should not be treated by dietary fat restriction alone because the resultant dietary energy content will be too low to meet energy needs. If symptoms of steatorrhoea are particularly troublesome, a proportion of dietary fat can be isocalorically substituted by either glucose polymers or medium chain triglycenides.

Anaemias Iron-deficiency anaemia is a particular risk following gastrectomy as a result of the common combination of poor iron intake and poor absorption. Haematological status should be regularly assessed and improved if necessary.

Pernicious anaemia can be a secondary consequence of gastrectomy as a result of the loss of intrinsic factor (produced by gastric parietal cells) and other local conditions necessary for the absorption of vitamin B_{12}. B_{12} will be given by injection at intervals to those considered to be at risk.

Megaloblastic anaemia may also result from folate deficiency, particularly if dietary intake is poor and malabsorption is present. Oral folate supplementation may be necessary.

Dietary guidance following gastric reconstruction should focus on the need for:

- small, frequent, regular meals
- avoiding large quantities of sugar-rich foods and drinks
- consuming fluids between meals rather than with them
- eating a variety of nutrient-dense foods (e.g. milk, dairy products, lean meat, eggs). Non-bulky (i.e. not high-fibre) cereal foods and small amounts of fruit and vegetables should also be included in the daily diet
- boosting nutrient intake via food enrichment strategies if food intake is, or has been, particularly poor
- taking recommended supplements (either energy/nutrient supplements or vitamin/mineral preparations) if these are indicated.

Text revised by: Briony Thomas

Acknowledgements: Hayley Wordsworth

References

Department of Health. *Nutritional Aspects of the Development of Cancer*. Report of the Working Group on Diet and Cancer of the Committee on Medical Aspects of Food and Nutrition Policy. London: The Stationery Office, 1998.

Galmiche JP, Letessier E, Scarpignato C. Treatment of gastro-oesophageal reflux in adults. *British Medical Journal* 1998; **316**: 1720–1723.

International Agency for Research on Cancer (IARC). Liver flukes and *Helicobacter pylori. IARC Monographs on the Evaluation of Carcinogenic Risk of Chemicals to Humans* 1994; **61**: 177–240. Lyons: IARC.

Kahrilas PJ. Gastro-oesophageal reflux disease. *Journal of the American Medical Association* 1996; **276**: 983–988.

Kitchin LI, Castell DO. Rationale and efficacy of conservative therapy for gastroesophageal reflux disease. *Archives of Internal Medicine* 1991; **151**: 448–454.

Nakane Y, Okumura S, Akehira K *et al*. Jejunal pouch reconstruction after total gastrectomy for cancer. A randomised controlled trial. *Annals of Surgery* 1995; **222**: 27–35.

Office of Population, Census and Surveys. *Occupational Mortality 1978–1980, 1982–1983*. Decennial Supplement, England and Wales. London: HMSO, 1986.

4.6 Disorders of the pancreas

Patients with pancreatic disease are particularly likely to have nutrition-related problems and be nutritionally depleted. Undernutrition is a high risk as a result of poor dietary intake (due to anorexia, sometimes compounded by alcohol abuse), malabsorption (caused by pancreatic exocrine insufficiency), hypercatabolic effects and the need for food withdrawal during acute episodes of the disease. Pancreatic damage may also affect endocrine function and result in the secondary development of diabetes mellitus.

4.6.1 Acute pancreatitis

The pancreas is normally protected against the proteolytic action of its own enzymes by their synthesis in the form of proenzymes. Acute pancreatitis develops when activated pancreatic enzymes are liberated within the pancreatic system, resulting in the autodigestion of tissue. The principal symptom is severe persistent pain in the upper left quadrant of the abdomen, and often accompanied by nausea and vomiting.

Acute pancreatitis is a serious disorder. Systemic complications include shock, renal failure and respiratory insufficiency, and local complications such as pancreatic necrosis, pseudocysts (collections of pancreatic secretions) and pancreatic fistulae may occur. Although many episodes of the disease will be mild, up to 20% of patients will have an attack which will be fatal (Mergener and Baillie 1998). Nor is the course of the disease always apparent on diagnosis; initially mild symptoms may worsen considerably before they improve. However, recent advances in pancreatic damage assessment and new methods of treatment may, in time, result in significant reductions in mortality and morbidity (Dervenis et al. 1999).

Acute pancreatitis most commonly results from:

- biliary tract disease (especially calculi in the common bile duct)
- alcohol abuse
- trauma or major abdominal surgery.

It can also be associated with other conditions such as hyperlipidaemia, hypercalcaemia, end-stage renal failure and viral infections, and in about 10% of cases may be idiopathic (Mergener and Baillie 1998).

The condition is diagnosed by the presence of elevated serum amylase and lipase concentrations (Dervenis et al. 1999). Imaging techniques such computed tomography (CT) and endoscopic retrograde cholangiopancreatography (ERCP) may also be used to identify the severity and underlying cause of the disease.

Acute pancreatitis is usually managed conservatively by withholding all oral nutrition in an attempt to reduce pancreatic enzyme secretion. Patients are maintained on a nil-by-mouth regimen with appropriate fluid replacement and analgesia. Severe cases may require aggressive intervention to correct fluid losses and electrolyte and glucose abnormalities and require renal, respiratory and cardiovascular support. Infected pancreatic necrosis may require surgical debridement.

The majority of patients with mild or moderate attacks of pancreatitis recover without the need for intensive or invasive therapy and will be able to resume an oral diet within 5–7 days.

However, if symptoms of nausea, vomiting or pain are still present, or recur when eating recommences, nutritional support must be instituted at this stage. In severely ill patients, or in those severely nutritionally depleted on admission, there may be benefits from commencing nutritional support as soon as is practicable to help offset the hypermetabolic consequences of the disease. Delay in providing nutritional support may slow recovery and prejudice the outcome of major surgery (Mergener and Baillie 1998).

Until fairly recently, parenteral nutrition was thought to be the feeding route of choice because even jejunal feeding was thought to result in some pancreatic stimulation (Cassim and Allardyce 1974). However, this is now less certain and a matter of current debate (Scolapio et al. 1999; Tesinsky 1999). Several studies have shown that jejunal enteral feeding is just as beneficial as parenteral nutrition and may even have a number of physiological advantages in addition to being safer and more cost-effective (Kale-Pradham et al. 1999; Kotani et al. 1999; Wyncoll 1999).

When the acute symptoms have remitted, oral fluids, and then oral foods, can gradually be reintroduced and the nutritional support regimen progressively reduced. Since dietary fat will be the least tolerated nutrient, patients are usually initially maintained on a low-fat diet but should gradually progress to a diet of normal fat content as soon as tolerance permits. Since appetite may remain poor and nutritional depletion as a result of the disease may be pronounced, the risk of energy inadequacy remains high. Oral nutritional support measures to maintain adequate energy intake, e.g. via food enrichment and supplementation, may be needed for some time (see Section 1.12, Oral nutritional support). Nutritional status should be monitored throughout the course of the disease.

Following recovery, patients should be encouraged to consume a normal, well-balanced diet which will maintain or continue to restore their nutritional status. Failure to regain appetite or weight is often indicative of continuing disease. Avoidance of alcohol for at least several months is usually mandatory for all patients; people with alcoholism will need specialist help. If permanent damage to the pancreas has resulted in diabetes or necessitates the use of pancreatic enzyme replacement, additional dietary guidance will be required (see below).

4.6.2 Chronic pancreatitis

This may follow repeated attacks of acute pancreatitis or may be associated with chronic inflammation of the biliary tract. There is a strong relationship between alcohol consumption and the risk of developing chronic pancreatitis.

The main features of the disease are severe weight loss and abdominal pain. Malabsorption is common and steatorrhoea will develop when 90% of exocrine function is lost. Appetite is often poor, thus exacerbating the nutritional depletion (Mergener and Baillie 1997).

Pancreatic enzyme supplementation is the cornerstone of treatment in long-term patient management and its function is twofold:

1 *To assist in pain control*: Negative feedback from exogenous pancreatic enzymes reduces exocrine pancreatic secretion and thus reduces pancreatic pain. Enzyme replacement therapy may therefore be used even if digestive function is normal. Enzyme supplementation may also aid the stabilization of insulin requirements among diabetic patients.
2 *To reduce malabsorption*: Pancreatic enzyme supplements contain amylase, trypsin and lipase, although the lipase content determines their effectiveness (average dose 10 000–12 000 units lipase/meal). The efficacy of these enzyme supplements is improved by simultaneous administration of H_2-receptor antagonists, since these enzyme preparations are known to become inactivated at a pH of less than 4.

Regular clinical, nutritional and biochemical assessments are all important in assessing the severity of disease and in establishing an appropriate treatment plan. Dietary management of chronic pancreatitis focuses on:

- The provision of sufficient energy and nitrogen to prevent further nutritional depletion. Fat restriction is not indicated even if steatorrhoea is present; pancreatic enzyme replacement should be used as a means of obtaining symptom relief. Oral nutritional support measures, possibly including the use of energy supplements, should be employed as necessary.
- Guidance on the use of pancreatic enzyme replacement therapy. Enzymes need to be taken with all meals and snacks, the amount taken at each meal adjusted according to the quantity of food eaten and its fat content. This is discussed in more detail in Section 4.7, Cystic fibrosis.

- Vitamin and mineral supplementation, particularly of fat-soluble vitamins, may be indicated if steatorrhoea has persisted for some time.
- Dietary measures to assist control of diabetes will be required if endocrine pancreatic insufficiency has developed. Primarily, these will need to focus on meal pattern and timing, and appropriate choices of carbohydrate foods (see Section 4.16, Diabetes mellitus).
- Alcohol avoidance is usually advised for all patients with chronic pancreatitis and is essential for those with a history of alcohol abuse.

Regular follow-up and assessment will be necessary to monitor compliance with and the effectiveness of dietary measures and pancreatic enzyme replacement therapy. Blood glucose should be measured at intervals to detect the development of diabetes.

Patients who suffer a recurrence of acute symptoms are normally managed by pancreatic rest and temporary cessation of oral feeding, as detailed above for acute pancreatitis.

4.6.3 Cancer of the pancreas

Pancreatic cancer accounts for about 2.5% of all malignancies in Great Britain and is slightly more common in men than women (DH 1998). The disease is often diagnosed at a stage when neither surgery nor chemotherapy or radiation will prolong survival time. The prognosis of the disease remains very poor, with high mortality rates within 1 year, and death within 5 years in 95% of cases, despite advances in diagnosis, surgical procedures and adjuvant therapy.

Many of the effects of pancreatic cancer are similar to those of chronic pancreatitis:

- pain
- progressive weight loss
- nausea and vomiting
- malabsorption and steatorrhoea
- secondary diabetes.

Additional effects may include:

- biliary obstruction and resulting jaundice
- pancreatic ascites, sometimes sufficient to mask severe weight loss.

As well as these consequences, patients with pancreatic cancer have to cope with the psychological effects of the diagnosis itself and its poor prognosis. The resulting depression and anxiety can profoundly impair the desire to eat. Since the rapid advancement of the disease can also result in high nutrient losses and poor nutrient intake if symptoms are not adequately controlled, the risk of debilitating malnutrition is high.

If pancreatic surgery is indicated, it is increasingly recognized that pre-operative and peri-operative nutritional support via jejunostomy or the parenteral route may make a considerable difference to recovery time and outcome. This aspect of care has often been overlooked in the past

(Ulander *et al.* 1991). Post-operatively, nutritional monitoring remains important. Since enzyme supplementation and insulin are commonly required following pancreatic resection, dietary guidance on these aspects is also likely to be needed.

If treatment is palliative, the aim of management is to improve quality of life via pain and symptom control. Nutritional support should be sufficient to prevent unnecessary nutritional debilitation while not being overinvasive. Proprietary supplements may be useful to help maintain adequate energy and nutrient intake. Dietary guidance to help to alleviate problems such as nausea, early satiety and loss of taste may be beneficial. The overall nutritional objective is to ensure that eating remains a pleasurable aspect of life for as long as possible while preserving as much of the patient's strength and well-being as is practicable.

Text revised by: Briony Thomas

Acknowledgement: Hayley Wordsworth

References

Cassim MM, Allardyce DB. Pancreatic secretion in response to jejeunal feeding of an elemental diet. *Annals of Surgery* 1974; **180**: 228–231.

Department of Health. *Nutritional Aspects of the Development of Cancer*. Report of the Working Group on Diet and Cancer of the Committee on Medical Aspects of Food and Nutrition Policy London: The Stationery Office, 1998.

Dervenis C, Johnson CD, Bassi XC *et al*. Diagnosis, objective assessment of severity, and management of acute pancreatitis. Santorini consensus conference. *International Journal of Pancreatology* 1999; **25**: 195–210.

Kale-Pradhan PB, Elnabtity MH, Park NJ, Laus M. Enteral nutrition in patients with pancreatitis. *Pharmacotherapy* 1999; **19**: 1036–1041.

Kotani J, Usami M, Nomura H *et al*. Enteral nutrition prevents bacterial translocation but does not improve survival during acute pancreatitis. *Archives of Surgery* 1999; **134**: 287–292.

Mergener K, Baillie J. Chronic pancreatitis. *Lancet* 1997; **359**: 1379–1385.

Mergener K, Baillie J. Fortnightly review: acute pancreatitis. *British Medical Journal* 1998; **316**: 44–48.

Scolapio JS, Malhi-Chowla N, Ukleja A. Nutrition supplementation in patients with acute and chronic pancreatitis. *Gastroenterology Clinics of North America* 1999; **28**: 695–707.

Tesinsky P. Nutritional care of pancreatitis and its complications. *Current Opinion in Clinical Nutrition and Metabolic Care* 1999; **2**: 395–398.

Ulander K, Grahn G, Sundahl G, Jeppsson B. Needs and care of patients undergoing subtotal pancreatectomy for cancer. *Cancer Nursing* 1991; **14**: 27–34.

Wyncoll DL. The management of severe acute necrotising pancreatitis: an evidence-based review of the literature. *International Care Medicine* 1999; **25**: 146–156.

Cystic fibrosis

Cystic fibrosis (CF) is an inherited disorder which causes widespread dysfunction of the exocrine glands, resulting in chronic lung disease and pancreatic insufficiency. The nutritional implications of CF are considerable because the effects of the disease tend to increase nutritional requirements but also impair food intake and nutrient absorption. Without effective dietary management, the risk of poor nutritional status, and inadequate growth and weight gain in children, is high. Since good nutritional status is clearly linked with pulmonary status and survival, it is essential that each patient receives expert dietetic care.

4.7.1 Features of cystic fibrosis

Prevalence

CF is the most common autosomal recessively inherited disease in the UK. The incidence of CF in Caucasians is approximately 1 in 2500 live births and 4% of the population are carriers (i.e. 1 in every 25 people) (Lewis 1995). However, the incidence of CF in non-Caucasians is much lower, and estimated to be around 1 in 20 000 in ethnic African populations and 1 in 100 000 in Oriental populations (Corey *et al.* 1988).

Causation

CF results from mutations in a single gene in the middle of chromosome 7. This affects the production of a protein [cystic fibrosis transmembrane regulator (CFTR)] which helps to control the movement of chloride across cell membranes, and hence the movement of sodium and water in and out of epithelial cells. As a consequence of this, exocrine secretions such as mucus have increased viscosity and tend to obstruct small airways and ducts.

Although 80% of the CF population in the UK share the same genetic defect (delta F508 mutation), more than 800 different mutations have now been identified (RCP 1990; CF Genetic Consortium 1996). As a result, there is considerable variability in the physical manifestations (see below); for example, the vast majority of CF patients have pancreatic insufficiency, but a small minority (about 5%) do not.

Consequences

The clinical consequences of CF vary in nature and severity. CF primarily affects:

- *Respiratory function*: The presence of thickened mucus in the lungs increases the risk of colonization by pathogens and respiratory infection. Repeated chest infections lead to progressive lung disease. Regular antibiotics and physiotherapy are required to help to maintain lung function.
- *Gastrointestinal function*: The exocrine ducts of the pancreas may become blocked, inhibiting the secretion of pancreatic enzymes into the gastrointestinal tract. This results in significant malabsorption, often characterized by severe steatorrhoea. Malabsorption is also exacerbated by pancreatic bicarbonate deficiency which results in reduced ability to buffer gastric acid reaching the duodenum, and causing pancreatic enzyme inactivation and bile salt precipitation. Altered bile salt composition, intestinal mucosal transport abnormalities and increased motility of the small intestine can be additional contributory factors (Littlewood and Wolfe 2000). CF can present as meconium ileus and be associated with intussception, increased gastro-oesophageal reflux and rectal prolapse in infants and young children.
- *Sweat gland function*: CF results in abnormally high concentrations of sodium and chloride in sweat. This is a diagnostic feature of the disease.

Longer term consequences of CF can include:

- *Liver disease*: Liver and bile salt metabolism may be affected leading to cholecystitis, cirrhosis or liver failure.
- *CF-related diabetes*: Progressive pancreatic damage leads to an increasing risk of diabetes with age.
- *Pancreatitis*: This may also be a consequence of pancreatic damage.
- *Impaired fertility*: Most men with CF are infertile as a result of congenital abnormalities associated with the disorder (such as bilateral absence of the vas deferens) or obstructive problems caused by the production of thickened mucus. In women, fertility tends to be reduced by the presence of thickened mucus in the cervix but this does not necessarily preclude the possibility of pregnancy.
- *Bone and joint disorders*: Chronic malabsorption increases the risk of osteoporosis and arthropathy.

Onset and diagnosis

Symptoms usually become apparent in infancy but, now that milder mutations are being identified, diagnosis may not be made until later in life. Symptoms which are suggestive of CF include:

- recurrent chest infections

- passage of large, pale, greasy, offensive-smelling stools
- failure to thrive in children or undernutrition in adults
- meconium ileus.

CF is usually confirmed by two positive sweat tests (which reveal the presence of excessive concentrations of sodium and chloride).

The condition is increasingly being identified by prenatal or neonatal screening (Wildhagen *et al.* 1998).

Prognosis

Life expectancy, although still reduced, has increased dramatically in recent decades. In the 1960s, many people diagnosed with CF survived for only a few years and rarely reached adulthood; currently, the expected survival following diagnosis is approximately 40 years and is continuing to rise (Elborn *et al.* 1991). This increased longevity has created new dietetic challenges such as the management of pregnancy, liver disease, diabetes or transplantation in people with CF, in addition to those which have long been recognized.

4.7.2 Nutritional implications of cystic fibrosis

The nutritional implications of cystic fibrosis are considerable because the disease tends to:

- *Impair nutrient absorption*: About 95% patients have pancreatic enzyme insufficiency, impairing the absorption of fat, nitrogen and fat-soluble vitamins, and compromising energy balance and nutritional status. These effects can be offset by pancreatic enzyme replacement therapy but not necessarily prevented altogether; Murphy *et al.* (1991) found that even patients who appear to be taking sufficient quantities of pancreatic enzymes may still lose as much as 10% of dietary energy via their stools. Other factors, particularly bicarbonate depletion, also compound malabsorption.
- *Impair food intake*: Loss of appetite is a common accompaniment to the chronically infected chest and may be worse during acute exacerbations. Phases of poor food intake increase the likelihood of energy and nutrient needs not being met.
- *Increase energy expenditure*: The pulmonary disease associated with CF increases energy requirements as a result of the increased energy cost involved in breathing, and the frequent infections associated with it (Buchdahl *et al.* 1988; Shepherd *et al.* 1988). The increase in resting energy expenditure is related to the severity of lung disease (O'Rawe *et al.* 1992). There may also be an inherent increase in energy expenditure resulting from a genetic defect of the disease itself (Buchdahl *et al.* 1988).

In older patients, there may be additional nutritional considerations as a result of diabetes, liver disease, heart–lung/lung transplant, pregnancy or bone disease.

The risk of nutritional inadequacy is therefore high and, in the past, underweight and poor growth in children were a common feature of CF. However, malnutrition should not be regarded as inevitable; with appropriate clinical and dietetic management, its effects can be minimized and good nutritional status, can be maintained. Furthermore, it is extremely important that this objective is achieved. Nutritional status has important prognostic significance (Gaskin *et al.* 1982; Corey *et al.* 1988.). Well-nourished patients have a better chance of maintaining good health and pulmonary status, and have prolonged survival (Levy *et al.* 1986; Dalzell *et al.* 1992). Correcting underweight by long-term nutritional support measures has been shown to decrease the prevalence of pulmonary infections and improve or stabilize lung function (Dalzell *et al.* 1992; Smith *et al.* 1994; Steinkamp and von der Hardt 1994). While good nutrition cannot cure lung damage, it can slow down the rate of deterioration in lung function. Dietetic and clinical objectives are therefore closely linked.

The dietetic treatment priorities are to:

1 minimize the effect of malabsorption by optimal pancreatic enzyme replacement therapy
2 ensure that all nutritional needs (particularly for fat-soluble vitamins) are met, and institute any necessary nutritional support or supplementation measures.

4.7.3 Pancreatic enzyme replacement therapy

Most patients with CF will require pancreatic enzyme replacement therapy (PERT) to minimize the symptoms and nutritional consequences of malabsorption. Pancreatic insufficiency should be confirmed by evidence of fat malabsorption before PERT is commenced (Littlewood and Wolfe 2000).

Types of enzyme preparation

PERT has improved considerably since the mid-1980s with the traditional powder-based and enteric-coated tablet formulations largely having been superseded by enteric-coated microsphere/minimicrosphere preparations. These have a pH-sensitive coating which only disintegrates when the pH rises above 5.5; the enzymes are therefore protected from stomach acid inactivation and only released into the duodenum. As a result, both fat and nitrogen absorption are improved and fewer malabsorptive symptoms are experienced (Leonard and Knox 1997). Types of pancreatic enzyme preparation available are listed in Table 4.7.

High-strength enzyme preparations

In recent years, high-strength enzyme preparations have become available. This is advantageous in terms of the number of capsules which need to be taken and hence convenience, compliance and cost. High-strength preparations may also achieve better control of symptoms such as stool frequency and consistency in some patients (Morrison *et al.* 1992).

Table 4.7 Pancreatic enzyme preparations available in the UK

Product (manufacturer)	Dosage	Enzyme content BP units per stated quantity (i.e. per capsule/tablet/sachet or per gram)		
		Lipase	Protease	Amylase
Granules				
Pancrex (Paines & Byrne)	Per gram	5000	300	4000
Powder1				
Pancrex V (Paines & Byrne)	Per gram	25000	1400	30000
Enteric-coated microspheres				
Pancrease (Janssen-Cilag)	Per capsule	5000	350	300
Nutrizym GR (Merck)	Per capsule	10000	650	10000
Creon 10000 (Solvay)	Per capsule	10000	600	8000
Enteric-coated minitablets				
Nutrizym 10 (Merck)	Per capsule	10000	500	9000
Higher strength enteric-coated minitablets				
Pancrease HL (Janssen-Cilag)	Per capsule	25000	1250	22500
Nutrizym 22 (Merck)	Per capsule	22000	1100	19800
Higher strength enteric-coated microspheres				
Creon sachets (Solvay)	Per sachet	20000	1125	22500
Creon 25000 (Solvay)	Per capsule	25000	1000	18000

Data compiled 2000.
[1]No longer recommended and rarely used.

Problems can sometimes arise when patients change from a standard strength to a high-strength preparation if they are given inappropriate dosage advice or are confused by different types of capsules. Some may have fears about overdosage and consequently take insufficient quantities to be effective. Others may need more than the theoretical one-third of a standard dose to obtain symptom relief; if more than half of their usual dose is required, treatment costs will increase.

There has also been concern over the safety of certain high-strength preparations which have been linked with the development of fibrosing colonopathy (colonic strictures), particularly in children (Smyth *et al.* 1994). This may be a consequence of an excessive lipase and/or protease dosage, or undissolved microspheres reaching the colon. As a result, the UK Committee on the Safety of Medicines (CSM 1995) has advised that:

- The total dose of pancreatic enzyme supplements should not normally exceed 10 000 units of lipase per kg body weight per day.
- Pancrease HL and Nutrizym 22 should not be used in children under the age of 15 years.

More recently it has been suggested that fibrosing colonopathy may be more closely related to the amount of methacrylic acid copolymer (MAC) coating present in some preparations, rather than to the enzyme strength *per se* (Prescott and Bakowski 1999).

Enzyme dosage and administration

The dosage of enzymes is usually based on body weight (up to 10 000 units lipase/kg per day), with the enzymes being distributed throughout the day to match the fat content of food and drinks consumed. In the USA, dosage is calculated as lipase units/kg body weight per meal (i.e. 1000 units/kg/meal for children <4 years; 500 units/kg/meal >4 years), with a recommended maximum of 2500 lipase units/kg/meal (Borrowitz *et al.* 1995). However, some centres feel that better control is achieved by basing dosage more closely on dietary fat intake and calculate dosage in terms of lipase units per gram of fat or per meal, or on a combination of dietary fat content and body weight (Leonard and Knox 1997). Recent guidelines from Australia (Anthony *et al.* 1999) recommend dosage levels of 500–1000 units of lipase/g fat for an infant and 500–4000 units lipase/g fat for a child or adult, up to a daily maximum of 10 000 units lipase/kg body weight per day (Anthony *et al.* 1999). The importance of using the lowest effective dose of enzymes is also stressed.

In practice, individual requirements for pancreatic enzymes can depend on a number of factors, such as:

- the degree of residual pancreatic function
- the type of enzyme preparation used: some patients respond better to one product than another
- the composition of the diet, particularly its content of fat
- the pH of food and drink consumed
- factors affecting pH within the gastrointestinal tract.

A certain amount of trial and error is usually necessary to find the dosage that best relieves stool frequency and bulk, and abdominal discomfort, but it is important to stress to patients that any self-adjustment of dosage should only be carried out in conjunction with dietetic or medical guidance, to avoid inappropriate or excessive dosage.

Enzymes should be taken with all meals and fat-containing snacks, drinks and oral supplements, the dose being appropriate for the fat content. Half the dose should be taken before the meal, and half during it. For overnight tube feeding, the enzyme capsules may be divided into two or three doses, although practice varies (see Enteral feeding, below).

The way in which the enzymes are administered is important. Microspheres must not be chewed or crushed as this will reduce enzyme efficiency (as will exposure to hot food or food with a pH of >5.5). Capsules need to be opened for infants and young children and the microspheres mixed with a little soft or semi-solid food (e.g. apple purée) so that they can be swallowed whole.

Guidelines on the use of pancreatic enzymes are summarized in Table 4.8. Readers are referred to the review by Littlewood and Wolfe (2000) for more detailed discussion on the subject.

Monitoring the effectiveness of enzyme replacement therapy

Even with modern PERT, maldigestion and malabsorption may still not be adequately controlled in some patients, especially in those not receiving regular review or attending specialist CF units. Factors that may contribute to inadequate PERT include:

- *Inadequate patient assessment of steatorrhoea*: Patients tend to become accustomed to what is a normal stool pattern for them and may fail to recognize symptoms of steatorrhoea or that their enzyme dosage needs to be adjusted (Littlewood and MacDonald 1987).
- *Inappropriate guidance*: Doctors may pay less attention to the nutritional aspects of CF than to pulmonary aspects of the disease. PERT may be overlooked or inadequately monitored.
- *Lack of regular dietetic assessment*: Dietetic supervision is essential if an appropriate balance between PERT and food intake is to be achieved (MacDonald *et al.* 1991). Such balance is not only essential to prevent unnecessary malabsorption, but may also be important to prevent the side-effects associated with overadministration of enzymes.
- *Poor compliance with guidance given*: Patients may not have followed, or may have misunderstood, advice given in respect of timing or dosage of enzymes.
- *Other factors*: Low duodenal pH (e.g. due to excessive production of gastric acid or reduced pancreatic bicar-

bonate) can result in inappropriate release or denaturation of enzymes.

The effectiveness of the regimen in terms of malabsorption can be assessed by measurement of faecal fat or stool weight, although in practice these are not usually carried out routinely. Stool weight is a good indicator of energy losses because stool energy content remains relatively constant at 8 kJ/g wet weight whereas stool lipid is poorly related to stool energy losses (Murphy *et al.* 1991). More usually, PERT's effectiveness is monitored by the level of malabsorptive symptoms or by weight change. Faecal fat microscopy, faecal chymotrypsin and steatocrit may also be used as indicators of PERT sufficiency.

4.7.4 Meeting the nutritional needs of people with cystic fibrosis

Every patient with CF requires a diet which achieves and maintains good nutritional status so that any potential for growth is realized, resistance to infection maximized and outcome optimized. Good nutritional education from diagnosis onwards is needed in order to achieve this. This requires:

- assessing individual nutritional requirements
- devising a dietary strategy by which they can be met
- monitoring the effectiveness of these measures and identifying failure to meet nutritional needs
- correcting nutritional inadequacy by appropriate nutritional support measures.

Assessing nutritional requirements

Energy

Dietary energy requirements in CF will usually be higher than normal as a result of the increased energy expenditure resulting from lung disease and the continuing energy losses via malabsorption (which is often present to some extent even with PERT).

As a rule of thumb, it is recommended in the UK that the diet should provide 120–150% of estimated average requirement (EAR) for energy (MacDonald 1996). However, as a result of the heterogeneity of the disease, individual needs will vary. Patients who are pancreatic suf-

Table 4.8 Guidelines on the use of pancreatic enzyme preparations

1 Enzymes should be taken with every meal, with ideally half the dosage being taken before the meal and half during it
2 Enzymes should be taken with all fat-containing snacks
3 Extra enzymes (e.g. 1–2 capsules or tablets) should be taken with particularly fatty meals
4 Enzymes should not be taken with fat-free snacks and drinks, e.g. soft drinks, fruit drinks, alcohol, fresh and tinned fruit, glucose polymer supplements, boiled or jelly sweets
5 Enteric-coated tablets or microspheres must be swallowed without being chewed (to avoid losing their effectiveness). With young children, or if swallowing is difficult, the capsules should be opened and the contents mixed with a little soft food, jam or honey or fruit purée. Granules must not be sprinked over a meal
6 Under medical or dietetic supervision, the enzyme dose should be increased (e.g. by 1–2 capsules or tablets) if the stools are loose or malodorous or occur more than twice daily
7 Adequate hydration is important, especially with higher strength enzyme preparations
8 In tube-fed patients, enzymes should not be added to the feed or administered via the feeding tube

ficient may be able to meet their needs for growth on average levels of energy intake (i.e. EAR), whereas those with more advanced pulmonary disease and/or uncontrolled malabsorption are likely to require considerably more.

Protein

Protein requirements have not been well researched but it is generally accepted that the protein intake should be higher than average to compensate for excessive loss of nitrogen in the faeces and sputum and ensure sufficiency for growth (Goodchild 1986; Dalzell *et al.* 1992). A target intake of 120% of the reference nutrient intake (RNI) for protein is commonly used (Dodge 1988).

Fat

Fat restriction as a means of reducing steatorrhoea and its associated symptoms is not recommended in the management of CF. Such a measure inevitably compromises intake of energy and fat-soluble vitamins and, with the advent of more effective PERT, is now considered unnecessary.

It is usually suggested that diets contain between 35 and 40% energy in the form of fat (MacDonald 1996), although in practice intakes of between 30 and 35% are more likely to be achieved (Buchdahl *et al.* 1989; Wootton *et al.* 1991). However, with increasing longevity, the relevance of dietary composition to long-term health should not be overlooked. A relatively high-fat intake does not always have to be achieved by an excessive intake of saturated fat. While in some instances it may be appropriate to increase the consumption of high fat foods such as full-fat milk, cream and cheese, fats such as spreads and oils can be derived from monounsaturated sources.

The use of medium chain triglyceride (MCT) oil preparations in cooking is no longer recommended. MCT oil is unpalatable, inconvenient to use and still needs the concurrent administration of pancreatic enzymes to aid absorption; it therefore confers no advantages.

Dietary fibre

The need for a diet of relatively high energy density means that the fibre intake of children with CF may be low, and this has been associated with gastrointestinal symptoms such as abdominal pain (Gavin *et al.* 1997). This aspect of the diet should not be overlooked and some patients may benefit from an increased fibre intake if energy requirements are met.

Vitamins

Vitamin supplements are routinely prescribed for pancreatic insufficient CF patients, although the amounts recommended vary widely (Peters and Rolles 1993). Much remains to be learnt about vitamin absorption, metabolism, losses and toxicity in the CF population.

Water-soluble vitamins CF does not increase the risk of water-soluble vitamin deficiency and supplementation is not routinely necessary (Peters and Rolles 1993).

Fat-soluble vitamins All pancreatic insufficient CF patients are at risk from deficiencies of fat-soluble vitamins and require supplements of vitamins A, D and E, and possibly vitamin K (Eid *et al.* 1990; Leonard and Knox 1997). However, the optimal supplementary dosage levels have not been adequately established and it is not known whether the historical recommendations are appropriate. Halford and Jackson (1993) have suggested that compensatory mechanisms may result in relatively good absorption of retinol and alpha-tocopherol, so high supplemental doses may not be necessary. Requirements are likely to be highest in those with poorly controlled malabsorption and impaired liver function (which affects vitamin metabolism, storage and transport) (Rayner 1992).

Vitamin A: Severe vitamin A deficiency in CF has been shown to result in night blindness (O'Donnell and Talbot 1987), xerophthalmia and bulging fontanelles, and to increase intracranial pressure (Eid *et al.* 1990). Such problems are relatively rare, but subclinical deficiency may be quite common and its consequences significant. Vitamin A is needed for the maintenance of the mucus-secreting epithelial lining of the lungs and hence it may be particularly important to avoid deficiency in people with CF. Vitamin A deficiency has been related to an increased susceptibility to pulmonary infection and more rapid progression of lung disease (Rayner and Littlewood 1992; Watkin *et al.* 1992).

As a general guide, appropriate levels of vitamin A supplementation are: 4000 IU (1200 μg)/day in infants, and 8000 IU (2400 μg)/day in children and adults. However, these will vary according to the degree of pancreatic sufficiency and fat-soluble vitamin status. Oral nutritional supplements may also provide significant quantities of the vitamin. Monitoring of plasma levels is advisable.

Particular caution is needed in women who are pregnant, or planning a pregnancy, because of the risk of teratogenesis (see Dietary guidance for pregnant women with cystic fibrosis, below).

Vitamin D: Although clinical deficiency (such as rickets) is rarely seen in CF, subclinical deficiency is a risk. Adolescents and adults with CF have been found to have low blood levels compared with age-matched controls. Inadequate vitamin D status may also be a factor in abnormal mineral metabolism and poor bone mineralization (Gibbens *et al.* 1988; Stead *et al.* 1988; Durie and Pencharz 1989) leading to osteoporosis. Most pancreatic insufficient CF patients require supplements to maintain blood levels of vitamin D within the normal range. A daily supplement of 10–20 μg (400–800 IU) is currently recommended. More may be required during pregnancy and in older patients.

Vitamin E: Vitamin E deficiency in CF has been associated with neurological malfunction and reduced haemoglobin levels (Kelleher 1987; Sitrin *et al.* 1987; Durie and Pencharz 1989). Vitamin E may also be important in controlling the progression of lung disease in CF; its scavenger role, together with that of other antioxidants, may help to protect lungs from damage during the inflammatory response to infection (Watkin *et al.* 1992). The vitamin E:lipid ratio should be monitored. Low plasma levels can be corrected by giving a daily supplement ranging from 50 mg for infants to 200 mg for adults.

Vitamin K: Severe lack of vitamin K prolongs bleeding time and increases the risk of haemorrhage. However, overt vitamin K deficiency in CF has been considered rare, and routine supplementation (other than that given to all newborn infants to prevent haemorrhagic disease) only thought necessary for CF infants with respiratory problems or meconium ileus, or in patients with liver disease or given prolonged antibiotic therapy (Durie and Pencharz 1989; Ramsey *et al.* 1992; Rayner 1992).

However, Rashid *et al.* (1999) found that many CF patients with pancreatic insufficiency or liver disease have evidence of vitamin K deficiency (as measured by immunoassay of PIVKA-II) and have suggested that people with CF should be given supplements. An additional reason for vitamin K supplementation may be because of its role in bone metabolism, and the fact that osteopenia and osteoporosis are being increasingly reported in children and adults with CF (Grey *et al.* 1993; Henderson *et al.* 1996).

Because of the increased risk of haemorrhage if vitamin K deficiency is present, it is recommended that the blood-clotting status of all CF patients is checked prior to any surgical procedure (Leonard and Knox 1997).

General aspects of fat-soluble vitamin supplementation
Vitamins A, D and E should be provided from diagnosis onwards in pancreatic insufficient CF patients; evidence of fat-soluble vitamin deficiency has been found in infants below the age of 3 months (Sokol *et al.* 1989). Because no single preparation is available which provides all these vitamins in sufficient quantities, regimens must combine a multivitamin preparation (or A and D capsules) and an additional vitamin E supplement. Fully comprehensive supplements (e.g. Ketovite liquid and tablets) are unnecessary and may not provide sufficient quantities of individual fat-soluble vitamins.

Intake of fat-soluble vitamins from fortified nutritional supplements should also be borne in mind, particularly in respect of vitamin A during pregnancy (see Dietary guidance for pregnant women with cystic fibrosis, below).

It is recommended that fat-soluble vitamin status should be assessed at an annual review by measuring plasma levels of vitamins (Kelleher 1987; Rayner 1992). It should be borne in mind that plasma vitamin reference ranges vary considerably and are not necessarily an accurate indication of vitamin status. Stool vitamin losses (Halford and Jackson 1993) are usually only measured for research purposes. Vitamin supplements should be commenced in pancreatic sufficient patients if deficiency is demonstrated.

Minerals and trace elements

Sodium CF results in an abnormally high concentration of sodium being excreted in sweat, and sodium loss will be increased in conditions causing excessive sweating, e.g. exposure to the sun or physical exertion. However, overt salt depletion is only a risk during heatwaves and in hot climates. In these circumstances consumption of extra salt or salt supplements may be necessary, but normally there is no need to encourage the consumption of salty foods or aggressive use of the salt pot.

Iron Serum iron levels are frequently low in CF patients (Erhardt *et al.* 1987; Pond *et al.* 1996) but routine iron supplementation is not usually given. However, patients should be aware of their increased iron requirements.

Devising a dietary strategy to meet nutritional needs

Individual assessment is imperative to determine the type of diet which is both appropriate and acceptable for each patient. Factors which need to be taken into account include age, clinical condition, pancreatic enzyme therapy, nutritional requirements, evidence of nutritional depletion, and food preferences and tolerances. Furthermore, the diet may need to be adjusted as necessary according to changing requirements for growth, clinical, nutritional and vitamin status, and changes in diet and bowel habit.

Because energy needs are often high but appetite is frequently poor, diets usually need to be relatively energy dense. While consumption of bulky, cereal fibre-rich foods should not be excessive, foods such as bread and breakfast cereals still have an important place in the diet in order to provide sufficient fibre to maintain bowel function.

Monitoring dietary effectiveness

It is essential that each patient receives regular nutritional assessment and review by an experienced CF dietitian. This should ascertain:

- dietary intake
- problems with appetite or other aspects of food intake
- the effectiveness of PERT, by considering its administration, compliance with guidance previously given and symptoms of malabsorption (see Section 4.7.3)
- nutritional status, especially change in body weight and, in children, parameters of growth
- the use of fat-soluble vitamin supplementation
- the use of other supplements.

Prior to an annual review, dietary diary records kept for 3–5 days, and ideally sent to the dietitian beforehand, can provide a useful basis for exploration of usual dietary intake and diet-related issues.

The reasons for any apparent shortfall between nutritional intake and requirements should be explored:

- *The diet may be too low in energy content or energy density*: Dietary studies show that patients rarely achieve recommended intakes of 120–150% of average energy requirements, with 35–40% of this energy being derived from fat. More typically, intakes are between 95 and 120% of the EAR (Tomezsko *et al.* 1992; Morrison *et al.* 1994), of which only 30–36% is derived from fat (Buchdahl *et al.* 1989; Wootton *et al.* 1991). While this may be sufficient to meet the requirements of some patients, such intakes may be inadequate for those with serious lung disease. Furthermore, it is in these patients that appetite is most likely to be poor and even this level of intake not achieved. In these circumstances, supplementary forms of nutrition are likely to be needed.

Other patients may be failing to meet their energy needs because their fat intake is too low. Although fat restriction as a means of mitigating steatorrhoea is no longer advocated, some older patients who have been on fat-restricted diets in the past may have become accustomed to, and prefer, low-fat foods. Others may adopt the low-fat, healthy-eating measures recommended for the general population but which are inappropriate for their particular needs.

- *Non-compliance with dietary guidance*: In the teenage years, changes in dietary habits and attitudes mean that compliance with dietetic guidance, PERT or use of vitamin supplements may become poor (Rayner 1992). Problems such as eating disorders, use of alcohol or teenage pregnancy may also compromise dietary adequacy.
- *Behavioural feeding problems*: These often result from undue pressure being exerted by overanxious parents understandably concerned to try and make sure that their child consumes sufficient food. The consequent tension can make meal times less pleasant and increases the likelihood of anorexia and food refusal on the part of the child. Overemphasis on the 'special diet' for CF and overuse of nutritional supplements can exacerbate this problem.
- *Failure to institute appropriate nutritional support measures early enough*: Dietetic vigilance is necessary to detect emerging nutritional problems and institute corrective measures (e.g. the use of energy supplements) at an early stage before significant nutrient depletion or weight loss has occurred.

Additional nutritional support measures

General strategies to improve poor food intake can be employed to boost energy intake, e.g. increasing meal frequency, choosing energy-dense foods and the use of food fortification measures (see Section 1.12, Oral nutritional support). In the USA, behavioural strategy programmes have been shown to improve oral intake in CF children (Stark *et al.* 1990), but as yet this approach has been little used in the UK.

If nutrient intake remains poor, or to compensate for poor nutrition during an acute infection, dietary supplementation with either modular products (such as glucose polymer liquids or powders, or fat plus carbohydrate products) or sip feed supplements may be appropriate (see Appendix 6.7). Use of high-fat, high-energy, milk-based oral supplements has been shown to be an effective way of improving nutritional status and weight gain in both adults and children with CF (Rettammel *et al.* 1995; Skypala *et al.* 1998).

Although oral supplements are widely prescribed for those with CF, their use and effectiveness are not always well monitored. Patients do not always receive adequate instruction, encouragement or supervision to use them appropriately, nor may attempts be made to find products which are acceptable and hence consumed. The quantity and timing of dietary supplements also need careful consideration so that appetite is not impaired and nutrient intake from normal foods decreased; it is not uncommon to find young children taking large quantities of glucose polymer drinks and then refusing solid foods. It is important that supplements are used as an adjunct to, and not a substitute for, other dietary measures designed to increase nutrient intake from ordinary foods and beverages. There should always be an emphasis on the use of normal foods rather than supplements.

If energy intake remains continuously inadequate, more aggressive nutritional support measures should be considered (Moore *et al.* 1986; Ramsey *et al.* 1992).

Enteral feeding

Artificial nutritional support can be successfully provided via overnight nasogastric (Smith *et al.* 1994) or gastrostomy/jejunostomy (Levy *et al.* 1985; Boland *et al.* 1986; Steinkamp and von der Hardt 1994) feeding. The choice of route depends largely on patient preference and the likely duration of the supplementary feeding (see Section 1.13, Artificial nutritional support). Nutritional support may need to be long term (for a period of months or even years) in order for there to be significant benefit in terms of nutritional status, growth and lung function. For example, it may take up to 6 months before there is an increase in linear growth velocity (Steinkamp and von der Hardt 1994).

Overnight enteral feeding usually aims to provide 30–50% of total requirements given in conjunction with enteric-coated pancreatic microsphere preparations (Steinkamp and von der Hardt 1994). Some patients may receive a greater proportion of their energy needs via this route if daytime intake is particularly poor.

Enzyme administration during enteral feeding Pancreatic enzymes are usually administered before starting the feed and sometimes during it as well. A survey by the UK Dietitians' Cystic Fibrosis Interest Group showed considerable variation in UK dietetic practice regarding the method of enzyme administration and assessment of required enzyme dose for enteral feeding. Since the fat present in an enteral feed is delivered in small increments rather than as a large dietary load (and hence is better tolerated), and because of concerns over the potential hazards of excessive doses of enzymes, many centres now use lower enzyme dosages than would normally be the case for a fat load of this size. The optimum pattern of enzyme administration remains to be established.

Feeding formulae Adults are usually given whole protein enteral feeds with a high energy density (1.5–2 kcal/ml); occasionally one of the specialist high-fat feeds formulated for people with pulmonary disease may be used (see Appendix 6.7). Children can be given paediatric whole-protein feeds providing 1.5 kcal/ml.

It has been hypothesized that low-fat elemental formulae are better absorbed in CF, but these feeds are expensive, have a high osmolality and generally have a lower energy density than whole protein feeds. Newer elemental formulae with a high proportion of fat from MCT are favoured by some CF centres, and have been shown to improve weight gain even in patients with advanced lung disease (Williams *et al.* 1999). Furthermore, these elemental MCT-based formulae may be given without concurrent PERT because it has been shown that their absorption may be equivalent to that of whole protein formulae with enzyme replacement (Erskine *et al.* 1998). However, this strategy is currently still controversial.

Problems associated with enteral feeding Tube displacement due to coughing, vomiting or physiotherapy has been reported to be a problem with feeding via the nasogastric route (MacDonald *et al.* 1991), although others have found that this only occurs rarely (Smith *et al.* 1994). Gastrostomy feeding can result in problems such as gastrostomy site infections, leakage or gastro-oesophageal reflux (MacDonald 1996). Artificial supplementary feeding is also associated with a high incidence of nocturnal hyperglycaemia which may require treatment with insulin, although this is not a contraindication to enteral feeding (Smith *et al.* 1994).

If patients find it difficult to accept or tolerate nasogastric or gastrostomy feeding, it may be possible to achieve a sufficient level of nutritional support by means of oral supplementation (Hayes *et al.* 1995).

Parenteral nutrition

Parenteral nutritional support is usually only indicated in special circumstances, and usually on a short-term basis, for example when enteral feeding is contraindicated as a result of meconium ileus or severe respiratory problems.

4.7.5 Specific considerations in the management of cystic fibrosis

Cystic fibrosis and pregnancy

The increased longevity of CF patients means that pregnancy in women with CF is becoming increasingly common. Although CF reduces fertility, it has been estimated that about 4% of women with CF become pregnant each year (Edenborough *et al.* 1995).

In a review of the outcome of pregnancy in women with CF, Edenborough *et al.* (1995) found that although pregnancy is generally well tolerated, there are increased risks to both mother and child. In general, maternal weight gain is lower than average and the risk of spontaneous abortion or delivery of a preterm or small-for-dates infant is higher (Kent and Farquharson 1993; Edenborough *et al.* 1995). Women with mild lung disease are more likely to be able to maintain their own weight and deliver a healthy term infant than women with moderate to severe lung disease. Poor outcomes have been associated with a weight gain of <4.5 kg and a forced vital capacity of less than 50%

of predicted values (Kent and Farquharson 1993). Attention to energy intake and pulmonary function during pregnancy is important (Kent and Farquharson 1993).

Dietary guidance for pregnant women with cystic fibrosis

Preconceptional dietary advice is important for all women who are planning a pregnancy (see Section 3.1, Pregnancy) but especially so for those with CF because the risk of suboptimal nutritional status is higher. Vitamin and mineral status should be checked and appropriate supplementation commenced if indicated.

Care should be taken to avoid oversupplementation with vitamin A because of the risk of teratogenicity, and the intake of vitamin A from routine use of proprietary energy supplements should be taken into account. In practice, supplemental vitamin A is usually continued at the normal level (i.e. up to 8000 IU/day), but plasma levels are closely monitored.

During pregnancy, the primary nutritional aims are to:

- *Minimize the impact of pregnancy-related problems on food intake*: Problems such as nausea, vomiting and gastro-oesophageal reflux can significantly reduce food intake. Guidance on ways to alleviate these problems and improve nutrient intake may be helpful, and energy supplements may be appropriate in some circumstances (see Section 1.12, Oral nutritional support).
- *Achieve adequate but not excessive weight gain*: Weight gain should be monitored regularly. Poor weight gain increases the risk of fetal undernutrition and also compromises the mother's own health. Excessive weight gain will also compromise respiratory function and result in debilitating breathlessness. Ideal weight gain is between 10 and 12 kg

Following the birth, breast feeding can normally be encouraged but it is important that women are aware of the need to meet their increased energy and nutrient needs (Michel and Mueller 1994). Breast feeding may be contraindicated in women whose CF necessitates the use of certain drugs.

Cystic fibrosis in infants

Although not yet routine, the increasing use of antenatal and neonatal screening to identify mutations in the CF gene means that many more infants with CF are being diagnosed (Cystic Fibrosis Trust 1998).

Studies have shown that the effects of CF are apparent at an early stage. Bronstein *et al.* (1992) found that 59% of CF infants diagnosed through a newborn screening programme had pancreatic insufficiency and that such infants gained less weight between birth and diagnosis despite higher energy and protein intakes. Fat malabsorption was evident in 79% of infants at 6 months and 92% at 12 months of age. Vitamin E and essential fatty acid status have also been found to be compromised (Mischler *et al.* 1991).

The advent of better pancreatic enzyme replacement therapy has meant that specially modified milks (high in protein and low in fat) are not usually necessary in the management of CF and that either breast milk or ordinary infant formula milk is suitable. However, the use of protein hydrolysate infant formulae remains common in the USA (Cannella *et al.* 1993). Breast feeding can be successful and should be encouraged, either on its own or in conjunction with an infant formula (Luder *et al.* 1990; Holliday *et al.* 1991).

Marcus *et al.* (1991) followed the progress of infants diagnosed through neonatal screening and found that normal growth patterns could be achieved with mean energy intakes of 112 and 102 kcal/kg body weight at 6 and 12 months, respectively. However, the amount consumed will vary on a daily basis, usually in response to hunger (Simmonds *et al.* 1994). Some infants with pancreatic insufficiency require a relatively high energy intake of 200 kcal/kg, necessitating either supplementation of normal infant formula milk with glucose polymers or glucose/fat emulsions, or the use of a high-energy infant formula (see Section 1.14.3 in Enteral feeding in paediatric patients). Once adequate enzyme therapy has been established, infants usually thrive on an energy intake of between 100–120 kcal/kg. Higher energy intakes are indicated if weight gain is inadequate, or if a meconium ileus has resulted in surgery and short bowel syndrome, when energy requirements are likely to be in the range of 150–200 kcal/kg (MacDonald *et al.* 1991).

If the infant has a temporary disaccharide intolerance following surgery for a meconium ileus, or is milk intolerant, a lactose-free, protein hydrolysate formula will be necessary (see Section 4.35, Food exclusion), with or without the use of additional energy supplements.

It is necessary to give pancreatic enzymes with all types of infant milk, including breast milk. Enteric-coated microspheres should be mixed with a little breast or formula milk and administered separately by spoon, not added directly to a bottle of feed. If the mixture of milk and microspheres tends to cause choking, the granules can instead be mixed with a small amount of fruit purée, which creates a more easily swallowed gel.

All pancreatic insufficient infants should be given fat-soluble vitamin supplements from the time of diagnosis (4000 IU vitamin A, 400 IU vitamin D, 50 mg vitamin E).

Because energy needs tend to be higher than normal in the infant with CF, early weaning (between the ages of 3 and 4 months) to a diet of average fat content (in conjunction with pancreatic enzymes) is often appropriate, provided that steatorrhoea is well controlled.

Cystic fibrosis-related diabetes mellitus

CF is associated with progressive deterioration in glucose tolerance, as a result of damage to the pancreatic islets and beta-cells and long-term use of steroids (Lanng *et al.* 1995). The prevalence of overt diabetes has been estimated to be between 7 and 15% (Finkelstein *et al.* 1988; Lanng *et al.* 1994), a figure which is rising as survival time increases.

The combination of diabetes and CF is a significant concern because it is associated with deterioration in both respiratory and nutritional status, increased mortality and the development of microvascular (but not macrovascular) diabetic complications (Lanng 1996; Wilson *et al.* 2000). Although CF-related diabetes differs in some respects from other types of diabetes (its onset is more likely to be insidious and asymptomatic) there are common aspects. Most patients will require insulin and hence need to observe dietary precautions to prevent hypoglycaemia. The clinical objective of maintaining good glycaemic control in order to prevent microvascular complications is also important. However, in order to avoid jeopardizing energy intake, the dietetic ways in which these objectives are achieved in the patient with CF are different:

- The proportion of energy derived from fat should not be restricted. Some substitution of monounsaturated fat with saturated fat can be made as long as this does not jeopardize total energy intake.
- The type of carbohydrate consumed may be different. In order to maintain a diet of high energy density, intake of fibre-rich starchy foods should not be excessive and some carbohydrate in the form of monosaccharides, glucose polymers or other concentrated form is likely to be required to meet energy needs. However, to minimize hyperglycaemia, such rapidly absorbed forms of carbohydrate should ideally be consumed in conjunction with other foods, rather than in isolation.
- Insulin dosage should be determined by the need for carbohydrate, not the other way round.

Closely monitored individualized advice is essential in order to maintain optimum control of both the diabetes and the CF.

If a patient with CF-related diabetes is malnourished, overnight enteral feeding with an adjusted insulin regimen can be given.

Distal intestinal obstructive syndrome (DIOS) (meconium ileus equivalent)

This is more common in adults (but can also occur in children) with pancreatic insufficiency and presents with abdominal pain, distension, vomiting and constipation. Following treatment, dietary management should review compliance with enzyme therapy and whether enzyme preparations are being used appropriately. Under medical guidance, an increased intake of fibre and fluid may be beneficial for some patients.

Cystic fibrosis-related liver disease

This can occur in up to 20% of patients with CF and can make it particularly difficult to meet nutritional requirements. Oral intake may be reduced as a result of:

- nausea
- early satiety (resulting from enlargement of the liver and/or spleen)

- abdominal pain
- steatorrhoea (which will also increase nutrient losses).

Nutritional support measures are likely to be necessary and close monitoring is essential, especially if the disease progresses to end-stage ascites and encephalopathy (see Section 4.13, Liver and biliary disease).

Lung or heart/lung transplantation

Lung or heart/lung transplantation is now an option for patients with severe pulmonary disease.

Pre-transplant, prolonged chronic illness is likely to have resulted in considerable nutritional depletion and efforts should be made to correct this as much as possible prior to surgery.

Post-transplant, restoring and maintaining optimal nutritional status is a priority and, since patients usually feel much better, they are able to eat much better than before. In the long term, other nutritional problems may emerge, e.g. steroid-induced diabetes following the use of immunosuppressive drugs, hypercholesterolaemia, hypertriglyceridaemia, obesity and osteoporosis.

Text revised by: Briony Thomas

Acknowledgements: Alison Morton, Sue Wolfe and the UK Dietitians' Cystic Fibrosis Interest Group.

Useful addresses

The Cystic Fibrosis Trust, 11 London Road, Bromley, Kent BR1 1BY
Tel: 020 8464 7211

UK Dietitians' Cystic Fibrosis Interest Group
c/o The British Dietetic Association, 5th Floor, Charles House, 148–9 Great Charles Street, Queensway, Birmingham B3 3HT

International Cystic Fibrosis Nutrition Group
Can be contacted via the UK Dietitians' CF Interest Group (see above)

Further reading

Anthony H, Paxton S, Catto-Smith A, Phelan P. Physiological and psychosocial contributors to malnutrition in children with cystic fibrosis: review. *Clinical Nutrition* 1999; **18**: 327–335.
Dodge JA. Nutrition in cystic fibrosis. In Davies DP (Ed.) *Nutrition in Child Health*, pp. 123–132. London: Royal College of Physicians of London, 1995.
Hill CM (Ed.). *Practical Guidelines for Cystic Fibrosis Care*. Edinburgh: Churchill Livingstone, 1998.
MacDonald A. Nutritional management of cystic fibrosis. *Archives of Disease in Childhood* 1996; **74**: 81–87.
Pencharz PB, Durie PR. Nutritional management of cystic fibrosis. *Annual Reviews of Nutrition* 1993; **13**: 111–136.
Schoni MH, Casaulta-Aebischer C. Nutrition and lung function in cystic fibrosis patients: review. *Clinical Nutrition* 2000; **19**: 79–85.

Abstracts and compilations of papers presented at the annual meetings of the International Cystic Fibrosis Nutrition Group are a useful source of recent research findings. Details of these and proceedings from other major symposia can be obtained from the UK Dietitians' Cystic Fibrosis Interest Group (address given above).

References

Anthony H, Collins CE, Davidson G *et al.* Pancreatic enzyme replacement therapy in cystic fibrosis: Australian guidelines. Pediatric Gastroenterological Society and the Dietitians Association of Australia. *Journal of Paediatrics and Child Health* 1999; **35**: 125–129.
Boland MP, Stoski DS, MacDonald NE *et al.* Chronic jejunostomy feeding with a non-elemental formula in undernourished patients with cystic fibrosis. *Lancet* 1986; **i**: 232–234.
Borrowitz DS, Gard RJ, Durie PR. Use of pancreatic enzyme supplements for patients with cystic fibrosis in the context of fibrosing colonopathy. Consensus Committee Review. *Journal of Pediatrics* 1995; **127**: 681–684.
Bronstein MN, Sokol RJ, Abman SH *et al.* Pancreatic insufficiency, growth, and nutrition in infants identified by newborn screening as having cystic fibrosis. *Journal of Pediatrics* 1992; **120**: 533–540.
Buchdahl RM, Cox M, Fulleylove C *et al.* Increased resting energy expenditure in cystic fibrosis. *Journal of Applied Physiology* 1988; **64**: 1810–1816.
Buchdahl RM, Fulleylove C, Marchant JL *et al.* Energy and nutrient intakes of cystic fibrosis. *Archives of Disease in Childhood* 1989; **64**: 373–378.
Cannella PC, Bowser EK, Guyer LK, Borum PR. Feeding practices and nutrition recommendations for infants with cystic fibrosis. *Journal of the American Dietetic Association* 1993; **93**: 297–300.
Committee on Safety of Medicines. *Report of the Pancreatic Enzyme Working Party*. Medicines Control Agency UK, 1995.
Corey M, McLaughlin FJ, Williams M, Levison H. A comparison of survival, growth and pulmonary function in patients with cystic fibrosis in Boston and Toronto. *Journal of Clinical Epidemiology* 1988; **41**: 583–591.
Cystic Fibrosis Genetic Analysis Consortium. *Consortium Newsletter* 1996; May issue.
Cystic Fibrosis Trust. *Genetics*. Kent: Cystic Fibrosis Trust, 1998.
Dalzell AM, Shepherd RW, Dean B *et al.* Nutritional rehabilitation in cystic fibrosis: a 5–year follow-up study. *Journal of Pediatric Gastroenterology and Nutrition* 1992; **15**: 141–145.
Dodge JA. Nutritional requirements in cystic fibrosis: a review. *Journal of Pediatric Gastroenterology and Nutrition* 1988; **7** (Suppl 1): S1–S11.
Durie PR, Pencharz PB. A rational approach to the nutritional care of patients with cystic fibrosis. *Journal of the Royal Society of Medicine* 1989; **82** (Suppl 16): 11–20.
Edenborough FP, Stableforth DE, Webb AK *et al.* Outcome of pregnancy in women with cystic fibrosis. *Thorax* 1995; **50**: 170–174.
Eid NS, Shoemaker LR, Samiec TD. Vitamin A in cystic fibrosis. Case report and reviews of the literature. *Journal of Paediatric Gastroenterology and Nutrition* 1990; **10**: 265–269.
Elborn J S, Shale D J, Britton JR. Cystic fibrosis: current survival and population estimates to year 2000. *Thorax* 1991; **46**: 881–885.
Erhardt P, Miller MG, Littlewood JM. Iron deficiency in cystic fibrosis. *Archives of Disease in Childhood* 1987; **62**: 185–187.

Erskine JM, Lingard CD, Sontag MG, Accurso FJ. Enteral nutrition for patients with cystic fibrosis: comparison of a semi-elemental and non elemental formula. *Journal of Pediatrics* 1998; **132**: 265–269.

Finkelstein SM, Wielinski CL, Elliott GR *et al.* Diabetes mellitus associated with cystic fibrosis. *Journal of Pediatrics* 1988; **112**: 373–377.

Gaskin K, Gurwitz D, Durie P *et al.* Improved respiratory prognosis in patients with cystic fibrosis and normal fat absorption. *Journal of Pediatrics* 1982; **100**: 857–862.

Gavin J, Ellis J, Dewar AL *et al.* Dietary fibre and the occurrence of gut symptoms in cystic fibrosis. *Archives of Disease in Childhood* 1997; **76**: 35–37.

Gibbens DT, Gilsanz V, Boechat MI *et al.* Osteoporosis in cystic fibrosis. *Journal of Pediatrics* 1988; **113**: 295–300.

Goodchild MC. Practical management of nutrition and gastrointestinal tract in cystic fibrosis. *Journal of the Royal Society of Medicine* 1986; **79** (Suppl 12): 32–35.

Grey AB, Ames RW, Matthews RD, Reid IR. Bone mineral density and body composition in adult patients with cystic fibrosis. *Thorax* 1993; **48**: 589–593.

Halford PJ, Jackson AA. Faecal losses of retinol and alpha-tocopherol in subjects with cystic fibrosis and healthy controls (Abstract). *Proceedings of the Nutrition Society* 1993; **52**: 2.

Hayes R, Kanga JF, Craigmyle L, D'Angela S. Nocturnal oral supplementation in patients with cystic fibrosis. *Pediatric Pulmonology Supplement* 1995; **12**: 266.

Henderson RC, Madsen CD. Bone density in children and adolescents with cystic fibrosis. *Journal of Pediatrics* 1996; **128**: 28–34.

Holliday K, Allen JR, Waters DL *et al.* Growth of human milk-fed and formula-fed infants with cystic fibrosis. *Journal of Pediatrics* 1991; **118**: 77–79.

Kelleher S. Laboratory measurements of nutrition in CF. *Journal of the Royal Society of Medicine* 1987; **80** (Suppl 15): 28–29.

Kent NE, Farquharson DF. Cystic fibrosis in pregnancy. *Canadian Medical Association Journal* 1993; **149**: 809–813.

Lanng S. Diabetes mellitus in cystic fibrosis. *European Journal of Gastroenterology and Hepatology* 1996; **8**: 744–747.

Lanng S, Thorsteinsson B, Lund-Anderson C *et al.* Diabetes mellitus in Danish cystic fibrosis patients: prevalence and late diabetic complications. *Acta Paediatrica* 1994; **83**: 72–77.

Lanng S, Hansen A, Thorsteinsson B *et al.* Glucose tolerance in patients with cystic fibrosis: five year prospective study. *British Medical Journal* 1995; **311**: 655–659.

Leonard CH, Knox AJ. Pancreatic enzyme supplements and vitamins in cystic fibrosis. *Journal of Human Nutrition and Dietetics* 1997; **10**: 3–16.

Levy LD, Durie PR, Pencharz PB, Corey ML. Effects of long-term nutritional rehabilitation on body composition and clinical status in malnourished children and adolescents with cystic fibrosis. *Journal of Pediatrics* 1985; **107**: 225–230.

Levy L, Durie P, Pencharz PB, Corey M. Prognostic factors associated with patient survival during nutritional rehabilitation in malnourished children and adolescents with cystic fibrosis. *Journal of Pediatric Gastroenterology and Nutrition* 1986; **5**: 97–102.

Lewis PA. The epidemiology of cystic fibrosis. In Hodson ME, Geddes DM (Eds) *Cystic Fibrosis*, pp. 1–13. London: Chapman and Hall, 1995.

Littlewood JM, Wolfe SP. Control of malabsorption in cystic fibrosis. *Pediatric Drugs* 2000; **2**: 205–222.

Littlewood JM, MacDonald A. Rationale of modern dietary recommendations in cystic fibrosis. *Journal of the Royal Society of Medicine* 1987; **80** (Suppl 15): 16–24.

Luder E, Kattan M, Tanzer-Torres G, Bonforte RJ. Current recommendations for breast feeding in cystic fibrosis centers. *American Journal of Diseases of Children* 1990; **144**: 1153–1156.

MacDonald A. Nutritional management of cystic fibrosis. *Archives of Disease in Childhood* 1996; **74**: 81–87.

MacDonald A, Holden C, Harris G. Nutritonal strategies in cystic fibrosis: current issues. *Journal of the Royal Society of Medicine* 1991; **84** (Suppl 18): 28–35.

Marcus MS, Sondel SA, Farrell PM *et al.* Nutritional status of infants with cystic fibrosis associated with early diagnosis and intervention. *American Journal of Clinical Nutrition* 1991; **54**: 578–585.

Michel SH, Mueller DH. Impact of lactation on women with cystic fibrosis and their infants: a review of five cases. *Journal of the American Dietetic Association* 1994; **94**: 159–165.

Mischler EH, Marcus MS, Sondel SA *et al.* Nutritional assessment of infants with cystic fibrosis diagnosed through screening. *Pediatric Pulmonology Supplement* 1991; **7**: 56–63.

Moore MC, Greene HL, Donald WD, Dunn GD. Enteral tube feeding as adjunct therapy in malnourished patients with cystic fibrosis: a clinical study and literature review. *American Journal of Clinical Nutrition* 1986; **44**: 33–41.

Morrison G, Morrison JM, Redmond AOB *et al.* Comparison between a standard pancreatic supplement and a high enzyme preparation in cystic fibrosis. *Alimentary Pharmacology and Therapeutics* 1992; **6**: 549–555.

Morrison JM, O'Rawe A, McCracken KJ *et al.* Energy intake and losses in cystic fibrosis. *Journal of Human Nutrition and Dietetics* 1994; **7**: 39–46.

Murphy JL, Wootton SA, Bond SA, Jackson AA. Energy content of stools in normal healthy controls and patients with cystic fibrosis. *Archives of Disease in Childhood* 1991; **66**: 495–500.

O'Donnell M, Talbot JF. Vitamin A deficiency in cystic fibrosis: case report. *British Journal of Ophthalmology* 1987; **71**: 787–790.

O'Rawe A, McIntosh I, Dodge JA *et al.* Increased energy expenditure in cystic fibrosis is associated with specific mutation. *Clinical Science* 1992; **82**: 71–76.

Peters AA, Rolles CJ. Vitamin therapy in cystic fibrosis – a review and rationale. *Journal of Clinical Pharmacy and Therapeutics* 1993; **18**: 33–38.

Pond MN, Morton AM, Conway SP. Functional iron deficiency in adults with cystic fibrosis. *Respiratory Medicine* 1996; **90**: 409–413.

Prescott P, Bakowski MT. Pathogenesis of fibrosing colonopathy: the role of methacrylic acid copolymer. *Pharmacoepidemiological Drug Safety* 1999; **8**: 377–384.

Ramsey BW, Farrell PM, Pencharz P, Consensus Committee. Nutritional assessment and management in cystic fibrosis: a consensus report. *American Journal of Clinical Nutrition* 1992; **55**: 108–116.

Rashid M, Durie P, Andrew M *et al.* Prevalence of vitamin K deficiency in cystic fibrosis. *American Journal of Clinical Nutrition* 1999; **79**: 378–382.

Rayner RJ. Fat-soluble vitamins in cystic fibrosis. *Proceedings of the Nutrition Society* 1992; **51**: 245–250.

Rayner RJ, Littlewood JM. Vitamin A status as a marker of prognosis in cystic fibrosis. In *Proceedings of the XIth International Cystic Fibrosis Congress*, Dublin, August 1992.

Rettammel AL, Marcus MS, Farrell PM *et al.* Oral supplementation with a high-fat, high-energy product improves nutritional status and alters serum lipids in patients with cystic fibrosis. *Journal of the American Dietetic Association* 1995; **95**: 454–459.

Royal College of Physicians. *Cystic Fibrosis in Adults. Recommendations for Care of Patients in the UK.* London: RCP, 1990.

Shepherd RW, Vasques-Velasquez L, Prentice A *et al.* Increased energy expenditure in young children with cystic fibrosis. *Lancet* 1988; **i**: 1300–1303.

Simmonds EJ, Wall CR, Wolfe SP, Littlewood JM. A review of infant feeding practices at a regional cystic fibrosis unit. *Journal of Human Nutrition and Dietetics* 1994; **7**: 31–38.

Sitrin MD, Lieberman F, Jensen WE *et al.* Vitamin E deficiency and neurologic disease in adults with cystic fibrosis. *Annals of Internal Medicine* 1987; **107**: 51–54.

Skypala IJ, Ashworth FA, Hodson ME *et al.* Oral nutritional supplements promote weight gain in cystic fibrosis patients. *Journal of Human Nutrition and Dietetics* 1998; **11**: 95–104.

Smith DL, Clarke JM, Stableforth DE. A nocturnal feeding programme in cystic fibrosis adults. *Journal of Human Nutrition and Dietetics* 1994; **7**: 257–262.

Smyth RL, van Velzen D, Smyth AR *et al.* Strictures of ascending colon in cystic fibrosis and high-strength pancreatic enzymes. *Lancet* 1994; **343**: 85–86.

Sokol RJ, Reardon MC, Accurso FJ *et al.* Fat soluble vitamin status during first year of life in infants with cystic fibrosis identified by screening newborns. *American Journal of Clinical Nutrition* 1989; **50**: 1064–1071.

Stark LJ, Bowen AM, Tyc VL *et al.* A behavioural approach to increasing calorie consumption in children with cystic fibrosis. *Journal of Paediatric Psychology* 1990; **15**: 309–326.

Stead RJ, Houlder S, Agnew J *et al.* Vitamin D and parathyroid hormone and bone mineralization in adults with cystic fibrosis. *Thorax* 1988; **43**: 190–194.

Steinkamp G, von der Hardt H. Improvement of nutritional status and lung function after long-term nocturnal gastrostomy feedings in cystic fibrosis. *Journal of Pediatrics* 1994; **24**: 244–249.

Tomezsko JL, Stallings VA, Scanlin TF. Dietary intake of healthy children with cystic fibrosis compared with normal control children. *Pediatrics* 1992; **90**: 547–553.

Watkin S, Bell SC, Wynn S *et al.* Vitamin A and E levels in cystic fibrosis. In *Proceedings of the XIth International Cystic Fibrosis Congress*, Dublin, August 1992.

Wildhagen MF, ten Kate LP, Habbema JD. Screening for cystic fibrosis and its evaluation. *British Medical Bulletin* 1998; **54**: 857–875.

Williams SG, Ashworth F, McAlweenie A *et al.* Percutaneous endoscopic gastrostomy feeding in patents with cystic fibrosis. *Gut* 1999; **44**: 87–90.

Wilson DC, Kalnins D, Stewart C *et al.* Challenges in the dietary treatment of cystic fibrosis related diabetes mellitus. *Clinical Nutrition* 2000; **19**: 87–93.

Wootton SA, Murphy SL, Bond SA *et al.* Energy balance and growth in cystic fibrosis. *Journal of the Royal Society of Medicine* 1991; **84** (Suppl 18): 22–27.

4.8 Malabsorption

Malabsorption has many different causes (Table 4.9). When present, dietary measures are likely to be required to alleviate symptoms and nutritional supplementation may be necessary to correct nutritional depletion or prevent further nutritional deterioration. It is, however, vital that the underlying cause of the malabsorption is identified and, if possible, treated.

4.8.1 Diagnostic features of malabsorption

Clinical features of malabsorption include some or all of the following:

- diarrhoea or change in stool consistency
- abdominal distension
- flatulence
- loss of weight.

Generalized nutrient deficiencies are likely and the risk of specific deficiencies is heightened by disease or resection in particular sites of the gastrointestinal tract (Fig. 4.4). Severe diarrhoea can result in dehydration and loss of electrolytes.

Diarrhoea is the most common presenting feature and the nature of the stool often indicates the type of malabsorption:

- *Fat malabsorption* results in steatorrhoea, where the stool is pale, malodorous, greasy and unformed.

- *Carbohydrate malabsorption* more typically results in diarrhoea which is watery and frothy owing to the presence of fermented sugars.

However, if more than one nutrient is malabsorbed (e.g. due to loss of absorptive surface or pancreatic insufficiency) this distinction is less clear-cut.

Fat malabsorption can be confirmed by faecal fat measurement (BSG 1996, Bo-Linn and Fordtran 1984). Ideally, 70 g fat should be taken for 6 days with isotopic or radio-opaque markers; misleading results, especially false negatives, can occur if stool collections are incomplete. The upper limit of daily fat excretion is normally 7 g or 20 mmol/24 hours. A very high faecal fat excretion (50 g or more) is suggestive of pancreatic insufficiency. The ^{14}C-triolein breath test can also be used to diagnose steatorrhoea (Newcomer et al. 1978), particularly in cases where fat malabsorption is part of a multiple malabsorption syndrome. Increasingly both these tests are being replaced by faecal fat microscopy or faecal chymotrysin measurement.

The most useful test for the diagnosis of carbohydrate malabsorption is the breath hydrogen test. Normally, cells do not produce hydrogen but many bacteria in gut flora will do so if a suitable substrate such as an unabsorbed disaccharide is present. The hydrogen then produced will be absorbed into blood and can be detected and measured as it is excreted in breath. Measurement of breath hydrogen following a test load of lactose is a particularly effective test for lactose malabsorption (Newcomer et al. 1975). In infants, unabsorbed lactose in the stool can be clearly

Table 4.9 Causes of malabsorption

Reason for malabsorption	Common causes
Reduced absorptive capacity	Intestinal resection Villous atrophy, e.g. coeliac disease; tropical sprue Gastrocolic and jejunocolic fistulae Infiltration, e.g. amyloid, scleroderma, lymphoma Vascular insufficiency Mucosal damage, e.g. by drugs or irradiation, or following surgery or serious gastroenteritic infection
Enzyme deficiencies	Disaccharidase deficiency, e.g. primary alactasia or secondary lactase deficiency Lipase and/or proteolytic enzyme deficiency, e.g. pancreatic insufficiency
Intralumenal factors	High pH in duodenum, e.g. achlorhydria Low pH in duodenum, e.g. Zollinger–Ellison syndrome Bile salt deficiency, e.g. obstructive jaundice
Infection	Deconjugation of bile salts by bacterial colonization of the small intestine, e.g. blind loop syndrome Competition for nutrients, e.g. parasitic infections Increased intestinal transit time, e.g. gastroenteritis
Impaired transport mechanisms	Impaired fat transport, e.g. congenital lymphangectasia, retroperitoneal fibrosis Impaired monosaccharide transport, e.g. congenital primary malabsorption of glucose and galactose; secondary glucose malabsorption following surgery, protein-energy malnutrition or gastroenteritis

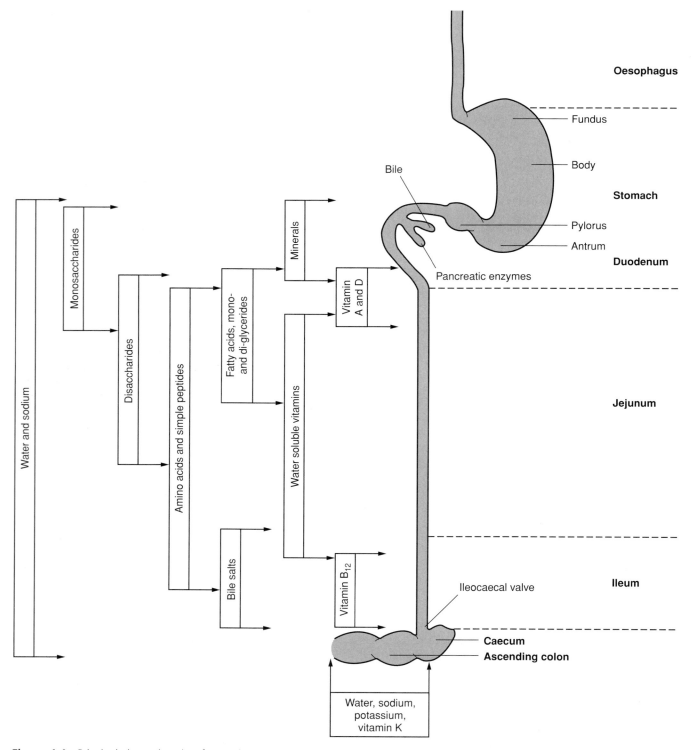

Figure 4.4 Principal absorption sites for nutrients.

identified by paper chromatography or other tests for faecal reducing substances.

Carbohydrate malabsorption can also be diagnosed by administering a test dose of a disaccharide (such as lactose) and measuring the subsequent rise in blood glucose. A flattened glycaemic curve compared with that produced by an equivalent glucose load is indicative of malabsorption. However, this test can give variable results and is now less used. Alternatively, direct measurement of disaccharidases (lactase, maltase and sucrase) can be made following endoscopic biopsy, and can help to identify congenital lactase deficiency, and disaccharidase deficiency in coeliac disease; however, the general use of these tests is limited because of high coefficients of variation (McIntyre *et al.* 1994).

4.8.2 Dietary treatment of malabsorption

Whatever the cause of malabsorption the principles of dietary therapy remain the same:

1 dietary treatment of the primary disorder, e.g. coeliac disease;
2 dietary measures to provide symptom relief;
3 the daily replacement of large losses of fluid and electrolytes;
4 the restoration of optimal nutritional status, by supplementation if necessary.

Specific aspects of particular types of malabsorption are considered below.

Fat malabsorption

The main nutritional significance of the loss of fat is the associated loss of energy and fat-soluble vitamins A, D, E and K. Unabsorbed fatty acids may also form complexes with minerals, such as calcium, thus inhibiting their absorption. This can increase the risk of complications such as anaemia or osteoporosis.

Steatorrhoea is no longer treated by marked restriction of dietary fat because this tends to compromise energy intake in patients who may already have suffered severe weight loss. Severe steatorrhoea due to pancreatic insufficiency can be treated with pancreatic enzymes. However, if, despite optimum drug therapy, the symptoms of steatorrhoea continue to be socially and personally unacceptable, or are causing electrolyte disturbances or mineral deficiencies, modification of fat intake may need to be considered. This is usually best achieved by reducing total fat intake by up to 50% and replacing energy via modular carbohydrate supplementation (see Section 1.12, Oral nutritional support).

Alternatively, or additionally, a proportion of long chain triglyceride (LCT) can be substituted with medium chain triglyceride (MCT). About one-third of ingested MCT can directly enter mucosal cells as a triglyceride and be hydrolysed by a mucosal lipolytic system, the medium chain fatty acids then passing into the portal vein. However, large amounts of MCT are not always well tolerated and can cause osmotic diarrhoea. Many people find it unpleasant to consume on its own and its taste usually needs to be disguised by mixing it with foods or beverages. If used for cooking, the oil must not be heated above 150–160°C or its palatability is further impaired. MCT sip feed supplements may be more acceptable (Section 1.12, Oral nutritional support).

For those requiring artificial nutrition support, MCT-containing enteral feeds (sometimes in conjunction with elemental or semi-elemental formulae) may be indicated for some severe forms of fat malabsorption (see Appendix 6.7).

In most cases, supplements of fat-soluble vitamins will be required to restore losses and prevent further deficiency. In cases of persistent malabsorption it may be necessary to administer these in water-soluble form or by injection.

Carbohydrate malabsorption

Lactose malabsorption

This results from varying degrees of deficiency of the enzyme lactase and consequent impaired ability to digest dietary lactose. Lactose remaining within the intestine can cause osmotic diarrhoea and is also fermented by colonic bacteria, resulting in symptoms such as abdominal distension, flatulence and explosive watery diarrhoea, often acidic in nature and causing perianal dermatitis.

Lactose intolerance occurs in three main forms: hereditary alactasia, and primary and secondary lactase deficiency.

Hereditary alactasia This is a severe and rare condition characterized by complete absence of lactase, and requires total and permanent lactose exclusion. The symptoms of profuse watery diarrhoea appear soon after birth following the first feeds of human or cow's milk. Breast feeding is contraindicated and the use of lactose-free infant formulae is essential (see Section 4.35, Food exclusion). Paediatric dietetic expertise will be required from weaning onwards to ensure that the diet remains both lactose free and nutritionally adequate.

Primary lactase deficiency This is an autosomal recessive disorder where a gradual reduction in lactase activity causes symptoms of lactose maldigestion in older children and adults. It is particularly common in people whose genetic origins lie in countries where milk consumption after infancy is traditionally uncommon, i.e. South-East Asia, India, the Middle East and parts of Africa. Prevalence studies suggest that over 50% of people of Indian origin and over 80% of African–Caribbean people have evidence of primary lactase deficiency, compared with only about 3% of white Western Europeans (Ferguson *et al.* 1984; Iqbal *et al.* 1993). In susceptible populations, the prevalence of lactose maldigestion is low in children under the age of 4 years but increases with age, reaching a plateau at the age of 13 years and beyond (Rosado 1997).

In lactase-deficient people, ingested lactose can cause abdominal distension, sometimes pain, flatus and diarrhoea, although not everyone with low lactase levels has physical symptoms of lactose intolerance (Iqbal *et al.* 1996). The clinical effects are dose related and only become marked at high levels of intake (e.g. 50 g loads); many malabsorbers can tolerate moderate intakes of milk and milk products (Suarez *et al.* 1995, 1997; Suarez and Levitt 1996; Vesa *et al.* 1996).

Complete avoidance of lactose is therefore unnecessary, and is also undesirable because of the risk of compromising calcium intake. Instead symptoms should be stabilized at a low intake and lactose-containing foods then reintroduced in gradually increasing amounts. The individual level of tolerance varies, but most people with low lactase levels can consume 12–15 g lactose/day (equivalent to about 250 ml or half a pint of milk) without discomfort (Johnson *et al.* 1993) and in some cases amounts up to 25 g/day may be well tolerated (Suarez *et al.* 1997).

Symptoms may also be less likely to occur if lactose is consumed with food rather than in isolated liquid form such as a glass of milk between meals, probably as a result of differences in the rate of gastric emptying (Martini and Saviano 1988). Lactose in fermented milk products such as yoghurt may also be better tolerated as a result of beneficial proliferation of colonic flora such as bifidobacteria which can metabolize lactose (Hertzler and Saviano 1996; Vesa *et al.* 1996). However, some people may adapt better than others in this way.

Since the clinical effects of lactose intolerance are similar to those of irritable bowel syndrome, the possibility of primary lactase deficiency should always be considered, particularly in people from genetically susceptible groups. Similarly, the possibility should also be considered in children complaining of recurrent abdominal pain (Ferguson *et al.* 1984). However, it should also be borne in mind that a considerable proportion of people (perhaps as many as 30%) claiming to be milk intolerant are in fact experiencing aversion, i.e. psychological rather than physical effects (Suarez and Levitt 1996; Rosado 1997).

Secondary lactase deficiency This is a common, usually temporary, consequence of damage to the intestinal brush border as result of severe gastroenteritis, intestinal surgery or untreated coeliac disease or cow's milk protein intolerance. The condition is characterized by diarrhoea which persists after the primary disorder has been treated and is particularly likely to occur in infants and children. Severe secondary lactose intolerance is sometimes accompanied by secondary sucrose intolerance.

Although transient in nature, it may take weeks rather than days for lactase secretion to be adequately re-established. Most lactase production takes place in the older cells at the tips of the villi rather than in the newer cells at the base. Lactase production is therefore the first disaccharidase to be affected by damage to the villi and the last to be restored.

Management depends on the severity of symptoms. In adults and children, avoidance of lactose for a few days will cause symptoms to subside and it can then gradually be reintroduced into the diet with the use of foods such as lactose-reduced milk, fermented milk products such as yoghurt and hard cheeses. As tolerance improves, the range of lactose-containing foods and their level of consumption can be increased. Because the condition is usually resolved within a relatively short period, the avoidance of milk and milk-based foods, even by children, is unlikely to pose a nutritional problem. However, if lactose (and hence milk) restriction is required for more than 3–4 weeks, the question of nutritional adequacy in terms of calcium, protein and energy will need to be addressed.

Formula-fed infants with secondary lactase deficiency may require a lactose-free infant formula as a temporary substitute for cow's milk. Breast milk is usually tolerated but, in severe cases, partial or total substitution by a lactose-free formula may be necessary. If the secondary lactase intolerance has resulted from an intolerance to cow's milk protein, a soya-based or alternative milk-free, lactose-free formula will be required (see Section 4.35, Food exclusion).

Malabsorption of other disaccharides

Primary disaccharidase deficiencies Congenital disorders such as sucrase–isomaltase deficiency can occur but are rare. Management requires total avoidance of the disaccharide substrate.

Secondary disaccharidase deficiency Production of enzymes such as sucrase and maltase is less likely to be affected by intestinal damage than lactase but severe enteropathies or infections, particularly in children, may result in malabsorption of disaccharides such as sucrose coexisting alongside lactose malabsorption. Temporary avoidance of major sources of sucrose followed by its gradual reintroduction may be necessary.

Monosaccharide malabsorption

Congenital monosaccharide malabsorption This is rare and requires specialist dietary management. It involves a disturbance in the active transport of the monosaccharides glucose and galactose. The diet must be free of all starch, disaccharides, glucose and galactose, and infants will require a fructose-based formula such as Galactomin 19 (SHS). All oral medicines must be carbohydrate free. The diet should be nutritionally adequate in all other respects, and vitamin and mineral supplementation may be necessary. Strict adherence to the diet is required during infancy, although in later years limited quantities of milk and sucrose may be added.

Secondary malabsorption of monosaccharides This may occur in infants following surgery, protein-energy malnutrition or gastroenteritis. An initial period of intravenous fluids is often necessary to correct water and electrolyte imbalances. This will be followed by a carbohydrate-free formula during which there should be careful monitoring for signs of hypoglycaemia. The problem is thought to be one of monosaccharide malabsorption, since disaccharidase activity is normal. The ability to tolerate carbohydrates slowly recovers and a monosaccharide such as glucose or fructose may be added to the diet in increasing increments of 1% of normal carbohydrate intake. These children are often underweight and gravely ill, and parenteral nutrition may be lifesaving if resumption of adequate oral nutrition is delayed.

The detailed dietary management of carbohydrate malabsorption in infants and children should be sought in paediatric dietetic textbooks.

Protein malabsorption

Malabsorption states in which there is a deficiency of enzymes involved in protein digestion, e.g. pancreatic proteolytic enzyme, trypsinogen or enterokinase deficiency, are not indications for the dietary restriction of protein. When increased protein losses occur as a result of an enteropathy or malabsorption, a high protein intake (1.0–1.5 g/kg/day) may be necessary to allow for the decreased efficiency of absorption. If fat malabsorption is present, high-protein foods must be selected which are also low in fat, although care must be taken not to compromise energy intake. Modular protein supplements can be used along with glucose polymers (see Section 1.12, Oral nutritional support).

Pancreatic enzyme replacement therapy (PERT) is often a cardinal aspect of management of such malabsorption states (see Section 4.7, Cystic fibrosis).

Text revised by: Briony Thomas

Further reading

Shaw V, Lawson M (Eds). *Clinical Paediatric Dietetics*, 2nd edn. Oxford: Blackwell Science, 2001.

References

Bo-Linn GW, Fordtran JS. Fecal fat concentration in patients with steatorrhoea. *Gastroenterology* 1984; **87**: 319–322.

British Society of Gastroenterology (BSG). *Tests for Malabsorbtion*. London: BSG, 1996.

Ferguson A, Macdonald DM, Brydon GW. Prevalence of lactase deficiency in British adults. *Gut* 1984; **25**: 163–167.

Flatz G. Genetics of lactose digestion in humans. *Advances in Human Genetics* 1987; **16**: 1–77.

Hertzler SR, Savaiano DA. Colonic adaptation to daily lactose feeding in lactose maldigesters reduces lactose intolerance. *American Journal of Clinical Nutrition* 1996; **64**: 232–236.

Iqbal TH, Wood GM, Lewis KO *et al*. Prevalence of primary lactase deficiency in adult residents of west Birmingham. *British Medical Journal* 1993; **306**: 1303.

Iqbal TH *et al*. Small intestinal lactase status, frequency of distribution of enzyme activity and milk intake in a multi-ethnic population. *Clinical Nutrition* 1996; **15**: 297–302.

Johnson AO, Semenya JG, Buchowski MS *et al*. Adaptation of lactose maldigesters to continued milk intakes. *American Journal of Clinical Nutrition* 1993; **58**: 879–881.

McIntyre AS, Smith JA, Amoah J *et al*. The use of small endoscopic biopsies to measure disaccharidase activities and the effect of duodenal ulceration. *European Journal of Gastroenterology* 1994; **6**: 229–234.

Newcomer AD, McGill DB, Thomas PJ, Hofmann AF. Prospective comparison of indirect methods for detecting lactase deficiency. *New England Journal of Medicine* 1975; **293**: 1232–1236.

Newcomer AD, Hofmann AF, di Magno EP. Triolein breath test: a sensitive and specific test for fat malabsorption. *Gastroenterology* 1978; **87**: 319–322.

Rosado JL. Lactose digestion and maldigestion: Implications for dietary habits in developing countries. *Nutrition Research Reviews* 1997; **10**: 137–149.

Suarez FL, Levitt MD. Abdominal symptoms and lactose: the discrepancy between patients' claims and the results of blinded trials. *American Journal of Clinical Nutrition* 1996; **64**: 251–252.

Suarez FL, Savaiano DA, Levitt MD. A comparison of symptoms after the consumption of milk or lactose-hydrolyzed milk by people with self-reported severe lactose intolerance. *New England Journal of Medicine* 1995; **333**: 1–4.

Suarez FL, Savaiano D, Arbisi P, Levitt MD. Tolerance to the daily ingestion of two cups of milk by individuals claiming lactose intolerance. *American Journal of Clinical Nutrition* 1997; **65**: 1502–1506.

Vesa TH, Marteau P, Zidi S *et al*. Digestion and tolerance of lactose from yogurt and different semi-solid fermented dairy products containing *Lactobacillus acidophilus* and bifidobacteria in lactose maldigestion – is bacterial lactase important? *European Journal of Clinical Nutrition* 1996; **50**: 730–733.

4.9 Coeliac disease

Coeliac disease is caused by an intolerance to gluten, a protein found in wheat and rye, and to similar proteins found in barley and, possibly, oats. The reaction to gluten damages the mucosal lining of the small intestine, flattening the villi and reducing the ability to absorb nutrients. As a result, symptoms of malabsorption commonly occur, although these can vary in nature and severity. The intolerance is permanent, and requires complete and life-long exclusion of gluten from the diet. This not only corrects the histological and clinical consequences but also reduces the risk of long-term detrimental effects on health.

Gluten intolerance can also manifest itself as the skin disorder dermatitis herpetiformis (see Section 4.33.4, in Disorders of the skin). Although this may also be associated with intestinal damage, dermatitis herpetiformis is less likely to result in gastrointestinal symptoms.

4.9.1 Features of coeliac disease

Causation

The word 'coeliac' is derived from the Greek word *koiliakos* which means 'suffering in the bowels'. The coeliac condition was first described nearly 1800 years ago in the writings of the Roman physician Aretaeus of Cappadocia. He mentioned fatty diarrhoea, loss of weight, pallor and food passing undigested through the body. He also said 'that bread is rarely suitable for giving (coeliac children) strength'. It was not until 1888 that Samuel Gee of St Bartholomew's Hospital in London gave the second classic description and a clear clinical account of the condition.

No real progress in understanding the disease was made until after the World War II. In 1950, Professor Dicke, a Dutch paediatrician, described how coeliac children had benefited dramatically during the war when wheat, rye and oat flours, which were unavailable, were replaced by maize or rice; while at the end of the war, the children relapsed when wheat flour was air-lifted into Holland. Dicke (1953) also went on to show that it was the protein fraction in wheat (gluten) which exacerbated the disorder.

Much remains to be learnt about how or why gluten harms the intestine. Coeliac disease results from an immune reaction to antigenic fractions within gluten. The fraction of gluten in wheat responsible for the damage is known to be gliadin, an alcohol-soluble prolamin, but gliadin is itself a mixture of proteins. The alpha, beta, gamma and omega fractions all appear to be harmful, although the alpha fraction is possibly the most antigenic. As well as gliadin in wheat, prolamins found in other cereals such as secalin in rye and hordein in barley also trigger the immunological response leading to coeliac disease. Until recently, the prolamin in oats, avenin, was thought to have the same deleterious effects and oats have traditionally been excluded from a gluten-free diet. However, the necessity for this is now less certain and a matter of current debate (see Oats toxicity, in Section 4.9.2 below).

Onset and prevalence

Symptoms of coeliac disease can develop at any age, and the condition is no longer regarded as primarily a paediatric disorder. The incidence of coeliac disease in children has declined, probably as a result of changes in infant feeding practices, in particular the use of gluten-free weaning foods and avoidance of exposure to gluten in the first few months of life (Challacombe *et al.* 1997). The peak age of onset is now between 40 and 50 years, with increasing numbers of people being diagnosed in later life as awareness of the condition and its variable presentation improves. The disease is more common in women than in men (by almost 3:1 in middle-aged adults) (Feighery 1999).

A commonly quoted figure for the prevalence of coeliac disease is 1 in 1000 but it now seems likely that the condition is underdiagnosed and that this figure is a considerable underestimate (Johnston *et al.* 1996; Hin *et al.* 1999). Screening studies suggest that as many as 1 in 300 Europeans may have coeliac disease (Mylotte *et al.* 1973; Catassi *et al.* 1994; 1995). The condition is rare in Oriental and African–Caribbean populations.

The risk of coeliac disease is increased in people with a family history of the disease. Although not dominantly inherited, coeliac disease is associated with a particular human leucocyte antigen (HLA) genotype, with the HLA-DQ heterodimer, appearing to confer disease susceptibility (Sollid and Thorsby 1993). The prevalence of coeliac disease may be at least 10% in families with a history of coeliac disease.

Genetic links may also account for an increased prevalence of coeliac disease in a number of immune-related disorders. A common genetic background, particularly in HLA type, is thought to explain its association with:

- *Type I diabetes*: The prevalence of coeliac disease is increased to between 2.0 and 7.8% in people with type I diabetes (Cronin and Shanahan 1997). For this reason, coeliac disease should be suspected in any diabetic patient with gastrointestinal symptoms or unexplained anaemia. It has also been suggested that type I diabetic patients should be screened for coeliac disease every few years (Saukkonen *et al*. 1996).

- *Autoimmune disorders*: Coeliac disease is more prevalent in people with autoimmune thyroid disease (5–5.8%) and primary biliary cirrhosis (3%) (Feighery 1999).
- Immune deficiency states: Between 2 and 2.6% of people with immunoglobulin A (IgA) deficiency have coeliac disease (Feighery 1999).

The high prevalence of coeliac disease in people with Down's syndrome (reported to be 7–16%; Jansson and Johansson 1995; George *et al*. 1996) is possibly explained by genetic factors, although the nature of the linkage remains to be determined (Morris *et al*. 2000).

There is also an association between coeliac disease and epilepsy (Macdonald and Playford 1996), although this may be a consequential rather than a causal link, possibly as a result of anaemia or the neurotoxic effects of antigliadin antibodies (Hadjivassiliou *et al*. 1996).

Osteoporosis can often be a marker of undiagnosed coeliac disease since this is a common chronic consequence of the condition (see Long-term consequences of coeliac disease, below); people with osteoporosis may be 10 times more likely to have coeliac disease than the general population (Lindh *et al*. 1992).

Clinical presentation

Coeliac disease can result in severe symptoms of malabsorption such as steatorrhoea (characterized by the passage of pale, bulky stools), abdominal discomfort and weight loss (or in children, growth failure). However, it is important to appreciate that this 'classic' presentation is in fact quite rare, and that 'atypical' presentation comprised of less specific symptoms is much more common, especially in adults.

Infants with coeliac disease are usually fit and well until after the introduction of gluten-containing solids, following which they produce pale, bulky, offensive-smelling stools, become miserable and lethargic and generally fail to thrive. Older children may exhibit poor growth and have other signs of malabsorption such as anaemia or vitamin deficiencies, complain of abdominal pain or discomfort, and pass stools which are softer, paler and more frequent than usual.

In adults, the clinical picture is much more variable (Maki and Collin 1997). Although the onset can be acute and cause severe diarrhoea and rapid weight loss, it is usually more insidious with less obvious symptoms resulting from chronic malabsorption, such as:

- tiredness
- irritability
- breathlessness
- anaemia
- abdominal discomfort
- mild gastrointestinal upsets
- unexplained weight loss

- recurrent mouth ulcers
- bone and joint disorders, arthralgia or osteoporotic fracture
- dental enamel defects
- neurological symptoms.

The nature of these symptoms explains why the condition is not always recognized. Many health professionals, particularly in the primary care setting, have only been taught the classic symptoms of coeliac disease and assume that it will always result in diarrhoea and weight loss. Yet, in a study of newly diagnosed adult patients, Dickey and Bodkin (1998) found that only about one-third (36%) had symptoms of diarrhoea. Nor was underweight an inevitable resenting feature, with only 22% of patients having a body mass index (BMI) <20; almost half (44%) of the patients were in the normal BMI range and 34% were overweight (BMI >25). In the absence of obvious signs of malabsorption, symptoms such as tiredness and anaemia are likely to be attributed to other causes (Hin *et al*. 1999). Diagnosis is therefore often missed or delayed, particularly in elderly people (Hankey and Holmes 1994).

In adults, anaemia may be a particularly important indicator of coeliac disease. In coeliac patients identified by serological screening (with subsequent confirmatory biopsy), over 80% did not have gastrointestinal symptoms but over half had anaemia (Hin *et al*. 1999). Coeliac disease should therefore be considered in any patients with anaemia or symptoms of tiredness, especially when there is a family history of the disease.

In addition to the classic and atypical forms of coeliac disease, the disease can also be clinically silent or latent (Ferguson *et al*. 1993):

- *Silent cases* have a flat intestinal mucosa but have no obvious symptoms.
- *Latent cases* have a normal intestinal mucosa and no symptoms, but do have laboratory markers of genetic susceptibility and an increased lifetime risk of developing the condition.

Diagnosis of coeliac disease

Diagnosis is by intestinal biopsy (usually of the duodenum) revealing mucosa with characteristic villous atrophy and crypt hyperplasia. Further confirmation can be obtained by a second biopsy showing normal mucosa after several months on a gluten-free diet. Doubt about a diagnosis can be resolved by a biopsy taken after a period of gluten consumption (gluten challenge).

More recently, less invasive serological diagnostic tests to measure blood antibodies have also been developed. Of these, the serum IgA endomysial antibody (EMA) test is the most reliable, identifying over 87% of cases (McMillan *et al*. 1991; Ferreira *et al*. 1992; Feighery *et al*. 1998). The IgG antigliadin antibody test is less reliable, with a typical sensitivity of 69% and a much higher proportion of false-positive results (Feighery *et al*. 1998), although it may be useful in people who are deficient in IgA who will always be negative for EMA (Feighery 1999). While serological tests are not infallible (although their sensitivity is likely to continue to improve), nor a substitute for histological diagnosis, they are particularly useful in the primary care setting to indicate whether people with symptoms such as anaemia, neurological symptoms or osteoporosis should proceed to biopsy. They can also be useful as a screening tool to identify silent or undiagnosed cases of coeliac disease in high-risk groups (e.g. those with a family history of the disease, type I diabetes or autoimmune thyroid disease).

Long-term consequences of coeliac disease

Intestinal malignancy

Coeliac disease is associated with an increased risk of malignant small intestinal lymphomas (Swinson *et al.* 1983; BSG 1996). Known as enteropathy-associated T-cell lymphomas (EATCLs), they represent approximately one-third of all cases of small bowel lymphoma. Long-term follow-up of coeliac patients who have adhered to a gluten-free diet suggests that the risk of small bowel lymphoma is reduced (Holmes *et al.* 1989). Coeliac disease also increases the risk of small bowel adenocarcinoma (BSG 1996).

Osteoporosis

Coeliac disease is a strong risk factor for osteoporosis. Untreated coeliac disease associated with significant malabsorption can result in severe metabolic bone disease manifesting as bone pain, deformity and fracture, although this is relatively rare. However, less obvious disturbances in bone metabolism are common, and both treated and untreated people with coeliac disease appear to have an increased risk of osteoporosis. Bone mineral density in newly diagnosed coeliac patients has been shown to be significantly lower than age- and sex- matched controls (McFarlane *et al.* 1996). Corazza *et al.* (1996) found that adults with subclinical or silent coeliac disease had a bone mineral density which was intermediate between those with overt coeliac disease and normal subjects. Among treated adult patients, approximately half have been found to have a bone mineral density indicative of osteoporosis (i.e. more than 2 standard deviations below mean peak bone mass) (McFarlane *et al.* 1995a). The incidence of fractures among coeliac patients is not known, but there is no reason to suppose that the reduction in bone mineral density is less predictive of fracture risk than in the general population (Scott *et al.* 2000).

The reduced bone mineral density is thought to be due to:

- chronic malabsorption of calcium prior to diagnosis leading to increased parathormone secretion which in turn increases bone turnover and cortical bone loss (Walters 1994);
- the reduced intake of calcium following diagnosis (McFarlane *et al.* 1995b). Since in the average UK diet, bread and cereals normally contribute about 25% of daily calcium intake (Gregory *et al.* 1990), avoidance of these foods can result in a considerable reduction of calcium

intake. Adult coeliacs with a low bone mineral density have been found to have a lower intake of calcium (860 mg/day) than those with normal bone mineral density (1054 mg calcium/day) (McFarlane *et al.* 1995a);
- not adhering strictly due to a gluten-free diet (so that subclinical malabsorption continues to occur).

Institution of a gluten-free diet helps to restore normal calcium absorption and improve bone mineral density (Corazza *et al.* 1996; Valdimarsson *et al.* 1996), although may not restore it to the level found in comparable non-coeliac people (McFarlane *et al.* 1996). A calcium rich gluten-free diet may achieve even better remineralization (Ciacci *et al.* 1997). Recently published guidelines for the prevention and treatment of osteoporosis in coeliac disease recommend a daily intake of at least 1500 mg calcium (Scott *et al.* 2000).

4.9.2 Management of coeliac disease

Treatment of coeliac disease is exclusively dietary and requires complete exclusion of gluten from the diet. This necessitates avoidance of all sources of wheat, rye and barley. Consumption of oats may need to be restricted or, in cases of individual sensitivity, avoided altogether (see Oats toxicity, below). A gluten-free diet is a major undertaking and always requires expert dietetic advice (BSG 1996). Exclusion of gluten necessitates avoiding a wide range of manufactured and processed foods and imposes considerable constraint on food choice and variety. As a result, without guidance, the overall diet can become unbalanced, thus increasing the risk of other health problems.

Dietary objectives

The dietary objectives are to ensure that people with coeliac disease:

- exclude all dietary sources of gluten
- know which foods and ingredients are naturally free from gluten
- substitute gluten-containing foods and ingredients with gluten-free alternatives to improve dietary acceptability and nutritional adequacy
- consume a balanced diet which helps to maintain health and protect against disease, particularly osteoporosis.

Excluding dietary sources of gluten

In practice, there are two sources of gluten in the diet: the obvious and the less obvious. Its presence in foods made from wheat flour such as bread, cakes, biscuits and pastry is easy to identify. However, gluten is also a hidden component of many manufactured foods and can be present in almost any type of product (e.g. even vending-machine drinks). These sources are much less apparent, and are also difficult to predict since some brands in a product range (e.g. baked beans) may contain gluten while others do not.

Manufactured foods may contain gluten as a result of:

- wheat flour added as an ingredient, processing aid,

binder, filler or a carrier for flavourings and spices. Although, in some cases, wheat flour will only be present in small amounts this will still be significant in terms of gluten content;

- wheat starches used as a carrier for spices, seasonings, flavourings or as a filler or binder, or for dusting during the manufacturing process. Since February 2000, manufacturers are required to state in the ingredients listing the origin of starch or modified starch if this is likely to contain gluten;
- other sources of wheat, rye, barley (or oats) used as an ingredient;
- contamination with wheat, rye, barley (or oats) during food production or storage (e.g. particles of flour from foods being made in one area can be suspended in the atmosphere and cross-contaminate supposedly gluten-free foods being produced in another).

While an ingredients list on a food product can confirm that a food does contain gluten, it cannot confirm that the food is gluten-free. Gluten may be present via compound ingredients (the individual constituents of which may not have to be declared) or cross-contamination during production. For this reason, any food that comes out of a can, packet or jar, or which has been coated or modified in some way has to be suspected of containing gluten unless it has been established that this is not the case. Even then, a particular brand may not be gluten-free at a later point in time owing to product reformulation. For example, as a result of the recent removal of genetically modified soya and maize from manufactured foods, many products which were previously 'gluten-free' now contain ingredients such as wheat starch, wheat flour or wheat protein.

The widening European market has also created some problems for people trying to avoid gluten. Some products with a single brand name (e.g. a particular type of chocolate bar) may be gluten-free if produced in the UK but contain gluten if made in another EU country. Since the latter may be freely available in the UK but there will be no indication of its country of production on the label, some branded products have to be avoided in case they are imported.

Many food manufacturers and supermarkets voluntarily identify gluten-free products by providing this information or a logo on the label. However, in the absence of such verification, it cannot be assumed simply by looking at the ingredients that a product is gluten-free.

In the UK, The Coeliac Society maintains a constantly updated database of manufactured foods-free from gluten and publishes an annual handbook for its members. Regular updates to this are made throughout the year via a telephone information line, their website or BBC Ceefax. It is essential that dietitians stress to patients the importance of using the latest information and not to rely on a handbook several years old.

Oats toxicity

Oats have traditionally been excluded from a gluten-free diet as a result of studies in the 1950s suggesting that they were deleterious to people with coeliac disease. However, many of these studies used large amounts of oats (140–150 g/day) and Moulton (1959) showed that smaller quantities (50–60 g/day) did not appear to have deleterious physiological effects. Subsequent studies tended to confirm this (Anderson *et al.* 1972; Hamilton and McNeill 1972; Dissanayake *et al.* 1974) although some doubts remained (Baker *et al.* 1976; Milne 1975).

Better understanding of the cereal components causing coeliac disease provided reasons why oats should be less harmful than wheat, rye or barley. The prolamin in oats (avenin) is biologically less like gliadin (the toxic fraction in wheat gluten) than the prolamins in rye (secalin) and barley (hordein). Avenin also only comprises a small proportion of the protein in oats (5–15%), whereas prolamins in wheat, rye and barley comprise about 40% of protein (Shewry *et al.* 1992).

More recently, carefully controlled studies suggest that moderate amounts of oats (40–60g /day) are not harmful to most patients with coeliac disease (Janutainen *et al.* 1995), even in patients who are particularly sensitive to gluten (Srinivasan *et al.* 1996). Oats challenge caused no change in parameters such as lymphocyte infiltration of the surface epithelium or the production of antibodies to endomysium and gliadin, in contrast to patients given only a microchallenge of gluten (Srinivasan *et al.* 1996).

There may nevertheless be a threshold effect whereby large amounts of oats consumed for long periods could provide sufficient loads of immunogenic components to trigger adverse reactions in coeliac patients. In a review of recent studies, Schmitz (1997) concluded that it is reasonable to assume that moderate amounts of oats may be consumed by most patients without risk, but that consuming large amounts of oats over long periods would be unwise until further research has been carried out.

If oats are not harmful, the ability to include them in the diet has benefits for the coeliac patient in terms of improving dietary variety and as a valuable source of fibre, especially soluble fibre. It should, however, be borne in mind that oatmeal can sometimes be contaminated with wheat flour and hence gluten during its production, and some physicians still recommend oats exclusion on these grounds (Ferguson 1997). Oats produced by dedicated oat millers are more likely to be wheat-free.

Interim guidelines from The Coeliac Society (1998) on the use of oats are summarized below.

- Moderate amounts of oats (up to 50 g/day, i.e. one reasonable serving) may be consumed by most coeliacs without risk. This applies also to patients with dermatitis herpetiformis. More caution may be advisable with coeliac children since there has been little research on the effects of oats in this age group.
- Severe coeliacs who are particularly sensitive to gluten should probably not, at present, be allowed oats.
- With due information and explanation, patient preference must be taken into account.
- Care must be taken to use oat products that are free from

contamination (listed in the Appendix section of The Coeliac Society's Annual Food List).

- Careful follow-up is necessary.

The Coeliac Society also advises people not to make significant changes to diet without prior discussion with their own consultant gastroenterologist and dietitian.

Foods and ingredients naturally free from gluten

Most foods which have not undergone additional processing, such as fresh meat, fish, eggs, milk, fruit and vegetables, can be safely included in a gluten-free diet. These are summarized in Table 4.10.

Use of proprietary gluten-free foods

The need to exclude most types of bread and cereals from a gluten-free diet imposes considerable constraints in terms of food choice and variety, and hence its acceptability. It also compromises nutrient intake since these foods are important sources of carbohydrate, fibre, vitamins and minerals, and conflicts with healthy-eating guidelines which encourage greater consumption of starchy foods as a substitute for those high in saturated fat.

These problems can be offset by the use of proprietary gluten-free products. Foods such as gluten-free bread, biscuits, crackers and pasta are ACBS prescribable for people medically diagnosed with coeliac disease or dermatitis herpetiformis. Prescribable gluten-free flours and flour mixes are also available to make cakes, biscuits and other baked goods. The types of gluten-free foods available are summarised in Table 4.11. More details can be found in the British National Formulary or Monthly Index of Medical Specialities (MIMS), or obtained directly from the manufacturers.

The taste and acceptability of proprietary gluten-free foods have improved enormously in recent years and coeliac patients should be encouraged to use them to reduce the risk of dietary imbalance or non-compliance. Some general practitioners (GPs), unaware perhaps of the extent of dietary constraints imposed by coeliac disease, may also need to be encouraged to prescribe them.

People with coeliac disease and dermatitis herpetiformis are not classified as 'chronically sick' and hence are not entitled to free National Health Service (NHS) prescriptions (although the usual exemptions apply, e.g. children under 16 years, those in full-time education under 19 years, men and women over 60 years, pregnant women and those in receipt of certain state benefits). Non-exempt people can use a prepayment facility, which is a single payment made in advance to cover charges for either 4 months or 1 year, and includes all prescriptions, not just those relating to gluten-free foods. This can represent a significant saving.

Luxury items such as gluten-free cakes, chocolate and fancy biscuits are also available but not prescribable (Table 4.11). They are expensive and not necessary, but their occasional use may make the diet more acceptable, particularly at festive times of the year. They can be bought from pharmacies, health-food shops and supermarkets, or by mail order.

The need for overall dietary balance

While gluten avoidance is the principal dietary objective, it should not be overlooked that people with coeliac disease probably have the same risk of developing the chronic disorders associated with ageing (such as heart disease) as the rest of the population. They are also known to have an increased risk of malignancy and osteoporosis. They therefore need to adopt diet and lifestyle measures which help to reduce these risks.

Dietary advice should be given in the context of *The Balance of Good Health*, with particular emphasis on food choices to ensure:

- at least five portions/day of fruit and vegetables
- an adequate intake of dietary calcium: people should consume a minimum of 1500 mg calcium/day, most of which should be of high bioavailability such as that from milk and dairy products. Some brands of gluten-free bread are now fortified with calcium and are an additional source. If this level cannot be achieved, supplemental calcium (500–1000 mg/day) should be considered (Scott *et al.* 2000).
- an adequate intake of vitamin D: supplements may be advisable in elderly people who have little exposure to sunlight and in some ethnic groups
- avoidance of excessive alcohol intake.

Adequate levels of weight-bearing exercise and cessation of smoking are additional important measures.

Practical aspects of dietary management

All newly diagnosed coeliac patients should be nutritionally assessed to establish overall dietary adequacy. At the time of diagnosis, as many as 85% of patients may have asymptomatic iron deficiency as a result of chronic malabsorption, and subclinical deficiencies of other vitamins and minerals, especially folate, vitamin D and calcium, are likely (BSG 1996). Immediately after treatment has started, there will be a phase of tissue growth and regeneration, and requirements for many nutrients will increase. It is important that the diet is sufficiently energy and nutrient dense to meet these increased needs and help to restore losses. Additional vitamin and mineral supplementation, particularly of iron, may be required for a period of weeks or months. South Asian people may need more prolonged supplements of calcium and vitamin D, and at higher doses.

Symptoms of coeliac disease such as tiredness and arthralgia usually improve within a few weeks of commencing a gluten-free diet. It can take several months for mucosal damage to the small bowel to be completely repaired and villi return to normal. After a year on a gluten-free diet, significant improvements in previously impaired parameters such as weight and blood haemoglobin, albumin, calcium and alkaline phosphatase values will have occurred (Hankey and Holmes 1994). Complete, and permanent, avoidance of gluten is essential in order to reduce the risk of bowel malignancy as well as other long-term consequences of the disease.

Table 4.10 Gluten and gluten-free foods

	Gluten-free	May contain gluten[1]	Gluten-containing
Cereals and flours	Manufactured gluten-free products (see Table 4.11) Rice (white, brown, wild, rice flour, ground rice) Maize (corn), maize starch/modified starch, maize flour Cornflour, corn starch/modified starch, cornmeal, popping corn Polenta Potato flour, potato starch Soya, soya flour Bean flours (chick-pea flour, split-pea flour) Sago, tapioca, cassava Arrowroot Amaranth Buckwheat Millet Quinoa Sorghum Teff Rice/maize/soya bran		Wheat, rye, barley Oats[1] Bulgar wheat, durum wheat Spelt, triticale, kamut wheat flour (eg plain/self-raising/strong flour) and other flours derived from rye, barley, spelt, triticale and oats[1] Wheat starch/modified starch Wheatgerm Wheat bran, oat bran[1] All types of bread (white, brown, wholemeal, chapattis, naan, paratha) Cakes, biscuits made with flour Desserts and puddings made with flour Pastry and pies Semolina, couscous Malt and malted barley
Bread, cakes and biscuits	Manufactured gluten-free products, e.g. bread, rolls, crispbread, biscuits Pastry, cakes, biscuits made with gluten-free flours or mixes Rice cakes Cakes made without flour (e.g. macaroons) Gluten-free pizza bases		Bread and bread products containing wheat, rye, barley and oats[1] (e.g. white/brown, wholemeal/ wholegrain bread and rolls, croissants, brioche, naan bread, pitta bread, chapattis, parathas, ciabatta, ryebread) Ordinary biscuits, crispbread, crackers, matzos, rusks Ordinary cakes and pastries, muffins and scones Pizza, pastry, croutons Batter, pancakes, Yorkshire pudding
Pasta	Manufactured gluten-free pasta Corn pasta, rice pasta Rice noodles		All other fresh, dried or canned pasta, including spaghetti, macaroni, lasagne, ravioli, pasta shapes Noodles
Breakfast cereals	Cornflakes Rice cereals Manufactured gluten-free muesli Buckwheat flakes	Other breakfast cereals	Wheat-based breakfast cereals (e.g. Weetabix, Shredded Wheat, Puffed Wheat, All-bran) Muesli Porridge oats and oatmeal[1]
Fruits, vegetables, pulses and nuts	Fresh/frozen/canned/dried whole or sliced fruit Fresh/frozen/canned vegetables Frozen and microwave chips Peas, beans, lentils Plain/roasted / salted nuts	Takeaway/restaurant chips (may be cross-contaminated with flour from a deep-fat fryer) Instant mashed potato Vegetables in sauce Canned fruit-pie fillings Canned baked beans Dry roasted nuts	Vegetables/potatoes/chips coated with batter, breadcrumbs or flour Potato croquettes/potato waffles or other flour-containing products Fruit pies, pasties or fruit coated with batter or flour
Milk and dairy products	Whole/semi-skimmed/skimmed milk Dried skimmed milk Evaporated and condensed milk Sterilized and UHT milk Soya milk Goat's milk Most yoghurts and fromage frais Cream Coffee and tea whiteners Cheese	Cheese spreads Processed cheese	Milk with added fibre Artificial cream Yoghurt and fromage frais containing muesli or cereals

Table 4.10 (Continued)

	Gluten-free	May contain gluten[1]	Gluten-containing
Meat and meat products	Fresh red meat, poultry, game and offal Meat canned or prepacked in its own juices or jelly Smoked or cured pure meat such as bacon or ham Gluten-free sausages Continental sausages that are 100% meat	Beefburgers Canned meat products Meat pastes and patés Fish products (e.g. fish fingers, coated fish, fish paste) Ready meals	Any type of meat coated in breadcrumbs or batter Meat pies and puddings Haggis Ordinary sausages and sausage meat Faggots and rissoles
Fish and shellfish	All fresh fish and other seafood Smoked, kippered and dried fish Fish canned in oil or brine	Fish in sauces Fish pastes and patés	Fish/shellfish in batter or breadcrumbs Fish cakes Fish finders Taramasalata Scotch eggs
Eggs	Whole eggs Egg yolk Egg white Meringue (free from flour)	Egg substitutes	
Desserts and puddings	Jelly Sorbets Milk puddings made with gluten-free ingredients, e.g. egg, cornflour, rice, ground rice, sage and tapioca Home-made puddings made from gluten-free ingredients	Ice-cream Instant desserts Custard powders Mousses	Puddings containing flour or breadcrumbs Semolina and macaroni milk puddings Trifles Sponge and suet puddings Pastry, pies and crumbles Shredded suet
Fats and oils	Butter Lard Vegetable oils Margarines and fat spreads	Vegetable suet	
Soups, sauces and seasonings	Soups, sauces or gravy made with gluten-free ingredients or thickened with gluten-free flours Salt, pepper, peppercorns Tomato purée Garlic, herbs and spices Wine and cider vinegars; malt vinegar Pickled vegetables in vinegar Gluten-free stuffing mix	Canned and packet soups Packet sauces and sauce mixes 'Cook-in' sauces Bottled sauces and ketchups Stock and stock cubes Gravy brownings and gravy mixes Mustard powder Curry powder Mayonnaise, salad cream, salad dressings Pickles and chutneys	Soy sauce Mixed seasonings and spices specifying flour on the label Stuffing and stuffing mixes
Savoury snack foods	Plain potato crisps Home-made popcorn	Flavoured crisps and snacks	Snack products made from wheat, rye, barley or oats[1] Pretzels
Preserves and spreads	Sugar, glucose, golden syrup, treacle, molasses Jam, conserves, honey, marmalade Peanut and other nut butters	Mincemeat Lemon curds and cheeses Chocolate or other sweet spreads	
Confectionery	Home-made sweets and chocolates made with gluten-free ingredients	Sweets, chocolate, toffee, etc. Iced lollies Chewing gum	Boiled sweets and seaside rock dusted with flour
Beverages	Tea, coffee Fruit juices, fruit squash Mineral water Clear fizzy drinks Cocoa Milk Spirits, wines, liqueurs, cider, sherry and port	Herbal teas Instant coffee containing barley Chocolate powders and drinks Milk shakes and mixes Sports and 'health' drinks	Vending-machine chocolate drinks Barley waters Cloudy fizzy drinks Malted milk drinks Beer, lager, ale and stout, home-brewed beers, low-alcohol beers and lagers
Miscellaneous	Gelatine Bicarbonate of soda, cream of tartar Fresh and dried yeast Tofu, Quorn Food colourings, essences and flavourings	Baking powder Cake coverings and decorations Marzipan Meat, vegetable and yeast extracts	Ice-cream cones and wafers Communion wafers
Medications		Some pharmaceutical preparations, both over-the-counter and prescription-only medicines; local pharmacies can provide guidance	

Adapted from The Coeliac Society, *The Gluten-free diet*.
[1]Some coeliac patients may be permitted to eat modest quantities of oats.

Table 4.11 Types of gluten-free foods available

Type of product	Gluten-free products available	Notes
Prescribable gluten-free foods		Some products are also wheat-free
Bread and rolls	White bread (sliced/unsliced)	Some breads and rolls are vacuum-packed either
	White rolls/baguettes	fully or partially baked; a few products are
	Brown/wholemeal bread (sliced/unsliced)	available fresh (and can be frozen)
	Brown/wholemeal rolls	
	High-fibre bread	
	Bread mixes	
Flour substitutes	Flour mixes (white/brown/fibre)	Can be used for home baking
Biscuits	Digestives	
	Tea biscuits	
	Crackers/savoury biscuits	
	Crispbread	
Pasta	Fusilli	
	Lasagne	
	Macaroni	
	Penne	
	Rigati	
	Spaghetti	
	Spirals	
	Tagliatelle	
Convenience foods	Pizza bases	
Non-prescribable gluten-free foods		Patients may like to buy these occasionally as a treat
Breakfast cereals	Muesli breakfast cereal	
	Hot breakfast cereal	
Biscuits	Wafers	
	Pretzels	
Cakes	Madeira cake	
	Ginger cake	
	Fruit cake	
	Rich fruit cake	
	Cake mixes	
Seasonal fare	Mince pies	
	Christmas pudding	
	Stuffing mix	
Confectionery	Chocolate bars	

Current manufacturers of gluten-free foods (together with brand names of their products) are: Brewhurst Health Food Supplies Ltd (Pleniday), Dr Schär (Schär), General Dietary Ltd (Ener-G, Valpiform, Tinkyada), Gluten Free Foods Ltd (Barkat, Clara's Kitchen, Glutano, Tritamyl), Jacobs (Liga), Larkhall (Trufree), Novartis Consumer Health (Bi-Aglut), Nutricia Dietary Care (Glutafin), Nutrition Point Ltd (Dietary Specialities), Scientific Hospital Supplies (Juvela), Ultrapharm Ltd (Aproten; Arnott, Bi-Aglut, Lifestyle, Polial, Ultra). Addresses of manufacturers are listed in Appendix 6.9.

It should be noted that the names of both the producers and product names are liable to change. A full list of all currently available proprietary gluten-free foods can be obtained from The Coeliac Society. Details of ACBS prescribable products can also be found in the British National Formulary or Monthly Index of Medical Specialities (MIMS).

The ideal is complete avoidance of gluten, but dietary advice also has to be pragmatic and achievable; over-stringent guidance can be counterproductive in terms of compliance. Guidance on oats will currently be determined by local practice and individual gluten sensitivity.

Guidelines on the management of patients with coeliac disease by the British Society of Gastroenterology (BSG 1996) recommends that treatment should be supervised by a dietitian and that follow-up is essential because of the potential long-term complications. Follow-up for a coeliac patient should also include:

- small intestinal biopsy 4–6 months after initiating treatment to establish normalization of the villi
- regular review at 6–12 monthly intervals to assess symptomatic improvement, nutritional state, dietary compliance and outcomes of routine blood tests

- review of patients at particular times of stress; both physical and emotional; pregnancy can lead to a deterioration in symptoms
- life-long monitoring because of the risk of long-term complications such as lymphoma and osteoporosis.

Good dietetic support, both initially and via regular follow-up, is essential for good compliance with a gluten-free diet and to ensure that the overall diet is balanced and appropriate for long-term health. Annual dietetic review is important because even experienced coeliac patients may be inadvertently consuming gluten or consuming a poorly balanced diet (McFarlane *et al.* 1995a). However, at present not all patients are offered this opportunity (McFarlane *et al.* 1995a).

4.9.3 Diet-related problems

Poor compliance

Evaluating compliance is a particularly important aspect of a dietary review. The difficulties in following a gluten-free diet, both in terms of family meals and eating away from home, should not be underestimated. Many patients are tempted to deviate from the dietary constraints in some circumstances, especially if there are no obvious penalties (such as unpleasant symptoms) for doing so. Compliance is particularly likely to be a problem in people found to have silent coeliac disease, where the benefits from gluten avoidance will be even less obvious.

In addition to knowingly breaking the rules, many people inadvertently consume gluten by mistakenly assuming a food to be gluten-free (perhaps by relying on an out-of-date food list) or as a result of cross-contamination within in the home (e.g. frying gluten-free foods in oil previously used to cook a flour-coated product, or using the same bread board to slice ordinary and gluten-free bread). These aspects should also be explored during a dietetic review.

While dietitians should remind patients of the reasons for compliance with a gluten-free regimen, it is important that they also help to foster a positive dietary outlook by emphasizing the many foods that can be eaten, by encouraging appropriate use of prescribable gluten-free foods and by suggesting ways in which particular difficulties can be overcome. Patients should also know where to obtain further advice on queries or problems so that they feel they have a constant source of support.

Extreme sensitivity to gluten

Some people are more sensitive to the effects of gluten than others and can react to minute amounts. Even proprietary 'gluten-free' foods can contain traces of gluten if wheat starch is an ingredient, because although this will have been specially treated to remove the gliadin, it is impossible to remove it altogether and, under Codex Alimentarius gluten-free standards, up to 200 ppm of gluten may remain.

It should also be borne in mind that the assay of gluten in some foods is still problematical and there is still no method that is completely acceptable in terms of sensitivity, specificity and reliability. Gluten which has been cooked or hydrolysed by enzymic action (e.g. in the production of malted barley used to make beer) can be particularly difficult to detect by conventional methodology, and hence a food may be assumed to be gluten-free when in reality this is not the case.

Some patients may therefore suffer reactions to foods that they believed to be free from gluten. In some instances, the food itself may have been gluten-free but was contaminated with gluten from another source (see Compliance, above). Dietitians should be alert to this possibility when exploring possible relationships between food intake and symptom recurrence.

Patients who are found to be highly sensitive to gluten will need to use proprietary gluten-free foods which are also 'wheat free' (i.e. free from wheatstarch and only containing starches derived from maize, potato, rice or soya). Other foods containing traces of gluten such as malt extract (normally considered suitable for most coeliac patients) and oats (see Oats toxicity, above) will need to be excluded.

Coexisting disorders requiring dietary intervention

The presence or subsequent development of other disorders such as diabetes or hyperlipidaemia can significantly complicate a gluten-free diet and it is imperative that such people receive expert dietetic guidance. Weight-reducing or vegetarian diets may also benefit from being checked by a dietitian to make sure that they are nutritionally adequate.

Constipation

Avoidance of gluten-containing cereal foods inevitably reduces consumption of cereal fibre and constipation can be a problem in some patients. Measures which may help to alleviate this include:

- increasing fibre intake from fruit and vegetables, especially dried fruit, potato skins and pulses (peas, beans and lentils)
- using higher fibre varieties of prescribable gluten-free bread, mixes and crackers
- increasing consumption of wholegrain gluten-free cereals such as cornmeal, brown rice and buckwheat.
- increasing fluid consumption
- in some circumstances, adding gluten-free soya or rice bran to the diet; however, these are not always well tolerated and are not generally recommended.

4.9.4 Dietary considerations in particular age groups

Preschool children

In this age group it is generally easier if the whole family eats gluten-free foods; difficulties at meal times are more likely if a young child sees that everyone else has different foods on their plate. Other children's parties need not be a problem if the situation is discussed with the host parent beforehand and a supply of gluten-free food provided (although its consumption by the right child may be harder to police). Food at their own parties should all be gluten-free.

Preschool groups present few problems since the children are usually only allowed to eat food under supervision, so it is not difficult to ensure that only gluten-free snacks are consumed. Playing dough used in such groups is sometimes made from ordinary flour and, although flavourings are usually added to give an unpleasant taste, can occasionally be a source of gluten consumption.

School-aged children

It is important that a coeliac child is not excluded from school activities as well as social events such as eating out, parties and holidays. Most children adapt surprisingly quickly to the idea that they cannot eat certain foods and are willing to take their own supply of suitable items to eat outside the home. There may, however, be some situations that pose temptations, e.g. the common practice of swapping snacks in the playground.

Growth needs to be carefully monitored in this age group and signs of poor growth investigated. The possibility of poor compliance with a gluten-free diet and resultant chronic malabsorption needs to be considered. However, an inadequate energy intake, particularly if the child is a faddy eater, is a more likely cause.

Teenagers

Rebellion against the dietary constraints of a gluten-free diet is common in this age group (Fabiani *et al.* 1996), and easier to accomplish as adult supervision lessens and fewer meals are consumed at home. There is a strong desire to be one of the crowd and choose the same takeaway or fast foods such as fish and chips, pies, hamburgers or pizzas. Those who become ill after doing so are usually wary of future indiscretions, but others with a higher degree of gluten tolerance may not suffer any immediate symptoms. Teenagers should be reminded that damage to the intestinal mucosa will still occur, but also offered as much positive advice as possible regarding what foods can suitably be eaten when eating out with friends. Parents should also bear in mind that the appetites of teenagers, particularly boys, can be voracious and that dietary indiscretions are more likely to occur when they are hungry; providing them with plenty of gluten-free snacks may help to counteract the temptation.

Adults

The greatest difficulties usually arise when eating away from home, but can be averted to some extent by advance planning. For example, when invited to eat with friends, the nature of the diet should be explained beforehand, not on arrival. At work, some canteens will, with notice, provide gluten-free meals and others will be willing to microwave a pre-prepared meal supplied by the coeliac person. Hotels and restaurants can be sounded out in advance and if necessary sent information about the diet. Many airlines will provide gluten-free meals on long-distance (not always short-haul) flights if sufficient notice is given. Nevertheless, carrying a supply of gluten-free rolls, crackers or similar foods is a wise precaution when travelling, on holiday or going to social functions, so that suitable foods are always available. 'Be prepared' is a useful motto.

The Coeliac Society is a useful source of advice in these and many other circumstances.

Elderly people

Elderly patients will always find it difficult to change the eating habits of a lifetime but many will do so successfully if given sufficient help in making suitable dietary substitutions. Some will also welcome feeling fitter on a gluten-free diet after perhaps years of having had undiagnosed coeliac disease with consequent chronic tiredness and feeling below par.

Gluten avoidance may be more difficult in those dependent on others for meals. Meals-on-wheels services may not provide gluten-free diets, although most will endeavour to provide suitable food choices (e.g. a piece of fruit instead of a pudding) once they understand the nature of the diet. Since the prevalence of coeliac disease among elderly people is increasing as awareness and diagnosis of the condition improves, educating residential and care homes regarding the needs of coeliac patients is particularly important.

Text revised by: Briony Thomas

Acknowledgements: Rae Ward and The Coeliac Society

Useful addresses

British Society of Gastroenterology
3 St Andrews Place, Regent's Park, London NW1 4LB
Tel: 020 7935 2815
Website: www.bsg.org.uk

The Coeliac Society
PO Box 220, High Wycombe, Bucks HP11 2HY
Tel: 01494 437278 Fax: 01494 474349
Hotline for recorded message of deletions to the Food list: 01494 473510
Website: www.coeliac.co.uk

Gluten-free communion wafers can be obtained from: Dumont Ltd, High Street, Lyminge, Folkestone, Kent CT18 8EL

Further reading and resources

The Coeliac Society produces a wide range of support information for people with coeliac disease and dermatitis herpetiformis, including:

The Diet Booklet (contains detailed information about the gluten-free diet)

The Food List (an annually updated list of manufactured foods free from gluten)

The Handbook (contains general information about coeliac disease)

The Coeliac Cookbook (providing suitable recipes)

Many information leaflets covering topics such as hospital admission, holidays, travel and vegetarianism are also available.

Details about these and other publications can be obtained from The Coeliac Society.

The following companies also provide information and advice on coeliac disease and gluten-free diets to both consumers and health professionals:

Coeliac Disease Resource Centre (Nutricia Dietary Care)
CDRC Careline: 01225 711566
Website: www.glutafin.co.uk

Juvela Nutrition Centre (SHS)
Advice Line: 0151 228 1992
Website: www.juvela.co.uk

References

Anderson CM *et al*. Coeliac disease: some still controversial aspects. *Archives of Disease in Childhood* 1972; **47**: 292–298.

Baker PG *et al*. Oats and barley toxicity in coeliac patients. *Postgraduate Medical Journal* 1976; **52**: 264–268.

British Society of Gastroenterology. *Clinical Guidelines for the Management of Patients with Coeliac Disease*. London: BSG, 1996.

Catassi C, Ratsch IM, Fabiani E *et al*. Coeliac disease in the year 2000: exploring the iceberg. *Lancet* 1994; **343**: 200–203.

Catassi C, Ratsch IM, Fabiani E *et al*. High prevalence of under-diagnosed coeliac disease in 5280 Italian students screened by antigliadin antibodies. *Acta Paediatrica* 1995; **84**: 672–676.

Challacombe DN, Mecrow IK *et al*. Changing infant feeding practices and declining incidence of coeliac disease in West Somerset. *Archives of Disease in Childhood* 1997; **77**: 206.

Ciacci C, Maurelli L, Klain M *et al*. Effects of dietary treatment on bone mineral density in adults with celiac disease: factors predicting response. *American Journal of Gastroenterology* 1997; **92**: 992–996.

The Coeliac Society. *Guidelines on Coeliac Disease and Oats*. A position paper for health professionals from the Society's Medical Advisory Council. High Wycombe: The Coeliac Society, 1998.

Corazza GR, DiSario A, Cecchetti L *et al*. Influence of pattern of clinical presentation and of gluten-free diet on bone mass and metabolism in adult coeliac disease. *Bone* 1996; **18**: 525–530.

Cronin C, Shanahan F. Insulin-dependent diabetes mellitus and coeliac disease. *Lancet* 1997; **349**: 1096–1097.

Dicke WK, Weijers HA, van de Kamer JH. Coeliac disease II. The presence in wheat of a factor having deleterious effect in cases of coeliac disease. *Acta Paediatrica* 1953; **42**: 34–42.

Dickey W, Bodkin S. Prospective study of body mass index in patients with coeliac disease. *British Medical Journal* 1998; **317**: 1290.

Dissanayake AS *et al*. Lack of harmful effect of oats on small intestinal mucosa in coeliac disease. *British Medical Journal* 1974; **4**: 189–191.

Fabiani E, Catassi C, Villari A *et al*. Dietary compliance in screening-detected coeliac disease adolescents. *Acta Paediatrica* 1996; **85** (Suppl 412): 65–67.

Feighery C. Coeliac disease. Clinical review. *British Medical Journal* 1999; **319**: 236–239.

Feighery C, Weir DG, Whelan A *et al*. Diagnosis of gluten-sensitive enteropathy: is exclusive reliance on histology appropriate? *European Journal of Gastroenterology and Hepatology* 1998; **10**: 919–925.

Ferguson A. Coeliac disease. *Prescribers' Journal* 1997; **37**: 206–212.

Ferguson A, Arranz E, O'Mahony S. Clinical and pathological spectrum of coeliac disease – active, silent, latent, potential. *Gut* 1993; **34**: 150–151.

Ferreira M, Lloyd Davies S, Butler M *et al*. Endomysial antibody: is it the best screening test for coeliac disease? *Gut* 1992; **33**: 1633–1637.

George EK, Mearin ML, Bouquet J *et al*. High frequency of celiac disease in Down syndrome. *Journal of Pediatrics* 1996; **128**: 555–557.

Gregory JR, Foster K, Tyler H, Wiseman M. *The Dietary and Nutritional Survey of British Adults*. London: HMSO, 1990.

Hadjivassiliou M, Gibson A, Davies-Jones GAB *et al*. Does cryptic gluten sensitivity play a part in neurological illness? *Lancet* 1996; **347**: 369–371.

Hamilton JR, McNeill M. Childhood celiac disease: response of treated patients to a small uniform daily dose of wheat gluten. *Journal of Pediatrics* 1972; **81**: 885–893.

Hankey GL, Holmes GKT. Coeliac disease in the elderly. *Gut* 1994; **35**: 65–67.

Hin H, Bird G, Fisher P *et al*. Coeliac disease in primary care: case finding study. *British Medical Journal* 1999; **318**: 164–167.

Holmes GK, Prior P, Lane MR *et al*. Malignancy in coeliac disease – effect of a gluten-free diet. *Gut* 1989; **30**: 333–338.

Jansson U, Johansson C. Down syndrome and celiac disease. *Journal of Pediatric Gastroenterology and Nutrition* 1995; **21**: 443–445.

Janutainen EK, Pikkarainen PH, Kemppainen TA *et al*. A comparison of diets with and without oats in adults with celiac disease. *New England Journal of Medicine* 1995; **333**: 1033–1037.

Johnston SD, Watson RGP, McMillan SA *et al*. Preliminary results from follow-up of a large scale population survey of antibodies to gliadin, reticulin and endomysium. *Acta Paediatrica* 1996; **85** (Suppl 412): 61–64.

Lindh E, Ljunghall S, Larsson K, Lavo B. Screening for antibodies against gliadin in patients with osteoporosis. *Journal of Internal Medicine* 1992; **231**: 403–406.

Macdonald CE, Playford RJ. Iron deficiency anaemia and febrile convulsions ... and coeliac disease (Letter). *British Medical Journal* 1996; **313**: 1205.

McFarlane XA, Bhalla AK, Reeves DE *et al*. Osteoporosis in treated adult coeliac disease. *Gut* 1995a; **36**: 710–714.

McFarlane XA, Marsham J, Reeves D *et al*. Subclinical nutritional deficiency in treated coeliac disease and nutritional content of the gluten free diet. *Journal of Human Nutrition and Dietetics* 1995b; **8**: 231–237.

McFarlane XA, Bhalla AK, Robertson DA. Effects of a gluten free diet on osteopenia in adults with newly diagnosed coeliac disease. *Gut* 1996; **39**: 180–184.

McMillan SA, Haughton DJ, Biggart JD *et al*. Predictive value for coeliac disease antibodies to gliadin, endomysium and jejunum in patients attending for jejunal biopsy. *British Medical Journal* 1991; **303**: 1163–1165.

Maki M, Collin P. Coeliac Disease. *Lancet* 1997; **349**: 1755–1759.

Milne D. Oats and coeliac disease (Letter). *British Medical Journal* 1975; **i**: 152.

Morris MA, Yiannakou JY, King AL *et al*. Coeliac disease and Down syndrome: associations not due to genetic linkage on chromosome 21. *Scandinavian Journal of Gastroenterology* 2000; **35**: 177–180.

Moulton ALC. The place of oats in the coeliac diet. *Archives of Disease in Childhood* 1959; **34**: 51–55.

Mylotte M, Egan-Mitchell B, McCarthy CF, McNicholl B. Incidence of coeliac disease in the west of Ireland. *British Medical Journal* 1973; **i**: 703–705.

Saukkonen T, Savilahti E, Reijonen H *et al*. Coeliac disease: frequent occurrence after clinical onset of insulin-dependent diabetes mellitus. *Diabetic Medicine* 1996; **13**: 464–470.

Schmitz J. Lack of oats toxicity in coeliac disease (Editorial). *British Medical Journal* 1997; **314**: 159.

Scott EM, Gaywood I, Scott BB, British Society of Gastroenterologists. Guidelines for osteoporosis in coeliac disease and inflammatory bowel disease. *Gut* 2000; **46** (Suppl 1): 1–8.

Shewry PR, Tatham AS, Kasada DD. Cereal proteins and coeliac disease. In Marsh MN (Ed). *Coeliac Disease*, pp. 305–348. Oxford: Blackwell Science, 1992.

Sollid LM, Thorsby E. HLA susceptibility genes in coeliac disease: genetic mapping and role in pathogenesis. *Gastroenterology* 1993; **105**: 910–922.

Srinivasan U, Leonard N, Jones E *et al*. Absence of oats toxicity in adult coeliac disease. *British Medical Journal* 1996; **313**: 1300–1301.

Swinson CM, Slavin G, Coles EC, Booth CC. Coeliac disease and malignancy. *Lancet* 1983; **i**: 111–115.

Valdimarsson T, Lofman O, Toss G *et al*. Reversal of osteopenia with diet in adult coeliac disease. *Gut* 1996; **38**: 322–327.

Walters JRF. Bone mineral density in coeliac children. *Gut* 1994; **35**: 150–151.

4.10 Inflammatory bowel disease: Crohn's disease and ulcerative colitis

Inflammatory bowel disease (IBD) manifests itself in a number of ways, the most common being as either Crohn's disease or ulcerative colitis. Although these are distinct disorders with differences in their presentation and management, they share a number of common features. As with many relapsing – remitting inflammatory disorders, the causes remain unknown.

4.10.1 General aspects of inflammatory bowel disease

Frequency

Crohn's disease affects about 50 people per 100 000 and ulcerative colitis about 160 per 100 000; it is estimated there are between 100 000 and 200 000 sufferers in the UK (British Society of Gastroenterology 1996). The incidence of Crohn's disease has increased about five-fold throughout northern Europe since the 1950s (Rose *et al*. 1988; Kyle 1992; Montgomery *et al*. 1998); the reason for this is unknown. There is an increased risk of ulcerative colitis among South Asian immigrants and of both types of IBD in Jewish people (Probert *et al*. 1992).

Clinical features

Crohn's disease and ulcerative colitis both result in chronic inflammation of the bowel wall, the consequences of which can significantly impair the quality of life. Crohn's disease most commonly affects the small bowel, usually the terminal ileum, although it can affect any part of the gastrointestinal tract from the mouth to the anus, whereas ulcerative colitis is confined to the large bowel.

Crohn's disease is characterized by distinct areas of inflammation, often associated with granulomas and deep fissuring ulceration, interspersed with areas of unaffected bowel tissue. It is also accompanied by thickening of the intestinal wall which may lead to strictures. Perforation of the wall can result in localized or widespread infection or the formation of a fistula. The inflammation may spread through the wall to involve neighbouring tissues.

Ulcerative colitis results in an area of continuously inflamed mucosa in a variable length of the colon and/or rectum. The intestinal lining becomes red and inflamed and bleeds readily. The disease course tends to be most severe over the first 2 years; however, the long-term risk of colorectal cancer is greatly increased (Langholz *et al*. 1992, 1994).

Symptoms and diagnosis

The main presenting symptoms of IBD are:

- weight loss
- abdominal pain
- diarrhoea, sometimes with blood and mucus in the stool.

Tiredness and anaemia are common additional features.

In ulcerative colitis, stool blood loss may be severe. Crohn's disease is more likely to result in steatorrhoea but blood loss may also occur if the disease is active in the colon. Complications such as abscesses, fistulae and strictures are common. During active phases of IBD, inflammation may also occur in other areas of the body such as joints, skin and eyes.

Diagnosis is confirmed by barium studies, endoscopy, radiolabelled leucocyte scintiscans and histology. Haematological tests such as the erythrocyte sedimentation rate (ESR) or levels of C-reactive protein, alpha-1-antichymotrypsin and orosomucoid may be used as markers of disease activity and severity of inflammation.

Management

Drug treatment

Drug treatment is used to suppress inflammation, the choice of drug depending on where the disease is active.

Crohn's disease is usually treated with oral corticosteroids such as prednisolone. Chronic inflammation may also be reduced by cytotoxic immunosuppressants such as azathioprine because of their steroid-sparing effect. Antibiotics such as metronidazole or ciprofloxacin are commonly given to control infection or bacterial overgrowth of the small bowel. Aminosalicylates are generally ineffective in Crohn's disease other than in cases of Crohn's colitis.

Acute attacks of ulcerative colitis are usually managed by local or systemic treatment with prednisolone. Aminosalicylate drugs (such as sulfasalazine, mesalazine and osalazine) are then usually used to maintain remission.

Surgery

Surgery is often necessary in Crohn's disease to remove severely diseased areas of bowel, relieve stricture or repair a fistula, but tissue resection is not curative and inflammation usually recurs nearby or in another part of the gastrointestinal tract.

In contrast, ulcerative colitis can be completely cured by total colectomy and this may be performed if severe complications occur or signs of malignancy are detected.

Bowel rest

In Crohn's disease, but *not* ulcerative colitis, elemental, peptide or polymeric liquid diets, or complete bowel rest via parenteral nutrition can be used to induce remission (Griffiths 1998; Seo *et al.* 1999). The reasons for this are not understood but may include benefits resulting from the removal of food debris, changes in bacterial flora, immunomodulatory effects of altered fatty acid substrates, or from improved nutritional status. Liquid diets now tend to be used in preference to parenteral nutrition because they are safer and more cost-effective. The relative merits of elemental, hydrolysed and polymeric formulae have not been established, but all appear to be effective (Lennard-Jones 1992; Verma *et al.* 2000).

4.10.2 Dietary implications of inflammatory bowel disease

IBD incurs a high risk of nutritional depletion (Table 4.12). As with many functional bowel disorders, food consumption is often poor and nutrient intake inadequate, particularly in respect of energy and micronutrients such as iron, folate and vitamin C. The effects of this are compounded by high nutrient losses as a result of malabsorption or gastrointestinal bleeding, and relatively high nutritional requirements due to the metabolic costs of inflammation and repair of tissue damage, and also – if patients are young – the nutrient needs for growth (Han *et al.* 1999).

Drug treatment may also impact on nutritional status. Prolonged use of steroids may cause growth retardation in children, muscle wasting, diabetes, osteoporosis, peptic ulcer and liver or renal damage. Both aminosalicylates and the cytotoxic immunosuppressant drugs commonly have nausea and diarrhoea among their side-effects. Sulfasalazine is a folic acid antagonist and long-term use can cause megaloblastic anaemia.

Food intolerance and inflammatory bowel disease

The nutrient intake of IBD patients may be further compromised by self-imposed food restrictions. Many patients relate their gastrointestinal symptoms to specific foods ingested and food avoidance is common; Ballegaard *et al.* (1997) found that 65% of patients with IBD considered themselves intolerant to one or more food items and restricted their diet accordingly. However, although suggested, it has never been convincingly documented that food sensitivity is of pathogenic importance in chronic IBD. Ballegaard's study found no difference in the frequency and pattern of reported food intolerance between patients with Crohn's disease or ulcerative colitis, and since the effects of food withdrawal are clearly different in the two forms of IBD, any genuine food intolerance is likely to be coincidental, or possibly consequential, rather than causative.

In Crohn's disease, although food reintroduction following liquid or parenteral regimens commonly results in symptom recurrence, there is little evidence to suggest this is due to food intolerance *per se* in most cases. Pearson *et al.* (1993), in a study monitoring the effects of food reintroduction after elemental diet, found that while food sensitivities are apparent, they are associated with a wide variety of foods, the effects of which cannot always be confirmed by challenge and are often temporary in nature. As in the general population, a minority of patients may have genuine food intolerances and if this is suspected should be investigated and managed appropriately, but there is no evidence to justify putting all Crohn's patients through the rigours of dietary diagnostic procedures for food intolerance.

Table 4.12 Common nutritional deficiencies in patients with inflammatory bowel disease

Nutritional deficiency	Common causes
Dietary energy	Poor appetite as a result of symptoms or drug side-effects
	Catabolic effects of chronic inflammation
	Malabsorption (as a result of ileal IBD or following ileal resection)
Protein	Increased nitrogen losses
	High requirements for tissue repair
Vitamins D and K	Bile salt deficiency
Iron	Poor intake
	Poor absorption
	Chronic blood loss (especially in ulcerative colitis)
Folate	Impaired absorption
	Use of sulphasalazine (in ulcerative colitis)
Vitamin C	Low consumption of fruit and vegetables
Vitamin B_{12}	Ileal resection
	Small bowel overgrowth
Calcium, magnesium and zinc	Malabsorption and chronic diarrhoea
	Short bowel syndrome
	Avoidance of dairy foods
Sodium and potassium	Persistent diarrhoea and vomiting

Many patients with IBD avoid milk and dairy foods, either because they believe these to exacerbate symptoms or because popular diet books or health professionals have suggested that their exclusion may be beneficial (Mishkin 1997). Lactose intolerance can occur in Crohn's disease where ileal damage or resection results in malabsorptive problems. It is much less likely to be associated with ulcerative colitis, other than in patients with primary lactose intolerance of ethnic origin. In all such patients, lactose intake may need to be limited but rarely needs to be excluded altogether (see Section 4.8.2 in Malabsorption). Avoidance of milk and dairy products greatly increases the risk of nutrient deficiencies and should only be advised when there are clear indications that this is necessary. Dietary measures to rectify any resulting shortfall in intake of energy, protein, calcium and other micronutrients may be needed, especially in adolescents and young adults.

4.10.3 Dietary management of inflammatory bowel disease

General aspects of dietary management

The aims of dietary management in IBD patients are to:

- achieve and maintain good nutritional status during both active disease and remission
- help to alleviate clinical symptoms in combination with medical treatment
- help to treat clinical complications in combination with medical treatment
- help to achieve remission in Crohn's patients.

Patients should be encouraged to follow as normal a diet as is possible for their clinical state, and which is balanced in terms of overall composition. Most will benefit from relatively small meals of high energy and nutrient density consumed at fairly frequent intervals. At times when appetite is poor, food fortification strategies or supplement use may be necessary (see Section 1.12, Oral nutritional support). The importance of adequate fluid intake in the presence of diarrhoea, pyrexia or fistulae should be stressed. Nutritional status should be assessed at regular intervals and the growth of children and young people closely monitored.

Additional dietary manipulations may be needed to help to alleviate the effects of the disease or the consequences of intestinal resection (see Section 4.12), or to achieve remission in Crohn's patients. Some IBD patients may need to avoid specific foods which appear to exacerbate symptoms (see Food intolerance, above) but unnecessary food avoidance should be discouraged; the justification for excluding specific foods to help to alleviate symptoms should always be carefully considered.

The anti-inflammatory potential of *n*3 fatty acids and possible benefits of supplementation have recently been of interest following a study which reported reduced relapse rates in Crohn's patients given enteric-coated fish oil capsules for 1 year (Belluzzi *et al.* 1996). However, other studies have yielded more equivocal results and further trials are needed (Young-In 1996).

Specific aspects of the dietary management of Crohn's disease

People with Crohn's disease are at particular risk of nutritional deficiencies because this form of IBD is more likely to:

- occur in children or young adults whose energy needs are high
- result in malabsorption as a result of ileal inflammation or resection
- necessitate repeated surgery to treat complications such as stricture or fistulae.

The general detrimental effects of IBD on food intake described above compound the impact of these effects on nutritional status. The nutritional intake of children and adolescents with Crohn's disease is often particularly inadequate (Thomas *et al.* 1993; Hendricks *et al.* 1994) and this can have marked effects in terms of delayed puberty and impaired linear growth (Kirschner 1990). Belli *et al.* (1988) found that as many as 30% of juvenile Crohn's patients have some degree of growth retardation.

Restoring and maintaining good nutritional status is a treatment priority at all stages of the illness. As much as possible, this should be achieved by means of a diet comprised of ordinary foods and which minimizes disruption to normal life. However, additional enteral, possibly parenteral, nutritional support measures are likely to be needed at times in some patients, particularly perioperatively in those who are malnourished, in those with short bowel syndrome resulting from extensive intestinal resection (see Section 4.12.1 in Intestinal resection) and in paediatric patients with growth failure (Kelly and Fleming 1995).

Since appetite tends to be poor, the diet needs to be of high energy and nutrient density, and various strategies can be deployed to help to achieve this (see Section 1.12.1 in Oral nutritional support). If fat malabsorption is resulting in problematical symptoms, fat restriction to tolerance levels may be necessary, but care must to be taken to avoid compromising energy intake. Substitution of some long-chain triglyceride with medium-chain triglyceride (MCT), or dietary fortification with carbohydrate polymers may be necessary. Additional fat-soluble vitamins are also likely to be required. A daily multivitamin supplement may be advisable if food intake remains inadequate or malabsorption is pronounced.

Most Crohn's patients can tolerate a normal fibre intake but, because Crohn's disease is often complicated by strictures causing fibrosis and narrowing, dietary fibre content will be influenced by the presence of these and must be determined on an individual basis. People with evidence of strictures need to avoid fibrous, indigestible foods such as orange pith, dried foods, gristle, mushrooms and nuts.

Fluid needs should not be overlooked, particularly in the presence of symptoms such as diarrhoea or pyrexia, or when complications such as fistulae occur. An intake of at least 35 ml/kg per day plus replacement of symptom-related fluid losses should be advised.

Dietitians should always consider the nutritional impact of any food restrictions imposed by the patient (see Food intolerance in Section 4.10.2, above). Many patients will avoid greasy, spicy or irritant foods in an attempt to minimize symptoms, and such measures are of little nutritional consequence. Avoidance of foods such as milk and dairy foods will have a much greater impact and the necessity for such exclusions should be carefully explored with the patient.

Use of diet to achieve remission in Crohn's disease

Withdrawal of normal food for 4–6 weeks and replacing it with a liquid formula diet or parenteral nutrition can induce a phase of remission in Crohn's patients, thus improving the quality of life. Meta-analysis of randomized trials suggests that this strategy may be almost as effective as corticosteroids at inducing remission in active Crohn's disease (Fernandez-Banares *et al.* 1995) and is particularly useful for patients who are refractory to steroid treatment or for whom steroids are contraindicated.

Liquid diets tend to be used to induce remission in preference to parenteral regimens for reasons of safety and cost. Although it is known that whole protein, oligopeptide and elemental formulae can all be effective (Lennard-Jones 1992; Husain and Korzenik 1998), it remains unclear whether one type of formula is more beneficial than others. Most of the early studies were carried out using elemental diets (O'Morain *et al.* 1984; Saverymutto *et al.* 1985; Teahon *et al.* 1990; O'Brien *et al.* 1991) and the comparative effectiveness of the later use of peptide-based and whole protein diets has been less well evaluated and is more controversial (Giaffer *et al.* 1990). However, there is growing evidence that both types of formula are as capable of inducing remission as elemental preparations (Fernandez-Banares *et al.* 1994; Mansfield *et al.* 1995) and that whole protein feeds may have advantages in terms of acceptability and cost (Verma *et al.* 2000). The choice of formula will therefore depend on local policy.

The feed should be consumed orally if possible, but nasogastric feeding may be indicated if the patient is unable or unwilling to consume sufficient for their nutritional needs. Percutaneous endoscopic gastrostomy (PEG) feeding is not usually appropriate in Crohn's patients because of the risks of fistula formation and possible placement difficulties as a result of previous surgery.

If elemental diets are used, the practical problems associated with such regimens have to be borne in mind. Elemental formulae are unpalatable and 30–40% of patients find an elemental diet intolerable (Farthing 1991). An elemental formula needs to be introduced gradually over a period of 3–4 days to minimize side-effects such as nausea and osmotic diarrhoea and requires considerable dietetic support. Food is replaced with about eight drinks/day of the elemental formula, each drink being consumed slowly over a period of about 30 minutes. Palatability can be improved by consuming it from a covered cup with ice and a straw. Alternatively (and often the best procedure in children) the elemental diet can be given by nasogastric tube. Additional fluid will be needed, especially during the adjustment period, to meet fluid needs. Management of problems associated with the use of elemental diets in Crohn's disease is discussed by Teahon *et al.* (1995) and a protocol for their use has been produced by Holt (1997).

A period of 4–6 weeks is usually sufficient to achieve remission. Sometimes the treatment is maintained for a longer period (e.g. 12 weeks) in order to restore nutritional status in severely malnourished or growth-compromised individuals. Patients may need to be hospitalized for the initial few days of treatment but, once established on the regimen, can subsequently be managed at home.

Close dietetic monitoring is essential to check:

- tolerance to the regimen
- volume of diet consumed
- symptoms
- fluid intake
- compliance.

Ideally this should be on a daily basis during the first week, if necessary by telephone.

Initial problems often encountered are:

- loss of weight, particularly in first week
- tiredness
- postural hypotension
- hunger
- passage of green liquid stool with elemental diets.

Adjustments to the strength and rate of consumption of the formula may be necessary if osmotic diarrhoea occurs. Patients with short bowel syndrome or extensive inflammation may not be able to tolerate large volumes of feed at any one time and may need to consume small amounts at frequent intervals throughout the day.

After 7–10 days some symptomatic relief will usually have occurred, and after 2 or more weeks patients often feel remarkably well. At this stage, the importance of continued compliance with the liquid diet may need to be stressed in order to maximize the benefits.

If weight loss is occurring as a result of nutritional needs not being met, the volume or concentration of formula may need to be increased or the energy content fortified with modular carbohydrate or fat supplements.

Following the period of food withdrawal, transition to normal foods needs to be made with care, as too rapid a return will result in recurrence of symptoms. Food should be reintroduced gradually over 2–4 weeks with gradual cessation of formula diet so that overall nutritional intake is maintained.

The protocol for food reintroduction suggested by Holt (1997) for patients on elemental diets is probably suitable for all types of liquid formula diets and comprises:

- days 1–3: clear fluids (no milk): black tea or coffee, fruit juice, squash, Oxo, sieved soups, boiled sweets, jelly and ice lollies
- days 4–8: a few soft foods such as fish, chicken, egg, rice and potato as small frequent snacks rather than large meals

- days 9–13: increase variety, keeping fibre and fat content low, e.g. lean meat, peeled/stewed fruit, very well-cooked vegetables. Portion size can be increased, meal frequency decreased
- days 14–16: bread and other gluten-containing foods can be introduced
- days 17–19: milk and milk derivatives can be included (unless known to be milk intolerant)
- day 20 onwards: gradual resumption of other foods and progression to a normal, well-balanced diet.

Symptoms should be monitored throughout the reintroduction period and any poorly tolerated foods should be withdrawn and retried later. Food-associated symptoms may indicate an intolerance or, more probably, a temporary sensitivity. Foods most likely to cause problems are those high in fat, fibre or lactose, but tolerance to these components often improves with time and modest consumption can ultimately be achieved without problems. Suspected food intolerance should ideally be confirmed by blind challenge before permanent exclusion is advised.

Specific aspects of the dietary management of ulcerative colitis

Although, in contrast to Crohn's disease, the use of liquid or parenteral regimens cannot induce remission (see Bowel rest in Section 4.10.1, above), nutrition is still of primary importance in preventing the detrimental effects of malnutrition (Burke *et al*. 1997).

Surgical removal of the colon is curative and employed if drug treatment is unable to control the disease sufficiently, if severe complications arise (e.g. toxic megacolon, haemorrhage) or if precancerous changes are detected. Dietary management following colectomy is discussed in Section 4.12.2 in Intestinal resection).

Management of an acute relapse of ulcerative colitis

Severe attacks can be fatal and require emergency hospital admission with intravenous fluid and electrolyte support, possibly blood transfusion and steroid administration to induce remission as quickly as possible. If symptoms fail to improve, surgery may be needed.

If time permits, pre-operative nutritional support may be indicated in severely depleted patients. Peri-operative and post-operative support to maintain adequate nutrition is very important. In the absence of massive bleeding, perforation, toxic megacolon or obstruction, enteral rather than parenteral nutrition should be the mode of choice. Dietary measures to alleviate the effects of colonic resection may be needed (see Section 4.12.2).

Patients suffering from a mild or moderate attack, or after recovery from a more severe attack, will usually have lost weight and need to increase dietary energy and protein content. Oral energy supplements may be necessary if this cannot be achieved by use of normal foods alone (see Section 1.12, Oral nutritional support).

Particular attention should be paid to micronutrient requirements and supplements should be given if need-

ed. Additional folate will be required by patients on sulfasalazine, and supplementary calcium and vitamin D may be advisable for those on long-term steroids.

Management during remission of ulcerative colitis

Patients in remission should be encouraged to consume a varied, well-balanced diet and unnecessary food exclusions should be discouraged. Lactase deficiency necessitating lactose restriction occurs in a minority of patients but clinical evidence of this should be obtained before milk and dairy products are excluded.

Ulcerative colitis is associated with a high risk of colorectal carcinoma, particularly if the disease affects most, or the whole, of the colon and has been present for some years. General dietary measures which offer carcinogenic protection should be encouraged as much as possible (see Section 4.11.5, Colorectal cancer).

Text revised by: Briony Thomas

Acknowledgements: Helen Reilly and Carole Middleton

Useful addresses

Digestive Disorders Foundation (formerly the British Digestive Foundation)
3 St Andrew's Place, London NW1 4LB
Tel: 020 7486 0341
Website: www.digestivedisorders.org.uk

British Society of Gastroenterology
3 St Andrews Place, Regent's Park, London NW1 4LB
Tel: 020 7387 3534
Website: www.bsg.org.uk

National Association for Colitis and Crohn's Disease (NACC)
4 Beaumont House, Sutton Road, St Albans, Herts AL1 5HH
Tel: 01727 830038
E-mail: nacc@nacc-org.uk

References

Ballegaard M, Bjergstrom A, Brondum S *et al*. Self-reported food intolerance in chronic inflammatory bowel disease. *Scandinavian Journal of Gastroenterology* 1997; **32**: 569–571.

Belli DC, Seidman E, Bouthillier L *et al*. Chronic intermittent elemental diet improves growth failure in children with Crohn's disease. *Gastroenterology* 1988; **94**: 603–610.

Belluzzi A, Brignola C, Campieri M *et al*. Effect of enteric-coated fish oil preparation on relapses in Crohn's disease. *New England Journal of Medicine* 1996; **334**: 1557–1560.

British Society of Gastroenterology. *Inflammatory Bowel Disease. Clinical Guidelines*. London: BSG, 1996.

Burke A, Lichtenstein GR, Rombeau JL. Nutrition and ulcerative colitis. *Baillieres Clinical Gastroenterology* 1997; **11**: 153–174.

Farthing MJG. Crohn's disease in childhood and adolescence. In *Inflammatory Bowel Disease*. London: Chapman and Hall, 1991.

Fernandez-Banares F, Cabre E, Gonzalez-Huix F, Gassull MA. Enteral nutrition as primary therapy in Crohn's disease. *Gut* 1994; **35** (Suppl): S55–S59.

Fernandez-Banares F, Cabre E, Esteve-Comas M, Gassull MA. How effective is enteral nutrition in inducing clinical remission in active Crohn's disease? A meta-analysis of the randomized clinical trials. *Journal of Parenteral and Enteral Nutrition* 1995; **19**: 356–364.

Giaffer MH, North G, Holdsworth CD. Controlled trial of polymeric versus elemental diet in treatment of acute Crohn's disease. *Lancet* 1990; **335**: 816–819.

Griffiths AM. Inflammatory bowel disease. *Nutrition* 1998; **14**: 788–791.

Han PD, Burke A, Baldassano RN *et al*. Nutrition and inflammatory bowel disease. *Gastroenterology Clinics of North America* 1999; **28**: 423–443.

Hendricks KM, Williams E, Stoker TW *et al*. Dietary intake of adolescents with Crohn's disease. *Journal of the American Dietetic Association* 1994; **94**: 441–444.

Holt A. *Protocol for the Use of Elemental Diets in Crohn's Disease*. Liverpool: SHS, 1997.

Husain A, Korzenik JR. Nutritional issues and therapy in inflammatory bowel disease. *Seminars in Gastrointestinal Diseases* 1998; **9**: 21–30.

Kelly DG, Fleming CR. Nutritional considerations in inflammatory bowel diseases. *Gastroenterological Clinics of North America* 1995; **24**: 597–611.

Kirschner B. Growth and development in chronic inflammatory bowel disease. *Acta Paediatrica Scandinavica* 1990; **366** (Suppl): 98–104.

Kyle J. Crohn's disease in the northeastern and northern isles of Scotland: an epidemiological review. *Gastroenterology* 1992; **103**: 392–399.

Langholz E, Munkholm P, Davidsen M, Binder V. Colorectal cancer risk and mortality in patients with ulcerative colitis. *Gastroenterology* 1992; **103**: 1444–1451.

Langholz E, Munkholm P, Davidsen M, Binder V. Course of ulcerative colitis: analysis of changes in disease activity over years. *Gastroenterology* 1994; **107**: 3–11.

Lennard-Jones JE. Inflammatory bowel disease: medical therapy revisited. *Scandinavian Journal of Gastroenterology* 1992; **192**: 110–116.

Mansfield JC, Giaffer MH, Holdsworth CD. Controlled trial of oligopeptide versus amino acid diet in treatment of active Crohn's disease. *Gut* 1995; **36**: 60–66.

Mishkin S. Dairy sensitivity, lactose malabsorption and elimination diets in inflammatory bowel disease. *American Journal of Clinical Nutrition* 1997; **65**: 564–567.

Montgomery SM, Morris DL, Thompson P *et al*. Prevalence of inflammatory bowel disease in British 26 year olds: national longitudinal birth cohort. *British Medical Journal* 1998; **316**: 1058–1059.

O'Brien CJ, Giaffer MH, Cann PA, Holdsworth CD. Elemental diet in steroid-dependent and steroid-refractory Crohn's disease. *American Journal of Gastroenterology* 1991; **86**: 1614–1618.

O'Morain C, Segal AW, Levi AJ. Elemental diet as primary therapy of acute Crohn's disease: a controlled trial. *British Medical Journal* 1984; **288**: 1859–1862.

Pearson M, Teahon K, Levi AJ, Bjarnason I. Food intolerance and Crohn's disease. *Gut* 1993; **34**: 783–787.

Probert CSJ, Jayanthi V, Pinder D *et al*. Epidemiological study of ulcerative proctocolitis in Indian migrants and the indigenous population of Leicestershire. *Gut* 1992; **33**: 687–693.

Rose JDR, Roberts GM, Williams G *et al*. Cardiff Crohn's disease jubilee: the incidence over 50 years. *Gut* 1988; **29**: 346–351.

Saverymutto S, Hodgson HJF, Chadwick VS. Controlled trial comparing prednisolone with an elemental diet plus non absorbable antibiotics in active Crohn's disease. *Gut* 1985; **26**: 994–998.

Seo M, Okada M, Yao T *et al*. The role of total parenteral nutrition in the management of patients with acute attacks of inflammatory bowel disease. *Journal of Clinical Gastroenterology* 1999; **29**: 270–275.

Teahon K, Bjarnason I, Pearson M, Levi AJ. Ten years' experience with an elemental diet in the management of Crohn's disease. *Gut* 1990; **31**: 1133–1137.

Teahon K, Pearson M, Levi AJ, Bjarnason I. Practical aspects of enteral nutrition in the management of Crohn's disease. *Journal of Parenteral and Enteral Nutrition* 1995; **19**: 365–368.

Thomas AG, Taylor F, Miller V. Dietary intake and nutritional treatment in childhood Crohn's disease. *Journal of Pediatric Gastroenterology and Nutrition* 1993; **17**: 75–81.

Verma S, Brown S, Kirkwood B, Gaiffer MH. Polymeric versus elemental diet as primary treatment in active Crohn's disease: a randomized, double-blind trial. *American Journal of Gastroenterology* 2000; **95**: 735–739.

Young-In K. Can fish oil maintain Crohn's disease in remission? *Nutrition Reviews* 1996; **54**: 248–257.

4.11 Disorders of the colon

4.11.1 Constipation

It is always important to establish what patients mean by 'constipation', since many mistakenly assume this to mean the absence of a daily bowel movement. As a result, patients frequently take laxatives or rectal preparations without need, and laxative abuse may lead to hypokalaemia and an atonic, poorly functioning colon. Constipation is the passage of hard stools less frequently than is usual for that individual, usually accompanied by excessive straining, abdominal pain or discomfort, and often resulting in problems such as soiling, haemorrhoids or anal fissure. The possibility of constipation being caused by obstruction or other underlying disease must also be considered.

Simple constipation (i.e. not due to an underlying pathological cause) most commonly results from an inappropriate diet and lifestyle resulting in an inadequate consumption of dietary fibre and fluid, and insufficient physical activity. It may also be a secondary consequence of illness or surgery due to the combination of reduced bowel motility from analgesic (or other) drugs, lowered food intake and immobility.

In the absence of medical contraindications, simple constipation should always initially be treated by dietary means. People with simple constipation should be advised to:

1 *Increase their consumption of dietary fibre*, particularly cereal fibre which increases stool bulk.
Food choices which should be encouraged include:
- wholewheat, wholegrain and bran-containing varieties of breakfast cereals, bread and flour
- porridge oats
- root vegetables
- potatoes with skins (e.g. jacket potatoes)
- fruit with skins, e.g. apples, pears, grapes
- dried fruit, e.g. currants, raisins, sultanas, prunes, dates, figs
- fibre-containing biscuits and cakes, e.g. digestive or garibaldi biscuits, fig rolls, fruit cakes or cakes containing wholemeal flour
- peas, beans, lentils and nuts.
2 *Increase their consumption of fluid*. Inadequate fluid intake is often overlooked as a cause of constipation. All healthy adults should drink 1.5–2 litres (3–4 pints) of liquids every day (more in hot weather or if they take vigorous exercise) and many people do not achieve this level of intake. In the absence of sufficient fluid, dietary fibre cannot expand and soften sufficiently to exert its bulk-forming and peristaltic effect, and the faeces will become hard and compacted. People with simple constipation should be encouraged to increase their usual fluid intake, ideally to about 2 litres per day. A hot or warm drink first thing in the morning may be helpful to stimulate bowel activity.
3 *Increase their level of physical activity*. Exercise improves muscle function in all parts of the body and even modest regular exercise such as a daily walk may improve peristaltic function.

Although it is relatively simple to increase the fibre intake of a motivated adult, it can be more difficult in those with conservative eating habits, in particular those who are young or elderly. Elderly people, especially those with dentures, may reject fibre-rich foods on the grounds that they are too difficult to chew and leave irritating residues in the mouth. Children whose diet consists largely of convenience and snack foods may not greet the sudden advent of fresh fruit and vegetables, wholemeal bread and bran-based breakfast cereals with much enthusiasm. However, since there are numerous ways in which fibre-containing foods can be incorporated in the diet, it is usually possible to suggest measures which are acceptable to the individual. If wholemeal bread is disliked, a high-fibre white bread may be more acceptable. Cooked and puréed fruit may be preferred to raw fruit. Vegetables can be 'hidden' in casseroles or pies, or salad vegetables added to sandwiches. Wholemeal flours and cereals can be incorporated into home-baked foods.

If dietary fibre intake cannot be increased sufficiently by dietary means alone (e.g. if food intake is poor), a bulk-forming laxative such as ispaghula, methylcellulose and sterculia may be necessary. These preparations increase the bulk of the stool and soften its consistency, and are useful in the management of patients with colostomy, haemorrhoids, anal fissure and the constipated form of irritable bowel syndrome. However, it is vital that sufficient fluid intake accompanies the use of all these bulking agents to avoid the risk of intestinal obstruction.

Unprocessed wheat bran or oat bran has a similar bulk-forming effect and can be added to foods such as breakfast cereals or used in baking. They do, however, need to be used with care. To avoid the risk of faecal impaction or obstruction, they must be introduced gradually into the diet (no more than two teaspoons per day initially, slowly increasing to a maximum of three tablespoons per day) and fluid intake must be increased as well. It should be borne in mind that since unprocessed bran impairs the absorption of iron, calcium, zinc and other trace elements, prolonged supplementation should be avoided in those whose intake of micronutrients is marginal or inadequate.

If bulk-forming preparations are contraindicated (e.g. in those with dysphagia or at high risk of intestinal obstruction) an osmotic laxative such as lactulose is a more appropriate alternative. Lactulose is an unabsorbed disaccharide and its mild osmotic action results in softer, bulkier motions within 1–2 days. It is particularly useful for re-establishing bowel habits in constipated children, in patients following treatment for an impacted bowel and in elderly people unable to consume much fibre. Its action is also dependent on sufficiency of fluid intake.

Other stronger osmotic laxatives such as magnesium hydroxide and magnesium sulphate (Epsom salts) which have a strong purgative action, or stimulant laxatives (such as senna, fig, castor oil, bisacodyl or danthron) which increase intestinal motility should only be used for specific medical reasons, and never as a routine means of promoting a daily bowel movement.

Faecal softeners (e.g. dioctyl sodium sulphosuccinate) or lubricants (e.g. liquid paraffin) are sometimes indicated in the management of haemorrhoids or anal fissure. However, patients should be strongly discouraged from the regular use of liquid paraffin without medical direction as it can cause a number of side-effects in addition to impairing the absorption of fat-soluble vitamins.

4.11.2 Diarrhoea

Diarrhoea is a symptom resulting from a wide variety of causes. An acute attack of diarrhoea most commonly results from:

- pathogenic infection of bacterial, viral or protozoan origin
- acute food allergy or intolerance
- drug side-effects
- acute anxiety
- excessive consumption of dietary constituents with osmotic effects, e.g. fructose or sorbitol.

Chronic episodes of diarrhoea may reflect:

- underlying disease, e.g. carcinoma or inflammatory bowel disease
- functional bowel disorders, e.g. irritable bowel disease
- malabsorption, e.g. lactose intolerance, coeliac disease, pancreatic insufficiency
- increased intestinal motility, e.g. short bowel syndrome, stress, anxiety
- overflow from impacted faeces
- drug side-effects or laxative abuse
- chronic infection, e.g. giardiasis, amoebic dysentery.

Acute diarrhoea

Isolated attacks are usually self-resolving and, in normally healthy adults, simply require the substitution of food by plenty of clear fluids such as savoury or soft drinks or thin soups until the symptoms resolve. Oral rehydration solutions may be helpful if symptoms are severe. Antidiarrhoeal drugs such as loperamide may be useful to get through an awkward situation such as a long journey, but are best avoided for infective episodes of diarrhoea as their use hampers the body's ability to eliminate the causative organism.

Acute diarrhoea poses a much greater risk in infants or young children, elderly people or those with chronic illness as dehydration can develop rapidly, particularly if accompanied by vomiting. Medical advice must be sought as fluid and electrolyte repletion will be required and hydration status will need to be closely monitored.

Chronic diarrhoea

This always requires investigation to determine the underlying cause, and its management will depend on the nature of the diagnosis and its treatment. Many conditions resulting in diarrhoea will require dietary manipulations as part of their primary treatment (e.g. coeliac disease, lactose intolerance, pancreatitis) or these may become necessary as a secondary consequence of treatment (e.g. following intestinal resection). Specific details of these can be found in the relevant sections of the manual.

If despite, or while awaiting, treatment, chronic diarrhoea remains a problem, dietary guidance should be given to help to mitigate its effect on nutrient and fluid losses. People should be encouraged to:

- Maintain a good fluid intake at times when symptoms are acute, i.e. 10–15 cups of fluids per day. The choice of drinks is a matter of individual tolerance and preference. Clear fluids such as sweetened soft drinks, clear soups or savoury drinks are likely to be better tolerated than milk or undiluted fruit juices, and cold drinks are less likely to trigger diarrhoea than hot ones. However, the important aspect is that good fluid intake is maintained in whatever way suits the patient. Provided that they do not worsen symptoms, any drink that helps to maintain energy or nutrient intake (e.g. glucose drinks, milk supplement drinks, diluted fruit juices) will always be an added nutritional bonus.
- As symptoms remit, gradually resume eating soft or easily digested foods, e.g. white bread or toast, white fish, mashed potato, plain biscuits, jelly, sorbets, low-fat yoghurt, milk puddings or ice-cream. Once these are tolerated, variety should gradually be widened as appropriate for the underlying condition. Highly fibrous foods such as wholegrain breads and fruit and vegetable skins will usually need to be avoided.

General measures which may help to prevent symptom recurrence and maintain nutritional adequacy are to:

- keep meals small in size but consume them at regular intervals
- eat slowly, chew food well and relax after meals
- eat as wide a variety of foods as possible but avoid irritant, spicy, greasy or fibrous foods or others known to exacerbate symptoms

- avoid consuming large quantities of undiluted fruit juices, fizzy drinks, alcohol, and strong tea and coffee
- boost nutrient intake by using over-the-counter supplement drinks, food-enrichment strategies or prescribed supplements if these are recommended.

4.11.3 Irritable bowel syndrome

Irritable bowel syndrome (IBS) is a common disorder, thought to affect at least 20% of the adult population in Western countries (Jones and Lydeard 1992) and probably affecting many more who never consult a doctor (Heaton *et al.* 1992). In itself, IBS is a harmless condition, although it can cause much misery to those who suffer from it. However, because its symptoms can mimic those of other more serious disorders, it always requires investigation to exclude the possibility of underlying disease such as malignancy, inflammation or coeliac disease. As a result, IBS accounts for about half of all referrals to gastroenterology clinics.

The condition is defined as a functional bowel disorder, i.e. one which results in characteristic symptoms but with no obvious structural or biochemical cause. It usually presents as a combination of disordered defecation (constipation, diarrhoea or both) together with abdominal pain and distension.

IBS most commonly starts in people aged 15–40 years but can occur at any age. The prevalence in men and women is probably similar, but women are more likely to seek medical attention (Farthing 1995).

Diagnosis of irritable bowel syndrome

There is no single pathophysiological marker for IBS and diagnosis is based on symptoms and the exclusion of organic disease. The symptom criteria for IBS (and other functional bowel disorders) were reached by consensus at an international working party of experts in Rome (Thompson *et al.* 1992) and replace the earlier diagnostic criteria devised for IBS by Manning *et al.* (1978). Subsequent minor modifications to the Rome criteria have been made (Neal *et al.* 1997; Thompson *et al.* 1999) but the most commonly used definition of IBS is:

1 Abdominal pain relieved by defecation or associated with change in frequency or consistency of stool
   and
2 An irregular pattern of defecation for at least 2 days a week (three or more of the following):
   - altered stool frequency (>3 times/day or <3 times/week)
   - altered stool form (hard/loose)
   - altered stool passage (straining, urgency, sense of incomplete evacuation)
   - passage of mucus
   - abdominal bloating or feeling of distension.

The severity of the symptoms varies; for some people they are extremely debilitating while in others they are no more than a minor inconvenience. The condition may also spontaneously appear and then disappear (Talley *et al.* 1992).

Causation of irritable bowel syndrome

The cause of IBS is unknown, although some abnormalities of intestinal motility and visceral sensation have been found in some patients. Psychological influences on bowel function are also thought to be important and about half of all patients seeking advice for IBS have clinical symptoms of anxiety, depression or both (Farthing 1995). However, it is also possible that signs of stress or emotional disturbance could be a consequence of having IBS, rather than being the cause of it (Maxwell *et al.* 1997).

It has been suggested that altered bacterial flora composition may play a part in the development of IBS (King *et al.* 1998) because the condition sometimes develops following an episode of bacterial gastroenteritis (Neal *et al.* 1997) or a course of antibiotics (Jones *et al.* 1984). Other factors such as increased production of inflammatory cytokines (Collins 1994), lack of fibre (Manning *et al.* 1977) or food intolerance (Alun Jones *et al* 1982; Nanda *et al* 1989) have also been suggested to have a pathogenic role (see below). However, at present there is little evidence that any factor has a consistently causative influence, or even that IBS has a single cause (Maxwell *et al.* 1997). Much remains to be learnt about the condition.

Management of irritable bowel syndrome

Because IBS is poorly understood and in the past has often been misdiagnosed, there is no universally agreed approach to treatment. As a result of variations in diagnostic criteria and consequent misdiagnosis, many of the early controlled clinical trials on its management have been shown to be flawed (Klein 1988).

Current treatment tends to adopt a combination of two strategies:

1 *Treating the gastrointestinal symptoms*:
   - giving antidiarrhoeal drugs such as loperamide to reduce bowel movement frequency
   - giving smooth muscle relaxants for pain
   - increasing fibre intake of those with constipation
   - exploring other possible dietary triggers
2 *Treating affective disorders and psychological symptoms*:
   - providing reassurance that, although unpleasant, the condition is harmless
   - identifying psychological factors which may be contributing to symptoms
   - using psychological and behavioural strategies to help people to cope with stress and symptoms
   - using drug treatment to relieve depression and anxiety as appropriate.

Some clinicians place greater emphasis on one of these approaches than the other.

Dietary influences on irritable bowel syndrome

The role of diet in the management of IBS remains poorly understood, complicated by the multifaceted nature of the disorder in terms of both origin and presentation, and the paucity of research that takes this into account.

The following dietary factors may have an influence on IBS symptoms.

Dietary fibre

In 1977, Manning *et al.* showed that the addition of 7 g of wheat bran to the diet of IBS patients for six weeks resulted in a significant improvement of symptoms. As a result of this, a high-fibre diet became a mainstay of IBS management for many years. However, recent review of this practice has shown that while it may help some patients, it is by no means a panacea for all and may worsen symptoms in some (Francis and Whorwell 1992; Hammonds *et al.* 1997). It now seems clear that fibre (both soluble and insoluble) is most likely to benefit IBS patients with symptoms of constipation, hard stools and urgency, but is unlikely to help those with abdominal distension, diarrhoea or flatulence (Lambert *et al.* 1991) and may make such symptoms worse (Rees *et al.* 1994).

Food intolerance

There has been much speculation that food intolerance may exacerbate the symptoms of some people with IBS, but this is difficult to establish from current evidence which presents a confusing picture. A systematic review of the literature on adverse food reactions in IBS sufferers (Niec *et al.* 1998) revealed considerable disparity among the seven studies examined. The proportion of IBS patients reported to benefit from an elimination diet ranged from 15 to 71%; confirmation of intolerance by double-blind placebo-controlled challenges was achieved in as few as 6% or as many as 58% of cases. Milk, wheat and eggs and, to a lesser extent, the salicylate and amine content of foods were most frequently associated with symptom exacerbation. There appeared to be a trend towards adverse food reactions being more likely in those with diarrhoea as a predominant symptom. However, since all of these studies were found to have limitations in terms of trial design, patient selection, nature and duration of exclusion diets and methods of food challenge, the role of food exclusion in IBS is hard to determine and remains to be clarified by carefully controlled clinical trials.

Dietitians should be aware of the possibility that specific food sensitivities may be present in some cases, but should not assume that they will be present in everyone. If a diet and symptom history is suggestive of food intolerance then trial exclusion measures should be considered. However, whether the disruption imposed by formal exclusion diets justifies the potential benefits is a balance which must always be weighed up on an individual basis (see Section 4.34, Food allergy and intolerance). Guidance for investigating food tolerance in IBS patients is given below (see Practical aspects of dietary management).

Lactose intolerance

The possibility of lactose intolerance coexisting with, or even being mistaken for, IBS should also be considered.

Unrecognized lactose intolerance has been found in a proportion of IBS patients following breath hydrogen and blood glucose measurements after administration of 50 g lactose (Bohmer and Tuynman 1996). There is also evidence that some patients have been mistakenly diagnosed as having IBS when in reality they have lactose intolerance (the symptom complexes of the two disorders can be similar) and that this may explain the refractory nature of some cases of IBS (Shaw and Davies 1999). The symptoms of such patients rapidly improve once the correct diagnosis is made and a reduced-lactose regimen instituted.

However, it should also borne in mind that many IBS patients simply assume that they are intolerant to milk and dairy products and exclude these foods for no good reason. Vesa *et al.* (1998) found that 60% of IBS sufferers believed themselves intolerant to lactose but evidence of this could only be found in 24%. Furthermore, even if lactose intolerance is present, complete avoidance of milk and dairy products is usually unnecessary; most lactose maldigesters can consume loads of up to 6 g lactose (equivalent to a small glass of milk) without experiencing any problems (Hertzler *et al.* 1996) (see Lactose malabsorption in Section 4.8.2).

Gut flora

Differences in the composition of intestinal flora of IBS patients, with a reduction in coliforms, lactobacilli and to a lesser extent bifidobacteria, compared with control subjects have been observed (Alun-Jones *et al.* 1984; Balsari *et al.* 1992), although whether this is a cause or consequence of IBS is unknown. As a result, malfermentation may contribute to IBS symptoms (Hunter 1991); colonic gas production, particularly of hydrogen, has been shown to be greater in patients with IBS than in controls (King *et al.* 1998). It is also possible that some of the improvements noted on exclusion diets are attributable to the resultant changes in bacterial flora and reduced gas production rather than to food intolerance *per se* (King *et al.* 1998). However, more research is required in this area.

The potential use of prebiotics (types of dietary fibre which reach the colon intact and may selectively encourage the growth of beneficial bacteria, e.g. fructo-oligosaccharides and inulin) and probiotics (foods containing beneficial live bacteria which may colonize in the gut, beneficially altering the floral balance) is currently an active area of investigation but their role in the management of IBS remains to be evaluated.

Practical aspects of dietary management of irritable bowel syndrome

Because of the variability of the disorder, no single dietary treatment strategy is likely to be uniformly effective in the management of IBS. Furthermore, given the general lack of research in this area, dietary management has to rely more on clinical experience and reasoned judgement than on a sound evidence base. Nevertheless, dietary guidance which is symptom led, based on sound healthy-eating principles, monitored and modified as necessary can significantly improve the quality of life for many patients (Francis and Whorwell 1997).

Initial patient assessment is essential to determine:

- the nature of the symptoms: which ones predominate and their pattern of occurrence
- whether they are exacerbated by stress, anxiety or other factors
- current clinical treatment including the use of preparations such as bulking agents, laxatives, analgesics and antispasmodic drugs.

Dietary assessment should focus on:

- previous dietary measures tried and with what degree of success
- suspected food intolerances or self-imposed food restrictions
- current meal pattern and overall dietary balance
- current fluid intake.

These factors determine the nature of the advice given. Obvious dietary imbalances in terms of meal pattern and dietary intake should be addressed. People who lead a stressed lifestyle with erratic meal patterns or prolonged periods without food should be encouraged to adopt a more sensible approach.

Dietary guidance should be based on healthy-eating principles but also incorporate specific measures that may help particular symptom profiles.

If symptoms of constipation, hard stools and urgency predominate

- Increased consumption of dietary fibre, both insoluble and soluble, may be helpful, particularly if the habitual intake is low. However, additional fibre should be introduced gradually into the diet, to avoid triggering problems of bloating and wind. If increased consumption of cereal fibre appears to cause problems, non-fermentable bulking agents such as methylcellulose or ispaghula may be better tolerated (Prior and Whorwell 1987; Kumar *et al.* 1987).
- As with all patients with constipation and hard stools, adequacy of fluid consumption should also be considered.

If symptoms of diarrhoea predominate

- Fibre consumption should not be increased and may need to be reduced.
- Food-related symptoms are more likely to be apparent and patients may benefit from avoiding items such as dried fruit, nuts, seeds, fruit and vegetable skins, and other irritant or spicy foods known to cause problems.
- Consideration should be given to the possibility of lactose intolerance or food intolerances, particularly to wheat.

If symptoms of bloating and wind are a problem

- Lactose intolerance should be considered.

- Flatus production may be reduced by limiting the consumption of peas, beans and legumes, onions and brassica vegetables such as cabbage and Brussels sprouts.

If food intolerance is suspected

The basis for any reported benefits from self-imposed food restrictions should be closely explored. Patients with IBS have often subjected themselves to commercial 'allergy tests' of dubious value, or have read popular books and articles suggesting dietary remedies for the condition. As a result, misinformation is common and dietary exclusions may be both extreme and unwarranted. An important role of the dietitian is to take people's food concerns seriously and assess the likelihood of genuine intolerance being present.

A food exclusion regimen to help to identify food intolerance in people with IBS has been described by Parker *et al.* (1995). This replaces cereals and dairy foods with rice and soya substitutes, the remainder of the diet being comprised of meat, poultry, fish, non-citrus fruits and vegetables (other than onions and potatoes). The diet is followed for 2 weeks with patients keeping a detailed food and symptom record so that the dietitian can ascertain whether the regimen has been correctly followed and evaluate its effectiveness. If no improvement occurs within 2 weeks, patients return to a normal diet. If symptom relief occurs, foods are then reintroduced singly, at 2 day intervals, in moderately sized portions. Any that provoke a reaction are excluded and no further foods reintroduced until symptoms have stabilized.

However, it should also be borne in mind that the placebo response rate to drug treatment is particularly high among IBS sufferers and the same may be true of dietary manipulations (Klein 1988). Identified food intolerances should be re-evaluated at intervals to see whether continued dietary exclusions are necessary.

If no evidence of food intolerance can be found, people can still benefit enormously from supportive general guidance to help restore dietary balance and mitigate symptoms.

All patients with IBS should have regular dietetic follow-up to monitor the effectiveness of remedial measures suggested and make adjustments if necessary.

4.11.4 Diverticular disease

A diverticulum is a protrusion through the muscular coat of the inner lining of the colon to form a small sac with a narrow neck. Diverticula occur as a result of localized pressure on a weak area of bowel wall and most commonly appear in the lower left part of the colon. They tend to develop in later life and the presence of diverticula (known as diverticulosis) is relatively common by the age of 70 years in Western societies. The condition is closely associated with constipation and a habitually low intake of dietary fibre.

Diverticulosis often remains asymptomatic and is only detected by chance during bowel investigations for other disorders. However, it may become apparent as a result of diverticulitis, when bacterial overgrowth and inflammation occur within the diverticula causing localized abdominal pain, diarrhoea and fever. Other complications such as abscess, rupture and haemorrhage can also occur (Thompson and Patel 1986).

Dietary management

Acute episodes of diverticulitis will require treatment with antibiotics and pain relief. While symptoms remain acute, the diet should be fairly bland, avoiding irritant or poorly digested foods such as onions, fruit and vegetable skins, seeds and nuts. Since the symptoms inevitably impair appetite at this time, most people will automatically adopt a diet of this type. As symptoms remit, normal food intake can gradually be resumed.

Following recovery, people should be encouraged to make long-term adjustments to their diet to minimize the risk of recurrence. In particular, people should be encouraged to increase their consumption of dietary fibre from both soluble and insoluble sources and also to increase their fluid intake.

It may be a sensible precautionary measure for people to continue to avoid items which are most likely to be poorly digested and lodge within diverticula such as skins, sweetcorn, seeds and nuts (although there is little evidence that this is necessary). However, other unnecessary food restrictions should be discouraged.

Since many people with diverticulosis are elderly, care should be taken to ensure that these measures are achieved in ways that do not compromise nutrient intake. If appetite is small, additional guidance on good choices of nutrient-dense foods or food-enrichment strategies may be necessary. If there are problems with continence or mobility, strategies for increasing fluid intake need to take account of such difficulties (see Section 3.7, Older adults).

4.11.5 Colorectal cancer

Colorectal carcinoma is (after lung cancer) the second most common cause of cancer in men and women in the UK and throughout much of the Western world (DH 1998). It is also one of the cancers whose development is most strongly associated with dietary factors, particularly a diet which is low in vegetables and fibre and high in red and processed meats (DH 1998). Much of the disease could probably be prevented by consumption of a more appropriate diet and avoidance of smoking (see Section 4.37, Cancer).

Such preventive measures may be especially important in those with a family history of the disease. There is a strong genetic predisposition to two forms of the disease, familial adenomatous polyposis (FAP) and hereditary non-polyposis colorectal cancer (HNPCC). Other types are termed sporadic colorectal cancer. Since people rarely know which form of the disease affected a relative, anyone with a family history of the disease should be considered at elevated risk.

Colorectal cancer usually presents with symptoms of change in bowel habit (constipation and /or diarrhoea), rectal bleeding and abdominal pain often accompanied by loss of weight. It most commonly occurs in people over the age of 45 years. If the disease is detected at an early stage, it can be completely cured by surgery. However, survival rates following late diagnosis remain poor.

The likely prognosis of a colorectal tumour and its treatment depend on the type and grade of tumour and its degree of spread as determined by the Duke's clinico-pathological classification:

- Duke's A: tumour is confined to the bowel wall and has not penetrated its full thickness
- Duke's B: tumour has breached the bowel wall
- Duke's C: regional lymph-node involvement
- Duke's D: presence of distant metastases.

Surgical resection for Duke's B and C is likely to be more extensive than for Duke's A and to be followed by chemotherapy. The use of radiotherapy is usually confined to those with rectal or rectosigmoid tumours or for palliation (Midgley and Kerr 1999). New surgical techniques and treatment modalities are continually being developed and it is being increasingly recognized that optimum outcomes for patients with colorectal cancer require specialized surgical management and multidisciplinary care (Midgley and Kerr 1999).

More detailed information about colorectal cancer and its management can be found in Midgley and Kerr (1999), SIGN (1997) and Neal and Hoskin (1997).

Dietary management

Some patients admitted for surgery following diagnosis may present in a nutritionally depleted state as a result of the effects of chronic symptoms on food intake, periods of starvation imposed for investigative procedures and the cancer process itself. In such patients, appropriate nutritional support measures should be instituted as soon as possible to help them to withstand the effects of surgery.

Patients who are well nourished on admission do not usually require artificial nutritional support measures following colorectal surgery. Nevertheless, their nutritional status during the recovery period should be monitored, particularly if post-surgical complications such as anastomotic breakdown occur or if resumption of oral food intake is slow, and evidence of depletion should be corrected at an early stage (see Section 5.6, Surgery). Adequate pain relief is important, as continuous pain or discomfort will markedly suppress appetite.

Specific dietary measures may be required during the initial phase of adjustment to the effects of intestinal resection and possible creation of a pouch or stoma (see Section 4.12, Intestinal resection). Others may need advice on maintaining a good nutritional intake during phases of radiotherapy or chemotherapy if these are given (see Section 4.37.2). However, in general the aim should be to encourage a food intake of high nutrient and energy density until normal appetite has been restored.

If pronounced weight loss has occurred as a result of surgery and food intake remains inadequate, additional oral nutritional support measures should be implemented (see Section 1.12, Oral nutritional support).

Following recovery, people should be encouraged to consume a varied and well-balanced healthy diet in order to optimize carcinogenic protection (see Section 4.37.1, Diet and the causation of cancer). The potential benefits from consuming at least five portions of fruit and vegetables per day in terms of both bowel function and carcinogenic protection should be particularly strongly stressed.

Text revised by: Briony Thomas

Acknowledgements: Hayley Wordsworth and Sue Acreman

Useful address

British Digestive Foundation
3 St Andrew's Place, London NW1 4LB
Tel: 020 7486 0341
Website: www.bdf.org.uk

References

Alun Jones V, McLaughlan P, Shorthouse M *et al*. Food intolerance: a major factor in the pathogenesis of irritable bowel syndrome. *Lancet* 1982; **ii**: 1115–1117.

Balsari A, Ceccarelli A *et al*. The faecal microbial population in the irritable bowel syndrome. *Microbiologica* 1992; **5**: 185–194.

Bohmer CJ, Tuynman HA. The clinical relevance of lactose malabsorption in irritable bowel syndrome. *European Journal of Gastroenterology and Hepatology* 1996; **8**: 1013–1016.

Collins SM. Irritable bowel syndrome could be an inflammatory disorder. *European Journal of Gastroenterology and Hepatology* 1994; **6**: 478–483.

Department of Health. *Nutritional Aspects of the Development of Cancer*. Report of the Working Group on Diet and Cancer of the Committee on Medical Aspects of Food Policy (COMA). Report on Health and Social Subjects 48. London: The Stationery Office, 1998.

Farthing MJG. Fortnightly review: irritable bowel, irritable body or irritable brain? *British Medical Journal* 1995; **310**: 171–175.

Francis CY, Whorwell PJ. Bran and irritable bowel syndrome: time for reappraisal. *Lancet* 1992; **344**: 39–41.

Francis CY, Whorwell PJ. The irritable bowel syndrome. *Postgraduate Medical Journal* 1997; **73**: 1–7.

Hammonds R *et al*. The role of fibre in IBS. *International Journal of Gastroenterology* 1997; **2**: 9–12.

Heaton KW, O'Donnell LJD, Braddon FE *et al*. Symptoms of irritable bowel syndrome in a British urban community: consulters and non-consulters. *Gastroenterology* 1992; **102**: 1962–1967.

Hertzler SR, Huynh BC, Savaiano DA. How much lactose is low lactose? *Journal of the American Dietetic Association* 1996; **96**: 243–246.

Hunter JO. Hypothesis; food allergy – or enterometabolic disorder? *Lancet* 1991; **338**: 495–496.

Jones R, Lydeard S. Irritable bowel syndrome in the general population. *British Medical Journal* 1992; **304**: 87–90.

Jones VA, Wilson AJ, Hunter JO, Robinson JE. The aetiological role of antibiotic prophylaxis with hysterectomy in irritable bowel syndrome. *Obstetrics and Gynaecology* 1984; **5** (Suppl 1): S22–S23.

King TS, Elia M, Hunter JO. Abnormal colon fermentation in irritable bowel syndrome. *Lancet* 1998; **352**: 1187–1189.

Klein KB. Controlled treatment trials in the irritable bowel syndrome: a critique. *Gastroenterology* 1988; **95**: 232–241.

Kumar A, Kumar N, Vij JC *et al*. Optimum dosage of ispaghula husk in patients with irritable bowel syndrome – correlation of symptom relief with whole gut transit time and stool weight. *Gut* 1987; **28**: 150–155.

Lambert JP, Brunt PW, Mowat NA *et al*. The value of prescribed 'high fibre' diets for the treatment of the irritable bowel syndrome. *European Journal of Clinical Nutrition* 1991; **45**: 601–609.

Manning AP, Thompson WG, Heaton KW, Morris AF. Towards positive diagnosis of the irritable bowel syndrome. *British Medical Journal* 1978; **11**: 653–654.

Manning AP, Heaton KW, Uglow P, Harvey RF. Wheat fibre and the irritable bowel syndrome: a controlled trial. *Lancet* 1977; **ii**: 417–418.

Maxwell PR, Mendall MA, Kumar D. Irritable bowel syndrome. *Lancet* 1997; **350**: 1691–1695.

Midgley R, Kerr D. Colorectal cancer. *Lancet* 1999; **353**: 391–399.

Nanda R, James R, Smith H *et al*. Food intolerance and the irritable bowel syndrome. *Gut* 1989; **30**: 1099–1104.

Neal AJ, Hoskin PJ. Carcinoma of the colon and rectum. In *Clinical Oncology: Basic Principles and Practice*, 2nd edn. London: Edward Arnold, 1997.

Neal KR, Hebden J, Spiller R. Prevalence of gastrointestinal symptoms six months after bacterial gastroenteritis and risk factors for development of the irritable bowel syndrome: postal survey of patients. *British Medical Journal* 1997; **314**: 779–782.

Niec AM, Frankum B, Talley NJ. Are adverse reactions linked to irritable bowel syndrome? *American Journal of Gastroenterology* 1998; **93**: 2184–2190.

Parker TJ, Naylor SJ, Riordan AM, Hunter JO. Management of patients with food intolerance in irritable bowel syndrome: the development and use of an exclusion diet. *Journal of Human Nutrition and Dietetics* 1995; **8**: 159–166.

Prior A, Whorwell PJ. Double-blind study of ispaghula in the irritable bowel syndrome. *Gut* 1987; **28**: 1510–1513.

Rees GA, Trevan M, Davies GJ. Dietary fibre modification and the symptoms of irritable bowel syndrome – a review. *Journal of Human Nutrition and Dietetics* 1994; **7**: 179–189.

Scottish Intercollegiate Guidelines Network (SIGN). *Colorectal Cancer*. Publication 16. Edinburgh: SIGN, 1997.

Shaw AD, Davies GJ. Lactose intolerance: problems in diagnosis and treatment. *Journal of Clinical Gastroenterology* 1999; **28**: 208–216.

Talley NJ, Weaver AL, Zinmeister AR, Melton LJ. Onset and disappearance of gastrointestinal symptoms and functional gastrointestinal disorders. *American Journal of Epidemiology* 1992; **136**: 165–177.

Thompson WG, Patel DG. Clinical picture of diverticular disease of the colon. *Clinical Gastroenterology* 1986; **15**: 903–916.

Thompson WG, Creed F, Drossman DA *et al*. Functional bowel disease and functional abdominal pain. *Gastroenterology International* 1992; **5**: 75–91.

Thompson WG, Longstreth GF, Drossman DA *et al*. Functional bowel disorders and functional abdominal pain. *Gut* 1999; **45** (Suppl 2): 43–47.

Vesa TH, Seppo LM, Marteau PR *et al*. Role of irritable bowel syndrome in subjective lactose intolerance. *American Journal of Clinical Nutrition* 1998; **67**: 710–715.

4.12 Intestinal resection

Resection of a part of the small and/or large intestine may be necessary for reasons of obstructive, neoplastic or inflammatory disease. Although the body can adapt remarkably well to the subsequent loss of absorptive tissue, resective procedures may have both short- and long-term effects requiring dietetic intervention. Patients who have had prolonged periods of ill health and poor food intake prior to surgery are at particular risk of nutritional depletion.

The consequences of intestinal resection depend on which part of the intestine is removed and the amount and type of intestinal tissue which remains. The large intestine absorbs water and sodium so if most or all of this is resected, these losses may be significantly increased and need to be replaced. Major resection of part of the small intestine results in the malabsorption of nutrients as well as fluid and electrolytes, the latter losses being compounded if the colon is removed as well. If less than 100 cm of small intestine remains (or 50 cm in conjunction with an intact colon), the digestive and absorptive capacity of the bowel is permanently impaired (Nightingale and Lennard-Jones 1993).

4.12.1 Resection of the small intestine

Minor resection

Resection may be confined to removal of a segment of ileum to remove diseased tissue or to relieve a stricture (e.g. in Crohn's disease), the two unaffected ends of intestine then being joined together. This only has relatively minor and short-term consequences in terms of impaired absorption; adaptation soon occurs via hypertrophy of the intestinal brush border.

Major resection and short bowel syndrome

More extensive resection may result in the remaining end of the small intestine being anastomosed to the colon (jejunocolic or ileocolic anastomosis) or ending at a stoma on the abdomen (jejunostomy or ileostomy). The loss of the ileum, and perhaps some of the jejunum, considerably impairs digestive and absorptive function, resulting in symptoms of short bowel syndrome. When the absorptive function of the colon is not available, even more sodium and water will be lost.

The residual jejunal length, and whether the colon is present or absent, determine the nutritional implications and hence management. Once less than 200 cm of small intestine remains, symptoms of short bowel syndrome are likely to occur. Once less than 100 cm jejunum remains (or <50 cm if colonic function is preserved), malabsorptive problems are likely to be permanent and require long-term parenteral support. Temporary parenteral support may be necessary in other cases of short bowel syndrome during periods of adaptation and if residual disease remains.

All patients with short bowel syndrome have problems with fluid and electrolyte balance, particularly in the immediate post-operative period. Nutrient requirements will also be increased as a result of malabsorption. The long-term risk of gall stones is increased.

Nutritional implications of jejunostomy

The loss of colonic function in addition to that of the ileum greatly increases the losses of water and sodium. The risk of fluid and sodium depletion is therefore high and needs to be monitored closely. Daily fluid balance and weight should be measured during the initial post-operative period until the patient is stable.

Following jejunostomy, the rate of gastric emptying and intestinal transit time are increased, thus enhancing stomal losses. Gastric antisecretory drugs or a somatostatin analogue such as octreotide may help to reduce this. Loperamide and/or codeine phosphate may also benefit some patients. These drugs may be needed in large doses and should be taken 30–60 minutes before meals.

In some people (known as 'secretors') stomal losses of water, sodium and sometimes magnesium may exceed the amount which can be taken in by mouth and parenteral replacement will be required. This is particularly likely to occur if the stoma is situated less than 100 cm along the jejunum (Lennard-Jones 1994). Secretors may be in constant negative sodium balance of up to 400 mmol/day.

Those who can maintain sodium balance will still lose considerable amounts of sodium (up to 200 mmol sodium daily). Patients with a stomal output of <1200 ml/day can usually maintain their sodium balance by adding extra salt at the table and in cooking. When the losses are greater than this, an oral sodium supplement will be required. This should be provided as a glucose electrolyte solution with a sodium content of at least 90 mmol sodium/l (the sodium concentration of stomal effluent) (Nightingale *et al*. 1992). Additional fluids with lower sodium concentrations, or water alone, should be avoided as they will increase stomal sodium losses (Lennard-Jones and Wood 1991). The benefits of glucose electrolyte solutions containing potassium and bicarbonate as well as sodium are unclear; there is little evidence that bicarbonate promotes sodium absorption, and potassium stomal losses are in any case small (Lennard-Jones 1990).

If the patient is receiving an enteral feed, sodium may need to be added to increase the sodium content to >90 mmol/l.

Magnesium deficiency can usually be corrected with oral magnesium oxide supplements.

After the immediate post-operative period, patients with a jejunostomy can usually consume a normal diet without fat reduction and there is no evidence that an elemental or hydrolysed diet is necessary (Lennard-Jones 1994). In contrast to short bowel patients with an intact colon (see below), medium-chain triglyceride (MCT)-based supplements are usually inappropriate because of their high osmolarity and tendency to increase jejunostomy output. Additional nutritional support measures such as modular carbohydrate supplementation or use of energy supplements may be necessary. If the residual small bowel length is less than 100 cm, patients usually require long-term parenteral support. In the future, intestinal transplantation may be able to obviate this need (Powell-Tuck 1994).

Nutritional implications of jejunocolic anastomosis

People with a preserved colon have a greater ability to absorb fluid and electrolytes than those with a jejunostomy, and hence can adapt to resection more easily. Gastric emptying also tends to be normal, making it easier for fluid and electrolyte balance to be maintained. Problems are only likely to remain when the residual length of the small intestine is less than 50 cm.

However, the presence of a colon does have other dietary implications. Malabsorption results in long-chain fatty acids and bile acids reaching the colon, causing watery diarrhoea. Patients usually benefit from a diet which is high in carbohydrate and low or moderately restricted in fat (depending on the individual level of tolerance). Unabsorbed carbohydrate reaching the colon is converted by bacterial fermentation to short-chain fatty acids (SCFA) which are readily absorbed as a source of energy. It has been shown that short bowel patients with a functional colon are able to increase their absorption of energy by 465 kcal/day (range 300–750 kcal/day) by increasing carbohydrate intake from 20% to 60% of total energy intake in an otherwise isocaloric diet (Nordgaard 1998). In addition, a sustained increase in the substrates available for colonic fermentation increases SCFA production as a result of bacterial adaptation. Use of glucose polymers or other modular carbohydrate supplements may be necessary to help to achieve the desired level of carbohydrate and energy intake.

Substituting long-chain triglyceride fat with MCT has also been shown to reduce faecal fat excretion in short bowel patients with colonic function (Jeppesen and Mortensen 1999). Malabsorbed long-chain fatty acids are not absorbed in the large intestine but medium-chain fatty acids are absorbed almost as effectively as SCFA. Fatty acid chain length is therefore an important consideration.

If, despite dietary and drug manipulation, steatorrhoea remains severe, temporary parenteral nutrition may be required to maintain nutritional status. A secondary consequence of steatorrhoea is a greater risk of calcium oxalate renal stones, due to increased colonic oxalate absorption and resultant hyperoxaluria (see Calcium stones in Section 4.15.2). A low-oxalate diet may be advisable in these circumstances (Lennard-Jones 1994).

Dietary management of short bowel syndrome following ileal resection

The above considerations will determine the nutritional management of a particular individual, but the general principles can be summarized as:

- Immediately post-surgery, parenteral nutrition will be required. Close attention should be paid to fluid, electrolyte and trace element balance (especially sodium and magnesium since losses may be very high).
- In order to stimulate gut adaptation, enteral feeding should be introduced as soon as possible with patients gradually being transferred to oral fluids and nutrients while still receiving some parenteral support. Initially, the patient's oral fluid intake should not exceed 500 ml/day.
- When fluids are tolerated, small meals and snacks can gradually be introduced. Fat, fibre and lactose are most likely to cause problems of malabsorption and significant quantities of these should initially be avoided. Soluble fibre may be useful to slow transit time; feeds and supplements containing fructo-oligosaccharides (FOS) have been successfully used to reduce and thicken stomal output.
- Parenteral support can be reduced as oral intake increases. However, intravenous fluids and/or oral glucose-electrolyte solutions are likely to be needed to meet fluid and sodium requirements until gut adaptation takes place. Additional nutritional support in the form of supplements or overnight feeding is likely to be required.
- Electrolyte status should be carefully monitored and supplemented as necessary.
- As adaptation occurs, gradual transition to a more normal diet can be made, with inadequacies in nutrition or fluid being compensated by nutritional support measures if indicated. People with an intact colon usually benefit from a diet high in carbohydrate and reduced in fat and oxalate content.
- Since restoration of intestinal lactase levels is one of the last adaptive mechanisms to occur, large lactose loads may need to be avoided for a period of some weeks, possibly longer in some people.
- Iron, folate supplements and vitamin B_{12} injections may be required to prevent anaemia. Bile salt malabsorption should be controlled by the use of cholestyramine.

Close dietetic supervision of these patients is vital during the early stages until intestinal adaptation has taken place and the patient is able to take a nutritionally adequate diet. Manipulation of the diet and changes in drugs should be staged, with several days allowed for each stage, to assess the impact of each change on intestinal output. Each patient is different and will need a lot of time and patience to find the combination which suits them. Short bowel patients benefit from a team approach with close liaison between doctors, nurses (especially the stoma nurse), dietitian and pharmacist.

Long-term nutritional monitoring should review:

- the severity of malabsorptive symptoms
- hydration and electrolyte status
- anthropometric status, particularly changes in body weight and body mass index (BMI)
- adequacy of nutritional intake
- micronutrient status, particularly that of magnesium, zinc, folate, iron and vitamin D.

Nutritional supplements or other support measures may be required if there is significant evidence of malnutrition. Severe symptoms of malabsorption such as profuse diarrhoea may necessitate resumption of parenteral support to maintain hydration and electrolyte status.

4.12.2 Resection of the large intestine

Until relatively recently, resection of the colon and rectum resulted in the creation of a permanent stomal exit, either an ileostomy (following complete removal of the colon and rectum) or a colostomy (after removal of the terminal segment of the colon and rectum). Intestinal effluent is collected in a bag fixed on to the stoma. These procedures are still performed if carcinogenic disease requires such extensive rectal resection that no functioning muscle tissue in the anal area remains.

However, where possible, panproctocolectomy with permanent ileostomy is increasingly being replaced by restorative proctocolectomy, a procedure which involves the creation of a pouch reservoir from a segment of ileum which is then joined to the anus. The pouch acts as an artificial rectum, thus conserving anal continence and avoiding the need for an external bag. This technique is commonly used to treat patients with ulcerative colitis or familial adenomatous polyposis and is much more acceptable to patients than a permanent ileostomy.

Ileal pouches derive their names from the number of limbs of ileum used in their fashioning (J-pouch, S-pouch and W-pouch). The surgical procedures which anastomose these different pouch types to the anal canal [ileal pouch – anal anastomosis (IPAA)] share common methodology. Ileal reservoirs can also be constructed without IPAA (e.g. the continent ileal reservoir or Kock pouch).

Pouch creation is complex and the operation is often done in two, or sometimes three, stages. Firstly, it involves colectomy (removal of the colon) and proctectomy (removal of diseased rectal mucosa), leaving the rectal muscular cuff and anal sphincter intact. A pseudorectum (pouch) is constructed by joining a portion of the terminal ileum to the anal canal and a temporary ileostomy created to divert bowel contents away from the newly formed pouch, allowing it to heal. A further operation then anastomoses the pouch to the intestine and reverses the ileostomy.

Following surgery, problems with stool frequency and/or consistency are likely to occur but continence is usually achieved after 10 days and, over a period of about 1 year, the pouch gradually adapts, with bowel movements becoming less frequent and more solid in consistency.

Nutritional implications of proctocolectomy with pouch or ileostomy creation

Removal of the colon results in considerable loss of absorptive capacity in respect of fluids and electrolytes, especially sodium. Initially, considerable quantities of both electrolytes and fluid will be lost (1200–2000 ml/day) and requirements for both will be increased for at least 6–8 weeks. After this time, the ileum appears to adapt and losses decrease, although will still remain in the order of 400–600 ml/day. However, in contrast to cases with accompanying ileal resection (see above), the digestive and absorptive capacity of the small intestine remains, so nutrient malabsorption is less likely to occur.

While the ileum is adapting and stools and stomal effluent remain liquid, fluid losses should be replaced by the consumption of not less than 1.5–2 litres fluid/day. Additional salt (e.g. up to one teaspoon added to food during the course of a day) may be necessary in hot weather or if excretal losses are particularly high. As the stool frequency and consistency improve, losses will decrease but it remains important to ensure fluid and salt adequacy. An episode of vomiting or diarrhoea can rapidly create an electrolyte imbalance, and extra potassium (via fruit juices) and sodium (via extra salt on food or salty beverages such as soup or meat extracts) is advisable. In severe cases, more intensive rehydration measures may be necessary.

Gradually, the range of foods consumed can be increased and patients encouraged to follow as normal a diet as possible. No foods are specifically contraindicated for ileostomy or pouch patients, but some foods can cause unpleasant symptoms such as stool odour or flatulence. Blockage, particularly of stomal exits, with undigested food residues can occur, especially if the anastomosis is tight. Occasionally a low-residue diet is required if obstruction regularly occurs. However, in most people this is unnecessary and avoidance of the few specific foods which typically cause the problem is sufficient to prevent it. There is little documented evidence on food-related problems in ileostomy/pouch patients, but commonly reported associations include:

- poorly digested foods (and most likely to cause blockage): mushrooms, sweetcorn, fruit or vegetable skins, lentils, peas, nuts, seeds, tomatoes, coconut, fibrous fruit and vegetables such as celery or pineapple, Chinese food;
- increased stool odour: onions, garlic, brassica vegetables (Brussels sprouts, cabbage, cauliflower and broccoli), beans, fish, eggs;

- increased flatulence/bloating: baked beans, lentils, peas, onions, garlic, brassica vegetables, fizzy drinks, beer and lager;
- increased stool frequency: fruit, fruit juice, vegetables, wine, beer, fried food, spicy food.

However, it should be borne in mind that individual tolerance may vary considerably, so people should be encouraged to discover for themselves on a trial-and-error basis which foods are best tolerated. They should also be warned that foods such as beetroot can change the colour of the stool to such an extent that it can be mistaken for bleeding.

Continuing problems with stool frequency may be treated with loperamide. Thirlby and Kelly (1997) found no evidence that supplementary fibre in the form of pectin or methylcellulose is helpful in this respect.

It should not be overlooked that many patients will be nutritionally depleted after colorectal surgery, particularly if they suffered chronic ill health beforehand and food intake was poor. If, as in the case of pouch patients, two, or even three, operations are required, this is a further strain on nutritional status. It will also take some time before normal appetite is restored. It is therefore important that patients are encouraged to consume small, frequent nutrient-dense meals and snacks and that additional oral nutritional support measures are instituted when necessary (see Section 1.12, Oral nutritional support).

Much less is known about the nutritional and metabolic implications of pouch procedures than those resulting in ileostomy (Tang 1997), but the long-term consequences in terms of faecal volume and chemistry appear to be similar in patients after restorative proctocolectomy with J-pouch and those with conventional panproctocolectomy and permanent ileostomy (Christie *et al.* 1990). However, owing to the kidney's attempt to conserve water and sodium, both groups of patients are at greater risk of uric acid stones as a result of producing urine which is low in volume and pH, and with a high concentration of calcium and oxalate compared with control subjects (Christie *et al.* 1996). J-pouch patients may additionally be at increased risk of calcium stones and abnormal bile acid metabolism.

Dietary guidance for ileostomy or pouch patients

Since the effects of proctocolectomy are broadly the same in both groups of patients, dietary guidance for ileostomy and pouch patients is similar. People should be encouraged to:

- adopt a regular meal pattern: some people may need smaller meals more frequently. Those with pouches may need to avoid eating late at night to avoid nocturnal stool production
- eat a varied, well-balanced diet
- consume meals slowly and chew foods well

- only avoid foods which cause unpleasant symptoms such as excessive flatulence, odour, unacceptable stool consistency or blockage
- drink plenty of fluids (not less than 6–8 cups/day) and more in hot weather
- consume extra fluid and salt if stool or stoma losses suddenly increase or during episodes of vomiting or fever. Medical advice may be needed if these losses are severe or persistent. Patients with pouches should be additionally warned of the symptoms of pouchitis and may be prescribed metronidazole for this eventuality.

All patients should receive regular dietary follow-up to ensure that diet-related problems are remedied, unnecessary food restrictions are avoided and good nutritional status is maintained via a well-balanced diet.

Text revised by: Briony Thomas

Acknowledgements: Helen Reilly and Carole Middleton

Useful address

IA (formerly the Ileostomy Association, now the Ileostomy and Internal Pouch Support Group)
PO Box 132, Scunthorpe DN15 9YW
Tel: 01724 720150
Helpline: 0800 018 4724
Website: www.ileostomypouch.demon.co.uk

References

Christie PM, Knight GS, Hill GL. Metabolism of body water and electrolytes after surgery for ulcerative colitis: conventional ileostomy versus J pouch. *British Journal of Surgery* 1990; **77**: 149–151.

Christie PM, Knight GS, Hill GL. Comparison of relative risks of urinary stone formation after surgery for ulcerative colitis: conventional ileostomy vs J-pouch. a comparative study. *Diseases of the Colon and Rectum* 1996; **39**: 50–54.

Jeppesen PB, Mortensen PB. Colonic digestion and absorption of energy from carbohydrates and medium-chain fat in small bowel failure. *Journal of Parenteral and Enteral Nutrition* 1999; **23** (5 Suppl): S101–S105.

Lennard-Jones JE. Oral rehydration solutions in short bowel syndrome. *Clinical Therapeutics* 1990; **12** (Suppl A): 138.

Lennard-Jones JE. Review article: practical management of the short bowel. *Alimentary Pharmacology and Therapeutics* 1994; **8**: 563–577.

Lennard-Jones JE, Wood S. Coping with the short bowel. *Hospital Update* 1991; October.

Nightingale JM, Lennard-Jones JE. The short bowel syndrome: what's new and old. *Digestive Diseases* 1993; **11**: 12–31.

Nightingale JM, Lennard-Jones JE, Walker ER, Farthing MJ. Oral salt supplements to compensate for jejunostomy losses: comparison of sodium chloride capsules, glucose electrolyte solution and glucose polymer electrolyte solution. *Gut* 1992; **33**: 759–761.

Noorgaard I. What's new in the role of the colon as a digestive organ in patients with short bowel syndrome? *Nutrition* 1998; **14**: 468–469.

Powell-Tuck J. Management of gut failure: a physician's view. *Lancet* 1994; **344**: 1061–1065.

Tang H. *Dietary Survey Among Subjects with Continent Ileal Reservoir with or without Ileal Pouch Anal Anastomosis*. Final year dissertation, School of Biological Sciences, University of Surrey, Guildford, 1997.

Thirby RC, Kelly R. Pectin and methylcellulose do not affect intestinal function in patients after ileal pouch – anal anastomosis. *American Journal of Gastroenterology* 1997; **92**: 99–102.

4.13 Liver and biliary disease

Nutritional support plays a major role in the clinical management of patients with liver and biliary disease. The objectives of nutritional support are to provide nutrients in the correct quantity and form, to restore and maintain nutritional status, correct specific deficiencies, treat clinical symptoms and promote hepatocyte regeneration.

Although there have been many recent advances in the medical aspects of liver disease, less attention has been given to nutritional management. However, it is widely recognized that malnutrition adversely affects outcome in both chronic and acute liver disease and that nutritional deficiencies commonly arise in patients with chronic hepatobiliary disease (Mendenhall *et al.* 1986; Lautz *et al.* 1992; Pikul *et al.* 1994; Merli *et al.* 1996).

The nutritional management of patients with liver disease is primarily concerned with ensuring that their nutrient intake meets requirements which are often increased. The specific dietary modifications which are needed in some patients to treat the complications of liver disease, for example, fluid retention and hepatic encephalopathy, are of secondary importance. This change in emphasis away from dietary restrictions and towards nutrition support has been brought about by an increasing awareness that some traditional dietary regimens are not evidence-based and may be associated with the impairment of nutri-

tional status (Madden 1992; Soulsby *et al.* 1997; Soulsby and Morgan 1999).

4.13.1 Anatomy and function of the liver

The liver is the largest organ in the body and comprises one-fiftieth of the total body weight. The liver has a double blood supply: the hepatic artery supplies the liver with arterial blood and the portal vein brings venous blood from the intestines and the spleen.

The liver cells (hepatocytes) comprise about 60% of the total liver weight. Bile canaliculi form a network between the hepatocytes, allowing bile produced in the liver to pass into the common hepatic duct before travelling via the cystic duct to the gall bladder for concentration and storage, or into the duodenum via the common bile duct.

The liver plays a central role in many essential body functions, including the metabolism of nutrients (Table 4.13). Irrespective of its aetiology, liver disease may impair nutritional function; the degree of nutritional impairment is related to the severity and duration of the liver disease.

4.13.2 Classification of liver disease

Liver disease is often categorized as either acute or

Table 4.13 Major functions of the liver

Digestion	Bile acid production
Carbohydrate metabolism	Maintenance of glucose homoeostasis
	Storage of glycogen
	Mobilization of glucose in response to hypoglycaemia
Protein metabolism	Utilization of amino acids for protein synthesis and gluconeogenesis
	Deamination of amino acids into urea for excretion
	Regulation of amino acid supply to peripheral tissues
	Synthesis of plasma albumin, prothrombin, fibrinogen and clotting factors
Lipids and lipoproteins	Production of triglycerides and lipoprotein formation
	Synthesis of phospholipids and cholesterol
	NEFA synthesis and degradation.
	Ketogenesis
Vitamins	Storage of vitamins A, B_2, B_3, B_6, B_{12}, K, folate
	Synthesis of prothrombin and factor VII requiring vitamin K
	Conversion of tryptophan to nicotinic acid
	Hydroxylation of vitamin D
Detoxification/deactivation	Oxidation of alcohol $\rightarrow$ acetaldehyde $\rightarrow$ acetate $\rightarrow$ CO_2 + fatty acids + H_2O
	Deactivation of drugs in the cytochrome P450 system
	Conjugation of oestrogens, corticosteroids and other steroid hormones for excretion
Excretion	Excretion of porphyrins, drugs, environmental toxins and heavy metals via bile secretion
Immune function	Cytokine production
	Kupffer cell formation (mononuclear phagocyte system)
Haematological function	Synthesis of haem
	Regulation of iron metabolism

Table 4.14 Some causes of acute liver disease

Viral infections	Virus A, B, D, E, G
	Epstein–Barr virus
	Cytomegalovirus
	Yellow fever virus
Alcohol	Alcoholic hepatitis
Drugs	Paracetamol
	Halothane
Non-viral infections	Toxoplasmosis
	Leptospira
Poison	*Amanita phalloides*
	Aflatoxin
	Carbon tetrachloride
Other	Acute fatty liver of pregnancy
	Wilson's disease

Table 4.15 Some causes of chronic liver disease.

Alcohol	
Infections	Viral hepatitis B, C, D
	Schistosomiasis
Autoimmune	Chronic active hepatitis
	Primary biliary cirrhosis
Metabolic disorders	Wilson's disease
	Haemochromatosis
	Alpha1-antitrypsin deficiency
	Type IV glycogen storage disease
	Organic acidaemias
	Abetalipoproteinaemia
	Porphyria
Drugs	Methotrexate
	Methyldopa
	Isoniazid
Biliary obstruction	Atresia
	Bile-duct occlusion by gall stones or strictures
	Sclerosing cholangitis
Vascular disorders	Chronic right heart failure
	Budd–Chiari syndrome
	Veno-occlusive disease
Miscellaneous	Neonatal hepatitis syndrome
	Intestinal bypass
	Sarcoidosis
	Cystic fibrosis
	Carolis syndrome
Cryptogenic	Unknown aetiology

chronic. An acute episode may also be superimposed on pre-existing chronic disease.

Acute liver disease

This may be caused by viruses, alcohol, drugs or other toxins (Table 4.14). Development of severe hepatic dysfunction occurs within 6 months of the first symptoms and in the absence of any pre-existing liver disease. When these features develop very quickly (within 8 weeks of the first symptoms), the condition is described as fulminant hepatic failure (FHF). This condition is rare but requires intensive nutritional support and has a high mortality rate; patients who survive FHF usually make a full recovery (Katelaris and Jones 1989).

Chronic liver disease

This may be caused by a variety of agents (Table 4.15) including alcohol, infections such as viral hepatitis and autoimmune disease. Chronic liver disease may give rise to cirrhosis, which reflects a state of irreversible liver damage characterized by fibrosis, nodular regeneration and disturbance of normal hepatic architecture. The severity of the cirrhosis is graded using Pugh's modification of Child's classification (Pugh *et al.* 1973; Table 4.16).

Cirrhosis does not always cause symptoms, in which case it is said to be well compensated, i.e. although the liver is damaged, it is still able to function adequately and the patient's condition is stable. However, further insults to the

liver, for example infection, gastrointestinal bleeding, dehydration or continued alcohol abuse may lead to decompensation and a number of complications including fluid retention and encephalopathy.

4.13.3 Nutritional assessment of patients with liver disease

Nutritional status must be assessed before initiating nutritional support. Regular evaluation is also necessary to monitor the effects of dietary intervention and ensure that deficiencies do not arise as a result of inadequate or ill-conceived dietary advice. It is difficult to assess nutritional status in these patients as liver disease may influence the validity and interpretation of standard tests. However, a satisfactory and useful evaluation can be made by combining the results from a clinical and diet history, a physical examination and anthropometric measurements.

Table 4.16 Severity of cirrhosis using Pugh's modification of Child's classification (Pugh *et al.* 1973)

Variable	Score 1	Score 2	Score 3
Bilirubin (μmol/l)	$\leqslant 33$	34–51	$\geqslant 52$
Albumin (g/l)	$\geqslant 36$	28–35	$\leqslant 27$
Prothrombin (s)	$\leqslant 16$	17–19	$\geqslant 20$
Ascites	None	Mild	Moderate/severe
Encephalopathy	None (EEG $\geqslant 7.5$ c/s)	Grade I/II (EEG 5.6–7.4 c/s)	Grade III/IV (EEG $\leqslant 5.5$ c/s)

Each of the variables is scored between 1 and 3 and the sum of the numbers calculated to provide a score within a range of 5–15. Patients scoring less than 7 (grade A) are generally well, between 7 and 9 (grade B) are moderately unwell and above 9 (grade C) are severely ill.
EEG: electroencephalogram.

A global assessment scheme incorporating these variables has been externally validated in patients with chronic liver disease and shown to be reliable (Madden *et al.* 1997):

- *Clinical observation* will indicate the presence of muscle wasting, loss of subcutaneous fat and the presence of ascites, oedema and jaundice. A history of the presenting complaint will give an indication of the duration and severity of the patient's illness and should include details of any recent weight changes and whether these reflect fluctuations in fluid retention or lean tissue. Patients who report a gain in weight associated with an increase in abdominal girth and swollen lower limbs often recognize that they are also losing 'flesh' even though they are becoming heavier.
- *A diet history* should be obtained, although in some patients with alcoholic liver disease this may be unreliable; relatives may be able to provide some clarification (Watson *et al.* 1984). Nevertheless, even a rough guide will facilitate the identification of nutrient deficiencies and serve as a useful guide for meal planning. When evaluating the adequacy of intake it must be borne in mind that most patients with liver disease have increased nutritional requirements.
- *Anthropometric measurements*: height and weight must be measured. In the presence of ascites and/or oedema an approximate 'dry weight' may be estimated by deducting an estimated weight for fluid retention. This figure should be derived using published guidelines (Mendenhall 1992) (Table 4.17), previously known accurate weight and clinical judgement. Although of limited accuracy in itself, an estimated dry weight will facilitate the calculation of an approximate body mass index (BMI) value and provide some indication of current body stores. Mid-arm circumference and triceps skinfold thickness (TSF) should be measured, and mid-arm muscle circumference (MAMC) calculated and compared with reference values (Bishop *et al.* 1981). Although peripheral oedema may confound the measurement of skinfold thickness, this is rarely a problem in upper arm anthropometry which, in the practized observer, provides one of the most useful and reliable measures of nutritional status in this patient population. TSF and MAMC measurements should be repeated at regular intervals to assess change
- *Biochemical values* must be interpreted with extreme caution. The transport proteins, including albumin, transferrin and retinol binding protein, are synthesized in the liver and, therefore, in the presence of liver disease are invalid markers of nutritional status. Hepa-

torenal failure and a compromised urinary output may affect the validity of nitrogen balance, while a low urinary creatinine excretion may reflect reduced hepatic degradation of its precursor, creatine, rather than loss of muscle. Laboratory evaluation of trace element and vitamin status is difficult and rarely available. Biochemical variables should not be used to assess nutritional status.

4.13.4 General nutritional aspects of liver and biliary disease

Malnutrition

Patients with chronic liver disease are often malnourished. The prevalence of malnutrition observed in this patient population varies between 10 and 100% (McCullough and Tavill 1991; Müller 1995; Kalman and Saltzman 1996). The severity of malnutrition is closely associated with the severity, length and clinical manifestations of the liver disease (Italian Multicentre Project 1994). In addition to the usual causes of malnutrition, the nutritional status of patients with liver disease may be adversely affected by the complications of the disease process itself, including hypermetabolism, ascites, encephalopathy, variceal bleeding and steatorrhoea, and also by the negative effects of inappropriate dietary advice (Table 4.18).

Energy and protein requirements

There is limited but increasing evidence to show that adults with liver disease have altered requirements of energy and protein. Few studies have evaluated total energy expenditure in this patient population but measurements of resting energy expenditure show a greater deviation from predicted values (Harris and Benedict 1919; Schofield 1985) than would be expected in a healthy population with more than 50% of patients outside the $\pm$ 10% range (Müller *et al.* 1992; Madden and Morgan 1999a). Although both hypometabolism and hypermetabolism exist in patients with chronic liver disease, increased resting energy expenditure has been more widely reported (Green *et al.* 1991; Campillo *et al.* 1992; Chang *et al.* 1997; Müller *et al.* 1999) and, consequently, energy intakes of

Table 4.17 Guidelines for estimating fluid weight in patients with ascites and peripheral oedema (Mendenhall 1992)

	Ascites	Oedema
Minimal	2.2 kg	1.0 kg
Moderate	6.0 kg	5.0 kg
Severe	14.0 kg	10.0 kg

Table 4.18 Factors adversely affecting nutritional status in patients with liver disease

Ascites, oedema
Encephalopathy
Steatorrhoea, diarrhoea
Hypermetabolism
Anorexia
Vomiting, nausea
Gastrointestinal bleeding
Alcohol withdrawal
Altered taste sensation
Inappropriate dietary advice
Unpalatable diets and treatment
Repeated investigations

up to 40 kcal/kg/day have been recommended (Plauth *et al.* 1997) (Table 4.19). Protein requirements have been clearly demonstrated to be increased in adults with chronic liver disease and are substantially higher than in healthy individuals (Swart *et al.* 1989a; Nielsen *et al.* 1995; Kondrup and Müller 1997) (Table 4.19).

Micronutrient requirements

All patients with liver disease may be at risk from frank or subclinical deficiencies of vitamins, minerals and trace elements, irrespective of the aetiology of their condition. However, limited work has been undertaken to elucidate the optimum requirements in this patient population. While circulating concentrations of specific micronutrients can be measured, the results must be interpreted with caution as circulating levels may not reflect tissue stores, plasma binding may be abnormal and function may be impaired by the deficiency of cofactors. As a result, multivitamin therapy, which is cheap and harmless if recommended doses are not exceeded, should be instigated. The administration of single agents should be avoided unless there is good evidence for a specific need, and then care should be taken to ensure that all other micronutrients are provided in adequate quantities.

Route of feeding

Nutrient intake should be provided orally wherever possible, supplemented, if necessary, by enteral tube feeding. Parenteral nutrition should only be used on the rare occasions when the gastrointestinal tract is non-functioning or inaccessible.

Oral supplementation

Standard sip feeds can be used to augment the nutrient intake of patients with uncomplicated liver disease. Monitoring of total nutrient intake should be undertaken regularly and consideration given to increased energy and protein requirements (see above).

Enteral feeding

Patients who have a functioning gut but are unable to consume an adequate oral intake should be tube fed (see Section 1.13.2, Enteral feeding). Standard 1 kcal/ml polymeric feeds are suitable for use in uncomplicated liver disease, but high-energy feeds, providing 1.5–2.0 kcal/ml, are preferable if patients are fluid restricted or have increased requirements. Enteral feeding is not precluded by the complications of liver disease, for example ascites, encephalopathy and varices (see below), and early instigation of an adequate feeding regimen is essential in patients with these problems. The initiation and increase in rate of enteral feeding should proceed in accordance with standard local feeding policies; routine monitoring procedures should be undertaken.

Table 4.19 Energy and protein intakes in chronic liver disease recommended by the ESPEN Consensus Group (Plauth *et al.* 1997)

Clinical condition	Non-protein energy (kcal/kg/day)	Protein (g/kg/day)
Compensated cirrhosis	25–35	1.0–1.2
Inadequate intake/ malnutrition	35–40	1.5
Encephalopathy grade I–II	25–35	Transiently 0.5, then 1.0–1.5
Encephalopathy grade III–IV	25–35	0.5–1.2

Parenteral nutrition

Parenteral nutrition should be reserved for patients who cannot be fed or fed adequately via the gastrointestinal tract. If patients with liver disease fulfil these criteria, parenteral support must be commenced. Standard regimens which provide energy in the form of 50% carbohydrate and 50% lipid should be used (Muscaritoli *et al.* 1986; Forbes and Wicks 1990). Nitrogen can be provided as either standard L-amino acids or branched-chain amino acids (BCAA); there is no evidence that BCAA formulae are nutritionally superior to (Plauth *et al.* 1997) or more effective in the management of hepatic encephalopathy than standard regimens (Morgan 1999). Volume and electrolyte provision may require restriction in some patients and should be decided on an individual basis.

Liver dysfunction may occur secondary to parenteral nutrition in patients with no previous history of hepatic disease. This may be manifest as increased serum concentrations of aspartate transaminase, alkaline phosphatase and bilirubin, fatty infiltration of the hepatocytes and intrahepatic cholestasis; in some cases, death may ensue. The risk of such complications may be reduced by avoiding the administration of excessive calories and, in particular, limiting the infusion of large amounts of glucose (Fisher 1989; Buchmiller *et al.* 1993).

4.13.5 Management of specific aspects of liver and biliary disease

Ascites

Ascites is the presence of a protein-rich fluid in the peritoneal cavity and is a common feature of liver disease caused by portal hypertension (increased pressure in the portal vein). The volume of ascitic fluid may exceed 25 litres in some patients, causing gross abdominal distension and severe discomfort, and compromising respiration, mobility and food intake. Ascites may be accompanied by oedema and, in up to 6% of patients, a pleural effusion.

Ascites may develop slowly over the course of several months or suddenly owing to decompensation of liver function, for example as a result of a variceal bleed or infection. Hospital admission is usually necessary for evaluation and treatment.

Patients with ascites are often malnourished and, as a consequence of severe abdominal distension, frequently have an inadequate intake (Wicks *et al.* 1995). Treatment consists of sodium restriction, diuretic therapy, paracentesis and bed rest.

Sodium restriction

While sodium restriction alone may not be effective in treating ascites, it will enhance and hasten the effects of diuretics. Levels of restriction vary between a low-sodium diet of 40 mmol Na$^+$/day and a No Added Salt regimen providing up to 100 mmol Na$^+$/day (Table 4.20). Restrictions below 40 mmol Na$^+$/day are rarely required even in the presence of gross ascites and, because of the detrimental effects on nutrient intake (Soulsby *et al.* 1997), should not be advocated for long-term use. If such diets are advised, it should be for a limited period and managed under strict hospital supervision so that the adequacy of nutrient intake and its effect on nutritional status can be closely monitored.

In some centres, total fluid intake may be restricted to between 1 and 1.5 litres per day, while in others up to 1.5 litres of oral fluid may be permitted in addition to prescribed intravenous fluid. Changes in fluid retention should be monitored using accurate fluid balance charts and by weighing the patients daily in minimal clothing at approximately the same time of day using the same scales. Serial measurements of abdominal girth may also be useful providing care is taken to standardize the measurement technique. Changes in serum sodium concentrations should not be used as an indication to modify dietary intake; concentrations below the lower limits of the reference range may have serious consequences and require medical rather than dietetic intervention. As with all critically ill patients, the optimum care of those with severe ascites requires close collaboration with medical colleagues.

Salt substitutes consisting of potassium compounds, for example Ruthmol (Larkhall Natural Health, Trowbridge, UK), are available and can be used to add flavour and improve palatability of a low-sodium diet. However, careful monitoring of serum potassium concentration is required and the use of salt substitutes is contraindicated in patients with hyperkalaemia and hepatorenal syndrome. All patients should be advised to avoid Lo Salt (Klinge, East Kilbride, UK) and other preparations which contain a substantial amount of sodium.

Prescribed and 'over-the-counter' medication, in particular antacids, effervescent tablets and some antibiotics, may also contribute a significant intake of sodium. The hospital pharmacist can advise on suitable alternatives.

The sodium content of most standard, 1 kcal/ml sip feeds, with the exception of some savoury flavours, does not exceed 4 mmol/100 ml of supplement and, therefore, small volumes can be incorporated into a No Added Salt restriction without exceeding the sodium restriction. However, severely ascitic patients with gross abdominal dis-

Table 4.20 Salt restricted diets.

No Added Salt
This restricts sodium intake to less than 100 mmol Na$^+$/day.
A pinch of salt may be used in cooking, but none should be added to food at the table.
The following foods must be avoided:
  Bacon, ham, sausages, paté
  Tinned fish and meat
  Smoked fish and meat
  Fish and meat pastes
  Tinned and packet soups
  Sauce mixes
  Tinned vegetables
  Bottled sauces and chutneys
  Meat and vegetable extracts, stock cubes
  Salted nuts and crisps
  Soya sauce
  Monosodium glutamate
  Cheese: up to 100 g/week
  Bread: up to four slices/day
40 mmol sodium diet
In addition to the foods listed above, the following restrictions apply:
  No salt to be used in cooking or at table
  Salt-free butter or margarine must be used
  Milk should be restricted to 300 ml/day
  Breakfast cereals must be salt free (e.g. Puffed Wheat, Shredded Wheat)

tension and a profoundly compromised food intake may require nutritional supplementation while restricted to a 40 mmol sodium diet. These patients require energy-dense supplements providing at least 2 kcal/ml with minimal sodium. Nepro (Abbott Laboratories, Maidenhead, UK) and Nutrison Concentrated LE (Nutricia, Trowbridge, UK) fulfil these criteria and can be used as both an oral supplement and an enteral feed. Alternatively, a standard feed supplemented with glucose polymers and/or a liquid fat source, or a home-made feed based on specific nutrient modules may be prepared for individual oral use. The adequacy of vitamin, mineral and trace element content must be considered.

Diuretics

The aim of diuretic therapy is to block sodium-conserving mechanisms within the kidney. Potassium-sparing diuretics, such as spironolactone and amiloride, are used initially but some patients with resistant ascites may also require a powerful loop diuretic such as frusemide or bumetanide. Body weight must be monitored daily during diuretic therapy to ensure that weight loss does not exceed 1 kg/day. Rapid fluid loss may precipitate complications such as hepatorenal syndrome, encephalopathy and electrolyte disturbance.

Paracentesis

Paracentesis is the therapeutic drainage of ascites from the abdomen using a transabdominal catheter. The volume of ascitic fluid removed may vary from 20 ml for diagnostic purposes to volumes exceeding 20 litres to relieve abdominal distension. In order to maintain the circulating blood volume and prevent rapid shifts of body fluid and hypovolaemic shock that would otherwise accompany large volume paracentesis, intravenous salt-poor albumin is infused simultaneously with drainage (Runyon 1997; Arroyo *et al.* 1999). The therapeutic benefits of large-volume paracentesis are immediate, with improvements in appetite, mobility and sense of well-being. However, the long-term nutritional consequences of repeated paracentesis have not been evaluated. It is unlikely that the protein content of the infused albumin adequately replaces that lost in the drained ascitic fluid, which may be as high as 60 g/l (Ginés *et al.* 1987), and over several months the net protein loss may be significant. It is, therefore, essential that the nutrient intake and protein stores of patients undergoing frequent large volume paracentesis are regularly assessed and that they are advised to increase their dietary protein intake.

Bed rest

Patients with moderate and severe ascites require bed rest to increase renal perfusion and maximize diuresis.

Other treatment

A small number of patients with refractory ascites but good hepatic function may undergo insertion of a Leveen shunt which connects the peritoneal cavity with the jugular vein, thus facilitating the internal recycling of ascitic fluid. Dietary sodium restriction should be relaxed if the shunt is functioning.

Hepatic encephalopathy

The term encephalopathy, or portal systemic encephalopathy (PSE), refers to a wide range of neuropsychiatric signs and symptoms which are associated with both chronic and acute liver disease. There is no consensus about the pathogenesis of hepatic encephalopathy, although three interrelated concepts are thought to be involved (Blei 1999):

- circulating neurotoxins which derive from the gastrointestinal tract
- neuroanatomical modification in the brain
- alterations in neurotransmission.

Encephalopathy may be either a chronic problem or arise acutely in response to precipitating factors (Table 4.21). Therapy consists of removing or treating the precipitants,

Table 4.21 Factors precipitating hepatic encephalopathy.

Gastrointestinal/variceal haemorrhage
Portocaval shunts
Infection
Diuretic therapy with or without electrolyte/fluid abnormalities
Drugs, e.g. sedatives
Constipation
Surgery
Diarrhoea/vomiting
Alcohol binge

bowel cleansing with enemata and medication with non-absorbable disaccharides such as lactulose. Dietary protein restriction, which was once considered a central pillar of treatment, is no longer considered optimum therapy.

Dietary treatment of encephalopathy.

Low-protein diets were first introduced in the 1950s in response to the implication of nitrogenous substances in the pathogenesis of encephalopathy (Sherlock *et al.* 1954). However, considerable variation was observed in the degree of tolerance of dietary protein and although only a small minority of patients were considered to be truly protein intolerant, dietary protein restriction became widespread. The subsequent development of non-absorbable antibiotics and disaccharides in the 1950s and 1960s provided effective alternative treatment for encephalopathy and yet low-protein diets continued to be widely advocated and strictly implemented. A growing awareness of the high prevalence of malnutrition in patients with chronic liver disease (Mendelhall *et al.* 1986; Lautz *et al.* 1992; Italian Multicentre Project 1994), the association between nutritional status and clinical outcome (Merli *et al.* 1996) and the accumulating evidence of increased protein requirements (Swart *et al.* 1989a; Nielsen *et al.* 1995; Kondrup and Müller 1997) brought about a questioning of routine protein restriction (Soulsby and Morgan 1999). There is increasing evidence that patients with hepatic encephalopathy can tolerate intakes of up to 100 g protein/day without exacerbation of their symptoms and that supplemented patients receiving a higher protein intake actually show a significant improvement in their mental symptoms compared with unsupplemented patients (Kearns *et al.* 1992; Morgan *et al.* 1995).

This evidence is reflected in the ESPEN guidelines for recommended protein intakes (Table 4.19). The recommendation of 0.5 g protein/kg body weight should be undertaken for a very limited period and only until an acute episode of hepatic encephalopathy resolves. If the patient is acutely ill, for example after a variceal bleed, they may remain without nutritional support for 24–48 hours and thus effectively be protein restricted for this period. On commencement of nutritional support it is, therefore, inappropriate to impose additional restrictions, and protein intake should be increased steadily to a target of 1.2 g/kg/day. Standard or high-energy enteral feeds should be used if patients require nasogastric feeding.

Truly protein-intolerant patients are rarely encountered; although it is difficult to provide exact figures, it is likely that most specialist liver centres will treat fewer than two such patients per year. Dietary manipulation rather than restriction may limit the need to impose strict low-protein regimens. Dairy and vegetable-derived protein may be tolerated better than meat protein (Fenton *et al.* 1966; Greenburger 1977; Bianchi *et al.* 1993) and a high-fibre diet will help to ensure that gastrointestinal transit time is reduced. Encouraging several smaller meals and a bedtime snack rather than a few larger meals may improve protein tolerance and optimize energy and nitrogen metabolism (Swart *et al.* 1989b; Zillikens *et al.* 1993; Verboeket-van de Venne *et al.* 1995; Chang *et al.* 1997). There is evidence that patients with cirrhosis already tend to follow this eating pattern (Madden and Morgan 1999b).

The use of BCAA in the treatment of encephalopathy remains controversial (Morgan 1991). A large number of studies have been undertaken to investigate the effects of BCAA, with varying results, and a recent meta-analysis was unsuccessful because insufficient data were available (Fabbri *et al.* 1996). Consequently, no recommendations can be made for the use of BCAA as treatment for encephalopathy. If they are used at all, they should be reserved for malnourished cirrhotic patients with hepatic encephalopathy who are unable to tolerate an adequate protein intake using the dietary manipulations described above.

Steatorrhoea

Bile is required for the emulsification of dietary fat, and bile acids act as cofactors for digestive lipases, protecting them from the proteolytic effects of other digestive enzymes (Carey and Hernell 1992). Fat malabsorption may occur if secretion of bile is significantly impaired (cholestasis). However, although up to 50% of adults with chronic liver disease have increased faecal fat excretion, far fewer experience steatorrhoea. The need to restrict dietary fat intake is, therefore, limited to a small minority of patients.

Dietary treatment of steatorrhoea

Malabsorption of dietary fat is idiosyncratic and highly individual. Patients should be initially advised to reduce their fat intake to approximately 20 g/day for 2 weeks so that any potential benefit from the diet can be confirmed. If malabsorption improves, dietary fat should be slowly reintroduced, with the patient keeping a food diary and recording their abdominal symptoms and bowel movements. A maintenance diet can then be developed by trial and error, supported by flexible advice. Restricting dietary fat may lead to an inadequate intake of energy and other nutrients and, therefore, additional advice and supplementation are required:

- *Total energy*: Carbohydrate and protein intake should be increased and, if necessary, the energy density of the diet augmented with additional sugar, glucose polymers or medium-chain triglycerides (MCT) (see Appendix 6.7); if enteral feeding is required, an MCT-based feed should be used, e.g. Nutrison MCT (Nutricia Clinical, Trowbridge, UK) or Fresubin 750 MCT (Fresenius, Warrington, UK) and feeding commenced slowly.
- *Fat-soluble vitamins*: Replacement therapy should be given orally or by intramuscular injection, depending on the degree of fat malabsorption (Table 4.22). Circulating concentrations of vitamins A and D and prothrombin time (associated with vitamin K) should be monitored in adults. In addition, children require supplementation with vitamin E.

- *Essential fatty acids*: If total fat intake is limited, it must include a good source of essential fatty acids. Parenteral or topical administration has been advocated for the treatment of deficiency but there is little evidence to support this.
- *Calcium*: Supplementation may also be required (Epstein *et al.* 1982).

Gastrointestinal varices

Portal hypertension is frequently associated with the development of varices (enlarged veins) in the oesophagus, stomach and, occasionally, lower gastrointestinal tract. Variceal haemorrhage is an acute medical emergency and carries a high risk of mortality. Treatment may include temporary compression using a Sengstaken–Blakemore tube, infusion of vasoconstrictive medication, endoscopic banding, sclerotherapy or surgery.

Patients are kept 'nil by mouth' while varices are actively bleeding and often until their clinical condition stabilizes. However, an oral intake should be established as soon as possible. Although there is no evidence to show that eating rough foods, for example toast or biscuits, increases the incidence of rebleeding, patients may prefer to take a softer diet initially or for short periods after endoscopic treatment. Some individuals may need help to overcome fears that eating will provoke further haematemesis, and regular monitoring of nutritional status is essential.

Transient, occasionally severe, encephalopathy may occur after variceal bleeding in some patients, caused by the effects of large quantities of endogenous blood-derived protein in the gastrointestinal tract. Suppression of bleeding followed by enemata to remove residual blood is the principal treatment; protein restriction is not required.

The presence of varices is no longer considered a contraindication to enteral feeding, as fine-bore tubes are well tolerated (Nompleggi and Bonkovsky 1994). Although a recent study failed to demonstrate the theoretical benefit of commencing nasogastric feeding on the first day after variceal bleeding, no significant differences in the incidence of rebleeding, mortality or length of hospital stay were found between patients who were enterally fed and those permitted oral intake on the fourth day after

Table 4.22 Supplementation of fat-soluble vitamins in adults with chronic liver disease and cholestasis (Morgan 1999)

Vitamin	Route of administration	
	Oral	Intramuscular
A	25 000 IU daily	100 000 IU 3-monthly
D	400–4000 IU daily	100 000 IU monthly
E	Alpha-tocopherol acetate 50–200 IU/kg daily[1]	DL-Alpha-tocopherol 1–2 IU/kg daily, then at intervals
K	2.5–5.0 mg daily	10 mg monthly

[1]Paediatric dose.

bleeding (de Lédinghen *et al.* 1997). Further studies are needed.

Liver transplantation

Liver transplantation is now an established treatment for patients with end-stage liver disease and fulminant hepatic failure (Balan *et al.* 1999). The indications for transplantation include acute and chronic liver disease but vary between different centres (Table 4.23). There are seven supraregional liver transplant centres in the UK which are based in Birmingham, Cambridge, Edinburgh, Leeds, London (Kings College and Royal Free Hospitals) and Newcastle.

Transplant candidates must undergo a detailed nutritional assessment as part of their pre-surgery work-up. Such candidates are frequently malnourished and, therefore, at risk (Shaw *et al.* 1985; Pikul *et al.* 1994; Ricci *et al.* 1997; Selberg *et al.* 1997). The identification of an individual as malnourished should provide an opportunity to instigate active nutritional support if time before transplantation permits; malnutrition alone does not provide a reason for withholding surgery.

The management of the liver transplant patient in the immediate post-operative period is similar to that of any critically ill patient after major surgery. Ventilatory support and immunosuppressive therapy are required. Many patients undergoing elective transplantation make a prompt recovery and are able to recommence oral intake by the third post-operative day and rapidly progress to a full diet. Nutritional support varies greatly between transplant centres (Weimann *et al.* 1998), with some commencing early jejunal feeding, either as routine practice or in selected patients, and others instigating parenteral support within the first 48 hours, continuing until an adequate oral intake is achieved; in some cases, nutritional support is deferred until it is apparent that the reintroduction of oral nutrients will be delayed. Current available evidence shows that jejunal feeding within 24 hours of surgery is practical and safe and may reduce the incidence of infection (Wicks *et al.* 1994; Hasse *et al.* 1995; Mehta *et al.* 1995). However, the start of enteral feeding may be delayed until the fifth post-operative day in patients who have undergone a Roux-en-Y anastomosis. Although this may not be the case at all transplant centres, no reports of safety or efficacy have been undertaken and further investigation is required.

If parenteral nutrition is instigated at all, it should not be continued for longer than necessary because of the additional risk of infection in immunosuppressed patients. A high-protein, high-energy oral diet should be commenced as soon as possible, but if the appetite is slow to return and intake is inadequate, tube feeding may be indicated. Patients should be encouraged to consume a free diet and reassured that it is safe for them to do so; pre-transplant dietary restrictions are rarely required after surgery.

Hyperglycaemia is common during the first 4–5 post-operative days and is controlled by insulin; no dietary

Table 4.23 Indications for orthotopic liver transplantation

Chronic liver disease	Chronic active hepatitis
	Primary biliary cirrhosis
	Sclerosing cholangitis
	Viral hepatitis
	Haemochromatosis
Acute liver failure	Viral hepatitis
	Drug induced (e.g. paracetamol overdose)
Metabolic disorders	Wilson's disease
	Alpha-1-antitrypsin deficiency
	Glycogen storage disease
Biliary disease	Biliary atresia
Malignant disease	Unresectable primary hepatic and bile-duct malignancy

restriction is necessary. In some patients, steroid-induced diabetes may develop and additional dietary measures may then be needed. Increased appetite due to steroid therapy and the relaxation of dietary restrictions may result in excessive weight gain and appropriate advice should be given. Unless implicated in the diagnosis of the liver disease, alcohol may be consumed within recommended safe limits. Obesity and hyperlipidaemia are common long-term problems which may require dietetic intervention (Munoz *et al.* 1991; Palmer *et al.* 1991).

4.13.6 Management of particular types of liver and biliary disease

Primary biliary cirrhosis

In primary biliary cirrhosis (PBC) small intrahepatic bile ducts are progressively destroyed, probably by an immunological process, leading to cholestasis. The condition usually affects middle-aged women and is associated with jaundice, pruritus and steatorrhoea, which may be severe. Depending on their symptoms, patients may require dietary advice about fat malabsorption and appropriate nutritional support.

Wilson's disease

Wilson's disease is an inherited disorder characterized by abnormal copper transport and storage mechanisms which result in the excessive deposition of copper in tissues, including the liver, and cirrhosis may result. D-penicillamine is used as a chelating agent to remove excess copper and prevent further accumulation. Low copper diets are rarely used, although still advocated in many textbooks.

Haemochromatosis

Haemochromatosis is a genetically transmitted autosomal recessive disease characterized by the progressive deposition of iron in the liver and other organs. Treatment is by regular venesection; dietary iron should not be restricted.

Liver cancer

Benign tumours are rare. Malignant tumours, such as hepatocellular carcinoma, commonly arise as a complication of long-standing cirrhosis. Patients may be considered for liver transplantation, surgical resection or embolization and require nutritional support according to their symptoms. The liver is a common site of metastatic deposits; again, nutritional support and advice given should be according to the individual's need.

Cholangiocarcinoma

Tumours of the biliary tract can be extrahepatic or intrahepatic giving rise to severe jaundice. Palliative therapy for the former consists of passing a stent (a thin plastic tube) during endoscopic retrograde cholangiopancreatography (ERCP). A free diet should be encouraged and fat restricted only if patients are symptomatic. Malnutrition is common and nutritional support often required.

Primary sclerosing cholangitis

This condition results from the inflammation and fibrosis of the bile ducts leading to multiple areas of narrowing throughout the biliary system. The cause is unknown and 70% of patients have inflammatory bowel disease. Patients, who are predominantly young, are often malnourished and require active nutritional support and, in some cases, advice about fat malabsorption.

Gall stones

Gall stones may be asymptomatic or may present as either acute or chronic cholecystitis or obstruction of one of the bile ducts. Patients may present with gastrointestinal symptoms, jaundice or pain. While dietary factors and body weight influence biliary cholesterol secretion and hence the formation of some gall stones, there is no good evidence that dietary restrictions, particularly low-fat diets, play a role in the management of patients with existing gall stones (Madden 1992). A healthy diet should be recommended for chronic sufferers and obese patients encouraged to reduce their weight gradually. Patients with impacted or intrahepatic stones may be acutely ill and therefore require nutritional support until the problem can be treated by surgical or other means.

Paediatric liver and biliary disorders

The fundamental aim in the nutritional management of infants and children with liver and biliary disorders is, as in adults, to achieve an adequate nutrient intake while minimizing therapeutic dietary restrictions. However, the consequences of malnutrition in paediatric patients are exacerbated by their high nutrient requirements and the presence of relatively small fat and protein stores. Appropriate and prompt nutritional support is, therefore, essential. Specific details, in particular regarding inborn errors of metabolism, are described in *Clinical Paediatric Dietetics* (Shaw and Lawson 1994).

Text revised by: Angela Madden

Useful addresses

British Liver Trust, Ransomes Europark, Ipswich IP3 9QG
Tel: 0808 800 1000
E-mail: info@britishlivertrust.org.uk
Website: www.britishlivertrust.org.uk

The British Liver Trust is the only national charity supporting adults with all forms of liver disease. The Trust provides help through its telephone information line and a network of local support groups, and by funding ongoing research into liver disease. It also distributes a wide variety of information leaflets, including one entitled *Diet and Liver Disease* which was written and endorsed by State Registered Dietitians working in the field.

British Association for the Study of the Liver (BASL)
BASL Secretariat, Ransomes Europark, Ipswich IP3 9QG
Tele: 01473 276326

BASL is a multidisciplinary society involving scientists and clinicians and has approximately 350 members. It holds an annual meeting, usually in September, and awards travel bursaries for other international meetings.

References

Arroyo V, Ginés P, Planas R, Rodés J. Pathogenesis, diagnosis, and treatment of ascites in cirrhosis. In Bircher B, Benhamou JP, McIntyre N *et al.* (Eds) *Oxford Textbook of Clinical Hepatology*, 2nd edn, pp. 697–731. Oxford: Oxford University Press. 1999.

Balan V, Marsh JW, Rakela J. Liver transplantation. In Bircher B, Benhamou JP, McIntyre N *et al.* (Eds) *Oxford Textbook of Clinical Hepatology*, 2nd edn, pp. 2039–2063. Oxford: Oxford University Press, 1999.

Bianchi GP, Marchesini G, Fabbri A *et al.* Vegetable versus animal protein diet in cirrhotic patients with chronic encephalopathy. A randomized cross-over comparison. *Journal of Internal Medicine* 1993; **233**: 385–392.

Bishop CW, Bowen PE, Ritchey SJ. Norms for nutritional assessment of American adults by upper arm anthropometry. *American Journal of Clinical Nutrition* 1981; **34**: 2530–2539.

Blei AT. Hepatic encephalopathy. In Bircher B, Benhamou JP, McIntyre N *et al.* (Eds) *Oxford Textbook of Clinical Hepatology*, 2nd edn, pp. 765–783. Oxford: Oxford University Press, 1999.

Buchmiller CE, Kleiman-Wexler RL, Ephgrave KS *et al.* Liver dysfunction and energy source: results of a randomized clinical trial. *Journal of Parenteral and Enteral Nutrition* 1993; **17**: 301–306.

Campillo B, Bories PN, Devanlay M *et al.* The thermogenic and metabolic effects of food in liver cirrhosis: consequences on the storage of nutrients and the hormonal counterregulatory response. *Metabolism* 1992; **41**: 476–482.

Carey MC, Hernell O. Digestion and absorption of fat. *Seminars in Gastrointestinal Disease* 1992; **3**: 189–208.

Chang WK, Chao YC, Tang HS *et al.* Effects of extra-carbohydrate supplementation in the late evening on energy expenditure and substrate oxidation in patients with liver cirrhosis. *Journal of Parenteral and Enteral Nutrition* 1997; **21**: 96-99.

de Lédinghen V, Beau P, Mannant PR *et al.* Early feeding or enteral nutrition in patients with cirrhosis after bleeding from esophageal varices? A randomized controlled study. *Digestive Diseases and Sciences* 1997; **42**: 536–541.

Epstein O, Kato Y, Dick R, Sherlock S. Vitamin D, hydroxyapatite, and calcium gluconate in treatment of cortical bone thinning in postmenopausal women with primary biliary cirrhosis. *American Journal of Clinical Nutrition* 1982; **36**: 426–430.

Fabbri A, Magrini N, Bianchi G *et al.* Overview of randomized clinical trials of oral branched-chain amino acid treatment in chronic hepatic encephalopathy. *Journal of Parenteral and Enteral Nutrition* 1996; **20**: 159–164.

Fenton JCB, Knight EJ, Humpherson PL. Milk and cheese diet in portal-systemic encephalopathy. *Lancet* 1966; **i**: 164–165.

Fisher RL. Hepatobiliary abnormalities associated with total parenteral nutrition. *Gastroenterology Clinics of North America* 1989; **18**: 645–666.

Forbes A, Wicks C. Fulminant hepatic failure, nutrition and fat clearance. *Recent Advances in Nutrition* 1990; **1**: 67A–69A.

Ginés P, Arroyo V, Quintero E *et al.* Comparison of paracentesis and diuretics in the treatment of cirrhosis with tense ascites. *Gastroenterology* 1987; **93**: 234–241.

Green JH, Bramley PN, Losowsky MS. Are patients with primary biliary cirrhosis hypermetabolic? A comparison between patients before and after liver transplantation and controls. *Hepatology* 1991; **14**: 464–472.

Greenburger NJ. Effect of vegetable and animal protein diets in chronic hepatic encephalopathy. *Digestive Diseases* 1977; **22**: 845–855.

Harris JA, Benedict TG. *Biometric Studies of Basal Metabolism in Man.* Publication No. 279. Washington, DC: Carnegie Institute of Washington, 1919.

Hasse JM, Blue LS, Liepa GU *et al.* Early enteral nutrition support in patients undergoing liver transplantation. *Journal of Parenteral and Enteral Nutrition* 1995; **19**: 437–443.

Italian Multicentre Cooperative Project on nutrition in liver cirrhosis. Nutritional status in cirrhosis. *Journal of Hepatology* 1994; **21**: 317–325.

Kalman DR, Saltzman JR. Nutrition status predicts survival in cirrhosis. *Nutrition Reviews* 1996; **54**: 217–219.

Katelaris PH, Jones DB. Fulminant hepatic failure. *Medical Clinics of North America* 1989; **73**: 955–970.

Kearns PJ, Young H, Garcia G *et al.* Accelerated improvement of alcoholic liver disease with enteral nutrition. *Gastroenterology* 1992; **102**: 200–205.

Kondrup J, Müller MJ. Energy and protein requirements of patients with chronic liver disease. *Journal of Hepatology* 1997; **27**: 239–247.

Lautz HU, Selberg O, Körber J *et al.* Protein-calorie malnutrition in liver cirrhosis. *Clinical Investigator* 1992; **70**: 478–486.

McCullough AJ, Tavill AS. Disordered energy and protein metabolism in liver disease. *Seminars in Liver Disease* 1991; **11**: 265–277.

Madden A. The role of low fat diets in the management of gallbladder disease. *Journal of Human Nutrition and Dietetics* 1992; **5**: 267–273.

Madden AM, Morgan MY. Resting energy expenditure should be measured in patients with cirrhosis, not predicted. *Hepatology* 1999a; in press.

Madden AM, Morgan MY. Patterns of energy intake in patients with cirrhosis and healthy volunteers. *British Journal of Nutrition* 1999b; **82**: in press.

Madden AM, Soulsby CT, Morgan MY. Assessment of nutrition in patients with cirrhosis (Abstract). *Hepatology* 1997; **26**: 125.

Mehta PL, Alaka KJ, Filo RS *et al.* Nutritional support following liver transplantation: comparison of jejunal versus parenteral routes. *Clinical Transplant* 1995; **9**: 364–369.

Mendenhall CL. Protein-calorie malnutrition in alcoholic liver disease. In Watson RR, Watzl B (Eds) *Nutrition and Alcohol*, pp. 363–384. Boca Raton: CRC Press, 1992.

Mendenhall CL, Tosch T, Weesner RE *et al.* VA cooperative study on alcoholic hepatitis II: Prognostic significance of protein-calorie malnutrition. *American Journal of Clinical Nutrition* 1986; **43**: 213–218.

Merli M, Riggio O, Dally L, Policentrica Italiana Nutrizione Cirrosi. Does malnutrition affect survival in cirrhosis? *Hepatology* 1996; **23**: 1041–1046.

Morgan MY. The treatment of chronic hepatic encephalopathy. *Hepatogastroenterology* 1991; **38**: 377–387.

Morgan MY. Nutritional aspects of liver and biliary disease. In Bircher B, Benhamou JP, McIntyre N *et al.* (Eds) *Oxford Textbook of Clinical Hepatology*, 2nd edn, pp. 1923–1981. Oxford: Oxford University Press, 1999.

Morgan TR, Moritz TE, Mendenhall CL, Haas R, VA Cooperative Study Group. Protein consumption and hepatic encephalopathy in alcoholic hepatitis. *Journal of the American College of Nutrition* 1995; **14**: 152–158.

Müller MJ. Malnutrition in cirrhosis. *Journal of Hepatology* 1995; **23** (Suppl 1): 31–35.

Müller MJ, Lautz HU, Plogmann B *et al.* Energy expenditure and substrate oxidation in patients with cirrhosis: the impact of cause, clinical staging and nutritional state. Hepatology 1992; **15**: 782–794.

Müller MJ, Böttcher J, Selberg O *et al.* Hypermetabolism in clinically stable patients with liver cirrhosis. *American Journal of Clinical Nutrition* 1999; **69**: 1194–1201.

Munoz SJ, Deems RO, Moritz MJ *et al.* Hyperlipidaemia and obesity after orthotopic liver transplantation. *Transplantation Proceedings* 1991; **23**: 1480–1483.

Muscaritoli M, Cangiano C, Cascino A *et al.* Exogenous lipid clearance in compensated liver cirrhosis. *Journal of Parenteral and Enteral Nutrition* 1986; **10**: 599–603.

Nielsen K, Kondrup J, Martinsen L *et al.* Long-term oral refeeding of patients with cirrhosis of the liver. *British Journal of Nutrition* 1995; **74**: 557–567.

Nompleggi DJ, Bonkovsky HL. Nutritional supplementation in chronic liver disease: an analytical review. Hepatology 1994; **19**: 518–533.

Palmer M, Schaffner F, Thung SN. Excessive weight gain after liver transplantation. *Transplantation* 1991; **51**: 797–800.

Pikul J, Sharpe MD, Lowndes R, Ghent CN. Degree of preoperative malnutrition is predictive of postoperative morbidity and mortality in liver transplant recipients. *Transplantation* 1994; **57**: 469–472.

Plauth M, Merli M, Kondrup J *et al.* ESPEN guidelines for nutrition in liver disease and transplantation. *Clinical Nutrition* 1997; **16**: 43–55.

Pugh RNH, Murray-Lyon IM, Dawson JL *et al.* Transection of the oesophagus for bleeding oesophageal varices. *British Journal of Surgery* 1973; **60**: 646–649.

Ricci P, Therneau TM, Malinchoc M *et al.* A prognostic model for the outcome of liver transplantation in patients with cholestatic liver disease. *Hepatology* 1997; **25**: 672–677.

Runyon BA. Treatment of patients with cirrhosis and ascites. *Seminars in Liver Disease* 1997; **17**: 249–260.

Schofield WN. Predicting basal metabolic rate, new standards and review of previous work. *Human Nutrition: Clinical Nutrition* 1985; **39C** (Suppl 1): 5–41.

Selberg O, Böttcher J, Tusch G *et al*. Identification of high- and low-risk patients before liver transplantation: a prospective cohort study of nutritional and metabolic parameters in 150 patients. Hepatology 1997; **25**: 652–657.

Shaw BW Jr, Wood RP, Gordon RD *et al*. Influence of selected patient variables and operative blood loss on six-month survival following liver transplantation. *Seminars in Liver Disease* 1985; **5**: 385–393.

Shaw V, Lawson M (Eds) *Clinical Paediatric Dietetics*. Oxford: Blackwell Scientific, 1994.

Sherlock S, Summerskill WHJ, White LP, Phear EA. Portal-systemic encephalopathy. *Lancet* 1954; **ii**: 453–457.

Soulsby CT, Morgan MY. Dietary management of hepatic encephalopathy in cirrhotic patients: survey of current practice in United Kingdom. *British Medical Journal* 1999; **318**: 1391.

Soulsby CT, Madden AM, Morgan MY. The effect of dietary sodium restriction on energy and protein intake in patients with cirrhosis (Abstract). *Hepatology* 1997; **26**: 382A.

Swart GR, van den Berg JWO, van Vuure JK *et al*. Minimum protein requirements in liver cirrhosis determined by nitrogen balance measurements at three levels of protein intake. *Clinical Nutrition* 1989a; **8**: 329–336.

Swart GR, Zillikens MC, van Vuure JK, van den Berg JWO. Effect of a late evening meal on nitrogen balance in patients with cirrhosis of the liver. *British Medical Journal* 1989b; **299**: 1202–1203.

Verboeket-van de Venne WPHG, Westerterp KR, van Hoek B, Swart GR. Energy expenditure and substrate metabolism in patients with cirrhosis of the liver: effects of the pattern of food intake. *Gut* 1995; **36**: 110–116.

Watson CG, Tilleslejor B, Hoodecheck-Schaw B *et al*. Do alcoholics give valid self reports? *Journal of Studies on Alcohol* 1984; **45**: 344–348.

Weimann A, Kuse ER, Bechstein WO *et al*. Perioperative and enteral nutrition for patients undergoing orthotopic liver transplantation. Results of a questionnaire from 16 European transplant units. *Transplant International* 1998; **11** (Suppl 1): S289–S291.

Wicks C, Somasundaram S, Bjarnason I *et al*. Comparison of enteral feeding and total parenteral nutrition after liver transplantation. *Lancet* 1994; **344**: 837–840.

Wicks C, Bray GP, Williams R. Nutritional assessment in primary biliary cirrhosis: the effect of disease severity. *Clinical Nutrition* 1995; **14**: 29–34.

Zillikens MC, van den Berg JWO, Wattimena JLD *et al*. Nocturnal oral glucose supplementation. The effects on protein metabolism in cirrhotic patients and in healthy controls. *Journal of Hepatology* 1993; **17**: 377–383.

4.14 Renal disease

Nutritional therapy plays a central role in the management of individuals with renal disease. In health, the major activities of the kidneys are involved with the maintenance of electrolyte and fluid homoeostasis, together with the excretion of metabolic waste products. The main consequences of renal disease are therefore a disordered fluid and electrolyte balance, with an accumulation of metabolic waste products. In addition, the kidneys have other important functions that are also of clinical and nutritional significance. They produce the hormone erythropoietin, which stimulates red blood cell production and also helps to maintain acid–base balance. Left untreated, the anaemia that develops in renal disease is debilitating, causes anorexia and can reduce food intake. In association with the acidosis and the resulting muscle degradation, the overall effect on nutrition is adverse.

Dietetic treatment will help to limit the consequences of declining renal function, thereby maintaining the patient's well-being. Several dietary elements require consideration, for a variety of reasons. These should be tailored to the individual's needs, bearing in mind their clinical condition, treatment and blood biochemistry (Table 4.24). An appreciation of the close link between clinical and dietetic management is helpful. This section of the Manual will cover both the medical and dietetic aspects of care using the following classifications:

- *acute renal failure (ARF)*, where the renal failure develops over a short time-span of hours or days
- *chronic renal failure (CRF)*, where the renal failure develops in the longer term, over months and years
- *end-stage renal failure (ESRF)*, where renal function has deteriorated to a point that renal replacement therapy (dialysis or transplantation) is required to maintain the well-being of the patient
- *the nephrotic syndrome*, in which patients experience excessive protein losses in the urine. Renal function may be either normal or deranged.

4.14.1 Acute renal failure

The definition of ARF is somewhat arbitrary and many different definitions appear in the literature (Thadani *et al.* 1996). A commonly used definition is 'a recent deterioration in renal function resulting in a rise in serum creatinine of more than 50% above the baseline value'. However, this assumes that the baseline creatinine was known, which is not always the case. A less rigid definition is 'a rapid deterioration in renal function sufficient to result in an accumulation of nitrogenous wastes in the body'.

Table 4.24 Dietary elements and renal failure

	Protein	Energy	Potassium	Phosphate	Sodium and Fluid
Significance in renal disease	Sufficient needed to avoid malnutrition Low intake may delay progression of CRF (contentious)	Sufficient required to prevent malnutrition	Hyperkalaemia may cause cardiac arythmias/cardiac arrest	Hyperphosphataemia involved with development of renal bone disease	Excess intake leads to fluid overload and hypertension
Acute renal failure	≥ 1.0 g/kg BW	Matched to requirements	As required (see text)	As required (see text)	As required (see text)
Pre-dialysis	0.8–1.0 g/kg BW or 0.6 g/kg BW	35 kcal/kg BW	Unrestricted unless hyperkalaemic	Restriction usually required (to approximately 30 mmol/day)	NAS if hypertensive NAS + fluid restriction if overloaded
Haemodialysis	1.0–1.2 g/kg IBW	≥ 35 kcal/kg IBW	Restriction usually required (1 mmol/kg BW)	Restriction usually required (to approximately 30 mmol/day)	NAS + fluid restriction usually required
Continuous ambulatory peritoneal dialysis	>1.2 g/kg IBW	>35 kcal/kg IBW (including glucose absorbed from dialysate	Unrestricted unless hyperkalaemic	Restriction usually required (to approximately 35–40 mmol/day)	NAS + fluid restriction usually required

CRF: chronic renal failure; BW: body weight; IBW: ideal body weight; NAS: no added salt.
All intakes are daily recommendations.

Causes of acute renal failure

Virtually all classifications use the terms pre-renal, renal and post-renal to divide ARF into those cases due to impaired renal perfusion (pre-renal), intrinsic renal pathology (renal) and obstruction to the outflow of urine (post-renal). However, there is an important overlap between the first two groups as any pre-renal cause, if uncorrected, can lead to ischaemic damage to the kidney, causing the pathological lesion of acute tubular necrosis. Major causes of ARF are listed in Table 4.25. It is important to bear in mind that ARF is often multifactorial, for example an elderly patient taking diuretics and/or angiotensin-converting enzyme (ACE) inhibitors who then becomes dehydrated owing to an episode of gastroenteritis. Patients with pre-existing chronic renal impairment from whatever cause are more vulnerable to ARF and the term acute-on-chronic renal failure is often used for such patients.

Clinical aspects of acute renal failure

A recent estimate of the number of patients with ARF in the UK is 70 patients per million population per year requiring dialysis, and perhaps another 130 per million per year needing input from a nephrologist but not requiring dialysis (Renal Association 1997). ARF becomes more common with increasing age. The overall mortality from ARF still exceeds 50%, with the highest mortality being in patients with multi-organ failure, in whom mortality can be as high as 80–90%.

ARF may be detected incidentally following blood tests performed either routinely or to investigate other complaints. Patients may present having noticed a reduction in urine volume or with general symptoms such as nausea and vomiting. More serious presentations include pulmonary oedema, pericarditis, confusion or depressed level of consciousness, in which case treatment is needed urgently.

Management of acute renal failure

General management

Providing the patient does not present with a life-threatening indication for urgent dialysis such as pulmonary oedema, severe hyperkalaemia or pericarditis, the initial management will be predominantly aimed at the underlying cause of renal failure and include efforts to preserve renal function. The initial management will include investigations to elucidate at least the broad category of renal failure, although this will often be apparent from the clinical setting.

The kidneys are critically dependent on an adequate blood supply and therefore in any cause of ARF, but particularly pre-renal ARF, measures to restore the circulating blood volume and blood pressure are important. This will generally entail intravenous fluid replacement and is more effective the earlier it is initiated. Assessment of hydration in critically ill patients is not always straightforward and often requires invasive monitoring with central venous pressure recordings. Accurate charting of all fluid intake

Table 4.25 Causes of acute renal failure

1. Pre-renal
Reduced intravascular volume
  Blood loss, gastroenteritis, diuretics, hypoalbuminaemia, burns
Cardiac failure
Vasodilatation
  Sepsis
Increased resistance to renal blood flow
  Renal artery disease
  Renal vein thrombosis
Hepatorenal syndrome[1]

2. Renal
Glomerular disease
  Primary renal disease or as part of a multi-system disorder
  (includes any cause of acute glomerulonephritis)
Intra-renal vascular disease
  Vasculitis
  Atheroembolic disease
  Haemolytic uraemic syndrome
Tubulointerstitial disease
  Acute tubular necrosis:
    Post-ischaemic (pre-renal)[2]
    Toxic agents: drugs, poisons, X-ray contrast
  Acute interstitial nephritis:
    Infective
    Infiltration, e.g. lymphoma
    Drug reaction

3. Post-renal
Obstruction to the flow of urine can be at any level from the
  intra-renal tubules to the urethra
Intra-renal obstruction
  Crystals (uric acid, oxalate, calcium)
  Abnormal proteins (e.g. myeloma)
Ureteric obstruction (needs to be bilateral unless only one
  functioning kidney)
Bladder outflow obstruction
  Prostate and bladder tumours
  Bladder calculi
Urethral obstruction
  Tumours, strictures

[1] The hepatorenal syndrome is an incompletely understood syndrome in which acute renal failure occurs in association with liver failure. The liver failure is the primary lesion and renal function generally improves as the hepatic failure recovers.
[2] Acute tubular necrosis can result from any pre-renal cause of renal failure if of sufficient duration and intensity. In hospital this is most commonly seen in the context of sepsis, trauma, major surgery and cardiac failure.

and output is also essential. Other important general measures include aggressive treatment of sepsis and measures to improve cardiac function if impaired.

Patients with an intrinsic renal cause for their ARF will generally need further investigation, often up to and including a renal biopsy, to ascertain whether specific therapy may be of benefit, an example being immunosuppressive agents for vasculitis. An important general aspect of management is to withdraw all potentially nephrotoxic agents from the patient's therapy. If the patient's urinary tract is obstructed, prompt relief of the obstruction may preserve renal function.

Renal replacement therapy in acute renal failure

Dialysis is discussed in detail in Section 4.14.3 (End-stage renal failure), below.

If the underlying cause of ARF cannot be reversed fairly rapidly, renal replacement therapy will be necessary to preserve the patient's well-being. There are several treatment options and the modality chosen will be a reflection of both clinical aspects of a particular case and facilities available locally.

Acute peritoneal dialysis is a theoretical treatment option for some ARF patients but in practice its use is only very occasional as it is less efficient than haemodialysis, and the excessive catabolism associated with ARF in most patients therefore mitigates against its successful use. Peritoneal dialysis has been used successfully in the case of patients with severe cardiac failure who do not tolerate the extracorporeal circulation associated with haemodialysis.

For patients with ARF, who do not have multiple-organ failure, the most common treatment modality is regular intermittent haemodialysis, which provides a very efficient clearance of waste products. In contrast to chronic dialysis patients, each treatment should be prescribed individually, paying attention to the amount of dialysis to be delivered and the volume of fluid to be removed. Haemodialysis will need to be on alternate days or in some cases daily. If the patient is oliguric, fluid balance becomes a critical aspect of management as dialysis provides the only opportunity for removal of fluid and there is a finite amount of fluid removal that any one patient will tolerate in a single dialysis session. This can be a major problem if other aspects of the patient's care such as blood transfusion or feeding involve the administration of large volumes.

Continuous haemofiltration techniques are continuous therapies in which a large volume of plasma is removed by passing the blood at high pressure across a haemofilter and replacing the filtrate so removed with sterile fluids. Waste products are removed from the body with the filtrate by convection. Fluid balance can be manipulated by varying the volume of fluid replaced each hour to allow net loss or gain of fluid. Originally, the technique relied on the patient's own arterial blood pressure to drive the circuit and required both arterial and venous cannulation [continuous arteriovenous haemofiltration (CAVH)]. Nowadays CAVH has been largely supplanted by continuous venovenous haemofiltration (CVVH), in which a blood pump is used to drive the circuit, which means that access is only required to the venous circulation. Over a 24 hour period the performance of CVVH matches or surpasses haemodialysis and it facilitates much better control of fluid balance. It is much easier to administer large volumes of total parenteral nutrition to a patient on continuous therapy than one treated intermittently. Most units regard continuous therapies as the treatment of choice for patients with multiple organ failure who need to be managed on an intensive care or high-dependency unit.

Dietetic considerations in acute renal failure

The aims of dietetic treatment in ARF are the same as for patients with a chronic deterioration in renal function, i.e. to maintain nutritional status and limit the complications of renal failure. However, the shorter time-scale in ARF means that changes in fluid, electrolyte and acid–base balance are more pronounced. Malnutrition can also develop rapidly following the onset of ARF, despite a patient's previous nutritional intake having been adequate until very recently. Therefore, dietetic input is desirable at an early stage.

The patients' altered metabolism, varied disease state and the treatment intervention complicate provision of nutritional support in ARF. However, their nutritional requirements can be broadly categorized according to the disorder precipitating the renal failure. Macronutrient requirements in ARF caused by a urinary tract obstruction or some other non-catabolic event are not elevated. In contrast, ARF from a catabolic cause such as sepsis or trauma is accompanied by increased protein turnover and nutritional needs. Management of these two groups is different and is considered separately.

Non-catabolic acute renal failure Treatment of patients in this group is straightforward. Energy and protein requirements are not increased, and can usually be met by oral diet alone or with addition of nutritionally dense (1.5–2 kcal/ml) supplementary sip feeds. There is no place for restricting protein intake. Where required, renal replacement therapy (RRT) will usually be provided by intermittent haemodialysis. Fluid and electrolyte intake should be individualized according to blood biochemistry and fluid status. Where serum levels are high, a low-potassium and low-phosphate diet should be implemented. In oliguric and fluid-overloaded patients, fluid intake should be restricted. Ideally, this should be limited to a volume equivalent to the previous day's urine output plus 500 ml. Limiting sodium intake to a 'No Added Salt' level will curb thirst and aid compliance.

The restrictions are likely to be required until renal function begins to improve. When this happens, patients may become polyuric and an increased fluid intake, adequate to cover the large urine volumes and insensible losses, must be maintained to avoid dehydration. As serum potassium and phosphate levels normalize, any dietary restrictions should be lifted.

Catabolic acute renal failure This group of patients will include people who are extremely ill. Frequently, they will have multiple organ failure and will be managed on an intensive care unit where the necessary support can be provided. Mortality rates are high (40–80%) but appropriate feeding is associated with improved survival (Rainford 1981; Bartlett *et al.* 1986).

Protein In the absence of exogenous nitrogen, amino acids are sourced from skeletal muscle. Negative nitrogen balance results and although this catabolism cannot be reversed, appropriate feeding will reduce muscle wasting. Therefore, nitrogen intake should be matched to the clinical condition (Elia 1990). However, the provision of more than 0.2 g N/kg body weight per day to septic or trauma patients confers no further benefit (Ishibashi *et al.* 1998).

Energy Individual assessment will help to prevent the harmful effects of both underfeeding and overfeeding.

Since there is considerable variation between predicted and measured energy expenditure in the critically ill (Makk et al. 1990), requirements are best estimated by indirect calorimetry. Unfortunately, in clinical practice the necessary equipment is rarely available and metabolic rate tables are likely to be used. ARF itself has no effect on the patient's metabolic rate (Schneeweiss et al. 1990) and use of excessively high stress and activity factors should be avoided. Even in individuals with ARF and multi-organ failure, measured requirements are found to be only 20% above resting values (Bouffard et al. 1987).

Electrolytes Requirements for electrolytes are variable, depending upon the individual's clinical condition and treatment. Frequent monitoring of blood biochemistry is essential to guide provision.

Micronutrients The requirements for trace elements and vitamins in ARF are not well documented and there are no specific recommendations. The plasma levels of vitamins A, E and D of individuals in ARF are lower than normal (Druml et al. 1998). Commercial parenteral preparations of multivitamins can be used where required. However, excessive amounts of ascorbic acid should be avoided, as megadoses of 1500 mg have been reported to cause oxalate deposition in ARF (Friedman et al. 1983). Care should also be taken when providing trace elements parenterally. There is the potential for toxicity since the normal means of maintaining trace element homoeostasis by varying gastrointestinal absorption rates and renal excretion are not in operation.

Influence of renal replacement therapy RRT will also influence the nutritional prescription. In oliguric patients on intermittent dialysis, low volumes of feed will be required to avoid fluid overload. This may result in the nutritional requirements not being fully met. Continuous RRT permits larger volumes of feed to be administered, allowing the patient to receive their full nutritional prescription.

Individuals in ARF being treated by conventional haemodialysis and receiving parenteral nutrition lose approximately 5 g of amino acids per session via the dialysate (Hynote et al. 1995). In continuous RRT, approximately 10% of infused amino acids are lost (Davenport and Roberts 1989; Davies et al. 1991) and nitrogen provision should be increased to compensate. Continuous treatments also have a positive effect on nutrition. Absorption of dextrose from the dialysate solutions used for haemofiltration (CAVH or CVVH) results in significant gains of energy (Bellomo et al. 1991). This, together with the energy derived from the metabolism of lactate, used as a buffer in the replacement solutions, should be taken into account when designing regimens.

Nutritional support route Wherever possible, nutrition support should be provided via the enteral route. In patients on continuous RRT, where potassium and phosphate levels have been normalized, standard commercial formulae can be used. However, specialist renal feeds with a reduced electrolyte content are useful where the control of serum phosphate and potassium or fluid balance proves difficult. If required the nitrogen:energy ratio of the feed can be increased by the addition of protein-rich (approx. 10 g protein/100 ml) sip feeds

Where parenteral nutrition is required, attention should be given to the balance of the energy substrates, as both carbohydrate and lipid metabolism are altered in ARF. Insulin resistance, coupled with accelerated gluconeogenesis from amino acid catabolism, leads to glucose intolerance. Lipid clearance is also impaired, a problem in ARF that is not overcome by the use of medium-chain triglyceride (MCT) fat emulsions (Druml et al. 1992). Therefore, energy should be provided from a balance of both dextrose and lipid, avoiding an excess of either. Special nitrogen-containing solutions have been developed for parenteral use. They aim to correct the abnormal amino-acid profile seen in the serum of individuals with renal failure. However, no clinical benefit has been demonstrated and a standard mixture of essential and non-essential amino acids is recommended (Kopple 1996). Glutamine-containing parenteral regimens have been safely administered in ARF (Griffiths et al. 1997).

4.14.2 Chronic renal failure

CRF is the state of irreversible (and usually progressive) renal impairment due to any cause. Definition in terms of plasma creatinine or glomerular filtration rate (GFR) is somewhat arbitrary, although the recent United Kingdom Renal Association standards document suggests that anyone with repeated plasma creatinine of greater than 150 μmol/l should be regarded as a potential CRF patient and be reviewed by a nephrologist (Renal Association 1997). Other important terms are frequently used in the management of CRF:

- *Uraemia* is the term used to describe the illness that results from impaired renal function and encompasses a whole host of symptoms.
- *End-stage renal failure*, the management of which is discussed in Section 4.14.3, is the state where renal function has declined to negligible levels and dialysis therapy is indicated. Again, there is no standard definition of ESRF, although a GFR <10 ml/minute is widely used.

Causes of chronic renal failure

CRF results from progressive loss of functioning nephrons and hence there are very many potential underlying pathologies. The main causes of chronic renal failure are listed in Table 4.26.

Management of chronic renal failure

Medical management of CRF can be divided into two broad categories, namely disease-specific therapy aimed at removing or abating the cause of renal dysfunction, and non-specific treatments common to most, if not all, causes of CRF.

Table 4.26 Causes of chronic renal failure

Glomerulonephritis
  Primary renal disease
  As part of a multisystem disorder (e.g. connective tissue
  diseases)
Diabetic nephropathy
Renal vascular disease/hypertension
Chronic pyelonephritis
Obstruction (subacute)
Chronic tubulointerstitial disease
Polycystic kidney disease
Multiple myeloma and related disorders

Disease-specific therapy

This includes strategies such as antibiotic therapy for urinary tract infections, improved blood sugar control in diabetic renal disease and immunosuppressive therapy for autoimmune disorders causing CRF.

Non-specific therapy

Hypertension   There is now evidence that, in virtually all causes of CRF, improved control of blood pressure will significantly delay the rate of progression of CRF. There is also evidence that the ACE inhibitor class of antihypertensive agent confers a particular benefit, at least in part from its antiproteinuric effect (Navis *et al.* 1997). Treatment of elevated blood cholesterol levels is also believed to be beneficial in this respect.

Anaemia   This is an important complication of CRF, as the kidneys produce the hormone erythropoietin which plays a key role in the production of red blood cells. Effective treatment of this anaemia improves the cardiovascular status of renal patients, improves quality of life and often delays the need to institute RRT. The mainstay of treatment is the use of recombinant human erythropoietin (Winnearls 1998). When treating patients with erythropoietin it is important to exclude other causes of anaemia and to ensure that the body's iron stores are adequate; this may require parenteral iron supplementation.

Renal bone disease   Renal bone disease is an important complication of CRF that can be associated with a high morbidity if untreated. Its aetiology is complicated but it is a consequence of both hyperphosphataemia (due to reduced renal excretion of phosphate) and hypocalcaemia (due mainly to reduced activation of vitamin D in the kidney). These two stimuli lead to hyperparathyroidism which, if not corrected, causes significant bone disease.

Phosphate levels are controlled by dietary phosphate restriction (see Phosphorus, below) and if this alone proves inadequate, by the use of phosphate-binding drugs which reduce the amount of phosphate absorbed from the gut. The most commonly used phosphate binder in the UK is calcium carbonate, although newer agents with potentially greater efficacy have recently become available. Aluminium hydroxide is rarely used now owing to problems of aluminium toxicity which can result in bone disease and also dementia (Tomson and Ward 1989).

To correct hypocalcaemia, activated vitamin D or a vitamin D analogue is given. With such therapy it is important to monitor the patient's plasma calcium level as iatrogenic hypercalcaemia can result, with potentially deleterious effects on renal function.

Acidosis   Metabolic acidosis is a consequence of reduced renal function. It can have deleterious effects on protein metabolism (Reaich *et al.* 1993) and also contributes to renal bone disease. It can be corrected or ameliorated by the use of oral sodium bicarbonate therapy (Cunningham *et al.* 1982).

Dietetic considerations in chronic renal failure

Protein

Low-protein diets have long been advocated for use with patients in CRF. However, their value is now questioned. Despite much research in this area, the issue remains contentious and the debate warrants close scrutiny.

Prior to dialysis being widely available as a chronic treatment, Giovannetti and Maggiore (1964) popularized the use of low-protein diets for patients with CRF. Their regimens were of a very low protein content (19–22 g protein) and were used to alleviate the symptoms of nausea and vomiting caused by advanced renal failure. Whilst a low protein intake will reduce blood urea levels, it should be remembered that urea itself is relatively non-toxic. Unless blood levels are exceptionally high, it is difficult to predict from blood results which patients will be symptomatic; some patients are asymptomatic with blood urea levels in excess of 35 mmol/l, whilst others will have severe symptoms with levels of less than 25 mmol/l. The best treatment for symptomatic uraemia is dialysis. Therefore, by the 1970s, as dialysis availability increased, the popularity of low-protein diets decreased.

Interest in low-protein diets was rekindled in the 1980s. New work in rats with experimentally induced renal failure showed that the diets improved survival and slowed the rate of decline in renal function. Several studies reported that low protein diets were similarly effective in humans (Maschio *et al.* 1982; Bennett *et al.* 1983; Rosman *et al.* 1984). However, on close examination many studies had methodological problems, casting doubt on their findings (El Nahas and Coles 1986). Studies have been criticized because of the failure to recognize that CRF does not always progress, inadequacies in the methods used to assess renal function, the fact that many studies were only short term and the lack of appropriate controls.

The 1990s saw the publication of two large, prospective, randomized trials which examined the effect of dietary protein restriction on the course of CRF in humans. Both the Northern Italian Co-operative Study (Locatelli *et al.* 1991) and the Modification of Diet in Renal Disease (MDRD) study from the USA (Klahr *et al.* 1994) were multicentre studies, following large numbers of patients for periods of at least 2 years. In the Italian study, no significant difference was seen in rate of CRF progression between the experimental low-protein diet of 0.6 g/kg and the controlled 'normal' diet of 1.0 g/kg body weight. Problems with dietary compliance were identified: the experimental group overconsumed and the control group underconsumed protein. As a result, the difference in protein intake between the two groups was not as great as designed and in theory may have accounted for why the rates of decline in renal function did not differ. However, analysis of achieved (rather than prescribed) intake across the experimental and control groups failed to find any correlation between protein intake and rate of decline in renal function.

The MDRD study was of a more complex design, consisting of two arms. In the first, individuals with moderate renal failure were randomized to either a 'usual' protein diet of 1.3 g/kg or a low-protein diet of 0.58 g/kg. No significant difference in the rate of decline of renal function was seen between the two groups. Individuals with more advanced renal failure were studied in the second arm of the MDRD study. These patients were randomized to a low-protein diet of 0.58 g/kg, or a 0.28 g/kg diet plus keto acid–amino acid supplements. Again, the rate of decline in renal function between the two groups did not significantly differ. However, as with the Northern Italian Co-Operative Study, the MDRD study suffered difficulties with dietary compliance, with individuals consuming more protein than prescribed. As a consequence, secondary analyses were undertaken to examine the relationship between the achieved protein intake and the rate of decline in renal function. In individuals with moderate renal failure, some evidence was found of an association between achieved protein intake and the rate of decline in GFR but, over the 3 years of the study, this failed to reach statistical significance (Levey *et al.* 1996b). In patients with advanced renal failure, a lower protein intake was associated with a significantly slower rate of decline in GFR (Levey *et al.* 1996a). Whilst these secondary analyses point to a relationship between a low protein intake and a decreased rate of decline in GFR, their therapeutic importance is unclear. Because the analyses were made by correlation, rather than by 'intention to treat', their findings cannot be directly applied to the clinical setting.

A major concern over the use of low-protein diets is that they may induce malnutrition. Even in the MDRD study which involved intense dietetic support of up to 200 minutes per patient per month from trained renal dietitians (Dolecek *et al.* 1995), nutritional status significantly deteriorated in patients prescribed a low-protein diet (Kopple *et al.* 1997). The prevention of malnutrition must be a major goal since patients who are poorly nourished at the onset of dialysis suffer poorer outcomes. In a review of the co-morbidity of over 800 haemodialysis patients, malnutrition was found to be an independent prognostic factor of outcome. The odds ratio of death within the first 6 months of dialysis was increased by a factor of 2.5 in patients who were poorly nourished at the onset of the dialysis (Barrett *et al.* 1997).

The use of low-protein diets remains contentious. In the USA there are strong advocates of their use (Walser *et al.*

1999) but in the UK they are used in only a small number of renal units (Gilmour and Hartley 1997). A protein intake of 0.8–1.0 g/kg body weight per day is recommended (Renal Association 1997).

If low-protein diets are to be used, careful control and regular supervision by the dietitian is required. Tight monitoring of dietary compliance and nutritional status is necessary to avoid the development of undernutrition. They are demanding for the patient and poor compliance is to be an expected problem. Conventionally, a restriction of 0.6 g/kg per day is applied. Although lower than the 0.75 g/kg per day recommended for healthy adults (FAO/WHO/UNU 1985), it is believed adaptive responses take place in CRF. Approximately two-thirds of the protein should come from high biological sources and an adequate energy intake (>35 kcal/kg) ensured. Alternatives to the conventional low-protein diet are regimens of a very low protein content (0.3 g/kg body weight per day) that are supplemented with mixtures of essential amino acids or ketoacids. They are not recommended for use in the UK (Renal Association 1997) because of compliance problems and the fact that they may lead to negative nitrogen balance.

Whilst the issue of protein restriction will continue to be debated, there is widespread agreement that the primary goal of any nutritional therapy must be to optimize the patient's nutritional status.

Energy

Energy intake influences the metabolism of nitrogen. Even with high protein intakes, nitrogen balance will remain negative unless energy intake is maintained at an adequate level. The resting energy expenditure of CRF patients is no different to that of control subjects (Schneeweiss *et al.* 1990) and confirms that renal failure *per se* does not influence energy requirements. Energy requirements will therefore be dependent upon activity levels as well as body size, but an intake of 35 kcal/kg per day will be adequate for most patients' needs (Kopple *et al.* 1986). Foodstuffs high in energy and low in protein, together with the prescribable low-protein products, will have to be taken if the desired energy intake is going to be achieved where low-protein diets are followed.

Some thought should be given to the energy substrates, as hyperlipidaemia is prevalent in over 20% of CRF patients. In general, triglyceride blood levels are increased secondary to the reduced clearance of lipid-rich particles by the liver and peripheral tissues. High-density lipoprotein (HDL)-cholesterol levels are also reduced. However, in renal disease, unlike in other patient groups, it is unclear whether hyperlipidaemia increases the risk of atherosclerosis. Whilst there are no conclusive data to show that lipid-lowering therapy is of any benefit in this patient group, equally there is no good reason not to treat the abnormality, especially as many patients will already have or will later develop cardiovascular and other vascular disease. In these circumstances it is reasonable to advise patients to follow 'healthy eating guidelines' providing that an overall nutritionally adequate intake can be achieved.

Potassium

The aim should be to maintain blood potassium levels within the normal range. Hyperkalaemia is to be avoided since potentially it is the most serious of electrolyte disturbances. It can lead to irregular heart rhythms and, in extreme cases, death from cardiac arrest. However, in the majority of patients, blood potassium levels will remain normal until CRF is well advanced and renal replacement therapy is imminent. Non-dietary factors that may contribute to hyperkalaemia include acidosis, constipation and medications such as ACE inhibitors or potassium-sparing diuretics.

Potassium cannot be completely eliminated from the diet because it is found in a wide range of foodstuffs, but a low-potassium diet can significantly reduce intake. This involves avoiding potassium-rich foods such as pure fruit juices, bananas and chipped or jacket potatoes, and limiting the consumption of other fruits and vegetables. Vegetables should be cooked by boiling, rather than by steaming, pressure cooking or in a microwave. The intake of milk, cheese, meat and fish should also be moderated. A dietary history will enable the dietitian to see where specific advice needs to be directed.

Phosphorus

Hyperphosphataemia occurs with advancing renal failure when the kidneys are no longer able to excrete sufficient phosphorus to maintain homoeostasis. It is a common problem in the pre-dialysis patient where GFR has declined to 15 ml/minute per m^2 or less (normal values 120 ml/minute per m^2), and is accompanied by changes in calcium metabolism. Hyperphosphataemia together with hypocalcaemia is characteristic of CRF and stimulates the parathyroid gland to produce more parathyroid hormone (PTH), a condition known as secondary hyperparathyroidism. In individuals with normal renal function, the increased levels of PTH restore normal phosphate and calcium blood levels which, in turn, feed back to suppress further PTH secretion. However, in renal failure the feedback loop fails and without therapeutic intervention, high levels of circulating PTH persist and lead to renal bone disease and soft tissue calcification.

Treatment is aimed at suppressing PTH activity. This involves:

- reducing phosphate blood levels to within the range of 0.8–1.5 mmol/l (Renal Association 1997)
- increasing calcium blood levels
- supplementing with active vitamin D.

Dietary phosphorus is restricted by avoiding an excessive intake of protein (since protein-rich foods are also rich in phosphate) and other foods with a high phosphate content. In addition, phosphate absorption in the gut is reduced by the prescription of phosphate binders. Aluminium hydroxide is a very effective binder but is now rarely used because of the dangers of aluminium toxicity. Calcium carbonate or calcium acetate is the first-choice binder with most patients, although newer agents are cur-

rently under investigation. They are most effective when taken prior to meals. Calcium salts offer the further benefit of providing additional calcium to help to increase calcium blood levels.

When phosphate levels are well controlled, active vitamin D can be given in the form of calcitriol or 1-alpha-hydroxycholecalciferol. Careful monitoring of blood biochemistry is necessary to titrate dosage to individual requirements and avoid hypercalcaemia.

Sodium and fluid

It is helpful to consider sodium and fluid together, since they are closely associated in the body and the mechanisms for regulating their balance are interrelated. The body's sodium and fluid status is a main determinant of blood pressure and is therefore of clinical importance. Individuals with renal failure lose their ability to adapt to changes in dietary sodium intake; high intakes may promote salt and water accumulation, while low intakes may lead to depletion and dehydration. Both extremes are to be avoided.

Restriction of dietary sodium intake to the level of No Added Salt (<100 mmol sodium per day) should be implemented if patients are hypertensive or oedematous or require a fluid restriction for other reasons. It should be remembered that medication may also contribute to sodium balance. For example, in the treatment of acidosis a typical day's dosage of 1500 mg sodium bicarbonate three times daily provides 54 mmol sodium.

Many patients will not require a fluid restriction until they are nearing ESRF, when their urine volume diminishes. At this point, daily intake should be limited to 500 ml plus the equivalent of the previous day's urine output.

Micronutrients

The metabolism and status of trace elements and vitamins are altered in renal failure. Factors involved include the degree of renal insufficiency, concurrent medication, the mode of renal replacement therapy (if any) and, importantly, the patient's nutritional status and food intake.

Absolute requirements for trace elements have yet to be established. Aluminium and copper status are increased in CRF and in ESRF patients on dialysis. Iron deficiency is a common occurrence, especially when erythropoietin therapy is used. Supplementation with oral iron is cheap and safe, but unfortunately its effectiveness is limited and parenteral iron is often required. Zinc and selenium levels are also reduced but routine supplementation is not recommended (Gilmour *et al.* 1998).

Deficiencies in ascorbic acid, thiamin (B_1), riboflavin (B_2) and pyridoxine (B_6) may occur in individuals in CRF adhering to low-protein diets and supplementation should therefore be considered. Plasma levels of vitamin A are high in all patient groups, primarily because of an increase in retinol-binding protein, but toxicity is rarely seen because the vitamin is bound to the protein and is therefore inactive. Studies of vitamin E status in renal failure report contradictory findings. There is no evidence that supplements of vitamin B_{12}, folic acid, biotin, pantothenic acid or vitamins A or E are required to correct deficiencies in any group of patients (Gilmour *et al.* 1998).

4.14.3 End-stage renal failure

As with CRF, the definition of ESRF is arbitrary but one definition is a creatinine clearance <10 ml/minute. In practical terms it is the point at which adequate well-being can no longer be maintained without RRT. RRT is the replacement of renal function by artificial means. The term is slightly misleading as normally only a fraction of the renal function that is lost is replaced and not all of the functions of the kidneys are replaced, particularly by dialysis.

Any cause of both acute and chronic renal failure can lead to ESRF. The most common causes in the UK at present are glomerulonephritis, renal vascular disease and diabetes.

Patients with untreated ESRF are likely to experience symptoms of uraemia. The exact point at which a particular patient may need to start RRT depends upon many factors including age, nutrition, co-morbidity, cause of renal disease and speed of onset. Diabetic patients will often suffer uraemic symptoms earlier and commence dialysis sooner than non-diabetics.

RRT can comprise:

- haemodialysis
- peritoneal dialysis
- renal transplantation.

Haemodialysis

The process of haemodialysis involves passing the patient's blood through an artificial kidney or dialyser. The dialyser contains a semi-permeable membrane which separates blood on one side from a dilute electrolyte solution (dialysis fluid) on the other side. During dialysis three processes occur:

- There is an equilibration of the electrolyte composition of the blood and the dialysis fluid.
- Products of metabolism are removed from the blood by diffusion across the membrane into the dialysis fluid and also by convective mass transport.
- Water is removed from the plasma at a controlled rate by ultrafiltration due to a pressure difference between blood and the dialysis fluid.

Vascular access

In order to carry out haemodialysis, access to the patient's circulation is required. The preferred access is usually an arterio-venous fistula created surgically by joining an artery to a vein at either the wrist or elbow. This is then cannulated by two large-bore needles for each treatment session. Alternatives are the placement of a large, indwelling, semi-permanent catheter in either the jugular or femoral vein or the use of an artificial shunt between an artery and vein. These latter forms of access place the patient at higher risk of infection. Creation, complications and failure of vascu-

lar access are major causes of hospital admission for haemodialysis patients (Manas and Talbot 1997).

In patients with diabetes there can be considerable problems in maintaining vascular access for haemodialysis, owing to the likelihood of arterial disease. Other disadvantages of this procedure for diabetic patients are the tight fluid restriction and generally poorer glycaemic control than can be achieved with peritoneal dialysis.

Adequacy of haemodialysis

Most haemodialysis patients receive a treatment of approximately 4 hours, three times a week, but there is still considerable debate as to how much dialysis is adequate and how to measure dialysis. Most renal units now assess dialysis by the technique of urea kinetic modelling (UKM). UKM is based upon the urea clearance rate and uses mathematical formulae to describe the changes that occur in the body's urea content between and during dialysis. The amount of urea removed during treatment is proportional to the 'dose' of dialysis and is defined as Kt/V, where K is urea clearance rate, t is treatment duration and V is patient volume (total body water). Between treatments blood urea levels rise as a function of the protein catabolic rate (PCR). In stable patients, PCR is equivalent to the individual's dietary protein intake. PCR underestimates protein intake in anabolism, and overestimates it in catabolism. Computer software simplifies the application of UKM.

Survival data link both Kt/V and nutrition to outcome on dialysis. Patient morbidity increases significantly with a low PCR or a low Kt/V (Gotch and Sargent 1985). Both parameters are useful audit tools: PCR provides valuable information regarding protein intake, highlighting to dietitians those individual patients who would benefit from further dietetic intervention, and Kt/V can be compared to the recommended minimum standards of a stable Kt/V >1.2 (Renal Association 1997). Treatment schedules can then be adjusted accordingly; however, there is no internationally agreed standard method of calculating Kt/V, nor is there a defined Kt/V above which no further advantage accrues.

A simpler measure of the dose of dialysis is the urea reduction ratio (URR), based upon predialysis and postdialysis urea levels. A URR of less than 60% significantly increases the risk of death (Owen *et al.* 1993). However, use of URR is limited by its failure to provide nutritional data and its inability to account for any residual renal function that the patient may have.

Dietetic considerations in haemodialysis

Malnutrition Malnutrition is prevalent in 40–50% of haemodialysis patients (Marckmann 1988; Aparicio *et al.* 1999) and is of particular concern since undernutrition is highly associated with increased patient morbidity and mortality (Lowrie and Lew 1990). Therefore, the detection and treatment of malnutrition in dialysis patients is a dietetic priority.

Diabetic patients who develop gastric neuropathy may be prone to develop malnutrition as a consequence of gastric stasis and poor food tolerance.

Regular review of the patient's nutritional status should be undertaken. However, no single method can be relied upon to diagnose malnutrition since many of the commonly used markers are unreliable in renal disease. Weight is influenced by fluid balance, low serum albumin levels are more likely to reflect an active acute-phase response rather than a poor protein intake (Kaysen *et al.* 1997), and prealbumin and transferrin metabolism are altered. It is recommended that nutritional assessment be undertaken using several parameters including body weight, height, upper arm anthropometry and serum proteins (NIH Consensus Statement 1993) (see Section 1.8, Assessment of nutritional status). The technique of Subjective Global Assessment can also be applied to renal patients.

Multiple factors have an adverse effect on the nutritional status of dialysis patients. Some, such as hormonal changes, acidosis and anorexia, are common to all CRF patients. Others are specific to the dialysis treatment. In haemodialysis there are losses of amino acids during dialysis, and the bioincompatability between blood and dialysis membranes stimulates protein catabolism. Underdialysis can also adversely affect nutritional intake.

Where malnutrition is identified, treatment should be aimed at removing any non-dietary causes together with efforts to promote an adequate nutritional intake. Nutritionally dense supplement drinks are useful where appetite is diminished but excessive volumes should be avoided to prevent the development of fluid overload. Nasogastric or gastrostomy feeding can also be utilized. Alternatively, nutrition support can be provided by intradialytic parenteral nutrition (IDPN). This usually involves administering a 1000 ml parenteral feed mixture over the course of dialysis and provides approximately 7 g nitrogen and 900 kcal three times per week. In malnourished patients, IDPN improves nutritional status (Cano *et al.* 1990) and is associated with lower mortality and morbidity rates (Chertow *et al.* 1994).

Protein Provision of protein and energy must be adequate to prevent the development of malnutrition. An intake of 1.0 g/kg ideal body weight per day has been recommended (Renal Association 1997) and appears adequate for stable patients. Others advocate 1.2 g/kg/day as a safer level. This would help to cover the needs of individuals with increased requirements.

Energy Energy requirements are not altered by haemodialysis, and a daily intake of at least 35 kcal/kg ideal body weight is recommended (Renal Association 1997). Diabetic dialysis patients may be less active if mobility is impaired by limited vision, severe peripheral neuropathy and/or vascular disease (see Section 4.16, Diabetes mellitus).

Hyperlipidaemia is relatively common and consideration needs to be given to the energy substrates. A pragmatic approach to balancing healthy-eating principles against the need to achieve an adequate intake is required to ensure that the patients are not confused.

Potassium The aim is to maintain pre-dialysis blood levels within the range of 3.5–6.5 mmol/l (Renal Association 1997). To avoid hyperkalaemia, dietary potassium should be restricted (see Potassium in Section 4.14.2). A more liberal potassium intake may be allowed in those patients in whom some residual renal function is maintained.

Phosphorus Hyperphosphataemia is a problem encountered in the majority of patients. Low phosphate diets, together with the use of phosphate binders (see Phosphorus in Section 4.14.2) will be needed to maintain pre-dialysis levels within the target range of 1.2–1.7 mmol/l (Renal Association 1997).

Fluid and sodium Soon after starting haemodialysis, urine output in the majority of patients will cease or reduce to very low volumes. Fluid and salt intakes will therefore require restriction if hypertension and oedema are to be avoided. Patients need reminding that foods such as jelly, ice-cream and milk puddings have to be included in their fluid allowance. Many find limiting fluid intake the most demanding aspect of their restrictive regimen. Helpful hints to limit fluid intake include using smaller cups and sucking ice cubes.

Patients with insulin-treated diabetes should be advised to use concentrated carbohydrates such as honey or glucose tablets to counteract hypoglycaemia, rather than liquids such as fruit juices and sugar-containing soft drinks.

Changes in body weight between dialysis treatments mirror changes in fluid balance and allow compliance to be monitored. Gains in excess of 1–2 kg over the interdialytic period indicate an excessive fluid intake.

Micronutrients (see also Micronutrients in Section 4.14.2 above). Thiamin status in haemodialysis has been reported both as low and normal, whereas riboflavin levels tend to be increased. Deficiency of pyridoxine has been reported in some patients but, if pyridoxine supplementation is given, it should be carefully monitored.

Ascorbic acid is removed by haemodialysis and low levels of plasma ascorbic acid have been reported in patients not taking supplements. Consequently, supplementation with 150–250 mg daily is recommended. Larger doses are potentially harmful and result in high serum oxalate concentrations.

Although the folate status of dialysis patients is normal, supranormal levels can improve the deranged metabolism of the amino acid homocysteine. The hyperhomocysteinaemia seen in dialysis patients is believed to be an atherogenic risk factor and may contribute to the high prevalence of cardiovascular disease. Supplementation with 5 mg folic acid daily reduces homocysteine levels in patients on haemodialysis and continuous ambulatory peritoneal dialysis (CAPD) by 30% (Arnadottir *et al.* 1993).

Pharmacological doses of vitamin E may protect against lipid peroxidation. Administration of 20 IU and 50 IU of vitamin E has been shown to reduce the susceptibility to oxidation of low-density lipoproteins in haemodialysis patients (Panzetta *et al.* 1995).

Peritoneal dialysis

The abdominal cavity is lined by the peritoneal membrane, which consists of mesothelial cells, peritoneal capillaries and an interstitium. In the process of peritoneal dialysis this membrane behaves as a semi-permeable membrane or dialyser, and if an electrolyte solution is infused into the abdominal cavity, solute will diffuse into this fluid from the blood until equilibration is achieved. If this solution is then drained from the peritoneal cavity, removal of solute from the body will have been achieved. By adding an osmotic agent (usually glucose) removal of water or ultrafiltration can also be performed. Based upon these basic principles, there are several different techniques of peritoneal dialysis.

Continuous ambulatory peritoneal dialysis (CAPD)

In CAPD, dialysis is continuous all day, every day to compensate for the lesser efficiency of this technique compared with haemodialysis. Between 1.5 and 2 litres of dialysis fluid is exchanged four or five times daily in a process that takes 20–30 minutes. The old fluid is discarded after drainage. At all other times the patients are free to carry out their normal daily activities. Different glucose concentrations are used depending on the need to remove fluid. The major difficulties for the patients are the necessity to store large quantities of dialysis fluid at home and the need for somewhere clean and quiet in which to carry out the exchange.

Intermittent peritoneal dialysis (IPD)

In IPD the patient is connected permanently for two 24 hour periods each week to a machine that automatically instills and removes dialysis fluid. The machine can be programmed to use a particular volume of fluid, and the 'dwell time' in which fluid is neither instilled nor removed. At the end of the dialysis period the fluid is drained out and the patient disconnected from the machine. This was the first peritoneal dialysis technique used as a treatment for CRF, but it is not very effective and in practice its use is restricted to small groups of frail patients unsuitable for other treatment modalities.

Automated peritoneal dialysis (APD)

APD patients have a machine at home similar to an IPD machine to which they connect themselves in bed every night. Their dialysis prescription in terms of numbers and volume of exchanges, together with the different dialysis fluids used, can be individualized. The advantage of this technique is that it frees the patients from the need to carry out daytime exchanges, although in order to achieve adequate dialysis they may need to spend rather longer than 8 hours in bed and may need to add in a solitary daytime exchange as well. For certain groups of patients APD is superior to CAPD in terms of the quantity of dialysis that can be delivered. However, the technique is more expensive and some patients suffer disturbed sleep by the presence of the machine, which is not completely silent.

Peritoneal dialysis access

To carry out peritoneal dialysis, permanent access is required to the peritoneal cavity. This is achieved by inserting a silastic catheter into the peritoneum (Tenchkoff catheter), which is held in place by dacron cuffs. After exit from the peritoneum the catheter is tunnelled a short distance through the subcutaneous tissue before coming out to the abdominal surface. This 'tunnel' forms an extra barrier to infection. The catheter can be inserted either percutaneously with or without the aid of a laparoscope or surgically at a mini-laparotomy.

Peritonitis

This is the major complication of peritoneal dialysis owing to the presence of an indwelling catheter which is frequently manipulated. Meticulous attention to asepsis during exchanges, or connection and disconnection in the case of APD, is the principal protection against peritonitis and it is vital that the patients understand the need for a clean environment in which to carry out these procedures.

The earliest sign of peritonitis is the appearance of cloudy dialysis fluid, which often precedes any symptoms and should permit early diagnosis and treatment. A straightforward episode of peritonitis should be treated successfully using intraperitoneal antibiotics without the need to interrupt peritoneal dialysis (Keane *et al.* 1996).

Peritoneal dialysis adequacy

As with haemodialysis, the amount of dialysis can be monitored and prescriptions individualized for each patient. There is no consensus about the best method to measure the dose of peritoneal dialysis and most units use UKM (see Adequacy of haemodialysis, above) and/or measured creatinine clearance. The clinical value is equivocal; some workers report Kt/V to be correlated with the clinical assessment of dialysis adequacy (Keshaviah *et al.* 1990; CANUSA Peritoneal Dialysis Study Group 1996) whilst others have failed to find any association between Kt/V and outcome (Blake *et al.* 1991; Harty *et al.* 1993). However, approximate minimal targets for weekly $Kt/V > 1.7$ in CAPD and $Kt/V > 2.0$ in APD have been set (Renal Association 1997).

Dietary considerations in peritoneal dialysis

CAPD is the most popular form of peritoneal dialysis. As a result, most work on nutritional status and dietary requirements has been undertaken in patients on CAPD and little information is currently available for those given other treatment modalities.

The popularity of APD is increasing and patients may move to it from CAPD to increase the dose of delivered dialysis. One approach to dietary management in APD is to continue with the CAPD diet until new research, or evidence from monitoring, suggests that changes are required.

Malnutrition in peritoneal dialysis patients Malnutrition is as prevalent with CAPD as with haemodialysis, with approximately half of the patients suffering from undernutrition (Jacob *et al.* 1995). Poor outcome has been linked to a poor nutritional status (CANUSA Peritoneal Dialysis Study Group 1996) and the detection and treatment of malnutrition remains a primary goal for the dietitian.

Many of the causes of malnutrition and the treatments used in peritoneal dialysis are common to those encountered in haemodialysis (see above). Important differences with CAPD include the average daily loss of 15 g protein across the peritoneum (Blumenkrantz *et al.* 1981). The amount of protein lost can vary greatly between patients, but during episodes of peritonitis protein losses increase significantly. A further effect that may limit food intake in CAPD is the feeling of satiety and bloating from the presence of infused dialysate in the abdominal cavity.

Use of supplements with a high protein content (approx. 10 g/100 ml), may be appropriate in CAPD. Amino acid-based dialysate can also be used to treat malnutrition although, while its use has been shown to improve serum protein levels (Kopple *et al.* 1995), its clinical benefit remains unproven.

Protein To compensate for the high losses of protein during dialysis, a dietary protein intake of >1.2 g/kg ideal body weight is recommended (Renal Association 1997). Patients who eat less than this may not be at risk, providing they are stable. In patients with a low protein intake, use of high-protein sip feeds may be helpful.

Energy Glucose absorption from the dialysate across the peritoneum will provide approximately 300 kcal daily. Energy intake from this source will increase with the use of hypertonic bags or more frequent exchanges. The energy gain may be of benefit to those who are undernourished. However, it may adversely affect glycaemic control in diabetics and energy intake may have to be reduced to avoid excessive weight gain. It is recommended that a combined (oral and dialysate) energy intake of >35 kcal/kg ideal body weight should be attained in all patients (Renal Association 1997).

Potassium The aim is to maintain serum levels within the range of 3.5–5.5 mmol/l (Renal Association 1997). Hyperkalaemia is less of a problem in CAPD than in intermittent forms of dialysis and a more liberal potassium intake is generally allowed. However, blood levels will require monitoring and dietary potassium intake should be restricted where appropriate.

Phosphorus Foods with a high protein content commonly also have a high phosphorus content. Consequently, the higher protein diet recommended with CAPD will contain more phosphorus. To achieve serum levels within the recommended range of 1.1–1.6 mmol/l (Renal Association 1997), a dietary phosphorus restriction will usually be required and phosphate binders should be prescribed.

Fluid and sodium Dietary intakes of both sodium and fluid will need to be limited to prevent excessive retention of fluid. Urine output is more likely to be maintained with CAPD, so the allowance of fluid may be larger than with haemodialysis. Patients should check their weight daily. Sudden changes in body weight reflect changes in fluid balance and indicate that fluid intake is too high.

Micronutrients (see also under Sections 4.14.2–4.14.3) Low thiamin status has been identified amongst CAPD patients and supplementation is recommended. Riboflavin levels are not reduced in CAPD. Pyridoxine deficiency occurs in some patients and can be corrected by supplementation. Some patients also have low ascorbic acid levels which can be treated by 100 mg ascorbic acid daily. However, even this low dosage can significantly increase the serum oxalate concentration in patients on peritoneal dialysis.

Renal transplantation

For the majority of ESRF patients, renal transplantation is the best RRT option (Goldberg and Teerlink 1997). This was the first solid organ transplant procedure to become established, having been performed since the 1960s. In the UK approximately 1500 renal transplant operations are performed each year and patients can anticipate a 1 year graft survival of 90% and a 5 year graft survival of approximately 75%. The main limiting factor to transplantation is the supply of donor organs, which has fallen in recent years as a result of improved road safety.

Medical aspects of transplantation

Most ESRF patients will be worked up for transplantation, the exceptions being those not considered medically fit enough to withstand the operation and subsequent therapy, for instance those with severe ischaemic heart disease. Donor kidneys come from two sources. In the UK by far the biggest source of kidneys is cadaveric donors: patients on intensive care units who have been declared brain dead and have expressed a wish to be organ donors. The other option is live donors, who are usually close relatives who have agreed to donate one of their kidneys.

The biggest threat to transplantation is rejection whereby the body recognizes the new kidney as foreign and tries to destroy it via the immune system. This is countered in two ways: through matching of donor and recipient tissue type, and through the use of immunosuppressive drugs to damp down the immune system.

Immunosuppression Despite attention to matching of tissue types, rejection of the transplant is still likely if drugs are not used to suppress the patient's immune system. Many immunosuppressive drugs are available and different combinations are used depending on an assessment of each patient's risk of rejection. The most widely used agents are corticosteroids, cyclosporin and azathioprine. It is important to remember that some, if not all, of these agents will need to be taken for the lifetime of the transplant and that they all have considerable side-effects. In addition, because of their immunosuppression, transplant patients are at great risk of infectious disease which can occasionally be life-threatening.

Post-transplant care Following successful transplantation the patients need to be monitored closely for signs of rejection, which is done principally by measuring plasma creatinine. Rejection, when it occurs acutely, can usually be treated successfully by augmenting the immunosuppression. As renal function normalizes, the patient will become less like an ESRF patient and may no longer need such treatments as erythropoietin, phosphate binders and vitamin D analogues. However, each patient needs to be treated individually, especially with regard to bone biochemistry as some patients may already have irreversible hyperparathyroidism.

Transplant failure The length of time for which a transplant will survive is very variable, ranging from less than 1 year to as much as 20 years or more. Many factors determine graft survival. Chronic rejection occurs over a long period as the graft is slowly damaged. The process is incompletely understood and means that it is not possible to predict how long a transplant will last in an individual patient. However, it would be inappropriate to permit patients, especially younger ones, to believe that their kidney will last forever. In reality, patients will require further dialysis support at some stage, hopefully prior to subsequent re-transplantation. It is important to remember that a patient with a transplant that is no longer functioning well is a patient with CRF and should be treated as such.

Dietetic considerations following transplantation

A well-functioning graft enables the restrictive dietary regimens imposed in the pre-dialysis and dialysis periods to be relaxed. Whilst patients can look forward to a more liberal diet following a transplant, nutrition remains an important aspect of their care. In both the peri-operative phase and over the longer term, there are nutritional concerns to be addressed.

Peri-operative considerations Undernutrition and overnutrition adversely affect outcome in renal transplant recipients. Death rates following transplant are significantly increased in patients with a body mass index (BMI) <18 kg/m^2 and the risk of graft failure rises with increasing BMI (Chertow *et al*. 1996). Obese recipients also suffer from significantly higher rates of delayed graft function, new-onset diabetes and higher mortality rates (Holley *et al*. 1990). These factors highlight the need to maximize the patient's nutritional status pre-operatively.

Some kidneys work immediately post-transplant, but most take a few days to function. As kidney function improves, patients become polyuric and need encouragement to drink large volumes. Intravenous therapy is frequently required to prevent dehydration. Hypophosphataemia can develop and additional supplementation may be needed. Urine volume reduces with time as the kidney's ability to concentrate the urine increases. Appetite usually improves in association with the patient's general well-being and previous dietary restrictions can be relaxed once blood biochemistry has normalized. For these and other reasons, weight gain can become a problem (see below).

Many of the immunosuppressive agents that are used to prevent graft rejection have side-effects which can alter nutritional requirements (Table 4.27). In the immediate post-operative period, hyperkalaemia may persist, despite good kidney function. In such cases dietary potassium should be restricted until serum levels reduce. Opportunistic mouth and throat infections are another problem related to immunosuppression. Modification of food texture and the use of sip feeds can help to maintain an adequate nutritional intake.

Longer-term considerations Weight gain following transplantation is well documented. Average weight increases of 14% in the first year post-transplant have been reported (Przygrodzka *et al*. 1992). In some patients this may be welcome and reflect an improving nutritional status. However, in others it may lead to worsening obesity and exacerbation of morbid conditions such as hyperlipidaemia or diabetes. Dietary intervention at an early stage has been shown to limit weight gain successfully in this patient group (Patel 1998).

Hyperlipidaemia occurs in 25% of transplant patients and is associated with an increased incidence of cardiovascular and cerebrovascular events. Forty per cent of deaths following transplant are attributed to cardiovascular disease. Since high blood cholesterol levels accelerate atherosclerosis, a cholesterol-lowering diet would be expected to be of benefit. However, while some studies suggest that dietary treatment improves lipid levels in transplant patients (Nelson *et al*. 1988), other work shows that although the patient's diet may improve, lipid profiles are not significantly changed (Lawrence *et al*. 1995). Nevertheless, for most patients with good graft function, a cardioprotective diet based on healthy eating principles is appropriate. High protein intakes should be discouraged because of the dangers of protein-induced hyperfiltration, and a protein intake of 1.0 g/kg ideal body weight should be encouraged.

Eventually, as transplant function declines, the patient will suffer symptoms of advancing renal failure. Like

Table 4.27 Effects of immunosuppressive agents in transplant patients

Corticosteroids	Glucose intolerance
	Weight gain
	Negative nitrogen balance (with high doses)
Cyclosporin	Hyperkalaemia
	Hypercholesterolaemia
	Weight gain
Mycophenolate mofetil (MMF)	Gastrointestinal disturbances
	Hypercholesterolaemia
Tacrolimus	Glucose intolerance
	Gastrointestinal disturbances

patients in CRF, dietary restrictions are likely to be required at some stage.

4.14.4 The nephrotic syndrome

The nephrotic syndrome is a term that describes the clinical consequences of excessive urinary protein losses. Proteinuria of >150 mg/24 hours is considered abnormal but to cause the nephrotic syndrome urinary protein loss needs to be 3.5 g/24 hours or greater. The cardinal features of the nephrotic syndrome are:

- proteinuria >3.5 g/24 hours
- peripheral oedema
- hypoalbuminaemia
- hypercholesterolaemia.

It should be stressed, however, that all of its clinical features are a consequence of the urinary protein losses.

Causes of the nephrotic syndrome

The nephrotic syndrome is not a disease entity but the presenting syndrome of a whole range of renal diseases. Common causes of the nephrotic syndrome are listed in Table 4.28. In children and young adults the most common cause is minimal change glomerulonephritis, which usually has a very good prognosis.

It is important to remember that some of the pathological conditions can be present without causing the nephrotic syndrome and that there is great heterogeneity in the extent to which these conditions lead to CRF and ESRF. In general, however, the nephrotic syndrome will, if long-standing, lead to significant renal impairment.

Medical management of the nephrotic syndrome

With the exception of children and adolescents, in whom a straightforward case of nephrotic syndrome is likely to be due to minimal change glomerulonephritis and likely to respond to oral steroid therapy, a specific diagnosis is needed in order to both predict outcome and to target precise therapy. In almost all cases this will involve renal biopsy together with other investigations such as serological tests for autoantibodies. Therapy can then be divided into disease-specific measures and management of the manifestations of the nephrotic syndrome itself.

Disease-specific therapy will often take the form of corticosteroids and other immunosuppressive agents. General

Table 4.28 Common causes of the nephrotic syndrome

Minimal change glomerulonephritis
Focal segmental glomerulosclerosis
Membranous glomerulonephritis
Mesangioproliferative glomerulonephritidies
Diabetic nephropathy
Amyloidosis and myeloma kidney

therapy in the nephrotic syndrome is primarily aimed at reducing the degree of oedema. The first-line therapy is generally loop diuretics such as frusemide and bumetanide, which may have to be given in large doses. The additional use of an ACE inhibitor may reduce the degree of proteinuria and hence improve the oedema. Oedema in the nephrotic syndrome can be very refractory to therapy, in which case additional options include adding in a thiazide diuretic or the administration of intravenous albumin in combination with diuretics, which acts to increase plasma oncotic pressure and hence promote a diuresis. Sometimes these measures contribute to a deterioration in renal function. This may be regarded as the lesser of two evils as the nephrotic syndrome is a hypercoagulable state associated with considerable risk of vascular thromboembolic events. For this reason most nephrologists would also recommend measures to reduce the plasma cholesterol, which will probably require drug therapy and dietary modification.

Dietary considerations in the nephrotic syndrome

Some diseases causing the nephrotic syndrome respond rapidly and successfully with pharmaceutical treatment. Where this is not the case, dietary therapy has an important role. Consideration should be given to the amount of protein prescribed, when to use salt restriction and whether lipid-lowering advice is indicated.

Protein

Traditionally, high-protein diets were advocated. However, work on hyperfiltration in the 1980s led to a suggestion that such diets might be harmful. Support for abandoning the use of high-protein diets is provided by studies comparing the effects of different protein intakes in nephrotic patients. Diets containing 0.8 g protein/kg ideal body weight daily were shown to increase serum albumin levels compared with 1.6 g/kg body weight diets (Kaysen *et al.* 1986). It has also been found that a high protein intake (2.0 g/kg ideal body per day) fails to increase serum protein levels and results in higher levels of proteinuria. Protein intakes of 1.0 g/kg ideal body weight are therefore advocated (Mansy *et al.* 1989).

Salt

Oedematous patients will benefit from a combination of fluid restriction and a reduction in their sodium intake with a No Added Salt restriction. In the long term, regular diuretics will usually enable strict fluid restriction to be relaxed.

Hyperlipidaemia

Most nephrotics are hypercholesterolaemic, with high LDL-cholesterol and low HDL-cholesterol levels. A proportion of patients will also have increased serum triglyceride levels. Hyperlipidaemia is closely linked to albuminuria; hence, where protein losses in the urine can be successfully treated the lipid abnormalities will rapidly resolve. Where hyperlipidaemia persists, dietary lipid-lowering regimens should be the first line of treatment. However, because serum lipids are often so high, in practice dietary methods alone may not be sufficient and lipid-lowering agents will also be required.

The use of dietary intervention in hyperlipidaemia in the nephrotic syndrome has not been fully investigated. Specially formulated diets have been shown to reduce serum cholesterol levels (Barsotti *et al.* 1991; Gentile *et al.* 1993) but the design of these studies can be questioned as well as whether the unconventional diets that were used are safe and palatable in the long term. Low-fat, low-cholesterol, high complex-carbohydrate diets, containing adequate amounts of energy (35 kcal/kg) and protein (0.8–1.0 g/kg), may be preferable (Kaysen 1992).

Renal failure in the nephrotic syndrome

Some nephrotic patients will develop renal failure. Serum biochemistry requires monitoring and, where appropriate, adjustments should be made to dietary intake. One advantage is that proteinuria losses will reduce with a declining GFR.

Text revised by: George Hartley and Russell Roberts

References

Aparicio M, Cano N, Chauveau P *et al*. Nutritional status of haemodialysis patients: a French national cooperative study. *Nephrology, Dialysis, Transplantation*. 1999; **14**: 1679–1686.

Arnadottir M, Brattstrom L, Simonsen O *et al*. The effect of high-dose pyridoxine and folic acid supplementation on serum lipid and plasma homocysteine concentrations in dialysis patients. *Clinical Nephrology* 1993; **40**: 236–240.

Barrett BJ, Parfey PS, Morgan J *et al*. Prediction of early death in end-stage renal disease patients starting dialysis. *American Journal of Kidney Diseases* 1997; **29**: 214–222.

Barsotti G, Morelli E, Cupisti A *et al*. A special supplemented 'vegan' diet for nephrotic patients. *American Journal of Nephrology* 1991; **11**: 380–385.

Bartlett RH, Mault JR, Dechert RE *et al*. Continuous arteriovenous hemofiltration:improved survival in surgical acute renal failure? *Surgery* 1986; **100**: 400–408.

Bellomo R, Martin H, Parkin G *et al*. Continuous arteriovenous haemodiafiltration in the critically ill: influence on major nutrient balances. *Intensive Care Medicine* 1991; **17**: 399–402.

Bennett SE, Russell GI, Walls J. Low protein diets in uraemia. *British Medical Journal* 1983; **287**: 1344–1345.

Blake PG, Sombolos K, Abraham G *et al*. Lack of correlation between urea kinetic indices and clinical outcomes in CAPD patients. *Kidney International* 1991; **39**: 700–706.

Blumenkrantz MJ, Gahl GM, Kopple JD *et al*. Protein losses during peritoneal dialysis. *Kidney International* 1981; **19**: 593–602.

Bouffard Y, Viale JP, Annat G *et al*. Energy expenditure in the acute renal failure patient mechanically ventilated. *Intensive Care Medicine* 1987; **13**: 401–404.

Cano N, Labastie-Coeyrehourq J, Lacombe P *et al*. Perdialytic parenteral nutrition with lipids and amino acids in malnourished hemodialysis patients. *American Journal of Clinical Nutrition* 1990; **52**: 726–730.

CANUSA Peritoneal Dialysis Study Group. Adequacy of dialysis and nutrition in continuous peritoneal dialysis: association with clinical outcomes. *Journal of the American Society of Nephrology* 1996; **7**: 198–207.

Chertow MN, Ling J, Lew NL *et al*. The association of intradialytic parenteral nutrition administration with survival in hemodialysis patients. *American Journal of Kidney Diseases* 1994; **24**: 912–920.

Chertow GM, Lazarus JM, Milford EL. Quetelet's index predicts outcome in cadaveric kidney transplantation. *Journal of Renal Nutrition* 1996; **6**: 134–140.

Cunningham J, Fraher LJ, Clemens TL *et al*. Chronic metabolic acidosis with metabolic bone disease. Effect of alkali on bone morphology and vitamin D metabolism. *American Journal of Medicine* 1982; **73**: 199–204.

Davenport A, Roberts NB. Amino acid losses during high-flux hemofiltration in the critically ill patient. *Critical Care Medicine* 1989; **17**: 1010–1014.

Davies SP, Reaveley DA, Brown EA, Kox WJ. Amino acid clearances and daily losses in patients with acute renal failure treated by continuous arteriovenous hemodialysis. *Critical Care Medicine* 1991; **19**: 1510–1515.

Dolecek TA, Olson MB, Caggiula AW *et al*. Registered dietitian time requirements in the modification of diet in renal disease study. *Journal of the American Dietetic Association* 1995; **95**: 1307–1312.

Druml W, Fischer S, Sertl S *et al*. Fat elimination in acute renal failure: long-chain vs medium-chain triglyerides. *American Journal of Clinical Nutrition* 1992; **55**: 468–472.

Druml W, Schwarzenhofer M, Apsner R, Horl WH. Fat-soluble vitamins in patients with acute renal failure. *Mineral and Electrolyte Metabolism* 1998; **24**: 220–226.

Elia M. Artificial nutritional support. *Medicine International* 1990; **82**: 3392–3396.

El Nahas AM, Coles GA. Dietary treatment of chronic renal failure: ten unanswered questions. *Lancet* 1986; **i**: 597–600.

Food and Agriculture Organization/World Health Organization/United Nations University Joint (FAO/WHO/UNU) Expert Consultation. *Energy and Protein Requirements*. Technical Report Series 724. Geneva: WHO, 1985.

Friedman AL, Chesnelof RW, Gilbert FF. Secondary oxalosis as a complication of parenteral alimentation in ARF. *American Journal of Nephrology* 1983; **3**: 248

Gentile MG, Fellin G, Cofano F *et al*. Treatment of proteinuric patients with vegetarian soy diet and fish oil. *Clinical Nephrology* 1993; **40**: 315–320.

Gilmour ER, Hartley GH. Managing malnutrition. *British Journal of Renal Medicine* 1997; **2**: 22–24.

Gilmour ER, Hartley GH, Goodship THJ. Trace elements and vitamins in renal disease. In Mitch WE, Klahr S (Eds) *Handbook of Nutrition and the Kidney*, 3rd edn, pp. 105–122. New York: Lippincott-Raven, 1998.

Giovannetti S, Maggiore Q. A low-nitrogen diet with proteins of high biological value for severe chronic uraemia. *Lancet* 1964; **i**: 1000–1003.

Goldberg L, Taube D. Adult renal transplantation. In: Hakim NS (Ed.). *Introduction to Organ Transplantation*, pp. 73–91. London: Imperial College Press, 1997.

Gotch FA, Sargent JA. A mechanistic analysis of the National Cooperative Dialysis Study (NCDS). *Kidney International* 1985; **28**: 526–534.

Griffiths RD, Jones C, Palmer TEA. Six-month outcome of critically ill patients given glutamine-supplemented parenteral nutrition. *Nutrition* 1997; **13**: 295–302.

Harty J, Boulton H, Heelis N *et al*. Limitations of kinetic models as predictors of nutritional and dialysis adequacy in continuous ambulatory peritoneal dialysis patients. *American Journal of Nephrology* 1993; **13**: 454–463.

Holley JL, Shapiro R, Lopatin WB *et al*. Obesity as a risk factor following cadaveric renal transplantation. *Transplantation* 1990; **49**: 387–389.

Hynote ED, McCamish MA, Depner TA, Davis PA. Amino acid losses during hemodialysis: effects of high-solute flux and parenteral nutrition in acute renal failure. *Journal of Parenteral and Enteral Nutrition* 1995; **19**: 15–21.

Ishibashi N, Plank LD, Sando K, Hill GL. Optimal protein requirements during the first 2 weeks after the onset of critical illness. *Critical Care Medicine* 1998; **26**: 1529–1535.

Jacob V, Marchant PR, Wild G *et al*. Nutritional profile of continuous ambulatory peritoneal dialysis patients. *Nephron* 1995; **71**: 16–22.

Kaysen GA. Nutritional management of nephrotic syndrome. *Journal of Renal Nutrition* 1992; **2**: 50–58.

Kaysen GA, Gambertoglio J, Jimenez I *et al*. Effect of dietary protein intake on albumin homeostasis in nephrotic patients. *Kidney International* 1986; **29**: 572–577.

Kaysen GA, Stevenson FT, Depner TA. Determinants of albumin concentration in hemodialysis patients. *American Journal of Kidney Diseases* 1997; **29**: 658–668.

Keane WF, Alexander SR, Bailie GR *et al*. Peritoneal dialysis-related peritonitis treatment recommendations. *Peritoneal Dialysis International* 1996; **16**: 557–573.

Keshaviah PR, Nolph KD, Prowant B *et al*. Defining adequacy of CAPD with urea kinetics. *Advances in Peritoneal Dialysis* 1990; **6**: 173–177.

Klahr S, Levey AS, Beck GJ *et al*. The effects of dietary protein restriction and blood-pressure control on the progression of chronic renal disease. *New England Journal of Medicine* 1994; **330**: 877–884.

Kopple JD. The nutrition management of the patient with acute renal failure. *Journal of Parenteral and Enteral Nutrition* 1996; **20**: 3–12.

Kopple JD, Monteon FJ, Shaib JK. Effect of energy intake on nitrogen metabolism in nondialyzed patients with chronic renal failure. *Kidney International* 1986; **29**: 734–742.

Kopple JD, Bernard D, Messana J *et al*. Treatment of malnourished CAPD patients with an amino acid based dialysate. *Kidney International* 1995; **47**: 1148–1157.

Kopple JD, Levey AS, Greene T *et al*. Effect of dietary protein restriction on nutritional status in the modification of diet in renal disease study. *Kidney International* 1997; **52**: 778–791.

Lawrence IR, Thompson A, Hartley GH *et al*. The effect of dietary intervention on the management of hyperlipidemia in British renal transplant patients. *Journal of Renal Nutrition* 1995; **5**: 73–77.

Levey AS, Adler S, Caggiula AW *et al*. Effects of dietary protein restriction on the progression of advanced renal disease in the modification of diet in renal disease study. *American Journal of Kidney Diseases* 1996a; **27**: 652–663.

Levey AS, Adler S, Caggiula AW *et al*. Effects of dietary protein restriction on the progression of moderate renal disease in the modification of diet in renal disease study. *Journal of the American Society of Nephrology* 1996b; **7**: 2616–2626.

Locatelli F, Alberti D, Graziani G *et al*. Prospective, randomised, multicentre trial of effect of protein restriction on progression of chronic renal insufficiency. *Lancet* 1991; **337**: 1299–1304.

Lowrie EG, Lew NL. Death risk in hemodialysis patients: the predictive value of commonly measured variables and an evaluation of death rate differences between facilities. *American Journal of Kidney Diseases* 1990; **25**: 458–482.

Makk LJK, McClave SA, Creech PW *et al*. Clinical application of the metabolic cart to the delivery of total parenteral nutrition. *Critical Care Medicine* 1990; **18**: 1320–1327.

Manas DM, Talbot D. Vascular access. In Jamison RL, Wilkinson R (Eds) *Nephrology*, pp. 895–909. London: Chapman and Hall, 1997.

Mansy H, Goodship THJ, Tapson JS *et al*. Effect of a high protein diet in patients with the nephrotic syndrome. *Clinical Science* 1989; **77**: 445–451.

Marckmann P. Nutritional status of patients on hemodialysis and peritoneal dialysis. *Clinical Nephrology* 1988; **29**: 75–78.

Maschio G, Oldrizzi L, Tessitore N *et al*. Effects of dietary protein and phosphorus restriction on the progression of early renal failure. *Kidney International* 1982; **22**: 371–376.

Navis G, de Zeeuw D, de Jong PE. ACE-inhibitors: panacea for progressive renal disease? *Lancet* 1997; **349**: 1852–1853.

Nelson J, Beauregard M, Gelinas M *et al*. Rapid improvement of hyperlipidemia in kidney transplant patients with a multifactorial hypolipidemic diet. *Transplantation Proceedings* 1988; **XX**: 1264–1270.

NIH Consensus Statement. *Morbidity and Mortality of Dialysis* 11, 2nd edn. Bethesda, MD: National Institutes of Health, 1993.

Owen WF, Lew NL, Liu Y *et al*. The urea reduction ratio and serum albumin concentration as predictors of mortality in patients undergoing hemodialysis. *New England Journal of Medicine* 1993; **329**: 1001–1006.

Panzetta O, Cominacini L, Garbin U *et al*. Increased susceptibility of LDL to *in vitro* oxidation in patients on maintenance hemodialysis: effects of fish oil and vitamin E administration. *Clinical Nephrology* 1995; **44**: 303–309.

Patel MG. The effect of dietary intervention on weight gains after renal transplantation. *Journal of Renal Nutrition* 1998; **8**: 137–141.

Przygrodzka F, Rayner HC, Morgan AG, Burden RP. Change in nutritional status after successful renal transplantation. *Journal of Renal Nutrition* 1992; **2**: 18–20.

Rainford DJ. Nutritional management of acute renal failure. *Acta Chirurgica Scandinavica* 1981; **507** (Suppl): 327–329.

Reaich D, Channon SM, Scrimgeour CM *et al*. Correction of acidosis in humans with CRF decreases protein degradation and amino acid oxidation. *American Journal of Physiology* 1993; **265**: E230–E235.

Renal Association (Ed.). *Treatment of Adult Patients with Renal Failure. Recommended Standards and Audit Measures*, 2nd edn. London: The Royal College of Physicians, 1997.

Rosman JB, Meijer S, Sluiter WJ *et al*. Prospective randomised trial of early dietary protein restriction in chronic renal failure. *Lancet* 1984; **ii**: 1291–1296.

Schneeweiss B, Graninger W, Stockenhuber F *et al*. Energy metabolism in acute and chronic renal failure. *American Journal of Clinical Nutrition* 1990; **52**: 596–601.

Thadani R, Pascual M, Bonventre JV. Acute renal failure. *New England Journal of Medicine* 1996; **334**: 1448–1460.

Tomson CRV, Ward MK. Aluminium toxicity in renal failure. In Maher JF (Ed.) *Replacement of Renal Function by Dialysis*, pp. 1004–1017. Dordrecht: Kluwer Academic, 1989.

Walser M, Mitch WE, Maroni BJ, Kopple JD. Should protein intake be restricted in the predialysis patients? *Kidney International* 1999; **55**: 771–777.

Winnearls CG. Recombinant human erythropoetin: 10 years of clinical experience. *Nephrology, Dialysis, Transplantation* 1998; **13** (Suppl 2): 3–8.

4.15 Gout and renal stones

4.15.1 Gout and hyperuricaemia

The importance of the role of purines in human disease has been realized since the discovery that uric acid (to which they are metabolized) is a component of some renal stones and that serum uric acid levels are elevated in patients with gout. Elevated serum levels can lead to deposition of urate crystals in joints, resulting in an acute inflammatory response, or in soft tissues such as cartilage without accompanying inflammation. Hyperuricaemia may be primary or secondary, but whatever its aetiology it reflects either overproduction of purines, reduced renal clearance of uric acid or a combination of both.

The most common manifestation of hyperuricaemia is gout, which for many years has been thought to be a familial disease. However, it does not follow any recognizable pattern of inheritance, with the majority of cases of hyperuricaemia resulting from individual variation in metabolic and renal function on which environmental influences are superimposed (Scott 1996).

Many factors affect the serum urate concentration, particularly those which lead to increased degradation of ATP to AMP, which is not then reused but degraded to adenosine and inosine and thus to the purine bases and urate. Such factors include alcohol or fructose ingestion, sustained exercise and tissue hypoxia from any cause, all of which can result in overproduction of urate. Asymptomatic hyperuricaemia can be regarded as the first phase of gout (Harris *et al*. 1999).

Acute gout most commonly presents with severe pain and inflammation in the first metatarsal joint of the foot, but other joints may also be involved. Definitive diagnosis can be made by the detection of crystals in synovial fluid aspirate, although in most cases the combination of hyperuricaemia and clinical symptoms is sufficiently diagnostic. If untreated, progressive crystal deposition can lead to chronic gouty arthritis and an increased risk of soft-tissue damage.

The condition is much more common in men than in women, with the peak incidence occurring between the ages of 30 and 50 years (Harris *et al*. 1999).

Treatment of gout

Acute episodes of gout are managed with non-steroidal anti-inflammatory drugs (NSAIDs) or colchicine. Once the acute phase has subsided, the condition can be kept under control by long-term drug treatment with:

- allopurinol, a xanthine-oxidase inhibitor, which reduces uric acid production: this drug has been used as the main treatment for gout for over 30 years
- uricosuric drugs such as probenecid or sulfinpyrazone: these increase urinary uric acid excretion.

Dietary intervention is no longer regarded as primary therapy but may still have an important subsidiary role, particularly in the management of asymptomatic hyperuricaemia where drug treatment is usually contraindicated. Dietary factors which can influence hyperuricaemia include:

- *Dietary purine content*: The contribution of dietary purines to uric acid production is only small and, in most people, purine restriction is of little benefit and unnecessary. However, regular or excessive consumption of purine-rich foods (typically those rich in cell nuclei such as yeast-rich foods or fish roes; see Table 4.29) will make more of an impact and some restriction is advisable.
- *Alcohol*: Excessive alcohol consumption has been associated with gout for centuries, although it is less certain whether this is a direct effect of alcohol *per se*, or an indirect effect of either the high purine content of some types of alcohol (particularly beer) or the contribution of alcohol to excessive energy intake and obesity. Whatever the mechanism, moderation of alcohol consumption to (or below) safe drinking levels is advisable.
- *Obesity*: This exacerbates hyperuricaemia and weight loss can significantly reduce serum urate levels (Emmerson 1996). However, any such weight loss should be gradual since fasting or strict dieting will result in lean tissue breakdown and an acute rise in serum uric acid level.
- *Fluid intake*: In order to lessen the risk of crystallization of urate in the urine, particularly if uricosuric drugs

Table 4.29 Principal dietary sources of purines (Clifford *et al*. 1976; Wood 1996)

Meat sources	Fish sources	Other sources
Liver	Anchovies	Yeast and extracts
Heart	Crab	Beer
Kidney	Fish roes	Asparagus
Sweetbreads	Herring	Cauliflower
Meat extracts (e.g. Oxo)	Mackerel	Mushrooms
	Sardines	Beans and peas
	Shrimps	Spinach
	Sprats	
	Whitebait	

are used, it is important that people consume sufficient fluid, possibly as much as 3–3.5 litres/day.

4.15.2 Renal stones

Most urinary stones found in patients in the majority of countries are renal stones; bladder stones are becoming less common. Diagnosis is rarely difficult because the symptoms are so painful, ranging from dull loin pain if the stone is in the renal pelvis to agonizing colic if it is lodged in the ureter.

In the UK the prevalence of urinary tract stone disease is relatively low at about 1.5% (Currie and Turner 1979). The annual incidence of stone formation is around 7 per 10 000 of the population, with a male:female ratio of about 2:1. Renal stones tend to recur and the recurrence rate is about 75% over 20 years (Pak 1998).

In most industrialized countries, 80% of stones are composed of calcium salts, usually as calcium oxalate (Daudon *et al.* 1995). The remaining 20% of stones are composed of uric acid, magnesium ammonium phosphate or cystine. Stones with any other composition are very rare (less than 1% of total stone occurrence).

The formation of stones requires supersaturated urine; the greater the concentration of ions, the more likely they are to precipitate. The concentration of ions depends on the urinary pH, ionic strength, solute concentration and complexation. Both environmental and nutritional factors have been shown to affect stone nucleation and growth by their effects on urinary constituents and pH.

Before aetiology and treatment can be specified, the type of renal stone must be determined. Stones are classified into four main types according to their chemical constituents:

- calcium stones
- uric acid stones
- 'infection' stones
- cystine stones.

The aetiology and management of each of these types of stone is discussed below.

4.15.3 Calcium stones

Calcium oxalate is the main component of 80% of all kidney stones (Lemann *et al.* 1996). Hypercalciuria contributes to calcium stone formation by increasing the urinary saturation of calcium salts and by inactivating urinary inhibitors. These inhibitors have been found to be lower in stone formers than the rest of the population (Robertson *et al.* 1976). Inhibitors identified include citrate, glycoproteins, glycosaminoglycans and Tamm–Horsfall glycoprotein.

In 80% of cases there is no underlying cause and the stone can be described as idiopathic. In the remaining 20%, the stone is secondary to some other renal factor. The causes of secondary stone disease are discussed later in this section.

Idiopathic calcium stone disease (idiopathic hypercalciuria)

This is a syndrome of unexplained hypercalciuria, which can be distinguished from primary hyperparathyroidism only by its normal serum calcium levels. Contributory factors include:

- *Gender*: Men are particularly susceptible and account for 85% of cases.
- *Age*: It occurs most commonly between the ages of 20 and 50 years but the incidence rises in the fourth decade.
- *Occupation*: The risk of stone formation is greater in people who work in hot climates or conditions, as a result of the increased likelihood of dehydration.
- *Social class*: The incidence is greater in social classes II and I, possibly associated with higher dietary protein intakes (Robertson *et al.* 1980, 1981).
- *Diet*: Dietary factors which have been suggested to be related to idiopathic hypercalciuria include high intakes of calcium, vitamin D, protein, sodium and refined carbohydrate, and low intakes of fluids and fibre. However, some of these associations remain equivocal (see Role of diet in idiopathic calcium stone formation, below).
- *Increased intestinal absorption of calcium*: The cause of increased calcium absorption in the intestine is unknown. It may result from either increased synthesis of 1,25-dihydroxycholecalciferol or the presence of more calcitriol intestinal receptor sites (Dretler 1998). Intestinal hyperabsorption of calcium raises serum calcium (remaining within the normal range), which reduces endogenous parathyroid hormone production. This leads to decreased renal tubular reabsorption of calcium and therefore excess calcium is excreted in the urine in order to maintain a normal serum calcium level.
- *Impaired tubular reabsorption of calcium*: Secondary hyperparathyroidism stimulates calcitriol synthesis and increases intestinal calcium reabsorption (Pak 1998).
- *Increased urinary oxalate*: Increased urinary oxalate excretion significantly increases stone risk. However, given the low oxalate content of most common foods and its low absorption rate (8–12%), the impact of dietary oxalate on urinary excretion is questionable (see below).
- *Urinary uric acid*: Total urinary uric acid output is usually normal in stone formers but the concentration is increased. This is thought to reduce the activity of the urinary inhibitors.

Role of diet in idiopathic calcium stone formation

Calcium   For many years it has been assumed that a high calcium intake increases the risk of stone formation. However, severe calcium restriction (<400 mg per day) does not appear to be beneficial in reducing the frequency of new stone formation in patients with recurrent urolithiasis (Wendland 1991) and may even be detrimental as negative calcium balance and secondary hyperoxaluria may occur. A major prospective study on a group of 45 619 men found a 34% lower incidence of stone occurrence among those on a high calcium diet (Curhan *et al.* 1993). However, this study was carried out on healthy subjects and may not be applicable to patients with existing stones.

Vitamin D The role of excessive vitamin D intake in stone formation has been studied for many years and continues to be an area of controversy. There is a direct correlation between plasma vitamin D and calcium excretion and for this reason patients may be discouraged from self-medication with multivitamin preparations or fish liver oil capsules containing vitamin D. However, a large-scale epidemiological study found a lower incidence of renal stones in men with a high intake of vitamin D (Curhan *et al.* 1993). A review by Parivar *et al.* (1996) found that there was no conclusive evidence to link excessive dietary vitamin D or prolonged exposure to sunlight with a higher incidence of urolithiasis (renal stones).

Protein The role of excessive protein has become clearer in recent years but the mechanism remains complex. Following a protein load there is brief period of metabolic acidosis and although urinary pH *per se* is not a major risk factor, calcium oxalate is less soluble in acid conditions. Dietary protein has also been found to increase oxaluria and uricosuria, which are associated with urolithiasis (Borghi *et al.* 1999).

Sodium Urinary sodium excretion correlates directly with urinary calcium excretion (Wasserstein *et al.* 1989). A high-sodium diet therefore increases calcium excretion and consequently the risk of stone formation. Hypercalciuric patients may be more sensitive to the calciuric effect of a sodium load. High sodium intake also increases the saturation of monosodium urate, the crystals of which can act as a basis for calcium crystallization.

Fluid The detrimental effects of a low fluid intake are obvious: a low fluid intake results in a low urinary output with an increase in the concentration of ionic particles and the saturation level of various salts.

Fibre There are conflicting epidemiological studies on the role of fibre intake on urolithiasis risk, largely as a result of the different definitions and analytical methods used to estimate 'fibre' intake. At present, no conclusions can be drawn.

Refined carbohydrate It has been suggested that a reduction in the intake of refined carbohydrate may be beneficial (Rao *et al.* 1982) but there is little confirmatory evidence to support this or to distinguish this observation from a possible link with lack of dietary fibre.

Diagnosis of idiopathic hypercalciuria

A range of tests and questions is required to establish the likely cause and type of stone:

- *24 hour urine collection*: An accurate 24 hour urine collection will provide information on the elevated amounts of excretory products. The urine must be

collected at home with the patient consuming their normal diet and fluid intake. Serum concentrations of calcium, uric acid, electrolytes and parathyroid hormone should also be measured.

- *Dietary history*: It is very important to determine the past and present intake of all relevant nutrients to establish whether hypercalciuria is of dietary origin or due to hyperabsorption. Hypercalciuria on a low or normal calcium diet (<700 mg/day) indicates hyperabsorption.

- *Social history*: Patients should be asked about past and present occupations to establish whether the working environment is likely to have caused long periods of dehydration (e.g. miners and heavy-metal workers). Caucasians who have worked abroad in a hot climate are at similar risk. Prolonged bed rest (e.g. following limb fracture) can also be a contributory cause since this can result in mobilization of calcium from the bones and thus hypercalciuria. Previous history is important as a stone may have formed in the past and been growing slowly.

Dietary treatment of idiopathic hypercalciuria

There are different schools of thought as to which dietary restrictions are necessary to treat idiopathic hypercalciuria and, more importantly, to prevent the recurrence of stones.

Calcium Calcium restriction is not indicated in patients with idiopathic hypercalciuria who have normal intestinal absorption of calcium. A decreased calcium intake will result in the preferential absorption of oxalate and hence increased oxaluria. Dietary compliance with calcium restriction has also been shown to be poor in the long term (Baker and Mallinson 1979). Many studies now support the theory that increasing calcium intake will beneficially decrease urinary oxalate excretion (Lemann *et al.* 1996; Coe *et al.* 1992).

Reduced bone mineral content (BMC) has also been reported in idiopathic stone formers who have been following a low-calcium diet (352 ± 20 mg) for about 10 years (± 0.7 years) (Fuss *et al.* 1990a). The reduction in BMC was as pronounced as that observed in hyperparathyroid stone formers. Although comparison with normal subjects showed that idiopathic renal stone formers had lower than average BMC whether or not they restricted calcium intake, those on a low-calcium diet were found to have lower BMC in the distal radius than those on a free diet (Fuss *et al.* 1990b). This may be caused by one or more of the following:

- Idiopathic hypercalciuria, if not compensated by an adequate calcium supply, will lead to negative calcium balance.
- Hypophosphataemia in idiopathic renal stone formation is associated with increased resorption and decreased formation of bone.
- Elevated circulating levels of 1,25-dihydroxyvitamin D (calcitriol) can induce bone resorption and result in negative calcium balance, especially if associated with a low-calcium diet (Fuss *et al.* 1990a).

The role of pharmacological doses of calcitriol remains uncertain. Studies have shown that calcitriol potentiates the loss of bone mineral by aggravating the negative calcium balance caused by a low-calcium diet (Coe *et al.* 1992). Calcitriol and its analogues are able to reduce the production of parathyroid hormone, which explains the failure of serum parathyroid hormone levels to rise if dietary calcium is low.

Oxalate The majority of urinary calculi contain oxalate and therefore it would seem logical that the dietary oxalate intake should be reduced. However, approximately 60% of urinary oxalate is produced from endogenous metabolism of glycine, glycolate and hydroxyproline, with 25–30% from the metabolism of ascorbic acid (Parivar *et al.* 1996) or via endogenous synthesis in the liver (Holmes *et al.* 1995). Therefore, only 10–15% of urinary oxalate is derived from dietary intake and in addition only 8–12% of dietary oxalate is absorbed (Tiselius 1980). The potential benefits from dietary oxalate restriction are therefore questionable. Goldfarb (1988) has suggested that restrictions should be confined to patients who normally have a high consumption of oxalate-rich foods (Table 4.30).

A recent study by Lemann *et al.* (1996) has also shown that body size is a major determinant of urinary oxalate excretion in healthy adults, presumably reflecting endogenous oxalate synthesis with tissue formation. Assuming that this is applicable to stone formers, modest weight reduction in those who are overweight may be beneficial. This should be carried out under guidance, as rapid or extreme weight gain or loss may precipitate stone development (Stoller and Bolton 1995).

Fluid There is consensus that an oral fluid intake sufficient to produce a urine output of at least 2 litres a day (ideally 3–3.5 litres of fluid intake) is adequate hydration for stone patients. A high intake of fluid has been shown to be effective when used as the only method of stone prevention (Borghi *et al.* 1996). A recent review by Kleiner (1999) stressed that dietitians should be encouraged to promote and monitor fluid intake among patients; this may be aided by a specified fluid intake plan. The importance of extra fluids in hot weather and when on holiday in a hot climate should be stressed. Patients do not need to purchase a water softener in order to reduce the calcium content of the water, and this may even be detrimental as softened water has a higher sodium content.

Protein and sodium A high dietary intake of protein can increase the excretion of calcium and uric acid and decrease the excretion of citrate. Protein restriction to 0.8 g/kg per day in patients with idiopathic hypercalciuria has been shown to reduce urinary excretion of urea, calcium, uric acid and oxalate but increase urinary citrate excretion (Giannini *et al.* 1999). These effects are thought to be due to a reduction in bone resorption and renal loss of calcium due to the decreased exogenous acid load. A high sodium intake leads to increased urinary sodium and calcium excretion as a result of their inhibited reabsorption in the proximal tubule and along the loop of Henle. Patients should be advised to consume a maximum of 1 g protein/kg body weight per day and follow a No Added Salt diet (80–100 mmol/day).

Sugar and refined carbohydrates There is some evidence that a reduction in the intake of sugar and refined carbohydrate is beneficial (Rao *et al.* 1982) but, rather than attempting to eliminate them from the diet, it is more conducive to compliance to recommend a reduction in intake in line with that advocated for the rest of the population. There is no evidence that aspartame or other artificial sweeteners have an adverse effect on oxaluria or increase the risk of stone formation (Nguyen *et al.* 1998).

Citrate The merits of a diet high in citrate have yet to be investigated. Citrate is a naturally occurring urinary stone inhibitor that binds calcium in solution to form a highly soluble calcium–citrate complex. This complex decreases the ionic concentration of calcium and hence the relative saturation of calcium oxalate and calcium phosphate in the urine. However, the benefits from large intakes of citrus fruits and vegetables are likely to be offset by the resultant hyperoxaluria caused by the consequent increased intake of dietary oxalate.

Fish oils Eicosapentanoic acid has predominantly been reported to decrease urinary calcium excretion in people with idiopathic hypercalciuria who, it is thought, have erythrocyte ion-transport abnormalities and different erythrocyte membrane lipid composition compared with healthy controls (Curhan and Curhan 1997). There may be a group of patients for whom fish oil supplementation could correct this defect; however, evidence to date is inconclusive.

Vitamin B_6 and vitamin C High intakes of vitamins B_6 and C have previously been thought to increase the incidence of stone formation. However, in a large study of 85 557 women, those on high intakes of vitamin B_6 were shown to have an inverse association with risk of stone formation and there was no increased risk associated with high intakes of vitamin C. Therefore, routine restriction of

Table 4.30 Principal dietary sources of oxalate (Kasidas and Rose 1980)

Food	Oxalic acid content (mg/100 g)
Beetroot	500
Carob powder	73
Chocolate (and other products containing cocoa)	117
Parsley (can be used in small amounts)	100
Peanuts[1]	187
Rhubarb	600
Spinach	600
Tea infusion (mg/100 ml)	55–78

[1]All nuts should be considered to be high in oxalates.
Foods which contain moderate amounts of oxalates and which should be taken in limited quantities include strawberries, celery and instant coffee.

vitamins B_6 and C appears to be unwarranted (Curhan *et al.* 1999).

Non-dietary treatment of idiopathic hypercalciuria

Thiazide diuretics or hydrochlorothiazide appear to act on the renal tubules, causing greater reabsorption of calcium and restoring parathyroid function, intestinal calcium absorption and urinary calcium excretion to normal. Potassium citrate or bicarbonate given with the thiazide prevents hypokalaemia and improves the excretion of citrate (Pak 1994).

Sodium cellulose phosphate, a calcium-binding resin, when taken with meals reduces calcium absorption but increases urinary oxalate excretion. It can also cause side-effects such as gastric discomfort and diarrhoea. Studies have not proven its effectiveness in reducing stone formation and it is no longer prescribed for this purpose.

Secondary calcium stone disease

Secondary calcium stone disease usually results from one of the following.

Primary hyperparathyroidism

The treatment of primary hyperparathyroidism is a parathyroidectomy. Parathyroid hormone levels should always be measured when assessing patients with stones. If parathyroidectomy is delayed or unsuccessful a low-calcium diet may be prescribed to lower plasma and urine calcium levels. In some cases surgical removal of the stone may be required.

Medullary sponge kidney

Because of the abnormal anatomy of the kidney, these patients make stones when the urinary calcium concentration is normal and should therefore reduce their calcium intake.

Renal tubular acidosis

This is a rare condition, caused by primary or secondary damage to the renal tubules. The patient cannot produce acid urine because of a failure of bicarbonate reabsorption and calcium phosphate stones are formed. Renal tubular acidosis can be treated by the use of alkalis to return the serum bicarbonate and pH to within the normal range and/or diet. A diet rich in animal protein will increase the urinary acidity, so a reduction in animal protein intake may be helpful. Some patients may choose to make radical changes to their diet and become vegan since such a diet can have a dramatic effect in reducing their symptoms. They should be given help to make sure that their diet is nutritionally balanced.

Primary hyperoxaluria

Type I primary hyperoxaluria is an autosomal recessive trait, which is caused by an inborn error of glyoxylic acid metabolism. Glyoxylic acid is normally transaminated to glycine or glycolic acid but, if the necessary enzymes are absent, oxalic acid will be produced. Two enzyme deficiencies, and hence two forms of primary oxaluria, have been identified: absence of alanine glyoxalate aminotransferase (type I) and absence of D-glycerate dehydrogenase (type II hyperoxaluria). The majority of cases are type I.

The full biochemistry of oxalic acid and glyoxylic acid metabolism is not known, but in patients with primary hyperoxaluria the production and excretion of oxalic acid is vastly increased. Calcium oxalate is insoluble, so renal stones readily occur and, in addition, oxalosis (oxalate deposition) in the heart, bones, joints, eyes and other tissues is common. When this occurs the prognosis is very poor.

Treatment of primary hyperoxaluria This comprises:

- *Pyridoxine supplements*: This is the only known effective treatment for primary hyperoxaluria. In doses of up to 1 g/day, pyridoxine has been shown to reduce urinary oxalate excretion from 1.4 mmol/24 hours to nearly normal (upper limit 0.5 mmol/24 hours; Rose 1979). Although not all patients respond to pyridoxine, it remains the cornerstone of treatment.
- *Increased fluid intake*: Increasing urinary volume to 3 litres/24 hours should be encouraged.
- *Diet*: Patients should be advised to follow a low-oxalate diet. A list of foods high in oxalate which should be avoided is given in Table 4.30.
- *Measures to increase the solubility of calcium oxalate*: In those with hypercalciuria, oral citrate supplements, given in conjunction with the use of thiazide diuretics, are beneficial. Oral phosphate supplements may also be considered.

Secondary hyperoxaluria

There are several causes of secondary hyperoxaluria:

- *Iatrogenic*: Hyperoxaluria may occur as a result of the treatment used for idiopathic hypercalciuria (see above).
- *Intestinal bypass and bowel disease*: Enteric hyperoxaluria can result from malabsorption by the small bowel from any cause, including resection, e.g. ileostomy formation, intrinsic disease as seen with Crohn's disease and jejunoileal bypass. If these result in steatorrhoea, calcium will bind with fatty acids in the gut and be unable to bind with oxalate; as a result, more oxalate will be passively absorbed. Treatment focuses on reducing dietary oxalate to reduce hyperoxaluria, and decreasing intake of fat to reduce the steatorrhoea. Medium-chain triglyceride (MCT) oil has no effect on oxalate absorption and can therefore be used to increase energy intake if required. Oral calcium supplements have also been used to precipitate oxalate in the intestinal lumen, and cholestyramine to bind fatty acids, bile acids and oxalate may be suggested. Oral citrate supplements and advice on how to achieve a high fluid intake can also be beneficial.

- *Excessive vitamin C intake*: Vitamin C intake in large doses has been implicated as a risk factor for stone formation as a result of ascorbate being metabolized to oxalate, which is then excreted in the urine (see Dietary treatment of idiopathic hypercalciuria, above)
- *Vitamin D overdose*: This will cause increased intestinal absorption of calcium.
- *Immobilization*: If prolonged, immobilization leads to bone resorption and consequent hypercalcaemia and hypercalciuria.

4.15.4 Uric acid stones

Uric acid is produced by the biochemical conversion of dietary and endogenous purines. The factors which lead to the formulation of uric acid calculi include:

- hyperuricosuria (>750 mg/day uric acid)
- persistently acidic urine
- low urine volume.

Treatment of uric acid stones

Dietary modification

Hyperuricosuria has been found to occur in conjunction with a high protein intake (Goldfarb 1988). A high protein intake increases the acid load for the kidneys to buffer. Patients with uric acid stone disease have a defect in the production of this buffer resulting in acid urine, which increases the amount of less soluble uric acid. The elderly often have a defect in this buffering process and hence have a higher incidence of uric acid stones (Radman 1991). Therefore, it is wise to recommend a decrease in protein consumption for all stone formers, particularly sources of protein that also have a high purine content.

Patients should be advised to avoid foods rich in purine (Table 4.29); however, the necessity for severe restriction has been superseded by the use of allopurinol and protein restriction.

Fluid intake

As with all types of stone, a high fluid intake sufficient to produce a daily urine output of at least 2 litres is desirable. Patients with chronic diarrhoea or high ileostomy outputs have an increased risk of uric acid stones owing to the loss of fluid and alkali which allows uric acid supersaturation. In patients with chronic diarrhoea syndromes, the use of potassium salts to replace alkali can cause intestinal irritation and therefore sodium bicarbonate may be the preferred treatment. The aim is to reach a urine pH of above 6, when uric acid is unlikely to be supersaturated.

In patients with an ileostomy, the amount of fluid required to maintain an adequate urine output may result in excessive stoma output; a balance may have to be achieved between the two.

Allopurinol

This drug inhibits the action of the enzyme xanthine oxidase in the pathway oxidizing hypoxanthine to urate and is very successful in preventing uric acid stone formation.

4.15.5 'Infection' stones or struvite stones

These stones contain magnesium ammonium phosphate and calcium phosphate. Chronic infection of the urinary tract with a urea-splitting organism is a very common cause of these types of stone. The organisms break down urea, producing ammonia and resulting in an alkaline urine. Magnesium ammonium phosphate and calcium phosphate are extremely insoluble in alkaline conditions and once urinary pH exceeds 7.2, struvite will precipitate spontaneously.

Treatment of infection stones

Surgery

The best treatment of struvite calculi is stone removal. However, bacterial penetration of small residual calculi may still occur and long-term antibiotics will be required (Michaels *et al.* 1988).

Eradication of the infection

The best prevention for struvite calculi is to eradicate the source of the infection by antimicrobial therapy. After clearance of the struvite calculi, 3 months of oral culture-specific antibiotic treatment is recommended.

Urease inhibitor

It has been shown that it is possible to inhibit the action of the urea-splitting enzyme, urease, in the bacteria in the kidney, thus preventing ammonia release. The substance used is acetohydroxamic acid (1 g/day). Data on usage for 2 or more years do not show a significant difference between patients and controls sufficient to recommend treatment for all patients. The inhibitor must be given with antibiotics as it has no antibacterial effect. Approximately 20–30% of patients are unable to tolerate acetohydroxamic acid because of reversible side-effects.

Diet

Drinking cranberry juice has been recommended for many years as a way of preventing and treating infections of the urinary tract, although there is no good-quality evidence for this (Jepson *et al.* 1999). Initially, it was thought that the acidity of the juice decreased the pH of the urine to nearer 5.5, which achieves bacteriosis, but *in vitro* studies suggest that the ability of proanthocyanidins present in the juice to inhibit bacterial adhesion to the uroepithelial-cell surfaces may be more significant (Howell *et al.* 1998). The main disadvantage of recommending cranberry juice is that oxalate and uric acid stones form in acidic urine and that an intake of more than 1 litre juice/day may result in uric acid stone formation (Rogers 1991). The high sugar content of the juice may also lead to weight gain. Patients with these problems should be advised to drink no more than 250 ml twice per day.

Table 4.31 Urinary concentration of cystine

Patient	Cystine concentration (μmol/l)
Normal	10–100
Heterozygous cystinurics	200–600
Homozygous cystinurics	1400–4200

4.15.6 Cystine stones

This is a very rare autosomal recessive genetic disorder affecting the renal tubular reabsorption of cystine, arginine and ornithine, resulting in increased concentration of cystine in the urine (Table 4.31). The limit of solubility of cystine at pH 7.5 and 37°C is 1250 μmol/l, so homozygous cystinurics readily precipitate cystine. Heterozygotes (asymptomatic carriers) may excrete up to 10 times as much cystine as normal but do not form cystine stones.

Treatment of cystine stones

Diet

A salt restriction may lower cystine excretion (Rodriguez *et al.* 1995), so patients should be advised to limit their intake to 80–100 mmol/day or lower. Cystine is a non-essential amino acid and is synthesized in the body from methionine. A diet low in methionine may reduce urinary cystine. However, the diet is restrictive, ineffective and difficult to follow. Animal protein has to be limited to 30 g/day from meat, fish, cheese and eggs, in addition to that contained in 300 ml milk. Additional protein requirements are met by vegetable protein. The diet should only be used as a last resort when other treatments have failed.

Dilution of urine

The patient should be advised to drink enough fluid to pass at least 3 litres of urine per 24 hours. This will include getting up during the night to pass urine. A fluid plan should be advised to ensure an adequate regular intake, particularly at bedtime and during the night. This treatment is seen as a very simple way of preventing recurrence of stones but, in practice, can be difficult for the patient to comply with.

Alkalinization of urine

Urine alkalinization increases the solubility of cystine and may decrease stone formation (Anderton 1998). Potassium citrate is preferred to sodium bicarbonate if salt restriction is imposed concurrently. This may be used when penicillamine therapy is not well tolerated.

Drugs

The sulphydryl group in D-penicillamine reacts with cystine to form a more soluble complex in urine. The treatment carries a risk of side-effects including rashes, thrombocytopenia, neutropenia, proteinuria and nephrotic syndrome.

Angiotensin-converting enzyme inhibitors have been used as an alternative form of treatment but may not be as effective (Chow and Streem 1996).

Text revised by: Julie Leaper and Jacki Bishop

References

Anderton JG. Cystinuria: an update. *Journal of the Royal Society of Medicine* 1998; **91**: 220–221.

Baker LRI, Mallinson JW. Dietary treatment of idiopathic calciuria. *British Journal of Urology* 1979; **51**: 181–183.

Borghi L, Mesci T, Amato F *et al.* Urinary volume, water and recurrences in idiopathic calcium nephrolithiasis: a 5-year randomised prospective study. *Journal of Urology* 1996; **155**: 839–843.

Borghi L, Meschi T, Guenra A *et al.* Essential arterial hypertension and stone disease. *Kidney International* 1999; **55**: 2397–2406.

Chow GK, Streem SB. Medical management of cystinuria: results of contemporary clinical practice. *Journal of Urology* 1996; **156**: 1576–1578.

Clifford AJ, Riumullo JA, Young VR, Scrimshaw NS. Effect of oral purines on serum and urinary uric acid of normal and gouty humans. *Journal of Nutrition* 1976; **106**: 428.

Coe FL, Parks JH, Asplin JR. The pathogenesis and treatment of kidney stones. *New England Journal of Medicine* 1992; **327**: 1141–1151.

Curhan GC, Curhan SG. Diet and urinary stone disease. *Current Opinions in Urology* 1997; **7**: 222–225.

Curhan GC, Wilett WC, Rimm EB, Stamfer MJ. A prospective study of dietary calcium and other nutrients and the risk of symptomatic kidney stones. *New England Journal of Medicine* 1993; **328**: 833–838.

Curhan GC, Willett WC, Speizer FE, Stampfer MJ. Intake of Vitamin B6 and C and the risk of kidney stones in women. *Journal of the American Society of Nephrology* 1999; **10**: 840–845.

Currie WJC, Turner P. The frequency of renal stones within Great Britain in a gouty and non-gouty population. *Lancet* 1979; **351**: 1797–1801.

Daudon M, Dosimoni R, Hennequin C *et al.* Sex and age-related composition of 10617 calculi analysed by infrared spectroscopy. *Urology Research* 1995; **23**: 319–326.

Dretler SP. The physiologic approach to the medical management of stone disease. *Urologic Clinics of North America* 1998; **25**: 613–623.

Emmerson BT. The management of gout. *New England Journal of Medicine* 1996; **334**: 445–451.

Fuss M, Pepersack T, Bergman P *et al.* Low calcium diet in idiopathic urolithiasis: a risk factor for osteopenia as great as in primary hyperparathyroidism. *British Journal of Urology* 1990a; **65**: 560–563.

Fuss M, Pepersack T, Van Geel J. Involvement of low-calcium diet in the reduced bone mineral content of idiopathic renal stone formers. *Calcified Tissue International* 1990b; **46**: 9–13.

Giannini S, Nobile M, Sartori L *et al.* Acute effects of moderate dietary protein restriction in patients with idiopathic hypercalciuria and calcium nephrolithiasis. *American Journal of Clinical Nutrition* 1999; **69**: 267–271.

Goldfarb S. Dietary factors in the pathogenesis and prophylaxis of calcium nephrolithiasis. *Kidney International* 1988; **34**: 544–555.

Harris MD, Siegel LB, Alloway JA. Gout and hyperuricaemia. *American Family Physician* 1999; **59**: 925–934.

Holmes RP, Goodman HO, Assimos DG. Dietary oxalate and its intestinal absorption. *Scanning Microscopy* 1995; **9**: 1109–1120.

Howell AB, Vorsa N, Der Marderosian A, Foo LY. Inhibition of the adherence of P-fimbriated *Escherichia coli* to uroepithelial cell surfaces by proanthocyanidin extracts from cranberries. *New England Journal of Medicine* 1998; **339**: 1085–1086.

Jepson RG, Mihaljevic L, Craig J. Cranberries for treating urinary tract infections (Cochrane Review). In *The Cochrane Library* Issue 2, 1999. Oxford: Update Software.

Kasidas GP, Rose GA. Oxalate content of some common foods: determination by an enzymatic method. *Journal of Human Nutrition* 1980; **34**: 255–266.

Kleiner SM. Water: an essential but overlooked nutrient. *Journal of the American Dietetic Association* 1999; **99**: 200–206.

Lemann J, Pleuss JA, Worcester EM *et al.* Urinary oxalate excretion increases with body size and decreases with increasing dietary calcium intake among healthy adults. *Kidney International* 1996; **49**: 200–208.

Michaels EK, Fowler JE Jr, Mariano M. Bacteriuria following extracorporeal shock wave lithotripsy of infection stones. *Journal of Urology* 1988; **140**: 254–256.

Nguyen UN, Dumoulin G, Henriet MJ, Reynard J. Aspartame ingestion increases urinary calcium but not oxalate excretion in healthy subjects. *Journal of Clinical Endocrinology and Metabolism* 1998; **83**: 165–168.

Pak CYC. Citrate and renal calculi: an update. *Mineral and Electrolyte Metabolism* 1994; **20**: 371–377.

Pak CYC. Kidney stones. *Lancet* 1998; **351**: 1797–1801.

Parivar F, Low RK, Stoller ML. The influence of diet on urinary stone disease. *Journal of Urology* 1996; **155**: 432–440.

Rao PN, Prendiville V, Buxton A *et al.* Dietary management of urinary risk factors in renal stone formers. *British Journal of Urology* 1982; **54**: 578–583.

Robertson WG, Peacock M, Marshall RW *et al.* Saturation-inhibitor index as a measure of the risk of calcium oxalate stone formation in the urinary tract. *New England Journal of Medicine* 1976; **294**: 249–252.

Robertson WG, Peacock M, Heyburn PJ, Hanes FA. Epidemiological risk factors in calcium stone disease. *Scandinavian Journal of Urology and Nephrology* 1980; **53** (Suppl): 15–28.

Robertson WG, Peacock M, Heyburn PJ *et al.* The risk of calcium stone formation in relation to affluence and dietary animal protein. In Brokis JG, Finlayson B (Eds) *Urinary Calculus*, pp. 3–12. Littleton, MA: PSG Publishing, 1981.

Rodman JS. Management of uric acid in the elderly patient. *Geriatric Nephrology and Urology* 1991; **1**: 129.

Rodriguez LM, Santos F, Malaga S, Martinez V. Effect of a low sodium diet on urinary elimination of cystine in cystinuric children. *Nephron* 1995; **71**: 416–418.

Rogers J. Pass the cranberry juice. *Nursing Times* 1991; **87**: 36–37.

Rose GA. In Wickham JEA (Ed.) *Urinary Calculus Disease*, p. 119. Edinburgh: Churchill Livingstone, 1979.

Scott JT. Gout: the last 50 years. *Journal of the Royal Society of Medicine* 1996; **89**: 634–637.

Stoller ML, Bolton DM. Urinary stone disease. In Tanagho EA, McAninch JW (Eds) *Smith's General Urology*, pp. 276–304. Englewood Cliffs, NJ: Prentice-Hall International, 1995.

Tiselius, HG. Oxalate and renal stone formation. *Scandinavian Journal of Urology and Nephrology* 1980; **53** (Suppl): 135–143.

Wasserstein AG, Stolley PD, Soper KA *et al.* Case – control study of risk factors for idiopathic calcium nephrolithiasis. *Mineral and Electrolyte Metabolism* 1989; **13**: 85.

Wendland BE. Nutritional management of patients with urolithiasis. *Nephrology News Issues* 1991; **5**: 32, 34, 40.

Wood AJJ. The management of gout. *New England Journal of Medicine* 1996; **334**: 445–451.

4.16 Diabetes mellitus

Diabetes mellitus is one of the most common chronic disorders and affects about 1.4 million people in the UK. Its incidence is rising throughout the world; the current global prevalence of diabetes is about 110 million and this is predicted to double to 221 million by 2010 (Amos *et al.* 1997).

Diabetes has major implications in terms of morbidity and mortality, not only from the acute effects of the disease itself but also because it significantly increases the risk of cardiovascular disease and damage to the microcirculation of the kidneys (nephropathy), nerves (neuropathy), eyes (retinopathy) and limbs (peripheral vascular disease). As a result, diabetes is a major contributor to heart disease, stroke, renal failure, blindness, gangrene and amputations. As well as the cost in human terms, the management of diabetes and its complications pose a considerable financial burden on the National Health Service (NHS), consuming an estimated 8% of its resources (Marks 1999). About half of this cost is associated with hospital treatment for diabetes complications, many of which could be avoided with earlier diagnosis and better preventive care.

4.16.1 Features of diabetes

Diabetes results from lack of the hormone insulin, which is essential for the transfer of glucose from the blood to the tissues. Insulin deficiency may result from inadequate insulin production or resistance to its action. Without sufficient insulin, the amount of glucose in the blood becomes abnormally high (hyperglycaemia) and, if this level exceeds the renal threshold, passes into the urine (glycosuria). This, is turn, increases the amount of urine which has to be produced (polyuria). At the same time, the effective lack of glucose as an energy substrate at the cellular level means that the body has to use its stores of fat and, if necessary, muscle tissue as an alternative energy source. This combination produces the classic symptoms of diabetes:

- excessive urine production
- thirst
- unexplained weight loss.

If the lack of insulin is severe, the use of fat as a metabolic fuel may result in diabetic ketoacidosis, characterized by excessive production of ketones, electrolyte disturbances and increasing metabolic derangement. If untreated this will lead to coma and eventual death.

Types of diabetes

There are two distinct forms of the disease: type 1 and type 2 diabetes.

- *Type 1* diabetes is characterized by partial or total failure of insulin production by the beta-cells of the pancreas. The factors which cause this are still poorly understood, but certain viruses, autoimmune disease and genetic factors may all contribute. The disease usually develops suddenly in children or adults under 40 years, although it can occur at any age. It always requires treatment with insulin.
- *Type 2* diabetes is an insulin-resistant form where insulin is produced but in amounts that are insufficient or in an ineffective form. It is much more common than Type 1 diabetes, accounting for at least 75% of cases. There are strong genetic links with this type of diabetes and its development is closely associated with obesity. It most commonly develops in middle age and later life but, with rising obesity levels in the population, is increasingly being seen in younger adults and even children. Its onset is often insidious and its presence sometimes only discovered during routine health checks. Diet and lifestyle measures (particularly reduced energy intake and increased physical activity) may be sufficient to control the disease, but most patients will also require medication, either oral hypoglycaemic drugs which increase insulin production (sulphonylureas) or enhance its effectiveness (metformin), or insulin.

The terms 'insulin dependent' and 'non-insulin dependent' diabetes are no longer used, partly because some of the latter group of patients are now treated with insulin, but also because classification based on pathogenesis rather than treatment method more accurately reflects the metabolic differences and implications of the two forms of the disease.

Diagnostic criteria

The diagnostic criteria for diabetes formerly in use (WHO 1985) have recently been revised (Expert Committee 1999; WHO 2000).

In the presence of classic diabetes symptoms, diagnosis is confirmed by:

- a random venous plasma glucose concentration ≥ 11.1 mmol/l
  or
- a fasting plasma glucose concentration ≥ 7.0 mmol/l

(whole blood ≥ 6.1 mmol/l)

or

- 2 hour plasma glucose concentration ≥ 11.1 mmol/l 2 hours after 75 g anhydrous glucose in an oral glucose tolerance test (OGTT).

In the absence of diabetes symptoms, diagnosis must not be based on a single glucose determination but confirmed by at least one of the above additional glucose tests, made on a different day, and with a result in the range indicative of diabetes.

Additional categories of abnormal glucose tolerance have also been defined:

- *Impaired glucose tolerance (IGT)* is a stage of impaired glucose regulation defined as a fasting plasma glucose <7.0 mmol/l and OGTT 2 hour value ≥ 7.8 mmol/l but below <11.1 mmol/l/.
- *Impaired fasting glycaemia (IFG)* has been introduced to classify individuals who have fasting glucose values above the normal range but below those diagnostic of diabetes (fasting plasma glucose >6.1 mmol/l but <7.0 mmol/l). Diabetes UK (formerly known as the British Diabetic Association) recommends that all those with IFG should have an OGTT to exclude the diagnosis of diabetes.

IGT and IFG are not clinical entities in their own right but rather risk categories for cardiovascular disease (in the case of IGT) and/or future diabetes (both IGT and IFG).

Type 1 and type 2 diabetes are usually distinguished by clinical presentation but, if necessary, pancreatic insulin production can be assessed by measuring blood C-peptide levels, which will be very low or absent in type 1 diabetes.

Diabetes may also be a secondary consequence of pancreatic disease, certain drug treatments, particularly glucocorticoids, and some endocrine disorders such as acromegaly.

4.16.2 Consequences of diabetes

At all ages, mortality rates are higher in people with diabetes than in their non-diabetic counterparts (Laing *et al.* 1999). Although some deaths still occur from the acute effects of diabetes (mainly ketoacidosis), most result from the chronic complications associated with disease.

Microvascular complications

Microvascular complications are a common, often devastating, consequence of diabetes.

Diabetic retinopathy

This is a highly specific vascular complication of both type 1 and type 2 diabetes which is strongly related to duration of the disease. Small haemorrhages and microinfarcts in the retinal blood supply can eventually result in blood vessel proliferation and retinal deposits which, if not treated at an early stage, can cause loss of sight. Diabetic retinopathy is the most common cause of blindness in people

aged 16–64 years. After 20 years of diabetes, most patients with type 1 and over 50% of those with type 2 will have some degree of retinopathy. In addition, nearly 20% of newly diagnosed type 2 diabetic patients have a significant degree of retinopathy at diagnosis because the condition has often remained undetected for some time (UKPDS 1998a).

Diabetic nephropathy

This is a major cause of premature death, largely from uraemia and associated cardiovascular disease. It affects about 30% of patients with type 1 diabetes, typically about 10–20 years after the onset of the disease. In people with type 2 diabetes it tends to appear after a shorter period and its incidence varies with ethnic origin, ranging from about 25% in Europeans to around 50% in people of African-Caribbean and Asian origin. It is characterized by proteinuria (defined as urinary albumin excretion >300 mg/day), hypertension and a decrease in glomerular filtration rate (GFR), and usually leads to end-stage renal disease within 5 years. Nephropathy is usually preceded by asymptomatic microalbuminuria, defined as a urinary albumin excretion rate of 30–300 mg/day. Microalbuminuria and proteinuria are also markers of increased cardiovascular risk in people with diabetes.

Diabetic neuropathy

This is a common but more polymorphic complication, appearing in many different forms, and its aetiology is less well understood. It leads to sensory deficit and autonomic dysfunction, resulting in a range of symptoms including numbness, pins and needles or neuritic pain in limbs, and impotence. The combination of neuropathy, ischaemia and infection leads to tissue breakdown in areas such as the foot, which can result in gangrene and limb amputation. Diabetic neuropathy is also strongly linked with duration of diabetes.

There is now unequivocal evidence from long-term prospective trials that the development of microvascular complications is strongly linked to the length and degree of exposure to hyperglycaemia and that tight control of blood glucose is essential for their prevention in both type 1 and type 2 patients (DCCT Research Group 1993; UKPDS 1998a). Good control of blood pressure may also be equally important in the prevention of some types of retinopathy and nephropathy (UKPDS 1998b).

Cardiovascular disease

Diabetes greatly increases the risk of premature death from cardiovascular disease, particularly in women. People with diabetes are at least twice as likely to develop heart disease as the non-diabetic population (Laing *et al.* 1999). Premenopausal women are four times more likely to develop the disease as their non-diabetic counterparts because the usual protection against heart disease in this age group is lost. People with diabetes also have an two to three fold increase in the risk of stroke (Bell 1994). The outcome from myocardial infarction and stroke is also worse in a person with diabetes (Yudkin *et al.* 1996).

The development of cardiovascular disease is associated with hyperglycaemia but, in contrast to microvascular complications, this is not so much due to the effects of the elevated blood glucose *per se* but to disturbances in other metabolic parameters such as blood lipids which occur in the presence of poor glycaemic control. Hypertension is particularly strongly associated with cardiovascular risk in this group, and long-term tight blood pressure control in hypertensive type 2 diabetic patients has been shown to result in a significant fall in the incidence of cardiovascular complications and stroke (UKPDS 1998c). As in the non-diabetic population, preventing cardiovascular disease therefore requires multiple risk-factor reduction, particularly from influences such as smoking, hypertension, dyslipidaemia, obesity and inactivity.

4.16.3 Aims of management of diabetes

The aims of treatment are to:

- alleviate the acute symptoms of the disease
- prevent extremes of glycaemia resulting in hypoglycaemia or ketoacidosis
- reduce the risk of cardiovascular disease and diabetic microvascular complications
- maintain quality of life.

In order to achieve these, the clinical objectives are:

- tight blood glucose control (preprandial blood glucose level between 4 and 7 mmol/l; glycosylated haemoglobin (HbA_{IC}) at 7.0% or below)
- correction of hypertension and maintenance of blood pressure at 140/80 mmHg or below
- correction of disordered lipids
- reduction in the risk from other known cardiovascular risk factors (particularly smoking, physical inactivity, obesity and atherogenic diet).

Diet is an essential component of diabetic management in order to achieve these objectives. In the short term, food intake needs to be regulated, and often counterbalanced with hypoglycaemic medication, in order to optimize blood glucose control. In the long term, dietary composition needs to be such that it offers maximum protection against cardiovascular disease and microvascular damage. In many patients, reduction of weight and other lifestyle risk factors are essential to achieve these goals.

4.16.4 Nutritional objectives in the management of diabetes

Nutritional recommendations

In the UK, nutritional guidelines for the management of diabetes have been produced by Diabetes UK (BDA 1992a, currently under revision) and similar recommendations have been made elsewhere (Franz *et al.* 1994; European Association for the Study of Diabetes 1995, 2000; Ha and Lean 1998; American Diabetes Association 1999). There is now broad consensus on the type of diet which is most beneficial for people with diabetes which, in general, is a diet similar in composition to that recommended for the non-diabetic population. There are, however, some important differences in emphasis for those with diabetes, warranting dietetic intervention and monitoring to ensure that nutritional objectives are met.

Dietary energy

Energy balance is an important aspect of diabetic management. Prolonged surplus energy intake increases endogenous glucose production and hence the body's need for insulin, while at the same time creating surplus fat stores which increase insulin resistance and diminish its effectiveness. The development of obesity, particularly central obesity, results in additional metabolic disturbances which exacerbate those of the diabetes (see Section 4.17, Obesity).

Some 80% of type 2 diabetic patients are overweight at diagnosis, and shifting energy balance in a negative direction (by a combination of dietary energy restriction and increased physical activity) has rapid benefits in terms of glycaemic control and other metabolic abnormalities. For many of these patients, weight loss (or stabilization) is the most important aspect of their diabetic treatment.

In people with type 1 diabetes, it is important to prevent obesity because of its adverse effects on blood pressure, dyslipidaemia and cardiovascular disease. However, in young type 1 patients (children and adolescents) it is equally important to ensure that energy needs for growth are met.

Regular physical activity is of particular benefit to everyone with diabetes, not just those who are overweight, and as well as its contribution to weight control also improves glucose tolerance, lipid profile and maintains muscle mass. Most people should be encouraged to engage in a moderate level of physical activity for at least 20–30 minutes/day.

Protein

In the general population, the proportion of energy derived from protein is typically 10–20% energy, equivalent to about 1 g/kg body weight per day. People with diabetes often consume more protein than this, in both proportional and absolute terms, as a result of their restricted intake of sugar and fat (Eeley *et al.* 1996; Toeller *et al.* 1996).

There have been concerns that high intakes of protein may contribute to the pathogenesis of diabetic nephropathy, possibly via its elevating effects on GFR (Brenner *et al.* 1982; Hostetter *et al.* 1982). Several studies have suggested that low-protein diets may slow down the rate of progression of both pre-clinical nephropathy (Mogensen *et al.* 1995) and overt diabetic renal disease (Friedman 1982; Zeller 1991).

However, at present there is still insufficient evidence on which to base precise recommendations regarding protein consumption (Waugh and Robertson 1997). The current consensus is that, for the general diabetic population, there is no justification for overt protein restriction but that protein intakes at the lower end of the normal range (0.8–0.9 g/kg body weight per day) may be advantageous (Ha and Lean 1998; ADA 1999; EASD 2000). Intakes significantly in excess of requirements should be discouraged.

In patients with overt nephropathy, it may be beneficial to limit protein intake to 0.8 g/kg body weight per day, i.e. about 10% of dietary energy. Once GFR begins to fall, further restriction to 0.6 g/kg per day may prove useful in slowing the decline of GFR in selected patients.

There is no convincing evidence that the origin of dietary protein (whether from animal or vegetable sources) has any specific effect on diabetic renal disease (Henry 1994).

Fat

Dietary fat intake has important implications in terms of blood lipids, weight management and cardiovascular risk, and most diabetic patients will need to make adjustments to both the amount and type of fat consumed. In order to reduce atherogenic risk, the proportion of dietary energy from fat should be reduced to <35%, as is recommended for the general population. A higher proportion than this is only appropriate if it is composed of monounsaturated fat (see below). Total fat energy restriction is usually essential for those who are overweight (EASD 2000).

Saturated fatty acids Most of the reduction in fat intake should be achieved by avoidance of saturated fatty acids, which should comprise no more than 10% energy intake. This is less than the amount currently consumed by many diabetic patients (Toeller *et al*. 1996).

Monounsaturated fatty acids These should comprise the largest component of dietary fat intake, and provide 10–25% dietary energy (depending on the desired proportion of dietary energy from carbohydrate). Monounsaturated fatty acids (MUFA) (found in olive oil and rapeseed/canola oil) are preferable to *n6* polyunsaturated fatty acids because they reduce total and low-density lipoprotein (LDL)-cholesterol without adverse effects on high-density lipoprotein (HDL)-cholesterol or triglyceride levels (Ginsberg *et al*. 1990).

In non-diabetic people, diets relatively rich in MUFA (the 'Mediterranean' diet) appear to have cardioprotective properties (see Section 4.21.5 in Cardiovascular disease) and may also be more palatable (and hence more acceptable) than low-fat diets. High-MUFA, low-saturated fat diets can also be effective in the management of hypercholesterolaemia (see Section 4.23.4 in Hyperlipidaemia). These benefits may well apply to people with diabetes, and substituting a proportion of carbohydrate energy with MUFA may be a useful measure in patients who find it difficult to consume a high-carbohydrate diet or have hypertriglyceridaemia (see Carbohydrate, below). However, the greater energy density of higher fat diets must be borne in mind, especially in overweight type 2 patients, and for this reason, total fat restriction is usually preferable (EASD 2000).

Omega-6 (n6) polyunsaturated fatty acids (PUFA) Total consumption of *n6* PUFA should not exceed 10% dietary energy (the level recommended for the general population) and lower levels than this (3–7%) may be more appropriate (WHO 1990). Although substituting saturated fatty acids with *n6* PUFA reduces total and LDL-cholesterol, it also tends to lower HDL-cholesterol. High intakes may also, in the absence of antioxidant vitamins, enhance undesirable lipid peroxidation.

Omega-3 (n3) fatty acids Diets rich in these fatty acids (from oily fish and fish oils) have been shown to have beneficial effects in terms of thrombogenesis and to be highly effective in the secondary prevention of cardiovascular disease in non-diabetic populations (see Section 4.21, Cardiovascular disease). It is suggested that people with diabetes should be encouraged to consume at least one helping of fish, preferably oily fish, each week. Additional plant sources of *n3* fatty acids (e.g. from rapeseed oil, nuts and some green leafy vegetables) may also be beneficial.

Although pharmacological doses of these fatty acids can lower triglyceride levels, they can also raise LDL-cholesterol levels in diabetic patients (Mori *et al*. 1989; Friedberg *et al*. 1998), so the use of fish oil supplements is not recommended.

Trans fatty acids These are mainly produced during the hydrogenation of unsaturated fats used in food manufacturing and their main dietary source is biscuits, cakes and chocolate. Although their contribution to total dietary fat intake is small, their adverse effects on lipoproteins (increasing LDL and lipoprotein a, and reducing HDL) suggest that their consumption should be limited as much as possible.

Dietary cholesterol The relationship between dietary cholesterol and serum cholesterol is hyperbolic rather than linear and only of significance at extreme ranges of intake (Hopkins 1992). Since restriction of saturated fat intake will also curtail excessive intakes of dietary cholesterol, additional constraints are not usually necessary (see Section 4.23.4 in Hyperlipidaemia).

Carbohydrate

Until the 1970s, the diabetic diet was markedly restricted in carbohydrate as this was believed to be essential for blood glucose control. Not only was this assumption shown to be wrong but it also became increasingly apparent that a diet low in carbohydrate and consequently high in fat was unlikely to benefit a group of people at increased cardiovascular risk. Current recommendations therefore are that a relatively high proportion of dietary energy should be derived from carbohydrate and a much lower proportion from dietary fat.

Intakes of 45–60% carbohydrate energy are compatible with good diabetic control, but a realistic objective in the UK is a diet containing about 50% carbohydrate energy. Most of this carbohydrate should be derived from complex, fibre-rich foods with a low glycaemic index, such as starchy cereal foods, fruit, vegetables and legumes (see Type of carbohydrate in Section 4.16.6).

Concerns that high-carbohydrate diets *per se* elevate triglyceride levels are generally unfounded. Usually such an effect only occurs when the diet contains large amounts of refined carbohydrates (or other high glycaemic index foods), when total energy intake is excessive or when diabetic control is poor (Ha and Lean 1998). In cases where hypertriglyceridaemia is exacerbated by carbohydrate, or for reasons of patient preference, a proportion of carbohydrate energy can be isocalorically substituted with that from monounsaturated fat (MUFA) (Garg 1998). However, this measure is less appropriate for those who are overweight, and it is very often these patients who are hypertriglyceridaemic.

Sugars

The belief still persists among the general public, diabetic patients and even some health professionals that a diabetic diet has to be sugar free. This is not the case. The glycaemic response to a food is affected by many factors, of which sugar content is just one, and not necessarily the most influential (see Type of carbohydrate in Section 4.16.6 below). Many sugar-containing carbohydrate foods produce a lower glycaemic response than those which contain starch alone.

Modest amounts of sugar can be included in a diabetic diet as long as most of it is consumed as part of a meal and not in isolation. Current guidance is that total sugar intake should not exceed that advocated for the general population, i.e. up to 10% dietary energy. Lower levels than this may be more appropriate for those who are overweight. Large quantities of isolated sources of sugars (such as sucrose-rich drinks) are normally contraindicated in diabetes because their rapid rate of absorption results in a sharp rise in glycaemia. However, precisely because of this effect, such drinks or foods may at times be essential to correct or avert hypoglycaemia in patients treated with insulin or sulphonylurea drugs.

Fibre

Sources of soluble fibre (gums, gels and pectins) are beneficial. Soluble fibre delays the rate of postprandial glucose absorption and foods rich in soluble fibre such as oats, legumes and fruit have a low glycaemic index (Aro *et al.* 1981; Vinik and Jenkins 1988). Soluble fibre may also have small but beneficial effects on lipid metabolism (Brown *et al.* 1999).

In contrast, cereal fibre (e.g. bran and cellulose) has minimal effects on glycaemia or lipidaemia (Ha and Lean 1998). It therefore has no specific benefits for people with diabetes over and above those which apply to everyone in respect of gastrointestinal health.

Alcohol

The benefits from modest consumption of alcohol in terms of cardiovascular disease and the harmful effects which result from excessive consumption appear to apply to the diabetic as well as the general population (Valmadrid and Klein 1999). However, alcohol can create additional hazards for those with diabetes and the recommended safe drinking limits advocated for the general population (a maximum of 3–4 units/day for men and 2–3 units/day for women) may be too high for many diabetic patients (Ha and Lean 1998).

Alcohol markedly suppresses gluconeogenesis and so has a hypoglycaemic effect (Lieber 1994). In patients on insulin or sulphonylurea drugs, alcohol can cause hypoglycaemia of such severity that it can result in death or brain damage (Laing *et al.* 1999). It is therefore vital that diabetic patients only consume alcohol in conjunction with carbohydrate (probably before, during and after its consumption), and in amounts which do not exceed recommended safe drinking limits (and probably less). Insulin-treated patients whose control is unstable and who are known to experience marked swings in glycaemia may be well advised to avoid alcohol completely.

In type 2 patients treated by diet alone, alcohol does not pose this risk but, since most of these patients are overweight, the high energy content of alcohol should not be overlooked. Alcohol will also tend to exacerbate hypertriglyceridaemia, common in many type 2 patients.

The sulphonylurea drug chlorpropamide can react with alcohol and cause facial flushing. This is not hazardous but can be unpleasant for patients.

Vitamins

There is no evidence that vitamin requirements differ between the diabetic and non-diabetic populations, although people with poorly controlled diabetes may be more at risk from deficiencies of water-soluble vitamins as a result of polyuria. However, given the elevated cardiovascular risk and additional oxidative stress from the metabolic effects of diabetes, a diet rich in natural antioxidants (particularly vitamins C, tocopherols, carotenoids and flavonoids) should be encouraged (EASD 2000). This should be achieved via increased consumption of fruit and vegetables (a measure which will convey additional benefits in terms of soluble fibre and dietary energy density). Antioxidant supplements are not recommended as an alternative because they cannot confer all of these benefits and may, in excessive quantities, be harmful (ATBC Study Group 1994).

Good folate status may also be important to minimize the risk of hyperhomocysteinaemia, a cardiovascular risk factor.

Minerals and trace elements

Sodium The relationship between sodium and hypertension remains controversial (see Section 4.24.3 in Hypertension). Some people are probably more sensitive to the hypertensive effects of sodium than others but at present there is no way of identifying those who are most susceptible. Given that sodium consumption greatly exceeds requirement, the advice given to the general public that sodium intake should be reduced from an average of 9 g to 6 g salt/day is sensible. For those with diabetes, such a measure may be especially beneficial given the clear links between hypertension and the development of both microvascular and macrovascular complications.

Diabetic patients should be encouraged to reduce their sodium intake by consuming more fresh foods (such as fruit and vegetables) and avoid overuse of manufactured convenience foods (the principal dietary source of sodium). Guidance on using nutrition labelling information to choose brands of staple foods such as bread and breakfast cereals with a lower sodium content may also be helpful.

Potassium Since potassium counterbalances the hypertensive effects of sodium, this is an additional reason for encouraging the consumption of fruit and vegetables.

Diabetic patients on thiazide and loop-acting diuretics may need potassium supplements to replace potassium losses. However, hyperkalaemia sufficient to warrant potassium restriction may occur in patients taking angiotensin-converting enzyme (ACE) inhibitors or potassium-sparing diuretics, or in those with renal failure.

Other minerals and trace elements As with water-soluble vitamins, there is little evidence that people with diabetes have increased requirements unless losses are excessive as a result of poor control and polyuria.

Zinc status has been reported to be lower in people with diabetes as a result of altered metabolic utilization and increased excretion. However, routine zinc supplementation is not recommended since high intakes may also impair glucose tolerance (Raz *et al.* 1989) and interfere with iron absorption.

Chromium is an essential component of glucose transport mechanisms but the only circumstances in which chromium deficiency has been shown to be severe enough to impair glucose tolerance in humans is in people on prolonged parenteral nutrition (Freund *et al.* 1979; Mooradian *et al.* 1994). There is no evidence that chromium supplementation improves glucose tolerance in people with diabetes (Rabinowitz *et al.* 1983).

Magnesium deficiency associated with diabetes may occur as a result of a specific renal tubular defect causing osmotic diuresis and excessive magnesium losses (Garland 1992). Some types of oral hypoglycaemic drug may also alter magnesium handling (McBain *et al.* 1988). There is no evidence that magnesium supplementation is necessary other than where specifically indicated, e.g. in patients on diuretics, with ketoacidosis or with certain arryhthmias (Mooradian *et al.* 1994).

Alternative sweeteners

Non-nutritive sweeteners Aspartame, saccharin, acesulfame-K and cyclamate are suitable for those who require additional sweetness in drinks or desserts.

Nutritive sweeteners Fructose is not recommended as an alternative sweetener to sucrose (BDA 1992b). Any advantage in terms of a smaller glycaemic effect in comparison with sucrose is insignificant in the context of the overall diet and outweighed by disadvantages in terms of relative cost and laxative effect.

Nutritive sweeteners (e.g. polyalcohols such as sorbitol, mannitol, xylitol) or sucrose coated with artificial sweetener are not recommended for similar reasons.

'Diabetic foods'

The use of specialist products containing non-sucrose nutritive sweeteners (see above) is not recommended (BDA 1992b). Most of these products offer minimal benefits in terms of glycaemia, no advantage in terms of energy or fat content, and may be disadvantageous for those with hypertriglyceridaemia. They are expensive, sometimes unpalatable and can induce osmotic diarrhoea. The types of products available – chocolate, preserves, cakes and biscuits – tend to be consumed by overweight diabetic patients in the mistaken belief that these products are low in calories, or by elderly people who believe that they need them but can ill-afford them. They also tend to prolong the widespread misconception that sugar avoidance is the most important aspect of the diabetic diet and distract attention away from more important dietary aspects, such as eating less fat and more fruit and vegetables.

Putting nutritional recommendations into practice

Dietetic skill is needed to apply the nutritional objectives of diabetes management in a way which is realistic and practical. While the desired aims in terms of dietary composition should underpin dietary guidance, they should not be regarded as rigid targets to be imposed on every diabetic individual. For most patients, the actual target will be to make specific dietary changes in the right direction, i.e. towards the ideal. The nature of these changes will vary according to individual nutritional and clinical priorities, habitual diet and lifestyle and prevalence of risk factors.

Dietary objectives rarely need to be precisely quantified (e.g. calories of energy or grams of a nutrient per day) since dietary guidance is no longer given in these terms. The focus should always be on modifying an individual's existing eating habits (food choice and the timing of its consumption) in a realistic and achievable way; standardized diet sheets have no place in modern diabetic dietary management.

Dietary management of diabetes involves the following stages:

- assessing the nutritional priorities for that individual
- modifying the existing diet to meet these priorities
- providing additional guidance to meet specific needs and circumstances
- providing support and follow-up
- monitoring progress and evaluating effectiveness.

4.16.5 Assessing the nutritional priorities

It is impossible to decide which aspects of an individual's diet need to be changed without having some idea of what the usual diet is. Dietary assessment is thus essential to ascertain:

- *meal pattern*: the usual distribution of meals and snacks throughout the day and the extent to which this varies from day to day, between weekdays and weekends, or is influenced by factors such as shift work or business travel
- *food choices*: the types of food which comprise these meals and snacks and the typical amounts consumed
- *overall dietary balance*: how closely the dietary pattern matches *Balance of Good Health* guidelines, e.g. the number of portions of fruit and vegetables consumed per day
- *nutritional adequacy*: the likelihood of dietary surplus or deficiency
- *alcohol consumption*: typical intake and whether this ever exceeds safe limits
- *beliefs or misconceptions held about diet and diabetes*: for example, that sugar is forbidden or that diabetic foods are essential.

Individual factors such as age, gender, socioeconomic circumstances, ethnic group and occupation will also be relevant.

This information has to be considered in conjunction with clinical factors such as:

- the type of diabetes and whether it will be treated with insulin, oral hypoglycemic drugs or diet alone
- body weight
- physical activity level
- lipid profile
- blood pressure
- presence of other cardiovascular risk factors, e.g. smoking, history of coronary heart disease (CHD) or stroke.

Only then is the dietitian able to assess the nutritional priorities for that particular patient and, in consultation with the multi-disciplinary team, discuss with the patient how aspects of their existing diet and lifestyle can be modified to meet the needs of their diabetes.

4.16.6 Dietary modification

Because the nutritional objectives for those with diabetes are very similar to those advocated for the entire population, dietary guidance should be based on a framework of healthy eating principles (such as *The Balance of Good Health*) on which the specific aspects relevant to the diabetes in terms of food choice and meal timing are superimposed (Table 4.32). It should be noted that this does not mean that dietary advice is simply a matter of healthy eating guidance; many other issues have to be borne in mind (Purnell 1999).

The amount, type and timing of carbohydrate intake are major considerations. In order to maintain glycaemia within an acceptable range there has to be a balance between glucose entering the blood from the gastrointestinal tract and the supply of exogenous (injected) or endogenous (pancreatically produced) insulin available to deal with it.

In the non-diabetic person this happens automatically; insulin is produced as needed in response to the ingestion of food. In diabetic people on hypoglycaemic medication, the situation is different. Once insulin is injected (or a hypoglycaemic drug ingested), its hypoglycaemic action will continue to operate irrespective of whether food is, or is not, consumed. If food is not consumed at the scheduled time, or in insufficient amounts, the action of the drug will cause the blood glucose level to fall too low, causing hypoglycemia. Conversely, consuming large amounts of carbohydrate at times of low activity of the insulin or drug will result in undesirably high levels of blood glucose. Ensuring that there is a balance between carbohydrate intake and hypoglycaemic medication is therefore vital.

Hypoglycaemia cannot occur in diabetic people treated by diet alone (or on metformin) where, like the normal person, insulin is produced when food is eaten. However, because the ability to produce insulin is limited, it is still important to ensure that carbohydrate intake is evenly spread and within the body's ability to handle it. In practice, this balance is achieved by regulating:

- the meal pattern
- the amount of carbohydrate consumed
- the type of carbohydrate consumed.

Meal pattern

In most people, carbohydrate intake will need to be fairly evenly distributed throughout the day. Patients with totally erratic eating habits or those who go for long periods without food will need to adopt a more regular meal pattern to ensure a better, and more constant, balance between supply and usage.

For many patients, a meal pattern of three evenly sized meals and three smaller snacks per day is ideal, but this will vary between individuals according to the demands of medication, lifestyle and individual preference (e.g. between-meal snacks may need to be discouraged in obese type 2 patients). The important aspect is that an appropriate meal pattern, whatever that is for a particular person, remains relatively constant from day to day.

Amount of carbohydrate consumed at each meal

Traditionally, the amount of carbohydrate consumed has been regulated by means of an exchange system where foods containing a defined amount of carbohydrate (usually 10 g) were substituted for one another. Patients were told how many 'exchanges' to consume at each meal and these were chosen from an exchange list which specified the amount of each food that provided 'one exchange'. This system had a number of weaknesses:

- It assumed that equal quantities of carbohydrate had equal glycaemic effects, and this is known not to be the case (see Type of carbohydrate, below). The system was therefore unrealistic in physiological terms.

Table 4.32 Adapting *The Balance of Good Health* model for people with diabetes

Food group	Points to emphasize
Bread, cereal foods and potatoes These should form the largest component of meals and snacks	Quantity and timing: These need to remain fairly constant from day to day Good food choices: pasta, rice, bread, chappatis, potatoes, breakfast cereals (especially oat-based) Reduce the amount of fat added to these foods: The amount of fat spread on bread, or chappattis, or used in pasta sauces, should be kept to a minimum Wholemeal/wholegrain bread and cereals are high in fibre and have advantages in terms of satiety and helping to prevent constipation
Fruit and vegetables At least 5 servings of a variety of these foods should be eaten every day	These foods have major health benefits for people with diabetes 1–2 servings of vegetables (excluding potatoes) should be eaten with main meals More use should be made of fresh fruit as a snack or dessert Frozen or canned fruits and vegetables are useful alternatives to fresh varieties Fruit juice should be regarded as a sugar-containing drink and so not consumed on its own, only with meals Encourage consumption of salad or vegetables with manufactured convenience foods or ready meals
Milk and dairy products 2–3 servings/day	Low/reduced-fat varieties of milk, yoghurt, fromage frais, etc. should be chosen Full-fat cheese should be used with care, especially by those who are overweight. It is best used as a main meal component rather than as a snack Cream should only be used as an occasional treat
Meat, fish, pulses and alternatives 2 servings/day	Greater use should be made of pulses (peas, beans and lentils), either as an alternative to meat or as a way of making a smaller quantity of meat go further. Fresh, canned or dried pulses are all suitable Ideally at least two portions of fish should be consumed every week, one of which should be oily fish Fat avoidance is important, e.g. meat should be lean: visible meat fat should be trimmed or drained off after cooking. Consumption of meat products (e.g. burgers, pies, sausage rolls) or high-fat meat mixtures (mince) should be kept to a minimum: poultry is only a low source of fat if the skin is removed and fat which appears during cooking discarded.
Fat-rich and sugar-rich foods These should be kept to a minimum	*Sugar-rich foods*: The diet does not have to be sugar free, but sugar-rich confectionery and drinks will impair glycaemic control if consumed at inappropriate times or in addition to meals Low-calorie 'diet' soft drinks are good alternatives to their higher sugar counterparts Either ordinary jam/marmalade or reduced-sugar varieties can be used in small amounts on bread Small amounts of sugar-containing biscuits or cakes can be eaten as scheduled snacks, but higher fibre, lower sugar choices are best, e.g. teabreads, fruit cake, English muffins, plain cakes and biscuits. Those who are overweight should be encouraged to make more use of fruit as snacks Intense artificial sweeteners should be used if sweet-tasting drinks are required *Fat-rich foods*: Sources of fat should be avoided as much as possible Food should be boiled, baked, grilled, dry roasted or microwaved, not fried Minimum amounts of fat should be spread on bread, added to food or used in cooking. Reduced-fat monounsaturated spread and small amounts of monounsaturated oils (olive or rapeseed/canola) are the best choices High-fat snack foods such as crisps and biscuits should be eaten less often and replaced by healthier alternatives such as fruit, low-fat yoghurt or wholewheat crispbread

- It made the diet unnecessarily prescriptive and sometimes impractical, e.g. a 10 g exchange might comprise 'two-thirds of a large thin slice of bread' or '14 tablespoons of milk'.
- It focused exclusively on dietary carbohydrate while other aspects of the diet (such as fat content) tended to be ignored.
- It tended to restrict carbohydrate intake rather than encourage its substitution for dietary fat.

Increasingly, therefore, the 10 g exchange system is being replaced by more qualitative guidance based on appropriate choice and portion size of carbohydrate-containing foods. As long as the diet has been properly assessed (as described above) this is relatively easy for the practitioner to do and for the patient to accept, as it only involves making relatively simple adjustments to the habitual meal pattern (i.e. guidance as to whether someone needs to eat more, less or about the same at a particular meal). If necessary, food models or pictures can be used to help to assess or describe portion size (see Section 1.5.2 in Dietary assessment).

Some quantitative guidance on carbohydrate intake (e.g. the amount typically needed at a main meal, late-night snack or to prevent/treat hypoglycaemia) is helpful for many patients so that they can interpret nutrition labelling information. However, this should be regarded as further education rather than first-line advice.

Dietitians should bear in mind that patients who have had diabetes for many years may still use the 10 g carbohydrate exchange system. While it is reasonable to encourage consumption of a diet which is better balanced in terms of overall composition, some patients find it disturbing to be told to abandon a system which they understand and gives them the confidence to manage their diabetes. People should not be forced to change the way in which they manage the dietary aspects of their diabetes if they do not wish to do so (although many will welcome a more liberal approach). Dietitians therefore need to be familiar with the 10 g exchange concept even if they do not use it in practice, otherwise they will be unable to interpret information from patients given in terms of 'I have two exchanges for breakfast'. In addition, the use of insulin pumps for some type 1 patients is creating the need to assess, and possible regulate, diet in exchanges of carbohydrate in order to gauge insulin boluses. For reference, a 10 g carbohydrate list is given in Appendix 6.2.

Type of carbohydrate

In broad terms, most of the carbohydrate in the diabetic diet should be derived from starchy or soluble fibre-containing foods (cereals, legumes, fruits and vegetables), and isolated amounts of large quantities of simple sugars avoided (other than to treat hypoglycaemia). However, the glycaemic effect of a carbohydrate food is determined by many physical and chemical characteristics, not just its sugar or fibre content. Attempts have been made to quantify this effect and classify carbohydrate foods according to their glycaemic index (GI). This is done by comparing the glycaemic effect of a particular food with that from an equal amount of carbohydrate from a standard source of carbohydrate (CH), usually white bread or glucose. GI is calculated as:

$$\frac{\text{Area under the blood glucose response curve for test food containing 50 g CHO}}{\text{Area under the glucose response curve after 50 g glucose or white bread}} \times 100$$

A table summarizing published work from GI studies and encompassing over 600 foods was produced by Foster-Powell and Brand Miller (1995). However, it is not a definitive guide as there was considerable variation in the way in which the studies were conducted, the test carbohydrate used and the subjects on whom they were performed (single or combined groups of type 1 and type 2 diabetic subjects).

In theory, the GI provides guidance on the amount of a carbohydrate food which needs to be consumed in order to keep the glycaemic impact of the diet constant. In practice, its application is not this simple (Wolever 1997). The GI of an individual food can vary as a result of the way it is cooked or processed or its degree of ripeness. For example,

newly ripened bananas have a high content of resistant starch and hence a lower GI than fully ripened ones, where the starch has been converted into sugars; it is thus difficult to assign a specific GI figure for 'a banana' (Wolever *et al.* 1988). The glycaemic response to a single food will also change when it is eaten in conjunction with other foods; for example, fat content and meal size affect the rate of gastric emptying; soluble fibre present in one carbohydrate food may impact on the absorption of another. It is clearly impossible to determine the glycaemic effect of a food in the context of an almost infinite number of meal combinations.

Nevertheless, the concept of GI is useful as a pointer to food choice (Brand *et al.* 1991; Fontvieille *et al.* 1992). Types of foods with a consistently low glycaemic effect can be promoted as particularly good choices and restraint advised with those of higher glycaemic potential (Table 4.33). Substituting habitually consumed higher GI foods such as corn-based breakfast cereals, fruit juices, bread or potato with lower GI alternatives such as oat-based breakfast cereal, fruit, pasta and legumes has been shown to be a useful adjunct to management (Brand *et al.* 1991; EASD 2000). It is, however, important that dietitians do not lose sight of other aspects such as practicality and compliance (e.g. older adults may regard pasta as an unacceptable alternative to potato; people may not have time to cook porridge in the morning). Nor should GI be emphasized to such an extent that other important messages concerning meal pattern and overall dietary balance are lost.

4.16.7 Specific considerations in people with type 1 diabetes

Insulin regimen

The nature of the insulin regimen has to be considered in order to ensure that food choice and meal timing are compatible with its hypoglycaemic activity. Many insulin

Table 4.33 Glycaemic effect of carbohydrate foods

As a general guide to good food choice, groups of foods can broadly be divided into the following categories of glycaemic index. However, it should be borne in mind that other factors such as the way in which a food is prepared or cooked, its degree of ripeness and other foods with which it is consumed may alter its glycaemic effect.

Lower glycaemic index foods	Pulses, peas, beans and legumes Oat-based cereals and oat products Pasta Raw fruit (not overripe) Milk and plain yoghurt
Intermediate glycaemic index foods	New potatoes Granary bread Rice
Higher glycaemic index foods	Bread (white and wholemeal) Corn or wheat-based breakfast cereals Instant potato, old potatoes (especially if mashed) Honey Fruit juices

preparations are available, each one having a different speed and duration of activity. They can broadly be categorized into short- or intermediate/long-acting insulins.

Short-acting insulins

- *Soluble insulin* starts to act within 30–60 minutes, and has a peak action between 2 and 4 hours and a duration of action up to 8 hours. Synthetic human sequence preparations ('human' insulins) tend to have a more rapid onset and a shorter duration than insulins from animal sources.
- *Rapid-acting insulin analogues* are a new type of short-acting insulin preparation. They are analogues of human insulin which act more quickly and for a shorter time than soluble insulin, and are useful for those with problems with pre-prandial or unexplained episodes of hypoglycaemia, or to cover meals taken at unusual times.

Intermediate- and long-acting insulins

These start to act within 1–2 hours of injection, and have a maximal effect between 4 and 12 hours and a duration of 16–36 hours:

- *Isophane insulin* is a suspension of insulin with protamine, and is usually given twice a day together with soluble insulin. In practice, bisphasic isophane insulin (ready-mixed combinations of a short- and longer-acting insulin) is often used.
- *Insulin zinc suspensions*, particularly in crystalline form, have more prolonged action and are often used to provide a background level of insulin with several small doses of short-acting insulin being given during the day to cover the glycaemic effect of meals. Various combinations of amorphous and crystalline insulin zinc suspensions are used; the greater the proportion in the crystalline form, the more prolonged the action.
- *Protamine zinc insulin (PZI)* also has prolonged action but is now rarely used.
- *Long-acting insulin analogues* which offer the potential of producing better long-term background control of glycaemia are currently under development.

Many people are maintained on a combination of preparations in order to optimize blood glucose control throughout the 24 hour period. Most are still managed on a combination of a short-acting and intermediate-acting insulin administered twice a day (usually half an hour before breakfast and the evening meal). However, there is increasing use of multiple-injection regimens where one dose of a long-acting insulin is injected (usually at bedtime) to provide a continuous background supply of insulin and small amounts of short-acting insulin are administered via a pen injector prior to meals during the day. This system (known as basal bolus) permits greater flexibility in terms of eating habits than was previously the case and is particularly suitable for adolescents and other people with variable lifestyles.

Insulin is administered either by conventional syringe and needle, or 'pen' injection devices which dispense a metered dose of insulin from a cartridge.

Insulin can also be delivered via portable insulin pumps, either subcutaneous insulin infusion (SCII) pumps or the newer implantable insulin infusion (IPII) devices. These provide constant background insulin plus patient-activated bolus doses at meal times. These devices are not widely used because of their cost, the high level of patient training and expert supervision required for their safe use. Currently, their use is usually confined to patients whose control is particularly unstable.

Balancing diet and insulin

The dietary measures needed to balance the effects of insulin action depend on the type and dosage of the insulin injected. Ideally, an insulin regimen should be chosen to suit the patient's lifestyle and usual dietary habits, but this does not always happen in practice.

The advent of easy-to-use blood glucose monitoring devices, together with patients being encouraged to take greater control over their own diabetic management, has resulted in greater flexibility in insulin administration, with patients being taught to alter the insulin dosage as circumstances dictate. Similar flexibility also applies to diet. Many patients learn to adjust their food intake as part of the overall process of achieving tight glycaemic control. It is, however, important that the overall diet remains appropriate in terms of energy content and balanced in overall composition.

Hypoglycaemia

Hypoglycaemia is an ever-present threat for diabetic patients on injected insulin (and some oral antidiabetic drugs) because it is possible for its activity to override the homoeostatic mechanisms which normally ensure that the blood glucose level never falls too low.

If the blood glucose level approaches 4 mmol/l, the body attempts to release stored glucose by secreting large amounts of adrenaline, producing the characteristic hypoglycaemic warning signs such as sweating, shakiness, nausea, increased heart rate and irritability. If the glucose level continues to fall, brain function begins to be impaired, causing confusion, disorientation, slurred speech and increasingly disturbed, often aggressive, behaviour (symptoms which can easily be mistaken for drunkenness). Eventually the person may become unconscious.

Hypoglycaemia is always unpleasant although usually causes no long-term harm. However, it can be fatal following excessive alcohol consumption (which impairs gluconeogenesis and potentiates hypoglycaemia) or if insulin has been injected in excessive quantities. There is also a risk that an unsupervised unconscious person may choke to death. Hypoglycaemia (usually alcohol-related) is a significant cause of diabetes-related death in people under the age of 30 years, particularly in young men (Laing *et al*. 1999).

Isolated incidences of hypoglycaemia are usually caused by:

- a missed or delayed meal

- not consuming enough carbohydrate at the last meal
- being more physically active than usual (exercise increases glucose uptake by tissues, so has a hypoglycaemic effect)
- too much insulin
- alcohol (particularly if consumed on an empty stomach). Alcohol also makes people less receptive to the warning signs of hypoglycaemia, making a severe attack more likely.

People who suffer severe or frequent hypoglycaemic attacks require review to consider whether the meal pattern or food choices are appropriate for the prescribed medication, and whether adjustments to either diet or dosage are needed.

Treatment of hypoglycaemia

In the early stages, hypoglycaemia is easily correctly by consuming 10–20 g of rapidly absorbed carbohydrate such as glucose tablets or glucose/sugar-containing drinks.

As hypoglycaemia becomes more severe, people are less able to treat it themselves, finding it difficult to remember what they need to do, and may need encouragement and assistance from others. Some people may become aggressive or uncooperative and need considerable persuasion to consume some carbohydrate. In these circumstances, an oral glucose-containing gel which is smeared inside the cheek and rapidly absorbed through the oral mucosa may be useful. If unconsciousness occurs, injected glucagon is necessary to mobilize hepatic glucose.

Following initial recovery from a hypoglycaemic attack, additional slower-acting carbohydrate such as a sandwich, or glass of milk with one or two biscuits, or the next meal if due, should be consumed to prevent blood glucose levels falling again. Blood glucose should be checked at subsequent intervals.

Prevention of hypoglycaemia

The increasing emphasis on achieving tight blood glucose control (maintaining fasting glucose at near-normal levels) in order to minimize the risk of complications means that there is a much smaller margin for error in maintaining the balance between insulin/drug action and diet. Intensive management therefore increases the likelihood of hypoglycaemia (DCCT 1993). In order to lessen the risks, patients on insulin should:

- check their blood glucose frequently and especially before going to sleep. The risk of nocturnal hypoglycaemia is increased when this is <6.0 mmol/l
- 'keep four the floor' and be extra vigilant if blood glucose approaches this level
- always carry an emergency supply of carbohydrate (e.g. glucose tablets) and also some form of diabetic identification (in case they are found in a confused or unconscious state)
- be aware that exercise reduces blood glucose and that extra carbohydrate may be needed before, during and after exercise (see below)

- be aware that alcohol must never be consumed on an empty stomach and never in amounts which exceed safe drinking limits. After drinking in the evening, extra carbohydrate at bedtime may be advisable.

Exercise

Exercise lowers blood glucose and so compounds the effects of injected insulin (and some oral drugs). This should not discourage people from taking regular exercise; the benefits in terms of cardiovascular disease, weight control and diabetes far outweigh these disadvantages. Nevertheless, some types of exercise require dietary measures in the form of additional carbohydrate to prevent hypoglycaemia.

The amount of additional carbohydrate depends on the intensity and duration of exercise to be undertaken. A 20 minute walk may not need any additional carbohydrate unless it is immediately prior to a scheduled meal. A short session of vigorous exercise, such as a game of squash, may necessitate 10–20 g carbohydrate beforehand. Prolonged exercise may require additional carbohydrate at the start and regular top-ups at intervals.

Additional carbohydrate may also be needed after the exercise has finished, particularly if it has been strenuous and a meal is not imminently due. The hypoglycaemic effects of exercise can persist for a considerable period after it has finished and people can be caught unawares by a hypoglycaemic attack many hours later, perhaps during the subsequent night or even the following day.

The type of carbohydrate needed similarly depends on the nature of the exercise undertaken. Rapidly absorbed carbohydrate (e.g. a glucose drink or tablets, small chocolate bar) is necessary before intense bursts of activity; more slowly absorbed carbohydrate (such as a sandwich or biscuits) is more appropriate before sustained exercise, and after it has ceased.

The advent of blood glucose monitoring has made it much easier for people to assess how much and what type of additional carbohydrate is required for their own particular needs. Nutrition labelling information has also made it easier for people to select brands of snack bars, biscuits, etc., which provide a particular amount of carbohydrate.

Sometimes insulin or drug dosage may need to reduced as well, either in the short term (for particularly strenuous forms of exercise) or in the longer term (if there is a permanent increase in the daily level of physical activity). However, such adjustments must only be done under clinical guidance; if exercise is undertaken in conditions of insulin insufficiency, glucose uptake by the tissues will be impaired and diabetic control will worsen.

Illness

Illness, even if minor, creates metabolic stress and a rise in blood glucose concentration. Hyperglycaemic symptoms such as excessive thirst and increased urination may appear which, if untreated, may progress to diabetic ketoacidosis and potentially fatal coma.

Ketoacidosis can develop in a matter of hours in young children and over a period of 1–2 days in adults. Deaths from ketoacidosis are rare but account for between half and two-thirds of diabetes-related deaths in people under the age of 30 years (Laing *et al.* 1999). Most of these are avoidable.

During illness, it is imperative that blood glucose is closely monitored and that hypoglycaemic medication is continued as usual, or possibly increased. It is equally important that sufficient carbohydrate is also consumed to balance insulin or drug action and prevent blood glucose levels falling too low. Since people who are unwell often do not feel like eating, this carbohydrate may need to be consumed in an easily assimilated form such as sweetened drinks, milky drinks, soups or yoghurt. All type 1 patients should be given written guidance to keep for reference in such circumstances summarizing the types and amounts of foods and drinks which are compatible with their insulin prescription. The importance of sufficient fluid intake to prevent dehydration also needs to be emphasized, particularly if the illness results in fever, vomiting or diarrhoea.

If blood glucose rises above 15 mmol/l, or if ketoacidotic symptoms develop, patients should seek medical advice immediately.

4.16.8 Specific considerations in people with type 2 diabetes

Most type 2 patients are initially controlled by dietary measures alone, principally adaptation of meal pattern and food choice in order to achieve a more even distribution of carbohydrate throughout the day within the framework of a healthy diet. About 80% of type 2 patients are overweight at diagnosis and weight reduction is a high priority (see below). Even moderate weight loss of 5–10 kg improves glycaemia, dyslipidaemia, hypertension and life expectancy (Lean *et al.* 1990).

Drug treatment

If dietary measures alone are insufficient to reduce fasting blood glucose to below 7 mmol/l within 3 months, it is recommended that oral hypoglycaemic drugs are prescribed in addition. These may comprise:

- *Sulphonylureas*: These stimulate insulin production and so are capable of causing hypoglycaemia if not counterbalanced with sufficient carbohydrate, although this usually only happens with prolonged action sulphonylureas such as chlorpropamide or glibenclamide and not the shorter acting preparations such as gliclazide or tolbutamide.
- *Metformin*: This biguanide drug increases glucose uptake rather than insulin production and does not cause hypoglycaemia. It is more suitable for those who are overweight but, because it is not always effective at

maintaining glycaemic control, often needs to be combined with other forms of hypoglycaemic therapy.

Recently, some newer classes of oral hypoglycaemic drugs such as glitazones (which enhance the action of insulin in the body) have become available.

Acarbose, an inhibitor of the intestinal enzyme alpha-glucosidase, is sometimes given in addition to oral hypoglycaemic agents to delay the digestion and absorption of carbohydrate.

If good glycaemic control is not achieved with oral drugs, type 2 patients should be managed with insulin. Additional dietary guidance in respect of hypoglycaemia, exercise and illness, as detailed for type 1 diabetes above, will be required. Since insulin treatment in type 2 patients often results in weight gain, dietary measures to help to prevent this are advisable; early intervention and structured dietetic care can help minimize iatrogenic weight gain (UKPDS 1998a).

Weight management in type 2 diabetes

Weight management should be achieved by a combination of reduced energy intake (particularly via reduction of fat consumption) and increased level of physical activity. Dietary guidance to achieve this should focus primarily on appropriate food choice, with particular emphasis on avoidance of fat-rich, energy-dense foods. This guidance should be incorporated into the general healthy eating framework appropriate for diabetes, along with any necessary advice on meal pattern and timing. As with every patient, these dietary adjustments should be achieved by modification of existing eating habits rather than by standardized diet sheets.

Weight management programmes should have an achievable, time-limited target, such as a 4–5 kg (10 lbs) weight loss over a period of 3 months. Patients find it helpful to have a clear objective of what they are trying to achieve, while the health professional has defined criteria by which the effectiveness of the programme can be assessed. The reasons for failure to meet the desired goal can then be explored. However, long-term weight control is the primary objective and so any weight loss and maintenance should be viewed in a positive light.

Compliance with diet and lifestyle interventions is notoriously poor. Additional strategies such as cognitive behavioural therapy or group support via slimming clubs may be useful supportive measures (see Sections 4.17, Obesity, and 4.18, Cognitive–behavioural therapy in obesity treatment). Psychological guidance to address underlying problems of low self-esteem and confidence may be appropriate for some patients.

Appetite-suppressant drugs are now rarely used in the management of obesity as a result of their hazardous side-effects. Newer antiobesity drugs such as orlistat (a pancreatic lipase inhibitor which reduces the absorption of dietary fat) may have a limited role but their benefits remain to be evaluated and, currently, strict conditions are attached to their use (Royal College of Physicians 1999).

The use of very low-calorie diets (VLCDs) may be considered in severe cases of obesity, i.e. a body mass index (BMI) >35, but their use should be supervised by specialist medical centres.

4.16.9 Specific considerations in people with additional disorders

Dyslipidaemia

Altered lipid metabolism occurs in both type 1 and type 2 diabetes, but the pattern of dyslipidaemia is different.

Provided that glycaemia is well controlled, lipid profiles of people with type 1 diabetes tend to be similar to those of the non-diabetic population and hence elevated levels of total and LDL-cholesterol are common (Yudkin *et al*. 1996). However, since the risk of cardiovascular disease is higher in the diabetic population, it is more important that these elevated cholesterol levels, or other abnormalities, are detected and corrected at an early stage, ideally by means of dietary adjustment in terms of fat content and composition.

In type 2 diabetes, mild to moderate elevation of VLDL triglyceride is common (often in association with low HDL-cholesterol), particularly if obesity or proteinuria is also present or glycaemic control is poor (Brown 1994). Type 2 diabetic patients also tend to have prolonged chylomicronaemia after eating and an increase in the highly atherogenic intermediate-density lipoprotein and small, dense LDL subclass (Stewart *et al*. 1993).

In most type 2 patients, weight loss is the key to lipid management since this produces rapid improvements in both glycaemia and dyslipidaemia. Reducing energy intake by means of total and saturated fat restriction is likely to have most benefit since this will have direct effects on the lipid profile as well.

In some patients, hypertriglyceridaemia may be exacerbated by high carbohydrate consumption, particularly if consumed in a refined form. In such patients a proportion of carbohydrate energy can be isocalorically substituted by monounsaturated fat. This measure is less appropriate for the overweight hypertriglyceridaemic patient because the increased dietary energy density will make the primary objective of weight loss less likely.

In all diabetic patients, blood lipid levels are closely related to the degree of glycaemic control. Correction of dyslipidaemia therefore requires review of blood glucose management as well.

General aspects of the management of hyperlipidaemia are discussed in Section 4.23 (Hyperlipidaemia).

Coeliac disease

People with type 1 diabetes have a greater risk of developing coeliac disease than the general population, possibly as a result of the presence of HLA-related autoimmune factors which are common to both conditions (Cronin and Shanahan 1997). The need for a gluten-free diet makes life considerably more difficult for those with diabetes because of the additional constraints on food choice, many of which are key dietary sources of carbohydrate such as bread, pasta, breakfast cereals, biscuits and many other manufactured foods. Expert dietetic guidance is essential to ensure that carbohydrate consumption is not compromised and that people have appropriate information on gluten avoidance, alternative food choices (such as rice or potatoes) or substitutes (such as specially manufactured gluten-free breads, flours and pasta) (see Section 4.9, Coeliac Disease).

4.16.10 Specific considerations in particular groups of the population

Pregnancy

The combination of diabetes and pregnancy incurs risk for both mother and fetus because of the increased likelihood of congenital malformation, miscarriage, ketoacidosis, pre-eclampsia, premature or difficult labour, and neonatal problems such as hypoglycaemia and respiratory distress syndrome. The risk of these problems can be considerably reduced with optimal control of diabetes from the time of conception.

Pre-pregnancy

Hyperglycaemia can cause congenital abnormalities during embryogenesis (i.e. within the initial weeks of pregnancy). Since the damage may occur before pregnancy is suspected, it is vital that women with diabetes take pre-conceptional measures to optimize diabetic control. This should include a dietary review so that dietary adjustments can be made if necessary, particularly if there are changes in the insulin regimen. Other general nutritional aspects of pregnancy, such as the need for folate supplementation, can also be discussed.

Once pregnancy is confirmed

Regular dietary follow-up will be needed to help to maintain near-normal glycaemia whilst ensuring that the nutritional demands of pregnancy are also met. A stable meal pattern, usually comprising smaller but more frequent meals, is important. Snacks are usually essential to avoid hypoglycaemic attacks. Food choice should focus on the need for micronutrient-rich foods (fruit, vegetables, low-fat dairy products and lean meat, fish or alternatives) rather than energy-dense, fat-rich foods. Greater consumption of low GI foods such as oats and legumes can be encouraged. Frequent blood glucose monitoring is vital.

Dietitians should make sure that women are aware that tighter glycaemic control increases the risk of hypoglycaemia and that they know how to avert or correct this. Written guidelines for coping with problems such as nausea or vomiting may also be helpful.

As pregnancy progresses

Weight gain should be closely monitored. If this becomes rapid, there should be further focus on food choice to try to replace energy-dense foods with nutrient-rich, lower energy alternatives. The aim should be to hold weight steady or reduce the rate of weight gain. Active weight reduction is not appropriate for any pregnant woman because of the risk of compromising nutritional intake and fetal development.

Following delivery

Breast feeding should be encouraged and infants offered a feed as soon as possible after birth, although in some cases this will be more difficult if the infant requires specialist care in a neonatal unit. Once lactation is established, an additional 40–50 g carbohydrate/day compared with the pre-pregnancy intake is likely to be required by the diabetic mother. Extra carbohydrate may be required before going to bed if the infant is still having nocturnal feeds.

Gestational diabetes

Gestational diabetes is a symptomless form of glucose intolerance which develops during pregnancy but resolves after delivery in the vast majority of cases. It is usually detected via routine urine testing at antenatal visits and confirmed by a fasting venous plasma glucose above 7 mmol/l (WHO 2000).

The significance and management of gestational diabetes are a matter of debate (Jardine Brown *et al.* 1996; Jarrett 1997), and local policy and practice therefore vary. Physiological changes in pregnancy always worsen glucose tolerance and it is difficult to define the point at which harmless change becomes pathologically significant. Gestational diabetes increases the likelihood of macrosomia (high birthweight infants) and hence a more difficult delivery. However, the extent to which this is due to maternal glycaemia *per se* is uncertain because the relationship is confounded by maternal fatness (Goldenburg and Tamura 1996), and macrosomia also occurs in the non-diabetic obstetric population (Ales and Santini 1989). No clear benefit has been shown from screening for glucose intolerance during pregnancy, while a number of disadvantages is attached to a diagnosis of 'gestational diabetes' such as the acquisition of disease status, increased likelihood of caesarian delivery and anxiety to the patient (Jarrett 1997). Nor can the diagnosis help to protect against any risk of hyperglycaemia-induced congenital abnormalities because by the time it is detected (via routine screening at the first antenatal visit) embryogenesis will be complete.

The role of diet in the management of gestational diabetes is also unclear. While it is known that reducing maternal obesity can reduce fetal weight, the level of energy restriction needed to produce such weight loss is normally considered inadvisable during pregnancy because of the risk of fetal undernutrition. Systematic review found no evidence that dietary advice given to pregnant women with abnormal glucose tolerance affected outcome in terms of birthweight or the need for caesarian delivery (Walkinshaw 1999), although the lack of comprehensive data was also noted.

The main significance of a diagnosis of gestational diabetes is that it is a very strong marker for the development of type 2 diabetes in later life, particularly if the person remains or becomes overweight (O'Sullivan 1982; Dornhorst *et al.* 1990). Diet and lifestyle intervention is therefore a high priority following pregnancy, and may be more appropriate at this stage rather than during pregnancy itself.

Children

Management of paediatric diabetes is a specialist dietetic area and its detailed management is discussed elsewhere (BDA 1989, 1993; ISPAD/IDF/WHO 2000). Service provision to this client group should include a paediatric dietitian with expertise in diabetes (Haines and Swift 1997). The general issues which need to be considered in this age group include:

- Energy and nutritional needs are constantly changing in accordance with the demands of growth.
- Dietary habits and meal patterns are likely to be more variable and unpredictable than in adults. Food likes and dislikes change with time and phases of food faddism or behavioural difficulties at meal times commonly occur.
- Levels of physical activity tend to fluctuate more than in adults and may be more spontaneous (e.g. sudden spurts of playground activity as well as anticipated exercise such as school physical education sessions).
- As a result of the combination of erratic activity levels and fluctuations in food intake, hypoglycaemia is much more likely in this age group. Everyone with responsibility of care for the child therefore needs to know how to prevent, identify and treat hypoglycaemia. This may include considerable numbers of people: other members of the family, relatives, friends, school staff, nursery and preschool staff, child minders, baby sitters, youth group leaders, and others.
- The psychological welfare of a child has to be considered. Children hate to feel different from their peers but having diabetes makes this inevitable to some extent. Dietary management has to find the best compromise between maintaining good diabetic control while keeping life as normal as possible.
- Parental anxiety has to be addressed. The diagnosis of diabetes in a child is a traumatic experience for parents who are often terrified at the prospect of having to cope with insulin injections and dietary manipulations. Initially they require a lot of support and reassurance. Hypoglycaemia is a major worry and, while use of a formal carbohydrate exchange system is no longer considered appropriate, parents of diabetic children will need to be able to identify carbohydrate-containing foods and know what portion sizes are appropriate for different circumstances. Establishing a close relationship and regular contact between the dietitian and the child's family is imperative. The availability of 24 hour access to either the dietitian or another member of the care team can do much to alleviate parental anxiety in the initial weeks after diagnosis.

- Healthy eating habits should be encouraged, but care should be taken not to compromise energy intake by the inclusion of too many bulky, fibre-rich cereal foods. Suitable and popular food choices include pasta, bread, potatoes, rice, chapattis, unsweetened breakfast cereals, baked beans and fresh fruit.
- Dietary fat content should not be overlooked as a result of undue focus on carbohydrate/glycaemia issues. It is important to ensure that dietary fat content and type is such that it will help to prevent obesity and cardio-vascular disease in later life. Both the diabetic child and the whole family will benefit from general measures to reduce fat intake via alternative cooking methods to frying, using smaller quantities of leaner meat, discarding poultry skin and using reduced-fat dairy products. Other fat-restriction measures should not be over-vigorous in young children, especially if they have a small appetite. Skimmed milk and very low-fat dairy products are not suitable for any children below the age of 2 or for faddy eaters below the age of 5 years.
- Sweets and chocolate are usually regarded as a pleasurable aspect of childhood and there is no reason for the child with diabetes to be denied this pleasure, other than for reasons of dental health. It is, however, important that their intake is regulated in some way, for instance using them as carbohydrate top-ups prior to or during exercise. It is not necessary to prepare sugar-free artificially sweetened desserts or cakes for the diabetic child. Sugar can be used in baking and consumed as part of an overall balanced diet. 'Diabetic' chocolate, Easter eggs and similar products provide no benefit over ordinary chocolate products and have a number of disadvantages (see Diabetic foods, above).

Teenagers

Most adolescents go through a phase of resenting the constraints of their diabetes and bending the rules as much as they can. At the same time, the nutritional needs for growth may alter rapidly and lifestyle changes combined with new food habits (e.g. more fast foods, snacking, vegetarianism) may alter food intake.

A certain amount of dietary 'turbulence' and poorer control are, to some extent, inevitable and threats from health professionals about long-term complications are, at this stage, unlikely to have much impact, and may even be counterproductive if contact between patient and health professional is lost as a result. With greater maturity, a more responsible attitude to diabetes management returns. Perhaps the most important dietary message to convey to this group, all of whom will be on insulin, is of the potential dangers from alcohol (see Alcohol, above). For the diabetic teenager, overindulgence is not just unwise; the hypoglycaemic consequences can be fatal. Providing guidance on safe drinking limits, the unit content of alcoholic drinks, particularly the high alcohol content of some of the beers and lagers popular with this age group, and carbohydrate sufficiency is important.

Elderly people

Since the risk of type 2 diabetes rises with age and the UK population is becoming increasing elderly in composition, diabetes is increasingly common in people over the age of 65 years.

Many people in this age group, and sometimes those who care for them, regard the condition as 'just a touch of diabetes' and not of great significance. This is far from being the case. The risk of loss of sight, limb amputations, renal failure, stroke and coronary heart disease is greatly increased, particularly if the diabetes has not been well controlled (e.g. based on symptom relief rather than good glycaemic control) or possibly not even diagnosed at all (polyuria may be dismissed as incontinence, or tiredness as 'old age', and other reasons for weight loss may be explored before diabetes is considered). Older people who have had diabetes for many years are also more likely to develop long-term complications as the duration of the disease increases.

About 50% of newly presenting type 2 patients already show evidence of complications (UKPDS 1998a). Diagnostic screening programmes for diabetes and effective monitoring and management with early interventions to reduce the impact of disability are important aspects of health promotion in this age group. The review process should explicitly include an examination of the feet and eyes to identify early changes.

Particular aspects of diabetes in older adults which should be considered are:

- Most new cases of diabetes in this age group will be of type 2, and most likely to be managed by a combination of dietary measures and oral hypoglycaemic drugs. However, if adequate glycaemic control, which is imperative to prevent complications, cannot be achieved by these means, insulin treatment will be instituted.
- It should also not be forgotten that some older people will have had type 1 diabetes since early life and already be treated with insulin, with all that this implies.
- Hypoglycaemia increases the risk of falls and fractures, so there has to be a compromise between tight glycaemic control and the risk of hypoglycaemia. In this age group, the treatment objective of preprandial blood glucose levels between 4 and 7 mmol/l may be too narrow a margin of safety against hypoglycaemia and the target range is often revised upwards, e.g. to between 5 and 9 mmol/l. If for any reason appetite falls significantly, hypoglycaemic medication (whether oral or injected) may need to be reduced.
- Declining renal function may result in reduced excretion of oral hypoglycaemic drugs, hence prolonging their activity and increasing the risk of hypoglycaemia. For this reason, long-acting sulphonylureas such as chlorpropamide and glibenclamide are contraindicated in older people; shorter acting sulphonylureas such as gliclazide or tolbutamide (which are metabolized and inactivated by the liver) are more appropriate. Metformin is also unsuitable for many older people because of the risk of lactic acidosis in those with renal impairment.

- Poor eyesight, as well as arthritis or neurological disease, can make it difficult to draw up the correct dose of insulin. The use of preset syringes or magnifiers attached to the syringe may help to prevent misdosage.
- With advancing age it becomes increasingly likely that other diseases such as transient ischaemic attacks (TIAs), stroke, cancer or dementia will develop in addition to the diabetes. These may increase the likelihood of chronic illness, poor appetite, disability, forgetfulness and confusion which, in turn, can affect food intake, physical activity level and the ability to monitor blood glucose levels.
- The presence of other conditions (whether related to diabetes or not) means that many patients will be taking multiple combinations of drugs. Some of these may have direct effects on food and fluid intake (e.g. by altering appetite or alertness) or the diabetes (diuretics have a dehydrating effect which elevates blood glucose levels).
- Many people with type 2 diabetes will be overweight and will benefit from weight reduction but care needs to be taken not to compromise micronutrient intake. The emphasis should be on a regular meal pattern and better food choice, i.e. nutrient-rich foods such as bread, breakfast cereals, fruit and vegetables and low-fat dairy products, rather than high-fat, energy-dense items such as fried foods, cream, cakes, biscuits, pies and puddings. Increased levels of appropriate physical activity should be encouraged (e.g. chair exercises for those with mobility problems).
- Quality of life must not be overlooked. Dietary guidance has to find the right balance between meeting the clinical needs of the diabetes and not diminishing people's ability to enjoy food. Any intervention must be viewed holistically.

Because many people in this age group live alone and are physically frail, community care mechanisms need to be in place to ensure that those with diabetes receive the treatment and support they need. Strategies involving diabetic liaison nurses, district nurses and practice nurses are being developed in primary care settings to support the delivery of an effective package of care to the older person with diabetes.

In contrast, it has generally been assumed that the needs of older people with diabetes in residential care or nursing homes will automatically be met. There is evidence that this is not the case and that such people are a particularly vulnerable and neglected group as a result of inadequate care planning or management, lack of health professional input including dietetic expertise, and poor medical follow-up (Benbow *et al*. 1997). A recent report (BDA 1999a) recommends that national standards of diabetes care for those in residential homes should be developed and should include:

- the appointment of at least one diabetes nurse specialist with responsibility for older adults within each health area, whose remit would include those in long-term care

- the establishment of a diabetes education and training programme for care home staff within each healthcare district
- a policy of screening for diabetes within each residential home
- the development of a care protocol within each residential home
- the use of an individualized care plan for each resident with diabetes
- appropriate monitoring procedures and referral to other health professionals as necessary.

These recommendations are in line with the government initiative *Fit for the Future*, describing the minimum standards of care that people living in residential and nursing homes should expect.

People from ethnic minority groups

In the UK, the prevalence of diabetes is about four times higher in people of South Asian origin, and about twice as high in those of African–Caribbean origin, than in the indigenous European population. The prevalence of secondary complications such as cardiovascular and renal disease is also higher. In addition, access to or uptake of healthcare services by this sector of the population tends to be poorer, with the result that diagnosis of diabetes may be delayed and its management less effective. This is particularly likely to be the case with those in older age groups or whose command of the English language is poor. These issues are beginning to be addressed at both national and local level by targeted programmes of outreach and health improvement.

While the aims of dietary management are the same for ethnic minorities as for anyone else, the nature of the advice given must be culturally appropriate and local resources should reflect this. These issues are addressed in Section 3.9 (People from ethnic minority groups). Organizations such as Diabetes UK, the British Dietetic Association and British Nutrition Foundation have developed resource material for people from ethnic minorities with diabetes.

4.16.11 Education and follow-up

The diagnosis of diabetes is a considerable shock to most people and it takes time to adjust to its demands and implications. Diabetic education is the gradual ongoing process of helping people to make these adjustments. Dietary education is an integral part of this process to facilitate the diet and lifestyle changes necessary to achieve tight diabetic control and optimize long-term health. There is no blueprint as to how this can be done; every patient is an individual in whom the nutritional priorities for change, achievable targets, degree of change and acceptable pace of change will vary. It is essential that all members of the diabetes care team, including dietitians, adopt a counselling, patient-centred rather than prescriptive approach (Tasker 1998) (see Sections 1.6, Dietary modification, and 1.7, Achieving behavioural change).

Dietary education will never be completed in a single session following diagnosis; in the early stages, people may only be able to assimilate a very limited amount of information. The process starts with one-to-one dialogue between dietitian and patient, where needs are assessed and nutritional priorities evaluated. Initial targets for change and how these may be met are explored with the patient. Written information summarizing the key messages which the patient can take home and refer to later is usually essential. Regular follow-up is then essential to evaluate the effectiveness of change achieved so far and continue the learning process.

A variety of educational strategies, targeted at individuals or groups, via verbal, written or audiovisual forms of information can be used to expand and reinforce dietary messages. The important aspect is to match the type and level of information to individual needs and abilities: some people like a lot of information, others can only cope with a little; those from ethnic minority groups may need oral or written information in a different language; and educational material for children will need to be different to that for elderly people.

Close liaison with other members of the diabetes care team, as well as training and updating colleagues in respect of nutritional aspects of management, are essential to ensure that dietary messages are always consistent.

4.16.12 Monitoring progress and evaluating effectiveness

Dietary success or failure has in the past mainly been assessed in terms of dietary compliance, i.e. the degree to which someone's dietary intake matched their dietary prescription. This approach now has little value in the clinical setting because diets are rarely described in quantitative prescriptive terms; patients are more likely to be given unquantified healthy eating guidance focusing on meal pattern and food choice. It is also increasingly realized that the effects of dietary change are more important considerations than the actual changes. Ultimately, it is the impact of a diet on clinical parameters (such as glycaemic control and lipid profile) and risk factors (such as degree of obesity and level of physical activity) that matters, not whether someone is consuming x% or y grams of a particular nutrient. The latter may be the means to an end but are not the end-points themselves.

Dietary evaluation therefore needs to consider the clinical picture alongside the dietary one, so that the effects of dietary change can be assessed and further adjustments made as necessary. The monitoring process needs to include both clinical and dietary parameters.

Clinical parameters

- Glycaemic control: day-to-day blood glucose measurements, glycosylated haemoglobin level and frequency of hypoglycaemic attacks
- lipid profile

- blood pressure
- renal function
- weight change
- cardiovascular risk factors.

Dietary parameters

- Overall meal pattern, dietary compositional balance and food choice
- the extent to which specific dietary targets have been achieved, e.g. eating five portions of fruit/vegetables per day, losing 5 kg body weight
- reasons for failure to meet targets and how barriers to change may be overcome
- patient's ability to interpret blood glucose measurements and make the necessary dietary adjustments
- acceptability of the dietary changes made and their impact on the patient's quality of life.

As a result of the combined dietetic and clinical review, modifications can be made to the care and treatment plan.

The frequency of follow up depends on the patient's ability and confidence to keep their diabetes well controlled; initially this may need to be monthly, then 6 monthly. A more extensive review should take place annually or if glycaemic control remains poor.

4.16.13 Diabetes care provision

Diabetes care has changed dramatically in recent years:

- Much more patient care, particularly of people with type 2 diabetes, takes place in the primary care setting.
- Care is increasingly provided by a multidisciplinary diabetes care team.
- There has been a move away from doctor-dominated management to patients being encouraged to take a more active role in their own care, in partnership with health professionals.
- Dietary guidance is also more patient centred, the role of the dietitian being to facilitate dietary change rather than instructing people what to do.

There has, however, been variability in the standard of diabetes care provision. In particular, the care of type 2 diabetes in primary care has sometimes been inadequate, either through a lack of expertise or staffing provision in a particular practice or because it was considered to be only a 'mild' form of diabetes (Greenhalgh 1998). Now that the long-term health risks of type 2 diabetes have been clearly established, it is increasingly recognized that there must be integrated care between the primary and secondary sectors so that each patient is managed according to need rather than type of diabetes.

Standards and the National Service Framework for diabetes

The Joint BDA/DH St Vincent Task Force for Diabetes report (BDA/DH 1995) sets out the standards of care required to reduce mortality and morbidity from the disease. The level and type of services needed to provide these standards of care will vary between areas according to the composition and needs of the local population in terms of age, socioeconomic and ethnic composition, proportions of type 1 and type 2 populations and prevalence of complications. However, it is essential that all people with diabetes receive equal access to comprehensive care of high quality.

The British Diabetic Association has published recommendations for the structure of diabetes care services in both the specialist and primary care sectors (BDA 1997, 1999b), and for children (Haines and Swift 1997). These include the provision of:

- local diabetes services advisory groups (LDSAGs), which should be established in every health authority to monitor and advise on diabetes services
- a register of everyone with diabetes within a particular health authority to determine the service provision needed and to audit the quality of care
- local guidelines for management of people with diabetes, which should be prepared and agreed by all local health providers, e.g. hospitals and general practitioners, according to national evidence-based guidelines
- a district diabetes care facilitator to integrate primary and secondary diabetes care services.

Recent NHS reforms such as the creation of Health Improvement Programmes and Primary Care Groups should help to establish better and integrated care (DH 1997). A National Service Framework for diabetes is also being developed.

Recommendations have been made regarding the provision of dietetic services by state registered diabetes dietitians and that these should include (BDA 1999b):

- a dietetic consultation within 4 weeks of diagnosis of diabetes
- dietetic advice to all patients with newly diagnosed diabetes and their carers
- continuing dietetic advice and education to patients with diabetes and their carers
- non-crisis dietetic review annually to patients with diabetes
- access to a paediatric dietitian with a specialist expertise in diabetes for care of children with diabetes
- education, advice and outreach support for primary care
- creation of links with other specialist services as necessary, i.e. renal, metabolic, specialist obesity, community, paediatric, mental health, elderly
- co-ordination of dietary policy and education in diabetes care.

In order to provide this level of care, it has been estimated that 1.5 whole-time equivalent (WTE) state registered dietitians providing solely diabetes services are required for an average health authority serving a population of 250 000 with an average prevalence and pattern of diabetes (CSAG 1994). Surveys of the provision of dietetic services to people with diabetes (BDA 1987; Nelson *et al.* 2000) show that staffing provision falls well below this level in

many areas and, as a result, the range of dietetic services that can be offered is very variable. For example, fewer than half the dietitians specializing in diabetes recently surveyed were able to give their patients an annual review. This issue needs to be addressed.

Text revised by: Briony Thomas

Acknowledgements: Brenda Purnell, Sheridan Waldron, Norma McGough, Sue Durrant, Denise Ellis, Gary Frost, Shereen Huth, Tracey Parkin, Bernice Tighe and other members of the British Dietetic Association's Diabetes Management and Education Group (DMEG), Diabetes UK.

Useful address

Diabetes UK (known as the British Diabetic Association prior to June 2000)
10 Queen Anne Street, London W1M 0BD
Tel: 020 7323 1531
Careline: 020 7636 6112
Website: www.diabetes.org.uk

Further reading

Airey CM, Williams DRR. Cochrane Collaborative Review Group: Diabetes. *Diabetic Medicine* 1995; **12**: 375–376.
Day JL. *Living with Diabetes. The British Diabetic Association Guide for those Treated with Insulin*. Chichester: John Wiley & Sons, 1998.
Day JL. *Living with Diabetes. The British Diabetic Association Guide for those Treated with Diet and Tablets*. Chichester: John Wiley & Sons, 1998.
MacKinnon M. *Providing Diabetes Care in General Practice*. A practical guide for the Primary Care Team, 3rd edn. London: Class Publishing, 1997.
Sonksen P, Fox C, Judd S. *Diabetes at your Fingertips: The Comprehensive Diabetes Reference Book for the Year 2000*. London: Class Publishing, 1998.

Resources

Diabetes UK (formerly The British Diabetic Association) provides a wide range of leaflets, books, videos and other resource material for both health professionals and people with diabetes.

References

Ales KL, Santini DL. Should all pregnant women be screened for gestational glucose intolerance? *Lancet* 1989; **i**: 1187–1191.
Alpha-Tocopherol, Beta Carotene Cancer Prevention Study Group (ATBC). The effect of vitamin E and beta carotene on the incidence of lung cancer and other cancers in male smokers. *New England Journal of Medicine* 1994; **330**: 1029–1035.
American Diabetes Association. Nutrition recommendations and principles for people with diabetes mellitus. *Diabetes Care* 1999; **22** (Suppl 1): S42–S45.
Amos AF, McCarty DJ, Zimmet P. The rising global burden of diabetes and its complications: estimates and projections to the year 2010. *Diabetic Medicine* 1997; **14** (Suppl 5): S1–S85.
Aro A, Uusitupa M, Voutilainen E *et al.* Improved diabetic control and hypocholesterolaemic effect induced by long-term dietary supplementation with guar gum in type II (insulin independent) diabetes. *Diabetologia* 1981; **21**: 29–33.

Bell DSH. Stroke in the diabetic patient. *Diabetes Care* 1994; **17**: 213–219.

Benbow SJ, Walsh A, Gill GV. Diabetes in institutionalised elderly people: a forgotten population? *British Medical Journal* 1997; **314**: 1868–1869.

Brand JC, Colagiuri S, Crossman S *et al*. Low-glycaemic index foods improve long-term glycaemic control in NIDDM. *Diabetes Care* 1991; **14**: 95–101.

Brenner BM, Meyer TW, Hostetter TH. Dietary protein intake and the progressive nature of kidney disease: the role of hemodynamically medicated glomerular injury in the pathogenesis of progressive glomerular sclerosis in aging, renal ablation and intrinsic renal disease. *New England Journal of Medicine* 1982; **307**: 652–659.

British Diabetic Association (BDA). *Recommendations for the Management of Diabetes in Primary Care*. London, BDA, 1997.

British Diabetic Association (BDA). *Guidelines of Practice for Residents with Diabetes in Care Homes*. London: BDA, 1999a.

British Diabetic Association (BDA). *Recommendations for the Structure of Specialist Diabetes Care*. London: BDA, 1999b.

British Diabetic Association/Department of Health. *Report of the St Vincent Task Force for Diabetes*. London: BDA/DH, 1995.

British Diabetic Association (BDA), Nutrition Sub-Committee. The provision of dietetic services to diabetics in the United Kingdom. *Human Nutrition: Applied Nutrition* 1987; **41A**: 13–22.

British Diabetic Association (BDA), Nutrition Sub-Committee. Dietary Recommendations for Children and Adolescents with Diabetes. *Diabetic Medicine* 1989; **6**: 537–547.

British Diabetic Association (BDA), Nutrition Sub-Committee. Dietary recommendations for people with diabetes: an update for the 1990s. *Diabetic Medicine* 1992a; **9**: 189–202.

British Diabetic Association (BDA), Nutrition Sub-Committee. Discussion paper on the role of diabetic foods. *Diabetic Medicine* 1992b; **9**: 300–306.

British Diabetic Association (BDA), Nutrition Sub-Committee. Dietary recommendations for recommendations for children and adolescents: an implementation paper. *Diabetic Medicine* 1993; **10**: 874–885.

Brown L, Rosner B, Willett WW, Sacks FM. Cholesterol-lowering effect of dietary fiber: a meta-analysis. *American Journal of Clinical Nutrition* 1999; **69**: 30–42

Brown WV. Lipoprotein disorders in diabetes mellitus. *Medical Clinics of North America* 1994; **78**: 143–161.

Clinical Standards Advisory Group. *Standards of Clinical Care for People with Diabetes*. Report of a CSAG Committee and the Government Response. London: HMSO, 1994.

Cronin C, Shanahan F. Insulin-dependent diabetes mellitus and coeliac disease. *Lancet* 1997; **349**: 1096–1097.

Department of Health. *The new NHS: Modern, Dependable*. London: DH, 1997.

Diabetes Control and Complications Trial Research Group (DCCT). The effect of intensive treatment of diabetes on the development and progression of long-term complications in insulin-dependent diabetes mellitus. *New England Journal of Medicine* 1993; **329**: 977–986.

Dornhorst A, Bailey PC, Anyaoku V *et al*. Abnormalities of glucose tolerance following gestational diabetes. *Quarterly Journal of Medicine* 1990; **284**: 1219–1228.

Eeley EA, Stratton IM, Hadden DR *et al*. UKPDS 18: estimated dietary intake in type II diabetic patients randomly allocated to diet, sulphonylurea or insulin therapy. *Diabetic Medicine* 1996; **13**: 656–662.

European Association for the Study of Diabetes (EASD), Diabetes and Nutrition Study Group. Recommendations for health care professionals in the nutritional management of patients with diabetes. *Diabetes, Nutrition and Metabolism* 1995; **8**: 186–189.

European Association for the Study of Diabetes (EASD), Diabetes and Nutrition Study Group. Recommendations for the nutritional management of patients with diabetes mellitus. *European Journal of Clinical Nutrition* 2000; **54**: 353–355.

Expert Committee on the Diagnosis and Classification of Diabetes Mellitus. Committee Report. *Diabetes Care* 1999; **22** (Suppl 1): S5–S19.

Fontvieille AM, Rizkalla SW, Penfornis A *et al*. The use of low glycaemic index foods improves metabolic control of diabetic patients over five weeks. *Diabetic Medicine* 1992; **9**: 444–450.

Foster-Powell K, Brand Miller J. International tables of glycaemic index. *American Journal of Clinical Nutrition* 1995; **62**: 871S–893S.

Franz MJ, Horton ES Sr, Bantle JP *et al*. Nutrition principles for the management of diabetes and related complications. *Diabetes Care* 1994; **17**: 490–518.

Freund H, Atamian S, Fischer JE. Chromium deficiency during total parenteral nutrition. *Journal of the American Medical Association* 1979; **241**: 496–498.

Friedberg CE, Janssen MJ, Heine RJ, Grobbee DE. Fish oil and glycaemic control in diabetes. A meta-analysis. *Diabetes Care* 1998; **21**: 494–500.

Friedman EA. Diabetic nephropathy: strategies in prevention and management. *Kidney International* 1982; **21**: 780–791.

Garg A. High monounsaturated fat diets for patients with diabetes mellitus: a meta-analysis. *American Journal of Clinical Nutrition* 1998; **67** (Suppl): 577S–582S.

Garland HO. New experimental data on the relationship between diabetes mellitus and magnesium. *Magnesium Research* 1992; **5**: 193–202.

Ginsberg HN, Barr SL, Gilbert A *et al*. Reduction of plasma cholesterol levels in normal men on an American Heart Association step 1 diet or a step 1 diet with added monounsaturated fat. *New England Journal of Medicine* 1990; **322**: 574–579.

Goldenburg RL, Tamura TT. Pre-pregnancy weight and pregnancy outcome. *Journal of the American Medical Association* 1996; **275**: 1127–1128.

Greenhalgh T (Ed.). Diabetes care: a primary care perspective. *Diabetic Medicine* 1998; **15** (Suppl 3): S1–S64.

Ha TK, Lean MEJ. Recommendations for the nutritional management of patients with diabetes mellitus. *European Journal of Clinical Nutrition* 1998; **52**: 467–481.

Haines LC, Swift PGF. Report of the 1994 BPA/BDA Survey of services for children with diabetes: changing patterns of care. *Diabetic Medicine* 1997; **145**: 693–697.

Henry RR. Protein content of the diabetic diet (Technical review). *Diabetes Care* 1994; **17**: 1502–1513.

Hopkins PN. Effects of dietary cholesterol on serum cholesterol: a meta-analysis and review. *American Journal of Clinical Nutrition* 1992; **55**: 1060–1070.

Hostetter TH, Rennke HG, Brenner BM. The case for intrarenal hypertension in the initiation and progression of diabetic and other glomerulopathies. *American Journal of Medicine* 1982; **72**: 375–380.

ISPAD/IDF/WHO (International Society for Paediatric and Adolescent Diabetes/International Diabetes Federation/World Health Organization). *Consensus Guidelines for the Management of Insulin Dependent (Type I) Diabetes Mellitus in Child-*

hood and Adolescence. Zeist: Medical Forum International, 2000; in press.

Jardine Brown C, Dawson A, Dodds R *et al*. Saint Vincent and improving diabetes care. Report of the Pregnancy and Neonatal Care Group. *Diabetic Medicine* 1996; **13** (Suppl 4): S43–S53.

Jarrett RJ. Should we screen for gestational diabetes? 'The concept of gestational diabetes was popularised before considerations of evidence based medicine came on the scene'. *British Medical Journal* 1997; **315**: 736–737.

Laing SP, Swerdlow AJ, Slater SD *et al*. The British Diabetic Association Cohort Study, II: Cause-specific mortality in patients with insulin-treated diabetes mellitus. *Diabetic Medicine* 1999; **16**: 466–471.

Lean MEJ, Powrie JK, Anderson AS *et al*. Obesity, weight loss and prognosis in type 2 diabetes. *Diabetic Medicine* 1990; **7**: 129–133.

Lieber CS. Alcohol and the liver: 1994 update. *Gastroenterology* 1994; **106**: 1085–1105.

McBain AM, Brown IRF, Menzies DG, Campbell IW. Effects of improved glycaemic control on calcium and magnesium homoestasis in type II diabetes. *Journal of Clinical Pathology* 1988; **41**: 933–935.

Marks L. *Counting the Cost: The Real Impact of Non Insulin Dependent Diabetes*. London: King's Fund Policy Institute, 1999.

Mogensen CE, Keane WF, Bennett PH *et al*. Prevention of diabetic renal disease with special reference to microalbuminuria. *Lancet* 1995; **346**: 1080–1084.

Mooradian AD, Failla M, Hoogwerf B *et al*. Selected vitamins and minerals in diabetes (Technical review). *Diabetes Care* 1994; **17**: 464–479.

Mori TA, Vandongen R, Masarei JR *et al*. Dietary fish oils increase serum lipids in insulin-dependent diabetics compared with healthy controls. *Metabolism* 1989; **38**: 404–409.

Nelson M, Lean MEJ, Connor H *et al*. Survey of dietetic provision for patients with diabetes. *Diabetic Medicine* 2000; **17**: 565–571.

O'Sullivan JB. Body weight and subsequent diabetes mellitus. *Journal of the American Medical Association* 1982; **248**: 949–952.

Purnell B. The role of the dietitian in diabetes care. *Diabetes and Primary Care* 1999; **1**: 84–87.

Rabinowitz MB, Gonick HC, Levin SR, Davidson MB. Effects of chromium and yeast supplements on carbohydrate and lipid metabolism in diabetic men. *Diabetes Care* 1983; **6**: 319–327.

Raz I, Karsai D, Katz M. The influence of zinc supplementation on glucose homeostasis in NIDDM. *Diabetes Research* 1989; **15**: 95–102.

Royal College of Physicians. Clinical management of overweight and obese patients with particular reference to the use of drugs. Report of a working party. *Journal of the Royal College of Physicians of London* 1999; **33**.

Stewart MW, Laker MF, Dyer RG *et al*. Lipoprotein compositional abnormalities and insulin resistance in type II diabetic patients with mild hyperlipidaemia. *Arteriosclerosis and Thrombosis* 1993; **1**: 1046–1052.

Tasker PRW. The organization of successful diabetes management in primary care. *Diabetic Medicine* 1998; **15** (Suppl 3): S58–S60.

Toeller M, Klischan A, Heitkamp G *et al*. Nutritional intake of 2868 IDDM patients from 30 centres in Europe. *Diabetologia* 1996; **39**: 929–939.

United Kingdom Prospective Diabetes Study Group (UKPDS). UK Prospective Diabetes Study 33: Intensive blood glucose control with sulphonylureas or insulin compared with conventional treatment and risk of complications in patients with type 2 diabetes. *Lancet* 1998a; **352**: 837–853.

United Kingdom Prospective Diabetes Study Group (UKPDS). UK Prospective Diabetes Study 38: Tight blood pressure control and risk of macrovascular and microvascular complications in type 2 diabetes. *British Medical Journal* 1998b; **317**: 703–713.

United Kingdom Prospective Diabetes Study Group (UKPDS). UK Prospective Diabetes Study 39: Efficacy of atenolol and captopril in reducing risk of macrovascular and microvascular complications in type 2 diabetes. *British Medical Journal* 1998c; **317**: 713–720.

Valmadrid CT, Klein R. Alcohol intake and the risk of coronary heart disease mortality in persons with older-onset diabetes mellitus. *Journal of the American Medical Association* 1999; **282**: 239–246.

Vinik AI, Jenkins DJA. Dietary fibre in the management of diabetes. *Diabetes Care* 1988; **11**: 160–173.

Walkinshaw SA. Dietary regulation for 'gestational diabetes' (Cochrane Review). In: *The Cochrane Library*, Issue 2. Oxford: Update Software, 1999.

Waugh NR, Robertson AM. Protein restriction in diabetic renal disease (Cochrane Review). In: *The Cochrane Library*, Issue 4. Oxford: Update Software, 1999.

Wolever TMS. The glycaemic index: flogging a dead horse? *Diabetes Care* 1997; **20**: 452–456.

Wolever TMS, Jenkins DJA, Jenkins LA *et al*. Effect of ripeness on the glycaemic response to banana. *Journal of Clinical Nutrition and Gastroenterology* 1988; **3**: 85–88.

World Health Organization, Expert Committee on Diabetes Mellitus. *Second Report*. WHO Technical Report Series 646. Geneva: WHO, 1985.

World Health Organization. *Diet, Nutrition and the Prevention of Chronic Disease*. WHO Technical Report Series 797. Geneva: WHO, 1990.

World Health Organization. *Definition, Diagnosis and Classification of Diabetes Mellitus and its Complications*. Geneva: WHO, 2000.

Yudkin JS, Blauth C, Drury P *et al*. Prevention and management of cardiovascular disease in patients with diabetes mellitus: an evidence base. *Diabetic Medicine* 1996; **13** (Suppl 4): S101–S121.

Zeller KR. Low protein diets in renal disease. *Diabetes Care* 1991; **14**: 856–866.

This section focuses primarily on obesity in adults. Some of the issues relating to obesity in children are discussed at the end of the section (4.17.11).

4.17.1 Classification of obesity

The World Health Organization (WHO) report on obesity, prepared by the International Obesity Task Force, classifies obesity using the Quetelet index or body mass index (BMI) (WHO 1998). This is defined as:

$$BMI = \frac{weight\ (kg)}{height^2\ (m)}$$

(measured in indoor clothing and without shoes).

The WHO classification of obesity is shown in Table 4.34. In the UK, a similar stratification has been in common use, although using terms such as overweight, moderately obese, severely obese and morbidly obese rather than pre-obese, and obese classes I, II and III, respectively.

The BMI is an imperfect index because it is essentially a measure of relative weight for height. It does not measure body fat specifically. Thus, individuals with a particularly well-developed musculature may be classified as obese using the BMI alone. However, on a population basis this classification system provides a robust guide to the health risks of obesity based on data from large-scale prospective cohorts. Other specific measurements of body fat may be used in research studies or to monitor changes in body fat in individual subjects during a period of treatment (Jebb 1998).

In recent years there has been growing interest in the use of waist circumference as an alternative classification system (Lean *et al.* 1995). This provides a guide to the extent of the abdominal fat stores and gives a more sensitive measure of long-term health risks. Current recommended cut-off points for waist circumference for Caucasians are shown in Table 4.35.

Table 4.34   The WHO classification of obesity (WHO 1998)

Category	BMI
Underweight	≤ 18.5
Healthy weight	18.5–24.9
Pre-obese (overweight[1])	25–29.9
Obese class I (moderately obese[1])	30–34.9
Obese class II (severely obese[1])	35–39.9
Obese class III[1] (morbidly obese[1])	≥ 40

[1] Terms more commonly used in the UK.

Table 4.35   Waist circumference cut-off points (WHO 1998)

	Increased risk	Substantially increased risk
Men	≥ 94 cm (≈ 37 inches)	≥ 102 cm (≈ 40 inches)
Women	≥ 80 cm (≈ 32 inches)	≥ 88 cm (≈ 35 inches)

4.17.2 Prevalence of obesity

Obesity is the most common nutritional disorder in the world and is increasing at an alarming rate (WHO 1998). In general, the prevalence is higher in developed than in developing countries, but the rate of increase in some areas, especially in countries undergoing a rapid economic transition, is especially marked. Even in the UK there has been a dramatic increase in recent years, from 6% of men and 8% of women in 1980 to the current level of 17% of men and 20% of women in 2000. Moreover, the latest UK figures from the Health Survey for England show that a further 45% of men and 33% of women are classified as overweight (DH 1997). Today, the prevalence of obesity in the UK is greater than in other parts of northern and western Europe (with the exception of Germany), owing to the rapid increase in recent years which has been less marked in neighbouring countries, such as The Netherlands (Seidell and Flegal 1997). Although the absolute prevalence of obesity in the UK is lower than in the USA, the rate of increase is very similar.

There are marked trends in obesity with age. Among 16–24 year olds only 7% are obese, rising to 29% in 55–64 year olds, after which there is a modest decline. There is also a clear social class gradient, especially in women, where more than twice as many women in social class IV and V are obese relative to professional women in social class I. Thus, the typical obese patient will be middle aged and from social class III or below. General management protocols for obesity should be targeted at this group.

4.17.3 Impact of obesity on health
Health risks of obesity

Obesity is an independent risk factor for premature death, but it is also strongly associated, probably causally, with a number of other serious medical conditions. Overall, obese people are two to three times more likely to die prematurely than their lean counterparts (Calle *et al.* 1999).

The morbidity associated with obesity can be broadly divided into metabolic, mechanical and psychosocial disorders (Bray 1985). Diabetes, hyperlipidaemia and hypertension are strongly associated with excess weight, especially in the abdominal region. The increase in the risk of developing type 2 diabetes (formerly known as non-insulin-dependent diabetes) is particularly striking (Chan *et al.* 1994; Colditz *et al.* 1995). Men with a BMI of 30 kg/m^2 have approximately 13 times the risk of developing type 2 diabetes and for women of similar BMI the risk is increased 20-fold, relative to a BMI of 22 kg/m^2. Other conditions such as strokes, gall stones, some cancers (such as breast and colon) and reproductive problems, including polycystic ovarian syndrome and infertility, are all increased in obese subjects.

Mechanical problems including osteoarthritis, chronic low back pain and breathlessness are rarely life threatening, but contribute to decreased mobility, reduced work productivity and impaired quality of life. Sleep apnoea is a particular problem for many obese patients. The health risks of obesity in young adults are particularly marked and there is a tendency for the relative risk to decrease with age. However, at no age is there a protective effect of excess weight, except for a modest reduction in the risk of osteoporosis due to the enhanced bone density associated with increased weight.

There is an association between obesity and decreased psychological well-being, but this is not a simple relationship (Stunkard and Sobel 1995). Obesity does not cause psychological problems, but the social stigma attached to excess weight can leave many obese people, especially those with morbid obesity, with significant psychological morbidity, including depression and low esteem. In some cases this may contribute to a downward spiral of increasing weight and declining psychosocial functioning. Dietitians are not isolated from prevailing cultural attitudes towards obese people, and establishing an empathic, non-judgemental relationship with an obese patient makes an important contribution towards effective therapy.

Benefits of weight loss

Although the health benefits of maintaining a healthy weight throughout life are clear, there is less evidence that losing excess weight reduces the risk of premature death. This is because of the dearth of long-term prospective studies in which weight has been successfully lost and maintained alongside data in relation to health outcomes. The ongoing Swedish Obese Subjects (SOS) study, which now has more than 5 years of follow-up, will soon be able to test whether successful weight loss improves life expectancy (Sjostrom *et al.* 1995). Previous epidemiological studies which have assessed weight at two or more points in time and related this to long-term health have sometimes suggested that weight loss, and especially weight cycling, may be disadvantageous (Lissner 1995). However, there are many drawbacks to this analysis, including the validity of occasional body-weight measurements to reflect accurately an individual's weight history and voluntary (e.g. controlled dieting) weight loss versus involuntary (e.g. disease-related) weight loss. There is no evidence that obese patients, undergoing medically supervised weight loss using conventional strategies, incur an increased health risk. Indeed, there is good evidence from measurements of intermediary risk factors for disease that their health profile is considerably improved (Allison *et al.* 1999). Many studies have examined changes in specific disease markers in patients losing weight. The precise benefits to individual patients will depend on the initial body weight and health status, the magnitude of weight loss and type of treatment. Typical benefits of weight loss with respect to cardiovascular risk factors are shown in Table 4.36 (Jung 1997).

In addition, most patients who successfully lose weight and maintain the loss, report enhanced physical and psychological well-being. This is clearly illustrated in a study in which patients who had successfully lost 45 kg or more following gastric surgery reported that they would rather be deaf, blind, diabetic, have severe acne or even have a limb amputated than return to their former obese state (Rand and MacGregor 1991). However, there is little evidence that short-term weight loss followed by regain is associated with any improvement in physical health, and it may even impair psychological well-being. Persistent cycles of weight loss and subsequent regain may contribute to the low self-efficacy experienced by many obese subjects.

Obesity is a serious medical condition associated with a considerable burden of ill health. First and foremost, obesity is a preventable condition, and effective treatment and secondary prevention are associated with significant health benefits.

4.17.4 Aetiology of obesity

Obesity is not a single entity, but a group of conditions with different causes, each of which results in excess body fat. This includes a handful of diseases in which obesity is a major feature, but only one part of the overall pathology. The most significant are the Prader–Willi and Bardet–Biedel syndromes. A further group of patients develops obesity as a consequence of an endocrine disorder. These patients represent a tiny proportion of all cases of obesity and usually present with additional symptoms that can

Table 4.36 Benefits of 10 kg weight loss in a 100 kg subject (Jung 1997)

Mortality	20–25% decrease in premature mortality
Blood pressure	10 mmHg decrease in systolic pressure
	20 mmHg decrease in diastolic pressure
Lipids	10% decrease in total cholesterol
	15% decrease in LDL-cholesterol
	8% increase in HDL-cholesterol
	30% decrease in triglycerides
Diabetes	Reduces risk of developing type 2 diabetes by 50%
	30–50% decrease in elevated blood glucose
	15% decrease in HbA$_{IC}$

LDL: low-density lipoprotein; HDL: high-density lipoprotein; HbA$_{IC}$: glycosylated haemoglobin.

be readily identified and usually successfully treated. These include hypothyroidism and Cushing's syndrome. In many other cases endocrine alterations occur as a consequence of obesity and can be reversed by successful weight loss.

In these and all other cases of obesity, excess weight arises as a consequence of a long-term excess of energy consumed relative to an individual's energy requirements. The causes of this imbalance can be traced to a number of factors including specific genetic traits, which may convey a metabolic predisposition, behavioural factors and environmental circumstances (Jebb 1997). These factors may act alone or in combination to modulate intake and/or expenditure and hence determine the likelihood of an individual becoming obese. Understanding the causes of obesity helps to provide a rational foundation for subsequent treatment.

Genetic factors

There are several ways in which genetic factors may influence the development of obesity; for example, via differences in leptin production or regulation. Leptin is a novel hormone that is secreted from body fat, approximately in proportion to the size of body fat stores. There are leptin receptors in a number of tissues but its role in energy balance is mediated primarily through the hypothalamic leptin receptors. Here, leptin acts to decrease energy intake. This provides a negative feedback loop: an increase in body fat leads to an increase in leptin production, which suppresses intake and should lead to a decrease in body fat and hence in leptin production.

In laboratory animals a number of monogenic disorders are associated with severe obesity. In recent years examples have been reported of human obesity syndromes characterized by similar gene defects, including defects in the *ob* gene, resulting in congenital leptin deficiency mutations in the leptin receptor, defective pro-opiomelaninocortin (POMC) processing and mutations in the MC4 receptor gene. In humans each of these syndromes is associated with marked hyperphagia and severe obesity, although in animal models there are additional effects on energy expenditure. These individuals have a powerful drive to eat and conventional management alone is rarely successful in achieving weight loss. However, once the specific mechanism driving food intake is identified it becomes a potential target for specific therapeutic interventions. For example, recombinant leptin therapy in children with mutations in the leptin gene has resulted in substantial weight loss (Farooqi *et al.* 1999). However, at a population level such cases are extremely rare.

A much greater proportion of the population is likely to exhibit polymorphisms in other genes which have a significant but less dramatic effect on body weight (e.g. mutations in uncoupling proteins or the beta-3-adrenergic receptor). These genes may influence a wide range of metabolic and behavioural characteristics that together determine an individual's susceptibility to obesity. Associations have been observed between a number of these candidate genes and an increased risk of obesity, but the results of such studies are not always consistent, reflecting the multiple other influences on an individual's body weight, alongside the specific gene under consideration.

Research into body weight of monozygotic and dizygotic twins, adoptees and their biological and adopted parents, and other heritability studies attribute between 20 and 80% of obesity to genetic factors. Clearly, genes have a powerful impact but their precise contribution depends on the specific gene or genes involved. Defects in the leptin gene have a powerful effect on body weight, making obesity almost inevitable in affected individuals, but other genes may have only a minor influence and their effect is easily dominated by other factors. For example, some polymorphisms may be associated with a small reduction in resting metabolic rate, but this could be overwhelmed by the energy cost of voluntary physical activity.

Metabolic factors

There has been extensive research into putative metabolic differences between individuals that may account for differences in susceptibility to obesity. Previous suggestions that obese persons have a lower metabolic rate than lean individuals have been categorically refuted, since increases in weight are associated with increased energy needs (Prentice *et al.* 1996). However, this does not preclude subtle differences between individuals in the pre-obese period. Studies in Pima Indians have shown that a relatively low metabolic rate is associated with an increased risk of future weight gain (Ravussin *et al.* 1988). Similarly, some studies of post-obese subjects have shown minor differences in energy expenditure compared with age- and weight-matched never-obese controls (Astrup *et al.* 1999). However, these studies are thwarted by difficulties in accounting for subtle differences in body composition. Defects in diet-induced thermogenesis and impairments in fat oxidation have also been suggested as metabolic defects which may increase the risk of obesity, but the net effects on energy expenditure are extremely small (Astrup *et al.* 1996).

In recent years increasing attention has been paid to metabolic control of appetite. Food intake is controlled by a hierarchy of mechanisms, including orosensory, gastrointestinal and neuroendocrine factors (Blundell and Tremblay 1995). Defects in any part of these complex pathways may lead to a dysregulation of appetite. This is an area of much current research, particularly given the finding that most of the monogenic obesity syndromes are characterized by metabolic defects in the appetite control system rather than in energy expenditure.

Behavioural factors

It is only in recent years that it has really been acknowledged that behavioural traits may have a genetic basis. However, it is also apparent that in humans behavioural patterns are also determined by cognitive mechanisms. Voluntary behaviour has the potential to override a genetic and metabolic susceptibility to obesity, by increasing energy expenditure through voluntary exercise and decreasing energy intake through dietary restraint.

Recent research has identified high-fat, energy-dense diets and sedentary lifestyles as critical behaviours associated with an increased risk of obesity. These studies have been reviewed extensively elsewhere (Prentice and Poppitt 1996; Jebb and Moore 1999). In brief, epidemiological studies show that, within populations, those consuming diets with the highest proportion of fat and lowest proportion of carbohydrate are the most likely to be obese (Bolton-Smith and Woodward 1994). In experimental studies fat is less satiating than carbohydrate and when eating *ad libitum*, subjects consume more energy on high-fat diets than on diets high in carbohydrate (Stubbs *et al*. 1995). This is due at least in part to the relatively high energy density of most high-fat diets. Subjects may consume the same bulk of food, but, since fat contains more than twice as much energy as carbohydrate or protein, they consume significantly more energy, a phenomenon described as 'passive overconsumption' (Stubbs *et al*. 1996). Subjects fed a low-fat diet usually lose weight, at least in the short term. However, in the longer term issues relating to compliance and the possible adaptation of the appetite control mechanisms mean that long-term weight loss is limited unless additional strategies are employed to restrict intake (Bray and Popkin 1998).

Physical activity tends to reduce the risk of obesity. Cross-sectional studies show an increased risk of obesity in those at very low levels of activity, although there is little additional reduction in the risk associated with very high levels of exercise. In prospective studies, individuals who maintain a high level of activity gain significantly less weight than inactive people (Coakley *et al*. 1998). Studies of exercise as part of a weight-loss programme have generally shown little or no increase in weight loss with increased activity, but there is a reduced risk of weight regain (Pavlou *et al*. 1989). Together, these data suggest that physical activity helps to attenuate the rate of weight gain rather than accelerate weight loss.

Environmental factors

On a global level the marked increase in obesity which accompanies urbanization and economic development provides strong evidence that environmental factors *per se* play a strong part in the aetiology of obesity or unleash a latent genetic predisposition to obesity (e.g. the 'thrifty gene' hypothesis). It is clear that the modern urban environment promotes consumption through the advertising, accessibility and affordability of food, while simultaneously decreasing energy needs through increasing reliance on the car, labour-saving devices in the home and garden, and a decline in manual occupations. In today's world it can reasonably be argued that weight gain is a natural response (Prentice 1997). Many countries have now accepted the need for environmental changes to facilitate weight control in the population at large, for example through schemes to promote walking and cycling, and in some countries this philosophy has been incorporated into public health strategies, although sadly not in the UK.

Behavioural and environmental factors play an important role in the aetiology of obesity. The recent rapid expansion in the prevalence of obesity has greatly exceeded the increase that would be predicted for any disorder that is fundamentally genetic or metabolic in origin. Analyses of obesity trends in the UK in recent years suggest that the decline in habitual physical activity has greatly outstripped the more modest decreases in energy intake (Prentice and Jebb 1995). In population terms this may be deemed to be an environmental phenomenon, but at an individual level it is clear that weight will only increase if energy intake is not down-regulated to match the present low levels of physical activity and energy needs. The social class gradient in obesity in the UK is evidence that some individuals can develop coping strategies to protect their weight even in the face of the adverse environmental circumstances which foster energy consumption and limit energy expenditure. This raises the realistic possibility that behaviourally based strategies can combat the epidemic of obesity.

4.17.5 Treatment of obesity

Assessment

The aim of any treatment regimen is to improve health through the achievement and maintenance of a healthy weight. Although there is evidence of health benefits even in those with only mild degrees of overweight, most active treatment is directed towards those people at highest risk. This can be determined by considering:

- current weight BMI
- waist circumference
- concurrent morbidity (e.g. type 2 diabetes, hypertension)
- family history of obesity-related morbidity.

Patients with the highest BMI, greatest abdominal fat, existing illnesses or a strong family history are at the greatest risk. This classification system can be used to prioritize patients for treatment, but it should not be forgotten that many other patients would also benefit from successful weight loss. Other factors associated with obesity such as physical inactivity or psychological disturbance also have their own health risks.

Obtaining background information

Losing weight is difficult and it is often helpful to try to establish as much general information as possible regarding the patient in order to provide the most relevant help. It is useful to try to address some of the following issues at the first appointment.

- *Background information about the patient*: Discuss their family circumstances, occupation, etc. These may all contribute to the success or otherwise of a weight-loss programme and can guide appropriate interventions.

- *Motivation*: Discuss why the patient wants to lose weight. Is it for him/herself or because of pressure from other family members or doctors? Are there health reasons? Motivation is the key to weight loss and has to come from the patient, although it can be influenced by the therapist. Many patients are ambivalent about change; this is normal and strategies are available to overcome this (see Section 4.18, Cognitive–behavioural therapy in obesity treatment). Helping patients to identify a strong motivating factor can greatly assist successful weight loss. Write it down as a reminder for use when reviewing the patient's progress.
- *Treatment expectations*: What does the patient hope to achieve by losing weight? How realistic are these expectations? Try to look beyond weight loss alone to other aspirations. Non-weight targets can be a useful incentive, especially during periods when weight loss is slow.
- *Confidence*: How confident is the patient that he or she will succeed? Ask patients what they feel might enhance their confidence and consider what you can offer in this respect. Helping patients to succeed in other areas of their life can boost their self-confidence to take responsibility for their weight.
- *Knowledge*: How knowledgeable is the patient in matters relating to his or her weight? This might include nutritional awareness, understanding of their medical condition and potential benefits of weight loss. Try to correct any unhelpful myths that the patient may be harbouring about his or her weight.
- *Weight*: Most patients are preoccupied with their weight and it is helpful to discuss some of these weight-related issues. Discuss the patient's weight history and how he or she feels about their weight. Discuss any current 'goal' weight and, if appropriate, agree a realistic target.
- *Previous dieting and weight-loss history*: In some, but not all, cases it may be useful to review the patient's prior history. Care must be taken not to dwell on past failures but to use them as a constructive experience to identify rational future strategies.

Obtaining dietary information

There is now abundant evidence that obese people tend to underreport their habitual intake when questioned by a dietitian (Black *et al*. 1993). This confounds an easy analysis of dietary intake, but it does not invalidate the importance of obtaining information on a patient's current dietary habits. This qualitative information can be obtained using interviewing techniques based on the dietary history, focusing on food choice and eating behaviour rather than specific quantitative details. Some points are particularly relevant to the assessment of the intake of obese people:

- meal pattern: regular meal eaters or snackers
- preferred foods: sweet or savoury?
- food dislikes
- 'hard to resist' or 'trigger' foods: explore the possibility of binge eating, night eating or emotional eating
- typical portion sizes: replica foods or food photographs can be useful here to provide a visual picture rather than relying on the recollection of specific weights
- catering arrangements at work: packed lunches, office canteen or the local pub?
- cooking arrangements at home: who shops and cooks?

Most people do not eat to satisfy hunger, but in response to other feelings. This may be particularly so in people who are overweight. Twenty women at a slimming club (BMI 26–34 kg/m^2) were asked why they ate and gave the following reasons: hunger, boredom, comfort, stress, tiredness, habit, availability, anger and to be sociable. On further discussion the majority of them decided that hunger came at the bottom of the list (Bowyer, personal communication). Recent research into binge-eating disorders suggests that up to 30% of patients in obesity clinics may suffer from a clinically defined binge-eating syndrome (Spitzer *et al*. 1992). This may not be evident at the first assessment, but dietitians should be vigilant to the possibility and provide opportunities for patients to discuss their eating habits in an open and non-judgemental manner.

Food diaries are of limited value for the purpose of energy or nutrient intake calculations, but they can be used therapeutically to explore why, where and what people eat and to increase self-awareness of eating habits. A record sheet suitable for recording this information is shown in Table 4.37. Patients can be asked to describe how they feel before and after eating, and with accurately kept records patients can begin to learn about their own eating behaviour. The dietitian must take time to discuss with the patient methods of dealing with some of the reasons given, such as boredom, socializing or habit. Strategies for managing inappropriate eating behaviours are discussed in Section 4.18 (Cognitive–behavioural therapy in obesity treatment). Ultimately, the aim should be to help patients

Table 4.37 Suggested format for recording eating patterns

Day Date Time	Where	Who with	Food and drink consumed	Comments and feelings, e.g. hunger, anxiety, enjoyment, boredom

to evaluate their own diaries to use as part of a future self-monitoring programme.

Treatment protocols

The overall management programme for an obese patient should ideally be developed by a multidisciplinary team with access to the full range of potential therapies. Outline treatment protocols have been developed as part of the SIGN guidelines and local protocols are in place in many areas (SIGN 1996). The specific dietary aspects of obesity management must be integrated into the broader treatment plan. However, some general principles can be identified.

A standardized diet sheet handed out to all obese patients irrespective of their problems is of no therapeutic value whatsoever. Instead, the dietitian must work from a basic dietary outline and employ different strategies in order to create an individualized dietary programme tailored to the needs of the patient. Dietitians must also be prepared to educate their obese patients, not only in nutrition, but also in relevant basic physiology, i.e. how their bodies work. Some patients have strong preconceived ideas about their obesity and may believe that no diet will work for them because their body 'defies the laws of physics' or 'has a slow metabolism' or because of their 'glands'. These obesity myths can create a barrier to effective management.

The basis on which any obesity treatment should be planned is one of long-term change; the concept of being 'on a diet' should be discouraged as it is the time of being 'off the diet' which causes the damage. The long-term goal is to change habits, attitudes and behaviour by encouraging the patient to maintain the short-term goals which have been achieved.

Responsibility

A patient's 'weight problem' is often presented in such a way as if it is the responsibility of the professional and not the patient to solve the problem. In part, this is due to the medical model in which obesity is managed, where patients look to the professional to provide the solution. Typically, an obese patient presents to the general practitioner (GP), who provides a low-energy diet sheet and on a return visit, if the patient has lost no weight, the GP refers the patient to a dietitian on the patient's insistence that the diet did not work. If the dietitian's advice does not work then the patient goes back to the GP for the next referral on to an obesity clinic and so the situation continues. The end result of these referrals is reaffirmation for the patient that his or her 'weight problem' cannot be solved by any dietary intervention given by any professional. Many chronic dieters have a long list of diets that they have tried which did not work. However, in many of these patients, little attempt will have been made to help them to discover the fundamental reasons for their weight problem. It is the responsibility of health professionals to take the time and effort to uncover the real nature of the problem and advise on how this can be remedied; the responsibility for acting on this advice then lies with the patient alone.

Conventional dietary management

There is an extensive literature continually trying to provide the avid obese reader with the 'diet that really works', published as books (many reaching the bestseller list), in women's magazines and in national newspapers. Many rely on gimmicks, and most food constituents in the nation's diet have been the focus of restraint at some time. However, ultimately the only diet that will achieve a sustained reduction in body weight is one which leads to a permanent reduction in habitual energy intake. If necessary, energy requirements of individual patients can be calculated from predicted basal/resting metabolic rate with an appropriate allowance for voluntary physical activity (see Section 1.10, Estimating nutritional requirements).

When prescribing a weight-reducing diet, the following factors must be borne in mind:

- The diet must provide a sustainable reduction in energy intake, to below energy requirements. A deficit of 500–1000 kcal/day below predicted energy requirements will lead to a weight loss of approximately 0.5–1 kg/week.
- With the exception of energy, which will be provided from the existing body fat stores, the eating plan must provide the full nutritional requirements necessary for good health. This is an important consideration since any cut in total food intake will make it increasingly difficult to meet all of the micronutrient needs. Some patients with borderline micronutrient status may benefit from a single daily vitamin and mineral supplement.
- The diet must be sufficiently flexible to take into account a patient's taste, financial status and religious restrictions and other aspects of their lifestyle.

Specific dietary considerations

Energy requirements

Many obese patients claim to be unable to lose weight on a daily intake of 1000 kcal (4.2 MJ). However, there is clear evidence that energy needs increase with body weight. At rest, there are increased metabolic demands to sustain a greater body weight and the energy cost of specific activities is also higher than for lean individuals. There is no evidence of any obese adult with a recorded energy expenditure of less than 1500 kcal/day. A patient who fails to lose weight with a dietary prescription of 1000 kcal/day is unlikely to benefit from further reductions in their dietary allowance. Instead, attention should be paid to the reasons for their non-compliance with the dietary regimen.

Meal frequency

Although there is no direct association between eating frequency and the risk of obesity, a structured eating plan can help patients to shop wisely and reduce the risk of unplanned eating episodes. Eating plans are usually based on the traditional three-meal model, but can be adapted to provide additional snacks for patients who are accustomed to a more frequent eating pattern. Skipping scheduled meals is unhelpful. Many obese patients feel that they are doing themselves good by missing a meal, whereas in practice the energy saving is usually more than compensated for by nibbling later in the day. Some patients try to accommodate between-meal snacks by cutting down at their next meal which, in turn, does not satisfy them sufficiently, leading to further between-meal eating or bingeing.

Portion size

A sustained cut in energy intake can be achieved either by changing the proportion of different foods consumed or by reducing habitual portion sizes. There is a general trend towards large, American-style portions which needs to be addressed. Portion size is a function of habit and it will take some time for patients to become accustomed to eating less. For most people the first and last few mouthfuls of a particular meal or food are the most satisfying, so they should be encouraged to leave out a few of the mouthfuls in between!

Dietary fat

Fat is the most energy-dense macronutrient, providing 9 kcal/g compared to only 4 kcal/g for carbohydrate or protein, and provides the lowest satiety value. A reduction in total fat intake is the easiest method by which to reduce total energy intake. The absolute requirements for essential fatty acids are very small indeed and there is a large store of these vital nutrients. Thus, the percentage of energy from fat in a weight-reducing diet can be as low as is practically achievable. All fat-rich foods should be avoided. Adding fat to food (e.g. butter on vegetables), cooking in fat (e.g. frying or roasting) or consuming fat-containing sauces, gravies or batter should be avoided. Ideas for alternative foods or cooking methods should also be given. Advice on foods containing 'invisible' fat, including ready-made meals, processed meat products, cakes, biscuits and confectionery is particularly important.

Use of low-fat foods

Low-fat products can be used to substitute for full-fat equivalents, although it may be necessary to provide additional restrictions for concentrated fat sources such as low-fat spreads. Low-fat foods with a low energy content are particularly useful, e.g. low-fat dairy products. However, it should be emphasized that low-fat products will only assist weight loss as part of an overall energy-restricted diet. In recent years there has been a marketing explosion of low-fat foods in which fat has been replaced by simple carbohydrates; these foods may contain less fat but they do not necessarily contain fewer calories. Many patients may be inappropriately seduced into believing that these foods can help them to lose weight.

Dietary carbohydrate

Starchy carbohydrates such as bread, cereals, pasta and potatoes should provide the bulk of each meal as they help to provide a sense of fullness. Unfortunately, they are still perceived as especially 'fattening' by many people and this misconception must be clarified. These foods have a low energy density, and are inexpensive, easily available and good sources of a range of important nutrients. However, it is important that they are not prepared or served with additional fat, e.g. butter or creamy sauces. The use of carbohydrate exchange lists is sometimes useful, not so much for the purpose of restricting intake but to ensure that adequate amounts of these foods are consumed. This cannot be overemphasized as many obese people have been 'brainwashed' into restricting these foods. Fibre-rich sources of carbohydrate such as wholemeal bread and cereals are particularly valuable in terms of satiety and can also help to reduce the risk of constipation, which is a common feature of weight-reducing diets.

Dietary protein

The protein content of the diet must be adequate to meet daily requirements. Typically, protein provides about 12–15% of total energy intake. Most people in the UK eat far more protein than they actually require and the excess is broken down to provide energy. A reduction in absolute protein intake is therefore warranted. However, in order to maintain the absolute protein requirements relative to the total energy intake, the proportion of protein in a reducing diet will usually be around 20%. All energy-restricted diets should provide a minimum of 15% of energy in the form of protein. Guidelines on recommended portion sizes of the protein-rich foods, e.g. meat, fish, cheese, eggs, milk, yoghurt and pulses, to be included in a low-energy diet may be helpful.

Fruit and vegetables

Fruit and vegetables are a vital part of any reducing diet. The energy density of most fruit and vegetables is low, such that they provide bulk to a meal to promote feelings of fullness and satiety, with relatively little added energy. They are also a good source of dietary fibre, micronutrients and phytochemicals, which have a protective effect on health.

Sugar-rich foods

While energy-rich foods such as sweets, chocolates and cakes cannot be recommended for a low-energy diet, their inclusion in carefully controlled quantities as part of an structured eating plan is sometimes helpful. Obese patients frequently regard these foods as especially 'fattening' 'bad' or 'forbidden', and this imagery is unhelpful in achieving a balanced attitude towards food. Eating these foods may be a minor lapse from their eating plan but it is not a major relapse. One bar of chocolate or one cake will not cause uncontrollable weight gain; it will only add a small amount of energy to that day's total intake. Weeks or even months of effort must not be abandoned simply because of lapses on one day. Excessive dietary restrictions of any kind run the risk of creating compensatory cravings for these foods. Whilst total abstinence may occasionally be the best tactic in those in whom certain foods trigger excessive consumption, for most patients it is important to learn how to control their intake of such foods in a rational manner.

Fluid intake

Restricting water intake is not a successful strategy for weight loss. Many obese patients suffer from oedema, but this will be resolved by successful long-term weight loss, not by short-term water restriction. Patients should be recommended to drink at least 2 litres of water a day. Drinking water with a meal will help to reduce the energy density of the meal and increase feelings of fullness (satiety).

Food choice guidance

Lists of both 'foods which can be eaten freely' and 'foods to avoid' based on low and high energy-dense food, respectively, are helpful to patients. However, these lists should be practical and reasonably balanced in length; a long list of pleasant-tasting 'foods to avoid' accompanied by an 'unrestricted' list consisting only of items such as salt, pepper, mustard and low-calorie squash will not help the patient's morale.

Snacks

Most patients will snack on occasions. In the first instance it is important to help patients to distinguish snacks precipitated by hunger from other factors such as boredom or stress. If patients are genuinely hungry it is important to help them to make appropriate food choices, for instance, a bowl of cereal with semi-skimmed milk rather than a cheese sandwich or a packet of crisps.

Practicality

Many dietary regimens fail not through lack of knowledge but through inadequate practical skills. Many patients need to be specifically taught how to implement their eating plan in everyday circumstances. This may require lessons in shopping or cooking skills, choosing from restaurant or takeaway menus, coping with social situations where there may be pressure to eat, how to decline food, etc.

For more detailed information on the dietary management of obese patients see Summerbell (1998).

Very low calorie diets and meal-replacement products

Very low calorie diets (VLCDs) are commercially produced nutrient preparations providing less than about 600 kcal (2.5 MJ) per day, which are marketed for use as a total food substitute. In 1989 COMA issued detailed recommendations for their use (COMA 1987). VLCDs should not be used by pregnant or breast-feeding women, children or elderly people. Their use is also contraindicated in individuals with:

- cardiac disorders
- cerebrovascular disease
- hepatic or renal disease
- hyperuricaemia
- psychiatric disturbance
- porphyria.

In the 1970s there were reports of some deaths in patients taking VLCDs as a result of cardiac arrythmias. However, this was due to a deficiency of tryptophan and there is no evidence that modern-day formulations are inherently unsafe. Concerns about the use of VLCDs centre on the rate of weight loss, and its effects on metabolic rate and body composition, although this varies depending on individual characteristics and compliance to the diet plan. Extreme dieting is associated with significant reductions in resting metabolic rate and in the longer term this may counteract the theoretical benefits of the larger energy deficit on actual weight loss. It has been suggested that there may be disproportionately large losses of lean tissue, but the evidence is inconsistent owing to differences in the methodology used to measure changes in body composition. Recent studies of changes in body composition using sophisticated multicompartment models in patients following a milk-based diet providing 800 kcal/day have found no evidence of excessive losses of lean tissue in overweight women. However, there is reason to suspect that greater losses of lean tissue may be incurred in subjects who are not initially overweight, and this reinforces the opinion that VLCDs should be reserved for the treatment of obese individuals. Perhaps the most serious issue against the use of VLCDs is the inability of subjects to maintain their weight loss when food is reintroduced (Wadden and Frey 1997). Most studies show significant weight regain as patients return to their former eating habits.

VLCDs are sometimes used to replace one or two meals, whilst consuming food on the remaining eating occasions. Used in this way they are broadly analogous to the drinks or bars sold as meal-replacement products. Patients following this type of regimen have a higher energy intake than those following a rigorous VLCD and there are fewer concerns about their safety. Indeed, it is arguable that these products provide a more nutritionally complete meal than often consumed by subjects following a conventional weight-reducing diet. There has been surprisingly little detailed research on the use of meal-replacement products, although one study has shown impressive weight maintenance in regular consumers of meal-replacement products (Ditschuneit et al. 1999).

Relatively few dietitians are involved in the use of commercial VLCDs. Instead, most are sold over the counter or through networks of counsellors. Patients who report taking these products should be encouraged to contact their GP to ensure appropriate medical supervision. Some obesity centres use a modification of this approach based on milk, usually including 3 pints (1.7 litres) of semi-skimmed milk per day (approximately 800 kcal/day), plus additional low-energy drinks, including at least one salty drink, and a multivitamin and mineral supplement. Like commercially prepared formulae this has the advantage of removing the patients from the usual processes of shopping and preparing food, providing an opportunity to break old eating habits and achieve the early rapid weight loss which can be very motivating. Milk diets do not have the novelty associated with the commercial VLCDs but the reported rates of weight loss are very similar. When combined with a gradual reintroduction of food and intensive dietary education this can provide a useful intervention in selected patients. Dietetic input is critical alongside medical supervision of the patients and ideally a behavioural therapy programme.

The use of VLCDs and meal-replacement products in the management of obesity has recently been reviewed in more detail (Jebb and Goldberg 1998).

Physical activity and exercise

It is generally acknowledged that some exercise is beneficial to general health and well-being and people are being encouraged to include regular exercise in their lives as part of an overall lifestyle strategy (Cowburn *et al.* 1997). To many obese people 'exercise' means either stripping down to a minimum of clothing in a gymnasium or swimming pool, wearing Lycra and joining a fitness class or jogging around the park and, not surprisingly, most are unwilling to contemplate any of these. However, most are unaware that significant amounts of 'exercise' can be performed by means of ordinary daily tasks, e.g. walking up the stairs rather than using a lift, walking to the shops instead of taking the bus or driving, and finding some household task to do instead of watching television. Describing these actions as 'physical activity' rather than 'exercise' can be less daunting.

The severely obese have particular problems because they have difficulty with breathing, joints and balance. Increasing the level of activity should be done slowly and the type of activity geared to each patient's capabilities. Once the patient starts to lose weight and adapts to the level of activity, the amount and degree of difficulty of the tasks performed can be increased, e.g. walking more quickly, walking further and using the stairs more. It is important to recognize that although their physical abilities are more limited, every action will require more energy and so the net effects can be considerable; moreover, with training their stamina will improve.

Although exercise will not in itself contribute a great deal to weight loss directly, it has been shown to play an important role in weight-loss maintenance (Pavlou *et al.* 1989). It also contributes a positive aspect to weight control inducing a sense of well-being and helping to divert attention away from food. Increasing the level of physical activity will also have independent health benefits. Some patients enjoy, as well as benefit from, a formalized exercise programme and this can be planned with the help and advice of a physiotherapist. Primary care 'exercise prescription' schemes have been successfully set up in some areas.

A comprehensive systematic review of the role of physical activity in the prevention and treatment of obesity and its co-morbidities has recently been prepared (American College of Sports Medicine 1999).

Behavioural programmes

In recent years there has been growing interest in the application of the 'stages of change' model and use of behavioural strategies to achieve dietary change, particularly in the management of obesity. These aspects of dietetic practice are discussed in greater depth in general terms in Section 1.7 (Achieving behavioural change) and in relation to the management of obesity in Section 4.18 (Cognitive-behavioural therapy in obesity treatment).

4.17.6 Other approaches to obesity treatment

Pharmacotherapy

In recent years there have been significant advances in our understanding of the physiological processes that regulate body weight, especially the control of food intake (Finer 1997). This has spawned enormous interest from pharmaceutical companies seeking a novel anti-obesity drug. Currently, two compounds, sibutramine and orlistat, have been developed to assist weight loss and other drugs are at various stages of the development process.

Orlistat

Orlistat is licensed for use in both the USA and Europe. It is a pancreatic lipase inhibitor, which blocks the digestion and absorption of dietary fat. At the recommended dose of 120 mg three times a day taken before meals, approximately 30% of dietary fat is unabsorbed and remains in the gastrointestinal tract and is excreted. Given its mode of action, dietary management of patients receiving orlistat is crucial. Patients must reduce the fat content of their habitual diet to less than 30% by energy in order to minimize the risk of any adverse gastrointestinal events. Failure to follow this dietary prescription will lead to large quantities of unabsorbed fat in the colon, leading to loose, fatty stools and in extreme cases faecal incontinence. Data from clinical trials suggest that although many patients experience some early side-effects, they quickly learn to modify their behaviour to prevent such incidents occurring, enhancing compliance to the dietary programme. Indeed, a considerable proportion of the weight loss can be attributed to changes in intake rather than the relatively modest losses of energy from the gastrointestinal tract in unabsorbed fat. Data from the European multicentre trial show weight losses of 10.3 kg over 1 year compared with 6.1 kg in placebo-treated patients, with enhanced weight maintenance in the second year (Sjostrom *et al.* 1998). This and other studies have demonstrated that the weight loss is associated with reductions in risk factors for chronic disease (Davidson *et al.* 1999).

Dietetic support for patients receiving orlistat must be focused on a low-fat diet. However, other dietary principles are similar to those described previously for patients treated with diet alone.

Sibutramine

This is currently licensed in the USA, where it is known as Meridia, and in Germany, as Reductil, and is likely to become more widely available across Europe. Sibutramine is a centrally acting appetite suppressant that blocks the re-uptake of serotonin and noradrenaline in the synaptic neurons of the brain. Serotonin is one of the neurotransmitters that are known to influence appetite. Increases in serotonin concentration decrease spontaneous intake, mostly by decreasing meal size. Sibutramine is also known to stimulate sympathetic nervous system (SNS) activity. In small animals it is associated with a small increase in metabolic rate, although in humans the effects on energy expenditure are minor and not wholly consistent. There is some evidence that sibutramine may slightly attenuate the decrease in metabolic rate associated with weight loss, but there is little doubt that its primary effect on body weight is via a reduction in food intake. One of the adverse consequences of the SNS effects of sibutramine is a small increase in heart rate and smaller decreases in blood pressure than patients losing similar amounts of weight while taking a placebo.

One of the principal limiting factors in the efficacy of sibutramine is that many people eat even when they are not hungry. Boosting sensations of fullness using appetite suppressants can only help patients to adhere to a reduced-energy diet; it does not automatically lead to weight loss. Good dietetic input is essential to the overall success of sibutramine. Although fewer data are available than for orlistat, preliminary evidence suggests that the observed weight losses are similar to those observed with orlistat (Bray *et al.* 1994; Apfelbaum *et al.* 1999). In many of the sibutramine trials dietetic advice has been based on a 600 kcal/day deficit diet. This involves calculating the individual's daily energy needs, subtracting 600 kcal and then prescribing a nutritionally balanced structured eating plan, sometimes using a series of food exchanges. The basic principles of dietary therapy all apply for patients treated with sibutramine.

Guidance on the use of drugs in the management of obesity has been produced by the Royal College of Physicians (1997).

Gastric balloons

The gastric balloon or bubble is another medical device which has been used in the treatment of obesity, although nowadays is an unusual procedure. It is placed in a deflated state into the stomach via an endoscope and then inflated using air, water or a combination of both. The aim is to reduce the gastric volume and consequently the intake of food. It remains in place for a temporary period and is then deflated and removed. Side-effects are often reported and these include nausea, abdominal pain and vomiting. These usually disappear in most (but not all) patients in the first 2 weeks.

Early satiety has been reported in obese patients with the inflated balloon; however, there was no significant difference in weight loss over a 3 month period between those patients with a balloon and others who had a sham procedure (Hogan *et al.* 1989). Each group took part in a weight-loss programme which included a weight-reducing diet, behaviour modification and exercise. In another trial, where obese patients had an inflated balloon for 6 months, only 20% could maintain their weight loss (Worner *et al.* 1989). Overall, there is little evidence of any additional benefits over standard weight-loss therapy (Hogan *et al.* 1989).

Surgical techniques

Several surgical procedures have been used in the treatment of severe obesity. Each presents particular dietetic issues, which need to be carefully considered within the context of a multidisciplinary team. The Swedish Obese Subjects (SOS) study is a major long-term randomized trial of obesity surgery (using gastric bypass or gastroplasty) versus conventional management (Karlsson *et al.* 1998). It has shown striking benefits of surgical management, including weight losses of around 30% of initial weight, accompanied by significant improvements in obesity related morbidity. The data from this study are forcing a reconsideration of the appropriate use of surgery in obesity treatment protocols and a growing interest in this approach. In the UK a new professional association for bariatric surgeons (BOSS) has recently been established and is currently developing guidelines for care. The surgical procedures for the treatment of obesity have been reviewed in detail (Kolanowski 1997).

Jaw wiring

Wiring the jaws together to allow drinking, but not chewing, is usually associated with weight loss and for a time was used to limit food intake in severely obese subjects. However, in most cases weight is rapidly regained when the wires are removed. Moreover, the procedure is not without its direct hazards, including difficulties in maintaining dental hygiene and the risk of choking, especially if vomiting occurs, and this procedure is rarely performed today.

Jejunoileal bypass

In this procedure a short length of the proximal jejunum is anastomosed to a short length of the terminal ileum, hence bypassing a large segment of the small intestine. However, such operations are rarely performed today because of the risk of medical and surgical complications, including 'bypass enteritis', electrolyte disturbances, renal stones, liver damage, inflammatory skin and joint disease, and mineral and vitamin deficiencies (e.g. iron, folic acid, vitamin B_{12} and vitamin D). Many of the complications are severe enough to warrant reversal of the operation and are not always confined to the early post-operative period. There is a mortality rate of 3–4% and this procedure has been largely discontinued.

Gastric bypass

This operation produces a combination of malabsorption and restricted intake. A small pouch is created in the upper portion of the stomach that is anastomosed to the proximal jejunum, thus excluding most of the stomach and a 50 cm stretch of the duodenum, sometimes described as the 'Roux-en-Y' arrangement. It provides a prolonged sensation of fullness combined with modest malabsorption and is associated with fewer complications than the more radical jejunoileal bypass. Intestinal dumping is the most common problem as the hypertonic contents of the stomach empty rapidly into the small bowel, especially after carbohydrate-rich meals. There is a risk of iron and calcium malabsorption due to the bypassing of the duodenum, increasing the risk of anaemia and osteoporosis. Long-term follow-up is therefore crucial.

Stapled gastroplasty

Today, the vertical stapled gastroplasty is one of the most common procedures undertaken to reduce the size of the stomach. This procedure uses stapling to create a small pouch (approximately 30 ml) in the upper part of the stomach with a reinforced stoma through the staple line. Foods and fluids then pass from the upper pouch through to the remainder of the stomach. As there is no interruption of the gastrointestinal tract, food is digested in the normal way. The aim of the procedure is to limit the quantity of food and fluids taken at any one time by producing early satiety. Complications associated with large upper pouches include vomiting and stomal ulcers. The average weight loss is somewhat less than following gastric bypass, but there may be fewer complications. Later weight regain is not uncommon owing to excessive calorie intake facilitated either by frequent, energy-dense meals or by disruption of the staples.

Dietary management following bariatric surgery The dietary management of patients following gastric bypass or gastroplasty is similar. Post-operatively, once patients are able to tolerate sips of fluid, they should commence on a soft, puréed diet. Small portions of food (one or two tablespoons) are essential to prevent disruption of the staple line and allow time for healing. Too large a portion may cause pain, discomfort or vomiting. Since the bulk of food that can be consumed is limited, patients must be instructed to consume a nutrient-dense diet consisting of foods such as puréed porridge, puréed meat or fish, runny soft-boiled eggs, strained yoghurt, mashed potato, puréed vegetables, fruit juice or puréed fruit, and strained soup. One pint of milk should be consumed daily and vitamin and mineral supplements are usually necessary. It is important to commence this regimen while the patient is still in hospital.

Once discharged from hospital, the patient should be encouraged to increase the variety of food, gradually introducing solids. The range of food should expand, although some patients may be unable to tolerate certain foods. Some find, for instance, that bread appears to 'stick', although they are able to manage crackers or toast. Many find that chocolates or crisps are readily tolerated whilst fruit is more difficult! Patients should be encouraged to find their food tolerances by trial and error. With time, the patient is able to tolerate larger portions and it is essential to ensure that this does not facilitate an increased energy intake to such a level that weight loss does not occur. Although early weight losses are often dramatic, many patients begin to regain weight 1–2 years later. Patients may need to be discouraged from choosing energy-dense foods and reverting to inappropriate eating habits.

The dietitian has an important role to play in the management of these patients. In the short term patients need support to adapt to the physical constraints of their operation, leading on to nutrition education to develop a well-balanced diet and to ensure appropriate rates of weight loss and long-term weight maintenance. Managing patients' expectations of this treatment is also important. It is preferable for the dietitian to meet the patient before the operation to explain the effect that the procedure will have on their eating habits. Patients need to understand that the only role of the surgery is to provide a physical limit to eating and is not as such a 'cure'. They must recognize the need for major changes in their eating habits. Stapling is not an easy way of losing weight.

4.17.7 Weight loss groups

Most dietitians tend to see patients individually and there are many reasons for this, including the difficulties in changing traditional practices, organizational problems of convening a group, patient reluctance and inter-patient differences in treatment. However, there is preliminary evidence that in some circumstances groups can provide an efficient and effective method for seeing large numbers of patients (Hayaki and Brownell 1996). They have the added benefits of allowing regular contact, a planned course of education, peer support and greater possibilities for developing practical coping skills. A format which allows small group discussions and workshops to draw on the experiences of other people in similar situations and encourage the patients to find their own solutions can be very valuable.

4.17.8 Measuring outcomes

Any analysis of the outcome of an obesity treatment programme should reflect the broad aims of treatment, including long-lasting changes in eating and exercise behaviours and reductions in co-morbid conditions. Factors such as improvement in functional capacity, self-esteem, body image and quality of life may also be relevant. Changes in weight are an important component of outcome analysis. However, it should also be remembered that the natural history of body weight is for increase with age. Weight stability therefore is the first sign of success.

Subsequent goals should focus on a sustained reduction in body weight over time, not the greatest weight loss in the shortest period.

In the early days of a reducing diet, weight will be lost relatively quickly. This reflects the mobilization of the liver glycogen stores. Since each gram of glycogen contains only 4 kcal and is bound with 3 g of water, 1 g of weight will be lost for each calorie deficit. However, since liver glycogen stores are only about 300 g in total this is a short-lived phenomenon. Thereafter, the rate at which weight is lost is related to the energy content of fat. Adipose tissue has an energy value of approximately 7000 kcal (29 MJ)/kg, so a deficit of 1000 kcal (4.2 MJ)/day below energy requirements will lead to a weight loss of approximately 1 kg per week. Many patients (and some professionals) are disappointed when they 'only' lose 1 kg per week, but this implies a naïve understanding of the physiology of weight loss and emphasizes the importance of setting realistic treatment targets. More rapid rates of weight loss are usually indicative of losses of lean tissue.

As weight is lost, the resting metabolic rate (RMR) will decrease and therefore energy requirements will fall (Prentice *et al.* 1991). This is due to the absolute reduction in body weight and an adaptive response to underfeeding. Thus, the rate of weight loss will tend to decline. However, the extent of the decrease in RMR should not be overestimated and patients should be encouraged to offset the reduction in RMR associated with weight loss through increases in voluntary physical activity. Diets providing more than 1000 kcal/day are associated with a suppression of RMR of only around 5%. Greater reductions are seen with more severe energy deficits and this is one reason why there is little evidence that greater energy deficits lead to greater weight loss in the longer term. In general, reductions in the rate of weight loss over time are usually more closely related to lapsed compliance with the diet than to reductions in RMR.

It should be impressed clearly upon patients that short-term (daily) fluctuations in weight are due to changes in water balance and that the changes in fat weight are small and slow. For this reason, patients should be discouraged from weighing themselves more than once a week. They should also not allow a sudden increase in weight (mainly fluid) after a dietary indiscretion to discourage them from continuing with the attempt to lose fat.

Successful weight loss is not easy and there are often setbacks and periods of weight plateau. The most successful dieters do not let these setbacks deflect them from their ultimate goal. Dietitians can play an important role in helping patients through these difficult periods. Identifying other non-weight markers of progress can be very valuable at these times, e.g. eating non-fried potato more often, eating less confectionery and more fruit, not skipping breakfast, having a television-free day or taking a walk every day.

4.17.9 Weight maintenance

Losses of 5–10% of body weight are usually associated with significant improvements in health (Jung 1997). At this stage it is often appropriate to consider a period of weight maintenance to allow patients to demonstrate their ability to sustain this reduced body weight. They should be aware that their new weight brings a lower RMR than their obese weight and that they will not be able to return to their previous eating habits. It may be some time before the patient feels confident about controlling his or her weight and support should be offered during this period. Formal relapse-prevention programmes are now being developed to support patients at this time. After a period of successful weight maintenance further weight loss may be considered. In this way, long-term weight loss becomes a series of achievable small steps.

4.17.10 Prevention of obesity

The primary prevention of obesity refers to the prevention of weight gain in lean subjects. Secondary prevention encompasses the prevention of further weight gain in those who are obese, or in formerly obese subjects who have successfully lost weight. A comprehensive and detailed review of all aspects of obesity prevention has been published by Gill (1997).

Many community dietitians will be involved in comprehensive obesity prevention programmes, possibly including inter-sectoral initiatives and broader environmental policies. However, all dietitians should be alert to the potential opportunities for health promotion in their everyday work. Decreases in dietary fat and increases in fruit, vegetable and fibre consumption will all help to reduce the risk of obesity or minimize the potential for the development of co-morbidities. Physical activity has been shown to be a key component in the prevention of weight gain and its importance should not be underestimated. These guidelines for the prevention of obesity are wholly consistent with those for the reduction of other chronic diseases.

4.17.11 Obesity in children

Unfortunately, there are fewer nationally representative data on overweight and obesity in children than in adults, and absolute values depend on the precise definition used to diagnose excess weight. However, there is convincing evidence from a number of studies that increasing numbers of children of all ages are becoming obese. In a cohort study of preschool children, Reilly *et al.* (1999) found that, by the age of 2 years, almost 16% of boys and girls could be classified as overweight and 6% as obese; by the age of 4 years, these figures had risen to 20% and 8%, respectively (Reilly *et al.* 1999). In the population as a whole, the proportion of 6 year olds who can be classified as obese has doubled (to 10%) since the mid-1980s, and in 15 years olds it has trebled (to 17% compared with 5% in the mid-1980s) (Reilly and Dorosty 1999).

The aetiology of obesity in children is broadly similar to that in adults, reflecting a combination of genetic susceptibility and lifestyle factors. There is no doubt that obesity tends to run in families. Children with two obese parents have about an 80% chance of becoming obese themselves, compared with only 20% in those with lean parents, but this does not distinguish nature from nurture. Tracking studies have shown that in babies and very young children, parental obesity is a stronger predictor of adult weight than the weight of the child itself, but as children grow older their own body weight becomes increasingly closely associated with their adult weight status and parental factors decline in importance (Whitaker *et al.* 1997).

There is particular concern about levels of physical activity in children. Most children take the car or bus to school, rather than walking or cycling, there is less time in the school curriculum for physical activity, and less time is spent playing outdoors and more time in front of the television, video or computer. However, there have also been marked changes in eating habits. Children today have more personal purchasing power than previous generations, more food is consumed outside the home, and there is a strong trend towards snacking and away from traditional meal eating. The precise impact of these factors on the weight of children is unclear. However, the general recommendations for a healthy lifestyle to reduce the risk of overweight and obesity are equally applicable to children as to adults.

Treatment of obese children

Detailed information on the treatment of obese children can be found in paediatric dietetic textbooks. In brief, the basic tenet of obesity treatment in children is to achieve and maintain a healthy weight, whist ensuring adequate nutrients for normal growth and development, especially during growth spurts. For many children with modest degrees of overweight, the emphasis can be on weight stability rather than weight loss, allowing a reduction in relative weight as the child becomes taller and effectively grows into their weight. This concept must be carefully explained to the parents and child, who can otherwise become very discouraged by the absence of any weight loss and apparent lack of progress. In more severe cases weight loss may be recommended to reduce the long-term risk to health of excess weight. However, very low-energy diets are not suitable for any child.

Treating excess weight in children demands professional assistance, but this needs to be handled with tact and sensitivity. Many children may have suffered bullying or other discrimination at school as a result of their size, yet may still be embarrassed by the prospect of treatment. It is important to try to develop a rapport with the child and they should be encouraged to take an active role in their treatment. Parents or carers cannot lose weight for the child and trying to impose dietary regimens is likely to lead to family difficulties. However, in many cases the child will also have obese parents and there is good evidence that a family-based approach yields the most effective results. Everyone needs to work to common goals, to understand the need to modify their family lifestyle and to recognize the benefits that it will bring.

Interventions must have a broad and balanced philosophy to encourage rational attitudes towards food and body weight and minimize the risk of precipitating eating disorders in vulnerable children. The dietary principles are similar to those in adults, although they need to be implemented with flair and imagination. Topics for discussion can include all aspects of healthy living and eating, and not just focus on weight loss. Providing practical activities such as food diaries, scrap books, paintings and posters, practical cookery, games or quizzes, geared to their educational level, will help to maintain the child's interest in the programme. There may be opportunities to link up with local schools to develop some of these ideas.

Some of the most extensive data on the treatment of obesity in children come from the work of Professor Epstein in New York, with outcome data extending over 10 years (Epstein 1996). He has successfully employed eating plans based on a traffic-light system of food coding to identify foods to be eaten freely (green), in moderation (yellow) or rarely (red). There is clear evidence of the added benefits of increased levels of physical activity. Interestingly, the most successful programmes have targeted a reduction in sedentary activities rather than prescribed periods of exercise. A system of agreed rewards has also proved effective.

Recently, a residential weight-loss summer camp for overweight children and adolescents has been set up in Leeds. This provides an opportunity for children to try different types of foods and active hobbies within an environment which promotes the concept of a healthy lifestyle. This type of residential course will not be suitable, or affordable, for the majority of children who need attention and it is optimistic to imagine that all children who attend will achieve and maintain a healthy weight. There is a significant risk that children will simply return to the lifestyle which contributed to their excess weight when they return home. However, this camp does represent one novel initiative to tackle the problem of excess weight in children, and careful follow-up of the attendees will demonstrate how effective this approach may be in the management of overweight children. Undoubtedly, more attention needs to be given to providing access to treatment for all overweight children, across the UK, and in particular in the state-funded sector.

Text revised by: Susan Jebb

References

Allison DB, Zannolli R, Faith MS *et al.* Weight loss increases and fat loss decreases all-cause mortality rate: results from two independent cohort studies. *International Journal of Obesity* 1999; **23**: 603–611.

American College of Sports Medicine. American College of Sports Medicine Roundtable. *Physical Activity in the Prevention and Treatment of Obesity and its Co-morbidities*. Blair SN, Bouchard C (Eds), 1999.

Apfelbaum M, Vague P, Ziegler O *et al.* Long-term maintenance of weight loss after a very-low-calorie diet: a randomized blinded trial of the efficacy and tolerability of sibutramine. *American Journal of Medicine* 1999; **106**: 179–184.

Astrup A, Buemann B, Toubro S, Raben A. Defects in substrate oxidation involved in the predisposition to obesity. *Proceedings of the Nutrition Society* 1996; **55**: 817–828.

Astrup A, Gotzsche PC, van-de-Werken K *et al*. Meta-analysis of resting metabolic rate in formerly obese subjects. *American Journal of Clinical Nutrition* 1999; **69**: 1117–1122.

Black AE, Prentice AM, Goldberg GR *et al*. Measurements of total energy expenditure provide insights into the validity of dietary measurements of energy intake. *Journal of the American Dietetic Association* 1993; **93**: 572–579.

Blundell JE, Tremblay A. Appetite control and energy (fuel) balance. *Nutrition Research Reviews* 1995; **8**: 225–242.

Bolton-Smith C, Woodward M. Dietary composition and fat to sugar ratios in relation to obesity. *International Journal of Obesity* 1994; **18**: 820–828.

Bray G. Complications of obesity. *Annals of Internal Medicine* 1985; **103**: 1052–1062.

Bray GA, Popkin BA. Dietary fat intake does affect obesity. *American Journal of Clinical Nutrition* 1998; **68**: 1157–1173.

Bray GA, Blackburn GL, Ferguson JM. Sibutramine – dose response and long term efficacy in weight loss, a double-blind study. *International Journal of Obesity* 1994; **18** (Suppl 2): 60.

Calle EE, Thun MJ, Petrelli JM *et al*. Body mass index and mortality in a prospective cohort of U.S. adults. *New England Journal of Medicine* 1999; **341**: 1097–1105.

Chan JM, Rimm EB, Colditz GA *et al*. Obesity, fat distribution and weight gain as risk factors for clinical diabetes in men. *Diabetes Care* 1994; **17**: 961–969.

Coakley EH, Rimm EB, Colditz G *et al*. Predictors of weight change in men: Results from The Health Professionals Follow-Up Study. *International Journal of Obesity* 1998; **22**: 89–96.

Colditz GA, Willett WC, Rotnitzky A, Manson JE. Weight gain as a risk factor for clinical diabetes mellitus in women. *Annals of Internal Medicine* 1995; **122**: 481–486.

COMA. *The Use of Very Low Calorie Diets in Obesity*. London: HMSO, 1987.

Cowburn G, Hillsdon M, Hankey CR. Obesity management by lifestyle strategies. *British Medical Bulletin* 1997; **53**: 439–408.

Davidson MH, Hauptman JMD, Foreyt JP *et al*. Weight control and risk factor reduction in obese subjects treated for two years with Orlistat. *Journal of the American Medical Association* 1999; **281**: 235–242.

Department of Health (DH). *Health Survey for England 1997. Summary of Key Findings*. London: DH, 1997.

Ditschuneit HH, Flechtner MM, Johnson TD, Adler G. Metabolic and weight-loss effects of a long-term dietary intervention in obese patients. *American Journal of Clinical Nutrition* 1999; **69**: 198–204.

Epstein LH. Family-based behavioural intrevention for obese children. *International Journal of Obesity* 1996; **20** (Suppl 1): S14–S21.

Farooqi S, Jebb SA, Cook G *et al*. Recombinant leptin induces weight loss in human congenital leptin deficiency. *New England Journal of Medicine* 1999; **341**: 879–884.

Finer N. Present and future pharmacological approaches. *British Medical Bulletin* 1997; **53**: 409–432.

Gill TP. Key issues in the prevention of obesity. *British Medical Bulletin* 1997; **53**: 359–388.

Hayaki J, Brownell KD. Behaviour change in practice: group approaches. *International Journal of Obesity* 1996; **20** (Suppl 1): S27–S30.

Hogan R, Johnston J, Long B *et al*. A double-blind, randomised, sham controlled trial of the gastric bubble for obesity. *Gastrointestinal Endoscopy* 1989; **35**: 381–385.

Jebb SA. Aetiology of obesity. *British Medical Bulletin* 1997; **53**: 264–285.

Jebb SA. Measurement of body composition – from the laboratory to the clinic. In Kopelman P, Stock M (eds). *Clinical Obesity*. Oxford: Blackwell Science, 1998.

Jebb SA, Goldberg GR. The use of very low energy diets and meal replacements in the treatment of obesity. *Journal of Human Nutrition and Dietetics* 1998; **11**: 219–225.

Jebb SA, Moore MS. Contribution of a sedentary lifestyle and inactivity to the etiology of overweight and obesity: current evidence and research issues. *Medicine and Science in Sports and Exercise* 1999; **31** (Suppl): S534–S541.

Jung R. Obesity as a disease. *British Medical Bulletin* 1997; **53**: 307–321.

Karlsson J, Sjostrom L, Sullivan M. Swedish obese subjects (SOS)- an intervention study of obesity. Two-year follow-up of health-related quality of life (HRQL) and eating behavior after gastric surgery for severe obesity. *International Journal of Obesity* 1998; **22**: 113–126.

Kolanowski J. Surgical treatment for morbid obesity. *British Medical Bulletin* 1997; **53**: 433–444.

Lean MJ, Han TS, Morrison CE. Waist circumference as a measure for indicating need for weight management. *British Medical Journal* 1995; **311**: 158–161.

Lissner L. Health effects of weight cycling. In Cottrell RC. (Ed). *Weight Control*, pp. 68–75. London: Chapman & Hall, 1995.

Pavlou KN, Krey S, Steffee WP. Exercise as an adjunct to weight loss and maintenance in moderately obese subjects. *American Journal of Clinical Nutrition* 1989; **49**: 1115–1123.

Prentice AM. Obesity – the inevitable penalty of civilisation? *British Medical Bulletin* 1997; **53**: 229–237.

Prentice AM, Jebb SA. Obesity in Britain: gluttony or sloth? *British Medical Journal* 1995; **311**: 437–439.

Prentice AM, Poppitt SD. Importance of energy density and macronutrients in the regulation of energy intake. *International Journal of Obesity* 1996; **20** (Suppl 2): S18–S23.

Prentice AM, Goldberg GR, Jebb SA *et al*. Physiological response to slimming. *Proceedings of the Nutrition Society* 1991; **50**: 441–458.

Prentice AM, Black AE, Coward WA, Cole TJ. Energy expenditure in affluent societies: an analysis of 319 doubly-labelled water measurements. *European Journal of Clinical Nutrition* 1996; **50**: 93–97.

Rand CSW, MacGregor AMC. Successful weight loss following obesity surgery and the perceived liability of morbid obesity. *International Journal of Obesity* 1991; **15**: 577–579.

Ravussin E, Lillioja S, Knowler WC *et al*. Reduced rate of energy expenditure as a risk factor for body weight gain. *New England Journal of Medicine* 1988; **318**: 467–472.

Reilly JR, Dorosty AR. Epidemic of obesity in UK children. *Lancet* 1999; **354**: 1874–1875.

Reilly JR, Dorosty AR, Emmett PM. Prevalence of overweight and obesity in British children cohort study. *British Medical Journal* 1999; **319**: 1039.

Royal College of Physicians. Clinical management of overweight and obese patients with particular reference to the use of drugs. Report of a working party. *Journal of the Royal College of Physicians of London* 1999; **33** (No. 1 Jan/Feb).

Seidell JC, Flegal KM. Assessing obesity: classification and epidemiology. *British Medical Bulletin* 1997; **53**: 238–252.

Scottish Intercollegiate Guidelines Network (SIGN). *Obesity in Scotland. Integrating Prevention with Weight Management*. Edinburgh: Royal College of Physicians of Edinburgh, 1996.

Sjostrom L, Narbro K, Sjostrom D. Costs and benefits when treating obesity. *International Journal of Obesity* 1995; **19** (Suppl 6): S9–S12.

Sjostrom L, Rissanen A, Andersen T *et al*. Randomised placebo-controlled trial of orlistat for weight loss and prevention of weight regain in obese patients. European Multicentre Orlistat Study Group. *Lancet* 1998; **352**: 167–172.

Spitzer RC, Devlin M, Walsh BJ *et al*. Binge eating disorder: a multisite field trial of the diagnostic criteria. *International Journal of Eating Disorders* 1992; **11**: 191–203.

Stubbs RJ, Harbron CG, Murgatroyd PR, Prentice AM. Covert manipulation of dietary fat and energy density: effect on substrate flux and food intake in men eating ad libitum. *American Journal of Clinical Nutrition* 1995; **62**: 316–329.

Stubbs RJ, Harbron CG, Prentice AM. Covert manipulation of the dietary fat to carbohydrate ratio of isoenergetically dense diets: effect on food intake in feeding men ad libitum. *International Journal of Obesity* 1996; **20**: 651–660.

Stunkard AJ, Sobel J. Psychological consequences of obesity. In Brownell KD, Fairburn CG (eds). *Eating Disorders and Obesity: A Comprehensive Handbook*, pp. 417–430. London: Guilford Press, 1995.

Summerbell CD. Dietary treatment of obesity. In Kopelman P, Stock MJ (Eds). *Clinical Obesity*, pp. 377–408. Oxford: Blackwell Science, 1998.

Wadden TA, Frey DL. A multicenter evaluation of a proprietary weight loss program for the treatment of marked obesity: a five year follow-up. *International Journal of Eating Disorders* 1997; **22**: 203–212.

Whitaker RC, Wright JA, Pepe MS *et al*. Predicting obesity in young adulthood from childhood and parental obesity. *New England Journal of Medicine* 1997; **337**: 869–873.

WHO. *Obesity. Preventing and Managing the Global Epidemic*. Geneva: WHO, 1998.

Worner H, Weschler JG, Wenzel H *et al*. Long term results after treatment of obesity with the intragastric balloon. *International Journal of Obesity* 1989; **13**: 210A.

4.18 Cognitive–behavioural therapy in obesity treatment

A wide range of weight-loss and weight-management programmes, ranging from self-help through to commercial groups, dietary, exercise, behavioural, drug- and hospital-based treatments, is used in the treatment of obesity (see Section 4.17, Obesity). In general, the main treatment orientations have consisted of:

- traditional dietary therapy (TDT) focusing on dieting and weight reduction (Bush *et al.* 1988; Hankey *et al.* 1997)
- traditional cognitive–behavioural therapy (CBT) focusing on dieting and weight reduction (Wing 1992; Brownell 1997)
- non-dieting approaches focusing on the psychosocial consequences of obesity (Higgins and Gray 1999)
- emerging 'new paradigm' treatments which combine elements of both non-dieting and traditional CBT, and may include risk factor management (Wardle and Rapoport 1998).

4.18.1 Traditional dietary therapy

TDT focuses on what dietary changes need to be made. Following a dietary assessment, an energy-restricted diet plan or regimen of approximately 5 MJ or 1200 kcal per day is prescribed. This is often backed up with a diet sheet giving details of meal recommendations. Direct persuasion is used to try to convince the person that they should make the recommended dietary changes to achieve weight loss. TDT provides limited tools to help people to implement these changes (Rapoport 1998).

Using this approach, how successful are dietitians at treating obesity? This question is difficult to answer. There is a dearth of randomized controlled trials evaluating the efficacy of dietetic management of obesity. Audit information from hospital obesity clinics offering dietary advice suggests that these clinics are characterized by outstandingly poor attendance rates (Gallagher 1984). Even when patients do attend, treatment results have been modest and follow-up periods have been limited. This may explain the widespread despondency in the dietetic world about therapeutic effectiveness in the area of obesity treatment. The high level of non-compliance and non-attendance at obesity clinics has led dietitians as well as other health professionals to feel that giving dietary advice to obese people is a 'waste of time' and that obesity treatment is professionally unrewarding (Cade and O'Connell 1991). Another factor underlying the lack of research in this area may be the negative attitudes held by many dietitians about those who are obese (Oberrieder *et al.* 1995), perhaps reflecting a societal stigmatization of the obese. Many

believe that the obese person is at fault for not being able to exert the necessary self-control to reduce his or her weight (Sobal 1991; Frank 1993). Where nutritionists are trained in behaviour modification, they achieve better weight losses with patients than in trials of TDT (McReynolds *et al.* 1976).

4.18.2 Traditional cognitive–behavioural therapy

Traditional CBT focuses on how to change eating behaviour. Behaviour therapy emerged in the late 1950s and early 1960s as a means of modifying behaviours related to maintaining obesity. Cognitive therapy evolved in the 1970s, proposing that dysfunctional thoughts and beliefs are the underlying cause of many disorders and that these can be identified and modified through a set of cognitive techniques. Contemporary CBT embraces behavioural and cognitive approaches to optimize safe dieting for weight loss and may be described as the 'state of the art' in obesity treatment. In contrast to TDT, it focuses on strategies to help people to implement behavioural changes, to change their diet and thereby reduce their weight (Wing 1992; Grilo 1996). CBT techniques may be effectively combined with TDT, to give a multicomponent intervention emphasizing modifying eating and exercise behaviour to achieve weight loss and, more recently, to improve overall health risk. The emphasis is on training the client in a range of specific skills and strategies (e.g. self-monitoring, goal setting, problem solving, stimulus control, response prevention, social support, self-reinforcement, identifying and challenging negative thinking, relapse prevention) to help them to make and sustain permanent lifestyle changes (Marlatt 1995; Grilo 1996; Brownell 1997).

Traditionally, CBT programmes consist of a 16–20 week intervention, usually carried out in small groups, but shorter and less intensive interventions are being developed.

Success rates of traditional cognitive–behavioural therapy

Although a long-term solution to the treatment of obesity remains elusive, better compliance has been achieved with CBT programmes than with TDT, with average drop-out rates of only 20% (SIGN 1996). Full-length CBT programmes reliably result in significant short-term weight loss of about 10% or more (approximately 0.5 kg weight per week) of pre-treatment body weight (compared with the approximate weight loss of 5% with TDT). This weight loss does not restore most patients to normal weight, but there is growing evidence that even modest weight losses in obese people may be sufficient to improve cardiovascular disease (CVD) risk factors (Blackburn 1995). Combining CBT with very low calorie diets (VLCD) leads to weight losses of 18–20 kg over a 12 week programme, with larger losses for a longer treatment period (Wadden and Bartlett 1992).

Long-term results of standard CBT programmes alone or combined with VLCDs have tended to be disappointing and CBT is undergoing continuous refinement (Wilson 1996). Patients tend to maintain approximately 60–70% of weight loss for a minimum period of 1 year following treatment. By 5 years post-treatment, however, about 95% of patients have returned to their pre-treatment weight (Brownell and Wadden, 1992).

The continuous-care model of obesity management views obesity as a long-term chronic condition requiring continuous support once treatment has ended. Studies where this model has been applied show longer-term maintenance of weight loss (Perri 1995). Factors identified as improving weight loss maintenance have included:

- self-help groups
- regular therapist contact
- booster and refresher sessions
- increased physical activity
- skills training in relapse prevention.

New perspectives on cognitive–behavioural therapy

The poor long-term results with CBT have resulted in new developments in an evolving field. Strategies such as matching problems to therapeutic readiness, treatment type and service delivery method may improve the effectiveness of obesity treatment (Wardle 1996). The application of the stages-of-change model has been another major development in health behaviour research (see Section 1.7, Achieving behavioural change). Matching specific treatments to particular subgroups of patients (Brownell and Wadden 1992) has also been suggested, for example, identifying obese binge eaters, who make up approximately 30% of obese patients, and offering them modifications of treatment programmes used for bulimia nervosa (Fairburn et al. 1993), although there is as yet no agreement as to whether this should be introduced before, after or in parallel with weight control.

Other approaches stress the importance of helping the patient to accept modest weight loss goals and acquire weight maintenance skills once a weight loss of 10–15% has been achieved (Fairburn and Cooper 1996). This includes addressing the cognitive barriers to accepting a modest weight loss by focusing on cognitive factors, in particular any tendency to evaluate self-worth in terms of weight. Newer approaches include interventions to improve body image in the obese (Rosen 1996).

It is likely that future obesity treatment will include broader definitions of treatment success (e.g. improve-

ments in metabolic profiles, physical activity, self-esteem, body image, self-efficacy, quality of life and functional capacity) rather than that of weight loss alone.

4.18.3 The evolution of a new weight paradigm

The traditional model for obesity treatment focuses primarily on dieting (restricting the total amount of food eaten) to achieve weight loss, often ignoring obesity-related psychosocial costs. In contrast, a 'new weight paradigm' has emerged which encompasses two main movements, 'size acceptance' and 'non-dieting' (Parham 1996). Size acceptance challenges the concept that being fat is bad, questions the idea that obese people need to change, and asserts that fat people can be attractive and fit, with active, rewarding lives. The non-dieting movement shares the idea that overweight people should accept themselves at their current weight and self-acceptance is viewed as an essential foundation on which to build a healthy lifestyle. CBT can be used in this context to enhance self-acceptance to achieve an improved quality of life (improved body image and self-esteem) as well as more lasting changes in health-relevant eating and exercise behaviour. Non-dieting approaches support the view that restrictive dieting can trigger overeating, which might explain why treatments based on dietary restriction are rarely effective in the long term, with failed attempts to lose weight often resulting in negative psychological effects (e.g. lower self-esteem, body dissatisfaction, depression and anxiety) (Higgins and Gray 1999). In most cases non-dieting treatments provide skills for stopping dieting (participants are encouraged to consider all foods as acceptable), regularizing their eating pattern and identifying and addressing triggers for inappropriate or overeating. Some of the newer programmes are also beginning to include an education in healthy eating.

Few controlled trials of non-dieting interventions exist. In existing trials, dieting is generally reduced, tendency to restrained eating is weakened, self-esteem and self-acceptance are increased, whilst depressive symptoms and the incidence of eating-related psychopathology are reduced (Higgins and Gray 1999). In general, programme participation is associated with weight maintenance or even slight weight reduction, although at an individual level weight problems appear to be exacerbated for some.

In patients where dieting approaches have been unsuccessful, there is a case for risk factor reduction without restrictive dieting, with or without weight loss. In studies where there is a focus on dietary quality change, modest improvements in CVD risk factors can be achieved and maintained without deliberate energy restriction (Brunner et al. 1997) and improvements in cholesterol profile have been shown to be more directly related to improved dietary habits than to amount of weight lost (Andersen et al. 1995). There is a need for more research on non-dieting approaches to determine whether, in addition to improving psychological functioning, patients achieve improved metabolic profiles and dietary quality, and increased physical activity and fitness, all of which are now agreed to be essential outcomes in obesity management.

4.18.4 New perspectives on obesity treatment

An emerging consensus during the late 1990s supports the view that a wider perspective on weight-management is needed than one that focuses on weight loss alone. It is widely agreed that the essential components for weight management programmes are dietary modifi-cation and alterations in physical activity, with CBT techniques incorporated to achieve the best outcome (SIGN 1996; ADA 1997; RCP 1997; WHO 1998). Within the context of long-term lifestyle change, it is recommended that the goal of obesity treatment is reformulated from simple weight loss

Table 4.38 Techniques of behaviour modification for weight management (adapted from Brownell 1997)

1. STIMULUS CONTROL

Shopping:
  Shop for food only on a full stomach
  Shop from a list
  Only buy appropriate foods
  Avoid ready-to-eat foods
  Only carry the amount of cash needed for foods on the
    shopping list
Plans:
  Plan to limit food intake
  Preplan meals and snacks
  Substitute exercise for snacking
  Eat meals and snacks at scheduled times
  Do not accept food offered by others
Activities:
  Use graphs, cartoons, pictures, etc., to remind yourself to eat
    properly
  Make nutritionally acceptable foods as attractive as possible in
    preparation and presentation
  Remove inappropriate foods from the house
  Store problem foods out of sight
  Keep healthier foods visible
  Eat all food in the same place
  Remove food from inappropriate storage areas in the house
Serving food:
  Keep serving dishes off the table
  Use smaller dishes and utensils
  Avoid being the food server
  Serve and eat one portion at a time
  Leave the table immediately after eating
  Save leftovers for another meal instead of finishing what is on
    your plate
Holidays and parties:
  Prepare in advance what you will do
  Drink fewer alcoholic beverages
  Plan eating habits before parties
  Eat a low-calorie snack before parties
  Practise polite ways to decline food
  Do not be discouraged by an occasional setback

2. SELF-MONITORING

Keep a dietary diary that includes:
  Time and place of eating
  Type and amount of food
  Who else (if anyone) is present
  How you felt before eating
  Activities that you are doing at the same time
  Calorie or/and fat content of foods
  Examining patterns in your eating

3. EATING BEHAVIOUR

Slow rate of eating:
  Take one small bite at a time
  Chew food thoroughly before swallowing
  Put fork down between mouthfuls

Pause in the middle of the meal and assess hunger
Do nothing else while eating:
  Concentrate on act of eating
  Concentrate on enjoying food
  Eat all food in one place
  Follow eating plan

4. REWARDS
  Solicit help from family and friends
  Ask family and friends to provide this help in the form of praise
    and material rewards
  Clearly define behaviours to be rewarded
  Use self-monitoring records as basis for rewards
  Plan specific rewards for specific behaviours
  Gradually make rewards more difficult to achieve

5. NUTRITION EDUCATION
  Use self-monitoring diary to identify problem areas
  Make small changes that can be continued
  Eat a well-balanced diet according to the *Balance of Good
    Health*
  Learn nutritional values of foods
  Decrease fat intake, increase complex carbohydrate intake

6. PHYSICAL ACTIVITY
Lifestyle activity:
  Increase lifestyle activity
  Increase use of stairs
  Walk where you would normally use a bus or car
  Keep a record of frequency, intensity and duration of time
    walking each day
Exercise:
  Start a mild exercise programme
  Keep a record of daily exercise
  Increase the amount of exercise very gradually

7. COGNITIVE RESTRUCTURING
  Develop realistic expectations for weight loss
  Set reasonable, realistic weight-loss and behaviour-change
    goals
  Focus on progress, not shortcomings
  Avoid imperatives such as 'always' or 'never'
  Keep a record of thoughts about self and weight
  Challenge and counter self-defeating thoughts with positive
    thoughts

8. RELAPSE MANAGEMENT
  Learn to see lapses as opportunities to learn more about
    behaviour change
  Identify triggers for lapsing
  Plan in advance how to prevent lapses
  Generate a list of coping strategies in high-risk situations
  Distinguish hunger from cravings
  Make a list of activities to do which make it impossible to give
    in to cravings
  Confront or ignore cravings
  Outlast urges to eat

to 'weight management', incorporating:

- modest weight loss
- risk factor reduction
- prevention of weight gain

Additional aims should be:

- to have success judged by the effects on the overall health of participants rather than weight loss alone
- to achieve the best possible weight via life-long adoption of healthy lifestyle behaviours
- to emphasize eating practices and daily physical activity that are sustainable and enjoyable
- to manage the psychosocial consequences of obesity (improve self-esteem, body image, decrease binge eating and reduce stress levels) so that patients can sustain the continuous effort needed for treatment success (Sobal 1991; Rosen 1996; Wilson 1996; Grilo 1996; ADA 1997; Wardle and Rapoport 1998).

These new recommendations demonstrate a move towards integrating aspects of traditional dieting with non-dieting approaches.

A range of treatment techniques used in the cognitive and behavioural management of obesity is summarized in Table 4.38. A general introduction to the use of cognitive and behavioural strategies in achieving dietary change can be found in Section 1.7 (Achieving behavioural change). For more detailed discussion of CBT strategies in the management of obesity see Wardle and Rapoport (1998), Grilo (1996) and Wilson (1996).

Text written by: Lorna Rapoport

References

American Dietetic Association (ADA). Position of the American Dietetic Association: weight management. *Journal of the American Dietetic Association* 1997; **97**: 71–74.

Andersen RE, Wadden TA, Bartlett SJ *et al*. Relation of weight loss to changes in serum lipids and lipoproteins in obese women. *American Journal of Clinical Nutrition* 1995; **62**: 350–357.

Blackburn GL. Effects of weight loss on weight-related risk factors. In Brownell KD, Fairburn CG (Eds) *Eating Disorders and Obesity. A Comprehensive Handbook*, pp. 406–410. London Guilford Press, 1995.

Brownell KD. *The Learn Programme for Weight Control*. Dallas, TX: American Health Publishing Company, 1997.

Brownell KD, Wadden TA. Etiology and treatment of obesity: understanding a serious, prevalent and refractory disorder. *Journal of Consulting and Clinical Psychology* 1992; **60**: 505–517.

Brunner E, White I, Thorogood M *et al*. Can dietary interventions change diet and cardiovascular risk factors? A meta-analysis of randomized controlled trials. *American Journal of Public Health* 1997; **87**: 1415–1422.

Bush A, Webster J, Chalmers G *et al*. The Harrow slimming club: report on 1090 enrolments in 50 courses, 1977–1986. *Journal of Human Nutrition and Dietetics* 1988; **1**: 429–436.

Cade J, O'Connell S. Management of weight problems and obesity: knowledge, attitudes and current practice of general practitioners. *British Journal of General Practice* 1991; **41**: 147–150.

Fairburn CG, Cooper Z. New perspectives on dietary and behavioural treatments for obesity. *International Journal of Obesity* 1996; **20** (Suppl 1): S9–S13.

Fairburn CG, Marcus MD, Wilson GT. Cognitive–behavioural therapy for binge eating and bulimia nervosa: a comprehensive treatment manual. In Fairburn CG, Wilson GT (Eds) *Binge Eating: Nature, Assessment and Treatment*, pp. 361–404. New York: Guilford Press, 1993.

Frank A. Futility and avoidance. Medical professionals in the treatment of obesity. *Journal of the American Medical Association* 1993; **269**: 2132–2133.

Gallagher C. A review of dietetic outpatient attendance. *Human Nutrition: Applied Nutrition* 1984; **38A**: 181–186.

Grilo C. Treatment of obesity: an integrative model. In Thompson JK (Ed.) *Body Image, Eating Disorders, and Obesity*, pp. 389–423. Washington DC: American Psychological Association, 1996.

Hankey CR, Rumley A, Lowe GDO *et al*. Moderate weight reduction improves red cell aggregation and factor VII activity in overweight subjects. *International Journal of Obesity*, 1997; **21**: 644–650.

Higgins L, Gray W. What do anti-dieting programs achieve? A review of research. *Australian Journal of Nutrition and Dietetics* 1999; **56**: 128–136.

Marlatt GA. Relapse: a cognitive–behavioral model. In Brownell KD, Fairburn CG (Eds) *Eating Disorders and Obesity. A Comprehensive Handbook*, pp. 541–545. London: Guilford Press, 1995.

McReynolds WT, Lutz RN, Paulsen BK, Kohrs MB. Weight loss resulting from two behaviour modification procedures with nutritionists as therapists. *Behaviour Therapy* 1976; **7**: 283–291.

Oberrieder H, Walker R, Monroe D, Adeyanju M. Attitude of dietetics students and registered dietitians toward obesity. *Journal of the American Dietetic Association* 1995; **95**: 914–915.

Parham ES. Is there a new weight paradigm? *Nutrition Today* 1996; **31**: 155–161.

Perri MG. Methods for maintaining weight loss. In Brownell KD, Fairburn CG (Eds) *Eating Disorders and Obesity. A Comprehensive Handbook*, pp. 547–551. London: Guilford Press, 1995.

Rapoport L. Integrating cognitive behavioural therapy into dietetic practice: a challenge for dietitians. *Journal of Human Nutrition and Dietetics* 1998; **11**: 227–237.

Rosen JC. Improving body image in obesity. In Thompson JK (Ed) *Body Image, Eating Disorders, and Obesity*, pp 425–440. Washington, DC: American Psychological Association, 1996.

Royal College of Physicians (RCP). *Overweight and Obese Patients. Principles of Management with Particular Reference to the Use of Drugs*. London: RCP, 1997.

SIGN. *Obesity in Scotland: Integrating Prevention with Weight Management. A National Clinical Guideline Recommended for Use in Scotland by the Scottish Intercollegiate Guidelines Network*, Pilot edn. Edinburgh: SIGN, 1996.

Sobal J. Obesity and nutritional sociology: a model for coping with the stigma of obesity. *Clinical Sociology Review* 1991; **9**: 125–141.

Wadden TA, Bartlett SJ. Very low calorie diets: an overview and appraisal. In Wadden TA, Van Itallie TB (Eds) *Treatment of the Seriously Obese Patient*, pp. 44–79. New York: Guilford Press, 1992.

Wardle J. Obesity and behaviour change: matching problems to practice. *International Journal of Obesity* 1996; **20** (Suppl 1): S1–S8.

Wardle J, Rapoport L. Cognitive–behavioural treatment of obesity. In Kopelman P, Stock M (Eds) *Clinical Obesity*. Oxford: Blackwell Science, 1998.

Wilson GT. Acceptance and change in the treatment of eating disorders and obesity. *Behaviour Therapy* 1996; **27**: 417–439.

Wing RR. Behavioural treatment of severe obesity. *American Journal of Clinical Nutrition* 1992; **55**: 545S–551S.

World Health Organization (WHO). *Obesity: Preventing and Managing the Global Epidemic. Report of a WHO Consultation on Obesity, Geneva, 3–5 June 1997*. Geneva: WHO, 1998.

4.19 Eating disorders

There is a wide spectrum of people with eating disorders, from the emaciated, restricting anorexia nervosa sufferer through the normal weight individual with bulimia nervosa to the overweight or obese binge eater. The first two groups are generally referred to psychiatrists, psychologists and multidisciplinary eating disorder teams for treatment. The overweight binge eater is more likely to be referred to a dietitian without any psychological intervention. However, all three groups require a similar approach from dietitians, to help them to understand the mechanics of their food disorder and the positive effects of change.

This section does not provide great detail on the various treatment methods employed to help people with eating disorders as these are well documented elsewhere (Brownell and Fairburn 1995; Szmukler *et al.* 1995; Garner and Garfinkel 1998). Instead, it focuses on the aetiology and features of eating disorders and summarizes the rationale behind, and methods of, dietetic treatment.

4.19.1 General aspects of eating disorders

Diagnostic criteria

Diagnostic criteria for anorexia nervosa and bulimia nervosa have been published by the American Psychiatric Association (APA) in *The Diagnostic and Statistical Manual of Mental Disorders* (4th edn, DSM-IV, 1994) and by the World Health Organization (WHO) in *The International Classification of Diseases* (10th edn, ICD-10, 1992). The APA has also published diagnostic criteria for use in the research of binge eating disorder. These criteria are summarized in Tables 4.39–4.41.

These strict definitions allow identification of patients for research purposes, but it is clear that many people suffer less severe symptoms or partial syndromes, and still need help to recover.

Table 4.39 Diagnostic criteria for anorexia nervosa

ICD-10 (WHO 1992)	DSM-IV (APA 1994)
For a definite diagnosis, all of the following are required: (a) Body weight is maintained at least 15% below that expected (either lost or never achieved), or Quetelet's body mass index is 17.5 or less. Prepubertal patients may fail to make the expected weight gain during the period of growth (b) The weight loss is self-induced by avoidance of 'fattening foods'. One or more of the following may also be present: self-induced vomiting; self-induced purging; excessive exercise; use of appetite suppressants and/or diuretics (c) There is body-image distortion in the form of a specific psychopathology whereby a dread of fatness persists as an intrusive, overvalued idea and the patient imposes a low weight threshold on him or herself (d) A widespread endocrine disorder involving the hypothalamic–pituitary–gonadal axis is manifest in women as amenorrhoea and in men as a loss of sexual interest and potency. (An apparent exception is the persistence of vaginal bleeds in anorexic women who are receiving hormonal replacement therapy, most commonly taken as the contraceptive pill.) There may also be elevated levels of growth hormone, raised levels of cortisol, changes in the peripheral metabolism of the thyroid gland and abnormalities of insulin secretion (e) If onset is prepubertal, the sequence of pubertal events is delayed or even arrested (growth ceases; in girls the breasts do not develop and there is primary amenorrhoea; in boys the genitals remain juvenile). With recovery, puberty is often completed normally, but menarche is late	(A) A refusal to maintain body weight at or above a minimally normal weight for age and height (e.g. weight loss leading to maintenance of body weight less than 85% of that expected; or failure to make expected weight gain during a period of growth, leading to a body weight less than 85% of that expected) (B) Intense fear of gaining weight or becoming fat, even though underweight (C) Disturbance in the way in which one's body weight or shape is experienced, undue influence of body weight or shape on self-evaluation, or denial of the seriousness of the current low body weight (D) In postmenarcheal females, amenorrhoea, i.e. the absence of at least three consecutive menstrual cycles. (A woman is considered to have amenorrhea if her periods occur only following hormone, e.g. oestrogen, administration) Type of anorexia nervosa is also specified as: *Restricting type*: during the current episode of anorexia nervosa, the person has not regularly engaged in binge eating or purging behavior (i.e. self-induced vomiting or the misuse of laxatives, diuretics or enemas) *Binge eating/purging type*: during the current episode of anorexia nervosa, the person has regularly engaged in binge eating or purging behavior (i.e. self-induced vomiting or the misuse of laxatives, diuretics or enemas)

Table 4.40   Diagnostic criteria for bulimia nervosa

ICD-10 (WHO 1992)	DSM-IV (APA 1994)
For a definite diagnosis, all of the following are required: (a) There is persistent preoccupation with eating, and an irresistible craving for food; the patient succumbs to episodes of overeating in which large amounts of food are consumed in short periods of time (b) The patient attempts to counteract the 'fattening' effects of food by one or more of the following: self-induced vomiting; purgative abuse; alternating periods of starvation; use of drugs such as appetite suppressants, thyroid preparations, or diuretics. When bulimia occurs in diabetic patients they may choose to neglect their insulin treatment (c) The psychopathology consists of a morbid dread of fatness, and the patient sets herself or himself a sharply defined weight threshold, well below the premorbid weight that constitutes the optimum or healthy weight in the opinion of the physician. There is often, but not always, a history of an earlier episode of anorexia nervosa, the interval between the two disorders ranging from a few months to several years. This earlier episode may have been fully expressed, or may have assumed a minor cryptic form with a moderate loss of weight and/or a transient phase of amenorrhoea	(A) Recurrent episodes of binge eating. An episode of binge eating is characterized by both of the following: 1. Eating in a discrete period of time (e.g. within 2 hours) an amount of food that is definitely larger than most people would eat during a similar period of time and under similar circumstances. 2. A sense of lack of control over eating during the episode (e.g. a feeling that one cannot stop eating or control what or how much one is eating) (B) Recurrent inappropriate compensatory behaviour in order to prevent weight gain such as self-induced vomiting; misuse of laxatives, diuretics, enemas or other medications; fasting or excessive exercise (C) The binge eating and inappropriate compensatory behaviours both occur, on average, at least twice a week for 3 months (D) Self-evaluation is unduly influenced by body shape and weight (E) The disturbance does not occur exclusively during episodes of anorexia nervosa

Table 4.41   Research criteria for binge eating disorder (American Psychiatric Association 1994)

(A) Recurrent episodes of binge eating. Binge eating is characterized by two of the following:
   Eating in a discrete period of time (e.g. 2 hours) an amount of food that is definitely larger than most people would eat during a similar period of time and in the same circumstances
   A sense of lack of control over eating during the episode (e.g. a feeling that one cannot stop eating or control how much one is eating)
(B) The binge-eating episodes are associated with three or more of the following:
   Eating much more rapidly than normal
   Eating until feeling uncomfortably full
   Eating large amounts of food when not feeling physical hunger
   Eating alone because of being embarrassed by how much one is eating
   Feeling disgusted with oneself, depressed or very guilty after overeating
(C) Marked distress regarding binge eating is present
(D) The binge eating occurs, on average, on at least 2 days per week for 6 months
(E) The binge eating is not associated with the regular use of inappropriate compensatory behaviours (e.g. purging, fasting, excessive exercise) and does not occur exclusively during the course of anorexia nervosa or bulimia nervosa

Development of eating disorders

It is still true that most cases of anorexia nervosa and bulimia nervosa occur in young women in Western societies. The disorder commonly develops during adolescence and a period of dieting usually precedes the onset. Whether an eating disorder will result, and persist, depends on the circumstances that activate and sustain the individual's susceptibility to risk factors.

The development of an eating disorder in an individual requires predisposing and precipitating factors. Once it is established, it may persist because of additional perpetuating factors. The relative contributions of these factors and the timing of their influence are not fully understood.

Predisposing factors

These may include:

- depression*
- low self-esteem*

- feeding difficulties when younger
- obesity*
- sexual abuse as a child
- first-degree relatives with an eating disorder
- substance misuse in family.

Factors marked with an asterisk are those which may cause sufferers to try dieting as a solution to their problems. The use of dieting behaviour is the major precipitant to the development of an eating disorder.

Life events may then combine with the predisposing trait to create precipitating factors which trigger the start of the condition.

Precipitating factors

These include:

- dieting behaviour
- puberty
- separation

- relationship changes or crises
- illness
- adverse comments on the individual from others or bullying.

Whether the eating disorder continues and develops into a full syndrome or chronic illness depends on perpetuating factors that maintain the illness.

Perpetuating factors

These include:

- cognitive events:
  the cognitive distortions of semi-starvation
  extreme over-valuation of shape and weight
- interpersonal events:
  change in relationships due to the illness
  enhancement of self-esteem
  positive reward for self-control
- physiological events:
  semi-starvation
  delayed gastric emptying
  regression of adult hormone function.

It is from the influence of the perpetuating factors that the eating disorder takes on the full characteristics of the illness as described in the classification.

Treatment of eating disorders

These groups of patients are best treated by a multidisciplinary team which includes a dietitian (American Dietetic Association 1994; Eating Disorders Association 1995). Although dietitians have a vital contribution to make to the treatment of eating disorders, the involvement of other professionals is essential to deal with the psychological and medical aspects of the illness. For a summary of the integration of dietetic treatment into the work of an eating disorders team, see Beumont *et al.* (1997).

However, not all dietitians who encounter people with eating disorders work in such a group. The treatment interventions discussed below therefore describe dietetic advice which can be integrated into the different circumstances in which the dietitian may work.

It is essential that dietitians who work with patients with eating disorders have effective counselling and communication skills (Omizo and Oda 1988). These are discussed in greater depth in Section 1.7 (Achieving behavioural change), but can be summarized as:

- attentive listening
- empathic responses
- verbal encouragement
- encouraging self-decision making
- providing support
- acceptance of thoughts, feelings and actions.

Dietitians must also understand the underlying psychological disturbances that occur in people with eating disorders. There are several features common to all eating-disordered individuals in terms of underlying thoughts and feelings which drive changes in behaviour, in particular fear of becoming fat, and fear of loss of control.

4.19.2 Anorexia nervosa

Features of anorexia nervosa

Anorexia nervosa is a condition in which the sufferer, although usually physically well, limits food intake, and so loses weight and becomes malnourished. The essential features include deliberate restriction of food intake resulting in weight loss and a widespread endocrine disorder, body image distortion, and fear of fatness. Binge eating, and purging behaviour such as self-induced vomiting, laxative abuse and excessive exercise, may also occur in anorexia nervosa.

Diagnostic criteria for anorexia nervosa (WHO 1992; APA 1994) are summarized in Table 4.39, although there may be some variation in the features at presentation (Russell 1995).

Anorexia nervosa is much more common in women than men, with only 5–10% of those affected being male (Hoek 1993). Those in situations where slimness is particularly valued, such as ballet dancing, fashion modelling, gymnastics and athletics, are especially vulnerable (Hoek 1995). The peak age of incidence is in mid to late adolescence (Hoek 1993), but anorexia nervosa is a chronic, relapsing condition so can continue throughout adult life, and may arise in older individuals (Beck *et al.* 1996). Among prepubertal children, anorexia is rarer but, when it does occur, a greater proportion of boys presents with the illness (Bryant-Waugh 1993).

Nutritional effects of anorexia nervosa

Chronically inadequate food intake has physical, psychological and social effects. These have been comprehensively described by Keys *et al.* (1950), who studied a group of male volunteers who were maintained on a low-energy diet for an experimental period. This study, published as The Minnesota Experiment, remains an important source of information.

Physical effects

The most striking effect is loss of weight. In the early stages of weight loss, glycogen and associated water are shed. Adipose tissue becomes depleted and muscle mass is lost, causing weakness and impaired function, although this may be denied by the patient, who may even persist with excessive exercise. As starvation progresses, there is loss of tissue from other organs, including the brain (Dolan *et al.* 1988).

A number of endocrine changes occurs with weight loss. Changes in brain neurotransmitters cascade via the hypothalamus and pituitary to distal glands (see Fichter and Pirke 1995 for a comprehensive review). Thyroid function is suppressed as an adaptive response in order to reduce energy expenditure and protein turnover, and thus lower metabolic rate. Cortisol production is increased, and that of adrenaline decreased, together with reduced activity of the sympathetic nervous system. This results in hypotension, bradycardia and hypothermia. Sleep tends to be disturbed. Production of sex hormones is suppressed to infantile levels in both genders. Amenorrhoea is a diagnostic criterion for anorexia nervosa in women of child-bearing age (see Table 4.39). The loss of normal oestrogen activity contributes to the osteoporosis which is a serious effect of anorexia nervosa (Serpell and Treasure 1997). It may also be a cause of the paradoxical hypercholesterolaemia found in some patients (Rock and Curran-Celentano 1994).

Although there are profound nutritional deficits, people with anorexia nervosa are often spared symptoms of frank vitamin and mineral deficiencies (Rock and Curran-Celentano 1994; Rock and Vasantharajan 1995). This may be partly a result of the quality of their diets. Many have a high intake of fruit and vegetables, and so have high intakes of water-soluble vitamins. Some may even have hyper-carotenaemia, with yellowing of the skin, although the causes of this are not entirely clear (Rock and Yager 1987). Many take commercial vitamin and mineral supplements. Amenorrhoea reduces iron loss, so gives some protection from anaemia, although haemoglobin level tends to be low (Rieger *et al.* 1978).

The nutritional factors that may contribute to osteoporosis include low intakes of calcium, magnesium, vitamin D, protein and energy (Serpell and Treasure 1997). The effects of subclinical deficiencies of micronutrients await further investigation.

Psychological effects

The subjects of The Minnesota Experiment suffered increased depression, anxiety and irritability and, as starvation progressed, apathy. They became preoccupied with food to the exclusion of other issues, and subjectively felt that concentration and memory were impaired.

These changes are also seen in anorexia nervosa. It can be greatly reassuring to patients and their families that these distressing changes are no more than the normal effects of starvation, which will respond to nutritional rehabilitation. They can, however, make treatment difficult, so allowances have to be made in therapy for the patient's mood and impaired cognitive ability.

Social effects

Social isolation can become a distressing effect of anorexia nervosa. The Minnesota volunteers lost interest in social relationships, and their depression, irritability and loss of sense of humour made such relationships difficult. Restriction of eating impairs social functioning because normal sharing of meals becomes stressful or impossible.

Dietetic intervention in anorexia nervosa

Dietitians can make important contributions to the assessment and rehabilitation of people with anorexia

nervosa. Because there is such a profound impact on nutrition and eating behaviour, management must include identifying and addressing nutritional deficits and risks, and providing the education and support needed to establish and maintain eating behaviour which is not only nutritionally adequate, but socially normal.

Dietetic assessment

The aims of assessment are to gather information about the patient's nutritional status and eating behaviour and to begin to develop a trusting relationship which can foster openness, promote motivation and contribute to progress (Hunt and Hillsdon 1996). Information gained can be shared with the patient, carers and professionals to inform decisions about care and management.

The assessment interview may need to be considerably longer than the average dietetic assessment, so may need to extend beyond one session. It should include:

- *detailed history of weight and eating*, in particular identifying times when eating and weight have been normal, the use of dieting to manipulate weight, and disordered eating
- *current eating habits*, including information about frequency of eating and meal pattern, amounts eaten, foods which are avoided, and information about episodes of uncontrolled or binge eating, in particular trigger foods and binge foods
- *areas of concern* for the patient or her carers
- *current weight, height and body mass index*
- *additional available information on body composition*, such as anthropometry or bone density
- *blood chemistry and haematology*: low potassium levels may be associated with vomiting or abuse of laxatives, and there may be nutritional anaemia
- *endocrine function*, in particular menstruation, as an indicator of underweight
- *nutritional stress*, such as growth or physical illness
- *cognitive and emotional effects*
- *motivation to change*
- *nutritional knowledge, attitude and beliefs*: although many people with anorexia nervosa may read a great deal about food and nutrition, the beliefs that they have about it are often selected and distorted to fit the psychopathology of the illness (Beumont *et al.* 1981; Laessle *et al.* 1988).

Once this information has been gathered, it is possible to make some estimation of nutritional requirements, and plan priorities and strategies for meeting them. Because eating is such a sensitive issue for people with anorexia nervosa, and their practices and beliefs are very variable, it is important to construct an individual plan which takes into account personal difficulties, concerns and needs.

Nutritional rehabilitation

The aims of nutritional rehabilitation are to restore normal weight and health in a way which is safe and effective, and as comfortable and acceptable to the patient as possible, and maintain these achievements in the long term. The skills of dietitians are needed to fulfil these objectives and to keep the process understandable for everyone involved. Dietitians can provide guidance on appropriate nutritional rehabilitation to the multidisciplinary team, and advise caterers on provision of suitable food for in-patient care. They can offer patients and their carers sound and relevant nutritional information, and education and support to help to change eating behaviour.

Because the age of onset of anorexia nervosa is typically early in life, most patients have little experience of eating normally as an adult, and need help to learn and practise the skills to feed themselves appropriately. They need education to understand and deal with the nutritional risks that they face, not only during weight restoration, but throughout life.

Dietitians may be concerned that the main issues in anorexia nervosa are not food related and it may be helpful to bear the following in mind: '…food *per se* is rarely the issue but, although support is paramount to recovery along with effective counselling, the food issue should not be forgotten!' (Brooks 1995).

In-patient rehabilitation In-patient rehabilitation is usually reserved only for those whose physical condition is very serious. Because of the urgency of weight restoration and the physical frailty of such patients, the risks associated with refeeding are greater, and the process may even be undertaken against the will of the patient if she or he is sufficiently at risk to require compulsory treatment under the Mental Health Act.

In the early stages of refeeding of a severely starved patient in hospital, there is a risk of refeeding syndrome (Birmingham *et al.* 1996). This results from the metabolic stress of processing nutrients in a starved state. The major symptoms are oedema, myocardial dysfunction, cardiac arrhythmia and congestive cardiac failure. The cardiac effects can cause death (Solomon and Kirby 1990). Particular care is needed to ensure that enough phosphate is available to produce ATP for metabolizing an increasing carbohydrate load, especially when using commercial tube feeding products. Milk has a high phosphate: carbohydrate ratio, so can be useful in oral refeeding.

Delayed gastric emptying makes eating food uncomfortable (Robinson and McHugh 1995), so amounts should be increased gradually, and adequate time allowed for meals. For most patients, about 1500 kcal/day, divided into small meals and snacks, is tolerable, increasing over the first 2 weeks of treatment to an amount that achieves appropriate weight gain. In wards staffed by experienced nurses, it is possible to achieve average weight gains of 1–1.5 kg/week by feeding 3000 kcal/day. In other settings, slower gain may be more appropriate, gradually increasing energy intake to maintain weight gain.

Eating normal food is very stressful for physically and mentally exhausted people, so liquid nutritional supplements or tube feeding may be helpful in achieving adequate intake. Bolus feeding is usually preferable to continuous feeding, as it makes mobility easier for the patient and makes nursing supervision more manageable. It is helpful to encourage the patient to continue to eat some food, as recommencing oral food after a period of exclusive tube feeding may be very difficult.

In-patient nutritional rehabilitation is very stressful for all concerned, and information about the process, provided before it begins and at every stage, can make it easier to accept and tolerate. Dietitians providing such education should bear in mind the limits to patients' concentration and memory while they remain at low weight.

Careful planning for eating following discharge is essential, as the transfer of responsibility from staff to patient and carers, and the change of environment may be very difficult. Continuing monitoring and support are needed to maintain the gains achieved and to make further progress, as the risk of relapse is high.

Out-patient rehabilitation Out-patient rehabilitation depends on developing and maintaining the motivation and effort of the patient and those providing supporting at home. It allows the patient to maintain a significant degree of control of the process, which is often a very serious personal concern. It may make it easier to tolerate weight gain if the patient is able to feel that it was achieved in the way that she or he felt best for herself or himself. However, this process may be slow, and so prolong the course of the illness and the nutritional risk. A day-patient programme can provide supervision and support with eating to promote weight restoration (Freeman 1992; Gerlinghof *et al.* 1998).

A central characteristic of anorexia nervosa is fear of weight gain. The dietitian can help the patient to manage the anxiety and tolerate weight gain. By including information on the health risks of poor nutrition, and the benefits of a healthy diet and normal social eating, aims can be broadened beyond weight gain. Careful calculation of individual energy requirement can help to promote confidence that weight gain can be controlled, and even halted if necessary. A food exchange system, using food groups, can help patients to maintain control while working to achieve an adequate intake, and move away from obsessive calorie counting.

Short-term goals can be set to improve the nutritional quality of the diet, to establish a more socially normal eating pattern or to experiment with difficult foods, as well as to increase energy intake. By taking small steps, negotiated and agreed with the patient, the process can be made manageable and tolerable (Treasure 1997).

4.19.3 Bulimia nervosa

Unlike anorexia nervosa, bulimia nervosa has only come to medical attention in recent years. Bulimia nervosa can arise from an existing anorexic illness or may develop from many years of restrictive eating. The repeated dietary restriction eventually leads to bouts of hyperphagia (binge eating) which are compensated by the use of vomiting or laxative abuse. This means that the individual maintains a relatively stable and often normal weight, despite these periods of binge eating. Intense feelings of guilt become the focus of the psychological disturbance.

Features of bulimia nervosa

The clinical picture of bulimia nervosa has four main features:

1 Overriding importance is placed on body image as an attempt to improve self-esteem.
2 Restrictive eating practices are adopted, often to an extreme degree, in an attempt to control weight.
3 This extreme restriction preoccupies thoughts with food and leads to binge eating.
4 Purging behaviour (e.g. self-induced vomiting, laxative abuse, diuretic abuse) develops as a means to control the discomfort and guilt felt after large binge-eating episodes. The resultant low self-esteem tends to perpetuate the cycle of eating behaviour (Fig. 4.5).

Treatment of bulimia nervosa

Cognitive–behavioural therapy (CBT) is the leading treatment for the disorder (Fairburn *et al.* 1992) and has three stages:

1 Helping people to gain control of their eating and establishing a pattern of regular eating. This is mainly behavioural and educational.
2 Procedures for tackling dieting and the main precipitants of binge eating. Problematic ways of thinking are also addressed using standard cognitive techniques.
3 Consolidating progress and maintenance of change.

Dietitians can assist clients through all three of these stages of treatment in conjunction with colleagues qualified to

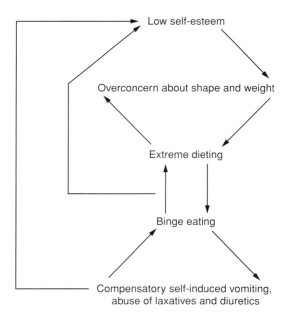

Figure 4.5 Cognitive maintenance of bulimia nervosa. Based on Fairburn and Cooper (1995); reproduced with permission of Oxford University Press.

conduct cognitive therapy. The use of the guided self-help manuals written specifically for the treatment of bulimia and binge eating disorder can be invaluable for those sufferers who cannot gain access to a qualified therapist (see Further reading at the end of this section).

Dietetic intervention in bulimia nervosa

Dietetic assessment

Dietetic assessment should be thorough and the assessment procedure described above for anorexia nervosa is appropriate. Additional information which should be ascertained includes:

- the importance attached to shape and weight
- the reaction to changes in weight
- desired weight
- previous attempts at dieting
- frequency of episodes of 'overeating'
- frequency of purging behaviour
- use of overexercising.

Dietetic treatment

This comprises the following:

- monitoring weight by recording it weekly
- monitoring behaviour
- introducing a meal plan and removing dieting behaviours
- establishing behavioural controls to overcome precipitants to binge eating
- eliminating dieting behaviours

Weight recording This should be completed weekly, either by the patient or by the dietitian. Individuals with bulimia may have been weighing themselves frequently throughout the day, recording minute changes in body weight, which are primarily due to shifts in fluid balance. The first part of education is to explore the mechanisms by which the body regulates weight, in order to encourage weighing only at weekly intervals.

Behaviour monitoring This is a vital part of the CBT. It enables clients to become aware of their behaviour, their patterns of dieting behaviour and precipitants to binge eating.

Introduction of a meal plan Many years of restrictive dietary practices will have left a mark. The sufferer will require education on their dietary needs and support in establishing a regular meal plan that excludes dietary rules.

Behavioural controls to binge eating The sheets used to self-monitor behaviour will highlight areas where binge eating becomes the behaviour 'norm'. Recognizing these patterns is important for their elimination. The use of behavioural techniques to overcome the urge to binge eat are valuable and self-help manuals , mentioned above, provide the individual with useful support.

Eliminating dieting behaviour Self-monitoring sheets will illustrate to the dietitian, as well as the sufferer, the patterns of dietary intake. The removal of dieting behaviours is essential. The dietitian needs to reassure the individual of the beneficial influence of a regular dietary intake.

4.19.4 Binge eating disorder

The term 'binge eating disorder' has come into being to describe those individuals who binge eat in the absence of compensatory behaviours, unlike in bulimia nervosa. It is thought that 20–30% of those presenting for the treatment of obesity have binge eating disorder (Bruce and Agras 1992; Spitzer *et al*. 1992). Binge eating disorder is therefore likely to be the most common eating disorder that dietitians will encounter.

Features of binge eating disorder

Binge eating is not an officially recognized eating disorder. However, a set of research criteria has been provided to help to define a disorder which is frequently encountered by clinicians but which is not a psychiatric condition in itself (Table 4.41). Nevertheless, binge eaters have a higher rate of concurrent psychiatric disorders such as anxiety, mood and personality disorders, and depression than people with bulimia nervosa.

Dieting has been implicated in the development of both binge eating and bulimia nervosa. However, in the latter, a period of dieting nearly always precedes an episode of binge eating, whereas only about 50% of obese people with binge eating disorder have restricted dietary intake prior to such episodes (Marcus 1995).

Treatment of binge eating disorder

Binge eating disorder in obesity presents two major treatment challenges:

- managing the binge eating
- addressing the obesity *per se* because of the health risks.

As with bulimia nervosa, the treatment of choice for those with binge eating disorder is CBT, which has been shown to have a similar success rate in terms of abstinence from binge eating (Telch *et al*. 1990; Smith *et al*. 1992). The behavioural therapy comprises three phases:

1 Altering chaotic eating habits
2 Identifying and changing attitudes to shape and weight
3 Preventing relapse.

There is, however, as yet no agreement as to whether the treatment for binge eating should be before, during or after the treatment for weight management (i.e. energy restriction).

Dietetic intervention in binge eating disorder

The self-help manuals (described above in Bulimia nervosa) are excellent resources for a description of the approach to treatment.

Education

It is important that dietitians remember that the individual with binge eating disorder is likely to be obese and, therefore, the removal of the dieting behaviour may well prove threatening for the individual. Education concerning the way in which the body uses food and 'normal nutrition' will prove valuable.

Exercise

It is also useful to discuss with the patient the benefits of exercise. An exercise programme consisting of three or four 20 minute walks each week is important (Agras 1995).

Self-monitoring

The use of a self-monitoring diary (Fig. 4.6) enables the dietitian and the patient to review eating and exercise behaviour. The aims should be to:

- remove dieting practices of eating infrequently and having long gaps between meals
- use behavioural techniques to help the individual to overcome the urge to binge eat, e.g. eat in a relaxed environment, eat 'in the open' rather than furtively
- help the individual to broaden their food choices, but to also provide information on the benefits of a lower dietary fat intake.

It is important to note that, unlike in bulimia nervosa, the dietary restraint in someone with binge eating disorder is less pronounced. Therefore, during the course of treatment, individuals may increase their degree of restraint over their eating. If the individual is obese, this is beneficial, and is primarily due to the lessening of chaotic eating patterns.

Other therapy

To overcome thoughts about shape and weight, sufferers ideally require help from a trained counsellor or therapist in order to improve their self-esteem. A group treatment

Fig. 4.6 An example of headings in a self-monitoring diary.

Time	Food Eaten	Quantity	Where Eaten	Who with	How did you feel?	Hunger?

programme for improving self-esteem in those with eating disorders has been described (Yellowlees 1997).

Text revised by: Kate Trotter and Denise Thomas

Useful address

The Eating Disorders Association
1st Floor, Wensum House, 103 Prince of Wales Road, Norwich NR1 1DW
Tel: 01603 621414

Further reading

Community Nutrition Group (CNG) of the British Dietetic Association. *Eating Disorders. Guidelines for Dietitians Working in Community Settings and GP Practice*. Birmingham: BDA, 1995.

Cooper PJ. *Bulimia Nervosa and Binge Eating. A Guide to Recovery*. London: Robinson, 1995.

Dewar H, Horvath R. *The Refeeding Syndrome: Guidelines*. Oxford: Radcliffe Hospital, 1996.

Fairburn CG. *Overcoming Binge Eating*. New York: Guilford Press, 1995.

Treasure J, Schmidt U. *Getting Better Bit(e) by Bit(e) – A Survival Kit for Sufferers of Bulimia Nervosa and Binge Eating Disorder*. Laurence Erlbaum Associates, 1993.

Trotter K. Nutrition and eating disorders. *Nursing Times* 1997; **93** (Suppl).

West R. *Eating Disorders, Anorexia Nervosa and Bulimia Nervosa*. London: Office of Health Economics, 1994.

References

Agras WS. Treatment of the obese binge eater. In Brownell KD, Fairburn CG (Eds) *Eating Disorders and Obesity*, pp. 531–535. New York: Guilford Press, 1995.

American Dietetic Association. The Position of the American Dietetic Association: nutrition intervention in the treatment of anorexia nervosa, bulimia nervosa and binge eating. *Journal of the American Dietetic Association* 1994; **94**: 902–907.

American Psychiatric Association (APA). *Diagnostic and Statistical Manual of Mental Disorders*, 4th edn. (DSM-IV). Washington, DC: APA, 1994.

Beck D, Caspar R, Andersen A. Truly late onset of eating disorders: a study of 11 cases averaging 60 years of age at presentation. *International Journal of Eating Disorders* 1996; **20**: 389–395.

Beumont PJV, Chambers TL, Rouse L, Abraham SF. The diet composition and nutritional knowledge of patients with eating disorders. *Journal of Human Nutrition* 1981; **34**: 265–273.

Beumont PJV, Beumont CC, Touyz SW, Williams H. Nutritional Counseling and Supervised Exercise. In Garner DM, Garfinkel PE (Eds) *Handbook of Treatment for Eating Disorders*. New York: Guilford Press; 1997.

Birmingham CL, Alothman AF, Goldner EM. Anorexia nervosa: refeeding and hypophosphataemia. *International Journal of Eating Disorders* 1996; **20**: 211–213.

Brooks R. Food is an issue. *Signpost, Newsletter of the Eating Disorders Association*, April 1995.

Brownell KD, Fairburn CG(Eds). *Eating Disorders and Obesity*, pp. 441–444. New York: Guilford Press, 1995.

Bruce B, Agras WS. Binge eating in females: a population based investigation. *International Journal of Eating Disorders* 1992; **12**: 365–373.

Bryant-Waugh R. Epidemiology. In Lask B, Bryant-Waugh R (Eds) *Childhood Onset Anorexia Nervosa and Related Eating Disorders*. Hove: Psychology Press, 1993.

Dolan RJ, Mitchell J, Wakeling A. Structural brain changes in patients with anorexia nervosa. *Psychological Medicine* 1988; **18**: 349–353.

Eating Disorders Association. *Eating Disorders: A Guide to Purchasing and Providing Services*. Norwich: Eating Disorders Association, 1995.

Fairburn CG, Cooper PJ. Eating disorders. In Hawton K, Salkovkis, PM, Kirk J, Clark DM (Eds) *Cognitive Behavioural Therapy for Psychiatric Problems*, p. 283. Oxford: Oxford University Press, 1995.

Fairburn CG, Agras S, Wilson GT. Research on treatment of bulimia nervosa: practical and theoretical implications. In Anderson GH, Kennedy SN (Eds) *The Biology of Feast and Famine: Relevance to Eating Disorders*, pp. 318–340. 1992.

Fichter MM, Pirke KM. Starvation models and eating disorders. In Szmukler G, Dare C, Treasure J (Eds) *Handbook of Eating Disorders: Theory, Treatment and Research*. Chichester: John Wiley, 1995.

Freeman CP. Day patient treatment for anorexia nervosa. *British Review of Bulimia, and Anorexia Nervosa* 1992; **6**: 1, 3–8.

Garner DM, Garfinkel PE (Eds). *Handbook of Psychotherapy for Anorexia Nervosa and Bulimia*. New York: Guilford Press, 1997.

Gerlinghof M, Backmund H, Franzen U. Evaluation of a day treatment programme for eating disorders. *European Eating Disorders*. Review 1998; **6**: 96–106.

Hoek HW. Review of the epidemiological studies of eating disorders. *International Review of Psychiatry* 1993; **5**: 61–4.

Hoek, HW. The distribution of eating disorders. In Brownell KD, Fairburn CG (Eds) *Eating Disorders and Obesity: A Comprehensive Handbook*. New York: Guilford Press, 1995.

Hunt P, Hillsdon M. Practitioner qualities. In *Changing Eating and Exercise Behaviour*, Chapter 5. Oxford: Blackwell Science, 1996.

Keys A, Brozek J, Henschel A *et al. The Biology of Human Starvation*. Minneapolis, MN: University of Minneapolis Press, 1950.

Laessle RG, Schweiger U, Daute-Herold U *et al.* Nutritional knowledge in patients with eating disorders. *International Journal of Eating Disorders* 1988; **7**: 1.

Marcus MD. Binge eating and obesity. In Brownell KD, Fairburn CG (Eds) *Eating Disorders and Obesity: A Comprehensive Handbook*. New York: Guilford Press, 1995.

Omizo A, Oda EA. Anorexia nervosa: psychological considerations for nutrition counselling. *Journal of the American Dietetic Association* 1988; **88**: 49–51.

Rieger W, Brady JP, Weisberg E. Hematologic changes in anorexia nervosa. *American Journal of Psychiatry* 1978; **135**: 984–985.

Robinson PH, McHugh PR. A physiology of starvation that sustains eating disorders. In Szmukler G, Dare C, Treasure J (Eds) *Handbook of Eating Disorders: Theory, Treatment and Research*. Chichester: John Wiley, 1995.

Rock CL, Curran-Celentano J. The nutritional disorder of anorexia nervosa: a review. *International Journal of Eating Disorders* 1994; **15**: 187–203.

Rock CL, Vasantharajan S. Vitamin status of eating disorders patients: relationship to clinical indices and effect of treatment. *International Journal of Eating Disorders* 1995; **18**: 257–262.

Rock CL, Yager J. Nutrition and eating disorders. *International Journal of Eating Disorders* 1987; **6**: 267–280.

Russell GFM. Anorexia nervosa through time. In Szmukler G, Dare C, Treasure J (Eds) *Handbook of Eating Disorders: Theory, Treatment and Research*. Chichester: John Wiley, 1995.

Serpell L, Treasure J. Osteoporosis – a serious health risk in chronic anorexia nervosa. *European Eating Disorders Review* 1997; **5**: 149–157

Smith DE, Marcus MD, Kaye W. Cognitive–behavioural treatment of obese binge eaters. *International Journal of Eating Disorders* 1992; **12**: 257–262.

Solomon SM, Kirby DF. The refeeding syndrome: a review. *Journal of Parenteral and Enteral Nutrition* 1990; **14**: 90–97.

Spitzer RC, Devlin M, Walsh BJ *et al*. Binge eating disorder: a multisite field trial of the diagnostic criteria. *International Journal of Eating Disorders* 1992; **11**: 191–203.

Szmukler GI, Dare C, Treasure J (Eds). *Handbook of Eating Disorders: Theory, Treatment and Research*. Chichester: John Wiley, 1995.

Telch CF, Agras WS, Rossiter EM *et al*. Cognitive–behavioural therapy for the non-purging bulimic: an initial evaluation. *Journal of Consulting and Clinical Psychology* 1990; **61**: 296–305.

Treasure J. *Anorexia Nervosa: A Survival Guide for Families, Friends and Sufferers*. Hove: Psychology Press, 1997.

World Health Organization. *The International Classification of Diseases*, 10th edn (ICD-10). Geneva: WHO, 1992.

Yellowlees A. *Working with Eating Disorders and Self Esteem*. Folens Publications, 1997.

4.20 Prader–Willi syndrome

The Prader–Willi syndrome (PWS) was first described in the 1950s in Switzerland (Prader *et al.* 1956) and in England a few years later (Laurance 1961). It is characterized by severe hypotonia, poor weight gain and feeding difficulties in early life, accompanied by learning disabilities, short stature and hypogonadism. Behavioural difficulties commencing in early childhood and including a characteristic tendency to overeat are frequently reported (Clarke *et al.* 1996). Severe obesity may develop, and diabetes mellitus and compromised respiratory function often occur.

The literature from the 1970s and earlier generally describes grossly obese, retarded patients with early death from obesity-related diseases. However, if obesity can be controlled, premature death is not inevitable (Carpenter 1994), although sudden early death is still frequently reported. Many older patients have hypertension, type 2 diabetes and peripheral oedema. Most have osteoporosis and marked psychiatric and/or behavioural problems (Cassidy 1998).

Early diagnosis and intervention is essential for successful management. Unfortunately, despite – or possibly because of – more awareness of the syndrome, many are not diagnosed until they are older. In such cases an appropriate regimen needs to be established as soon as possible and frequently involves major lifestyle changes as well as diet modifications.

4.20.1 Incidence and prevalence

Estimates of incidence and prevalence differ. The estimate of incidence is 1 in 10 000–20 000 (Holm *et al.* 1993) and there are estimated to be at least 3000 people with PWS in the UK. Increased awareness of the syndrome, with a consequential increase in diagnostic rate, should not be confused with an increase in prevalence. The condition appears in both genders and all ethnic groups.

4.20.2 Causation

PWS is a genetic disorder, the phenotype resulting from the absence of normally expressed paternally inherited genes on chromosome 15 (q11-q13); maternally inherited genes are normally inactive owing to genomic imprinting (Cassidy 1997). Should the deletion be on the maternally inherited chromosome 15, a very different condition – Angelman syndrome – results, also as a consequence of genomic imprinting.

Approximately 70–75% of those with clinically typical PWS have a deletion in the paternally contributed chromosome 15. The majority of the remainder have maternal uniparental disomy (UPD) of chromosome 15. About 5% of those with PWS have a translocation or other structural abnormality causing either a deletion or maternal UPD, while 1% (including virtually all families where there is a recurrence of PWS) have neither deletion nor UPD. More than one type of genetic test is needed to confirm or exclude an abnormality.

4.20.3 Clinical features and characteristics

Clinical features and characteristics are summarized in Table 4.42. Some patients display many of the described features, others fewer, and there is considerable variation in severity.

During pregnancy, mothers carrying a PWS infant frequently report lack of fetal movements. Almost without exception, neonates are severely hypotonic at birth. Respiratory support is rarely required, a feature helping to differentiate PWS from other causes of neonatal hypotonia such as Werdnig–Hoffman's disease (Zellweger 1988). Although infants with PWS are grossly hypotonic there is potentially good underlying muscle power, e.g. the ability to lift a limb against gravity spontaneously or in response to stimulation.

Two distinct phases of the syndrome occur:

- *Phase 1 (neonates, infants and young children)*: Neonates and infants. (occasionally even up to 12 months of age) are often unresponsive to either their own needs, e.g neither awakening nor crying for feeding, or to their environment, e.g. remaining undisturbed by a loud noise, a painful stimulus or a frightening experience. Failure to thrive is common during the first 1–2 years of life, although there is an indication that, for reasons unknown, weight increase may occur in the latter half of the first year prior to the onset of hyperphagia (Laurance 1990).
- *Phase 2 (older children, teenagers and adults)*: The second phase is characterised by a bizarre change to an apparently insatiable appetite resulting in weight increase and obesity. This tendency to overeat may be observed from 2 years of age (or occasionally earlier), although is generally of later onset. Without energy restriction, weight increases extremely rapidly and obesity becomes the major problem. It is important for dietitians to understand that the hyperphagia primarily results from a physiological malfunction, i.e. failure to

Table 4.42 Main clinical features of Prader–Willi syndrome (Alexander and Greenswag 1995; Waters 1996)

Regulatory abnormalities	Hyperphagia
	Hypoactivity
	Hypotonia
	Hypogonadism
	Higher vomiting threshold
	Decreased pain responsiveness
	Decreased motor skills
	Poor thermoregulation
	Rumination
	Sleep and respiratory disturbances (e.g. apnoea, excessive daytime sleepiness
Cognitive features	Behavioural manifestations:
	Argumentative or oppositional behaviours
	Emotional lability
	Compulsions
	Food seeking
	Obsessions
	Resistance to change
	Skin picking (which may be related to insensitivity to pain)
	Stubbornness
	Temper outbursts and tantrums
	Violent aggressive behaviour to objects, self and others
	Learning disabilities
	Speech and language problems, e.g. perseveration, poor articulation
Structural features	Distinctive facial features:
	High forehead
	Almond-shaped eyes
	Prominent nasal bridge
	Small, down-turned, slightly open mouth
	Central obesity
	Short stature (usually below the third centile)
	Small hands and feet
	Dental deformities
	Eye problems, e.g. myopia, strabismus
Secondary effects	Diabetes mellitus
	Heart and respiratory compromise
	Epilepsy
	Mental illness, e.g. depression, psychosis, schizophrenia
	Oedema
	Bowel function irregularities (constipation or diarrhoea)
	Bone disorders, e.g. osteoporosis, scoliosis
	Increased bruising
	Thick, sticky saliva
	Narcolepsy
	Menstrual irregularities
	Undescended testes

satiate, and not from lifestyle factors or the psychological disturbances associated with other forms of obesity.

Other features and abnormalities associated with PWS are outlined below.

Behavioural abnormalities

The placid infant usually progresses to a naïvely charming child. Children and adults with PWS are warm, friendly and loving, but occasionally have uncontrollable (frequently short-lived) temper tantrums, outbursts or rages. Many maladaptive behaviours have been reported in PWS and include temper outbursts, self-injury (particularly skin-picking), lethargy, impulsiveness, lability of mood, irritability, hyperactivity and stubbornness (Clarke *et al.* 1996). For many, the word 'diet' is enough to start an outburst and alternative terminology such as 'healthy eating' can overcome the inherent problem.

Obsessional behaviours are frequently displayed and may relate to food, aggression, hoarding, rituals, ordering and arranging (Dykens *et al.* 1996), and be directed at people or pets.

Learning disabilities

Learning disabilities associated with PWS range from very mild to severe (Waters 1996). Intelligence quotient (IQ) levels, particularly in young children, may underestimate cognitive levels as a result of motor and speech delays (Levine and Wharton 1995). Older children and adults are often extremely articulate and parents and professionals may fail to realize that functioning is not at the level that speech and practical abilities indicate.

Mental illness

Psychoses must be distinguished from behavioural phenotypes (Clarke 1993). Whether perseveration has an underlying physical or psychiatric basis or whether it is primarily a communication disorder has not yet been elucidated. Dietitians must avoid argument or confrontation when conversing with a person with PWS who exhibits this trait.

Abnormal body composition

People with PWS have an abnormal body composition resulting in:

- *Altered ratio of fat:fat free body mass*: The most outstanding abnormality in PWS is a high fat to lean body mass ratio (Brambilla *et al*. 1997). Increased fat stores are often present even before the child becomes overweight (Laurance 1990). Reduction in resting metabolic rate in adult PWS females can be explained by the reduction in lean tissue and increase in adipose tissue (Goldstone *et al*. 1999).
- *Altered bone density*: Body size has a major influence on total body mineral scan results in children, probably caused by an increased bone volume (Brismar *et al*. 1998). Bone mineral content in older adults with PWS has been found to be significantly lower than in normal weight subjects (Brambilla *et al*. 1997). Decreased bone mineral density can contribute to an increase in risk of fractures and to osteoporosis. Bone age in PWS can exceed chronological age, possibly related to high body mass index (BMI) (Whitman and Myers 1996). This finding has implications for growth hormone treatment because final height may well be reached at a younger age than normal, thus emphasizing the need for weight control from an early age.
- *Poor muscle function*: Muscle hypotonia in PWS is thought to be due to central nervous system abnormalities. Abnormalities in primary muscle pathology have also been noted (Sone 1994).

Facial and dental abnormalities

The specific facial features and muscular hypotonia in PWS frequently cause dysfunction of orofacial muscles, resulting in a high arched palate, shorter dental arches and crowding of front teeth (Storhaug 1998). Unusual dentition (eruption and/or arrangement of teeth) is common and contributes to an increased risk of dental caries. Reduced salivary flow and thick, sticky saliva are frequently observed.

Hypothalamic abnormalities

The number of alterations to the body's homeostatic mechanisms in PWS implicates the hypothalamus as the probable site of major brain dysfunction (Swaab 1997).

Altered levels of neurotransmitters and peptides

Current research suggests a number of abnormalities in PWS:

- Cholecystokinin (CCK) is reported to be raised (Holland *et al*. 1993).
- Gamma-aminobutyric acid (GABA) levels are two or three times higher than controls (Ebert *et al*. 1997).
- Neuropeptide Y is decreased, the opposite to what is expected (Swaab 1998).
- Oxytocin is reduced (Swaab *et al*. 1995; Swaab 1997).
- Serotonin (5-hydroxytryptamine, 5-HT) levels appear to be reduced, in indirect studies examining 5-HT activity. Interest in serotonin levels in PWS centres on its role in some personality traits in the general population (Holland *et al*. 1993).

PWS may also be associated with abnormalities in leptin levels (Weigle *et al*. 1996).

Endocrine abnormalities

Growth hormone

Many studies have shown that both growth hormone (GH) and insulin-like growth factors (IGF) are low in PWS (Lee 1995). GH replacement in PWS has many positive effects in addition to rapid acceleration of linear growth:

- Body composition is altered significantly by increasing the fat-free mass to fat ratio.
- Alteration in body shape is observed; abnormal truncal obesity diminishes, resulting in a more 'normal' appearance.
- Increase in muscle tone is significant.
- Bone density is increased.
- Respiratory function is improved (Lindgren *et al*. 1998a).

As a result of these improvements, levels of physical activity may increase, thus permitting consumption of a higher energy intake (Boyle and Boyle 1993).

Gonadal hormones

Because of the abnormal function of hypothalamic luteinizing hormone-releasing hormone (LHRH) neurons, gonadotrophins (follicle stimulating hormone and LH), oestrogen and/or testosterone levels are usually low in PWS (Crino 1998).

Testosterone replacement therapy can improve secondary sexual characteristics and improve quality of life, although this treatment, particularly when given as monthly injections, may exacerbate behavioural problems.

Oestrogen replacement may be indicated in older females as a preventive measure to delay the development of osteoporosis.

Diabetes mellitus

PWS is associated with an increased prevalence of type 2

diabetes as a result of obesity (Lee 1995). Weight reduction improves the degree of glucose intolerance.

4.20.4 Clinical diagnosis

Consensus diagnostic criteria in three categories – major, minor and supportive findings – have been agreed by international experts (Holm *et al.* 1993) with later modifications (Cassidy 1997; see Table 4.43). However, Smith *et al.* (1998), in formulating a case definition for PWS, used different scores. Livieri *et al.* (1998) suggested that the prevalence of minor criteria is not clearly defined and the importance of this category might be under estimated.

As knowledge about the syndrome increases, it is clear that patients can present with a wider clinical spectrum than previously recognised, e.g. lack of infantile hypotonia, normal puberty, and normal or tall stature (Harty *et al.* 1993; Cassidy et al 1998).

Some clinical differences are also beginning to emerge between those with PWS resulting from deletion and those resulting from UPD (Gillessen-Kaesbach *et al.* 1995, Mitchell *et al.* 1996; Cassidy *et al.* 1998). PWS phenotypes may also differ between racial groups (Cassidy *et al.* 1996).

Table 4.43 Summary of clinical diagnostic criteria

Major criteria (1 point each)	Characteristic facial features Developmental delay/mental retardation Hypogonadism: genital hypoplasia, pubertal deficiency Infantile central hypotonia Infantile feeding problems/failure to thrive Rapid weight gain between 1 and 6 years
Minor criteria (½ point each)	Decreased fetal movement and infantile lethargy Esotropia, myopia Hypopigmentation Narrow hands with straight ulnar border Short stature for the family by 15 years of age Skin picking Sleep disturbances/sleep apnoea Small hands and feet for height/age Speech articulation defects Thick, viscous saliva Typical behavioural problems
Supportive criteria (0 points)	Decreased vomiting Early andrenarche High pain threshold Normal neuromuscular studies Osteoporosis Scoliosis/kyphosis Temperature control problems Unusual skills with jigsaw puzzles

Diagnosis should be strongly suspected in those:
<3 years of age with 5 points, of which 3 are from major criteria;
>3 years of age with 8 points, of which 4 are from major criteria.

4.20.5 Dietary management

General dietary aspects

Dietetic treatment encompasses both extremes of the feeding continuum, i.e. failure to thrive in infancy, but weight gain in childhood, adolescence and/or adulthood due to hyperphagia. Additional problems that an individual with PWS may have, such as mental health, physical or learning disability, must be considered.

Energy requirements

The abnormal body composition in PWS explains why children and adults with PWS require a lower energy intake than normal: 1kg of adipose tissue metabolizes approximately 4.5 kcal/hour compared with muscle metabolizing 66 kcal/hour (Boyle and Boyle 1993).

A lower energy requirement was established in 1973 by Pipes and Holm, who later derived a formula which is still in use (Holm and Pipes 1976): 'normal' children grow if they receive 11–14 kcal/cm height, while those with PWS only need 10–11 kcal/cm height.

Nutritional assessment

Regular assessment of nutritional intake is essential, both during the failure-to-thrive phase and later, when energy restriction is needed, even when there is considerable over-eating.

Although the need for adequate intake of essential fatty acids is well documented, little attention has been given to omega-3 and omega-6 intake in PWS patients (Van Calcar 1998). Care must be taken that an adequate intake is achieved when very low fat regimens are followed. Small quantities of walnut oil will overcome any shortfall.

Specific study of vitamin and mineral requirements in the PWS population has not been reported. The general consensus amongst dietitians working with patients with PWS is that these should be as for dietary reference values (DRVs) of an age-equivalent child, adolescent or adult, and to achieve this, supplementation may be necessary.

Dietary management during phase 1: failure to thrive

Feeding neonates and infants

Many neonates with PWS have a low birthweight, despite being full term or of longer gestation. Appropriate early feeding patterns need to be established, not just for adequate nutrition but to ensure the development of oral muscles, essential for later speech development. While some mothers have attempted breast feeding, this is rarely successful owing to the poor sucking and swallowing ability of the infant with hypotonia.

Almost without exception, assisted feeding is essential. However, nasogastric feeding should progress to bottle feeding as soon as possible, a process which may be accelerated by the use of special bottles and/or teats, e.g. Haberman, Rosti, Mead Johnson soft bottle (Campbell and Trenouth 1987; Haberman 1988). Details of such feeding aids and their availability can be obtained from The Cleft Lip and Palate Association (their address is given at the end of this section). Unless there are medical contraindications, oral feeding should also be attempted to stimulate oral muscles and tactile feeding sensations. Good oral muscle movement patterns may also help to prevent the development of a high palatal arch. Alternatively, oral play should be introduced, e.g. use of a dummy or placing the child's fingers in their mouth.

Cup feeding should always be considered. This feeding method is recommended by the World Health Organization (WHO) and the United Nations Children's Fund (UNICEF) for use with sick and low birthweight infants, and complies with the baby-friendly hospital initiative (Lang *et al.* 1994). While a special cup has been developed by Ameda (Moody 1993), a small, flexible cup with a smooth edge, such as those supplied with liquid medications may be suitable (Whyte F 1998, unpublished observations). Mag-Mag or Avent mugs which have soft spouts, thus enabling milk to be tipped into the baby's mouth (avoiding the need to suck), are also suitable and available from larger pharmacies.

In order to develop safe feeding, attention needs to be given to lip closure, sucking support and swallowing. Supporting the cheeks strengthens facial muscles, while tapping the bottom of the bottle not only helps milk flow, but may assist in keeping the baby awake. Stimulation of the lips and tongue prior to introducing the nipple, teat or cup may help.

Weaning

The simple tasks of sucking, chewing and swallowing are hard work for the PWS infant and occasionally food can become trapped in the roof of the mouth when there is a high palatal arch. Reduced saliva secretion may be a major contributory factor to delayed chewing. However, it is vital that good weaning practices are encouraged; the introduction of new tastes and textures helps mouth muscle development and, without quality feeding skills, children are unlikely to demonstrate good articulation skills.

Poor feeding contributes to failure to thrive. Within this population, signs of poor feeding are subtle and include one or more of those listed in Table 4.44.

Toddlers and children

Feeding and eating skills Hypotonia and poor saliva production place children with PWS at high risk of not having a safe, efficient swallow. The addition of a moist (binding) food helps children to chew foods which they may have previously rejected, e.g. 1 cm pieces of raw celery, carrots, apple with peel and chicken. A low-energy binding food is advised, e.g. thick fruit purée, plain low-fat unflavoured yoghurt or fromage frais, low-fat gravy, low-calorie mayonnaise or salad dressing.

Observations of children with PWS suggest that there may be an extended period of poor eating skills characterized by a delay in transition from infant to adult-textured foods (Morris 1993) (Table 4.45).

Table 4.44 Signs associated with poor feeding in Prader–Willi syndrome (Adapted from Morris 1993)

Change in voice or cry quality
Chronic constipation
Coughing while swallowing
Difficulty in advancing to new textures, e.g. moving from baby-food green beans to fork-mashed green beans
Excessive drooling
Excessive weight gain attributable to texture sensitivity and consequent limited variety of foods
Excessive wet burps
Family fatigue from special food preparation and excessive time spent feeding the child
Frequent respiratory infections, bronchitis or pneumonia
Irritability during feeding
Multiple swallows to clear mouth
Poor weight gain in infancy
Slow intake

Table 4.45 Observations of the feeding skills of 11 children with Prader–Willi syndrome aged from 6 months to 5 years (Adapted from Morris 1993)

Standard	Percentage of PWS children not meeting standard
Normal infants take commercial infant food by 6 months	50% at 6 months 10% at 12 months 2% at 18 months
Normal infants eat soft family food by 1 year	33% at 1 year 10% at 1 ½ years
By 5 years children eat any texture:	
Meat loaf	8% at 5 years
Raw carrots	42% at 5 years
Raw celery	62% at 5 years
Apple with peel	41% at 5 years

Fluids Inadequate consumption of fluids is common in toddlers and children with PWS. It may be necessary to offer extra drinks or increased quantity to make up for loss. Fluids may need to be thickened.

Provided the toddler is eating a wide range of food and growing appropriately, semi-skimmed milk may be used from 2 years and, for some, the use of skimmed milk is preferable even from this early age.

Avoiding starvation Throughout phase 1, attention must be given to ensure that energy intake is adequate. Some parents exert an overzealous approach during part, or all, of phase 1. In their desire to prevent obesity they 'starve' the child, who then not only fails to gain expected weight but also fails to show linear growth. A dietitian faced with a toddler or older child who appears to be failing to thrive should immediately assess actual energy intake and compare with theoretical needs. Almost without exception, the failure to thrive is due to too low an energy intake. Usually 50–100 kcal more each day is all that is needed to reverse the situation, but sometimes energy supplements are needed.

Dietary management during phase 2: obesity

Understanding the nature of the eating disorder is essential for any dietitian involved with a PWS patient and they should be aware that many doctors, parents and indeed the older patients themselves have a poor understanding of hyperphagia and its associated problems.

PWS is the most common example of genetic obesity secondary to an impaired satiety response (Holland *et al.* 1995) and unrestricted access to food usually leads to excessive intakes (Kyriaxides *et al.* 1980). A controlled energy level is needed for life once the failure-to-thrive phase is over. With appropriate care, obesity need not necessarily result.

The principle of 'no weight loss but grow into weight' does not apply to children with PWS and it is cruel to adhere to it, unless excess weight is less than 4 kg. This population fails to exhibit a pubertal growth spurt. To achieve weight loss, as little as 7 kcal/cm height may be needed, regardless of age. In those with PWS, advising too high an energy level simply results in excessive weight gain, and possibly also loss of confidence in the professional by the parent or carer. When GH treatment is prescribed, energy intake needs to be adjusted to compensate for height increase and alteration in body composition.

Dietary regimens

Many dietary regimens have been used, including strict energy control, exchange systems, ketogenic diets, very low calorie diets and low-fat healthy eating. As a result of media coverage of the possible link between behavioural difficulties and the consumption of certain foods, some parents have also attempted to use elimination type diets.

The regimen of choice is that which suits the individual, is nutritionally balanced and has an appropriate energy intake. The whole family should be encouraged to follow healthy eating practices so that the PWS patient does not feel different or ostracized. Nevertheless, dietitians will find that the majority of parents are unhappy with the concept 'healthy eating' without specific advice about energy content. To help overcome the problems which commonly arise, PWSA (UK) has published a dietary management booklet, *Prader–Willi Syndrome: Food and Health* (Gellatly 1996). The regimen is centred on the food groups of *The Balance of Good Health* and is based on 50 and 100 kcal food exchanges.

'Free foods' and fluids

Care must be taken by dietitians when discussing these with PWS patients. Many will interpret statements such as 'as much as you like' quite literally. Dietary advice may need to be tempered, for example, 'not more than can be put on a plate and the plate lifted' or 'you may have two vegetables at any one meal'.

Similarly, fluid intakes may need to be specifically stated, for example, 'you may not have more than 2 litres of fluid a day'. Water intoxication is a risk with some types of medication if fluid intake is grossly excessive (Ritzen 1997; Robson *et al.* 1997).

As is so often the case when working with PWS, the other extreme is also deleterious, so that the consumption of a high-fibre diet must be accompanied by sufficient fluid intake.

Caution needs to be demonstrated in relation to both foods and fluids containing artificial sweeteners to ensure that acceptable daily intakes are not exceeded.

Food preferences

Despite their hyperphagia, people with PWS have food preferences and these must be reflected in the dietary advice offered (Holland *et al.* 1993; Glover *et al.* 1996).

Dietary compliance

Because of hyperphagia, adherence to a dietary regimen is difficult, but not impossible. Teaching children from an early age about healthy eating and acceptable behaviour is helpful, e.g. that fruit is better than chocolate or crisps for a snack, what 'appropriate' portion sizes look like, and that it is acceptable to want food shortly before the next meal or snack is due, but not half an hour after a meal.

Weight loss and control

The reasons for failing to lose weight in the general population are well documented. PWS patients not only have these common problems to overcome but must face the additional characteristics and features of the syndrome. Of particular importance, especially in the older child or adult, is the failure to satiate, which makes it physically impossible not to want to eat (Pipes 1993).

Nevertheless, dietitians should be optimistic even when faced with a PWS patient of 120 kg or heavier. With appropriate advice and the right environment, such patients can achieve a BMI of 30, or even less.

Parents may find it more helpful to weigh all food initially and not rely on guesswork when learning about the diet. Meals should be prepared so that they appear as large as possible in visual terms (e.g. by using smaller, 20 or 23 cm (8 or 9 inch), plates in place of the usual 25 cm (10 inch) size, cutting meat very thinly or spreading the food out rather than piling it up).

Dietitians need to be imaginative with advice: e.g. chopped vegetables on their own do not have much appeal but if the same vegetables are served as crudités with a herb and low-fat, low-calorie yoghurt dip the end product sounds, and is, considerably more attractive.

Many parents lose heart when their PWS child or adult is discharged from follow-up because little or no weight loss has been achieved. Dietitians and doctors often lose patience with the child and parents or carers for perceived lack of effort, especially when the professional is subjected to outcome scrutiny and audit procedures.

Food seeking and stealing

The phenomenon of food stealing is a major problem (Holm and Pipes 1976; Stadler 1995). Any food left unguarded, including items normally accepted as unappetising (e.g. food waste in dustbins, pet food, plants, berries, frozen products, packets of butter and margarine, and plate waste) may be devoured.

Dietitians are frequently faced with a PWS patient vehemently claiming adherence to the prescribed regimen, yet still gaining weight. Certainly this may well be the case, but only at meal times! The dietitian needs skill in handling such a consultation. Lateral thinking helps, e.g. what opportunities exist for extra food to be eaten or money obtained. By working through the normal day from waking to retiring, such times and places can be identified. People with PWS have a remarkable ability to find food and consume it rapidly. The majority do not get rid of wrappings, e.g. sweet papers are found in a pocket or under the bed, or no attempt has been made to hide the boxes from home-delivery pizzas (paid for perhaps via unauthorized use of a parent's credit card). Those travelling on a school bus may use the opportunity to eat their own (and even other children's) packed lunch and maintain at lunchtime that 'Mum forgot to give me any today'

Strategies to help the PWS person should be implemented e.g. food should only be available at meal times, and items such as crisps, sweets and fruit should be inaccessible at other times; a meal being prepared in the kitchen should not be left unattended, nor a table set with food left unsupervised. At the end of a meal all food should be cleared and dishes washed immediately. Many PWS individuals are best not left alone in the kitchen. Siblings, other family members or residents should be discouraged from keeping food in their rooms.

Excessive intakes can be consumed in a short time; rarely does the person with PWS vomit. An individual can easily consume 4000 kcal in a couple of hours and weight increase of 4–6 kg over a weekend of respite care is not unknown (Gellatly, personal communication).

Many with PWS will quickly take advantage of loopholes in the system, or lack of awareness of newcomers to obtain extra food (Waters 1996). Blame and punishment should never be directed at the PWS person. Their insistence that they have not consumed extra is an indication of their cognitive functioning, not simply an untruth. There is an inherent inability to link two events, e.g. a patient may deny taking the biscuits from the cupboard but their face is covered with crumbs and the wrappers are found in a pocket. Rather, the parent or carer should ask themselves, 'Have I set [X] up for failure?' i.e. what is it I have done or not done? Programmes which have had a limited effect in reducing food stealing have been described (Page *et al.* 1983a, b).

Environmental controls

For successful management, parents and carers may need to accept environmental controls. Food cupboards, freezers and refrigerators may need to be locked or made inaccessible (Stadler 1995). It may be preferable to keep the kitchen locked. As keys must be hidden carefully and hiding places changed regularly, digital punch-type locks are easier to use. Other entries to the food-storage areas or kitchens such as back doors, hatches and open windows may also need guarding.

Raising awareness

Friends, neighbours, relations, school and day centre staff need to have the condition explained so that they co-operate fully with the diet. As the child grows so do the problems, including pocket money, collecting shopping, or attending youth groups and clubs where there is a 'tuckshop'. Parents often find it a wise measure to let 'normal' children have a limited amount of spending money; PWS parents need even greater wisdom.

There have been instances of shoplifting, money stealing or eating large meals in restaurants and cafés without the means to pay. It is important for others such as the police, local shopkeepers or assistants to understand the nature of the disorder and for all to remember how stressful these situations can be for both the individual and family.

Consistency of advice and support

Parents and carers must accept that control of energy intake is vital. Most people with PWS will indicate that they do not want to be overweight or obese. As far as possible and practical, the syndrome sufferer should be included in decision making and discussion and helped to make appropriate choices. Anything that they are taught should be accurate, as they find it difficult, if not impossible, to accept change. The majority have difficulty with cognitive reasoning, including following sequential instructions, requests or questions, so many respond much better when given a choice of A or B rather than being given an open-ended question (Dykens *et al.* 1992).

Routine

People with PWS like routine, so this characteristic can be used to advantage. A daily meal pattern can readily be established and adhered to, for example, three meals a day with or without between-meal snacks, depending on individual circumstances and need. Rules must be made and kept by everyone involved.

Most with PWS react badly to situations that are unplanned and unexpected. Professionals, parents and carers must recognize this, for instance, by adhering to the preplanned menu and not swap an apple for an orange, and serving meals at the anticipated time and not 30 minutes later. There are times when a parent or carer may consider a menu change to be desirable or perhaps 'kind', e.g. serving pancakes on Pancake Day. The right approach will prevent or minimize behaviour problems, the carer could explain before the meal it is Pancake Day and this was overlooked when the menu was planned, so 'today there is a choice of a pancake instead of a yoghurt'.

If a dietary regimen needs alteration, the PWS patient should be included in discussion if at all possible, although frequently a parent or carer may need to be seen without the PWS patient being present.

Regular events such as Christmas or birthdays, when food is an important part of the celebrations, can also be approached routinely. For example, an energy intake reduction of 50 kcal/day some 14 days beforehand will allow saving up and 'banking' of 700 kcal in advance. This is preferable to coping with a large increase in weight afterwards.

Reinforcers and treats

The use of reinforcers is often seen as outmoded, but they can be particularly helpful with PWS people. While it may be desirable to choose non-food items such as toiletries, quiz or colouring books, outings or posters, food may be the choice of the person with PWS and can be used to their advantage (Caldwell *et al.* 1986). As far as possible, food reinforcers should be confined to low-energy foods or included as part of the daily energy intake.

There are times when, like everyone, PWS patients need and benefit from treats – they may have had a bad day and need mollycoddling. On such an occasion a suitable treat may be a fun-size chocolate bar.

Parents welcome suggestions for imaginative approaches, for instance, something simple such as a 'sparkler' or cocktail umbrella stuck into an eating apple, or a 'face' made with fruit slices instead of being served in a bowl.

The needs of siblings and other members of the household

The dietary needs of the non-PWS members of the family, particularly other children, should not be overlooked. Parents and carers often need reassuring about meeting their needs, particularly if they are underweight or very active and consequently require higher energy intakes.

Similarly, for those in a residential setting, it is imperative that the needs of the person with PWS do not dominate to the detriment of others. In PWS-specific group homes this problem tends not to arise.

Pica

Some with PWS consume non-food items, which parents find particularly hard to accept. Non-food items may be harmful; the absence of vomiting may mean that the person becomes very ill rapidly, yet does not complain of feeling unwell. Duker and Nielen (1993) described a successful strategy using negative practice each time the target behaviour occurs.

4.20.6 Monitoring progress

Height and weight

Growing children should have their height measured at least every 3 months. Weight may need to be checked monthly. These data can be recorded on standard height/weight charts (Buckler and Tanner 1997). It must be appreciated that length/height development is likely to be on a low centile. Weight should be not more than two centiles higher than the height centile.

With teenagers and adults the need for regular weighing remains important. For some, daily measurements are needed, while for others weekly or even monthly weigh-

ing is more appropriate. The use of standard charts is less helpful in the adolescent phase, as PWS teenagers do not undergo the pubertal growth spurt. PWS-specific growth standards have been produced for 14 physical parameters and provide a means to detect deviant growth in PWS patients (Butler and Meaney 1995).

Body composition

This can be assessed in several ways but the method used depends on factors such as the severity of the obesity, age, cost and technical equipment available. The results must be interpreted with caution:

- *Body mass index*: BMI is not a true predictor of adiposity but despite this shortcoming it may be the only practical option.
- *Skinfold calipers*: The practicality and accuracy of using skinfold calipers, particularly with children with PWS and adults unwilling to co-operate, is questionable (Davies and Joughin 1992). Stadler (1995) provided a useful summary of the results of different studies using this method.
- *Bioelectrical impedance*: Davies and Joughin (1992) suggested assessing body composition from bioelectrical impedance because of its simplicity. However, prediction and regression equations used in calculations need to be for a PWS-specific population in order to avoid a bias towards underestimation of total body water.
- *Dual-energy X-ray photon absorptiometry (DEXA)*: DEXA can measure bone mineral content, fat mass and fat free body mass in three regions (arms, trunk and legs) and may be the best technique to use with patients who are reluctant to co-operate (Brambilla *et al.* 1997). Results using this technique are more accurate than those mentioned above, but DEXA cannot distinguish between muscle and viscera when measuring lean body mass, and this may be relevant when considering underlying hypotonia. The method is also costly and not widely available.
- *Magnetic resonance imaging (MRI)*: This accurately measures adipose tissue *in vivo* (Goldstone *et al.* 1999) and overcomes problems of other techniques such as hydration of lean tissue in extreme obesity, differences in the relationships between subcutaneous and total body fat, body shape and visceral fat content. However, MRI is a costly and scarce resource.

4.20.7 Other aspects of management

The role and effects of exercise

Individuals with PWS are naturally sedentary and have a reduced total energy expenditure to basal metabolic rate ratio (Davies *et al.* 1992). Exercise should therefore be part of the daily routine from an early age. Most with PWS respond well to positive input from parents, e.g. family swimming sessions, bicycle rides, walks or organized group activity such as discos, barn dances, club or school outings. Aerobic exercises are especially beneficial for a person with PWS (Silverthorne and Hornak 1993).

Non-dietary interventions

Pharmacological treatments

Appetite suppressants such as fenfluramine (now withdrawn in the UK) and opiate antagonists have not been shown to have any long-term benefits in the PWS population, although short-term use has proved successful (Selikowitz *et al*. 1990). It is not yet known whether newer antiobesity drugs such as orlistat offer any benefit to people with PWS. Although the use of benzodiazepines for anxiety normally increases appetite, this effect may not occur in PWS patients (Fieldstone *et al*. 1998).

Surgical interventions

Intestinal bypass operations have been tried, both jejunoileal and gastric, but such procedures are not readily acceptable to parents and are by no means always successful.

Jaw wiring

This has been tried, but not in sufficient numbers of cases to establish whether it is a realistic option.

Hospital in-patient treatment

Hospital admissions can cause trauma and distress for all concerned, particularly if admission is to a busy ward and the reason for admission is not primarily related to dietary management.

It is imperative that medical advisers, nurses, therapists, dietitians, support staff and others coming into direct or indirect contact with the patient (ward or health care assistants, volunteers who staff shops, trolleys and snack bars) should be included in preadmission in-service awareness training. This allows all to appreciate the importance of dietary control and understand the peculiarities of PWS. If dietary control is overlooked weight can increase by several kilograms in 2 or 3 days.

Education

Integration into mainstream schools is not without difficulty, particularly after the infant school stage. Many are better placed in special day or boarding schools. After leaving school a wide variety of college courses, either residential or day release, may be accessed.

When statutory full-time education ceases, individuals are particularly vulnerable to rapid weight gain, primarily because supervision of dietary intake is more difficult.

Normalization and independence

As a normal lifespan may be possible, care in the community is essential. Parents of teenagers or young adults with PWS find relinquishing responsibility particularly difficult when weight control has been successful in the home environment because they know that weight gain is likely to happen with this change of lifestyle (Holland *et al*. 1995). As part of the preparation for moving from the family home, it is essential that all concerned with the care of the person, including the community dietitian, are fully conversant with the potential problems so that appropriate long-term arrangements can be made. The consequences of inappropriate placements can be severe and even life threatening. Crisis placements rarely work and the trauma to an individual whose placement breaks down must not be underestimated.

The need for ongoing support in some areas of life must not be misinterpreted as a failure. For some people with PWS, normalization may be living in a supported environment where all needs, including meaningful daytime activity, can be met.

Individuals should be given responsibility for areas of life where appropriate choices can be made, such as leisure activities and hobbies, and where and when they shop for clothing or toiletries. How much, or how little, input the PWS adult will have into meal planning, food shopping, cooking, and so on, will depend on the individual.

Ethical and legal issues

Excessive weight gain can affect quality of life and as the overeating behaviour is physiological, not motivational, the individual has no control over it (Dykens *et al*. 1997). Thus, the dietitian must acknowledge that the patient with PWS may be incapable of exerting autonomy in relation to food and accept that they are in need of care and protection (Holland and Wong 1999).

The need for integrated management

Successful management of PSW requires a multidisciplinary approach. Any management programme and strategy must be fully inclusive and based on close teamwork, support and co-ordination.

The literature describes several different approaches to management. The dietitian's attention is drawn to two methods:

- Descheemaeker *et al*. (1994) developed an integrated programme for children. The numbers in the study were small – the programme continues to be developed – but results appear encouraging so far. The dietary component of the programme is based on food exchanges.
- Hardwell and Hawke (1985) described a strategy developed for an individual which was remarkably successful: all food and drink had to be 'paid' for with tokens which could be earned through completion of, or co-operation in, a range of daily tasks. It illustrates the principle of behaviour management rather than behaviour modification, which is unsuccessful in PWS.

Holland (1998) devised a conceptual model to aid in the development of strategies to prevent obesity in PWS, which dietitians may also find helpful.

The only 'treatment' at present is to establish a sheltered and regulated lifestyle in a loving and understanding environment where each individual may develop and reach their full potential.

Text revised by: Margaret Gellatly

Ackmowledgement: Dr Anthony Holland

Useful addresses

Prader–Willi Syndrome Association (UK)
33 Leopold Street, Derby DE1 2HF
Website: www.pwsa-uk.demon.co.uk

International Prader–Willi Syndrome Organisation (IPWSO)
Contact via PWSA (UK)

The Cleft Lip and Palate Association (CLAPA)
235–237 Finchley Road, London NW3 6LS

Further reading

Greenswag LR, Alexander RC. *Management of Prader–Willi Syndrome* 2nd edn. New York: Springer, 1995.

Hanchett J, Greenswag LR. *Health Care Guidelines for Individuals with Prader–Willi Syndrome*. PWSA (USA), 1998.

James TN, Brown RI. *Prader–Willi Syndrome: Home, School and Community*. London: Chapman and Hall, 1992.

Waters J. *Prader–Willi Syndrome and the Younger Person*. Derby: PWSA (UK), 1992.

Waters J. *A Handbook for Parents and Carers of Adults with Prader–Willi Syndrome*. Derby: PWSA (UK), 1995.

Waters J. *Beyond the Veneer. A Guide to the Essential Features of Residential Care and Supported Living for Adults with Prade–Willi Syndrome*. Derby: PWSA (UK), 1997.

References

Alexander RC, Greenswag LR. Medical and nursing interventions. In Greenswag LR, Alexander RC (Eds) *Management of Prader–Willi Syndrome*, pp. 66–80. New York: Springer, 1995.

Boyle IR, Boyle JM. Improved quality of life with growth hormone in Prader–Willi syndrome. *Prader-Willi Perspectives* 1993; **1**(2): 7–8.

Brambilla P, Bosio L, Manzoni P *et al*. Unusual body composition in Prader–Willi syndrome. *American Journal of Clinical Nutrition* 1997; **65**: 1369–1374.

Brismar TK, Lindgren A-C, Ringertz H *et al*. Total bone mineral measurements in children with Prade–Willi syndrome: the influence of the skull's bone mineral content per area (BMA) and of height. *Pediatric Radiology* 1998; **28**: 38–42.

Buckler JMH, Tanner JM. Growth and development records. *European Journal of Paediatrics* 1997; 156.

Butler MG, Meaney FJ. Growth standards for Prader–Willi syndrome individuals. *Prade–Willi Perspectives* 1995; **4** (1): 11–21.

Butler MG, Moore J, Morawiecki A, Nicolson M. Comparison of leptin protein levels in Prader–Willi syndrome and control individuals. *American Journal of Medical Genetics* 1998; **75**: 7–12.

Caldwell ML, Taylor RL, Bloom SR. An investigation of the use of high and low-preference food as a reinforcer for increased activity of individuals with Prader–Willi Syndrome. *Journal of Mental Deficiency Research* 1986; **30**: 347–354.

Campbell AN, Trenouth MJ. A new feeder for infants with cleft palates. *Archives of Disease in Childhood* 1987; **62**: 1292–1293.

Carpenter PK. Prader–Willi syndrome in old age. *Journal of Intellectual Disability Research* 1994; **38**: 529–531.

Cassidy SB. Prader–Willi syndrome. *Journal of Medical Genetics* 1997; **34**: 917–923.

Cassidy SB. Aging in Prader–Willi syndrome (Abstract). *IPWSO III*, 1998.

Cassidy SB, Geer JS, Holm VA, Hudgins L. African–Americans with Prader–Willi syndrome are phenotypically different. *American Journal of Human Genetics* 1996; **59**: A21.

Cassidy SB, Forsythe M, Heegar S *et al*. Comparison of phenotype between patients with Prader–Willi syndrome due to deletion 15q and uniparental disomy 15. *American Journal of Medical Genetics* 1997; **68**: 433–440.

Cassidy SB, Heegar S, Schwartz S. Clinical spectrum and phenotype–genotype correlations for PWS (Abstract) *IPWSO III*, 1998.

Clarke DJ. Prade–Willi syndrome and psychoses. *British Journal of Psychiatry* 1993; **163**: 680–684.

Clarke DJ, Boer H, Chung MC *et al*. Maladaptive behaviour in Prader–Willi syndrome in adult life. *Journal of Intellectual Disability Research* 1996; **40**: 159–165.

Crino A. Gonadal function in Prader–Willi syndrome (Abstract). *IPWSO III*, 1998.

Davies PSW, Joughin C. Assessment of body composition in the Prader–Willi syndrome using bioelectrical impedance. *American Journal of Medical Genetics* 1992; **44**: 75–78.

Davies PSW, Joughin C, Livingstone MBE, Barnes ND. Energy expenditure in the Prader–Willi syndrome. *NATO ASI Series* 1992; **H61**: 181–187.

Descheemaeker MJ, Swillen A, Plissart L *et al*. The Prader–Willi syndrome: a self-supporting program for children, youngsters and adults. *Genetic Counselling* 1994; **5**: 199–205.

Duker PC, Nielen M. The use of negative practice for the control of pica behavior. *Journal of Behavior and Experimental Psychiatry* 1993; **24**: 249–253.

Dykens EM, Hodapp RM, Walsh K, Nash L. Profiles, correlates and trajectories of intelligence in Prader–Willi syndrome. *Journal of the American Academy of Child and Adolescent Psychiatry* 1992; **31**: 1131–1136.

Dykens EM, Leckman JF, Cassidy S. Obsessions and compulsions in Prader–Willi syndrome. *Journal of Clinical Psychology and Psychiatry* 1996; **37**: 995–1002.

Dykens EM, Goff BJ, Hodapp RM *et al*. Eating themselves to death: have 'personal rights' gone too far in treating people with Prader–Willi syndrome? *Journal of Mental Retardation* 1997; 312–314.

Ebert MH, Schmidt DE, Thompson T, Butler MG. Elevated plasma gamma-aminobutyric acid (GABA) levels in individuals with either Prader–Willi syndrome or Angelman syndrome. *Journal of Neuropsychiatry and Clinical Neuroscience* 1997; **9**: 75–80.

Fieldstone A, Zipf WB, Sarter MF, Bernston GG. Food intake in Prade–Willi syndrome and controls with obesity after administration of a benzodiazepine receptor agonist. *Obesity Research* 1998; **6**: 29–33.

Gellatly MSN. *Prader–Willi Syndrome: Food and Health*. Derby: PWSA (UK), 1996.

Gillessen-Kaesbach G, Robinson W, Lohmann D *et al*. Genotype–phenotype correlation in a series of 167 deletion and non-deletion patients with Prade–Willi syndrome. *Human Genetics* 1995; **96**: 638–643.

Glover D, Maltzman I, Williams C. Food preferences among individuals with and without Prader–Willi syndrome. *American Journal of Mental Retardation* 1996; **101**: 195–205.

Goldstone AP, Byrnes AE, Thomas EL *et al*. Body composition using whole body magnetic resonance imaging and resting metabolic rate in Prader–Willi syndrome adults. 1999 (in press).

Haberman A. A mother of invention. *Nursing Times* 1988; **84**: 2.

Hardwell A, Hawke M. Ten tokens to the 1 lb. *Nursing Mirror* 1985; **160** (17): 36–38.

Harty JR, Hollowell JG, Sieg KG. Tall stature: an atypical phenotype in Prader–Willi syndrome. *Clinical Paediatrics* 1993; **32**: 179–180.

Holland AJ. Understanding the eating disorder affecting people with Prade–Willi syndrome. *Journal of Applied Research in Intellectual Disabilities* 1998; **11**: 192–206.

Holland AJ, Wong J. Genetically determined obesity in Prader–Willi syndrome: the ethics and legality of treatment. *Journal of Medical Ethics* 1999; **25**: 230–236.

Holland AJ, Treasure J, Coskeran P *et al*. Measurement of excessive appetite and metabolic changes in Prader–Willi syndrome. *International Journal of Obesity* 1993; **17**: 527–532.

Holland AJ, Treasure J, Coskeran P, Dallow J. Characteristics of the eating disorder in Prade–Willi syndrome: implications for treatment. *Journal of Intellectual Disability Research* 1995; **39**: 373–381.

Holm VA, Pipes PL. Food and children with Prade–Willi syndrome. *American Journal of Diseases in Childhood* 1976; **130**: 1063–1067.

Holm VA, Cassidy SB, Butler MG *et al*. Prader–Willi syndrome: consensus diagnostic criteria. *Paediatrics* 1993; **91**: 398–402.

Kyriaxides M, Silverstone T, Jeffcoate W, Laurance B. Effect of naloxone on hyperphagia in Prade–Willi syndrome. *Lancet* 1980; 876–877.

Lang S, Lawrence CJ, Orme RL. Cup feeding; an alternative method of infant feeding. *Archives of Disease in Childhood* 1994; **71**: 365–368.

Laurance BM. Hypotonia, obesity, hypogonadism and mental retardation in children. *Archives of Disease in Childhood* 1961; **36**: 690.

Laurance BM. Questionnaire re timing of weight and appetite increase. *News PWSA (UK)* 1990; **27**: 10.

Lee PDK. Endocrine and metabolic aspects of Prader–Willi syndrome. In Greenswag LR, Alexander RC (Eds). *Management of Prader–Willi Syndrome*, pp. 32–57. New York: Springer, 1955.

Levine K, Wharton RH. Educational considerations. In Greenswag LR, Alexander RC (Eds) *Management of Prader–Willi Syndrome*, pp. 156–169. New York: Springer 1995.

Lindgren AC, Ritzen ME, Mileerad J. Growth hormone treatment increases ventilation and central respiratory drive in Prader–Willi syndrome (Abstract). *IPWSO III*, 1998a.

Lindgren AC, Hagenas L, Muller J *et al*. Growth hormone treatment of children with Prader–Willi syndrome affects linear growth and body composition favourably. *Acta Paediatrica* 1998b; **87**: 28–31.

Livieri C, Migliavacca D, Piasenti C *et al*. Prevalence of minor criteria and supportive findings in patients with Prader–Willi syndrome (Abstract). *IPWSO. III*, 1998.

Mitchell J, Schinzel A, Langlois S *et al*. Comparison of phenotype in uniparental disomy and deletion Prader–Willi syndrome: sex specific differences. *American Journal of Medical Genetics* 1996; **65**: 133–136.

Moody J. A revolution in baby feeding. *New Generation* 1993; **12** (2): 41.

Morris M. Feeding the young child with PWS. *The Gathered View PWSA (USA)* 1993; **XVIII** (1): 6–7.

Page TJ, Finney JW, Parrish JM, Iwata BA. Assessment and reduction of food stealing in Prader–Willi children. *Applied Research in Mental Retardation* 1983a; **4**: 219–228.

Page TJ, Stanley AE, Richman GS *et al*. Reduction of food theft and long term maintenance of weight loss in a Prader–Willi adult. *Journal of Behavior Therapy and Experimental Psychiatry* 1983b; **14**: 261–268.

Pipes PL. Nutrition and weight management for individuals with Prader–Willi syndrome. *Prader–Willi Perspectives* 1993; **1** (4): 3–6.

Pipes PL, Holm VA. Weight control of children with Prader–Willi syndrome. *Journal of the American Dietetic Association* 1973; **62**: 520–524.

Prader A, Labhart A, Willi H. Ein Syndrom von adipositas, kleinwuchs, kryptorchismus, und oligophrenie nach myatonieartigem zustand im neugeborenenalter. *Schweizerische Medizinische Wochenschrift* 1956; **86**: 1260–1261.

Ritzen ME. Can water be harmful? *Wavelength IPWSO* 1997; **6** (1): 15.

Robson WLM, Shashi V, Nagaraj S, Norgaard JP. Water intoxication in a patient with the Prader–Willi syndrome treated with desmopressin for nocturnal enuresis. *Journal of Urology* 1997; **157**: 646–647.

Selikowitz M, Sunman J, Pendergast A, Wright S. Fenfluramine in Prader–Willi syndrome: a double blind, placebo controlled trial. *Archives of Disease in Childhood* 1990; **65**: 112–114.

Silverthorne KH, Hornak JE. Beneficial effects of exercise on aerobic capacity and body composition in adults with Prader–Willi syndrome. *American Journal of Mental Retardation* 1993; **97**: 654–658.

Smith A, Warne G, Haan E *et al*. Prader–Willi syndrome: establishing a case definition. A new study of the Australian Paediatric Surveillance Unit (APSU) (Abstract). *IPWSO III*, 1998.

Sone S. Muscle histochemistry in the Prader–Willi syndrome. *Brain and Development* 1994; **16**: 183–188.

Stadler D. Nutritional management. In Greenswag LR, Alexander RC (Eds). *Management of Prader–Willi Syndrome*, pp. 88–114. New York: Springer, 1995.

Storhaug K. Oral and dental findings in Prader–Willi syndrome (Abstract). *IPWSO III*, 1998.

Swaab DF. Prader–Willi syndrome and the hypothalamus. *Acta Paediatrica* 1997; **423** (Suppl): 55–57.

Swaab DF. The hypothalamus in Prader–Willi syndrome (Abstract). *IPWSO III*, 1998.

Swaab DF, Purba JS, Hofman MA. Alterations in the hypothalamic paraventricular nucleus and its oxytocin neurons (putative satiety cells) in Prader–Willi syndrome: a study of five cases. *Journal of Clinical Endocrinology and Metabolism* 1995; **80**: 573–579.

Van Calcar S. Essential fatty acids. *The Gathered View PWSA (USA)* 1998; **XXIII** (1): 9.

Waters J. *A Handbook for Parents and Carers of Adults with Prader–Willi Syndrome*, pp. 13–19. Derby: PWSA (UK), 1996.

Weigle DS, Ganter SL, Kuijper JL *et al*. Effect of regional fat distribution and Prade–Willi syndrome on plasma leptin levels. *Journal of Clinical Endocrinology and Metabolism* 1996; **82**: 566–570.

Whitman BY, Myers SE. A survey of bone ages in children and teenagers with Prader–Willi syndrome (Abstract). *PWSA (USA) 11th Scientific Workshop*, 1996.

Zellweger H. Differential diagnosis in Prader–Willi syndrome. In Greenswag LR, Alexander RC (Eds) *Management of Prader–Willi Syndrome*, pp. 20–21. New York: Springer, 1988.

4.21 Cardiovascular disease: general aspects

Cardiovascular disease (CVD) is a term used to encompass the following conditions involving the vascular systems:

- coronary heart disease (CHD)
- stroke
- peripheral vascular disease (PVD).

Its origin is multifactorial and strongly associated with risk factors such as hypertension, hyperlipidaemia, renal disease and diabetes mellitus. The cardiovascular diseases and risk factor conditions have similarities in their aetiology and dietary management.

4.21.1 Prevalence

Cardiovascular disease is one of the most common causes of death in the entire British population, and the major cause of premature death.

CHD is the major cause of mortality in patients presenting with stroke, diabetes and renal disease. For example, patients receiving renal replacement therapy are 16–19 times more likely to develop CHD than matched controls, and the rate in diabetics with nephropathy is even greater (Wheeler 1997). Everyone with renal disease and diabetes should be regarded as being at increased risk of CHD, whether or not they have other risk factors, such as hyperlipidaemia, hypertension or obesity.

4.21.2 Causation

The interrelationship between these diseases appears to have a metabolic basis, but is not yet fully understood. Syndrome X, or the metabolic syndrome, is one condition in which several symptoms are grouped; it may include some or all of the following features: hypertension, raised plasma insulin, central obesity and dyslipidaemia [raised triglycerides and low HDL-cholesterol] (British Nutrition Foundation 1997; Trevisan *et al*. 1998). The root of syndrome X appears to be vascular endothelial dysfunction, but the understanding of the syndrome is still developing and insulin resistance has also been seen as the key feature.

The endothelium is the lining membrane of blood vessels and therefore has a huge surface area with an important role in controlling functions such as vasoconstriction and dilatation, the passage of metabolites across its surface area, and ultimately the process of atherosclerosis. Maintenance of the integrity of the endothelium is crucial to vascular health and the prevention of CVD.

4.21.3 Global risk assessment for cardiovascular disease

CVD risk is determined by a combination of genetic, risk factor and lifestyle elements.

In the past the decision to reduce CVD risk has depended on assessment of one or two individual risk factors (such as cholesterol level or blood pressure), largely as a result of the National Health Service (NHS) being organized into specialist areas. It is gradually being appreciated that a more global view of risk factor assessment is essential. As a result, cardiovascular risk assessment is becoming much more sophisticated, generally using lifestyle and risk data from analysis of the Framingham study to bring together the important risk predictors and give an overall measure of the risk of a cardiovascular event within a set number of years. To date, the best risk assessment (Wood *et al*. 1998; see below) is still based on these American population data, although some are now based on German populations, but there are indications that they are applicable to British populations as well. It is not known to what extent these data are applicable to population subgroups, for example people of South Asian origin.

A number of British specialist medical groups (the British Cardiac Society, British Hyperlipidaemia Association, British Hypertension Society and British Diabetic Association) have produced joint guidelines on cardiovascular risk assessment and prevention of CVD (Wood *et al*. 1998). These can be summarized as follows:

- *Patients with existing angina, myocardial infarction or other coronary heart disease, stroke or peripheral vascular disease* are considered to be at high risk of further CVD. All of these people should receive cardioprotective dietary advice and support, as well as dietary advice to reduce other risk factors (optimal control of body weight, lipids, blood pressure, diabetes). Other lifestyle and pharmacological interventions to optimize control of these risk factors are also warranted.

- *Patients without existing CVD but with any of the following risk factors: hypertension, dyslipidaemia, diabetes mellitus, family history of premature CHD or obesity*, should have their global CVD risk assessed. Information on gender, age, systolic and diastolic blood pressure, smoking status, serum total cholesterol and HDL-cholesterol, diabetic status and presence or absence of left ventricular failure (LVF) on electrocardiogram (ECG), if known, are used to calculate the percentage possibility of developing CVD in the next 10 years (i.e. the number of people out of 100 who would be expected to have a CVD event over the next 10 years at this level of risk). This risk can be calculated using the Joint British Societies CHD Risk Prevention Chart (Wood *et al*. 1998), or a simple computer program.

It is likely that national and local guidelines will establish at what level of absolute CVD risk specific types of treatment should be instituted. At present, recording of the relevant risk factors and action to reduce their impact is limited even in those with existing CVD (ASPIRE 1996). Adequate risk factor assessment and control in those with existing CVD is likely to be the initial priority in the short term, and should involve ongoing patient review including dietary assessment and cardioprotective advice.

Where this high risk group is adequately controlled, the next priority will be a commitment to assess and optimize the management of those at high risk but without manifest disease. Initially, it may be that only those with greater than 30% risk over 10 years will be treated pharmacologically, but lifestyle advice may be provided and reinforced in those with a lower risk level. An example of assessment of two patients without existing CVD is given in Table 4.46.

As awareness of these guidelines increases, global risk assessment will becomes a standard feature of CVD pre-

vention and management and it is important that dietitians are familiar with its concept and application.

4.21.4 Prevention

Primary prevention of CVD involves suitable lifestyle and risk factor control. The important aspects of lifestyle to assess (and improve) are:

- diet (aim for the cardioprotective diet)
- smoking (aim for non-smoking)
- physical activity (aim for physical activity and some aerobic exercise)
- stress levels and mental health (aim to help with relaxation, by referral if appropriate).

Risk factors to optimize, by lifestyle modifications and also with medication if appropriate, are:

- hypertension
- hyperlipidaemia
- diabetes
- obesity
- renal disease.

It is important that dietitians treat the whole person, not simply their diet, and are able to advise or refer for advice on all of the lifestyle factors. Risk factor control should be added to lifestyle optimization; further details can be found in the sections on Coronary heart disease (Section

---

Table 4.46   Example of global risk assessment in two primary care patients

Patients A and B have their cholesterol levels determined by their GP:

- Patient A is female, aged 35, with a total cholesterol of 7.9 mmol/l.
- Patient B is male, aged 55, with a total cholesterol of 5.9 mmol/l.

On the basis of this information alone it is likely that patient A will be referred for dietetic advice, while patient B will not. However, closer examination of their global risk (using the computer program issued with the Joint Recommendations, Wood *et al*. 1998) reveals the following data:

Factor	Patient A	Patient B
Gender	Female	Male
Age (years)	35	55
Total cholesterol (mmol/l)	7.9	5.9
HDL-cholesterol (mmol/l)	1.64	0.72
Smoking status	Non-smoker	Smoker
Systolic blood pressure (mmHg)	120	160
Diastolic blood pressure (mmHg)	80	95
Diabetic status	No	No
ECG-LVH data if available	No data	No data
% risk of CHD over 10 years	0.7	34.5
% risk of stroke over 10 years	0.2	6.6
Overall assessment	Low risk	High risk

Global risk assessment clarifies the situation:
- Patient A's risk is clearly low; that of patient B is high.
- Patient B should receive immediate cardioprotective dietetic advice including help with reduction of total cholesterol, boosting HDL-cholesterol and reduction of blood pressure. He may also require medication for lipids and blood pressure and should be helped to stop smoking.
- Patient A should receive 'healthy-eating' dietetic advice but she is low priority if resources are scarce.

4.22), Hyperlipidaemia (4.23), Hypertension (4.24), Stroke (4.25), Diabetes mellitus (4.16), Obesity (4.17) and Renal disease (4.14).

4.21.5 The cardioprotective (Mediterranean) diet

The cardioprotective diet is the first line of dietary advice in protection against the main cardiovascular diseases. It can be used in primary or secondary prevention and in conjunction with specific dietary advice on individually relevant risk factors (diabetes, renal disease, dyslipidaemia, hypertension, overweight). This diet should be encouraged in all those at increased risk of CHD, not just in those referred with additional risk factors such as dyslipidaemia or obesity.

Evidence of effectiveness of the cardioprotective diet

The concept of the cardioprotective diet arose from epidemiological work which highlighted the lower risk of cardiovascular disease in the Mediterranean area. Several elements of this diet have been proposed as being especially protective, and there is now good experimental evidence, from randomized controlled trials, to support its protective role in high risk populations. The three trials which provide the evidence base for the cardioprotective diet are summarized in Table 4.47. It should be noted that the benefits were achieved in these trials without significant changes in weight or serum lipids; other mechanisms appear to be operating.

The DART trial isolated oily fish as a protective factor. The two subsequent trials have included an oily fish component plus additional advice to increase fruits, vegetables, pulses, nuts and starchy foods, and moderate fat reduction with the use of monounsaturated fats and modest amounts of alcohol. This appears to have increased the protective effects of the diet. It is not entirely clear which of these additional dietary elements are responsible for the extra protection but, looking at the evidence as a whole, a picture of the rounded 'Mediterranean' or cardioprotective diet appears (British Dietetic Association 1998). The cardioprotective diet is very similar to the cancer-protective diet proposed in several recent reviews (World Cancer Research Fund 1997; DH 1998).

Further support for the protective effect of fish oils in people with cardiovascular disease has come from the GISSI-P trial (GISSI-Prevenzione 1999), in which 11 324 people who had had a myocardial infarction were randomized to receive fish oil capsules (0.9 g/day of omega-3 fats) or not and followed for 3.5 years. Those receiving fish oil capsules were significantly less likely to die from any cause over that period.

The cardioprotective diet appears highly effective in high risk populations (see Table 4.48) and cost-effectiveness appears very good relative to other common interventions (NHS CRD 1998). The effectiveness of the cardioprotective diet in primary prevention has not yet been established, but evidence to date suggests that similar benefits are likely (DH 1994).

Influence of the diet on cardiovascular disease

The cardioprotective diet probably exerts its effects on CVD by altering a wide range of risk factors in a positive way. These may include effects on blood pressure, lipid oxidation

Table 4.47 The trials which provide the evidence base for the cardioprotective diet

Trial name	Participants	Control group	Intervention group	Outcomes measured	Methodology	Conclusion
DART trial (Burr *et al.* 1989	2033 British men who had recovered from a MI	No advice on fish	Advised to eat > 2 portions oily fish[1] per week *or* fish oil supplements	Deaths and MI	RCT (factorial design with two other types of dietary advice)	Intervention group had 29% reduction in all-cause mortality (*p* <0.05)
Lyon Diet Heart Study (de Lorgeril *et al.* 1994)	605 French men and women following a first MI	No dietary advice	Provided with rapeseed margarine. Advised to eat more bread, fish, vegetables, fruit (daily), olive/rapeseed oils, and more poultry/less red meat	CVD deaths and non-fatal MI	RCT	After 27 months: *Control group*: 16 cardiac deaths, 17 MI; *Intervention group*: 3 cardiac deaths, 5 MI
Indian cardio-protective diet trial (Singh *et al.* 1992)	406 Indian men and women with definite or possible MI, or unstable angina	Reduced fat diet similar to American Heart Association Guidelines	Reduced-fat diet plus 400 g fruit/vegetables per day, plus pulses, nuts and fish	Deaths and cardiac events	RCT	After 1 year: Control group: 38 deaths 82 cardiac events; Intervention group: 21 deaths, 50 cardiac events

[1]200–400 g portions of mackerel, pilchard, sardine, salmon or trout.
MI: myocardial infarction; RCT: randomized controlled trial.

Table 4.48 Alternative treatments for the secondary prevention of coronary heart disease.

Number needed to treat (NNT) for 5 years to avoid one cardiovascular death in people with a 30% risk of CHD over 10 years (Adapted from NHS CRD 1998)

Treatment	NNT
Aspirin	37
Beta-blockers	30
Statins	26
Oily fish advice	19
Mediterranean diet	9

The information in this table needs to be used with caution as the data from which it is derived are limited, and further dietary trials in particular are required (Table 4.47). However, the data suggest that the cardioprotective diet, along with appropriate medication, can make an important contribution to reducing future cardiovascular events in those at moderate to high levels of risk.

Explanation of NNT: The number needed to treat is the number of patients who must be treated to prevent one adverse outcome. The smaller the NNT, the better the treatment. The smallest NNT is 1, which would mean that every patient treated was cured by the treatment.

For example, 200 patients have a nasty illness. Traditionally, they have been treated with carrot juice, but to test whether this is indeed helpful they are randomized to being given either healthy eating dietary advice, or healthy eating advice plus carrot juice advice. One hundred patients receive each treatment and the outcome is as follows:

	Unfavourable outcome (dead after 4 weeks)	Favourable outcome (alive after 4 weeks)	Total
Treatment (carrot juice)	5 *(a)*	95 *(b)*	100
Control (no carrot juice)	10 *(c)*	90 *(d)*	100
Total	15	185	200

The absolute risk reduction (ARR) is $c/(c + d) - a/(a + b) = 10/100 - 5/100 = 0.1 - 0.05 = 0.05$.
The NNT is $1/ARR = 1/0.05 = 20$, which means that for every 20 patients treated with carrot juice advice one life will be saved.

and inflammation (reducing injury to coronary arteries), lipid profile, homocysteine levels and insulin resistance (reducing fibrous plaque formation), platelet aggregation, clotting factors and arrhythmias (reducing the occurrence of thrombosis leading to heart attack and stroke). The effects of the diet on the cardiovascular system are summarized in Table 4.49 (British Nutrition Foundation 1997).

A summary of evidence for other dietary changes which are sometimes advocated to help to protect against CVD is presented in Table 4.50. Table 4.51 provides a reminder of the effects of various fatty components of the diet on factors related to CVD.

Practical aspects of the cardioprotective diet

The main elements of the cardioprotective diet are shown in Table 4.52. Further dietary modification relevant to specific risk factors is summarized in Table 4.53. Practical dietary details are given in Tables 4.54–4.57.

Cardioprotective dietary advice should always be set in the context of healthy eating guidance such as *The Balance of Good Health* (see Section 1.2, Healthy eating) to ensure that the overall diet is balanced. Over-focus on one nutrient (such as saturated fat) can risk compromising the

Table 4.49 Summary of the effects of a cardioprotective diet (British Nutrition Foundation 1997)

Omega-3 fatty acids (oily fish, rapeseed oil)	Anti-inflammatory effects, protecting the endothelium from damage Anti-thrombotic effects Reduced triglycerides Improved insulin sensitivity Anti-arrhythmic effects
Other fatty acids	The action of omega-3 polyunsaturates is improved by lower intakes of saturated fats (and omega-6 polyunsaturates in the case of rapeseed oil). Lower saturated fat intakes also reduce the risk of thrombosis and reduce serum lipids
Fruit and vegetables, plus pulses and nuts	Contain a variety of antioxidants (vitamins A, C and E, other compounds such as flavonoids and minerals such as selenium) to help to protect against the formation of oxidized LDL Are rich in potassium, which may help to control blood pressure Are rich in folic acid, which inhibits possibly damaging homocysteine formation Contain soluble fibre, which reduces fat absorption and improves cholesterol levels
Alcohol	Improved HDL levels Possible antioxidant effects

Table 4.50 Evidence for other dietary changes relating to cardiovascular disease

Dietary change advocated	Evidence	Evidence score[1]	References
Garlic/garlic capsule	Systematic review found trial quality to be poor; more research needed before any conclusion can be reached	1B	Silagy and Neil (1994)
Folate	Systematic review suggests that folate reduces serum homocysteine levels, but only observational studies link homocysteine with CVD risk	3A	Homocysteine Lowering Trialists Collaboration (1998)
Red wine	Systematic review of observational studies suggests that all alcoholic drinks are associated with lower risk	3A	Rimm et al. (1996)
Salt	Systematic review suggests that lowering salt intake will lower blood pressure (no trials with morbidity/mortality outcomes)	1B	Law et al. (1991)
Tea	Observational studies suggest that flavonoids are protective against CVD	3A	Hertog et al. (1989, 1993, 1997)
Vitamin A and beta-carotene	Randomized controlled trials suggest that taking these as a supplement may *increase* risk of CVD	1A	ATBC (1994), Omenn et al. (1994)
Fibre	Randomized controlled trial suggests that added fibre has no significant effect on risk of CVD	1A	Burr et al. (1989)
Lycopenes	Trials link increased dietary lycopenes with serum levels; observational studies link increased serum lycopene levels with lower CVD risk	3A	Kristenson et al. (1997)
Weight reduction	Trials show positive effects from weight loss on risk factors such as blood pressure, lipids and glucose tolerance; no evidence for overall CVD reduction	1B	Dattilo and Kris-Etherton (1992), Hadden et al. (1975), Stamler et al. (1980)
Coffee	Observational studies suggest no effect on CVD	3A	Myers and Basinsky (1992)
Oats	Intervention trials of high intakes show modest effects on lipids	1B	Ripsin et al. (1992)
Dietary cholesterol	Intervention trials show modest effects on lipids, but the relationship is not linear; most effect is seen in individuals with very high or very low cholesterol intakes	1B	Hopkins (1992)
Soy protein	Systematic review suggests that high intakes lead to modest total and LDL-cholesterol reductions	1B	Anderson et al. (1995)
Vitamin E (alpha-tocopherol)	Intervention trials to date show a non-significant effect on CVD (with a trend towards being harmful); further large trials are in progress	1A	ATBC (1994), Omenn et al. (1994), Stephens et al. (1996), GISSI-P (1999)

Where evidence is non-significant it is impossible to tell whether this is due to a shortage of trials, or because the intervention really has no effect.
[1]Evidence scores: 1, excellent (evidence from randomized controlled trials, or systematic reviews of randomized controlled trials); 2, good (evidence from non-randomized trials); 3, moderate (evidence from observational studies such as case-controlled or cohort studies); 4, poor (relying on opinions of authorities); A, evidence of an intervention effect on morbidity or mortality; B, evidence only for an intervention effect on a related risk such as lipid levels or blood pressure.

Table 4.51 Effects of different types of dietary fatty acids

Type of fatty acid	Effect on CVD and risk factors	Usual sources
Omega-3 polyunsaturates	↓ Thrombosis ↓ Inflammation ↓ Arrhythmia ↓ Triglycerides ↓ Insulin resistance	Oily fish and fish oil capsules, cod liver oil, rapeseed and linseed oils
Omega-6 polyunsaturates	↓ Total cholesterol ↓ LDL-cholesterol ↓ HDL-cholesterol (Compete with omega-3)	Sunflower, corn, safflower, soya, cottonseed oils
Monounsaturates	↓ Total cholesterol ↓ LDL-cholesterol ↔ HDL-cholesterol ↑ Thrombosis ↑ Insulin resistance	Olive, peanut (groundnut), rapeseed oils
Saturates	↑ Total cholesterol ↑ LDL-cholesterol ↔ HDL-cholesterol ↑ Thrombosis ↑ Insulin resistance	Animal fats, coconut oil
Trans fatty acids	As for saturates	Hydrogenated vegetable oils

↓: decrease; ↑ increase; ↔ unchanged.

intake of others (such as iron and calcium) if dietary advice is not comprehensive. Other dietary therapeutic objectives (such as maintenance of tight glycaemic control in the management of diabetes) may also be relevant.

There is little evidence on long-term outcomes for children on the cardioprotective diet; it is, however, a balanced diet and leads to healthy adults in Mediterranean countries. Total fat restriction is inappropriate for young children, but substituting saturated fat with monounsaturated or omega-3 fats, encouraging the consumption of small, varied portions of fruit and vegetables, and including some oily fish in the diet are all appropriate measures in this age group, provided they are achieved with foods which the child enjoys.

For frail or elderly people (who are at risk of being nutritionally compromised, especially if appetite and food intake are poor) oily fish, fruit and vegetables can be encouraged, but dietary fat content and composition should only altered if this can be achieved with no loss of enjoyment or reduction in dietary energy density.

Table 4.52 The cardioprotective diet

Dietary advice for the general population	Dietary advice for those at moderate risk	Dietary advice for those at high risk
0–14% risk of CVD over 10 years. Primary prevention via healthy-eating guidance based on COMA recommendations (DH 1994)	15–29% risk of CVD over 10 years. Usually primary prevention but may include those with diabetes, hypertension and renal disease	≥ 30%+ risk of CVD over 10 years. Usually people who have had CVD events or in whom they are likely to occur
2+ portions of fish weekly, one of which should be oily	3+ portions of oily fish per week	3+ portions of oily fish per week (fish oil capsules encouraged where oily fish is not acceptable)
At least 5 portions of a mixture of fruit and vegetables per day	At least 5 portions of a mixture of fruit and vegetables per day. Inclusion of pulses and nuts	At least 5 portions of a mixture of fruit and vegetables per day. Inclusion of pulses and nuts
Saturated fats replaced primarily by monounsaturates (rapeseed or olive oils)	Saturated fats replaced primarily by monounsaturates (rapeseed or olive oils)	Saturated fats replaced primarily by monounsaturates (rapeseed or olive oils)
Some dietary fat energy replaced by increased complex starch intake	Some dietary fat energy replaced by increased complex starch intake	Some dietary fat energy replaced by increased complex starch intake
Fat intake divided evenly between at least three regular daily meals	Fat intake divided evenly between at least three regular daily meals	Fat intake divided evenly between at least three regular daily meals
Avoidance of excessive alcohol intake (≤ 3 units daily for women, ≤ 4 units daily for men)	Modest alcohol (1–2 units per day) advocated (unless risk of addiction); ensure not excessive	Modest alcohol (1–2 units per day) advocated (unless risk of addiction); ensure not excessive
Salt intake limited	Salt intake limited	Salt intake limited

Table 4.53 Additional advice to the cardioprotective diet

Lifestyle factors to check: Adequate aerobic exercise. Not smoking	
Features to stress where other risk factors are present:	
Raised LDL-cholesterol	Reduce saturated and *trans* fatty acid intake. Correct overweight (especially elevated waist circumference)
Raised triglycerides	Correct overweight (especially elevated waist circumference). Ensure alcohol is not excessive. Reduce excessive intake of simple sugars
Low HDL-cholesterol	Ensure adequate aerobic exercise. Encourage modest alcohol if not contraindicated. Ensure moderate intake of unsaturated fats
Hypertension	Correct overweight (especially elevated waist circumference). Encourage salt restriction. Encourage increased potassium intake via fruit and vegetables. Ensure adequate aerobic exercise
Diabetes	Correct overweight (especially elevated waist circumference). Ensure tight glycaemic control via regular meal pattern and appropriate carbohydrate
Renal disease	Ensure diet is appropriate for disease management. Encourage weight control measures if appropriate

Specific considerations

Alcohol

The role of alcohol in the cardioprotective diet remains equivocal because of the lack of intervention studies to establish its benefits but there is clear evidence of its hazards at excessive levels of intake. However, epidemiological evidence suggests that for those at medium or high cardiovascular risk, a modest amount of alcohol is protective (Rimm *et al.* 1996). The benefits for those at low risk (for example, young women) are more doubtful. For those at increased cardiovascular risk a regular intake of 1–2 units per day of any alcohol probably confers maximal protection without adverse effects on triglycerides or blood pressure. However, this is only appropriate in people with no history of addictive behaviour.

Gout

Some people at high cardiovascular risk will also have gout and may need to avoid high intakes of purines, particularly if symptoms are severe or medication is only used intermittently (see Section 4.15.1, Gout). Since oily fish is rich in purines, increased consumption is contraindicated. In these circumstances fish oil capsules, which do not contain purines, should be advocated.

Table 4.54 Comparison of three types of diet: traditional high-fat, low-fat and cardioprotective

	Traditional high fat diet	Cardioprotective diet	Low fat-diet
Food intake for 1 day	1 pint whole milk 30 g butter 35 g instant coffee 20 g cornflakes, 90 g white bread 15 g digestive biscuit 90 g white bread, 20 g cheese 100 g pork chops (grilled, lean), 150 g mashed potato, 30 g canned peas, 50 g fruit pie, 10 g cream	1 pint skimmed milk 25 g olive-based spread 20 g rapeseed oil 35 g instant coffee 50 g muesli, 1 banana, 60 g wholemeal bread, 40 g mushrooms 25 g cashew nuts 90 g wholemeal bread, 20 g turkey, 30 g tomato 100 g mackerel, 100 g new potatoes, 50 g corn on the cob, 30 g mixed peppers and onion, 100 g mango, small glass red wine	1 pint semi-skimmed milk 45 g low-fat spread 35 g instant coffee, 70 g sugar 30 g cornflakes, 60 g wholemeal bread, 25 g marmalade 1 apple, 15 g ginger biscuit 60 g wholemeal bread, 40 g ham, 30 g tomato 100 g steamed haddock, parsley sauce (skimmed milk, cornflour), 150 g mashed potato, 50 g corn on the cob, 80 g stewed apples, 50 g low-fat yoghurt
Energy	1930 kcal	1930 kcal	1970 kcal
Total fat	92 g (43% energy)	79 g (37% energy)	59 g (27% energy)
Saturated fat	21% energy	6% energy	7% energy
Monounsaturated fat	13% energy	17% energy	7% energy
Polyunsaturated fat	2% energy	11% energy	7% energy
Omega-3 fatty acid	0.2 g	1.3 g	0.1 g
Sugars	23 g	62 g	131 g
Carbohydrate	200 g	217 g	295 g
Fibre	15 g	29 g	22 g
Potassium	3.7 g	5.3 g	4.5 g
Sodium	2.2 g	1.7 g	2.5 g
Vitamin C	29 mg	109 mg	66 mg
Folate	109 μg	212 μg	164 μg

Table 4.55 Oily fish

Suitable oily fish are those with high levels of omega-3 fatty
  acids. These include:
Herring and kippers
Mackerel
Pilchards, sardines and sild
Salmon
Trout
Sprats or brisling
Rock salmon (dogfish)
Fresh tuna (not canned tuna, which has a much lower omega-3
  fatty acid content)
Swordfish
Bloaters
Conger eel
Whitebait
Crab is also a good source of omega-3 fatty acids

Those at high risk of cardiovascular disease should aim to
consume 200–400 g of oily fish per week, i.e. about 3 portions
of at least 100 g (3–4 ounces) in weight

For those at high risk who are unable or unwilling to eat oily fish
regularly, fish oil supplements (fish body oil, *not* fish liver oil)
provide a useful alternative. A suitable dosage level is one that
provides approximately 0.5–1.0 g of omega-3 fatty acids per day
(usually as DHA and EPA)

For example, Brand X fish oil supplement:
  Each capsule contains 125 mg DHA and 176 mg EPA
  Total omega-3 fatty acids per capsule = 125 + 176 = 301 mg
  Therefore, 2 capsules per day (providing 602 mg omega-3 fatty
  acids/day) should be taken

Table 4.56 Portions of fruit and vegetables

One portion can be taken to be:
1 apple, 1 banana or 1 piece of other fresh fruit
1 raw carrot
3 tablespoons of cooked vegetables or beans
A handful of dried fruit (raisins, apricots, etc.)
A cup of salad
1 small glass of fruit juice (100 ml)
A handful of nuts (unroasted, unsalted)
A bowl of home-made vegetable soup or stew

Potatoes and processed foods with only a small fruit and
vegetable content (e.g. fruit cake, fruit yoghurt, canned vegetable
soups) do not count as a portion (see Section 1.2.1 in Healthy
Eating)

Table 4.57 Alcohol, units and limits

1 unit[1] of alcohol is provided by:
½ pint of standard strength (3–4% alcohol by volume) beer, lager
  or cider
1 small glass of wine (7–8 units per 75 cl bottle)
1 pub-sized measure of spirits

Optimal intake for those at moderate or high cardiovascular risk:
1–2 units of any type of alcohol per day
For people with a history of addiction, alcohol is
  contraindicated

Recommended maximum safe limits
3–4 units per day for men
2–3 units per day for women

[1]But see Using the unit system in Section 1.2.4 (Sensible use of
alcohol).

Safety

Concern has been expressed over the relatively high levels of dioxins and polychlorinated biphenyls (PCBs) present in fish and fish oils (MAFF 1999). These environmental pollutants, which are acquired from a variety of sources, are known to have carcinogenic potential and, being fat-soluble, accumulate in the body. The significance of this in terms of human health is unknown but cannot be ignored. The likely balance of benefit and risk from increased consumption of fish and fish oils therefore has to be considered. In those at high risk of CVD, there seems little doubt that the immediate benefits far outweigh any possible longer term risks. The risk–benefit balance is more difficult to assess in those at low or moderate risk of CVD, particularly in children who will have more years of exposure to potential hazards than adults. To keep the problem in perspective, it should be borne in mind that levels of these contaminants in fish have fallen in recent years and that the population exposure to all sources of these pollutants is closely monitored and where possible minimized. Dietitians should also note that levels of dioxins and PCBs are higher in fish liver oil supplements, i.e cod or halibut liver oils, than in fish body oils (MAFF 1997). Therefore, if fish oil supplementation is indicated, fish body oil rather than fish liver oil (which also has a lower omega-3 fatty acid content) should be recommended. This, and the distinction between them, usually needs to be explained.

Lifestyle

The cardioprotective diet should always be discussed in the context of a healthy lifestyle and reference should be made to activity and exercise levels, smoking cessation and continued use of prescribed medication. More information on these aspects of lifestyle can be obtained from local cardiac rehabilitation programmes or the British Heart Foundation.

Dietetic participation in cardiac rehabilitation helps to ensure a consistent message, with dietitians reinforcing the other lifestyle messages and other team members well informed on dietary issues.

Acceptability

Patients are often apprehensive about the perceived restrictions of a cardioprotective diet and may be visibly relieved when the positive changes are described and encouraged. The approach to the patient should be determined by the 'stages of change' model (see Section 1.7, Achieving behavioural change); those who have never contemplated change will need a different approach to those who have already started to make changes, or have previously made changes but slipped back.

Whilst many people enjoy the cardioprotective diet there are also some who find particular elements very difficult. Many people struggle to increase their intake of fruit and vegetables, and of oily fish, as well as to reduce or modify fat intake and cut down on salt. With fruit and vegetables, it is often useful to stress the wide variety of fruits, fresh and frozen vegetables, salads, dried fruit, unsalted nuts and fruit juices available, and to suggest that those which are enjoyed are eaten more frequently.

Similarly, people may recoil at the mention of oily fish, but are actually quite happy to eat tinned salmon, sardines or kippers. For those for whom this is not acceptable, fish oil capsules (fish body oil, not fish liver oil) are available and appear to provide most of the protection provided by the fish. An appropriate dosage level is 0.5–1.0 g omega-3 fatty acids per day. Fish oil capsules are best taken with a cold drink just before or during a meal to prevent the flavour repeating. Vegetarians, those allergic to fish or those who cannot take to the capsules can optimize their omega-3 intake by using vegetable omega-3 sources such as rapeseed (canola) or flax (linseed) oils, but the conversion rate is low and other polyunsaturates compete, so it is important to ensure that most fat intake is in the form of these oils. Rapeseed is the most practical as it can be used for cooking, whereas linseed can only be bought as a supplement.

The cardioprotective diet, like exercise and non-smoking, is protective as long as it is continued. To have eaten well or been fit last year is not helpful now. To help people to maintain their healthier habits, regular review is advisable. This may involve dietetic review in a central location or the community, or be delegated to other community staff, who must be trained, updated and provided with appropriate support materials.

Table 4.58 Possible factors to consider for monitoring and evaluation purposes

Dietary factors	Portions of oily fish per week
	Portions of fruit and vegetables per day
	Appropriate fats in cooking?
	Appropriate fat spread?
	Appropriate milk?
	Units of alcohol taken per day/ week
	Level of fat intake
	Level of salt intake
Emotional factors	Acceptability of diet
	Barriers to change
	Stages of change
Lifestyle factors	Smoking
	Exercise levels
	On medication for lipids?
	On medication for blood pressure?
Risk levels	Waist circumference
	Body mass index
	Weight change
	Total cholesterol
	Triglycerides
	HDL-cholesterol
	LDL-cholesterol
	Cholesterol/HDL ratio
	Blood pressure (systolic, diastolic)
	Factors relevant to diabetic or renal control
Outcomes	Myocardial infarction
	Angina frequency
	Stroke
	Coronary artery bypass graft
	Angioplasty
	Hospital admissions
	Death

Motivation can also be boosted by involving the whole family (Cousins *et al*. 1992). Where this occurs the sense of isolation is reduced and the whole family group, who may also be at increased genetic or lifestyle risk of CHD, will reap the benefits in risk reduction.

Monitoring and outcomes

Appropriate relevant factors to monitor are included in Table 4.58. It should be borne in mind that the benefits from dietary change depend on the extent to which other lifestyle changes have been achieved. These two aspects therefore need to be considered in conjunction with each other in order to assess the effectiveness of risk reduction measures.

Text written by: Lee Hooper in conjunction with the UK Heart Health and Thoracic Dietitians

Useful addresses

American Heart Association
National Center, 7272 Greenville Avenue, Dallas, Tx 75231, USA
Website: www.amhrt.org

American Stroke Association, address as American Heart Association
Website: www.amhrt.org/stroke/index.html

British Association for Cardiac Rehabilitation
c/o Dr Paul Bennett, PO Box 24, Newport NP9 4XP (regular newsletter, annual conference, other useful publications)

British Cardiac Society
9 Fitzroy Square, London W1P 5AH
Tel: 020 7383 3887
Website: www.cardiac.org.uk

British Heart Foundation
14 Fitzhardinge Street, London W1H 4DH
Website: www.bhf.org.uk

British Hyperlipidaemia Association
c/o DMC, AG 7&8, B&IC, Aston Science Park, Birmingham B7 4BJ
Tel: 0121 693 8338
E-mail: ebc@dircon.co.uk

Coronary Prevention Group
102 Gloucester Place, London W1H 3DA
Tel: 020 7935 2889

Family Heart Association
7 North Road, Maidenhead SL6 1PL
Tel: 01628 522177

National Heart, Lung and Blood Institute (USA)
Website: www.nhlbi.nih.gov/nhlbi/nhlbi.htm

National Stroke Association (USA)
96 Inverness Drive East, Suite 1, Englewood, Colorado, USA
Website: www.stroke.org
The Stroke Association
CHSA House, Whitecross Street, London EC1Y 8JJ
Tel: 020 7490 7999

UK Heart Health and Thoracic Dietitians
via British Dietetic Association
Elizabeth House, 22 Suffolk Street, Queensway, Birmingham B1 1LS
Tel: 0121 643 5483.
Website: www.vois.org.uk/bda/

Further reading

Systematic reviews in this area are available from the Cochrane Library (there are specialist interest groups on heart disease, peripheral vascular disease, stroke, hypertension, renal disease and tobacco addiction). Website: www.update-software.com/cochrane.htm

References

Alpha-Tocopherol, Beta Carotene (ATBC) Cancer Prevention Study Group. The effect of vitamin E and beta carotene on the incidence of lung cancer and other cancers in male smokers. *New England Journal of Medicine* 1994; **330**: 1029–1035.

Anderson JW, Johnstone BM, Cook-Newell ME. Meta-analysis of the effects of soy protein intake on serum lipids. *New England Journal of Medicine* 1995; **333**: 276–282.

ASPIRE Steering Group. A British Cardiac society survey of the potential for the secondary prevention of coronary disease: ASPIRE principal results. *Heart* 1996; **75**: 334–342.

British Dietetic Association. Dietary treatment of people at high coronary risk. Position Paper. *Journal of Human Nutrition and Dietetics* 1998; **11**: 273–280.

British Nutrition Foundation. *Diet and Heart Disease: A Round Table of Factors*. London: Chapman and Hall, 1997.

Burr ML, Fehily AM, Gilbert JF *et al*. Effects of changes in fat, fish, and fibre intakes on death and myocardial reinfarction: diet and reinfarction trial (DART). *Lancet* 1989; **ii**: 757–761.

Cousins JH, Rubovits DS, Duncan JK *et al*. Family versus individually oriented intervention for weight loss in Mexican American women. *Public Health Reports* 1992; **107**: 549–555.

Dattilo AM, Kris-Etherton PM. Effects of weight reduction on blood lipids and lipoproteins: a meta-analysis. *American Journal of Clinical Nutrition* 1992; **56**: 320–328.

De Lorgeril M, Renaud S, Mamelle N *et al*. Mediterranean alpha-linolenic acid-rich diet in secondary prevention of coronary heart disease. *Lancet* 1994; **343**: 1454–1459.

Department of Health, Committee on Medical Aspects of Food Policy. *Nutritional Aspects of Cardiovascular Disease*. Reports on Health and Social Subjects 46. London: HMSO, 1994.

Department of Health, Committee on Medical Aspects of Food Policy. *Nutritional Aspects of the Development of Cancer*. Reports on Health and Social Subjects 48. London: The Stationery Office, 1998

GISSI-Prevenzione Investigators. Dietary supplementation with *n*-3 polyunsaturated fatty acids and vitamin E after myocardial infarction: results of the GISSI-Prevenzione trial. *Lancet* 1999; **354**: 447–455.

Hadden DR, Montgomery DA, Skelly RJ *et al*. Maturity onset diabetes mellitus – response to intensive dietary management. *British Medical Journal* 1975; **iii**: 276–278.

Hertog MGL, Kromhout D, Aravanis C *et al*. Flavonoid intake and long-term risk of coronary heart disease and cancer in the Seven Countries Study. *Archives of Internal Medicine* 1989; **155**: 381–386.

Hertog MGL, Feskens EJ, Hollman PC *et al*. Dietary antioxidant flavonoids and risk of coronary heart disease: the Zutphen Elderly Study. *Lancet* 1993; **342**: 1007–1011.

Hertog MGL, Sweetnam PN, Fehily AM *et al*. Antioxidant flavonols and ischaemic heart disease in a Welsh population of men: the Caerphilly Study. *American Journal of Clinical Nutrition* 1997; **65**: 1489–1494.

Homocysteine Lowering Trialists Collaboration. Lowering blood homocysteine with folic acid based supplements: meta-analysis of randomised trials. *British Medical Journal* 1998; **316**: 894–898.

Hopkins P. Effects of dietary cholesterol on serum cholesterol: a meta-analysis and review. *American Journal of Clinical Nutrition* 1992; **55**: 1060–1070.

Kristenson M, Zieden B, Kucinskiene Z *et al*. Antioxidant state and mortality from coronary heart disease in Lithuanian and Swedish men: concomitant cross sectional study of men aged 50. *British Medical Journal* 1997; **314**: 629.

Law MR, Frost CD, Wald NJ. By how much does dietary salt reduction lower blood pressure? III – Analysis of data from trials of salt reduction. *British Medical Journal* 1991; **302**: 819–824.

MAFF. Dioxins and PCBs in fish oil dietary supplements and licensed medicines. *Food Surveillance Information Sheet* 1997; No. 106. (maff.gov.uk/food/infsheet/index.htm).

MAFF. Dioxins and PCBs in UK and imported marine fish. *Food Surveillance Information Sheet* 1999, No. 184. (maff.gov.uk/food/infsheet/index.htm)

Myers MG, Basinski A. Coffee and coronary heart disease. *Archives of Internal Medicine* 1992; **152**: 1767–1772.

NHS Centre for Reviews and Dissemination. Cholesterol and coronary heart disease: screening and treatment. *Effective Health Care* 1998; **4**: 1–16.

Omenn GS, Goodman GE, Thornquist MD *et al*. Effects of a combination of beta carotene and vitamin A on lung cancer and cardiovascular disease. *New England Journal of Medicine* 1996; **334**: 1150–1155.

Rimm EB, Klatsky A, Grobbee D, Stampfer MJ. Review of moderate alcohol consumption and reduced risk of coronary heart disease: is the effect due to beer, wine or spirits? *British Medical Journal* 1996; **312**: 731–736.

Ripsin CM, Keenan JM, Jacobs DR Jr *et al*. Oat products and lipid lowering. A meta-analysis. *Journal of the American Medical Association* 1992; **267**: 3317–3325.

Silagy C, Neil A. Garlic as a lipid lowering agent – a meta-analysis. *Journal of the Royal College of Physicians of London* 1994; **28**: 39–45.

Singh RB, Rastogi SS, Verma R *et al*. Randomised controlled trial of cardioprotective diet in patients with recent acute myocardial infarction: results of one year follow up. *British Medical Journal* 1992; **304**: 1015–1019.

Stamler J, Farinaro E, Mojonnier LM *et al*. Prevention and control of hypertension by nutritional–hygienic means. Long term experience of the Chicago Coronary Prevention Evaluation Program. *Journal of the American Medical Association* 1980; **243**: 1819–1823.

Stephens NG, Parsons A, Schofield PM *et al*. Randomised controlled trial of vitamin E in patients with coronary disease: Cambridge Heart Antioxidant Study (CHAOS). *Lancet* 1996; **347**: 781–786.

Trevisan M, Liu J, Bahsas FB, Menotti A. Syndrome X and mortality: a population based study. Risk Factor and Life Expectancy Research Group. *American Journal of Epidemiology* 1998; **148**: 958–966.

Wheeler DC. Cardiovascular risk factors in patients with chronic renal failure. *Journal of Renal Nutrition* 1997; **7**: 182–186.

Wood D, Durrington P, Poulter N *et al*. Joint British recommendations on prevention of coronary heart disease in clinical practice. *Heart* 1998; **80**: S1–S29.

World Cancer Research Fund. *Food, Nutrition and the Prevention of Cancer: A Global Perspective*. Washington DC: American Institute for Cancer Research, 1997.

4.22 Coronary heart disease

Coronary heart disease (CHD) is the most common form of cardiovascular disease. A broad overview of cardiovascular disease and the cardioprotective diet is given in Section 4.21 (Cardiovascular disease). This section focuses on the aetiology and management of CHD, and the role of the dietitian in its prevention.

4.22.1 Definitions and prevalence

CHD can present clinically in a number of different ways, which may include:

- stable angina
- unstable angina
- acute myocardial infarction (MI; 'heart attack')
- sudden death, with or without a history of angina or infarction.

The term CHD also encompasses heart failure and cachexia, which are the end stages of the disease.

CHD is a major contributor to morbidity and mortality; in the UK, more than 1.4 million people suffer from angina, and every year 300 000 have a MI and 110 000 die as result of heart disease (DH 2000). CHD is the most common cause of premature mortality in the UK, accounting for 26% and 16% of deaths under the age of 65 years in men and women, respectively (BHF 1999). It is also one of the leading causes of death for all ages, although the difference in overall mortality rate between men and women is not as great, with values 25% and 20%, respectively. Although CHD mortality rates fell over the latter part of the twentieth century, this did not occur as rapidly as in other countries. Thus, although deaths from CHD fell by 42% in adults aged 16–64 years during the 1990s, the UK continues to have one of the highest CHD mortality rates in the world (BHF 1999).

Within the UK, CHD is not distributed evenly. National statistics mask important and significant regional, socioeconomic and other variations in its prevalence and mortality. CHD is more common in Scotland, Northern Ireland and northern England, and there are substantial geographical variations within each of these areas, with particularly high rates being found in urban communities with a disproportionate number of people living on a low income (National Heart Forum 1998; Acheson 1998).

Dietary factors may contribute to these differences. Although there are only small regional differences in consumption of total and saturated fat consumption, there is much greater disparity in intakes of fruit and vegetables which are lower in Scotland, Northern Ireland and northern England. There are also significant differences in fruit and vegetable intake between socio-economic groups, with consumption being much greater in the highest income households than in the lowest (MAFF 1999). However, other influences are also clearly relevant, such as higher rates of smoking, lower physical activity levels and a greater prevalence of mental health problems among more disadvantaged groups (see Section, 3.8 People in low income groups).

Because rates of CHD are higher in men, they receive a greater proportion of available services and treatments, and this has tended to disguise the fact that CHD in women is also a serious problem. There are also difference in resources and treatments available in different geographical areas of the UK (National Heart Forum 1998).

4.22.2 Pathogenesis of coronary heart disease

The pathogenesis of CHD lies in the complex interaction of a number of processes. Both atherosclerosis and thrombosis are fundamental to the development of the disease and each is affected by diet. For ease of understanding, these two processes are described separately but in reality they are interlinked.

Atherosclerosis

The first step in the development of atherosclerosis is believed to be injury to arterial endothelium (the metabolically active 'lining' of the artery). In areas of damage, macrophages ingest low-density lipoprotein (LDL) and other atherogenic particles to form foam cells. When the macrophages die, the lipid remains in the arterial wall, accumulating over time to form a lipid core or pool (Fig. 4.7). The formation of this fatty streak is the first stage in plaque development.

Subsequent proliferation of smooth muscle cells, development of collagen strands, minor thrombi and calcification in this area of lipid accumulation then result in the formation of atherosclerotic plaque. As the plaque grows it protrudes into the lumen of the artery; it can rise above the surface plane between the ages of 20 and 30 years. The plaques are covered by a fibrous cap, which can rupture. If this happens, it triggers platelet aggregation and the formation of a blood clot.

The narrowing of the lumen of the coronary arteries as a result of plaque can lead to an inadequate oxygen supply to the myocardium (heart muscle) at times of stress

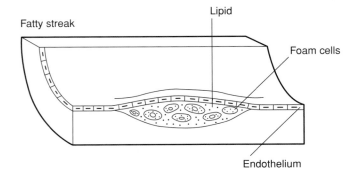

Fatty streak

Lipid

Foam cells

Endothelium

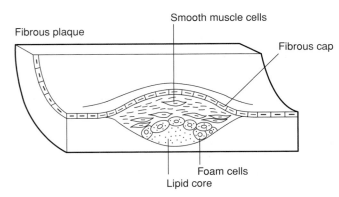

Fibrous plaque

Smooth muscle cells

Fibrous cap

Foam cells

Lipid core

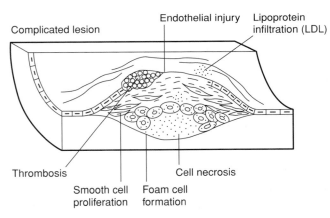

Complicated lesion

Endothelial injury

Lipoprotein infiltration (LDL)

Thrombosis

Cell necrosis

Smooth cell proliferation

Foam cell formation

Fig. 4.7 Stages of atherosclerosis.
© J. Farrington; reproduced with permission.

A description of lipoprotein metabolism and its influence on atherogenesis is given in Section 4.23 (Hyperlipidaemia). More detailed discussion of this subject can be found in Gotto and Pownall (1998).

Thrombosis

Damage to the endothelium at the micro-level, or to the cap of a plaque at the macro-level, can trigger platelet activation and coagulation. As well as being a cause of acute coronary events, thrombosis is an integral part of plaque development as thrombi can become incorporated into the structure.

The repair system is complex because the clot needs to be assembled at the site of damage and then removed when the repair is complete. Over 50 different chemicals are involved in the process, all of which are present in plasma all of the time. A shift in the balance of their activation determines whether the anticoagulants or procoagulants dominate.

There are four stages in the coagulation process (Simmons 1997):

- *Stage 1 – Vasoconstriction*: In smaller vessels this is caused by release of thromboxane A_2 and serotonin from platelets. Thromboxane also activates other platelets.
- *Stage 2 – Platelet plug formation*: Platelets become sticky when activated and form plugs which can close minute ruptures in small blood vessels. They also release active compounds such as growth factors, which promote smooth muscle cell proliferation, a stage in the process of atherosclerosis.
- *Stage 3 – Clot formation*: Platelet aggregation combines with the extrinsic and intrinsic pathways to produce a clot (Fig. 4.8). Prothrombin activator catalyses the split of prothrombin to form thrombin. This in turn causes the polymerization of fibrinogen to form fibrin threads. These form a mesh, which entraps platelets, plasma and blood cells to form the blood clot. This retracts, expressing the serum.
- *Stage 4 – Fibrinolysis*: Plasminogen is activated to produce plasmin, a proteolytic enzyme which digests the fibrin threads. A raised level of plasminogen activator inhibitor (PAI-1), which binds with the plasmin and so inhibits the process of clot breakdown, is a known risk factor for CHD.

4.22.3 Risk factors for coronary heart disease

There is no single cause of CHD and many factors can contribute to its development. Epidemiological studies and clinical trials have identified many of the major risk factors for CHD and these include physical and biochemical parameters as well as features of lifestyle and behaviour. Some risk factors, such as genetic influences, are unalterable, but many are potentially modifiable and hence are the focus of disease prevention. The principal risk factors are listed below; for more detail, the reader is referred to Ashwell (1998).

such as physical exertion. This is the cause of 'stable' angina.

Complete occlusion of the blood vessel by a thrombus (clot) will cut off the supply of oxygen to a section of the myocardium. According to the location and the extent of the occlusion this can cause 'unstable' angina or, if severe, MI, which is the death of an area of heart muscle tissue.

Plaques can vary considerably in their composition and stability and these factors are important in determining the risk of rupture and MI. Atherosclerotic plaques that are most vulnerable to rupture appear to be those which occupy an eccentric position in the arterial lumen and contain fewer collagen strands, hence making the structure less rigid.

Unmodifiable risk factors

The main unmodifiable risk factors for CHD are:

- *Age*: The risk increases with age.
- *Gender*: As a result of the protective effects of oestrogen, premenopausal women (and possibly postmenopausal women given hormone replacement therapy) have a lower prevalence of CHD than men of the same age, although this difference can disappear in some circumstances such as the coexistence of diabetes. There may also be gender differences in the clinical presentation of CHD and in the extent to which different risk factors influence its development (Schenck-Gustaffson 1996).
- *Genotype*: A family history of CHD is strongly associated with increased risk, probably due in part to genetic differences in lipid metabolism or somatotype (e.g. propensity to central or peripheral fat distribution). CHD risk is also enhanced in certain racial groups (see Section 3.9, People from ethnic minority groups).

Other unalterable environmental factors such as climate, season (CHD incidence rises in cold weather) or hardness of drinking water may also be relevant.

The risk of CHD is elevated in a number of disease states, particularly:

- diabetes mellitus
- renal disease and microalbuminuria
- stroke.

Modifiable risk factors

Modifiable factors known to influence the development of CHD include:

- smoking
- diet
- lack of physical activity
- hypertension
- hyperlipidaemia
- thrombogenic factors
- obesity, especially central obesity. Waist measurement may be a better indicator of risk than body mass index (BMI) as a high waist measurement is associated with syndrome X and endothelial dysfunction (see Section 4.21, Cardiovascular disease)
- hyperinsulinaemia
- hyperhomocysteinaemia.

Not all of these risk factors are directly causal in influence; for example, much of the effect of obesity on CHD is secondary to its consequences in terms of blood pressure, triglycerides and hyperinsulinaemia. With others such as hyperhomocystinaemia, although there is epidemiological evidence that this is a strong marker for cardiovascular disease (CVD) risk, it remains to be proven that measures which reduce blood homocysteine have a direct impact on cardiovascular morbidity and mortality (Eikelboom *et al.* 1999).

It should also be borne in mind that different risk factors confer different degrees of risk (e.g. smoking, hypertension, dyslipidaemia and diabetes have the greatest impact) and that the significance of a risk factor is affected by the presence or absence of others (e.g. the harmful effects of smoking may be compounded by a low dietary intake of antioxidants). Reducing CHD risk therefore requires multifactorial risk assessment and management (e.g. by using the chart produced by the Joint British Societies to assess the 10 year risk of CHD; Wood *et al.* 1998). Correcting one risk factor alone may have little impact on CHD risk if other risk factors are ignored (e.g. correcting raised cholesterol will be less beneficial if that person continues to smoke and be hypertensive). The benefits of diet and lifestyle change must also be considered in this context and it is vital that dietitians take a broad perspective of CHD risk which encompasses all contributory factors. The use of global risk assessment is discussed in Section 4.21.3 (Global risk assessment for cardiovascular disease).

4.22.4 Role of diet in the development of coronary heart disease

Many dietary factors may impact on the pathogenesis of CHD, although the significance of some of them remains to be determined (see Table 4.46 in Section 4.21, Cardiovascular disease). A detailed review of the subject can be found in the COMA report *Nutritional Aspects of Cardiovascular Disease* (DH 1994). The key influences are briefly summarized below.

Diet and blood lipids

Dyslipidaemia is a key risk factor in the development of CHD. The composition and concentration of the lipoprotein fractions and hence their atherogenic capacity are affected by diet. This is described in more detail in Section 4.23 (Hyperlipidaemia).

Diet and thrombogenesis

While blood cholesterol, total cholesterol: high-density lipoprotein (HDL)-cholesterol ratio and triglyceride level are all known risk factors for the development of heart disease, the levels of blood clotting factors, particularly factor VII, have been found to be better predictors of fatal MI (Meade *et al.* 1986, 1993).

The majority of blood clotting factors are inactive proteolytic enzymes which are converted into active enzymes during the process of coagulation. Once the active enzyme is formed it goes on to activate another coenzyme which in turn activates another, thus creating a cascade process which, along with a number of positive feedback loops, allows the process of coagulation to accelerate. Fig. 4.8 provides an overall summary of the process, which can be regarded as having two main components: the

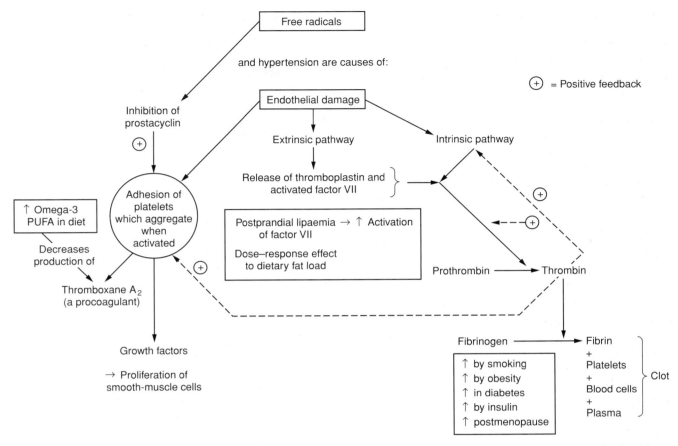

Fig. 4.8 Diet and haemostasis. This involves the complex interaction of processes. Clotting involves a number of positive feedback loops which combine to make the process fast. © J. Farrington; reproduced with permission.

aggregation of platelets and the coagulation cascade, which produces the fibrin threads that link and pull the clot together. Dietary factors that are known to influence this process include:

- *The type of fat consumed*: Omega-3 fatty acids decrease the effective concentration of thromboxane A_2, a procoagulant, and probably have other beneficial effects on thrombogenic mechanisms. The anticoagulant effect of aspirin is also achieved by inhibition of thromboxane A_2 production.
- *The amount of fat consumed*: The ingestion of dietary fat directly affects factor VII coagulant activity (a strong predictor of fatal MI in middle-aged men) (Meade *et al.* 1986), an effect which occurs for several hours postprandially and with a clear dose–response relationship (Miller 1998). However, the clinical significance of this observation remains to be established.
- *Weight loss and consequent decrease in plasma triglyceride concentration* are associated with a decrease in PAI-1 and improved fibrinolytic (clot breakdown) capacity (Marckmann *et al.* 1998).
- *Vitamin K* has long been known to have a role in haemostasis and vitamin K antagonists such as warfarin are used as anticoagulant drugs (Simmons 1997).

Vitamin K is a cofactor for the synthesis of prothrombin and the clotting factors VII, IX and X, although its impact on these factors within the normal range of dietary intake appears to be minimal. However, severe vitamin K deficiency significantly impairs blood coagulation and increases the risk of haemorrhage.

There is scant evidence of any direct impact of a dietary component on fibrinogen concentration; some of the other influences known to affect this risk factor are shown in Fig. 4.8.

Diet, antioxidants and free radicals

Free radicals are implicated in the processes of both atherosclerosis and thrombosis. The main mechanisms are currently believed to be those described in Fig. 4.9 and include:

- damage to the endothelium
- inhibition of prostacyclin and hence increase in platelet activation and aggregation
- oxidation of LDL and other atherogenic lipoproteins leading to preferential uptake by macrophages to form foam cells.

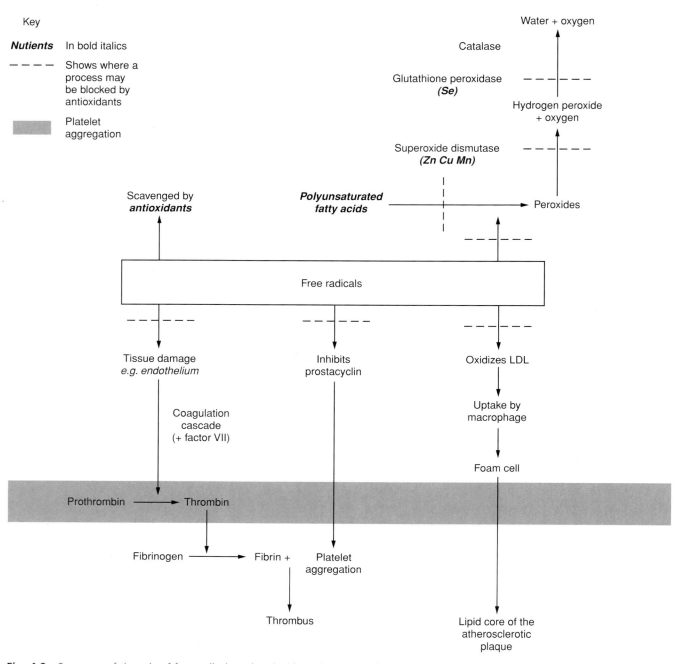

Fig. 4.9 Summary of the role of free radicals and antioxidants in coronary heart disease. © J. Farrington; reproduced with permission.

Figure 4.9 also illustrates the process by which polyunsaturated fatty acids under the influence of free radicals produce pro-oxidants.

The epidemiological and clinical trial evidence for the protective effect of antioxidant nutrients and biologically active non-nutrients such as carotenoids and flavonoids is growing. Section 4.21 on cardiovascular disease and the cardioprotective diet discusses the role and importance of fruit and vegetables in the diet and summarizes the trial evidence on antioxidant supplementation. More detail on antioxidant nutrients and biologically active non-nutrients

such as carotenoids and flavonoids can be found in Section 2.9 of the Manual.

Indirect dietary influences

As well as having direct effects on CHD development, diet can have important indirect influences, particularly as a result of its contribution to obesity and the consequent development of other risk factors such as hypertension, hypertriglyceridaemia or type 2 diabetes.

4.22.5 Management of coronary heart disease

The dietary management of CHD depends on the extent to which the disease has progressed and the way in which it is clinically treated. In the early stages, the main priority will be to achieve change to a cardioprotective diet in conjunction with other lifestyle risk reduction measures (see Section 4.21.5, The cardioprotective diet). Following a major coronary event, this objective remains the same but will need to be achieved as part of the stepwise process of cardiac rehabilitation (see Section 4.22.6, below). Invasive surgical procedures may temporarily alter dietetic priorities in favour of nutritional repletion. The development of heart failure or cachexia may necessitate permanent change in these priorities (see Section 4.22.7 and 4.22.8, below).

Understanding the medical and surgical management of CHD in terms of physical and psychological consequences (e.g. on nutritional status or patient motivation) can help to determine what these priorities should be. The types of investigation that are commonly carried out on people with suspected or confirmed CHD are summarized in Table 4.59.

Medical management of coronary heart disease

The main classes of drugs used in the prevention and management of angina and myocardial infarction are:

- antithrombotics: anticoagulants, antiplatelets, fibrinolytics
- anti-arrythmics: beta-blockers, digitalis drugs, calcium-channel blockers, amiodarone, disopyramide
- vasodilators: nitrates, angiotensin-converting enzyme (ACE) inhibitors, calcium-channel blockers
- anti-angina drugs: beta-blockers, nitrates, calcium-channel blockers
- antihypertensives: diuretics, ACE inhibitors, beta-blockers, calcium-channel blockers (see Section 4.24 Hypertension)
- antihyperlipidaemics: statins, fibrates (see Section 4.23, Hyperlipidaemia)

- management of heart failure: diuretics, ACE inhibitors, digoxin, beta-blockers.

Digitalis drugs

Digitalis drugs, such as digoxin and digitoxin are derived from the leaves of plants in the foxglove family. They are cardiac glycosides and give symptomatic relief for arrhythmias, e.g. atrial fibrillation, and for heart failure. They reduce the flow of electrical impulses in the heart and so reduce the heart rate. They also increase the force of contraction in the myocardium. These drugs are potentially toxic, more so in hypokalaemia, thus careful monitoring is required particularly when they are taken in conjunction with diuretics.

Beta-blockers

These are used in the treatment of hypertension, angina, arrythmia and heart failure. As they block the stimulating action of noradrenaline they reduce the force and speed of myocardial contraction and cause peripheral vasoconstriction. They have a number of side-effects including an adverse effect on the lipid profile.

Vasodilators

An effect of vasodilatation is to reduce the workload for the heart, thus these drugs are used in the treatment of hypertension, angina and heart failure. The main types of vasodilators are:

- nitrates, e.g. isosorbide dinitrate, glyceryl trinitrate (GTN), which can be taken as a sublingual tablet or spray as a prophylactic or for symptomatic relief of angina
- ACE inhibitors
- calcium-channel blockers.

The nitrates and calcium-channel blockers work by inhibiting smooth muscle contraction in the vessel walls. The ACE inhibitors act by reducing production of angiotensin II, a potent vasoconstrictor, and increasing bradykinin, a vasoconstrictor and growth promoter. Side-effects of vasodilators may include flushing, headaches and dizziness.

Antithrombotics

These may comprise drugs which:

Table 4.59 Investigative procedures for coronary heart disease

Investigation	Description
Electrocardiogram (ECG)	Monitors the progressive electrical stimulation of the heart muscle
Exercise stress testing	ECG recorded whilst the patient is exercising and having symptoms. It can assess whether pain on exertion is due to heart disease
24 hour ECG recording or 'Holter monitoring'	Monitoring during everyday activity including that which produces symptoms
Echocardiography	Ultrasound is used to provide a picture of the heart. It can also be used to measure the speed of blood flow
Electrophysiology studies	Used to study arrhythmia
Angiogram	Radio-opaque fluid is infused into the heart and major vessels. It reveals the outline of the lumen of the coronary arteries and hence the extent of atheromatous disease. It is used in the process of decision making about coronary artery bypass grafting and angioplasty

- *Reduce platelet aggregation*: Aspirin inhibits thromboxane production via inhibition of the enzyme cyclo-oxygenase and hence has an antiplatelet action. Clopidogrel, which inhibits platelet ADP receptors, and dipyridamole also reduce platelet aggregation.
- *Inhibit blood coagulation*: An anticoagulant can prevent formation of a blood clot or stabilise an existing clot to prevent embolism. Heparin may be given intravenously in acute situations e.g. post-surgery. Oral anticoagulants such as warfarin are used on a longer term basis for those at risk of thrombosis; dosages have to be carefully calculated and clotting times monitored.
- *Have a thrombolytic effect*: Thrombolytic drugs are used to dissolve existing clots and are routinely administered to people immediately post-MI to treat coronary thrombosis. They can also be administered directly into a blocked vessel. Both streptokinase and tissue plasminogen activator (tPA) act by increasing plasmin, the enzyme which breaks down fibrin. Alteplase, administered intravenously, is also used.

Surgical management of coronary heart disease

Following an angiogram (see Table 4.59) patients may be referred on for angioplasty and coronary artery bypass graft (CABG).

Angioplasty

A balloon is inflated at the site where blood flow through the arterial lumen has been significantly reduced as a result of atherosclerotic plaque. Once in position the balloon is inflated to increase the size of the arterial lumen. In some cases a small stent (a mesh tube that can be expanded to hold the artery open) is inserted.

Coronary artery bypass graft

In this surgical procedure, one or more diseased coronary arteries are bypassed. Blood vessels, usually taken from the leg, are grafted on to the existing coronary arteries to bypass the occluded section. Access to the heart is gained via the sternum, which is broken in the process. The procedure usually lasts for 3–4 hours. CABG is a major surgical procedure with all the metabolic and nutritional consequences which this implies (see Section 5.6, Surgery). It should also be borne in mind that, since some people will be advised by the surgical team to lose weight prior to the procedure, some will undergo surgery in a nutritionally depleted state as a result of inappropriate crash dieting.

4.22.6 Cardiac rehabilitation

Following a MI and/or corrective procedures such as angioplasty or CABG, patients undergo cardiac rehabilitation. This can be divided into a four phase process, as described by the British Association for Cardiac Rehabilitation (Coats and McGee 1995):

1 The in-patient stay
2 Immediate post-discharge phase
3 Intermediate post-discharge phase
4 Long-term maintenance.

The length of each phase will vary according to individual clinical needs and circumstances.

Phase 1: The in-patient stay

Post-myocardial interaction

A. In the Coronary Care Unit (CCU)	timescale: 24–48 hours
B. On a medical ward	timescale: variable, typically 3 days.

Post-coronary artery bypass graft

A. In cardiac surgical unit (intensive care)	timescale: 24 hours +
B. On the cardiac surgical ward	timescale: 5–7 days.

At this stage, dietary education can begin to some extent, but the ability of both patients and their families to assimilate information will be severely impaired by trauma. Immediately following a cardiac event or surgery, a patient is likely to be too unwell or too anxious to be receptive to dietary advice. Diet and lifestyle guidance is often given after 4 or 5 days, or immediately prior to discharge, but it should be borne in mind that many patients will be unable to recall information given to them at this time and may not even remember having seen a dietitian at all. People seen initially at this stage require follow-up. The carers may be very interested in information at this stage but the learning process is also likely to be hampered by stress and anxiety.

Following major cardiac surgery, the immediate dietary objectives (to restore recent energy and nutrient losses) may be quite different from the longer term aims (e.g. to reduce fat intake). Some patients may require oral nutritional support measures and hence 'healthy heart' food choices from the hospital menu may not be appropriate at this stage. Good communication between dietetic and nursing/medical staff is essential to ensure that the nutritional objectives are understood and that patients are given food which is appropriate for their nutritional needs.

Following MI, blood glucose levels are likely to be raised but this is not indicative of diabetes. Blood lipid concentrations are also likely to be adversely affected and a fasting lipid profile should be repeated at least 10 weeks post-MI.

Phase 2: Immediate post-discharge phase

This will last for 4–6 weeks and is a time of adjustment in which the patient begins to come to terms with events and their consequences for the family. In addition to their physical condition, people are concerned about the impact of events on employment and their economic circumstances. There may be little contact at this time with the cardiac rehabilitation team, particularly the dietitian.

Phase 3: Intermediate post-discharge phase

A formal cardiac rehabilitation outpatient programme typically lasts for 6 weeks; it is usually, but not exclusively, hospital based. A dietitian may see the patient in group sessions and individually. The patient's partner or carer should also be involved since they have an important role in helping the patient to implement and maintain the diet and lifestyle measures necessary for secondary prevention.

Cardiac rehabilitation programmes vary in their content according to the clinical circumstances and age and gender profile of the group being targeted. As well as a controlled exercise programme, most will also include sessions encompassing information about their condition and therapy, stress management and lifestyle changes, including dietary therapy.

Phase 4: Long-term maintenance

The role of the dietitian at this stage is to:

- monitor the effectiveness of the advice given in the context of overall risk factor reduction
- continue to facilitate change to a cardioprotective diet by helping to overcome barriers to change or difficulties experienced.

In many areas, lack of dietetic services may mean that there is little direct contact between patient and dietitian at this stage of follow-up. In these circumstances dietetic input should focus on the nutrition education of health professionals to ensure that dietary aspects of cardiac rehabilitation are not overlooked. Close liaison with primary health care teams is particularly important.

Details of the cardioprotective diet for the secondary prevention of CHD are given in Section 4.21.5.

4.22.7 Congestive cardiac failure

This is the end stage of diseases of the heart including CHD and is a significant cause of morbidity and mortality. It is estimated that up to 2% of the population may be affected, the incidence rising exponentially over the age of 65 years and approximating doubling in each subsequent decade of age. Heart failure currently accounts for about 5% of medical ward admissions in the UK, a figure which is increasing (BHF 1999).

Heart failure results from damage to the heart and may be caused by:

- myocardial infarction and ischaemic heart disease
- viral damage
- prolonged hypertension
- injury

- valvular heart disease
- alcohol abuse.

The physical effects include:

- inadequate cardiac output
- fluid imbalance
- pulmonary and other oedema
- dyspnoea
- fatigue.

Heart failure is a progressive condition and is classified into four stages according to the severity of symptoms. The annual mortality rate of people in the highest stages is 25–50%. The prognosis of congestive cardiac failure can be determined by the concentration of atrial naturetic peptide (ANP), a hormone released by the failing heart (Gibbs *et al*. 2000).

Medical management of heart failure

Medical management is by a variable combination of oxygen and drug therapy, typically ACE inhibitors, diuretics, beta-blockers and digitalis drugs.

ACE inhibitors improve morbidity, quality of life and exercise tolerance, and prolong survival when the heart failure arises from left ventricular systolic dysfunction. They can prevent or delay the onset of symptomatic heart failure in those with asymptomatic left ventricular systolic dysfunction. Angiotensin II type 1 receptor agonists have similar effects and can be used if people have unacceptable side-effects to ACE inhibitors.

Diuretics remove fluid that has accumulated in the tissues and lungs, so reducing blood volume, this in turn reduces the workload for the heart. They provide symptomatic relief but do not appear to improve prognosis.

Digoxin can be used to control ventricular rate in those with atrial fibrillation and heart failure, and also in those people whose heart failure is secondary to impaired left ventricular systolic function.

Beta-blockers may be used in conjunction with ACE inhibitors and diuretics in those with a chronic stable condition.

Surgical management of heart failure

This may involve:

- *Heart transplantation*, although a shortage of donor organs means that many potential recipients are unable to benefit from this.
- *Cardiomyoplasty*: This involves the transposition of electrically transformed, fatigue-resistant skeletal muscle on to the heart.
- *Mechanical support*: In a small proportion of patients whose condition is life threatening or who are on a waiting list for transplantation, a mechanical device may be implanted to assist cardiac function.
- *Dialysis*: This can be used to reduce left ventricular volume. Acute peritoneal dialysis or CAPD may be used in patients awaiting transplantation.

Dietetic management of congestive heart failure

The combination of reduced nutrient intake and increased requirements places the person with heart failure at risk of malnutrition. The therapeutic aims of dietary management are to:

- reduce the workload for the heart
- provide a nutritionally adequate diet
- be appropriate for the management of any underlying disease processes as well as heart failure

The principal dietary features are likely to include:

- *Sodium restriction*: This can usually be confined to the avoidance of high salt foods and not adding salt to food. In some circumstances further restrictions may be necessary but should not be imposed lightly because of the likely reduction in dietary palatability and possibly compromised intake of energy and essential nutrients.
- *Fluid restriction*: Patients who require fluid restriction are often severely anorexic, and the combination of the two increases the risk of nutritional needs not being met. Dietitians need to work closely with the other members of the care team to ensure that nutrition is an integral part of management, not an after-thought.
- *Maintaining an appropriate energy intake*: Energy intake needs to be sufficient to meet nutritional needs and prevent deterioration in nutritional status. However, excessive body mass increases the cardiac workload, and weight gain from increased fat stores should be avoided. Gain in adiposity should be distinguished from short-term fluctuations in body weight caused by changes in fluid balance (see Section 1.8.2, in Assessment of nutritional status).
- *Maintaining nutritional adequacy*: Particular attention should be paid to micronutrient intake since the use of diuretic and other drugs may result in significant urinary losses of potassium, water-soluble vitamins, etc. Since appetite is often poor, the diet may need to be relatively nutrient dense and meal frequency may need to be increased. Social factors such as support for food purchasing and preparation, particularly if the patient lives alone, should not be overlooked.

4.22.8 Cardiac cachexia

Prolonged cardiac insufficiency and heart failure can lead to cardiac cachexia with resulting malnutrition. The enlarged and labouring heart cannot maintain a sufficient blood and hence oxygen and nutrient supply for normal cellular function. For example, there may be insufficient oxygen supply to the bone marrow for adequate red blood cell production or to fuel respiratory function. The cachectic state is a strong independent risk factor for patients with chronic heart failure (Anker *et al.* 1997).

Dietary management of cardiac cachexia

These patients require active nutritional support measures;

an increase of 20–50% in basal energy requirements may be indicated. The levels of sodium and fluid restriction and micronutrient needs should be discussed with the referring clinician. Micronutrient requirements are affected by the hypermetabolic state, malabsorption and requirements for tissue rebuilding. The loss of lean body mass can lead to an increase in symptoms and decrease in capacity for exercise.

Anorexia is a feature of the condition that is exacerbated by

- dyspnoea: increases fatigue during eating, and swallowing exacerbates the symptoms of dyspnoea
- oedema
- palatability of food
- drug reactions
- depression.

Dietitians are gradually becoming more involved in the management of heart failure, and at an earlier stage, but this is variable across the country. Since the number of hospital admissions is increasing, it is likely that its management will adopt a rising profile in the clinical dietetic caseload. There is a need for further investigation and research into the role of diet therapy in the management of heart failure.

4.22.9 Public health prevention strategies for coronary heart disease

The multifactorial nature of CHD is reflected in public health strategy. In 1999, the government's report *Our Healthier Nation* (DH 1999) set out the national policy on public health. This included the target: 'To reduce the death rate from coronary heart disease and stroke and related diseases in people under 75 years by at least two fifths by 2010'.

The key features of *Our Healthier Nation* are that:

- It states the need to tackle the root causes of ill health.
- It recognizes that social and economic factors affect health and that government has to take action as some factors affecting risk of heart disease are out of people's control.
- Inequalities exist in morbidity and mortality, with poorer people suffering disproportionately.
- It outlines a national contract including the role of government, local agencies and communities, and people in addressing the environmental, lifestyle, social and economic factors in CHD.

The recognition of the considerable inequalities that exist in the prevalence of CHD and the need to tackle these represent a shift in policy from the previous national strategy for health outlined in *The Health of the Nation* (DH 1992).

The National Service Framework

The National Service Framework (NSF) for CHD (DH 2000) describes the programme for achieving the *Our Healthi-*

er Nation targets on CHD and stroke. It encompasses both clinical and public-health approaches to addressing CHD prevention.

The NSF defines 12 standards covering primary and secondary prevention, diagnosis and treatment. It sets out the milestones and goals to enable the programme to be monitored. The role of diet, but not the dietitian, is highlighted as a factor in population-based strategies, in work with high risk populations and in cardiac rehabilitation. The NSF requires the development and implementation of effective local policies to promote healthy eating and to reduce overweight and obesity. The standards on primary prevention highlight the importance of reducing inequalities in the risk of developing CHD and supports the use of community development strategies and projects to address this.

The NSF states that people with existing CVD or a risk greater than 30% should receive information and personalized advice on diet, which should be systematically documented. Cardiac rehabilitation services should have staff trained in dietary interventions. Other dietary aspects of management such as the need to avoid 'aggravating' dietary factors such as salt and alcohol in people with heart failure are briefly mentioned, although others such as the role of diet and nutritional support following surgical procedures are not. The focus is primarily on medical management.

Primary Care Groups, Health Authorities and Trusts are required to develop action plans for tackling CHD which are related to a 'local equity profile'. This includes the provision of dietetic services. For example, do referral rates for diet therapy match patterns of prevalence of CHD? Are proportionally more patients referred from practices in areas with higher standardized mortality rates for premature CHD? The NSF standard requiring that CHD registers be developed will enhance the ability to evaluate the provision of dietetic services.

Dietitians clearly have a role in supporting the implementation of the NSF at a policy and strategy level and in the organization and delivery of clinical services. Guidance for implementing the preventative aspects for the NSF has been produced by the Health Development Agency for the Department of Health (HDA 2000).

Health improvement programmes

Health improvement programmes define a local action plan for tackling heart disease. They are to be agreed and shared by local authorities, voluntary agencies, health authorities and health service providers alike.

An understanding of public health strategy is of particular relevance to a NHS dietetic department when

- planning standards, audit and clinical governance
- reporting on service provision to Primary Care Group and Health Authority
- setting priorities and objectives for service devel-opment.

It is important that dietetic departments examine whether their services are provided on an equitable basis, and are driven by patients' needs and health priorities.

The role of the dietitian in prevention of coronary heart disease

Dietitians have a multifaceted role in CHD prevention, which may include:

- advising on public health policy and strategy
- planning and implementing health promotion campaigns
- supporting food projects using principles of community development
- multi-agency work to enhance the local food economy
- training other health professionals involved in the care of cardiac patients
- organizing cardiac rehabilitation programmes for groups of people
- providing diet and lifestyle guidance for individuals at risk of, or with existing, heart disease
- ensuring that the nutritional management of surgical patients and people with cardiac failure and cachexia is appropriate and that appropriate nutritional support measures are implemented when necessary.

Text revised by: Jo Farrington and Briony Thomas in conjunction with the UK Heart Health and Thoracic Dietitians

Useful addresses

See Section 4.21, Cardiovascular disease.

Further reading

Department of Health. *Low Income, Food, Nutrition and Health, Strategies for Improvement*. Report by the Low Income Project Team for the Nutrition Task Force. London: DH, 1996.

Kinney MR, Packa DR. *Andreoli's Comprehensive Cardiac Care*, 8th edn. St Louis: Mosby, 1996.

McGlone P, Dobson B, Dowler E, Nelson M. *Food Projects and How they Work*. York: Joseph Rowntree Foundation, 1999.

National Food Alliance. *Food Poverty: What are the Policy Options?* Discussion Paper. London: NFA (now Sustain), 1998.

National Food Alliance. *Making Links, A Toolkit for Local Food Projects*. London: NFA (Sustain), 1999.

Roe L, Hunt P, Bradshaw H, Rayner M. *Health Promotion Interventions to Promote Healthy Eating in the General Population: A Review*. Health Promotion Effectiveness Reviews 1997, No. 6. London: Health Education Authority. (This is one of a series of effectiveness reviews produced by the Health Education Authority, which became the Health Development Agency in 2000.)

Vaughan A. *The Food Indicators Toolkit*. London: NFA (Sustain), 1999.

References

Acheson D. *Inequalities in Health: An Independent Inquiry*. London: The Stationery Office, 1998.

Anker SD, Ponikowski P, Varney S *et al*. Wasting as independent risk factor for mortality in chronic heart failure. *Lancet* 1997; **349**: 1050–1053.

Ashwell M (E.d.) *Diet and Heart Disease: A Round Table of Risk*

Factors, 2nd edn. London: Chapman and Hall for the British Nutrition Foundation, 1998.

British Heart Foundation (BHF) Statistics Database. *Coronary Heart Disease Statistics*. London: BHF, 1999.

Coats A, McGee H. *BACR Guidelines for Cardiac Rehabilitation*. Oxford: Blackwell Science, 1995.

Department of Health. *Health of the Nation: A Strategy for Health in England*. London: HMSO, 1992.

Department of Health, Committee on Medical Aspects of Food Policy. *Nutritional Aspects of Cardiovascular Disease*. Reports on Health and Social Subjects 46. London: HMSO, 1994.

Department of Health. *Our Healthier Nation: Saving Lives*. London: DH, 1999.

Department of Health. *National Service Framework for CHD: Modern Standards and Service Models*. London: DH, 2000.

Eikelboom JW, Lonn E, Genest J Jr *et al*. Homocyst(e)ine and cardiovascular disease: a critical review of the epidemiologic evidence. *Annals of Internal Medicine* 1999; **131**: 363–375.

Gibbs CR, Davies MK, Lip GYH. *ABC of Heart Failure*. London: BMJ Books, 2000.

Gotto AM, Pownall H. *Manual of Lipid Disorders – Reducing the Risk for CHD*, 2nd edn. New York: Lippincott, Williams and Wilkins, 1998.

Health Development Agency (HDA) *Coronary Heart Disease – Guidance for Implementing the Preventative Aspects of the National Service Framework*. London: HDA, 2000. Available from: www.hda-online.org/pubhealth.htm

MAFF. *The National Food Survey, 1998*. London: The Stationery Office, 1999.

Marckmann P, Toubro S, Astrup A. Sustained improvement in blood lipids, coagulation and fibrinolysis after major weight loss in obese subjects. *European Journal of Clinical Nutrition* 1998; **52**: 329–333.

Meade TW, Mellows S, Brozovic M *et al*. Haemostatic function and ischaemic heart disease: principal results of the Northwick Park Heart Study. *Lancet* 1986; **ii**: 533–537.

Meade TW, Ruddock V, Stirling Y *et al*. Fibrinolytic activity, clotting factors, and the long-term incidence of ischaemic heart disease in the Northwick Park Heart Study. *Lancet* 1993; **342**: 1076–1079.

Miller GJ. Effects of diet composition on coagulation pathways. *American Journal of Clinical Nutrition* 1998; **67** (3 Suppl): 542S–545S.

National Heart Forum. *Social Inequalities in CHD, Opportunities for Action*. Sharp I (Ed.). London: The Stationery Office, 1998.

Schenck-Gustafsson K. Risk factors for cardiovascular disease in women: assessment and management. *European Heart Journal* 1996; **17** (Suppl D): 2–8.

Simmons A. *Hematology – A Combined Theoretical and Technical Approach*, 2nd edn. London: Butterworth-Heinneman (now Arnold), 1997.

Wood D, Durrington P, Poulter N *et al*. Joint British recommendations on prevention of coronary heart disease in clinical practice. *Heart* 1998; **80**: S1–S29.

4.23 Hyperlipidaemia

Hyperlipidaemia (dyslipidaemia or hyperlipoprotein-aemia) means the presence of abnormal blood concentrations of lipids (cholesterol and/or triglycerides) or the lipoproteins that transport them. The clinical significance of hyperlipidaemia depends on the total level of lipids in the blood, the lipid level associated with particular lipoprotein fractions and the overall cardiovascular risk.

4.23.1 Lipid metabolism

Lipids such as cholesterol and triglyceride are essential substrates for many body processes. Cholesterol is a structural component of cell membranes and nerve sheaths and is required for the synthesis of steroid and adrenocortical hormones and bile acids. Triglyceride is required as an energy source, its constituent fatty acids and glycerol either being immediately metabolized or reconstituted into triglyceride and stored to meet future energy needs.

Lipids such as cholesterol and triglyceride are insoluble in water and are therefore transported in blood bound to proteins (apoproteins or apolipoproteins). These water-soluble complexes are called lipoproteins. Lipid metabolism is the process by which the initially large, lipid-filled, low-density complexes transporting either diet derived or endogenously synthesized lipids undergo gradual conversion to smaller, denser particles rich in protein and phospholipid prior to their utilization or excretion. Lipid metabolism is a complex process under the control and influence of many factors, the details of which are beyond the scope of this book but are summarized in Fig. 4.10. Measurement of blood lipids reveals much about the way in which the process is operating, and the concentrations found have pathological implications.

Since lipoprotein particles change in lipid content during the course of their metabolism, they can be classified by density:

- *Chylomicrons* are the form in which lipids consumed in the diet are absorbed from the gastrointestinal tract. As these large, lipid-rich particles circulate round the body, their triglyceride is gradually removed by skeletal muscle cells and adipose tissue under the influence of lipoprotein lipase. The chylomicron remnants are taken up by the liver and reassembled into new lipoproteins.
- *Very low-density lipoproteins (VLDL)* are constructed by the liver from chylomicron remnants and comprised mainly of triglyceride. VLDL maintain a supply of triglyceride for energy production to body tissues in the fasting state.

- *Intermediate-density lipoproteins (IDL)* are derived from partially degraded VLDL. They are short-lived intermediates.
- *Low-density lipoproteins (LDL)* are derived from VLDL. As the triglyceride is removed by body cells, the remaining cholesterol is concentrated within LDL for transfer to the peripheral tissues. Sixty per cent of total circulating cholesterol is contained within LDL. High concentrations of LDL cholesterol are a risk factor for coronary heart disease (CHD).
- *High-density lipoproteins (HDL)* are small, dense particles derived from chylomicron hydrolysis, and comprised of protein, cholesterol and phospholipid. They have an important role transporting cholesterol from cells back to the liver. Because HDL is associated with cholesterol removal, high concentrations are beneficial and inversely related to CHD.

Although convenient, this system of classification can give the impression that VLDL and LDL are completely different entities, whereas in reality they are artificial cut-off points in a continuous process of triglyceride removal and cholesterol accretion. Recently, subclassifications have been introduced to define and identify the more atherogenic subfractions of these particles. For example, within the classification of LDL there are some smaller, denser particles whose uptake into the endothelium is independent of receptors, thus bypassing an important control mechanism. These particles are also preferentially taken up by macrophages, particularly if oxidized, thus increasing the formation of foam cells, an initial step in the process of atherogenesis (see Section 4.22, Coronary heart disease). This type of small, dense LDL is often associated with elevated triglyceride levels, and may be one means by which high triglycerides become an independent risk factor for cardiovascular disease (Stampfer *et al.* 1996).

4.23.2 Prognostic significance of hyperlipidaemia

Both the total amounts of lipids in the blood, and the amounts associated with the various lipoprotein fractions, have prognostic significance.

Blood cholesterol

Raised blood cholesterol is, along with smoking and hypertension, one of the three principal risk factor for cardiovascular disease (Martin *et al.* 1986). Reducing total

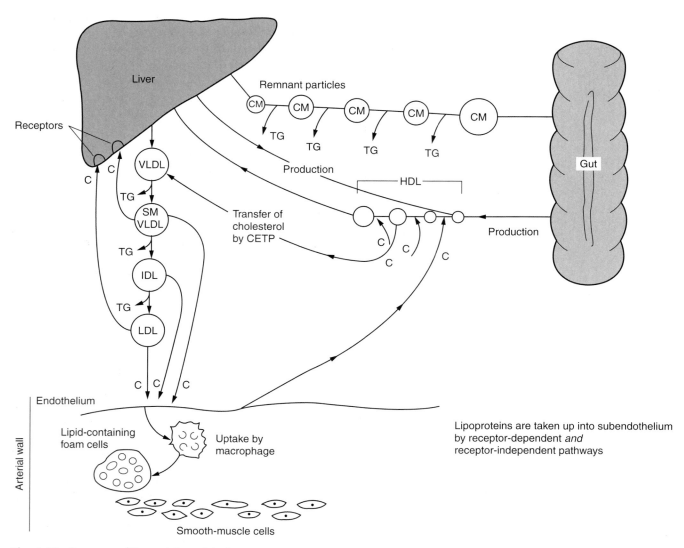

Fig. 4.10 Summary of lipoprotein metabolism.
C: cholesterol; TG: triglyceride; CM: chylomicron; VLDL: very low-density lipoprotein; SMVLDL: small very low-density lipoprotein; IDL: intermediate-density lipoprotein; LDL: low-density lipoprotein; HDL: high-density lipoprotein; CETP: cholesterol ester transfer protein.
© J. Farrington; reproduced with permission.

cholesterol level reduces cardiovascular risk. On a population basis, a 1% reduction in blood cholesterol is associated with a 3% reduction in CHD risk (DH 1994). The magnitude of this relationship is affected by age: a 10% reduction in blood cholesterol (equivalent to 0.6 mmol/l) has been associated with a 54% reduction in the incidence of CHD at 40 years and a 19% reduction at 80 years (Law *et al*. 1994). However, this does not negate the potential benefits of cholesterol reduction in older people because the risk of CHD also rises with age; in absolute terms, the benefits may be as great as in younger people (British Dietetic Association 1998).

However, since blood cholesterol concentration is only one of many factors which influences the development of CHD, it is not always a good predictor of individual CHD risk. A raised level poses a greater threat to an individual at high CHD risk than to someone at low risk. Similarly,

the benefits from cholesterol reduction in a particular individual will be affected by whether, for example, that person continues to smoke or have high blood pressure. It is increasingly recognized that effective prevention of cardiovascular disease requires multifactorial risk assessment and intervention (see Section 4.21, Cardiovascular disease). For this reason, blood lipid measurements must always be considered in the context of other risk factors and not in isolation.

The prognostic significance of blood cholesterol is primarily with that carried in the LDL fraction, as this reflects the level of cholesterol being transported to the tissues. HDL-cholesterol (a much smaller proportion of total blood cholesterol) reflects cholesterol removal, and high levels are therefore beneficial. The ratio of total: HDL-cholesterol is an important indicator of CHD risk (Wood *et al*. 1998).

Triglyceride

Until fairly recently it was thought that observed associations between blood triglyceride concentration and CHD risk simply reflected the more powerful predictive value of low HDL-cholesterol levels (which are inversely related to VLDL triglyceride). There is now evidence of a significant and independent association between serum triglyceride concentrations and the incidence of major coronary events (Assmann *et al*. 1996; Stampfer *et al*. 1996). A meta-analysis controlling for HDL-cholesterol suggested that for every 1 mmol/l rise in serum triglyceride concentration, the relative risk of CHD increased by 14% in men and 37% in women (Hokanson and Austin 1996). LDL particle size may be an additional important factor (Austin *et al*. 1998). Angiographic studies have shown that reducing triglyceride levels can slow the rate of progression of atheroma (Ericsson *et al*. 1996). Primary prevention trials to ascertain the clinical significance of such interventions are in progress.

4.23.3 Diagnosis and classification of hyperlipidaemia

Measurement of blood lipids

Analytical methods of determining blood lipid levels have improved in recent years, reducing measurement error within laboratories. However, significant differences can still occur between laboratories, so dietitians need to be aware of local reference ranges. The type and number of lipid measurements made will depend on the clinical circumstances. Measurements may be confined to the total levels of cholesterol and triglyceride in the blood. A more detailed picture will be provided by a lipid profile which provides information on the concentration of lipid associated with each lipoprotein fraction.

Total blood cholesterol

Measurements can be made in either the fed or fasted state since the level is relatively unaffected by a meal. However, if the triglyceride concentration or lipoprotein cholesterol is to be measured as well, fasting samples will be required (see below).

Total cholesterol fluctuates over the course of days or weeks, so a diagnosis of hypercholesterolaemia should not be based on a single measurement. It is recommended that three separate cholesterol measurements are made before the diagnosis is confirmed (Wood *et al*. 1998).

Illness can also affect blood cholesterol. A recent myocardial infarction, infection and surgery can reduce total cholesterol levels by as much as 2–3 mmol/l. Both mental and physical ill health can lead to a reduced food intake, which in turn can decrease blood cholesterol concentration over a period of time.

LDL and HDL

Fasting samples are advisable for the measurement of lipoprotein cholesterol measurements because the small amount of cholesterol contained in chylomicrons and VLDL may influence the results.

LDL cholesterol can be estimated using the Friedwald formula:

$$\text{LDL cholesterol} = \text{Total cholesterol} - \text{HDL-cholesterol} - \frac{(\text{Triglyceride})}{2.2}.$$

This formula is applicable when triglyceride levels are less than 4.5 mmol/l. If triglyceride levels are significantly above this level, the cholesterol present in VLDL and chylomicron particles will distort the calculation.

Total blood triglycerides

These are raised following a meal so measurements need to be made in a fasting or pre-prandial state. Repeated measurements are also advisable since transitory changes in triglyceride concentration can follow recent alteration in alcohol or carbohydrate consumption.

Normal and desirable reference ranges for blood lipids are shown in Table 4.60.

Interpretation of lipid measurements

Blood lipid measurements must not be interpreted on the basis of numerical values alone but always in the context of overall cardiovascular disease (CVD) risk (Betteridge *et al*. 1993). This is particularly important in the primary care setting where routine health checks will often discover a 'raised total cholesterol', with no additional information on triglyceride level or lipoprotein profile. All patients with an elevated lipid level should be assessed for CVD risk (e.g. using the Joint British Societies CHD Risk Assessment Chart; Wood *et al*. 1998), and diet and lifestyle advice (and possibly other therapeutic indications) tailored to these needs.

The possibility of secondary factors either causing or exacerbating the hyperlipidaemia should also be considered. Some of these influences are summarized in Table 4.61.

Clinical features of hyperlipidaemia

Hyperlipidaemia is usually symptomless and hence often remains undiagnosed. Specific signs and symptoms usually only occur if the elevation in lipid level is particularly severe.

Table 4.60 Blood lipid reference ranges

	Normal reference range (mmol/l)	Suggested ideal level[1] (mmol/l)
Total cholesterol	3.5–7.8	<5.0
LDL-cholesterol	2.3–6.1	<3.0
HDL-cholesterol	0.8–1.7	>1.0
Triglycerides	0.7–1.8	<2.3

[1]Joint British Guidelines (Wood *et al*. 1998).

Table 4.61 Secondary causes of disordered lipid metabolism

Secondary causes	Associated with raised cholesterol	Associated with raised triglyceride
Dietary factors	High intake of saturated fatty acids	Obesity Excessive energy intake Diet high in refined carbohydrate Excessive alcohol intake
Hormonal disorders/influences	Hypothyroidism Cushing's syndrome Oral contraception	Hypothyroidism Diabetes mellitus (either poorly controlled or undiagnosed) Pregnancy Oral contraception/hormonal replacement therapy
Disease	Chronic liver disease Nephrotic syndrome Cholestasis	Chronic renal failure Pancreatitits
Eating disorders	Anorexia nervosa	Bulimia nervosa
Therapeutic drugs	Beta-blockers Diuretics	Glucocorticoids

Very high cholesterol levels may result in:

- *xanthomata*: small soft deposits of cholesterol, sometimes seen as a uniform thickening of the Achilles tendon or as nodules in the tendons of the fingers (tendon xanthomata). Palmar xanthomata may be seen as yellow lines in the palmar creases. Tuberose xanthomata occur in the form of masses around the elbows or knees
- *corneal arcus*: a white ring visible around the coloured part of the eye
- *xanthelasma*: small, soft, yellow deposits of cholesterol and other fatty substances found in the skin, often on the eyelids
- *premature CHD* and/or peripheral vascular disease.

Very high triglyceride levels may result in:

- *eruptive xanthomata*: small, yellow, skin nodules on faintly erythematous base
- *lipaemia retinalis*: plasma lipids visible in the retinal veins
- *acute pancreatitis*.

Classification of hyperlipidaemia

The classification and definitions of hyperlipidaemia vary. Primary disorders of lipid metabolism are still sometimes categorized on the basis of elevated lipoprotein fraction by the Frederickson classification (Table 4.62), but this is now used less often.

More commonly, primary hyperlipidaemias are classified into three main types:

- familial hypercholesterolaemia (FH)
- polygenic hypercholesterolaemia
- familial combined hyperlipidaemia (FCH).

Familial hypercholesterolaemia

This is a genetic disorder caused by an autosomal polymorphic dominant gene and which dramatically increases the risk of premature CHD. Its effects can usually be detected in early childhood. The LDL-cholesterol concentration is typically elevated two- to three-fold as a result of genetic failure of LDL receptors, reducing their functional capacity to around 50% of normal. In homozygous individuals, plasma cholesterol levels may be as high as 30 mmol/l; in the more common heterozygous form, the typical LDL-cholesterol range is 10–20 mmol/l. FH is often accompanied by evidence of cholesterol deposition in tissues such as xanthomata.

The prevalence of heterozygous FH is believed to be 1 in 500. Many of these patients remain undiagnosed until CHD becomes clinically evident, sometimes as early as the age of 35 years. FH accounts for about 5% of the premature mortality from CHD in Europe and the USA.

Polygenic hypercholesterolaemia

This is the most common form of raised total and LDL-cholesterol levels (with normal HDL-cholesterol and triglyceride levels). Its prevalence is greater than that of FH but LDL-cholesterol is elevated to a lesser extent and clinical manifestations such as xanthomas are rare.

Familial combined hyperlipidaemia (FCH)

This is a common disorder characterized by raised VLDL triglycerides and LDL-cholesterol. The condition is associated with an increased risk of CHD and is usually diagnosed in adulthood. People with FCH are often hypertensive and overweight and may also have diabetes or gout.

4.23.4 Dietary influence on blood lipids

Many aspects of diet affect blood lipids and can contribute to hyperlipidaemia.

Dietary fat and fatty acids

In the short term, the consumption of a fat-containing meal has most effect on blood triglycerides. Triglyceride-rich chylomicrons will enter the bloodstream and VLDL triglyceride production by the liver will temporarily cease. Depending

Table 4.62 The Frederickson classification of hyperlipoproteinaemias

Type	Lipoprotein(s) elevated	Serum cholesterol	Serum triglyceride	Primary (genetic) causes	Secondary causes	Notes
I	Chylomicrons	Normal or slightly raised	Very high	1 Lipoprotein lipase deficiency 2 Apoprotein C II deficiency (Apoprotein C II activates lipoprotein lipase)	Alcoholism	Rare As a result of 1 and 2, chylomicrons cannot be broken down, so levels are grossly elevated
IIA	LDL	Raised	Normal	Familial hypercholesterolaemia 1 Homozygous form is severe 2 Heterozygous form mild to moderately severe Apoprotein beta-receptor deficiency	1 Hypothyroidism 2 Nephrotic syndrome	1 Heterozygous from relatively common 2 Enhanced risk of CHD in both types but especially in homozygous form which has a poor prognosis As a result of apoprotein beta-receptor deficiency, the removal of LDL by cells is impaired causing raised circulating LDL and thus raised total cholesterol
IIB	LDL and VLDL	Raised	Raised	Familial combined hyperlipoproteinaemia	1 Hypothyroidism 2 Nephrotic syndrome 3 Affluent living	1 Most common form of hyperlipoproteinaemia 2 Carries enhanced risk of CHD
III	IDL ('broad beta')	Raised	Raised	Familial dysbetalipoproteinaemia Apoprotein E_3 deficiency (accumulation of remnant particles, partially degraded VLDL or IDL)		Uncommon
IV	VLDL	Normal or slightly raised	Raised	1 Mild familial hypertriglyceridaemia 2 Tangier disease	1 Diabetes or glucose intolerance 2 Obesity 3 Excessive alcohol 4 Renal failure 5 Advanced liver disease	1 Common 2 May predispose to atherosclerosis
V	Chylomicrons and VLDL	Moderately raised	Very high	Severe familial hypertriglyceridaemia	1 Diabetes (poorly controlled) 2 Uraemia	Rare

on the amount of fat consumed, the total triglyceride level will rise.

In the longer term, the amount and type of dietary fat in the diet have a greater influence on total and LDL-cholesterol levels. Reducing both the absolute and proportional amount of total fat in the diet, particularly saturated fat, will reduce total and LDL-cholesterol and is considered to be a key measure for reducing CHD risk (DH 1994).

Recently, it has been suggested that, while restriction of saturated fat intake remains crucial, reduction of the total amount of dietary fat may not always be necessary to achieve these benefits. The same reduction in cholesterol levels can be achieved by replacing saturated fatty acids with either polyunsaturated or monounsaturated fatty acids (Keys *et al.* 1957; Gardner and Kraemer 1995). This may have some advantages. Low-fat diets can increase plasma triglyceride and lower HDL concentrations, thus potentially increasing CVD risk (Mensink and Katan 1992; Katan

et al. 1997). Substituting saturated fat with unsaturated alternatives may also make a lipid-lowering diet more palatable and improve compliance. Since diets containing a high proportion of monounsaturated fatty acids (the 'Mediterranean' diet; see Section 4.21.5 in Cardiovascular disease) appear to be advantageous to health, while a high intake of polyunsaturates may have adverse effects in terms of lipid peroxidation, monounsaturates would appear to be the preferable substitute. A high monounsaturated lipid-lowering diet has been shown to compare favourably with other cholesterol-lowering regimens (Kris-Etherton *et al.* 1999).

However, there are still circumstances when reduction of total fat intake is desirable (Connor and Connor 1997). Many people with hypercholesterolaemia will need to lose weight in order to treat hypertriglyceridaemia, hyperinsulinaemia, hyperglycaemia or other CVD risk factors such as hypertension, and weight loss may be easier to achieve on a diet of low energy density (Schaefer *et al.* 1995). A reduced total fat intake may also have benefits in terms of blood clotting factors (Miller *et al.* 1995). The optimal intake and composition of dietary fat must therefore be assessed on an individual basis.

Carbohydrate

Although carbohydrate has no direct effect on blood cholesterol levels, an increase in the proportion of energy derived from carbohydrate is usually encouraged as a means of keeping the proportion of saturated fat low.

Increasing the total amount of dietary carbohydrate consumed, particularly if energy intake is excessive, can elevate the VLDL triglyceride level, although this is usually transitory. Of more significance is the type of carbohydrate consumed. High consumption of rapidly absorbed refined carbohydrates exacerbates hypertriglyceridaemia, possibly mediated in part by their contribution to hyperinsulinaemia and obesity, and all patients with raised triglycerides should be encouraged to choose foods with a low glycaemic index (see Section 4.16.5 in Diabetes mellitus). Some people with endogenous hypertriglyceridaemia may be sensitive to all types of carbohydrate and require further restrictions.

Soluble fibre

Soluble fibre reduces total and LDL-cholesterol but the effect is small within the practical range of intake (Brown *et al.* 1999) and the physiological significance of this remains to be established. However, although an increased intake of soluble fibre can only be expected to have a small impact on cholesterol levels, the cardioprotective properties of foods rich in soluble fibre (particularly fruit and vegetables) are sufficient justification to advocate their increased consumption by hyperlipidaemic patients (see Section 4.21.5, *The cardioprotective diet*).

Dietary cholesterol

The influence of dietary cholesterol on blood cholesterol is relatively small because cholesterol is also synthesized by the liver and increased dietary intake tends to be offset by decreased endogenous production (Hopkins 1992). Only extreme levels of intake (e.g. atypically high consumption of eggs, shellfish or liver) are likely to have a significant elevating effect. Conversely, severe restriction to below 300 mg/day (which requires avoidance of most animal products) is necessary to reduce it. For most people, dietary measures which reduce intake of saturated fat will also prevent excessive consumption of dietary cholesterol and no additional restriction is necessary. The exceptions are people with familial hypercholesterolaemia who will require dietary cholesterol restriction to <300 mg/day (Betteridge *et al.* 1993).

n3 fatty acids

Fish oils rich in *n*3 fatty acids have been shown to reduce both fasting and postprandial blood triglyceride levels, although relatively large quantities (e.g. up to 7 g/day) may be required to produce a significant effect (Harris 1997; Adler and Holub 1997). The effect of fish oils on blood cholesterol is more equivocal: some studies have found that supplemental doses elevate LDL-cholesterol and reduce HDL-cholesterol, while others have found no effect (BNF 1999).

Alcohol

Alcohol exacerbates hypertriglyceridaemia and heavy drinking may actually cause the condition. Consumption may need to be reduced to 1–2 units per day or, in people with particularly high concentrations or severe obesity, avoided altogether.

Plant sterols

Plant sterols such as stanol esters inhibit the reabsorption of cholesterol from bile acids, thus reducing the amount of circulating cholesterol and lowering blood cholesterol levels (Miettinen and Gyling 1999). Various products such as fat spreads containing plant sterols have been recently marketed in the UK. While their ability to lower blood cholesterol is not in doubt, it remains to be established whether the physiological benefits are sufficient to justify their high cost.

Obesity

Hypertriglyceridaemia is commonly associated with, and exacerbated by, excessive body weight. If people are obese, weight (or waistline) reduction is always a treatment priority.

4.23.5 Dietary management of hyperlipidaemia

Diet should always be a central part of the management of hyperlipidaemia, either as a first-line treatment or as an adjunct to drug therapy, because the dietary measures used to lower lipid levels also reduce the elevated risk of CVD associated with all lipid disorders. Effective dietary measures are also a safer and cheaper option than drugs.

Role of diet in the management of hyperlipidaemia

Metabolic studies have shown that dietary measures can lower blood cholesterol levels by as much as 10–15% (Clarke *et al.* 1997), although this level of reduction is very difficult to achieve in free-living people. From a variety of trials of high- and low-risk individuals, a systematic review (Tang *et al.* 1998) suggested that dietary measures typically result in only an average 3% fall in total cholesterol. The main reason for this is lack of compliance with the guidance given. It is therefore important that dietary advice is given in a way which addresses barriers to change and uses counselling techniques to help to overcome these (see Section 1.7, Achieving behavioural change). Denke

(1995) demonstrated that, with good dietary counselling, it was possible to achieve a 10% reduction in blood cholesterol concentrations in people at high risk of CHD. However, even smaller levels of reduction in blood cholesterol may still be worthwhile (Law *et al.* 1994).

Dietary measures are also essential in the management of hypertriglyceridaemia, particularly weight reduction and avoidance of excessive alcohol and refined sugars.

Patients requiring lipid-lowering advice will not always be seen by a dietitian; in the primary care setting advice is more likely to be given by a practice nurse. Dietitians therefore have an important role as educators of other health professionals to ensure that appropriate, and consistent, dietary advice is given to people with mildly or moderately raised cholesterol. Primary care teams should also be given guidance on when dietetic referral is indicated. People with severe hyperlipidaemia (e.g. FH) should always receive expert dietetic advice.

Dietary treatment of specific patterns of hyperlipidaemia

Irrespective of the type of hyperlipidaemia, correcting blood lipid levels should not be the only dietary focus. It is important that the overall diet is one which is both balanced and helps to reduce cardiovascular risk. Advice should therefore be given in the context of the *Balance of Good Health* and the cardioprotective diet. Within this framework, the following points should be emphasized for particular patterns of dyslipidaemia.

Raised total and LDL-cholesterol (with normal HDL-cholesterol and triglyceride levels)

- Reduce saturated fat intake.
- Partially substitute with monounsaturated fat, to a level of energy intake appropriate for body weight.
- Encourage the consumption of sources of soluble fibre, e.g. fruit, vegetables, oats and pulses.
- Moderate intake of dietary cholesterol if excessive.

Raised triglyceride levels (with normal total, LDL- and HDL-cholesterol)

- If obese, weight loss is the overriding treatment priority and should be achieved by reduction of saturated and total fat.
- Replace high intakes of refined carbohydrates with more complex sources of carbohydrate.
- Reduce or avoid alcohol intake.

Raised total and LDL-cholesterol and raised triglyceride levels

- If obese, weight loss is the overriding treatment priority
- Reduce saturated and total fat intake.
- Partial substitution with monounsaturated fat to a level of energy intake appropriate for body weight.

- Replace high intakes of refined carbohydrates with more complex sources of carbohydrate.
- Reduce or avoid alcohol.
- Moderate intake of dietary cholesterol if excessive.

Low HDL-cholesterol

- Encourage regular aerobic exercise.
- Modest alcohol intake (1–2 units/day) can be encouraged.
- Ensure that total fat intake is not reduced too low (i.e. that some saturated fats are replaced with monounsaturated fats).

Dietary treatment of rare hyperlipidaemias

Type 1 (Familial Chylomicronaemia)

This results from congenital deficiency of lipoprotein lipase or C-II (an apoprotein) and is characterized by the presence of chylomicrons in fasting plasma. The aim of treatment is to reduce chylomicron formation, which necessitates severe fat restriction to 10–25% of dietary energy. The following dietary aspects will also need to be considered:

- *Energy*: Such a low fat content inevitably compromises energy intake. For normal weight adults and children this deficit will need to be rectified, possibly with the use of medium-chain triglycerides (MCT) which do not require lipoprotein lipase for metabolism, or modular carbohydrate supplements such as glucose polymers.
- *Essential fatty acids*: To prevent deficiency, supplements of linoleic acid and alpha-linolenic acid are likely to be required.
- *Fat-soluble vitamins*: Supplementation will be necessary to ensure sufficiency.
- *Protein*: Use of skimmed milk may be helpful to ensure protein adequacy.
- *Acceptability*: This is a particularly important aspect to be addressed as diets of such low fat content can be very unpalatable. Dietitians will require considerable motivational skills, as well as ingenuity, in order to find a dietary strategy compatible with long-term compliance. Some individuals may find the use of fat exchanges for preferred foods helpful.

4.23.6 Drug treatment of hyperlipidaemia

Lipid-lowering drugs are being increasingly used in the treatment of hyperlipidaemia, particularly for patients with established CHD or those at high risk of developing CHD on account of multiple risk factors. They are also used in the treatment of severe hyperlipidaemia inadequately controlled by dietary measures. However, drug therapy is never a substitute for dietary therapy, only an adjunct to it.

Statins (hydroxymethlglutaryl coenzyme A reductase inhibitors)

Statins are now the treatment of choice in the management

of hypercholesterolaemia, following the findings of two major studies showing their effectiveness in reducing CHD (Scandinavian Simvastatin Group 1994; Shepherd *et al.* 1995). Commonly used statins are atorvastatin, simvastatin, pravastatin, fluvastatin and cerivastatin.

These drugs reduce cholesterol biosynthesis in the liver by inhibiting the enzyme hydroxymethylglutaryl coenzyme A reductase. The reduced intracellular cholesterol consequently leads to an increased expression of LDL receptors, increasing LDL uptake and reducing total cholesterol. As well as reducing both total and LDL-cholesterol, statins result in a moderate reduction in triglyceride concentration and a small increase in HDL-cholesterol.

To ensure that these drugs are used to maximum effectiveness and to prevent over-prescription, the Department of Health (1997) has produced guidance on their use:

1 Use of diet and other lifestyle means of reducing CHD risk should be considered first.
2 Statins should not be used for the treatment of high cholesterol alone, only in those at high risk of major coronary events.
3 Statin use is indicated for:
   - patients who have had a myocardial infarction and with a total cholesterol of 4.8 mmol/l or more, (or LDL-cholesterol of 3.2 mmol/l or more)
   - patients with angina or other clinically overt atherosclerotic disease with a total cholesterol of 5.5mmol/l or more (or LDL-cholesterol of 3.7 mmol/l or more)
   - people with a high risk of developing CHD owing to unmodifiable factors such as diabetes, hypertension or familial hyperlipidaemia, and with a total cholesterol of 5.5 mmol/l of more (or LDL-cholesterol of 3.7 mmol/l or more).

Fibric acid derivatives (fibrates), e.g. bezafibrate, gemfibrozil

These drugs are generally used for mixed hyperlipidaemias, and are often used in conjunction with statins in diabetic patients where serum triglycerides are significantly raised. They function systemically and are thought to increase the excretion of cholesterol into the bile (thus also predisposing the patient to gall stones), increase lipoprotein lipase activity, decrease endogenous cholesterol synthesis and increase LDL receptor activity. The effects on the lipid profile are:

- reduction in VLDL triglyceride and hence total triglyceride level
- moderate reduction in total and LDL-cholesterol
- increase in HDL-cholesterol.

Other lipid-lowering drugs

Other classes of lipid-lowering drugs include:

- *Nicotinic acid (niacin)* and its derivatives: This is not commonly used in the UK because of its serious side-effects.

- *Bile acid sequestrants* such as cholestyramine and colestipol: These used to be widely used to treat hypercholesterolaemia but tend to be poorly tolerated by patients and their use has largely been superseded by more effective preparations such as statins.
- *Fish oil supplements*: Although these have beneficial effects on serum triglyceride levels, they are poorly tolerated owing to the large dosages required.

Text revised by: Briony Thomas and Fiona Moor in conjunction with Lee Hooper, Jo Farrington and the UK Heart Health and Thoracic Dietitians

Further reading

Gotto AM, Pownall H. *Manual of Lipid Disorders*, 2nd edn. New York: Lippincott, Williams and Wilkins, 1998.

References

Adler AJ, Holub BJ. Effect of garlic and fish oil supplementation on serum lipid and lipoprotein concentrations in hypercholesterolaemic men. *American Journal of Clinical Nutrition* 1997; **65**: 445–450.

Assmann G, Schulte H, von Eckardstein A. Hypertriglyceridaemia and elevated lipoprotein (a) are risk factors for major coronary events in middle-aged men. *American Journal of Cardiology* 1996; **77**: 1179–1184.

Austin MA, Hokanon JE, Edwards KL. Hypertriglyceridaemia as a cardiovascular risk factor. *American Journal of Cardiology* 1998; **81** (4A): 7B–12B.

Betteridge DJ, Dodson PM, Durrington PN *et al.* Management of hyperlipidaemia: guidelines of the British Hyperlipidaemia Association. *Postgraduate Medical Journal* 1993; **69**: 359–369.

British Dietetic Association. Dietary treatment of people at high coronary risk. Position Paper. *Journal of Human Nutrition and Dietetics* 1998; **11**: 273–280.

British Nutrition Foundation. *n-3 Fatty Acids and Health*. Briefing Paper. London: BNF, 1999.

Brown L, Rosner B, Willett WW, Sacks FM. Cholesterol-lowering effect of dietary fiber: a meta-analysis. *American Journal of Clinical Nutrition* 1999; **69**: 30–42.

Clarke R, Frost C, Collins R *et al.* Dietary lipids and blood cholesterol: a quantitative meta-analysis of metabolic ward studies. *British Medical Journal*. 1997; **314**: 112–117.

Connor WE, Connor SL. Should a low-fat, high-carbohydrate diet be recommended for everyone? The case for a low-fat, high-carbohydrate diet. *New England Journal of Medicine* 1997; **337**: 562–563, 566–567.

Denke DA. Cholesterol-lowering diets. A review of the evidence. *Archives of Internal Medicine* 1995; **155**: 17–26.

Department of Health, Committee on Medical Aspects of Food Policy (COMA). *Nutritional Aspects of Cardiovascular Disease*. Report on Health and Social Subjects 46. London: HMSO, 1994.

Department of Health. *Standing Medical Advisory Committee Advice on the Use of Statins*. London: DH, 1997.

Ericsson CG, Hamsten A, Nilsson J *et al.* Angiographic assessment of effects of Bezafibrate on progression of coronary heart disease in young male post-infarction patients. *Lancet* 1996; **347**: 849–853.

Gardner CD, Kraemer HC. Monounsaturated versus polyunsaturated dietary fat and serum lipids. A meta-analysis. *Arterio-*

sclerosis, Thrombosis and Vascular Biology 1995; **15**: 1917–1927.

Harris WS. *n*-3 fatty acids and serum lipoproteins: human studies. *American Journal of Clinical Nutrition* 1997; **65** (Suppl): 1645S–1654S.

Hokanson JE, Austin MA. Plasma triglyceride level is a risk factor for cardiovascular disease independent of high-density lipoprotein cholesterol level: a meta-analysis of population-based prospective studies. *Journal of Cardiovascular Risk* 1996; **3**: 213–219.

Hopkins PN. Effects of dietary cholesterol on serum cholesterol: a meta-analysis and review. *American Journal of Clinical Nutrition* 1992; **55** (6): 1060–1070.

Katan MB, Grundy SM, Willett WC. Should a low-fat, high-carbohydrate diet be recommended for everyone? Beyond low-fat diets. *New England Journal of Medicine* 1997; **337**: 563–566.

Keys A, Anderson JT, Grande F. Prediction of serum-cholesterol responses of man to changes in fats in the diet. *Lancet* 1957; **ii**: 959–966.

Kris-Etherton PM, Pearson TA, Wan Y *et al*. High monounsaturated fatty acid diets lower both plasma cholesterol and triacylglycerol concentrations. *American Journal of Clinical Nutrition* 1999; **70**: 1009–1115.

Law MR, Wald NJ, Thompson SG. By how much and how quickly does reduction in serum cholesterol concentration lower risk of ischaemic heart disease? *British Medical Journal* 1994; **308**: 367–373.

Martin MJ, Hulley SB, Browner WS *et al*. Serum cholesterol, blood pressure and mortality: implications from a cohort of 361,622 men. *Lancet* 1986; **ii**: 933–936.

Mensink RP, Katan MB. Effect of dietary fatty acids on serum lipids and lipoproteins. *Arteriosclerosis and Thrombosis* 1992; **12**: 911–919.

Miettinen IA, Gyling H. Regulation of cholesterol metabolism by dietary plant sterols. *Current Opinions in Lipidology* 1999; **10**: 9–14.

Miller GJ, Stirling Y, Howarth DJ *et al*. Dietary fat intake and plasma factor VII antigen concentration. *Thrombosis and Haemostasis* 1995; **73**: 893.

Scandinavian Simvastatin Survival Study (4S) Group. Randomised trial of cholesterol lowering in 4444 patients with coronary heart disease: the Scandinavian Survival Study (4S). *Lancet* 1994; **344**: 1383–1389.

Schaefer EJ, Lichtenstein AH, Lamon-Fava S *et al*. Body-weight and low-density lipoprotein cholesterol changes after consumption of a low-fat ad libitum diet. *Journal of the American Medical Association* 1995; **274**: 1450–1455.

Shepherd J, Cobbe SM, Ford I *et al*. Prevention of coronary heart disease with pravastatin in men with hypercholesterolaemia. *New England Journal of Medicine* 1995; **333**: 1301–1307.

Stampfer MJ, Krauss RM, Ma J *et al*. A prospective study of triglyceride level, low density lipoprotein particle diameter, and risk of myocardial infarction. *Journal of the American Medical Association* 1996; **276**: 882–888.

Tang JL, Armitage JM, Lancaster T *et al*. Systematic review of dietary intervention trials to lower blood total cholesterol in free-living subjects. *British Medical Journal* 1998; **316**: 1213–1220.

Wood D, Durrington P, Poulter N *et al*. on behalf of British Cardiac Society. Joint British recommendations on prevention of coronary heart disease in clinical practice. *Heart* 1998; **80**: S1–S29.

4.24 Hypertension

Hypertension (raised blood pressure) is a major risk factor for cardiovascular disease (CVD), both coronary heart disease (CHD) and stroke. In people with diabetes, it significantly increases the risk of both cardiovascular and microvascular complications, particularly diabetic nephropathy. Hypertension is usually a primary disorder but can be secondary to renal disease, liver disease and cardiac failure, and a complication of pregnancy.

4.24.1 Definitions and prevalence

Blood pressure is a measurement of the force exerted by the blood circulating in the arteries. It is influenced by the force at which the heart pumps blood, the diameter of the blood vessels and the volume of circulating blood. When taking a blood pressure reading two figures are recorded:

- systolic pressure, indicating the force during contraction of the heart ventricles
- diastolic pressure, which measures the blood pressure during ventricle relaxation

Readings will vary from day to day, and repeated measurements on two or more separate occasions are necessary to establish the usual blood pressure for a particular individual.

In young, healthy adults, normal systolic blood pressure is considered to be about 120 mmHg and diastolic pressure about 80 mmHg (120/80). Women tend to have a lower blood pressure than men and, in Westernized societies, blood pressure increases markedly with age (a trend which is much less apparent in populations from more deprived parts of the world). There are also genetic influences on blood pressure and the susceptibility to hypertension, and these may be particularly marked in some ethnic groups, particularly people of African–Caribbean origin (Beevers and Beevers 1993). Within the UK population, people from more deprived socioeconomic groups tend to have higher mean blood pressure than those from more affluent groups, largely as a result of differences in the prevalence of obesity and smoking (DH 1999a).

Hypertension occurs when the vessels through which the blood flows become too narrow or the volume of circulating blood becomes too high. Raised blood pressure increases the workload on the heart and can damage the endothelial lining of blood vessels. It also increases the infiltration of blood components such as lipids into the arterial wall, exacerbating endothelial damage, enhancing atherosclerotic deposition and ultimately increasing cardiovascular risk.

The point at which raised blood pressure becomes clinically significant depends on a patient's age and overall cardiovascular risk. Hypertension requiring investigation and possible treatment is usually defined as systolic blood pressure $\geq$ 140 mmHg and/or a diastolic pressure $\geq$ 90 mmHg (Ramsay et al. 1999). Systolic blood pressure $\geq$ 160 mmHg or diastolic $\geq$ 100 mmHg usually requires active antihypertensive treatment.

Based on the criteria of systolic blood pressure $\geq$ 140 mmHg and/or diastolic $\geq$ 90 mmHg, the 1998 Health Survey for England (DH 1999a) found that 40.8% of men and 32.9% of women were hypertensive, or on hypertensive medication. An earlier Health Survey for England (White et al. 1993) had found that 16% of men and 17% of women had a systolic blood pressure above 160 mmHg and/or a diastolic pressure above 95 mmHg.

4.24.2 Prognostic significance of hypertension

The risk of CVD, particularly stroke, increases across the whole range of blood pressures and is directly associated with both diastolic and systolic pressures (Stamler et al. 1989; MacMahon et al. 1990). Reducing blood pressure reduces the risk of both CHD and stroke, but the benefits in respect of stroke are more rapid (Collins et al. 1990). This is probably because reducing blood pressure has an immediate effect in terms of lessening the risk of rupture of microaneurysms (DH 1994). In people with diabetes, treatment of hypertension also reduces the risk of diabetic microvascular complications as well as CVD (UK Prospective Diabetes Study 1998).

For the majority of individuals, whether hypertensive or normotensive, a lower blood pressure should eventually confer a lower risk of cardiovascular disease (MacMahon et al. 1990). In prospective observational studies, a long-term difference of 5–6 mmHg in usual diastolic blood pressure has been found to be associated with about 35–40% less stroke and 20–25% less CHD (Collins et al. 1990). For this reason, reducing the mean blood pressure of the population by at least 5 mmHg by the year 2005 was one of the *Health of the Nation* targets (DH 1992). Reducing the mortality from CHD and stroke remains one of the principal objectives of *Our Healthier Nation* (DH 1999b).

However, when hypertension is detected, its prognostic significance in respect of cardiovascular disease cannot be considered in isolation; taking account of the presence or absence of other cardiovascular risk factors is an integral part of its management (Figure 4.11).

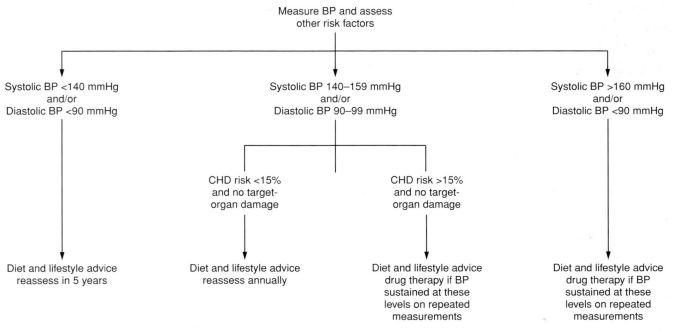

Figure 4.11 Management of blood pressure (BP) in conjunction with assessment of cardiovascular risk. Adapted from Wood *et al*. (1998).

4.24.3 Dietary influences on blood pressure

Diet and lifestyle factors which tend to raise blood pressure include:

- obesity
- low level of physical activity
- high alcohol intake
- high sodium intake
- low potassium intake.

Dietary calcium and *n*3 fatty acids may have the ability to lower blood pressure.

Obesity

There is a strong and direct relationship between obesity and increased blood pressure (DH 1995a), the prognostic significance of which may be greater if the excess fat is centrally distributed (Ashwell 1996).

In obese people, weight loss (or waistline reduction) has beneficial effects on blood pressure (Tuck *et al*. 1981; Rissanen *et al*. 1985). A high-quality systematic review suggests that dietary measures which achieve 3–9% reduction in body weight are likely to reduce systolic and diastolic pressures by about 3 mmHg (Brand *et al*. 1999). Although modest, these changes may be sufficient to decrease dosage requirements for those on hypertensive medication.

Physical activity

As well as the benefits of physical activity in terms of energy balance and obesity, aerobic exercise may have direct hypotensive effects. Increasing the level of physical activity has been shown to reduce both systolic and diastolic pressure in hypertensive individuals (Nelson *et al*. 1986; Hagberg *et al*. 1989; Martin *et al*. 1990), and these effects are reversed by a return to lower levels of exercise (Somers *et al*. 1991). In order to be beneficial, exercise needs to be aerobic rather than of a calisthenic or stretching nature (Martin *et al*. 1990), but does not have to be of high intensity; regular, low intensity exercise may be as effective as exercise of moderate intensity (Roman *et al*. 1981; Hagberg *et al*. 1989).

Alcohol

At intakes above 1–2 units per day, alcohol begins to raise both systolic and diastolic pressure, an effect which appears to be dose related (DH 1995b). Regular heavy consumption of alcohol or binge drinking is associated with significant rises in blood pressure (Marmot *et al*. 1994). Alcohol consumption should be reviewed in a person with hypertension and if necessary curtailed or excluded.

Sodium

The relationship between sodium and blood pressure is complex and difficult to establish for a number of reasons. Accurate estimates of sodium intake (or excretion, another marker of intake) are notoriously difficult to obtain in large-scale population studies, thus tending to obscure any relationship. Furthermore, in Western societies, the variation in sodium intake within an individual may be greater than the variation between individuals, thus diminishing the statistical power to detect significant associations (Liu *et al.* 1979). Smaller, more accurate studies are confounded by the heterogeneity of risk from other factors impacting on hypertension, such as age, body mass index (BMI), alcohol intake, level of physical activity and genetic susceptibility.

Nevertheless, epidemiological studies have repeatedly shown an independent, positive relationship between dietary intake of sodium and blood pressure both within and between populations (Intersalt Cooperative Research Group 1988; Frost *et al.* 1991; Law *et al.* 1991; Elliott *et al.* 1996; He and Whelton 1997). There is evidence that this has pathological significance; a large prospective cohort study has shown that, in overweight people, high sodium intake is strongly and independently associated with cardiovascular mortality (He *et al.* 1999). Sodium intake may also account for much of the rise in blood pressure associated with ageing; in societies where mean sodium intake is habitually low, there is little upward trend in blood pressure with age (Intersalt Cooperative Research Group 1988). Randomized controlled trials have demonstrated that reduced sodium intake leads to a reduction in blood pressure in both hypertensive and normotensive individuals (Trials of Hypertension Prevention Collaborative Research Group 1992; Midgley *et al.* 1996; Cutler *et al.* 1997; He and Whelton 1997; Whelton *et al.* 1998).

The magnitude of the association between sodium and blood pressure remains a matter of debate (Swales 1991; Elliott 1994). The elevating effect is probably smaller than that of obesity or alcohol, and salt restriction appears to have greater effect in older people and in those with highest blood pressure. It has been estimated (DH 1994) that reducing the average salt intake of the population from 9 g to 6 g/day (or 3.6 g sodium/day to 2.4 g/day) would reduce mean systolic blood pressure by about 3.5 mmHg, and a larger effect could be expected in the long term as the rise in blood pressure with age was reduced. Although the size and impact of this remain to be proven, there are good reasons for advocating such a measure as part of healthy-eating guidance. In affluent societies, sodium intake greatly exceeds physiological requirements, largely as a result of the high consumption of processed foods (in the UK, about 60–70% of sodium is derived from this source), and there is no evidence that this is in any way beneficial. Conversely, there is no evidence to suggest that moderate reduction in intake might be harmful. Since some individuals are undoubtedly more sensitive to the hypertensive effects of sodium than others but, at present, there is no way of identifying who such people might be, everyone should be encouraged to moderate their sodium intake.

Potassium

Potassium has a beneficial effect on blood pressure, partly as a consequence of its reciprocal physiological relationship with sodium. Blood pressure is negatively associated with potassium intake (or excretion) and directly associated with the ratio of dietary sodium:potassium (Intersalt

Cooperative Research Group 1988). An increased potassium consumption has been shown to lower blood pressure, especially in people who are hypertensive (Cappuccio and MacGregor 1991).

The COMA report on Cardiovascular Disease (DH 1994) recommended that, alongside a reduction in sodium intake, average potassium intake should increase from its current level of about 3 g/day to 3.5 g/day. This should primarily be achieved by increased consumption of fruit and vegetables, foods which will coincidentally confer additional cardioprotection as a result of their content of antioxidants and soluble fibre.

Calcium

Calcium is involved in the control of blood pressure via its effects on the regulation of smooth muscle tone and contraction, including that of blood vessel walls. The possible relationship between dietary calcium and blood pressure has been a subject of interest for many years, following studies in the 1960s and 1970s suggesting that mortality from CVD was inversely associated with the hardness of drinking water (Schroeder 1960; Stitt *et al.* 1973). Both cross-sectional and prospective studies have shown an inverse relationship between dietary calcium and blood pressure which is independent of age and may be particularly strong in some subgroups, such as people with low serum calcium and/or high parathyroid levels, or with abnormal calcium metabolism (Osborne *et al.* 1996). It has also been suggested that abnormalities in calcium metabolism may explain why some, but not all people, are sensitive to the hypertensive effect of sodium (Sowers *et al.* 1991; Osborne *et al.* 1996).

Calcium supplementation has been shown to lower the risk of pregnancy-induced hypertension (Bucher *et al.* 1996a) but, in the general population, trials of calcium supplementation have produced more mixed findings, possibly because not all studies have taken dietary calcium intake into account. Systematic review of the evidence suggests that while calcium supplementation can result in a statistically significant decrease in systolic blood pressure (but not diastolic pressure) in both hypertensive and normotensive individuals, the effect is too small to support the use of calcium supplements for preventing or treating hypertension *per se* (Scott 1996; Allender *et al.* 1996; Bucher *et al.* 1996b). It is conceivable that the effect may be greater in those with low calcium intakes (and negligible if calcium intake is adequate), but further research is required to clarify this. At present, dietary guidance should focus on ensuring that the diet contains sufficient calcium to meet nutritional needs and prevent osteoporosis.

Omega-3 fatty acids

Meta-analyses suggest that omega-3 (*n*3) fatty acids (found in fish oils) may have an independent hypotensive effect (Morris *et al.* 1993; Lawrence *et al.* 1993; Appel *et al.* 1993), possibly as a result of the increased synthesis of prostacyclin (a vasodilator) and reduced synthesis of thromboxane (a vasoconstrictor) from eicosapentaenoic acid. The effect is greatest in those with highest blood pressure and may not be apparent at all in normotensive people (Morris *et al.* 1993). Furthermore, the quantity of *n*3 fatty acids needed to achieve an effect is large: a minimum of 3 g/day may be needed for a significant reduction (Appel *et al.* 1993; Morris *et al.* 1993), which is equivalent to about 10 portions of oily fish per week or 9–10 fish oil capsules per day. Even higher supplemental doses of 5–6 g of *n*3 fatty acids have been used in some studies (de Deckere *et al.* 1998). Such levels may be neither realistic nor acceptable because of the side-effects of eructation and fishy taste associated with supplements in the region of 3 g/day (Appel *et al.* 1993). Concerns have also been expressed over the dioxin content of some fish oil supplements (see Section 4.21.5 in Cardiovascular disease).

Nevertheless, even if the effect of fish oils on hypertension is, for all practical purposes, insignificant, the protective effects of modest consumption of oily fish in a group of people who, as a result of their hypertension, are at high cardiovascular risk, should not be overlooked.

4.24.4 Management of hypertension

The management of hypertension is determined by the extent to which other cardiovascular risk factors are present (Fig. 4.11). Individual cardiovascular risk assessment now forms a central part of the decision-making process for the treatment of hypertension, and this is usually estimated using the chart produced by the Joint British Societies (Wood *et al.* 1998) to assess the 10-year risk of CHD. The presence of other risk factors such as renal disease, diabetes and hyperlipidaemia should also be taken into account, and it is recommended that all hypertensive people should be routinely screened via blood and urine tests for evidence of these, and should also undergo electrocardiography (ECG). Cardioprotective dietary measures should be adopted by all patients, irrespective of whether drug treatment is required.

Guidelines for the management of hypertension have been produced by the British Hypertension Society (Ramsay *et al.* 1999). These recommend that:

1 Non-pharmacological measures (diet and lifestyle change) are an important aspect of management of all hypertensive people, and should be used for those with borderline hypertension.
2 Antihypertensive drug treatment is indicated in people with sustained systolic blood pressure ≥ 160 mmHg or diastolic blood pressure ≥ 100 mmHg
3 In people where systolic blood pressure is between 140 and 159 mmHg or diastolic blood pressure is between 90–99 mmHg, treatment should be determined according to the presence or absence of target organ damage, CVD or a 10 year CHD risk ≥ 15% (as assessed by the Joint British Societies CHD risk assessment chart (Wood *et al.* 1998).

The optimal blood pressure treatment targets are systolic blood pressure <140 mmHg and diastolic blood pressure <85 mmHg.

The minimum recommended standard of acceptability for audit purposes is <150/90 mmHg. In people with diabetes, maintaining blood pressure at or below 140/80 mmHg is now recognized as being as important an aspect of treatment as tight blood glucose control (see Section 4.16.2 in Diabetes mellitus).

Dietary management of hypertension

Advice on diet and lifestyle changes should be offered to all hypertensive people, and to those with a strong family history of hypertension. If implemented, such measures have been shown to avoid the need for drug treatment, or to reduce the dosage of antihypertensive drugs required (Appel *et al.* 1997; Whelton *et al.* 1998).

Dietary advice should be given in the context of general cardioprotection (see Section 4.21, Cardiovascular disease), and tailored to individual risk factors and nutritional priorities. Diet and lifestyle measures which should be strongly recommended to people with hypertension are:

• If overweight, weight loss is of primary importance and weight-reducing measures are a priority.
• Sodium intake should be reduced. This can be achieved by using less salt in cooking or adding less to food, eating fewer salty foods, and decreasing the consumption of processed foods (the main dietary source of sodium for most people).
• Intake of fruit and vegetables (which elevate potassium intake in addition to their cardioprotective properties) should be significantly increased.
• Alcohol consumption should not exceed 1–2 units/day and less may be advisable in people who are overweight. Binge drinking must be avoided.
• Regular physical activity is important.
• The diet should be a balanced and cardioprotective one. The importance of foods such as oily fish (for thrombogenic protection) and low-fat dairy foods (to meet calcium needs) should not be overlooked.

Drug treatment of hypertension

Many of the drugs used to treat hypertension are also used in the management of CHD (see section 4.22.5 in Coronary heart disease) and the choice of drug will therefore be influenced by the nature of any clinical symptoms present as well as other factors such as age and renal function. Preferred first-line antihypertensive drugs of choice are:

• low dose thiazide diuretics (e.g. bendrofluazide) which inhibit sodium reabsorption from the distal tubules of the kidney, thus increasing fluid loss and reducing blood volume;
• beta-blockers (e.g. atenolol) which reduce the stimulating action of noradrenaline by blocking beta-adrenoreceptors in the heart and peripheral vasculature.

Beta-blockers lower blood pressure primarily by reducing the force and rate of cardiac output. For these reasons, these drugs are also commonly used in the management of angina and arrythmias.

Other drugs such as calcium-channel blockers (e.g. verapamil), which inhibit smooth muscle contraction in blood vessel walls, and angiotensin-converting enzyme inhibitors (e.g. captopril), which reduce the production of the vasoconstrictor angiotensin II, may be used if thiazides and beta-blockers are contraindicated or ineffective. A combination of hypertensive drugs may be needed to achieve optimal levels of control. Other drugs which reduce cardiovascular risk such as aspirin and statins may also be indicated.

4.24.5 Prevention of hypertension

Hypertension is usually symptomless and often only discovered as a result of routine health screening or when overt signs of CVD develop. For this reason, it is recommended that all adults should have their blood pressure measured every 5 years until the age of 80 years (Ramsay *et al.* 1999). Those with 'high normal' values (135–139/85–89 mmHg), or who have previously had high readings, should have annual measurements. Blood pressure readings should be taken twice using recommended procedures, and on at least two separate occasions before a diagnosis of hypertension is made.

Promoting diet and lifestyle measures which reduce the prevalence of hypertension in the whole population is an important aspect of prevention.

Text revised by: Briony Thomas and Fiona Moor in conjunction with the UK Heart Health and Thoracic Dietitians

Useful address

British Hypertension Society
Website: www.hyp.ac.uk/bhs

Further reading

British Nutrition Foundation. *Salt in the Diet*. Briefing Paper. London: BNF, 1994.
Ramsay LE, Williams B, Johnston GD *et al*. British Hypertension Society guidelines for hypertension management 1999: summary. *British Medical Journal* 1999; **319** 630–635.

References

Allender PS, Cutler JA, Follmann D *et al*. Dietary calcium and blood pressure: a meta-analysis of randomized controlled trials. *Annals of Internal Medicine* 1996; **124**: 825–831.
Appel LJ, Miller ER, Seidler AJ, Whelton PK. Does supplementation of diet with fish oil reduce blood pressure? A meta analysis of controlled clinical trials. *Archives of Internal Medicine* 1993; **153** 429–438

Appel LJ, Moore TJ, Obarzanek E *et al.*, for the DASH Collaborative Research Group. A clinical trial of the effects of dietary patterns on blood pressure. *New England Journal of Medicine* 1997; **336**: 1117–1124.
Ashwell M. Leaping into shape. In Sadler MJ (ed.) *Bodyweight and Health*. Proceedings of the British Nutrition Foundation Conference, pp. 47–54. London: BNF, 1996.
Beevers G, Beevers M. Hypertension: impact upon black and ethnic minority people. In Hopkins A, Bahl V (Eds). *Access to Health Care for People from Black and Ethnic Minorities*. London: Royal College of Physicians, 1993.
Brand HB, Mulrow CD, Chiquette E *et al*. Weight-reduction through dieting for control of hypertension in adults (Cochrane Review). In *The Cochrane Library*, Issue 1. Oxford: Update Software, 1999.
Bucher HC *et al*. Effect of calcium supplementation on pregnancy-induced hypertension and pre-eclampsia: a meta-analysis of randomised controlled trials. *Journal of the American Medical Association* 1996a; **275**: 1113–1117.
Bucher HC, Cook RJ, Guyatt GH *et al*. Effect of calcium supplementation on pregnancy-induced hypertension and pre-eclampsia: a meta-analysis of randomised controlled trials. *Journal of the American Medical Association* 1996b; **275**: 1016–1022.
Cappuccio FP, MacGregor GA. Does potassium supplementation lower blood pressure? A meta-analysis of published trials. *Journal of Hypertension* 1991; **9**: 465–473.
Collins R, Peto R, MacMahon S *et al*. Blood pressure, stroke and coronary heart disease. Part 2, short-term reductions in blood pressure: overview of randomised trials in their epidemiological context. *Lancet* 1990; **335**: 827–838.
Cutler JA, Follmann D, Allender PS. Randomized trials of sodium reduction: an overview. *American Journal of Clinical Nutrition* 1997; **65** (2 Suppl): 643S–651S.
de Deckere EAM, Korver O, Verschuren PM, Katan MB. Health aspects of fish and *n*-3 polyunsaturated fatty acids from plant and marine origin. *European Journal of Clinical Nutrition* 1998; **52**: 749–753.
Department of Health. *Health of the Nation: A Strategy for Health in England*. London: HMSO, 1992.
Department of Health. Report of the Cardiovascular Review Group of the Committee on Medical Aspects of Food Policy (COMA). *Nutritional Aspects of Cardiovascular Disease*. Report on Health and Social Subjects 46. London: HMSO, 1994.
Department of Health. *Obesity. Reversing the Increasing Problem of Obesity in England*. Report from the Nutrition and Physical Activity Task Forces. London: DH, 1995a.
Department of Health. *Sensible Drinking*. Report of an Inter-departmental Working Group. London: DH, 1995b.
Department of Health. *Health Survey for England: Cardiovascular Disease 1998*. Vol. 1: *Findings*. Erens B, Primatesta P (Eds). London: The Stationery Office, 1999a.
Department of Health. *Saving Lives: Our Healthier Nation*. London: The Stationery Office, 1999b.
Elliott P. Nutritional factors in blood pressure. *Journal of Human Hypertension* 1994; **8**: 595–601.
Elliott P, Stamler J, Nichols R *et al*. for the Intersalt Co-operative Research Group. Intersalt revisited: further analyses of 24 hour sodium excretion and blood pressure within and across populations. *British Medical Journal* 1996; **312**: 1249–1253.
Frost CD, Law MR, Wald NJ. By how much does dietary salt reduction lower blood pressure? II: Analysis of observational data within populations. *British Medical Journal* 1991; **302**: 815–818.

Hagberg JM, Montain SJ, Martin WH, Ehsani AA. Effect of exercise training in 60–69 year old persons with essential hypertension. *American Journal of Cardiology* 1989; **64**: 348–353.

He J, Whelton PK. Role of sodium reduction in the treatment and prevention of hypertension. *Current Opinions in Cardiology* 1997; **12**: 202–207.

He J, Ogden LG, Vupputuri S *et al*. Dietary sodium intake and subsequent risk of cardiovascular disease in overweight adults. *Journal of the American Medical Association* 1999; **282**: 2027–2034.

Intersalt Cooperative Research Group. Intersalt: an international study of electrolyte excretion and blood pressure. Results for 24 hour urinary sodium and potassium excretion. *British Medical Journal* 1988; **297**: 319–328.

Law MR, Frost CD, Wald NJ. By how much does dietary salt reduction lower blood pressure? I: Analysis of observational data among populations. *British Medical Journal* 1991; **302**: 811–819.

Lawrence J *et al*. Does supplementation of diet with 'fish oil' reduce blood pressure? *Archives of Internal Medicine* 1993; **153**: 1429–1438.

Liu K, Cooper R, McKeever J *et al*. Assessment of the association between habitual salt intake and high blood pressure: methodological problems. *American Journal of Epidemiology* 1979; **110**: 219–226.

MacMahon S, Peto R, Cutler J *et al*. Blood pressure, stroke and coronary heart disease. Part 1, Prolonged differences in blood pressure: prospective observational trials corrected for the regression dilution bias. *Lancet* 1990; **335**: 765–774.

Marmot MG, Elliott P, Shipley MJ *et al*. Alcohol and blood pressure: the INTERSALT study. *British Medical Journal* 1994; **308**: 1263–1267.

Martin JE, Dubbert PM, Cushman WC. Controlled trial of aerobic exercise in hypertension. *Circulation* 1990; **81**: 1560–1567.

Midgley JP, Matthew AG, Greenwood CMT, Logan AG. Effect of reduced dietary sodium on blood pressure. A meta-analysis of randomised controlled trials. *Journal of the American Medical Association* 1996; **275**: 1590–1597.

Morris MC, Sacks F, Rosner B. Does fish oil lower blood pressure? A meta-analysis of controlled trials. *Circulation* 1993; **88**: 523–533.

Nelson L, Jennings GL, Esler MD, Korner PL. Effect of changing levels of physical activity on blood pressure and haemodynamics in essential hypertension. *Lancet* 1986; **ii**: 473–476.

Osborne CG, McTyre RB, Dudek J *et al*. Evidence for a relationship of calcium to blood pressure. *Nutrition Reviews* 1996; **54**: 365–381.

Ramsay LE, Williams B, Johnston GD *et al*. Guidelines for management of hypertension: report of the third working party of the British Hypertension Society. *Journal of Human Hypertension* 1999; **13**: 569–592.

Rissanen A, Pietinen P, Siljamaki-Ojansuu U *et al*. Treatment of hypertension in obese patients: efficacy and feasibility of weight and salt reduction programmes. *Acta Medica Scandinavica* 1985; **218**: 149–156.

Roman O, Camuzzi AL, Villalon E, Klenner C. Physical training programme in arterial hypertension: a long-term prospective follow-up. *Cardiology* 1981; **67**: 230–243.

Schroeder HA. Relation between mortality from cardiovascular disease and treated water supplies: variations in states and 163 largest municipalities of the United States. *Journal of the American Medical Association* 1960; **172**: 1902–1908.

Scott P *et al*. Dietary calcium and blood pressure: a meta-analysis of randomized clinical trials. *Annals of Internal Medicine* 1996; **125**: 825–831.

Somers VK, Conway J, Johnston J, Sleight P. Effects of endurance training on baroflex sensitivity and blood pressure in borderline hypertension. *Lancet* 1991; **337**: 1363–1368.

Sowers JR, Zemel MB, Zemel PC, Standley PR. Calcium metabolism and dietary calcium in salt sensitive hypertension. *American Journal of Hypertension* 1991; **4**: 557–563.

Stamler J, Neaton JD, Wentworth DN. Blood pressure (systolic and diastolic) and risk of fatal coronary heart disease. *Hypertension* 1989; **13** (Suppl 5): I2–I12.

Stitt, FW, Clayton DG, Crawford MD, Morris JN. Clinical and biochemical indicators of cardiovascular disease among men living in hard and soft water areas. *Lancet* 1973; **i**: 122–126.

Swales JD. Dietary salt and blood pressure: the role of meta-analyses. *Journal of Hypertension* 1991; **9** (Suppl 6): S42–S46.

Trials of Hypertension Prevention Collaborative Research Group. The effects of nonpharmacological interventions on blood pressure of persons with high normal levels: results of the Trials of Hypertension Prevention, Phase 1. *Journal of the American Medical Association* 1992; **267**: 1213–1220.

Tuck ML, Sowers J, Dornfield L *et al*. The effect of weight reduction on blood pressure, plasma renin activity and plasma aldosterone levels in obese patients. *New England Journal of Medicine* 1981; **304**: 930–933.

United Kingdom Prospective Diabetes Study Group (UKPDS). UK Prospective Diabetes Study 38: Tight blood pressure control and risk of macrovascular and microvascular complications in type 2 diabetes. *British Medical Journal* 1998; **317**: 703–713.

Whelton PK, Appel LJ, Espeland MA *et al*., for the TONE Collaborative Research Group. Sodium reduction and weight loss in the treatment of hypertension in older persons. A randomised controlled trial of nonpharmacologic interventions in the elderly (TONE). *Journal of the American Medical Association* 1998; **279**: 839–846.

White A *et al*. *Health Survey for England 1991: A Survey Carried out by OPCS on Behalf of the Department of Health*. London: HMSO, 1993.

Wood D, Durrington P, Poulter N *et al*. Joint British recommendations on prevention of coronary heart disease in clinical practice. *Heart* 1998; **80**: S1–S29.

4.25 Stroke

A stroke or cardiovascular accident (CVA) results from a sudden interruption in the blood supply to an area of the brain, depriving the affected part of oxygen and causing death of brain tissue. Stroke is the third major cause of death in the UK, after coronary heart disease (CHD) and cancer, accounting for 12% of all deaths. People of West African, Caribbean and South Asian origin are at greater risk than the general UK population (DH 1999; Stewart *et al.* 1999).

While not always fatal, the neurological consequences may be profound and result in long-term disability, especially in elderly people. Approximately 350 000 people in the UK may be affected at any one time, of whom only half can expect to make a full recovery leaving no obvious sign of brain damage.

4.25.1 Types of stroke

There are two main types of stroke: ischaemic and haemorrhagic.

Ischaemic stroke

This is the most common type of stroke, accounting for 80–85% of cases and resulting from an obstruction in a cerebral blood vessel. Most of these, and about 50% of all strokes, are caused by cerebral thrombosis, i.e. the formation of a thrombus (blood clot) on the wall of a cerebral artery blocking the flow of blood and supply of oxygen to the brain. These types of strokes are subclassified into different types depending on the area of the infarction (Bamford 1991). The remainder of ischaemic strokes results from cerebral embolism when occlusive material (usually a blood clot but sometimes tissue debris or an air bubble) enters the circulation elsewhere in the body and causes a blockage when it is swept into a blood vessel supplying the brain.

Small, temporary blockages in cerebral blood vessels may also occur, resulting in transient ischaemic attacks (TIAs) or 'mini strokes', characterized by dizzy spells or temporary loss of awareness which resolve within 24 hours. TIAs can cause small but cumulative amounts of brain damage and often herald a major stroke.

Haemorrhagic stroke

This results from the rupture of a weakened or damaged blood vessel causing bleeding within or on the surface of the brain. This type of stroke has a high mortality rate and is more likely to occur in younger people. It accounts for about 15–20% of all cases.

A reduction in the level of ill health and death caused by stroke is one of the priorities identified in the Government's White Paper *Saving Lives: Our Healthier Nation* (DH 1999). This set a target of reducing the combined death rate from CHD and stroke in people under 75 years of age by at least two-fifths, before the year 2010.

4.25.2 Causation of stroke

Ischaemic stroke is a form of cardiovascular disease (CVD) and of similar multifactorial origin, its development strongly associated with hypertension and cigarette smoking (Shinton and Beevers 1989; Menotti *et al.* 1990). Excessive alcohol intake is an additional major risk factor for stroke (Hart *et al.* 1999). The risk of ischaemic stroke increases sharply with age and is increased in those with existing CVD or a previous history of stroke or TIAs.

The influence of cardiovascular risk factors on different subtypes of haemorrhagic stroke can vary (Vartiainen *et al.* 1995), but all types are closely associated with hypertension.

Dietary factors which affect the development of stroke are thus very similar to those of CVD in general, i.e. those which enhance the risk of atherogenesis and thrombogenesis via dyslipidaemia, hypertension and glucose intolerance, often compounded by obesity and physical inactivity (see Sections 4.21, Cardiovascular disease, and 4.22, Coronary heart disease).

4.25.3 Consequences of stroke

The consequences of survivable stroke depend on the location and extent of damage to the brain. Some stroke patients may be left with permanent paralysis and mental impairment. Others may, in time, make a good recovery.

Clinical effects of the brain damage can include:

- weakness or paralysis of muscles on one side of the body
- impaired movement
- loss of balance
- difficulties with communication, including speech
- difficulties with mastication
- dysphagia
- impaired vision
- incontinence
- impaired cognitive function or confusion
- memory loss

- inability to concentrate
- emotional instability.

Many of these factors can affect nutritional intake and management (see below).

4.25.4 Management of stroke

The Royal College of Physicians (2000) has produced national clinical guidelines for the management of stroke which set out the minimum basic standards of care based on graded evidence. They emphasize the importance of specialist multidisciplinary care and the need for early disability assessment and management in order to optimize recovery. Similar guidelines are in use in Scotland (SIGN 1997).

The RCP guidelines state that, as soon as is practicable after admission, every stroke patient should be formally assessed, using locally agreed procedures based on validated methods and applied by trained personnel, for:

- consciousness level (on admission)
- swallowing ability (within 24 hours)
- risk of pressure sore development (on admission)
- nutritional status (within 48 hours)
- cognitive impairment (within 48 hours of regaining consciousness)
- the patient's needs in relation to moving and handling (within 48 hours of admission).

Additional guidance is given regarding positioning to prevent respiratory and other complications such as contractures or pressure sores, on the prevention of venous thromboembolism, and on bladder and bowel management. The establishment of local guidelines setting out appropriate interventions for problems such as dysphagia or malnutrition is also recommended.

All patients should be referred to a specialist rehabilitation team as soon as possible, preferably within 7 days of admission. Guidelines are given on the assessment and management of problems related to:

- psychological impairment
- communication difficulties
- motor impairment
- sensory impairment and pain
- drug side-effects
- functional activities of daily living.

Issues relating to rehabilitation back into the community such as discharge planning, further rehabilitation and secondary prevention are also considered.

4.25.5 Nutritional aspects of stroke management

The provision of adequate nutrition has not always been recognized as being an integral part of stroke management, and one which may be as important as other forms of treatment. Multidisciplinary management of stroke in desig-

nated units has been shown to improve long-term survival and functional state (Indredavik *et al*. 1997).

The prognosis of stroke is unpredictable during the first 2–3 days and about one-quarter of cases will worsen significantly during this time. As soon as is practicable (and within 48 hours), the patient's nutritional needs and the factors which are likely to impact on them should be assessed to ensure that they can be incorporated into the patient's care plan.

The nutritional priorities following a stroke are:

In the acute phase, to:

- assess individual nutritional needs and underlying nutritional status
- consider the degree to which an individual's ability to self-feed and/or swallow is impaired
- ensure an individual's nutrient and fluid needs are met, if necessary by nutritional support measures via an appropriate route.

In the rehabilitation phase, to:

- help the patient to resume as near-normal eating habits as possible, given the constraints of any persisting neurological deficits
- minimize the risk of another stroke
- ensure nutritional adequacy and address any persisting nutritional problems (which at this stage may take the form of either undernutrition or overnutrition).

Nutritional requirements

The nutritional effects of acute stroke have many similarities with those of acute head injury (see Section 5.3). Stroke is followed by a phase of hypermetabolism and hypercatabolism as part of the body's response to injury, the extent of this response being roughly proportionate to the degree of brain damage. As a result there will be:

- increased energy requirements (due to hypermetabolism and pyrexia)
- increased nitrogen requirements (as a result of high nitrogen losses)
- insulin resistance and glucose intolerance (due to the effects of catabolic hormones)
- fluid and electrolyte imbalance
- acid–base imbalance.

These catabolic effects usually persist for about 4 weeks following the stroke and then slowly remit during the following month, although may not have completely returned to normal within 6 months (Smithard *et al*. 1996).

However, unlike most patients admitted with traumatic head injury, many stroke patients will be elderly and possibly frail and already malnourished (Axelsson *et al*. 1988). The combination of increased nutritional requirements, negative nitrogen balance and poor nutritional status can result in rapid nutritional deterioration. If this persists unchecked, changes in body composition and function will be profound and the risk of malnutrition high (Finestone *et al.* 1995). This risk is particularly acute in those with eating and swallowing problems, but other factors may also be relevant; Axelsson *et al.* (1989) found that stroke patients with poor nutritional status 3 weeks after admission were more likely to be those with low self-care performance, paralysis of the right arm, given intravenous fluids, who had poor nutritional status on arrival, and who were of advanced age or male. Malnourished patients with acute stroke have been shown to have an increased frequency of infections and pressure sores compared with their adequately nourished counterparts (Davalos *et al.* 1996), the presence of which may increase nutritional requirements. Malnutrition is also associated with a worse outcome and a slower rate of recovery from stroke (Finestone *et al.* 1996; Gariballa and Sinclair 1998). It is therefore important that appropriate nutritional support is instituted at an early stage in order to offset catabolic losses and reduce the risk of complications.

Dysphagia

Up to half of all cases of acute stroke are complicated by dysphagia (Gordon *et al.* 1987). The presence of dysphagia in stroke increases the risk of chest infection and is an independent predictor of mortality (Smithard *et al.* 1996). Silent aspiration, with its associated risk of pneumonia, may occur (Teasell *et al.* 1996; Daniels *et al.* 1998). Patients with dysphagia are also at greatest risk from nutritional and fluid depletion (Gordon *et al.* 1987; Unosson *et al.* 1994; Smithard *et al.* 1996). Dysphagia after stroke may involve difficulties with both the oral and pharyngeal phases of swallowing. At the oral stage, problems may occur with:

- bolus formation in the mouth due to poor lip seal
- poor tongue movement
- poor jaw movement and mastication
- pocketing food in the cheek.

The involuntary pharyngeal stage of swallowing may be absent or delayed.

All stroke patients should have their swallowing ability assessed as soon as possible, and before being given food or drink, by a simple validated bedside testing protocol carried out by trained personnel (RCP 2000). This is normally a simple water swallow test considered in conjunction with other parameters such as conscious level and respiratory status (SIGN 1997). Tests such as the absence of a gag reflex are not a reliable indicator of swallowing ability since many fit elderly people do not have a gag reflex (Davies *et al.* 1995). Suspected abnormalities should be assessed by a speech and language therapist and the nature and implications of the dysphagia ascertained. Some patients will be dysphagic to liquids but will be able to swallow those of a thicker consistency (see Section 4.3, Dysphagia). Others will not be able to manage safely any food or liquid via the oral route and will require some form of artificial nutritional support.

If oral feeding is contraindicated, feeding by alternative route needs to be commenced as soon as possible, and within 5 days (Taylor 1993). Intravenous fluids may be necessary during the initial period of stabilization (usually 2–4 days). Nasogastric feeding, using full-strength feed administered in gradually increasing quantities, may then be introduced. If gastric stasis remains a problem, nasojejunal feeding may need to be considered.

Because aspiration remains a risk with nasogastric feeding, it has been suggested that percutaneous gastrostomy (PEG) feeding may be an even better route of administration as it permits continuous and adequate nutritional support and results in better nutritional intake and better prognosis (Norton *et al.* 1996). However, several criticisms have been levelled at this particular study (Duncan *et al.* 1996; Esmonde 1996; Kerr *et al.* 1996) and it can also be questioned whether the invasiveness and resource implications of the PEG procedure can be justified on a routine basis. PEG feeding may be the method of choice if dysphagia is likely to be persistent, necessitating long-term enteral feeding. It may be more acceptable to the patient, and also preferred by ward and nursing home staff because it is a less time-consuming procedure than nasogastric feeding.

Whatever the feeding route, it is important that the chosen feeding route meets the nutritional requirements of the patient (see Section 1.13, Artifical nutritional support). Dietitians should be closely involved in the multidisciplinary management of nutritionally supported stroke patients.

Unlike dysphagia associated with many other neurological disorders, swallowing ability usually improves with time, many problems resolving within days and most having disappeared within 6 months. However, Smithard *et al.* (1997) found that problems persisted for more than 6 months in 8% of cases and recurred in others or developed later in the course of their recovery from stroke.

Before oral feeding is resumed, swallowing ability should be reassessed to ensure that this route is safe, and to determine the most appropriate consistency of foods and fluids (see Section 4.3, Dysphagia).

As dysphagia resolves and oral intake resumes, nutritional support should not be stopped until it is clear that nutritional needs can be met via oral feeding alone. Many patients will initially be unable to consume a sufficient volume of food in order to do this. It is also important to ensure that sufficient time and assistance can be given to those unable to self-feed.

Overnight feeding is often a useful intermediate support measure in those who are in the process of resuming an oral intake. People are then able to try eating 'normal' foods during the day, and often feel encouraged that they are 'making progress' as a result, but without compromising nutritional adequacy.

Other dietary measures to help to maximize the intake of nutrients from ordinary foods (e.g. food fortification) may also be appropriate (see Section 1.12, Oral nutritional support).

Neurological impairment

Some of the neurological consequences of brain injury are summarized in Table 4.63. Many of these can affect nutritional intake, in either the acute or rehabilitation phase.

Communication difficulties are likely. Problems with speech may make it difficult for stroke patients to indicate their needs or wishes, e.g. that they are thirsty or dislike the taste of a particular food. Patients may also have language difficulties (particularly following left side brain damage, i.e. right side paralysis), calling things by a wrong name or using nonsense words. They may also have problems in understanding what is said to them and answer 'yes' or 'no' to questions that they have not understood, which can be confusing for health professionals and carers.

People with damage to the right side of the brain (i.e. left side paralysis) are more likely to have perception problems, finding it difficult to recognize people or things. Some are only aware of one side of their body, eating food only on one side of the plate, or brushing only one side of their hair.

After a stroke, a person's ability to switch their attention or to do two things at once may be damaged. They may stop walking or talking, or fail to follow a conversation when several people are speaking. They often feel tired and irritable and have a short attention span.

Psychological effects may also be profound. As with any acute life-threatening illness, people who have suffered a stroke are likely to experience feelings of anxiety and/or depression which may affect the desire to eat. However, the effects of the stroke itself are likely to create additional psychological barriers to eating such as tiredness, emotional lability and frustration, perhaps over difficulties with movement, swallowing or communication. Encouragement to eat may provoke irritability or anger.

All of these factors can compromise nutritional intake and are discussed in greater depth in Section 4.28 (Neurorehabilitation).

4.25.6 Prevention of stroke

Secondary prevention

Patients who have suffered a stroke remain at high risk of a subsequent stroke (about 7% per annum), other forms of cardiovascular disease (about 7% per annum) and epilepsy (about 5% in 2 years) (Dennis *et al.* 1993; Burn *et al.* 1994; RCP 2000). The risk of further stroke is highest in the early period following the initial stroke (RCP 2000). Secondary prevention is therefore a high priority and will focus on antihypertensive measures to keep blood pressure below 140/85 mmHg, anticoagulation control and on reducing other factors associated with cardiovascular risk. Patients with a history of myocardial infarction and blood cholesterol >5 mmol/l may be given statins (see Section 4.23.6 in Hyperlipidaemia). Carotid endarterectomy may be indicated in some cases.

Table 4.63 Possible neurological consequences of stroke on nutritional intake (see also Section 4.28, Neurorehabilitation)

Neurological deficit	Influence
Perception	Cannot process information
	Unable to identify meal time
Visual perception	Cannot recognize or define food on the plate
Spatial deficits	Unable to analyse position of the plate
Planning and sequencing	Unable to match object and action
Neglect	Only half of the food will be seen, therefore only half will be consumed
Behaviour	Food may be thrown around or played with rather than consumed
Apraxia	Unable to self-feed
	Unable to recognize cutlery
Aphasia	Unable to fill out a menu or order food
Memory	Forget to eat
	Forget they have eaten
Hemiplegia	Can only use one hand to self-feed
Ataxia	Unable to self-feed
Psychological influences	Reduced appetite

Dietary objectives for the secondary prevention of stroke are the same as for primary prevention (see below). However, the nature of the advice given, and the way in which it is given, may need to differ as a result of disabilities incurred as a result of having had a stroke (Table 4.63). For example, if cognitive impairment results in a short attention span, dietary guidance will need to be given in short sessions; if there is an inability to understand words, dietary messages may need to be conveyed pictorially; if the patient is forgetful, written dietary reminders may be necessary. Physical disabilities, and the consequent difficulties with shopping, food preparation and consumption, may also influence the type of the advice given and necessitate close liaison with carers or occupational therapists.

Primary prevention

Primary prevention of stroke is very much that of reducing overall cardiovascular risk (Vartiainen *et al.* 1995) (see Section 4.21, Cardiovascular disease). For those who appear to be at particularly high risk of stroke (e.g. people with previous TIAs, diabetes or a strong family history of stroke) there is likely to be particular emphasis on:

- *Management of hypertension*: The benefits of reducing blood pressure in terms of stroke mortality are substantial and occur rapidly. Within a population, a fall in mean diastolic blood pressure of 5–6 mmHg is associated with a 35–40% fall in mortality from stroke (Collins *et al.* 1990). It has been shown that a blood pressure below 150/90 mmHg is essential for optimal stroke prevention (Du *et al.* 1997); the recommended clinical objective is to maintain blood pressure below 140/85 mmHg (Ramsay *et al.* 1999; RCP 2000). Even if this is not achievable, reduction in blood pressure will still significantly reduce the stroke risk (MacMahon *et al.*

1990). This is particularly important in elderly people as the net gain is greater than in younger individuals.

- *Smoking cessation*: Cigarette smoking is implicated in about one-third of strokes and cessation is followed within 1 or 2 years by substantial reduction in risk (Wolf *et al.* 1988).

Dietary measures to prevent stroke are those recommended to reduce cardiovascular risk (see Section 4.21.5 in Cardiovascular disease). For those at high risk of stroke, particular points to emphasize within the overall framework of the cardioprotective diet framework are:

- *The importance of preventing or reducing overweight*: Advice on curtailing intake of fat-rich and sugar-rich foods, and increasing consumption of cereal foods and fruit and vegetables is particularly pertinent to those who are overweight. It may be equally important to encourage an increase in physical activity because, apart from assisting weight loss, there is some evidence that regular exercise may be specifically beneficial in terms of stroke prevention (Gillum *et al.* 1996).
- *Increasing intake of fruit and vegetables*: Reviews of the literature are consistent with a strong protective effect of fruit and vegetables for stroke (Ness and Powles 1997; Appel 1999), particularly cruciferous and green leafy vegetables and citrus fruits and juices (Joshipura *et al.* 1999). This may reflect the combined benefits from their high content of antioxidants (which reduce cardiovascular risk) and potassium (which is antihypertensive).
- *Avoiding excessive consumption of sodium*: The role of sodium in the development of hypertension remains to be clearly established (see Section 4.24.3 in Hypertension) but there is some evidence that modest salt restriction may be beneficial in the treatment of hypertension (Cappuchio *et al.* 1997) and hence in the prevention of stroke (DH 1994). However, what is beyond doubt is that the typical UK diet contains salt at a level which is far in excess of physiological need, and that some reduction in this level will not be harmful and may well be beneficial to those at high risk of CVD and stroke. Since the vast majority of dietary sodium is obtained from processed manufactured foods, greater use of fresh or frozen unprocessed foods, especially fruit and vegetables, should be encouraged.
- *Increasing the consumption of fish, especially oily fish*: Omega-3 fatty acids in oily fish have beneficial antithrombogenic effects and possibly other cardioprotective effects (de Deckere *et al.* 1998). White fish is useful as a main meal component which is low in fat and energy.
- *Keeping alcohol consumption within safe limits*: Although modest consumption of alcohol may be protective in terms of CVD, excessive alcohol intake dramatically increases the risk of stroke (Hart *et al.* 1999).

More specific dietary guidance may be required for those with overt clinical problems such as:
- hypertension (see Section 4.24)
- hyperlipidaemia (see Section 4.23)
- diabetes: the importance of tight blood glucose control in the prevention of stroke in these patients has now been clearly established (UKPDS 1998) (see Section 4.16).

Text revised by: Briony Thomas

Acknowledgements: Helen Molyneux, Kathryn Morton, June Copeman, Dimple Thakrar, Alison Boyd and the British Dietetic Association's NAGE and DINT Groups.

Useful address

The Stroke Association, CHSA House, Whitecross Street, London EC1Y 8JJ
Tel: 020 7490 7999 Fax: 020 7490 2686
There are local support groups of this association in many areas.

Further reading

Laidler P. *Stroke Rehabilitation: Structure and Strategy*. London: Chapman and Hall, 1994.

Mulley GP. *Practical Management of Stroke*. London: Chapman and Hall, 1985.

Reviews by the Cochrane Stroke Research Group. (Available at www.dcn.ed.ac.uk/csrg)

Royal College of Physicians, The Intercollegiate Working Party for Stroke. *National Clinical Guidelines for Stroke*. London: RCP, 2000. (Available at www.rcplondon.ac.uk)

SIGN (Scottish Intercollegiate Guidelines Network). *Management of Patients with Stroke*. Edinburgh: SIGN Network, 1997. (Available at www.show.scot.nhs.uk/sign/clinical.htm)

The Stroke Association. *Reducing the Risk of Stroke*. London: The Stroke Association, 1996.

Wood VA, Hewer RL. The prevention and management of stroke. *Journal of Public Health Medicine* 1996; **18**: 423–431.

References

Appel IJ. Nonpharmacologic therapies that reduce blood pressure: a fresh perspective. *Clinical Cardiology* 1999; **22** (7 Suppl): III1–III5.

Axelsson R, Asplund K, Norberg A, Eriksson S. Eating problems and nutritional status during hospital stay of patients with severe stroke. *Journal of the American Dietetic Association* 1989; **89**: 1092–1096.

Axelsson R, Asplund K, Norberg A, Alafuzoff I. Nutritional status in patients with acute stroke. *Acta Medica Scandinavica* 1998; **224**: 217–224.

Bamford J, Sandercock P, Dennis M *et al*. Classification and natural history of clinically identifiable subtypes of cerebral infarction. *Lancet* 1991; **337**: 1521–1526.

Burn J, Dennis M, Bamford J *et al*. Long-term risk of recurrent stroke after a first-ever stroke. The Oxfordshire Community Stroke Project. *Stroke* 1994; **25**: 333–337.

Cappuchio FP, Markandu RGN, Carney C *et al*. Double-blind randomised trial of modest salt restriction in older people. *Lancet* 1997; **350**: 850–854.

Collins R, Peto R, MacMahon S *et al*. Blood pressure, stroke and coronary heart disease. Part 2, short-term reductions in blood pressure: overview of randomised trials in their epidemiological context. *Lancet* 1990; **335**: 827–838.

Daniels SK, Brailey K, Priestly DH *et al.* Aspiration in patients with acute stroke. *Archives of Physical Medicine and Rehabilitation* 1998; **79**: 14–19.

Davalos A, Ricart W, Gonzalez-Huix F *et al.* Effect of malnutrition after acute stroke on clinical outcome. *Stroke* 1996; **27**: 1028–1032.

Davies AE, Kidd D, Stone SP, MacMahon J. Pharyngeal sensation and gag reflex in healthy subjects. *Lancet* 1995; **345**: 487–488.

de Deckere EAM, Korver O, Verschuren PM, Katan MB. Health aspects of fish and *n*-3 polyunsaturated fatty acids from plant and marine origin. *European Journal of Clinical Nutrition* 1998; **52**: 749–753.

Dennis MS, Burn JP, Sandercock PA *et al.* Long-term survival after first-ever stroke: the Oxfordshire Community Stroke Project. *Stroke* 1993; **24**: 796–800.

Department of Health, Committee on Medical Aspects of Food Policy (COMA). *Nutritional Aspects of Cardiovascular Disease.* Report on Health and Social Subjects 46. London: HMSO, 1994.

Department of Health. *Saving Lives: Our Healthier Nation* London: HMSO, 1999.

Du X, Cruickshank K, McNamee R *et al.* Case–control study of stroke and the quality of hypertension control in north west England. *British Medical Journal* 1997; **314**: 272–276.

Duncan HD, Walters E, Silk DBA. Percutaneous endoscopic gastrostomy feeding after acute dysphagic stroke. Mortality associated with nasogastric tube feeding was high (Letter). *British Medical Journal* 1996; **312**: 973.

Esmonde T. Percutaneous endoscopic gastrostomy feeding after acute dysphagic stroke. Study's methods were inadequate (Letter). *British Medical Journal* 1996; **312**: 973.

Finestone HM, Greene-Finestone LS, Wilson ES, Teasell RW. Malnutrition in stroke patients on the rehabilitation service and at follow-up: prevalence and predictors. *Archives of Physical Medicine and Rehabilitation* 1995; **76**: 310–316.

Finestone HM, Greene-Finestone LS, Wilson ES, Teasell RW. Prolonged length of stay and reduced functional improvement rate in malnourished stroke rehabilitation patients. *Archives of Physical Medicine and Rehabilitation* 1996; 77 340–345.

Gariballa SE, Sinclair AJ. Assessment and treatment of nutritional status in stroke patients. *Postgraduate Medical Journal* 1998; **74**: 395–399.

Gillum RF, Mussolino ME, Ingram DD. Physical activity and stroke incidence in women and men: the NHANES I Epidemiologic Follow-up Study. *American Journal of Epidemiology* 1996; **143**: 860–869.

Gordon C, Hewer RL, Wade DT. Dysphagia in acute stroke. *British Medical Journal* 1987; **295**: 411–414.

Hart CL, Smith GD, Hole DJ, Hawthorne VM. Alcohol consumption and mortality from all causes, coronary heart disease and stroke: results from a prospective cohort study of Scottish men with 21 years of follow up. *British Medical Journal* 1999; **318**: 1725–1729.

Indredavik B, Slordahl SA, Bakke F *et al.* Stroke unit treatment. Long term effects. *Stroke* 1997; **28**: 1861–1866.

Joshipura KJ, Ascherio A, Manson JE *et al.* Fruit and vegetable intake in relation to risk of ischaemic stroke. *Journal of the American Medical Association* 1999; **282**: 1233–1239.

Kerr J, Butterworth R, Bath P. Percutaneous endoscopic gastrostomy feeding after acute dysphagic stroke. Speech and language therapists should have participated in the study (Letter). *British Medical Journal* 1996; **312**: 972.

MacMahon S, Peto R, Cutler J *et al.* Blood pressure, stroke and coronary heart disease I. Prolonged differences in blood pressure: prospective observational trials corrected for the regression dilution bias. *Lancet* 1990; **335**: 765–774.

Menotti A, Keys A, Blackburn H *et al.* Twenty-year stroke mortality and prediction in twelve cohorts of the seven countries study. *International Journal of Epidemiology* 1990; **19**: 309–315.

Ness AR, Powles JW. Fruit and vegetables, and cardiovascular disease: a review *International Journal of Epidemiology* 1997; **26**: 1–13.

Norton B, Homer-Ward M, Donnelly MT *et al.* A randomised prospective comparison of percutaneous endoscopic gastrostomy and nasogastric tube feeding after acute dysphagic stroke. *British Medical Journal* 1996; **312**: 13–16.

Ramsay LE, Williams B, Johnston GD *et al.* Guidelines for management of hypertension: report of the third working party of the British Hypertension Society. *Journal of Human Hypertension* 1999; **13**: 569–592.

Royal College of Physicians, The Intercollegiate Working Party for Stroke. *National Clinical Guidelines for Stroke.* London: RCP, 2000.

Shinton R, Beevers G. Meta-analysis of relation between cigarette smoking and stroke. *British Medical Journal* 1989; **298**: 787–794.

SIGN (Scottish Intercollegiate Guidelines Network). *Management of patients with Stroke. III Identification and Management of Dysphagia.* Edinburgh: SIGN, 1997.

Smithard DG, O'Neill PA, Parks C, Morris J. Complications and outcome after acute stroke. Does dysphagia matter? *Stroke* 1996; **27**: 1200–1204.

Smithard DG, O'Neill PA, England RE *et al.* The natural history of dysphagia following a stroke. *Dysphagia* 1997; **12**: 188–193.

Stewart JA, Dundas R, Howard RS *et al.* Ethnic differences in incidence of stroke: prospective study with stroke register. *British Medical Journal* 1999; **318**: 967–971.

Taylor SJ. Audit of nasogastric feeding practice at two acute hospitals: is early enteral feeding associated with reduced mortality and hospital stay? *Journal of Human Nutrition and Dietetics* 1993; **6**: 477–489.

Teasell RW, McRae M, Marchuk Y, Finestone HM. Pneumonia associated with aspiration following stroke. *Archives of Physical Medicine and Rehabilitation* 1996; **77**: 707–709.

UK Prospective Diabetes Study Group (UKPDS). Tight blood pressure control and risk of microvascular and microvascular complications in type 2 diabetes: UKPDS 38. *British Medical Journal* 1998; **317**: 703–713.

Unosson M, Ek A, Bjurulf P, van Schenck H, Larsson J. Feeding dependence and nutritional status after acute stroke. *Stroke* 1994; **25**: 366–371.

Vartiainen E, Sarti C, Tuomilehto J, Kuulasmaa K. Do changes in cardiovascular risk factors explain changes in mortality from stroke in Finland? *British Medical Journal* 1995; **310**: 901–904.

Wolf PA, D'Agostino RB, Kannel WB *et al.* Cigarette smoking as a risk of stroke. The Framingham study. *Journal of the American Medical Association* 1988; **259**: 1025–1029.

4.26 Neurodegenerative disorders

4.26.1 Parkinson's disease

Parkinson's disease is a chronic progressive neurological disorder in which the body's ability to control voluntary movements (such as walking, talking, writing and swallowing) becomes increasingly impaired. The condition was first described by James Parkinson in 1817 and is still not completely understood. It results from a loss of dopamine-producing nerve cells in the substantia nigra area of the brain. Dopamine is the neurotransmitter which relays signals between the substantia nigra and the corpus striatum area of the brain, resulting in smooth, purposeful muscle activity. Loss of dopamine causes the nerve cells of the striatum to fire out of control, leaving people unable to direct or control their movements in a normal manner.

Parkinson's disease is the most common form of parkinsonism, the name for a group of disorders with similar symptoms and all resulting from the loss of dopamine-producing brain cells. Parkinson's disease itself is sometimes referred to as idiopathic or primary Parkinson's disease because the reason for the death or impairment of dopamine-producing brain cells is unknown. Current research suggests that the condition may result from a combination of factors such as oxidative damage, environmental toxins, genetic predisposition and accelerated ageing. Other types of parkinsonism are usually secondary to another primary neurological disorder.

Parkinson's disease affects about 1 in 500 of the general population, its prevalence increasing with age to about 1 in 100 over 65 years and 1 in 50 over 80 years. There are about 120 000 sufferers in the UK and 10 000 new cases are diagnosed every year. Onset is usually between the ages of 55 and 65 years but between 5 and 10% of patients are under the age of 40.

Its progression is slow and life expectancy is not significantly reduced. It can, however, significantly impair the quality of life.

Features of Parkinson's disease

Parkinson's disease can be difficult to diagnose because the onset is usually gradual and the early symptoms such as stiffness, unsteadiness or slowness may be attributed to, or genuinely result from, the general ageing process. However, as the disease progresses the symptoms will worsen and begin to interfere with daily life. When about 80% of dopamine-producing cells have been lost, the following symptoms usually appear, although not all of these are present in every case:

- *Tremor*: An involuntary shaking of the limbs, head or entire body, which is most apparent when the affected part is at rest or the person is under stress. The typical tremor of Parkinson's is a rhythmic back and forth 'pill-rolling' movement between the thumb and forefinger at about 3 beats per second. Tremor decreases during deliberate movement and disappears during sleep. Initially it may only affect one side of the body, becoming more general in time. Although tremor is rarely disabling, it is one of the symptoms that bothers patients most.
- *Rigidity*: This describes the resistance to movement which results from involuntary muscle contraction. Normal movement depends on the contraction of one muscle being counterbalanced by relaxation in an opposing muscle. In Parkinson's disease, muscles remain in a constantly contracted state, causing symptoms such as muscle stiffness, weakness or aching. Patients are less aware of impaired movement and this may be obvious to a carer; for example, raising the patient's arm results in rachet-like jerky movements (cogwheel rigidity).
- *Bradykinesia*: This is slowness of movement and is often the most disabling feature of the disease. Normal activities such as washing and dressing may take hours. There may also be slowness in speech and delayed reaction to conversation. Bradykinesia may also be frustratingly unpredictable, with the affected person finding that they can move easily one moment but need help the next.
- *Postural instability*: Impaired balance and co-ordination results in general unsteadiness in movement, particularly while turning, and increased risk of falls. Patients often develop a forward or backward lean, or sometimes a stooped posture with the head bowed and the shoulders dropped. Gait disturbance becomes more obvious; some patients may halt in mid-stride, sometimes toppling over as a result, others may shuffle along with knees flexed and ultimately some may be unable to walk unaided.

The nature and intensity of symptoms vary between affected individuals. Other symptoms may include psychiatric or emotional disturbances, changes in bowel function or sleep pattern, and problems with eating, swallowing or speech. Tiredness and depression are common accompaniments to the disease, as is constipation. Drooling of saliva is common owing to failure to swallow and dysphagia may be a problem. Cognitive problems and dementia may occur later in the disease. Initially, symptoms may be predominantly one-sided but eventually progress to involve the other side of the body.

There are no simple tests for Parkinson's disease and diagnosis is based on clinical signs and symptoms and the exclusion of other possible causes for them. As a result, there is lack of uniformity in diagnostic criteria and study methods (Mutch 1995) and misdiagnosis may be relatively common (Hughes *et al.* 1992). Other conditions that can cause parkinsonian symptoms include:

- encephalitis
- drug side-effects, e.g. chlorpromazine and haloperidol prescribed for psychiatric disorders
- striatal degeneration of the brain
- arteriosclerotic disease of the brain resulting in small multi-infarcts
- exposure to toxic substances, e.g. carbon monoxide
- Wilson's disease, Huntington's disease, Alzheimer's disease and Creutzfeldt–Jakob disease.

Management of Parkinson's disease

Currently, there is no cure for Parkinson's disease, although drug therapy can relieve many of its symptoms. The type of medication used varies between individuals according to the nature and severity of symptoms. Since many of the available drugs have significant side-effects, the aim of drug therapy is to find a balance between effective symptom control and avoidance of side-effects.

Drugs commonly used in the management of Parkinson's disease are:

- *Levodopa (L-dopa)*: This is the cornerstone of treatment. L-dopa, a derivative of the amino acid tyrosine, crosses the blood–brain barrier and is converted to dopamine, resulting in significant improvement in many symptoms. However, because of the side-effects associated with its prolonged use, L-dopa is only given when the symptoms of the disease compromise normal functioning. It is usually taken in combination with a dopa-decarboxylase inhibitor (e.g. benserazide or carbidopa), which results in a better therapeutic response and also helps to minimize side-effects.
- *Dopamine agonists (e.g. bromocriptine, pergolide, lysuride and apomorphine)*: Younger patients are often initially started on a dopamine agonist to avoid the side-effects of protracted L-dopa therapy. Dopamine agonists stimulate dopamine receptors and thus potentiate the effect of dopamine.
- *Selegiline*: This is a monoamine oxidase B inhibitor which inhibits dopamine degradation, thus augmenting the effects of L-dopa. It may be given in the early stages to delay introduction of L-dopa therapy. It is also used in severe parkinsonism to reduce 'end-of-dose' deterioration to L-dopa.
- *Amantadine*: This enhances L-dopa release from presynaptic storage vesicles and results in modest improvements for about 1 year, after which L-dopa usually becomes necessary.
- *Anticholinergic agents (antimuscarinics), e.g. benzhexol, orphenadrine, benztropine and procyclidine*: These block acetylcholine receptors and may help to reduce tremor and rigidity. They are less effective than L-dopa but may usefully supplement its action or be used as an alternative to L-dopa in those with mild symptoms.

The effectiveness of drug therapy in Parkinson's disease tends to diminish with time and the duration of benefit after each dose becomes progressively shorter; this is known as 'end-dose failure'. Side-effects of L-dopa such as dyskinesia (abnormal involuntary movements) may also begin to appear.

Patients on long-term therapy may also suffer from 'on/off syndrome', causing sudden alterations in or loss of functional ability. These 'off' states are unpredictable and may last for only a few minutes or many hours. Different dosages or combinations of drugs are usually tried to overcome the problem.

There has recently been a resurgence of interest in the use of surgery or implantation of electrodes into the brain to control symptoms such as tremor and dyskinesia in cases proving intractable to drug therapy.

Nutritional aspects of Parkinson's disease

Many of the symptoms of Parkinson's disease can affect nutritional intake:

- *Tremor* in the hands does not usually prevent the action of getting food to the mouth but it does tend to increase spillage, thus tending to make the sufferer feel embarrassed and perhaps reluctant to eat in the company of others. This can result in social isolation, perhaps for a partner or carer as well.
- *Rigidity* and stiffness in muscles can inhibit a range of movements, particularly those requiring fine control such as cutting up food. Assistance may be required which, again, may be demoralizing to the sufferer if this becomes necessary in public. Difficulties with chewing and sometimes swallowing food may also develop.
- *Slowness of movement* can significantly prolong the time taken to eat a meal. Food may be abandoned either because it has become cold and unappetizing or because of fatigue arising from the sheer effort involved in eating. Part of a meal may also be abandoned in order not to keep others waiting.
- *Mood changes* such as anxiety, depression, irritability and restlessness may impair appetite. Side-effects of some anti-parkinsonian drugs may also exacerbate these problems (see below).
- *Drug side-effects*: Many of the side-effects of antiparkinsonian drugs have nutritional implications. Most of the dopaminergic drugs can have serious neuropsychiatric side-effects such as confusion, hallucinations or psychosis, all of which may affect food intake. Gastrointestinal side-effects may include nausea, vomiting, dry mouth or constipation.

Patients with Parkinson's are thus at considerable risk of undernutrition as a result of both the symptoms of the disease and the side-effects of its treatment (Beyer *et al.* 1995). Following the onset of the disease, about half of all sufferers will experience weight loss and about three-quarters will experience eating difficulties of some kind (Abbott *et al.* 1992).

The nutritional effects of poor food intake may also be exacerbated by increased energy expenditure as a result of tremor or rigidity.

Dietary management of Parkinson's disease

Since both the treatment and effects of Parkinson's disease may compromise nutritional intake, dietary management aims to:

- identify nutritional inadequacies at an early stage: simple screening and assessment tools can be used to detect nutritional status and identify patients at risk of malnutrition
- implement measures to correct deficiencies or nutrition-related problems
- find ways to minimize any practical difficulties associated with eating or swallowing
- prevent undesirable weight gain or loss
- lessen the impact of drug-therapy side-effects on dietary intake
- monitor the patient's nutritional status as the disease progresses.

These aspects are discussed in general terms in Section 4.28 (Neurorehabilitation).

Early stages of the disease

People should be encouraged to:

- eat a well-balanced diet along *Balance of Good Health* guidelines
- consume plenty of fluids and fibre
- adopt measures to make eating easier, e.g. the use of non-slip mats.

As the disease progresses

Specific guidance may be needed to help to overcome the following problems.

Poor food intake Guidance on ways of improving nutrient intake via the use of nutrient dense foods, food fortification measures or dietary supplements may be necessary. Other strategies to overcome problems such as anorexia, sensory impairment and fatigue may also be helpful (see Section 1.12, Oral nutritional support).

Swallowing difficulties These need to be addressed promptly to prevent weight loss and malnutrition. Significant problems with swallowing require expert assessment from a speech and language therapist and guidance regarding food texture modification (see Section 4.3, Dysphagia). Since altered texture diets may be nutritionally dilute, additional use of supplements may be indicated.

Tremor causing spillage or difficulties with eating Measures which may help include:

- use of a non-slip mat or damp cloth underneath the plate or bowl

- large-handled cutlery
- two-handled cups to reduce spillage
- a 'stay-warm' plate to keep food hot if it takes a long time to eat meals.

Drug-related side-effects Dietary measures which alleviate problems such as anorexia, nausea and vomiting may be helpful (see Section 1.12, Oral nutritional support).

Constipation This is a common feature of Parkinson's as a result of:

- reduced peristalsis causing delayed gut transit time
- lack of fibre intake due to difficulties in eating fibrous foods requiring a lot of chewing
- lack of fluid intake as a response to problems with urgency and frequency of micturition or incontinence
- reduced mobility
- a side-effect of some anti-parkinsonian drugs.

Patients should be encouraged to consume:

- sufficient fluid: about 2 litres of fluid per day (about 8–10 cups or 6–8 mugs) in the form of fluids such as water, soft drinks, fruit juice, tea or coffee
- sufficient fibre: in the form of fibre-rich foods which are easy to manage, e.g. high-fibre choices of breakfast cereals, wholemeal bread, easy to peel fruit such as bananas or satsumas, or dried fruit, and by including vegetables, peas, beans and lentils as meal components. However, the common practice of adding bran to foods should not be encouraged as this is more likely to create problems than solve them.

Overweight A reduction in activity level combined with inappropriate food choice can result in excessive weight gain. Dietary guidance should focus on the need to reduce fat-rich and sugar-rich food choices rather than more nutrient-dense foods. Consumption of fruit and vegetables should be increased and the use of reduced-fat milk and dairy foods encouraged.

End-stages of the disease

Cognitive dysfunction becomes increasingly likely. Confusion is common and may be accompanied by delusions and hallucinations. Drug dosage to control motor dysfunction may have to be reduced in order to produce a more settled psychological state. The consequent worsening of motor symptoms is likely to increase the risk of eating and swallowing difficulties necessitating dietetic involvement and possibly active nutritional support. This should be prescribed on an individual basis in consultation with the rest of the multidisciplinary team.

The needs of carers should not be overlooked. Looking after a person with Parkinson's disease can be stressful and often lead to social isolation. Ensuring that there is a key worker who is available to offer information, advice and support is essential (O'Reilly *et al.* 1996).

Dietary implications of drug therapy

L-Dopa should be taken after meals to lessen the likelihood of gastrointestinal side-effects such as nausea and vomiting. L-Dopa absorption is reduced by iron supplements. Its action is also antagonized by vitamin B_6 unless the drug is given without a dopa decarboxylase inhibitor.

Anticholinergic drugs can cause a dry mouth, in which case they should be taken before food is eaten. If gastrointestinal side-effects are problematical, the drugs should be taken after food.

Dietary manipulation and Parkinson's disease

Protein   It has been suggested that high protein intakes, in particular of neutral amino acids (phenylalanine, tyrosine and tryptophan), may compete with the receptor sites where L-dopa is converted to dopamine and hence reduce its effectiveness. As a result, it has been suggested that reduction or manipulation of dietary protein intake may help to counteract the decrease in the long-term effectiveness of the drug and so help to provide symptom relief.

Measures which have been advocated include restricting protein intake to 7–10 g during the day in order to maximize absorption of the drug and minimize motor fluctuations, and consuming most in the evening when poorer motor functions are less likely to disrupt a person's lifestyle. Riley and Lang (1998) report that this approach is well tolerated and beneficial. Pare *et al.* (1992) maintained that healthy, well-motivated individuals could maintain an adequate intake of most nutrients despite restricting dietary intake in the daytime as long as they received sufficient dietetic education and support.

Alternative strategies include reducing protein intake to 0.5 g/kg ideal body weight per day (25–35 g protein per day), distributing intake evenly throughout the day (Carter *et al.* 1989) and increasing the proportion of dietary carbohydrate to protein to a ratio of 5:1, thought to yield an optimum ratio between plasma neutral amino acids and L-dopa (Berry *et al.* 1991).

Karstaedt and Pincus (1992) suggested that the long-term use of a protein-restricted diet is a safe and simple technique to extend the usefulness of carbidopa/L-dopa therapy in advanced Parkinson's disease. However, it should be borne in mind that these are experimental techniques and that the benefits have not been sufficiently established for them to be regarded as standard practice. They may be a viable option in some instances when symptom control on medication is failing or inadequate but, in any patient where nutritional intake is already inadequate (particularly likely in patients with advanced disease) there is a considerable risk that such dietary manipulations could seriously compromise nutritional status.

Antioxidants   Oxidative stress and lipid peroxidation may play an important role in the pathogenesis of Parkinson's disease and it has been suggested that high dietary intakes of antioxidants may be protective against the development of the disease. However, at present this remains speculative; while some studies have reported findings consistent with this effect (de Rijk *et al.* 1997) others have failed to confirm this (Logroscino *et al.* 1996; Morens *et al.* 1996). Further research is needed (Ben-Shlomo 1997).

Once the disease has developed, there is no evidence that taking supplemental doses of antioxidants slows the progression of the disease or enhances the effects of antiparkinsonian drugs. Patients who are concerned about their intake of these nutrients should be reassured that a well-balanced diet will meet their antioxidant needs, and that food sources of these nutrients (particularly fruit and vegetables) may be better, and probably safer, than supplements.

4.26.2 Motor neurone disease

Motor neurone disease (MND) is the name given to a group of closely related disorders characterized by degeneration of motor neurones. The consequences of the disease are profound and highly distressing as the progressive loss of muscle movement may impair not only limb movement but ultimately the ability to speak, eat or swallow. In contrast, sensory neurones are usually unaffected so the patient remains fully aware of his or her surroundings and situation.

MND affects about 1 in 50 000 people every year, and its prevalence in the population is about 5–10 cases per 100 000. The vast majority of cases are sporadic and the cause of the disease is unknown. In about 5% cases the disease appears to be genetic in origin as a result of one or more mutations on certain genes, and several generations of one family may be affected.

The course of the disease varies according to the form of the disease, but prognosis is poor. About 40% of patients survive for 5 years and only 10% survive for 10 years. In some, the course of the disease is very rapid, and survival may only be a matter months.

Features of motor neurone disease

Types of motor neurone disease

The physical effects of the disease depend on which motor neurones are affected. Neurological lesions may primarily occur in the upper motor neurones (from the brain to the spinal cord), lower motor neurones (from the spinal cord to muscles), or both. MND is therefore broadly classified into three types, although as the disease progresses they become less distinguishable in terms of their symptoms.

Amyotrophic lateral sclerosis   This is the most common form of the disease (about two-thirds of cases), typically occurring after the age of 55 years. Men are affected more than women in the ratio 3:2.

It involves both upper and lower motor neurone lesions, causing:

- muscle weakness
- spasticity (stiffness)
- hyperactive reflexes (jerking of limbs).

Symptoms commonly appear first in the hands or feet, with people tending to drop things unaccountably or trip when walking.

Survival time from diagnosis is approximately 3–5 years.

Progressive muscular atrophy   This is a much rarer form of the disease, accounting only about 7.5% of MND cases. It tends to occur at a younger age (often below the age of 50 years) and is much more common in men than women. It is predominantly a degeneration of lower motor neurones, causing:

- muscle weakness and wasting
- weight loss
- fasciculation (muscle twitching), often starting in the small muscles of one hand.

Survival time usually exceeds 5 years.

Progressive bulbar palsy   This accounts for about 25% of cases of MND, mostly occurring in people over the age of 70 years, and is slightly more common in women than men.

It affects the upper motor neurones and causes a paralysis of the bulbar muscles which control speech, chewing and swallowing. It therefore tends to present in a different way from the other two forms of the disease. Early symptoms are:

- slurred speech
- inexplicable choking on certain foods.

Speech may gradually deteriorate to a point where other forms of communication are necessary. Chewing and swallowing foods and liquids becomes increasingly difficult and saliva tends to pool in and dribble out of the mouth.

Most people with progressive bulbar palsy retain the ability to walk. Progression is often rapid, with survival time from diagnosis being in the range of 6 months to 3 years.

Diagnosis

MND is difficult to diagnose in the early stages as its initial symptoms may be indistinguishable from those of other neurological disorders. As the disease progresses, diagnosis may confirmed by measuring electrical activity in muscles by electromyography or by muscle biopsy.

Management of motor neurone disease

There is no cure for MND, although several drugs which may slow the progression of the disease are at various stages of trial. Unlike some neurodegenerative disorders, there are no remissions, although there may be plateaus of weeks or months when no further deterioration occurs.

Nutritional aspects of management

MND affects each sufferer differently in terms of its effects and progression. Nutritional management will therefore depend on the nature of the individual problems. Malnutrition is a considerable risk, even in those without swallowing difficulties (Worwood and Leigh 1998).

In the early stages of the disease, the symptoms may be relatively slight and factors which are most likely to affect food intake are:

- anorexia as a result of depression or anxiety following the diagnosis
- fatigue
- side-effects of drug treatment such as nausea.

Suggested measures to help to overcome these effects in order to maintain good nutrition may be helpful (see Section 1.12, Oral nutritional support).

Emotional lability is a common consequence of the disease, causing inappropriate laughing or crying. Both patients and carers may find this distressing.

As the disease progresses, eating and swallowing difficulties become more likely. Increasing difficulties with communication are also likely to become a source of frustration to both patients and those trying to interpret their needs or wishes. Dietitians should not forget that the patient's ability to taste, smell and feel the texture of food (as well the senses of sight and hearing) are likely to be unimpaired even in the most debilitated patient.

Bowel and bladder function are not usually directly affected, but bowel problems may result from restricted fibre and fluid intake and immobility. Dehydration may result from limited fluid intake.

As the disease progresses, problems such as dysphagia are likely to necessitate more active nutritional intervention (see Section 4.3, Dysphagia). In the latter stages of the disease, complete artificial nutritional support may be required (see Section 1.13, Artificial nutritional support).

4.26.3 Huntington's disease

Huntington's disease (sometimes known as Huntington's chorea) is a genetic neurodegenerative disorder caused by a faulty copy of a gene on chromosome 4. It affects 4–8 people per 100 000 in European populations (Harper 1992) and results in progressive movement disorders, speech difficulties, mental deterioration and cognitive decline, usually resulting in dementia.

The disorder usually manifests itself in adulthood, typically between the age of 40 and 50 years when initial symptoms such as clumsiness, forgetfulness and mood swings become accompanied by chorea, i.e. random involuntary movements caused by overactive dopaminergic neurons. Worsening chorea eventually affects the orofacial region, affecting speech and swallowing ability. Progressive mental decline further impairs the ability to perform the activities of daily living.

Nutritional aspects of Huntington's disease

Huntington's disease inflicts many of the worst aspects of both neurodegenerative disease and dementia, and consequently has a number of nutritional implications:

- *The psychological consequences of the diagnosis*: The realization that the sufferer faces rapid physical decline and premature dementia, that only palliative care can be offered and that (being a dominantly inherited genetic disorder) any children of the affected individual have a

50% risk of inheriting the disease, not surprisingly induces profound anxiety and depression. Appetite and food intake are likely to be impaired.

- *Increased energy requirements*: People with Huntington's disease often exhibit marked weight loss despite high energy intakes (O'Brien *et al.* 1990; Kremer and Roos 1992). Originally this was assumed to reflect the energy costs of the choreic movements, but this is no longer thought to be the case; dystonic patients in the later stages of the disease may be even more hyperkinetic than those with motor dysfunction in the early stages. It has been suggested that defective mitochondrial energy metabolism as an integral part of the disease is more likely to be the cause (O'Brien *et al.* 1990).
- *The ability to self-feed*: Choreic movements may make it physically difficult to transfer food and liquids to the mouth without spillage and create psychological stresses such as loss of self-esteem and hence reluctance to eat in the company of others.
- *Dysphagia*: Poorly co-ordinated or unexpected involuntary movements of the mouth and pharynx result in severe swallowing difficulties. Aspiration pneumonia is the most common cause of death in these patients (Haines and Conneally 1986).
- *Mental decline*: Progressive cognitive impairment may result in many of the behavioural difficulties associated with dementia (see Section 4.29, Dementias). These are likely to be particularly distressing to the relatives and carers and it is they who are often in most need of appropriate dietetic guidance and support.

Dietetic objectives therefore comprise:

- *Helping to maintain the patient's quality of life* by suggesting strategies which help to overcome physical or psychological difficulties associated with feeding, thus maintaining the patient's dignity and enjoyment of food.
- *Ensuring that the patient's nutritional needs, particularly for energy, are met*: A body mass index (BMI) <20 at diagnosis has been shown to be a strong predictor for the rate of disease progression (Myers *et al.* 1991). Achieving an energy intake which helps to prevent or correct weight loss may be important. In some people, guidance on energy-dense food choices and food-fortification strategies may be sufficient (see Section 1.12, Oral nutritional support). Others may require more active nutritional support measures at an early stage (see Section 1.13, Artificial nutritional support).
- *Minimizing the risks from dysphagia* by ensuring that oral food and liquid intake is of a texture and consistency which minimize the risk of choking and aspiration (see Section 4.3, Dysphagia). This usually requires close liaison with a speech and language therapist.
- *Supporting relatives and carers* by providing practical dietetic guidance for coping with any of the physical and behavioural eating difficulties which arise.
- *Monitoring the patient's nutritional progress*, particularly in terms of weight stability and dysphagic problems

so that problems can be identified at an early stage and steps taken to rectify them.

Text written by: Briony Thomas

Acknowledgements: Karen Hyland, Dimple Thakrar, June Copeman, Helen Molyneux, and members of the British Dietetic Association's NAGE and DINT Groups.

Useful addresses

Parkinson's Disease Society of the United Kingdom
United Scientific House, 215 Vauxhall Bridge Road, London SW1V IEJ
Tel: 020 7931 8080 Fax: 020 7233 9908
Helpline: 020 7233 5373
Website: http://glaxocentre.merseyside.org/pds.html
E-mail: mailbox@pdsuk.demon.co.uk

Parkinson's Disease Scottish Resource
10 Claremont Terrace, Glasgow G3 7XR
Tel/Fax: 0141 332 3343

Motor Neurone Disease (MND) Association
PO Box 246, Northampton NN1 2PR
Tel: 01604 250505

Useful resources

The British Dietetic Association's NAGE Group has produced some useful resource material for dietitians dealing with patients with Parkinson's disease and other neurodisabilities. Details of current publications and availability can be obtained via the BDA website at www.bda.org.uk or directly from the British Dietetic Association.

Further reading

Parkinson's Disease

Kempster PA, Wahlqvist ML. Dietary factors in the management of Parkinson's disease. *Nutrition Reviews* 1994; **52** (2 Pt 1): 51–58.

Robertson DR, George CF. Drug therapy for Parkinson's disease in the elderly. *British Medical Bulletin* 1990; **46**: 124–146.

Motor neurone disease

Skelton J. Caring for patients with motor neurone disease. *Nursing Standard* 1996; **10** (32): 33–36.

Skelton J. Dysphagia in motor neurone disease. *Nursing Standard* 1996; **10** (33): 49–53.

Huntington's disease

Kimball France J. Huntington's disease: helping the patient retain function. *American Journal of Nursing* 1993; **93** (8): 62–64.

Skirton H, Glendinning N. Using research to develop care for patients with Huntington's disease. *British Journal of Nursing* 1997; **6** (2): 83–90.

References

Abbott RA, Cox M, Markus H, Tomkins A. Diet, body size and

micronutrient status in Parkinson's disease. *European Journal of Clinical Nutrition* 1992; **46**: 879–884.

Ben-Shlomo Y. The epidemiology of Parkinson's disease. *Bailleres Clinical Neurology* 1997; **6**: 55–68.

Berry EM, Growdon JH, Wurtman JJ *et al*. A balanced carbohydrate: protein diet in the management of Parkinson's disease. *Neurology* 1991; **41**: 1295–1297.

Beyer PL, Palarino MY, Michalek D *et al*. Weight change and body composition in patients with Parkinson's disease. *Journal of the American Dietetic Association* 1995; **95**: 979–983.

Carter JH, Nutt JG, Woodward WR *et al*. Amount and distribution of dietary protein affects clinical response to levodopa in Parkinson's disease. *Neurology* 1989; **39**: 552–556.

de Rijk MC, Breteler MM, den Breeijen JH *et al*. Dietary antioxidants and Parkinson's disease. The Rotterdam Study. *Archives of Neurology* 1997; **54**: 762–765.

Haines JL, Conneally PM. Causes of death in Huntington's disease, as reported on death certificates. *Genetic Epidemiology* 1986; **3**: 417–423.

Harper PS. The epidemiology of Huntington's disease. *Human Genetics* 1992; **89**: 365–376.

Hughes AJ, Daniel SE, Kilfod L, Leas AJ. Accuracy of clinical diagnosis of idiopathic Parkinson's disease: a clinico-pathological study. *Journal of Neurology, Neurosurgery and Psychiatry* 1992; **55**: 181–184.

Karstaedt PJ, Pincus JH. Protein redistribution diet remains effective in patients with fluctuating parkinsonism. *Archives of Neurology* 1992; **49**: 149–151.

Kremer HPH, Roos RAC. Weight loss in Huntington's disease. *Archives of Neurology* 1992; **49**: 349.

Logroscino G, Marder K, Cote L *et al*. Dietary lipids and antioxidants in Parkinson's disease: a population-based, case–control study. *Annals of Neurology* 1996; **39**: 89–94.

Morens DM, Grandinetti A, Waslien CI *et al*. Case–control study of idiopathic Parkinson's disease and dietary vitamin E intake. *Neurology* 1996; **46**: 1270–1274.

Mutch WJ Parkinson's disease. *Journal of Neurology, Neurosurgery and Psychiatry* 1995; **57**: 672–681.

Myers RH, Sax DS, Koroshetz WJ *et al*. Factors associated with slow progression in Huntington's disease. *Archives of Neurology* 1991; **48**: 800–804.

O'Brien CF, Miller C, Goldblatt D *et al*. Extraneuronal metabolism in early Huntington's disease. *Annals of Neurology* 1990; 78: 300–301.

O'Reilly F, Finnan F, Allwright S *et al*. The effects of caring for a spouse with Parkinson's disease on social, psychological and physical well-being. *British Journal of General Practice* 1996; **46**: 507–512.

Pare S, Barr SI, Ross SE. Effect of daytime protein restriction on nutrient intakes of free-living Parkinson's disease patients. *American Journal of Clinical Nutrition* 1992; **55**: 701–707.

Riley D, Lang AE. Practical application of low protein diet for Parkinson's disease. *Neurology* 1998; **38**: 1026–1031.

Worwood AM, Leigh PN. Indicators and prevalence of malnutrition in motor neurone disease. *European Neurology* 1998; **40**: 159–163.

4.27 Multiple sclerosis

Multiple sclerosis (MS) is a degenerative disorder of the central nervous system characterized by autoimmune destruction of the myelin sheath of nerves in the brain and spinal cord. As a result, conduction of nerve impulses is impaired. MS can result in considerable disability but this is not inevitable in every case; only about 50% of patients become confined to a wheelchair.

MS is the most common neurological disease among young adults and the chance of developing it is approximately 1 in 1000. The disease most commonly strikes between the ages of 20 and 40 years, although it can occur at any age. It affects women more than men (in the ratio 3:2). There are estimated to be about 85 000 sufferers in the UK (Multiple Sclerosis Society 1999).

4.27.1 Features of multiple sclerosis

There are two main forms of the disease:

* *Relapsing–remitting*: This is the most common form of MS, where periods of acute worsening of symptoms are followed by spontaneous improvement, leaving the sufferer either as they were before the relapse, or sometimes slightly worse. What triggers the relapse (or permits the remission) is unknown.
* *Chronic progressive*: In this type of MS there are no clear-cut attacks; the symptoms just become steadily worse. Occasionally this form can progress very rapidly, causing severe disability and premature death within a few years.

In some people, the relapsing–remitting form may become progressive in nature and is then described as *secondary progressive MS*.

The condition may also be classified as *benign*, where an initial attack is never followed by another one. The first 5 years after the onset of symptoms are the most indicative of prognosis; if the disease has not progressed much in that time it is likely to remain benign.

Symptoms

The symptoms of MS depend on the extent and location of the demyelination and may include:

* numbness
* pins and needles
* muscle weakness and impaired co-ordination
* visual disturbances, particularly double or blurred vision, and eye pain
* extreme fatigue
* bladder dysfunction and loss of bladder control
* vertigo
* mood changes
* spasticity or tremor
* paralysis.

Diagnosis is based on the clinical presentation, neurological tests and magnetic resonance imaging (MRI, which can reveal the presence of demyelinated plaques).

Causation

The cause of the autoimmune destruction of myelin is unknown, although several theories have been proposed. There appears to be an increased genetic susceptibility to the disease and some environmental links with the disease have also been observed (Murrell *et al*. 1991). The most striking and consistent of these is the relationship between MS prevalence and climate; the disease is rare in equatorial regions and increases with latitude. Hutter (1993) has suggested that exposure to solar radiation (related to latitude but also affected by altitude) is even more closely associated with MS prevalence.

Dietary links have also been reported. MS is more common in countries where saturated fat intake is high and consumption of long-chain polyunsaturated fatty acids, particularly from fish oils, is low (Murrell *et al*. 1991; Lauer 1994) and various theories have been proposed to explain this. However, for a variety of reasons, their significance remains to be established (see Nutrition and multiple sclerosis, below).

Vitamin D has been implicated in MS aetiology. Animal studies have suggested that the hormonal form of vitamin D_3 may be a selective enzyme regulator inhibiting this autoimmune disease (Hayes *et al*. 1997) and it is conceivable that, in conditions of low sunlight, insufficient vitamin D_3 is produced, limiting production of 1,25-hydroxyvitamin D and increasing the risk of MS. This is compatible with the geographical distribution of MS noted above. It also could explain the apparent protective effect of fish oils, since these are one of the few foods rich in vitamin D_3. However, the apparent immunosuppressant effects of sunlight could be related to other factors (Hutter and Laing 1996).

4.27.2 Management of multiple sclerosis

Treatment is primarily symptom led with pharmacological and other measures to alleviate problems such as limb spasticity, bowel or bladder dysfunction. Steroid therapy is likely to be used to reduce inflammation, particularly during phases of acute relapse.

There is some evidence that patients with the relapsing –remitting (but not the chronic progressive) form of the disease may benefit from treatment with interferon betas. Interferon beta-1a and interferon beta-1b have been reported to reduce the relapse rate in relapsing–remitting MS by about one-third (Interferon Beta Study Group 1995; Jacobs *et al*. 1996) and may delay disease progression (PRISMS Study Group 1998), although may not prevent it altogether. However, this form of treatment is extremely expensive and its cost-effectiveness is, at the time of writing (2000), under review by the National Institute of Clinical Excellence (NICE).

Other potential treatments include intravenous immunoglobulin which, like interferon betas, reduces the relapse rate (Fazekas *et al*. 1997), use of copolymer 1 (Johnson *et al*. 1995) and other immunomodulating therapies.

4.27.3 Nutrition and multiple sclerosis

The epidemiological associations observed between dietary fat intake and MS prevalence led to speculation that the amount and type of dietary fat consumed could influence the development and course of the disease. Early studies focused on the possible effects of either dietary fatty acid imbalance or essential fatty acid deficiency on the composition of the myelin sheath or the inflammatory process involved in its destruction. It was suggested that some MS patients may have an impaired ability to convert parent essential fatty acids (linoleic and alpha-linolenic acids) into their respective long-chain derivatives [gammalinolenic acid (GLA), dihomogammalinolenic and arachidonic acid, or eicosapentaenoic acid (EPA) and docosahexaenoic acid]. As a result, synthesis of prostaglandins, leukotrienes and other inflammatory mediators could be affected.

The effects of various types of dietary fat manipulations in MS patients have therefore been explored. The results have been interesting but far from conclusive. Some studies suggested that supplementation with linoleic acid decreased the frequency and duration of relapse (Millar *et al*. 1973; Bates *et al*. 1977) but only in patients in the early stages of disease (Dworkin *et al*. 1984). A 5 year trial of the use of fish oil supplements (in conjunction with increased linoleic acid intake) (Bates *et al*. 1989) showed trends towards decreased duration, frequency and severity of relapses, but the results were not statistically significant. Moreover, this entailed taking large numbers of fish oil capsules (more than 20 per day) and the cost, practicality and even safety of this can be questioned.

Diets of extremely low fat content (<20 g/day) have also been claimed to reduce the rates of both neurological deterioration and mortality in MS patients (Swank and Grimsgaard 1988; Swank and Duggan 1990), an effect explained on the grounds that people with MS may be very sensitive to, or intolerant of, saturated fatty acids. However,

most people would find it extremely difficult to adhere to, or meet their energy needs on the restrictive diet used in this study.

A more acceptable regimen, low in saturated fat but with an increased content of both omega-6 and omega-3 (*n*6 and *n*3) fatty acids, and comprised of foods which ensured a good intake of vitamins, minerals, trace elements and fibre, was devised by the organization Action for Research for Multiple Sclerosis (ARMS), and hence known as the ARMS diet. A 3 year study of its effectiveness suggested that patients who complied with the regimen (assessed by serial blood lipid analyses) had less deterioration in neurological status than those who did not (Fitzgerald *et al*. 1987). However, further research is needed to confirm these findings.

The problem with all the dietary intervention studies carried out to date is that the evaluation of improvement has been mainly subjective (more objective means of assessment such as MRI scanning have only recently become available), and the observed effects tend to be confounded by the relapsing–remitting nature of the disease in some, but not all, people. In addition, the power of the placebo effect in a group of people who made marked changes to their diet may have been considerable. Nor can it be assumed that dietary factors associated with the aetiology of MS will necessarily be involved in the progression of the disease, particularly if the underlying cause is a metabolic defect.

The current consensus is that extreme dietary manipulations have no place in management of MS and that people should be encouraged a follow a varied, well-balanced diet based on *The Balance of Good Health* principles. However, in view of the tenuous evidence which exists, particular emphasis can be placed on those features of the ARMS diet which are compatible with healthy-eating objectives, i.e. low consumption of saturated fat, moderately high intake on both *n*6 and *n*3 fatty acids and micronutrient-rich food choices (see below).

4.27.4 Dietary management of multiple sclerosis

Dietary management of people with MS centres around trying to achieve a healthy pattern of eating together with any additional measures needed to alleviate nutrition-related problems associated with the disease. Guidance to alleviate any adverse effects of self-imposed dietary restrictions or supplementation may also be appropriate. An important role of the dietitian is to convince patients that following a sensible, well-balanced diet is a positive step that they can take towards maintaining their health. It is equally important to ensure that any recommended changes in eating habits do not cause the patient any more difficulty with regard to shopping or cooking than is already encountered; fatigue is a debilitating feature of the disease and additional stress will not be helpful.

General dietary guidance

The general aim is to encourage the consumption of a well-balanced diet that is compatible with both the consequences of the disease and long-term health. For most people, guidance can be based on *The Balance of Good Health* principles, with particular emphasis on food choices which ensure:

- low consumption of saturated fatty acids (e.g. choosing low-fat/lean dairy foods and meat; substituting butter and lard with polyunsaturated alternatives; avoidance of fat-rich foods and snacks such as meat products, pastry, cakes and biscuits);
- moderately high intake of both *n*6 and *n*3 long-chain fatty acids:
  - *linoleic acid* is present in polyunsaturated spreads and oils derived from sunflower, safflower, soya, sesame seed, cotton seed, corn, rapeseed, grapeseed and walnut. Pulses, seeds, legumes and beans are also good sources of linoleic acid
  - *arachidonic acid*, the long-chain derivative of linoleic acid, is present in lean meats, offal and poultry
  - *alpha-linolenic acid* is derived from green leafy vegetables (such as broccoli, spinach or green beans) and legumes
  - *docosahexaenoic acid and eicosapentaenoic acids*, the long-chain derivatives of alpha-linolenic acid, are present in greatest quantities in oily fish, but all types of fish and seafood can be encouraged;
- micronutrient-rich food choices (plenty of fruit, vegetables, pulses, legumes and cereals; not too many choices from the sugar-rich/fat-rich food group).

The importance of an adequate fluid intake should also not be overlooked and people should be encouraged to consume at least 8–10 cups (6–8 glasses) of fluid per day.

Nutritional problems associated with multiple sclerosis

Nutrition-related problems associated with MS vary according to the symptoms associated with it and the degree of physical disability which has resulted, but those most likely to be encountered are listed below.

Undernutrition

Loss of interest in, or inadequate consumption of, food can result from:

- anorexia or depression as a result of the diagnosis
- side-effects of drug treatment
- fatigue: lack of energy to shop, prepare, cook or even eat food
- difficulties in food procurement or preparation as a result of physical disability (see Section 3.11.1, Physical disabilities)
- inadequate energy and/or nutrient intake as a result of following a very low-fat diet or an unbalanced alternative regimen.

Overweight

This can be associated with:

- decreased level of physical activity due to mobility problems
- comfort eating
- increased appetite due to use of corticosteroids.

Constipation

This is a common symptom as a result of:

- bowel spasticity resulting from the disease
- reduced mobility
- restricted fluid intake due to problems with micturition or continence
- consumption of a low-fibre diet.

The principles of management of these problems can be found elsewhere in the Manual, but the way in which they are applied to people with MS has to take account of individual needs, circumstances and difficulties.

Alternative diets and complementary therapies in multiple sclerosis

Many people with a progressive illness are keen to try alternative dietary remedies which offer a prospect of cure or remission particularly if, as is often the case with MS sufferers, they are still young, have family commitments and mortgages, or are developing a career. As a result, alternative therapies such as acupuncture, hyperbaric oxygen, osteopathy and homoeopathy have become popular among MS patients. Dietary therapies advocated in books, newspaper or magazine articles or on the internet may be adopted. Supplement usage is common. Therapies which are most likely to create nutritional problems include the following.

Gluten-free diets (either with or without animal fat restriction)

These diets (often known as Roger McDougall and Rita Greer diets) are often followed by MS patients. There is no evidence that they are beneficial (Hunter *et al*. 1984; Hewson 1984) but many MS sufferers claim to be helped by them. Such diets can be nutritionally unbalanced and also expensive if proprietary gluten-free foods are purchased.

'Allergy' diets

As a result of commercial 'allergy' testing, MS patients may be advised to avoid 'cytotoxic' foods in order to alleviate their symptoms. As a result, patients may be avoiding a wide range of foods, or even entire food groups such as milk and dairy products. Dietitians should attempt to restore more balanced eating habits, although they should also be mindful of the fact that MS patients are just as likely to have a genuine food intolerance as any other member of the population. Symptomatic evidence suggestive of this should therefore be properly investigated (see Section 4.34, Food allergy and intolerance).

Wholefood diets

Diets heavily reliant on wholegrain, raw and unrefined foods tend to be high in fibre and low in energy density and, as a result, people may not consume sufficient to meet their energy and nutrient needs.

Supplement usage

Patients may be taking combinations of different supplements in large doses, sometimes risking overdosage with fat-soluble vitamins. Types of supplements likely to be used include:

- *Evening primrose oil*: This is a source of GLA, which is not normally derived from food but by conversion of linolenic acid. It is expensive and not obtainable on prescription for MS (only for mastalgia and atopic eczema). Supplements of blackcurrant seed oil and borage oil contain an even higher proportion of GLA but there has been little evaluation of their effects or safety.
- *Fish oil capsules*: These are rich in EPA. They are expensive and concerns have been expressed over the dioxin content of some of these supplements (MAFF 1999). Eating fatty fish two or three times weekly may be a safer way of obtaining EPA.
- *Cod liver oil*: This is an alternative but less concentrated source of marine fatty acids. It is also a concentrated source of retinol and may be contraindicated if other vitamin A-rich foods such as liver are being eaten regularly.
- *Linseeds*: These may be used as a source of alpha-linolenic acid and sprinkled over a foods such as breakfast cereals, salads and casseroles. In large quantities they have a laxative effect and intake should be confined to 1 dessertspoonful per day.

If a well-balanced diet containing dietary sources of *n*3 and *n*6 fatty acids as outlined above is consumed, additional supplements of evening primrose oil (or other sources of GLA), fish oils, vitamins and minerals are unlikely to be necessary or beneficial. If people wish to take supplements as additional 'insurance', they should be advised to confine this to one multiple multivitamin/mineral preparation providing no more than the recommended dietary allowance, rather than taking several different types of supplement. Preparations containing vitamin A should be avoided if liver is a regular component of the diet.

Some of the general issues concerning the role of the dietitian in the management of people with chronic illness who choose to follow alternative dietary regimens are discussed in Section 4.37.3 (Alternative diets and cancer).

Text revised by: Briony Thomas

Useful addresses

The Multiple Sclerosis Society
25 Effie Road, Fulham, London SW6 1EE
Tel: 020 7736 9861
Helpline: 0808 800 8000
Website: www.mssociety.org.uk

Federation of Multiple Sclerosis Therapy Centres
Bradbury House, 155 Barkers Lane, Bedford MK41 9RX
Tel: 01234 325781

Further reading

Federation of Multiple Sclerosis Therapy Centres. *Healthy Eating for Multiple Sclerosis*. Bedford: Multiple Sclerosis Therapy Centres, 1998.

References

Bates D, Fawcett PRW, Shaw DA, Weightman D. Polyunsaturated fatty acids in treatment of acute remitting multiple sclerosis. *British Medical Journal* 1977; **ii**: 1390–1391.

Bates D, Cartlidge NEF, French JM *et al.* A double-blind controlled trial of long chain *n*-3 polyunsaturated fatty acids in the treatment of multiple sclerosis. *Journal of Neurology, Neurosurgery and Psychiatry* 1989; **52**: 18–22.

Dworkin RH, Bates D, Millar JHD, Paty DW. Linoleic acid and multiple sclerosis: a reanalysis of three double-blind trials. *Neurology* 1984; **34**: 1441–1445.

Fazekas F, Deisenhanner F, Strasser-Fuchs S *et al.* for the Austrian Immunoglobulin in Multiple Sclerosis Study Group. Randomised placebo-controlled trial of monthly intravenous immunoglobulin therapy in relapsing–remitting multiple sclerosis. *Lancet* 1997; **349**: 589.

Fitzgerald G, Harbige LS, Forti A, Crawford MA. The effect of nutritional counselling on diet and plasma EFA status in multiple sclerosis patients over 3 years. *Human Nutrition: Applied Nutrition* 1987; **41A**: 297–310.

Hayes CE, Cantorna MT, DeLuca HF. Vitamin D and multiple sclerosis. *Proceedings of Experimental Biology and Medicine* 1997; **216**: 21–27.

Hewson DC. Is there a role for GF diets in MS? *Human Nutrition: Applied Nutrition* 1984; **38A**: 417–420.

Hunter L, Rees BWG, Jones LT. Gluten antibodies in patients with MS. *Human Nutrition: Applied Nutrition* 1984; **38A**: 142–143.

Hutter C. On the causes of multiple sclerosis. *Medical Hypotheses* 1993; **41**: 93–96.

Hutter CD, Laing P. Multiple sclerosis: sunlight, diet, immunology and aetiology. *Medical Hypotheses* 1996; **46**: 67–74.

Interferon Beta Multiple Sclerosis Study Group/University of British Columbia MS/MRI Analysis Group. Interferon beta-1b in the treatment of multiple sclerosis: final outcome of the randomized controlled trial. *Neurology* 1995; **45**: 1277–1285.

Jacobs LD, Cookfair DL, Rudick RA *et al.* Intramuscular interferon beta-1a for disease progression in relapsing multiple sclerosis. *Annals of Neurology* 1996; **39**: 285–294.

Johnson KP, Brooks BR, Cohen JA *et al.* Copolymer 1 reduces relapse rate and improves disability in relapsing – remitting multiple sclerosis: result of a phase III multicenter, double-blind placebo-controlled trial. *Neurology* 1995; **45**: 1268–1276.

Lauer K. The risk of multiple sclerosis in the USA in relation to sociogeographic features: a factor-analytic study. *Journal of Clinical Epidemiology* 1994; **47**: 43–48.

MAFF. Dioxins and PCBs in fish oil dietary supplements and licensed medicines. *Food Surveillance Information Sheet* 1997; No. 106 (maff.gov.uk/food/infsheet/index.htm, internet).

Millar JGD, Zilkha KJ, Langman MJS *et al.* Double blind trial of linoleate supplementation of the diet in multiple sclerosis. *British Medical Journal* 1973; **i**: 765–768.

Multiple Sclerosis Society. *What is MS?* London: The Multiple Sclerosis Society, 1999.

Murrell TG, Harbige LS, Robinson IC. A review of the aetiology of multiple sclerosis: an ecological approach. *Annals of Human Biology* 1991; **18**: 95–112.

PRISMS (Prevention of Relapses and Disability by Interferon-1a Subcutaneously in Multiple Sclerosis) Study Group. Randomised double-blind placebo-controlled study of interferon-1a in relapsing/remitting multiple sclerosis. *Lancet* 1998; **352**: 1498–1504.

Swank RL, Dugan BB. Effect of low saturated fat diet in early and late cases of multiple sclerosis. *Lancet* 1990; **336**: 37–39.

Swank RL, Grimsgaard A. Multiple sclerosis: the lipid relationship. *American Journal of Clinical Nutrition* 1988; **48**: 1387–1393.

4.28 Neurorehabilitation

Rehabilitation is the process by which patients with brain injury or neurological damage are assisted to achieve their maximum potential in terms of quality of life. Such damage may result from:

- external trauma (head injury patients)
- stroke
- brain tumour or surgical removal of a tumour
- neurodegenerative disease such as Parkinson's or motor neurone disease.

In patients who suffer acute brain injury (e.g. following head injury or stroke), rehabilitation can be said to start from the moment the patient is admitted to hospital, although in practice the term is usually applied to the period subsequent to acute post-injury care. In those who develop chronic neurodegenerative disease, rehabilitation techniques help both patients and carers to mitigate or cope with problems and disabilities which exist or subsequently arise.

4.28.1 The neurological rehabilitation team

All patients with neurodisability resulting from brain injury or progressive neurological disease should receive multidisciplinary care from a neurological rehabilitation team. This comprises a number of health professionals who work closely together in conjunction with the patient and/or carers to assess the patient's needs, devise an individual plan of care, and monitor its implementation and progress. As well as medical and nursing personnel, this team may include expertise from a:

- dietitian
- physiotherapist
- speech and language therapist (SLT)
- occupational therapist
- continence adviser
- podiatrist
- psychologist
- social worker
- dentist.

One of these team members is usually assigned as the keyworker to co-ordinate an individual patient's care within the team, be a general point of contact for general issues regarding the patient, enlist the help of other team members when specific problems arise and liaise with district nursing or other support services as necessary. Clerical assistance is essential to carry out the necessary administration in terms of processing referral requests, arranging patient appointments, providing information to team members and liaising with other health professionals or agencies as necessary. A co-ordinator, who should be an active member of the team, will ensure that the team works effectively and efficiently.

Each team member has an influence on a person's nutritional status. Dietitians therefore need to be aware of the role of other team members in order to make appropriate inter-team referrals and facilitate quality of care.

4.28.2 Consequences of brain injury

Damage to the brain as a result of acute injury or chronic disease can have profound effects on an individual's physical and mental capabilities. The nature of the effects depends on the location, nature and extent of the damage.

Damage to the left hemisphere of the brain is most likely to affect:

- language
- speech
- reading and writing ability.

Damage to the right hemisphere is more likely to affect:

- the processing of visual and spatial information
- recognition
- co-ordination.

Although damage to brain tissue is irreversible since the body has no ability to regenerate brain cells, in some types of brain injury, particularly stroke, the body does seem able to adapt to some types of damage by 'rerouting' the way in which information is processed and hence enabling the individual to recover some or all of an ability (e.g. speech or swallowing) in time. This is termed neuroplasticity.

Alternatively, in progressive neurological disorders, physical and mental functioning may deteriorate with time.

4.28.3 Nutritional implications of brain injury

The neurological effects of brain injury can have significant implications in terms of nutritional intake and it is essential that dietitians are aware of the extent and nature of these effects in a particular individual before attempting to make nutritional assessment or provide dietary guidance.

Nutritional intake may be affected as a result of the following effects.

Effects on perception and cognition

Perception is the process by which sensory information conveyed to the brain is received in the cortex and transmitted to the parietal lobes for interpretation.

Cognition is the way the perceived information is used, enabling a person to learn, remember, plan, problem solve and monitor situations.

Perceptual and cognitive skills are directly interlinked and injury to some parts of the brain can result in:

- *Impaired visual perception*: People's faces or objects (such as items of food on a plate) may not be recognized. This is particularly likely to occur following brain injury in the occipital lobes and the right cerebral hemisphere.
- *Impaired spatial perception*: An individual's ability to analyse their position in relation to objects around them is impaired. Spatial perception requires intact visual fields and disruption to any part, from the retina up to the occipital lobe, can result in 'blind areas'.
- *Neglect*: Damage to the non-dominant parietal lobe may result in the phenomenon of 'neglect', in which the side of the body and environment opposite to the lesion do not seem to exist for the individual. As a result, an affected person may neglect to dress, wash or shave this side of the body. Neglect may also affect food intake because only half of the contents on a plate will be perceived to be there and so only half will be eaten.
- *Impaired planning and sequencing*: If cognition is impaired, an individual may not be able to carry out planned and sequenced tasks such as making a cup of tea, even if they are physically capable of doing so. Such a seemingly simple task involves complex mental processes requiring knowledge of which objects are the kettle, teapot, cup, saucer and milk jug, the ability to match each object to its appropriate function, and the logical capacity to carry out the task in an appropriate series of steps.

Impaired perception and cognition may considerably affect intake of food and fluid.

Effects on memory

Memory impairment as a result of brain injury is very common and can affect:

- sensory memory (where information is received by the sense organs and which only lasts for a few milliseconds)
- short-term memory (which holds information from the sensory store for several seconds, allowing a response to be formulated or the memory to be passed to the long-term memory)
- long-term memory (which holds information for periods from a few minutes to many years).

In the presence of cognitive impairment, memory problems can be very complex and have significant effects on nutritional intake. Patients may overeat as a result of forgetting that they have just had a meal, or undereat because they forget to eat at all (Richards-Hall 1994). Information such as dietary guidance may be forgotten or only partly remembered.

Memory loss can also create communication difficulties. Patients may not be able to remember information they have been given just minutes before, or, for example, that the person speaking to them is a dietitian.

Effects on the ability to communicate

Aphasia (damage to the language centre in the left hemisphere of the brain) may result in loss of or difficulties with speech (expressive aphasia). The ability to read or even interpret pictures may also be impaired (receptive aphasia). As a result of dysphasia, patients may be unable to communicate their wishes (for example that they are hungry or thirsty) or express their likes and dislikes. Aphasic patients may also have difficulty in completing a hospital menu or making sense of dietary information provided in a written or even pictorial form.

Effects on eating behaviour

Behavioural alteration

Frontal damage often results in altered behaviour, which may include:

- antisocial behaviour, e.g. poor table manners, spitting or throwing food
- aggression
- physical and/or verbal abuse
- disinhibition: hyperphagia may not be kept in check to the extent that it would normally be (Henson *et al.* 1993)
- disinterest or apathy.

Mood alteration

Alteration in brain function or sometimes drugs used to treat brain injury may have a direct effect on neurotransmitters and result in short- or long-term alteration in mood, for example depression or withdrawal.

Effects on appetite

Damage to the hypothalamus may result in loss of appetite control, resulting in hyperphagia (Henson *et al.* 1993) or hyperphagia of particular foods such as a craving for sweet carbohydrate foods. Drug therapy, particularly the use of mood-altering drugs, may also affect appetite.

Effects on the physical ability to eat

Ataxia

This describes tremor or shakiness, usually as a result of damage to the cerebellum, brainstem or pyramidal tracts causing poor motor control. It can result in considerable difficulties in getting food to the mouth, possibly to such an extent that the patient has to be fed. Equipment has been devised which enables the ataxic patient to self-feed (by creating a resistance against tremor, hence allowing a smooth transit from plate to mouth), but some individuals find the equipment large and unwieldy to use; others feel that it draws attention to their disability and prefer to be discreetly fed by a carer.

Apraxia

This is the term used to describe disordered purposeful movement. Apraxia is often associated with left hemisphere damage and may appear in a number of forms.

People with *ideomotor apraxia* may be unable to perform a specific task on request, despite understanding the concept and having the physical ability to do so. However, the individual may be able to carry out the task automatically.

Individuals with *ideational apraxia* may be unable to select the appropriate tool to carry out a particular task, e.g. may try to use a fork as a straw.

Hemiplegia

This results in paralysis of limbs on the one side of the body, opposite to the site of lesion in the brain. Other physical consequences may be muscle wasting, limb oedema and slowing of nail growth on the affected side. Hemiplegia is particularly likely to compromise nutritional status because energy requirements may be increased as a result of the reduced efficiency of movement and the presence of spasticity (Potempa *et al.* 1995), but food intake is often limited in both type and amount because of the difficulties of manipulating food with just one hand. Measures such as the use of antislip mats and adapted cutlery may be helpful (see Section 3.11.1, Physical disabilities).

Effects on the ability to swallow

Dysphagia is a common consequence of many types of brain injury. Not only may damage to cranial nerves have affected the swallowing reflex but other aspects necessary for the normal swallow such as the ability to visualize and recognize the food, achieve and maintain an appropriate posture of the head, neck and body, and have good lip and tongue movement may also be affected by brain injury. Posture tetany, often seen with Steele–Richardson syndrome (progressive supranuclear palsy), in which the whole body may become rigid, can profoundly affect the ability to swallow. Abnormal oral reflexes, e.g. tongue thrust and bite reflex, inability to concentrate, fatigue and fear of choking, may further compound a problem.

Any loss in swallowing ability is likely to compromise nutritional intake as a result of:

- insufficient consumption of food (intake of energy and nutrients may be inadequate)
- limited choice of food (dietary intake may be imbalanced)
- losses as a result of drooling and leakage of food from the mouth.

The management of dysphagia is discussed in detail in Section 4.3 (Dysphagia).

Psychological effects of the injury or disease

As well as physical effects, the psychological consequences of having suffered acute brain injury or having been diagnosed with a serious neurological disorder can affect nutritional intake.

Emotional reactions

Awareness of the nature of the injury or disease and the prospect of permanent or progressive disability is likely to be followed by an emotional reaction similar to that of bereavement, involving:

- shock
- emotional lability and depression
- realization (which may can result in further depression)
- adjustment.

Relatives may go through a similar process, so both patient and family need support.

Depression may also result from, or be compounded by, chemical changes following the brain injury. Depression can have a profound effect on food intake; patients may, for a while, simply 'not want to get better'. Physical difficulties with eating or swallowing may be compounded by fatigue and poor concentration. The consequent problems may make people feel frustrated or resentful and consequently irritable, even angry, with carers and health professionals. Alternatively, the inability to cope with what can be a stressful situation can make people withdrawn or tearful.

Social isolation

Embarrassment because eating is accompanied by spillage as a result of tremor, drooling or dribbling, or simply as a result of having to be fed, may make people reluctant to eat with others or in public. As a result, both patients and their relatives or carers can be very isolated (Osborn and Marshall 1993). Every effort should be made to help people to overcome the problems that cause them most distress and to retain as much independence as possible.

4.28.4 Nutrition management in neurorehabilitation

Many patients who have suffered acute injury to the brain such as head injury or stroke will commence the phase of rehabilitation in a state of undernutrition as a result of the hypercatabolic effects of acute trauma and the likelihood of energy and nitrogen needs not having been met (see Sections 5.3, Head injury, and 4.25, Stroke). Undernutrition is particularly likely if the injury was severe (which will result in a greater and more prolonged catabolic response) or the patient was malnourished prior to the injury (as may be the case in some elderly people who have suffered a stroke).

The initial nutritional priority in such patients is thus to restore nutritional status. As rehabilitation progresses this objective gradually changes to helping patients to overcome, or mitigate, their neurological difficulties affecting food intake and ensuring that nutrient intake is adequate. With further recovery but persisting disabilities the aim may be to prevent weight gain and overnutrition. The ultimate aim is to optimize nutritional intake in a way that maximizes the individual's rehabilitation potential.

For those with progressive neurological disorders, the process may operate in reverse. Gradually increasing immobility but relatively normal food intake may increase the likelihood of weight gain. As neurodisability increases, feeding and swallowing problems may become more pronounced and the risk of undernutrition gradually increases.

Nutritional assessment

Because many factors impact upon nutritional intake in the brain-injured patient, it is essential that nutritional assessment is carried out within the confines of a multidisciplinary team so that expert opinion on other parameters which impact on food intake (as outlined above) can be taken into account. Factors that need to be considered as part of a nutritional assessment are:

- the cause of the brain injury, its management and likely prognosis or progression;
- the physical and psychological consequences of the disease or injury on:
  - the desire to eat
  - the ability to eat
  - the ability to swallow
  - bowel function
  - the ability to carry out everyday tasks;
- the patient's nutritional intake;
- the patient's hydration status;
- the patient's nutritional status and whether this is likely to improve, worsen or remain stable.

The aim is to identify individuals who are:

- malnourished and in need of nutritional support
- at risk of malnutrition and whose nutritional status needs to be monitored
- at risk of dehydration and whose fluid intake and hydration status needs to be monitored
- in need of remedial measures to help to alleviate diet-related problems.

Assessing the extent of nutritional depletion

Weight loss This is usually the best way of assessing the degree of nutritional depletion in brain-injured patients. Comparison of the patient's weight at the start of rehabilitation with the patient's usual pre-morbid weight provides a good indication of the extent of energy depletion. This can be calculated as:

$$\% \text{ Usual body weight} \frac{\text{Current weight (kg)} \times 100}{\text{Usual weight (kg)}}$$

However, measurement of weight is often difficult in brain-

injured patients as appropriate scales may not be available if the patient is severely disabled. Hoist or weigh-bridge scales can be used to weigh an immobile patient, but such specialist equipment is not always available.

An additional problem may be that a reliable estimate of pre-morbid weight may not always be obtainable from either the patient or relatives.

Adiposity measurements These indicate the level of body fat stores but can be either difficult to measure or inappropriate in some types of brain-injured patients.

Body Mass Index (BMI) can only be calculated if measurements of body weight and height are available. As well as practical problems in measuring weight (see above), measurement of height is particularly difficult in brain-injured patients because even if standing is possible, they may not be able to stand erect or immobile for long enough. Alternative body measurements such as demispan and knee height from which height can be derived (see Table 1.16 in Section 1.8, Assessment of nutritional status) are not always appropriate alternatives since brain-injured patients may be unable to able to stretch their arms sufficiently for a measurement of demispan or to achieve the correct position for measurement of knee height. However, it is often possible to obtain an estimate of height directly from the patient or relative.

Skinfold thickness measurements, particularly triceps skinfold thickness, are fraught with problems in many brain-injured patients. In those with hemiplegia, the arm on the affected side may be oedematous, have abnormal muscle wasting and be flaccid or spastic, all of which may distort skinfold measurements. Skinfold measurements at other sites may be affected by poor posture or immobility.

Estimates of muscle mass Measurements such as mid-arm muscle circumference can be useful but inappropriate for patients with limb paralysis; in addition to the likelihood of muscle wasting in the affected arm, there is usually a compensatory increase in muscle mass in the unaffected arm. Immobility will also result in muscle wasting.

Biochemical and haematological indices Levels of blood glucose, electrolytes, serum urea and urinary nitrogen are used to monitor the degree of catabolism in an acute post-injury phase, but in the rehabilitation phase provide little information about a patient's nutritional status other than the state of hydration (Labbe 1986). Haematological indicators may be relevant if anaemia is suspected.

Assessing dietary intake

It can be difficult to obtain accurate dietary information from brain-injured patients. Many patients will have memory and cognitive impairments or dysphasia (receptive and expressive), which limit their ability to understand or communicate. Behavioural and mood changes may result in hostility or aggression towards the questioner, or alternatively withdrawal and lack of response.

It is essential to understand the patient's capabilities as well as limitations and to draw on the expertise and advice from other members of the care team. Communication problems may be overcome by the dietitian working in conjunction with the SLT. The amount, and degree of reliability, of dietary information which the patient is able to provide will vary considerably and the dietitian will need to be adaptable and innovative to make best use of the relevant circumstances. A skilled dietitian may be able to build up a useful diet history from no more than single-word responses to the display of food photographs or food models.

One of the most valuable ways of obtaining additional dietary information is by observing meal times. Not only does this give an estimate of the quantity of food and fluid consumed, but it also reveals any physical difficulties associated with eating or swallowing, together with any behavioural problems.

Assessment tools designed to evaluate problems such as food refusal, antisocial behaviour or assistance needed with feeding have been devised for patients with dementia (Watson 1994a, b; Watson and Deary 1994; VOICES 1998) but as yet no such assessment tool has been devised for brain-injured patients, whose behaviour and care needs are very different.

Managing dietary problems

Inadequate food intake is most likely to result from:

- physical difficulties with eating or swallowing
- anorexia (often as a result of depression, anxiety or medication)
- frustration or fatigue over the effort involved in eating
- food refusal, as a result of behavioural change or because people find it degrading to have to be fed
- drug-induced side-effects such as nausea and vomiting.

Some of these problems may be remedied by quite simple measures, such as smaller, more frequent, energy-dense meals for those suffering from anorexia or nausea, or the use of various aids to help to overcome the physical difficulties of getting food to the mouth, or it may be possible for the timing of drugs to be changed to reduce their effects on food intake (see Sections 1.12, Oral nutritional support, and 3.11.1, Physical disabilities).

Patients with evidence of malnutrition or at high risk of malnutrition will require a greater level of nutritional support via:

- food enrichment (see Section 1.12.3)
- energy and protein supplements (see Section 1.12.4)
- enteral feeding (either overnight supplementary or total support, via the nasogastric or gastrostomy route) (see Section 1.13.2).

The extent, means and route of support will depend on the level of nutritional depletion, the physical and psychological effects of the neurological lesions, whether the condition is relapsing–remitting or chronically progressive, and the preferences of the patient and carers.

The following problems may also have to be addressed.

Dysphagia

Management of dysphagia is discussed in Section 4.3. Measures that are likely to be needed in dysphagic brain-injured patients are:

- Assessment by the SLT and appropriate assistance, e.g. helping patients to convey food to the back of the mouth to trigger the swallowing reflex.
- Changes in food consistency and texture: This may necessitate either a uniform, soft consistency (e.g. puréed foods) or appropriately thickened fluids, depending on the nature of the dysphagia. As altered texture diets are nutritionally dilute, nutritional supplements may be required to meet energy needs.
- Maximization of sensory input: Foods may become more palatable and easier to swallow if they are served either 'hot' or 'cold', rather than just 'warm' or at room temperature. Chilled foods and drinks are often particularly well accepted. Main meals which are initially served as hot as possible are also more likely to remain at an acceptable temperature throughout what may be a long meal time. Flavourings should be used to make food as appetizing as possible.

Dehydration

Hydration status is particularly likely to be inadequate in those with poor oral or swallowing abilities. The problem often results from patients not being encouraged to consume fluids (either in liquid or semi-solid form) at regular intervals throughout the day, either because of lack of time by care staff or lack of awareness of the importance of this.

Constipation

This is extremely common in neurological disorders and may result from:

- inadequate fluid intake
- low fibre intake (especially on a modified consistency diet)
- reduced gut motility (as a result of reduced neurological signals from the brain, or muscle wasting in the gastro-intestinal tract)
- reduced mobility of the patient
- side-effects of medication (particularly opiates or levodopa).

Symptoms may be alleviated by:

- increasing fluid consumption to, ideally, 2 litres of fluid intake per day
- increasing consumption of fibre-rich foods which are compatible with the individual's eating or swallowing difficulties. Foods such as porridge, Weetabix, banana, peeled oranges or satsumas, prunes and dried fruits may be suitable possibilities.

All patients with nutritional problems, or identified as being at risk of nutritional problems should be regularly monitored and reviewed by the dietitian and other members of the care team.

4.28.5 The needs of carers

Providing day-in, day-out care for someone with serious physical or psychological difficulties is exhausting and emotionally demanding, and people who have this responsibility require considerable support if they are to maintain their own physical and mental health. The needs of carers have been increasingly recognized in recent years and strategies are being put in place to provide better support measures (DH 1999). The neurorehabilitation team can play an important part in ensuring that carers know about, and make use of, any available local support services which could make life easier or help them to feel less isolated.

The needs and problems faced by those who care for people with chronic illness are discussed further in Section 4.29.7 in Dementias).

Text written by: Briony Thomas

Acknowledgements: Helen Molyneux, Kathryn Morton, June Copeman, Dimple Thakrar, Sheila Merriman and other members of the British Dietetic Association's DINT and NAGE Groups.

Useful addresses

Disabled Living Foundation
380–384 Harrow Road, London W9 2HU
Tel: 0870 603 9177
Website: www.dlf.org.uk

Royal Association for Disability and Rehabilitation (RADAR)
12 City Forum, 250 City Road, London EC1V 8AF
Tel: 020 7250 3222

Further reading

Grieve J. *Neuropsychology for Occupational Therapists*. Oxford: Blackwell Science, 1993.

Laidler P. *Stroke Rehabilitation: Structure and Strategy*. London: Chapman and Hall, 1994.

Muir-Giles G, Clark-Wilson J. *Brain Injury Rehabilitation – A Neurological Approach*. London: Chapman and Hall, 1993.

Nocan A, Baldwin S. *Trends in Rehabilitation Policy*. London: King's Fund, 1998.

Robinson J, Turnock S. *Investing in Rehabilitation*. London: King's Fund, 1998.

Rose FD, Johnson DA. *Brain Injury and After*. Chichester: John Wiley and Sons, 1996.

Sinclair A, Dickinson E. *Effective Practice in Rehabilitation*. London: King's Fund, 1998.

Turner-Stokes L, Tonge P, Nyein K *et al*. The Northwick Park Dependency Score (NPDS): a measure of nursing dependency in rehabilitation. *Clinical Rehabilitation* 1998; **12**: 304–318.

References

Department of Health. *Caring about Carers: A National Strategy for Carers*. London: DH, 1999 (Available from Department of Health, PO Box 410, Wetherby LS23 7LN.)

Henson MB, DeCastro JM, Stringer AY, Johnson C. Food intake by brain injured humans who are in the chronic phase of recovery. *Brain Injury* 1993; 7: 169–178.

Labbe RF. Laboratory monitoring of nutritional support. *Archives of Pathology and Laboratory Medicine* 1986; **110**: 775–776.

Osborn CL, Marshall MJ. Self feeding performance in nursing home residents. *Journal of Gerontological Nursing* 1993; **19**: 7–14.

Potempa K, Lopez M, Brown LT *et al*. Physiological outcome of aerobic exercise training in hemiparetic stroke patients. *Stroke* 1995; **26**: 101–105.

Richards-Hall G. Chronic dementia – challenges in feeding a patient. *Journal of Gerontological Nursing* 1994; **20**: 21–30.

VOICES (Voluntary Organisations Involved in Caring in the Elderly Sectors). *Eating Well for Older People with Dementia*. VOICES, 1998. (Available from PO Box 5, Manchester M60 3 GE.)

Watson R. Measuring feeding difficulties in patients with dementia: developing a scale. *Journal of Advanced Nursing* 1994a; **19**: 257–263.

Watson R. Measuring feeding difficulties in patients with dementia: replication and validation of the Ed Fed Scale #1. *Journal of Advanced Nursing* 1994b; **19**: 850–855.

Watson R, Deary IJ. Measuring feeding difficulty in patients with dementia: multivariate analysis of feeding problems, nursing intervention and indicators of feeding difficulty. *Journal of Advanced Nursing* 1994; **20**: 283–287.

4.29 Dementias

Dementia is the collective term for conditions resulting from destructive pathological changes in brain tissue causing progressive loss of intellectual function. Dementia is characterized by:

- a progressive decline in the ability to remember, learn, understand, communicate and reason
- a gradual loss of skills, including those needed for everyday activities
- changes in personality or behaviour.

In time people, may lose the ability to care for themselves and become totally dependent on the help of others.

In some cases the decline may be rapid, while in others it may occur over a long period. Dementia is not in itself fatal and many sufferers can remain in good physical health for years. Eventually the effects of the disease lead to increasing weakness, and death normally results from infections such as pneumonia or gradual organ failure.

At present there is no effective treatment for dementia. Anticholinesterase drugs (which inhibit the breakdown of acetylcholine, a neurotransmitter) may be given to improve cognitive function in those in the early stages of dementia but will not prevent disease progression. There is no convincing evidence that supplements of lecithin (a dietary source of choline from which acetylcholine is synthesized) are of any clinical benefit to people with Alzheimer's or parkinsonian dementia (Higgins and Flicker 2000).

It is estimated there are about 650 000 people with dementia in the UK (Alzheimer's Disease Society 1996). Dementia usually occurs after the age of 40 years and the incidence increases sharply with age. Below the age of 65 years, only about 1 person in 1000 is affected but above this age about 4–5 people per 100 are affected. Over the age of 80, the risk is 1 in 5.

4.29.1 Types of dementia

Alzheimer's disease

Alzheimer's disease (formerly known as senile dementia) is the most common form of dementia, accounting for 50–60% of cases. It was first identified by Alzheimer in 1907 and results from the loss of neurones from the cortical areas of the brain, resulting in reduced production of acetylcholine and other neurotransmitters, and hence impaired transmission of messages connected with thought and memory.

The brain atrophies and decreases in weight, and microscopic examination reveals large numbers of neurofibrillary tangles (nerve cells become bunched together) and neuritic plaques (deposits of amyloid protein and other cellular debris). Alzheimer's can only be diagnosed with 100% certainty by post-mortem examination of the brain.

The cause of Alzheimer's disease is unknown. There appear to be genetic links with the early-onset form of the disease such as a defective gene on chromosome 14 (presenilin-1 or PS-1) or abnormalities in the amyloid producing gene in chromosome 21. Late-onset Alzheimer's disease appears to be associated with the epsilon 4 allele of apolipoprotein E (Polvikoski *et al.* 1995). However, how this genetic predisposition influences the development of Alzheimer's remains to be determined.

A considerable amount of research is being carried out into possible links between diet and other environmental factors and dementia, but there is as yet no convincing evidence that these influence either the onset or course of the disease. Following observations such as high levels of aluminum in the brain of some patients with the disease (McLachlan 1986) and increased prevalence of the disease in areas with high concentrations of aluminium in drinking water (Martyn *et al.* 1989), there has been speculation that environmental aluminium could be linked with the development of Alzheimer's. However, the significance of these findings has been a matter of debate, particularly in view of the fact that dietary aluminium is poorly absorbed and rapidly excreted (Priest 1993). In a detailed review of the experimental, clinical and epidemiological evidence, Doll (1993) concluded that, while aluminium is neurotoxic, it does not appear to be a cause of Alzheimer's disease, although further understanding of the neuropathophysiology of the disease is required to exclude the possibility altogether.

Vascular dementia

This term is applied to a number of different types of dementia associated with cerebrovascular disease causing impaired supply of blood to the brain, and hence oxygen starvation and damage to brain tissue (Amar and Wilcock 1996).

Multi-infarct dementia (MID) is the most common type of vascular dementia and accounts for about 20% of all dementia cases. A series of small infarctions in the brain (often manifested as 'dizzy spells') leads to increased areas of brain damage, causing symptoms of confusion which gradually worsen to dementia.

In contrast to Alzheimer's disease, mental decline in MID is likely to start more abruptly and symptoms tend to worsen in a stepwise manner following each attack. Since brain damage also tends to occur in localized areas rather than being widespread as in Alzheimer's, some mental abilities or the patient's personality may remain relatively unaffected, although short-term memory loss is nearly always pronounced. MID sufferers are more likely to be aware of their condition and often anxious and depressed as a result.

Other forms of vascular dementia include *stroke-induced dementia*, in which progressive confusion and mental impairment follow a stroke. Symptomatic stroke increases the risk of dementia more than nine-fold (Tatemichi *et al.* 1992). *Binswanger's disease* is a rare, slowly developing dementia caused by diseased blood vessels in the subcortical white matter of the brain. It is often associated with hypertension.

Treatment to control high blood pressure may be given to try to prevent further cerebral infarcts, and generalized cardiovascular disease risk reduction measures may be protective. However, there is no treatment that can reverse the dementia once it has occurred.

Diffuse Lewy body disease

This is characterized by the presence of Lewy bodies (small, spherical, protein-containing structures) in brain tissue, which are thought to be associated with the destruction of brain cells. It is difficult to diagnose pre-mortem and, because it has similar features to both Alzheimer's and Parkinson's disease, has often been classified as one of these forms or a variant of them. However, it is now thought to be a distinct form of dementia.

Creutzfeldt–Jakob disease

There are four main types of Creutzfeldt–Jakob disease (CJD), each differing in cause and symptoms, but all of which result in the production of an abnormal prion protein in the brain, causing progressive dementia and fatal brain disease. CJDs usually have a long latency period but, once symptoms appear, tend to progress rapidly, often causing death within a matter of months.

Sporadic CJD (spCJD)

Although rare, this is at present the most common form of CJD, affecting about one person per million per year (about 50–60 cases/year in the UK). The cause is unknown but probably results from a spontaneous genetic mutation resulting in production of abnormal prion protein. It causes an extremely rapid progressive dementia.

Genetic CJD (gCJD)

This is an inherited form of CJD, so there is usually a family history of the disease. It is extremely rare, affecting only about three people in the UK each year.

Iatrogenic CJD (iCJD)

This results from inadvertent transmission to a healthy person of the abnormal prion protein from someone with CJD. In the past this has most commonly occurred via injections of human growth hormone (hGH) extracted from human cadaver brain tissue, and occasionally following corneal transplant or human gonadotrophin injections used in fertility treatment. The use of synthetic hGH and other precautionary measures to prevent transmission should have reduced this risk.

Variant CJD (vCJD)

This is the form of CJD transmitted from cattle with bovine spongiform encephalopathy (BSE). It was first identified in 1996 and by August 2000, 83 cases had been confirmed or suspected in the UK, with the numbers being projected to rise, possibly substantially. Fourteen deaths from vCJD occurred in 1999, many of them young adults. vCJD typically begins with psychiatric or behavioural symptoms such as depression, social withdrawal and anxiety, sometimes followed by delusions, hallucinations or paranoia. Progressive neurological deterioration results in increasing physical inco-ordination and eventually fatal dementia. To date, the average duration of the illness has been about 14 months.

Dementia associated with other conditions

A number of conditions have an increased risk of dementia:

- *Parkinson's disease*: This increases the risk of dementia and as many as 15–20% of all dementia cases are secondary to Parkinson's disease (see Section 4.26.1).
- *Huntington's disease*: This genetically determined progressive neurodegenerative disorder results in movement disturbances (chorea), depression and dementia (see Section 4.26.3).
- *Down's syndrome*: Dementia is much more common in middle-aged people with Down's syndrome than in the rest of the population (Janicki and Dalton 2000).
- *Frontal lobe dementia*: This typically occurs in people in their early 50s and has about an 8 year survival span. Changes in personality and social behaviour are early symptoms.
- *Pick's disease*: This is a rare presenile dementia which resembles Alzheimer's disease, except that memory remains relatively intact and changes in personality and behaviour predominate. There is evidence of frontal lobe damage or atrophy.
- *Wernicke–Korsakoff syndrome*: This form of dementia is usually associated with alcoholism.
- *Chronic brain injury*: Repeated blows to the head resulting in periods of unconsciousness (as may occur among boxers) can lead to progressive brain damage, resulting in symptoms of dementia.

Dementia symptoms can also result from brain tumour or other cause of increased cranial pressure but, unlike other forms of dementia, can sometimes be cured by surgery.

4.29.2 Symptoms of dementia

Early stages of dementia

Dementia usually begins gradually with minor changes in the person's abilities or behaviour. Early symptoms may include:

- mild confusion, forgetfulness (often with words or names), repetition, indecision, impaired judgement
- narrowing of interests, loss of interest in other people or activities, social withdrawal
- slowness to grasp ideas and unwillingness to try new things
- increased agitation, irritability or low mood
- readiness to blame others for 'stealing' mislaid items.

Symptoms vary between individuals and with the type of dementia.

Middle stages of dementia

As dementia progresses, short-term memory loss and other changes are likely to become more pronounced and affect daily functioning. People may:

- have difficulties in understanding and communication
- forget recent events or what has just been said or done
- need reminders or help to eat, dress, wash or use the toilet
- be confused about where they are or wander and become lost
- become muddled about time and confuse night and day
- put themselves or others at risk by forgetfulness, e.g. turning on a gas appliance but failing to light it
- become easily upset, angry, aggressive or clinging
- fail to recognize people or confuse them with others.

Advanced stages of dementia

In the later stages, the person with dementia will require increasing amounts of help, eventually becoming totally dependent on others for care. They may:

- have little speech and little awareness of what is going on
- be unable to find their way around
- be generally unable to recognize even familiar objects or close relatives and friends, although there may be flashes of recognition
- be anxious, agitated, distressed or aggressive
- seem to be searching for something or someone from their past
- be incontinent
- have generalized and focal neurological signs such as tremor and lack of co-ordination resulting in immobility
- require 24 hour nursing care.

4.29.3 Diagnosis and management

Diagnosis of dementia depends primarily on measure-

ments of memory and mental ability, which are then repeated at intervals to see whether there is any decline. Brain scans can only to be used to exclude other possible causes of the symptoms.

Because the diagnosis can usually only be confirmed after death, misclassification of the type of dementia probably occurs in 10–20% of cases. Furthermore, some people, particularly those who are very elderly, may have a combination of both Alzheimer's and MID.

To some extent this is academic since there is at present no cure for any type of dementia and management is primarily symptom-led, using medication to help to alleviate neuropsychiatric disturbances and any associated movement disorders (e.g. as a result of parkinsonism). New treatments are being developed to try to protect messenger chemicals in the brain from being destroyed and so slow down the rate of mental decline.

However early diagnosis of dementia is important because in some cases it may be possible to prevent it becoming worse. It is particularly important that patients with evidence of vascular dementia receive any indicated treatment (e.g. for hypertension) that may reduce the risk of further infarctive damage. Diet and lifestyle measures such as losing weight, taking exercise and reducing salt intake are also important. People who have had strokes should receive specialist treatment and rehabilitation from a multidisciplinary team so that as much mental and physical ability as possible can be restored (see Section 4.28, Neurorehabilitation).

4.29.4 Nutritional implications of dementia

The effects of dementia on food and fluid intake and hence nutritional status may be considerable.

Early stages of dementia may result in:

- difficulty in shopping, cooking and storing food
- failing to recognize (and hence eating) spoiled foods
- forgetting to eat
- forgetting having eaten
- eating food which is too hot
- changes in food preferences (e.g. a strong liking for sweet, salty or spicy foods)
- unusual food choices (e.g. consuming a whole bottle of tomato ketchup)
- gorging, particularly of sweets.

Patients with MID or dementia associated with Parkinson's disease may, in addition, have physical problems affecting their ability to prepare and cook food, eat, chew and swallow.

These problems are likely to be exacerbated if the sufferer lives alone.

As dementia progresses:
- food may be hoarded in the mouth but not swallowed.
- food may not be chewed sufficiently

- non-foods may be eaten
- activity level (and hence energy requirements) may increase as a result of pacing or agitation
- appetite may increase, but loss of ability to use cutlery or even self-feed may prevent energy needs being met.

In advanced dementia problems may include:

- food not being recognized
- patients refusing to open their mouth and turning away when food is offered
- aphasia: the patient cannot ask for food or fluids
- apraxia: the patient cannot initiate movement to open the mouth and cannot chew
- dysphagia: the patient cannot swallow.

As a result of these problems, underweight and weight loss are common in demented patients. This is nearly always a consequence of an inadequate energy intake due to poor eating habits (Prentice *et al.* 1989; Sutherland *et al.* 1990) rather than a result of the disease itself, and can be corrected by energy supplementation (Carver and Dobson 1995). However, in some cases the energy deficit may be exacerbated by a relatively high energy expenditure as a result of agitation and pacing (Litchfield and Wakefield 1987; Rheaume *et al.* 1987).

In addition, infections (e.g. of the chest or urinary tract) are a frequent occurrence and further increase nutritional requirements and so increase the likelihood of malnutrition. This in turn enhances the risk of infection, so compounding the situation (Sandman *et al.* 1987).

Impacted faeces, dehydration and electrolyte imbalance, protein, energy or vitamin deficiencies may also occur.

4.29.5 Nutritional assessment in patients with dementia

Assessment of food intake usually depends on a combination of obtaining information from relatives or care staff and observing actual practice at meal times. Features that increase the likelihood of inadequate nutritional intake are:

- anorexia or loss of interest in food due to depression or decline in sensory perception, especially smell and taste
- food refusal due to paranoia or confusion
- physical difficulties in chewing or swallowing
- dependence on being fed
- behavioural disturbance involving food, e.g. spitting or throwing food
- medications resulting in side-effects of dry mouth and altered taste (e.g. antidepressants and antipsychotics) or heavy sedation

Assessment tools have been devised for patients with dementia (Watson 1994a, b; Watson and Deary 1994) which evaluate patients' behaviour at meal times and the level of help needed with feeding. The expert working group VOICES (1998) has also developed a meal time behaviour-assessment checklist with suggestions for dealing with each behaviour. By itemizing each potential behav-

iour at an early stage, specific strategies can be developed to help to resolve the issue (Table 4.64).

It is also important to check:

- the nutritional adequacy of the food being offered
- the frequency with which food is offered: in institutions there may be short intervals between daytime meals and long gaps (e.g. between tea-time and the next morning) when nothing is offered
- the time available for assisting people to eat and drink: if institutions are short-staffed or carers have additional family or work commitments, it is very difficult to devote sufficient time to coax the reluctant or slow eater to take sufficient nourishment. The need to encourage the consumption of fluids at frequent intervals may also be overlooked.

4.29.6 Dietary management of dementia

A number of strategies can be employed to optimize nutritional intake. These will vary according to the individual circumstances and stage of the disease, and perhaps additional clinical problems such as diabetes and depression.

People who live alone in their own homes should be encouraged to:

- keep a store of foods that do not require cooking and can be opened easily (i.e. not canned or heavily

Table 4.64 Mealtime behaviour assessment of people with dementia (Adapted from *Eating Well for Older People with Dementia*, VOICES, 1998)

Style of eating and pattern of food intake
Incorrectly uses spoon, knife or fork
Unable to cut meat
Difficulty getting food on to utensils
Eats dessert/sweets first
Eats too quickly
Plate wanders on table
Eats other people's food
Incorrectly uses cup or glass
Mixes food together
Slow eating, prolonged meal times

Resistive or disruptive behaviour
Hoards, hides or throws food
Verbally refuses to eat
Interrupts servers, or wants to help
Plays with food
Distracted from eating
Stares at food without eating
Demonstrates impatient behaviour during or before meal time
States 'I can't afford to eat' or wants to pay for meal
Eats small amount and leaves table, unable to sit still for meals

Oral behaviour
Difficulty chewing
Difficulty swallowing
Prolonged chewing without swallowing
Does not chew food before swallowing
Holds food in mouth
Bites on spoon
Spits out food
Refuses to open mouth

packaged food); suitable foods include bread, breakfast cereals, milk, cheese, sliced ham and bananas
- keep a good supply of cold drinks if preparation of hot drinks is a problem
- make use of meals provided by organizations such as meals-on-wheels or in day-care centres.

Advice to carers should focus on the need to:

- offer small meals and snacks at regular intervals: not only does this help to meet nutritional and fluid needs, but the routine of a regular meal pattern also seems to provide comfort and reassurance to many dementia patients
- provide a variety of foods which the person likes
- help to maintain the person's independence by providing foods of a consistency which they can manage themselves. Plate guards and adapted utensils may be helpful. If there is difficulty with using utensils, they may be able to cope with finger foods, e.g. sandwiches, chips, hard-boiled eggs, bananas
- make the most of 'good' times of day (usually breakfast and lunch-time) to provide foods which are good sources of nutrients and energy
- encourage fluid intake by providing it in the form of soup, sauces or jelly as well as conventional drinks. Cups should not be filled to the brim in an attempt to maximize fluid intake, as this will only result in spillage which the sufferer may find degrading.

If confusion is a particular problem, this may be minimized by:

- presenting only one course at a time and associated cutlery for only that course
- not adding extraneous objects such as flowers and cruets to a tray or table
- serving foods of a single composition (e.g. macaroni cheese; casserole with pre-added vegetables) or finger foods rather than offering several different foods on the same plate. Foods of mixed texture (e.g. peach slices in jelly or minestrone soup) may also be best avoided (see Section 3.7, Older adults)
- minimizing external distractions at meal times (e.g. television or background music).

If food intake is poor, nutrient intake can be boosted by fortifying foods and beverages with other foods (e.g. milk powder, grated cheese) or, if this proves insufficient, by providing supplemental drinks (see Section 1.12, Oral nutritional support). Finger foods may also be a useful way of helping Alzheimer's patients to maintain weight (Soltesz and Dayton 1993).

Guidance for staff who care for those in institutions should emphasize the:

- importance of adequate nutrition in preventing weight loss and malnutrition and the prevention of pressure sores
- importance of adequate amounts of fluid being consumed at frequent intervals

- need to recognize individual variation in terms of nutrient needs and personal likes and dislikes
- benefits of simple food-fortification measures and use of energy supplements for those with poor energy intake or increased energy requirements.

Nutritional objectives are more likely to be met if:

- foods offered are nutrient and energy dense and of an appropriate consistency for that individual
- attention is paid to individual likes and dislikes
- food is offered in portion sizes that are appropriate to the individual and second helpings are available to patients who will take them
- finger foods are offered to people with short attention spans who tend to wander during meal times
- sufficient time is allocated for feeding patients and for patients to feed themselves
- patients eat or are fed in an appropriate environment: some patients eat better in groups and some alone. Patients with deteriorating table manners should be separated from others who may be distressed by their behaviour
- food and fluid intake is monitored
- specific measures are taken to minimize or rectify problems impairing food intake, e.g. avoiding distractions in easily confused patients, not serving food in covered containers to patients with severe memory loss (who may be unable to find the food), and encouraging restless and wandering patients to finish their meals by seating them at a table which is less easily vacated (e.g. in a corner of the room)
- the patient's dignity is preserved as much as possible, e.g. by using plastic tablecloths which are easily wiped after spillage and disposable napkins instead of geriatric 'bibs'.

If the patient is unable to self-feed, guidance should be given on appropriate feeding technique, food choice and consistency.

In the final stages of the illness, multidisciplinary decisions involving the family may need to be made concerning the use of enteral feeding or intravenous hydration. The ethical issues involved are discussed in Section 1.19 (Healthcare ethics) and by BAPEN (1998).

General guidance for helping people with dementia

It is important that both health professionals and carers:

- Treat the person as an individual:
  - respect their right to privacy
  - make sure that their cultural and religious beliefs are respected and catered for
  - take account of their likes and dislikes
  - show affection, where appropriate.
- Communicate in an appropriate manner:
  - speak to the person as an adult, not a child

- make sure that they are called by a name they prefer
- never talk over their head as though they were not there
- speak in short sentences
- use calm movements and a reassuring tone
- encourage them to talk about the past.
- Encourage their strengths:
  - look for activities that they can still enjoy and manage
  - praise them for any achievement and for the way they look
  - encourage independence and let them take acceptable risks
  - do things with the person rather than for them
  - find ways to aid their memory, e.g. by putting things in the same place
  - let them do things at their own pace
  - do not scold, criticize or make them feel that they have failed.

4.29.7 The needs of carers

The needs of those who care for dementia sufferers in the domestic setting have been increasingly recognized. Accompanying guidance to the NHS and Community Care Act, 1990, made it clear that the preferences of carers should be taken into account and that their willingness to continue caring should not be assumed. In addition, the 1995 Carers (Recognition and Services) Act made it clear that carers who provide regular substantial care are entitled to a separate assessment of their needs. More recently, the Department of Health has published a national strategy to provide carers with more support, recognition and rights, both now and in the future (DH 1999).

Health professionals should work closely with the carers of someone with dementia because:

- carers know the sufferer best and are more likely to be able to identify or interpret any needs and problems
- carers have to implement any guidance given by health professionals.

If the carers are relatives, they too will need a lot of support from the healthcare team. Caring for someone with dementia is extremely demanding, both physically and emotionally. Carers may feel:

- unappreciated: that they are giving a lot for little return
- resentful: that their lives are dominated by this situation
- guilty: that they feel like this
- impatient and angry: often a sign of the strain they feel
- depressed and bereft: at the loss of the person they once knew and whose company they will be unable to enjoy again
- isolated: particularly if they are trying to cope alone
- frightened: of the difficulties ahead.

Carers need to be given the opportunity to express their feelings and be reassured that these are normal and understandable in these circumstances. Practical support should be offered in terms of:

- specific advice on how to deal with particular problems, e.g. aggression, wandering, feeding problems or incontinence
- the availability of local support services, e.g. social services departments may run carer support teams; there may be local groups for carers organized by professional or voluntary organizations such as the Alzheimer's Disease Society. The latter also has a national telephone advice line
- ensuring that they are receiving any benefits to which they are entitled by seeking advice from appropriate professionals, e.g. local advice agencies or the Benefits Enquiry line
- encouraging carers to accept help offered by family, friends, neighbours or the carer's religious/community organization, or to make use of respite care to enable them to have a break and make contact with other people
- advising carers to contact the general practitioner if there is any sudden change in the patient's physical or mental condition. Sometimes they may also need to be encouraged to ask for a specialist referral for expert assessment of the patient's needs and access to support measures.

Text written by: Briony Thomas

Acknowledgements: Helen Molyneux and the British Dietetic Association's NAGE Group.

Useful addresses

Alzheimer's Disease Society
Gordon House, 10 Greencoat Place, London SW1P 1PH
Tel: 020 7306 0606

CJD Support Network
E-mail: cjdnet@aizheimers.org.uk

National CJD Surveillance Unit, Edinburgh
Website: www.cjd.ed.ac.uk

VOICES (Voluntary Organisations Involved in Caring in the Elderly Sector).
c/o Association of Charity Officers, Beechwood House, Wyllyotts Close, Potters Bar, Herts EN6 2HN

Further reading

VOICES (Voluntary Organisations Involved in Caring in the Elderly Sectors). *Eating Well for Older People with Dementia.* VOICES, 1998. (Available from PO Box 5, Manchester M60 3GE.)
Copeman J. *Nutritional Care of Older People.* Age Concern, 1999.

Useful resources

The British Dietetic Association's NAGE Group has produced useful support material for dietitians who have patients with dementia and other diseases associated with ageing. Details of their current publications and availability can be obtained from the BDA website at www.bda.org.uk or from the BDA office.

References

Alzheimer's Disease Society. *No Accounting for Health: Health Commissioning for Dementia*. London: Alzheimer's Disease Society, 1996.

Amar K, Wilcock G. Fortnightly review: vascular dementia. *British Medical Journal* 1996; **312**: 227–231.

British Association of Parenteral and Enteral Nutrition (BAPEN). *Ethical and Legal Aspects of Clinical Hydration and nutritional Support*. Maidenhead: BAPEN, 1998.

Carver AD, Dobson AM. Effects of dietary supplementation of elderly demented hospital residents. *Journal of Human Nutrition and Dietetics* 1995; **8**: 389–394.

Department of Health. *Caring about Carers: A National Strategy for Carers*. London: DH, 1999. (Available from Department of Health, PO Box 410, Wetherby LS23 7LN.)

Doll R. Review: Alzheimer's disease and environmental aluminium. *Age and Ageing* 1993; **22**: 138–153.

Higgins JP, Flicker L. Lecithin for dementia and cognitive impairments (Cochrane Review). *Cochrane Database of Systematic Reviews* 2000; **4**: CD001015.

Janicki MP, Dalton AJ. Prevalence of dementia and impact on intellectual disability service. *Mental Retardation* 2000; **38**: 276–288.

Litchfield M, Wakefield L. Nutrient intakes and energy expenditures of residents with senile dementia of the Alzheimer's type. *Journal of the American Dietetic Association* 1987; **87**: 211–213.

McLachlan DRC. Aluminium and Alzheimer's disease. *Neurobiology of Aging* 1986; **7**: 525–532.

Martyn CN, Barker J, Osmond C *et al*. Geographical relationship between Alzheimer's disease and aluminium in drinking water. *Lancet* 1989; **i**: 59–62.

Polvikovski T, Sulkava R, Haltia M *et al*. Apolipoprotein E, dementia, and cortical deposition of beta-amyloid protein. *New England Journal of Medicine* 1995; **333**: 1242–1247.

Prentice AM, Leavesley K, Murgatroyd PR *et al*. Is severe wasting in elderly mental patients caused by an excessive energy requirement? *Age and Aging* 1989; **18**: 158–167.

Priest ND. The bioavailability and metabolism of aluminium compounds in man. *Proceedings of the Nutrition Society* 1993; **52**: 231–240.

Rheaume Y, Riley M, Volicer L. Meeting the nutritional needs of Alzheimer's patients who pace constantly. *Journal of Nutrition for the Elderly* 1987; **7**: 43–52.

Sandman P, Adolfsson R, Nygren C *et al*. Nutritional status and dietary intake in institutionalised patients with Alzheimer's disease and multi-infarct dementia. *Journal of the American Geriatric Society* 1987; **35**: 31–38.

Soltez KS, Dayton JH. Finger foods help those with Alzheimer's maintain weight. *Journal of the American Dietetic Association* 1993; **93**: 1106–1108.

Sutherland R, Rucker J, Woolton S. Energy intakes and weight loss in institutionalised psychiatric patients. *Proceedings of the Nutrition Society* 1990; **49**: 16A.

Tatemichi TK, Desmond DW, Mayeux R *et al*. Dementia after stroke: baseline frequency, risks, and clinical features in a hospitalized cohort. *Neurology* 1992; **42**: 1185–1193.

VOICES (Voluntary Organisations Involved in Caring in the Elderly Sectors). *Eating Well for Older People with Dementia*. VOICES, 1998. (Available from PO Box 5, Manchester M60 3GE.)

Watson R. Measuring feeding difficulties in patients with dementia: developing a scale. *Journal of Advanced Nursing* 1994a; **19**: 257–263.

Watson R. Measuring feeding difficulties in patients with dementia: replication and validation of the Ed Fed Scale #1 *Journal of Advanced Nursing* 1994b; **19**: 850–855.

Watson R, Deary IJ. Measuring feeding difficulty in patients with dementia: multivariate analysis of feeding problems, nursing intervention and indicators of feeding difficulty. *Journal of Advanced Nursing* 1994; **20**: 283–287.

4.30 Mental illness

Mental illness can develop at any age in any individual and may be completely curable or require continuous treatment and support. Since food habits are greatly influenced by psychological influences as well as physical signals such as hunger, alterations in a person's mood, emotions and behaviour can have marked effects on their nutritional intake. This may well be a contributory factor to the greater prevalence of morbidity and mortality observed in people with mental illness (DH 1993). Government strategies to improve the care and health of people with mental illness outlined in the document *Modernising Mental Health Services* (DH 1998) are in the process of being implemented in accordance with the principles and standards set out in the *National Service Framework for Mental Health* (DH 1999a). Promoting mental health is one of the priority areas identified in the government's action plan to improve the nation's health (DH 1999b).

Mental illness is distinct from learning disability (see Section 3.11.2, Learning disabilities). Learning disability is a permanent impairment of intellectual ability, either inherited or acquired as a result of damage to the brain. Mental illness can develop for many reasons and is often the result of a combination of factors such as:

- organic changes in the brain, e.g. altered production of neurotransmitters, alcohol or drug-induced brain damage
- environmental influences, e.g. the effects of stress, social isolation or major life events such as bereavement or redundancy may result in disordered mental function
- genetic influences: there may be a genetic predisposition to some types of mental illness.

The division between health and illness is not as clear in psychiatry as in other branches of medicine. Many of the symptoms are behavioural and it is not always easy to distinguish the cut-off point between normal and abnormal behaviour because the definition of 'acceptable behaviour' varies with the context in which the behaviour occurs.

4.30.1 Types of mental illness

The diagnostic criteria for mental illnesses can be found in the World Health Organization's *International Classification of Diseases*, 10th ed (ICD-10; WHO 1992) and in the American Psychiatric Association's *Diagnostic and Statistical Manual of Mental Disorders*, 4th edn (DSM IV; APA 1994). However, in broad terms, mental illness can be classified into neuroses and psychoses (Table 4.65). In both of these, normal emotional response changes to the extent that it interferes significantly with the sufferer's ability to function socially, professionally or personally, or causes physical illness. However, people with a neurosis usually maintain contact with reality. Those who suffer from a psychosis often have no insight into the fact that many of their experiences are unreal. Understanding the nature and effects of a particular form of mental illness is essential in order to identify and manage the types of nutritional problems that may result.

Although classified as organic psychoses, the management of dementias is not included in this section but discussed in depth in Section 4.29 (Dementias).

Mood disorders (depression and mania)

Depression and mania are collectively known as affective or mood disorders. ('Affect' is the term used in psychiatry when the mood is a symptom of the illness.) Mood may be classified as:

- dysphoric: feeling sad, hopeless, miserable or low
- euthymic: normal or premorbid mood
- euphoric: elated, happy, excited, irritable or high.

Depression is characterized by dysphoric mood; mania by euphoric mood. Hypomania is used to describe an elevated mood or slight degree of mania. The illness may be unipolar, presenting as depression or mania only, or bipolar when there are both manic and depressive episodes (manic-depression psychosis).

Table 4.65 Classification of mental illness

Neuroses	Psychoses	
	Functional psychosis (no abnormal pathology)	Organic psychosis (abnormal brain pathology)
Depressive neurosis	Manic-depressive psychosis	Acute confusional state
Anxiety neurosis	Schizophrenia	Alzheimer's disease
Obsessional neurosis		Multi-infarct dementia
Phobic neurosis		
Hysteria		
Post-traumatic neurosis		

Depression is the most common psychiatric illness, affecting an estimated 5% of the population to a significant degree and accounting for about a quarter of all general practitioner (GP) consultations (DH 1993). Depression is thought to result from an imbalance of the neurotransmitters that carry messages between brain cells. This can be disturbed by many factors such as the effects of stress, trauma or relationship breakdown, hormonal changes, or as a side-effect of some types of medication such as tranquillizers, steroids, antihypertensive and antihyperthyroid drugs. Genetic influences on brain function may also make some people more susceptible to the condition.

Types of depression may include:

- *Endogenous depression (functional psychosis)*: This has no apparent external cause and is thought to be biochemical in origin. Anorexia, constipation, indigestion and fluid refusal may be nutritionally important consequences.
- *Reactive, neurotic or secondary depression (psychoneurosis)*: This is far more common than endogenous depression and presents as a morbid sadness which relates to a stress or loss such as bereavement or unemployment. It may be secondary to other physical or mental illnesses. Either anorexia or excessive eating (or alcohol consumption) may result. Neurotic depression should be distinguished from *grief*, which is an appropriate, healthy feeling of sadness in response to a personal loss.
- *Postpartum depression*: This has elements of both endogenous and reactive depression. Some clients may also have puerperal psychosis, including psychotic depression.
- *Seasonal affective disorder (SAD)*: This condition is characterized by depression in autumn and winter, alternating with non-depressed periods in spring and summer (Rosenthal *et al.* 1984). During the phases of depression, symptoms of fatigue, overeating, carbohydrate craving and weight gain are commonly reported.
- *Pseudodementia*: Depression may present with confusion and cognitive deficits mimicking dementia. However, no organic changes in the brain can be detected and treatment of the underlying depression resolves the dementia symptoms.
- *Agitated depression*: The illness presents as anxiety or agitation but the underlying mood disturbance is dysphoric.

Nutritional implications of mood disorders

The nutritional consequences depend on the nature and severity of the disorder but some of the most common effects are summarized in Table 4.66. Disorders such as depression can alter food consumption, appetite and food preference in a variety of ways, and the effects can range from apathy and disinterest in food to disordered eating habits and excessive energy intake. Prior to treatment, a reduced food intake, comprised of a disproportionately high intake of carbohydrate, especially sweet foods, is common (Kazes *et al.* 1994; Christiansen and Somers 1996).

During or following treatment, increased appetite and weight gain, sometimes excessive, may occur. Depression associated with pre-existing obesity is often closely associated with eating dysregulation and results in a pattern of co-morbidity where all three factors are closely interlinked and impact on each other (Musante *et al.* 1998).

Nutrition and neurotransmitters   The role of nutrition in the aetiology of mood disorders has been a matter of considerable speculation but has been little researched in humans and remains poorly understood. Brain serotonin (5-hydroxytryptamine, 5-HT) is known to affect mood, and low levels of serotonin contribute to the aetiology of depression in some people (Young 1993). The possible effects of diet on serotonin production have therefore been of interest. Artificially induced depletion of the amino acid tryptophan (necessary for serotonin synthesis) has been shown to reduce serotonin production and result in a lowering of mood in some, although not all, subjects (Young 1993). High carbohydrate intake increases serotonin production, possibly by increasing the rate at which tryptophan enters the brain (Wurtman 1993), and may elevate mood (Markus *et al.* 1998). This effect may account for carbohydrate craving in some depressed people or those exposed to stress (Wurtman and Wurtman 1995). However, others have suggested that the benefit could also result from endorphin release as a result of the pleasurable experience of eating carbohydrate foods such as chocolate (Benton and Donohoe 1999). Other nutrients may also have an influence: folic acid deficiency has also been shown to lower brain serotonin in rats and may have some effects in

Table 4.66   Nutritional consequences of mood disorders

Mood disorder	Possible influences on food intake	Possible nutritional consequences
Depression	Apathy and disinterest in food Anorexia Sense of guilt or worthlessness causing feelings of 'not deserving food' Food refusal	Undernutrition Weight loss
	Loss of thirst sensation Fluid refusal	Dehydration Constipation, impacted faeces
	Distorted food intake Carbohydrate craving	Unbalanced diet, weight gain, obesity
Anxiety	Frequent loose stools Abdominal pain or discomfort	Selective food avoidance Food refusal
Mania	Drug side-effects causing dry mouth or altered taste	Difficulties in chewing or swallowing Altered taste sensation
	Increased appetite	Weight gain
	Hyperactivity	Increased energy requirements
	Erratic eating habits	Unbalanced diet, weight gain

humans (Young 1993), thiamin status has been shown to be associated with mood (Benton and Donohue 1999) and deficiency of *n3* fatty acids has been suggested to result in changes in membrane structure that could impair serotonin release and uptake (Edwards *et al.* 1998; Maes *et al.* 1999).

However, while of interest, the significance of these findings in terms of the management, or even prevention, of mood disorders remains unknown. Mechanisms observed under laboratory conditions, or in rats, may not be of significance in humans eating typical meals (Young 1991; Fernstrom 1994; Benton and Donohue 1999). Furthermore, most of the studies conducted to date have been confined to serotonin production, which is not the only, or necessarily always the most important, factor involved in psychiatric disturbance (Young 1993). Relationships between diet and psychopathology are undoubtedly complex and require further exploration before conclusions can be drawn.

Nutrition and drug treatment   Many of the drugs used to treat mood disorders have nutritional implications (Table

4.67). Those arising from the use of lithium in the management of mania, and for the prophylaxis of manic depression and recurrent unipolar depression, are particularly important. Lithium salts have a narrow range between therapeutic effectiveness and toxicity; they are therefore used with caution and usually not for longer than necessary owing to concern over their possible long-term effects on renal function. There is also an inverse relationship between sodium intake and serum lithium levels. Lithium toxicity (which can be fatal) can therefore be precipitated by sodium depletion. This is most likely to result from use of diuretics or other contraindicated drugs, but a sudden reduction in salt intake could have the same effect. Conversely, a sudden marked increase in salt intake could reduce serum lithium to a level where it becomes therapeutically ineffective. Patients on lithium therapy should therefore be advised to:

- maintain an adequate fluid intake: thirst is a common side-effect and people should be advised to drink as

Table 4.67   Possible effects of centrally active drugs on nutrition

Drug type	Examples	Uses	Potential nutritional side-effects
Antidepressants Tricyclic	Amitriptyline Imipramine Lofepramine Dothiepin Doxepin	Depressive illness	Dry mouth Sour metallic taste Constipation or rarely diarrhoea Nausea and vomiting, epigastric distress Increased appetite and weight gain due to carbohydrate craving Anorexia (rarely)
5-Hydroxytryptamine (5-HT) re-uptake inhibitors	Citalopram Fluoxetine Fluvoxamine Paroxetine Sertraline	Depressive illness	Anorexia Nausea and vomiting Weight loss Dry mouth Dyspepsia, diarrhoea 'Serotonin syndrome': restlessness with agitation and GI distress with tryptophan 1–4 g/day
Monoamine oxidase inhibitors (MAOI)	Isocarboxazid Phenelzine Tranylcypromine	Depressive illness Atypical depression Depression with phobic symptoms	Nausea and vomiting Dry mouth Constipation Increased appetite and weight gain Potentiation of action of insulin or oral hypoglycaemic with lowered blood glucose Hypertensive crisis if foods containing tyramine are ingested
Antipsychotics Phenothiazines	Chlorpromazine Fluphenazine Thioridazine Trifluoperazine	Psychoses Schizophrenia	Dry mouth Constipation Photosensitivity leading to low vitamin D levels Appetite increase and weight gain High doses reduce response to hypoglycaemic agents, causing elevated blood glucose
Butyrophenones	Haloperidol Droperidol	Psychoses Mania Schizophrenia	Nausea, dyspepsia Loss of appetite Less effect on appetite than phenothiazines
Thioxanthines	Flupenthixol decanoate Zuclopenthixol decanoate	Psychoses Schizophrenia	Increased appetite and weight gain Less commonly weight loss May affect diabetic control

(Continued overleaf)

Table 4.67 (*Continued*)

Drug type	Examples	Uses	Potential nutritional side-effects
Antipsychotics (continued) Substituted benzamides	Pimozide Sulpiride (fewer side-effects)	Mania Psychoses Schizophrenia	Nausea, dyspepsia Abdominal pain, constipation Changes in body weight Glycosuria
Dibenzodiazepines	Loxapine	Schizophrenia	GI disturbances Nausea and vomiting Weight gain or loss Dry mouth or hypersalivation Polydipsia
Atypical antipsychotics	Clozapine Olanzapine Quetiapine Risperidone	Psychoses	Increased appetite and weight gain (Likelihood of weight gain greatest with clozapine and then in decreasing order as listed)
Hypnotics and anxiolytics Benzodiazepines	Diazepam Chlordiazepoxide Lorazepam	Short-term anxiety Alcohol withdrawal	These symptoms have been reported both before and up to 6 weeks after withdrawal: GI upsets, nausea and vomiting Diarrhoea or constipation Appetite and weight changes Dry mouth, metallic taste Dysphagia
	Temazepam Nitrazepam	Short-term sleep disturbance	As above
	Zopiclone	Short-term sleep disturbance	Metallic taste changes
Mood stabilizers Lithium salts	Lithium carbonate Lithium citrate	Treatment of mania and hypomania and prophylactic treatment of recurrent affective disorders	*Early side-effects*: Nausea, metallic taste Increased thirst, polyuria Loose stools *Later*: Weight gain, mild oedema Polyuria Metallic taste Possible hypothyroidism *Toxic effects (can result from sodium depletion, see text)*: Loss of appetite Vomiting, diarrhoea
Anticonvulsants Benzodiazepines	Clonazepam Clobazam	All forms of epileptic seizure	As under Benzodiazepines, above
Barbiturates	Phenobarbitone Primidone (80% of its activity is phenobarbitone)	Grand mal and focal seizures	Decreased vitamin D levels Decreased folate levels Rarely, GI upsets
Other antiepileptics	Carbamazepine	Temporal lobe, tonic clonic and partial seizures (Mood regulation as an alternative to lithium)	Mimics action of ADH on kidney, causing water retention Nausea, loss of appetite, vomiting Diarrhoea or constipation (high dose) Dry mouth Lowered sodium levels in blood
	Sodium valproate	All types of seizures	Nausea and vomiting, anorexia, gastric irritation or increased appetite and weight gain
	Phenytoin	Tonic clonic seizures Following head injury or surgery	*Early*: Nausea and vomiting *Later*: Decreased absorption of vitamin D leading to osteomalacia Increased turnover and decreased absorption of folic acid leading to megaloblastic anaemias Gum hyperplasia and soreness, tooth decay

GI: gastrointestinal; ADH: antidiuretic hormone.

much as they feel they need to. If weight gain is a problem, suitable low-energy drinks can be suggested
- avoid dietary changes that might significantly reduce or increase sodium intake.

Schizophrenia

Schizophrenia is the most severe form of functional psychosis, producing the greatest disorganization of personality. It results in loss of contact with reality and usually follows a chronic course punctuated by relapses.

Schizophrenia is relatively common, affecting as many as 1 in 100 people (DH 1993). It usually starts in the late teens or early twenties, although can occur in later life. The onset of symptoms can be sudden or gradual and symptoms are complex in nature, being classified either as positive or negative.

Positive symptoms include:

- delusions
- hallucinations
- paranoia
- agitation
- hostility.

These symptoms often develop suddenly and are usually frightening for both sufferers and their families, but tend to respond well to treatment.

Negative symptoms may comprise:

- emotional withdrawal
- social withdrawal
- lack of motivation
- inability to cope with daily living tasks
- difficulty in rational thinking
- poor rapport.

Negative symptoms often develop more slowly, are less likely to respond well to drug treatment, and hence are more likely to be associated with poor outcomes and prolonged admissions.

Although stressful life events can trigger schizophrenia, the fundamental cause is not understood. Genetic factors contribute to a proportion of cases and there are racial differences in the prevalence of the disease. African–Caribbean people in the UK have a higher risk of developing psychosis, particularly schizophrenia, than the rest of the population (McDonald and Murray 2000), but the reason for this is unknown.

Diagnosis is based on a person's symptoms and there is at present no confirmatory diagnostic test, although a skin test is being developed that may fulfil this role (Ward *et al*. 1998). Early recognition is vital because of the high risk of suicide among untreated sufferers (DH 1993). The condition is particularly likely to be missed in teenagers because emerging symptoms such as mood swings, muddled thinking and strange beliefs may be attributed to nothing more than 'adolescence', and even more obvious symptoms such as hallucinations and delusions may be wrongly assumed to result from the use of drugs such as Ecstasy or LSD.

Treatment of schizophrenia usually comprises drug therapy together with psychotherapy and social and practical support, and most sufferers can lead a normal, or near-normal life (SANE 1993). Approximately 25% of people who present with schizophrenia recover fully in a few months and experience no recurrence. About 50% recover but have recurrent episodes throughout life. The remaining 25% may be seriously disabled by the illness and require ongoing care and treatment (DH 1993). Currently, one in seven sufferers commits suicide.

Nutritional implications of schizophrenia

The dietary intake of people with schizophrenia may be directly influenced by the symptoms of the disease and/or its treatment. In addition, schizophrenia may affect the ability to communicate and interact with a healthcare professional such as a dietitian, thus making assessment and management more difficult. Some of the most important dietary consequences of schizophrenia are listed below.

Effects of positive symptoms

Paranoia and delusions: Persecutory delusions may involve beliefs that certain foods or drinks are poisoned or harmful in some way. Bizarre demands for 'special diets' and/or very restricted food intakes may result from delusional beliefs about food. It is important for health professionals to understand that a delusion cannot be changed by logical argument or scientific evidence.

Hallucinations are sensory experiences which occur without external stimuli. Auditory hallucinations are common and the 'voices' may tell the person what to eat or drink. An acutely ill patient will pay attention to internal voices rather than to a dietitian.

Agitation and hostility may mean that it is very difficult for a dietitian to ask questions or create a rapport with the client.

Effects of negative symptoms

Withdrawal and lack of motivation may result in anorexia and an inadequate intake of food and fluids. They are also likely to make it difficult for a health professional to communicate and interact with a client.

Inability to cope with everyday tasks: Aspects of self-care such as shopping and meal preparation may be seriously impaired.

Difficulty in rational thinking: Normal associations between words and ideas may break down. There may be thought blocking, when thoughts stop abruptly, or an inability to think in abstract terms. When thought disorder is severe, speech may become incomprehensible.

Poor rapport: A schizophrenic person may speak fluently for some time before the health professional realizes that little, if any, information has been conveyed and that there is no emotional link or understanding between client and listener.

Socioeconomic consequences Many people with chronic schizophrenia live in disadvantaged circumstances and are thus vulnerable to the nutritional problems associated with low income and poor housing (see Section 3.8,

People in low-income groups). It has been estimated that as many as one in three homeless people may be schizophrenia sufferers (SANE 1993), many of whom are not receiving adequate professional psychiatric care (Sclare 1997). As a result, the physical health of people with long-term schizophrenia is often neglected. Cardiovascular and respiratory disorders are common (partly due to a high prevalence of smoking) and standardized mortality rates are two and a half times greater than for the general population (CSAG 1995).

Drug side-effects Anti-psychotic drugs such as chlorpromazine block the action of dopamine and help to control hallucinations and delusions, while other neuroleptic drugs such as clozapine and risperidone, which primarily act on other transmitters such as acetylcholine, histamine and serotonin, may be used to control hostile and aggressive behaviour. Antipsychotic drugs may have a number of side-effects (see Table 4.67). Problems such as drowsiness or nausea may reduce food intake. Dry mouth may make eating or swallowing difficult and taste changes may result in food avoidance or refusal. Inhibition of dopamine may result in parkinsonian side-effects such as tremor, shakiness or muscle spasms, creating physical difficulties in getting food to the mouth. Conversely, some combinations of psychotropic drugs increase appetite and can cause significant weight gain (Blackburn 2000) (see Obesity under Common problems, below).

Schizophrenia and gluten The suggestion that there may be a link between schizophrenia and coeliac disease remains controversial (Vlissides *et al.* 1986; Reichelt *et al.* 1996). Schizophrenia appears to be less common in societies that consume few cereal foods and it has been suggested that grain glutens may provoke schizophrenia in those with the appropriate genotype for the disease (Dohan 1966, 1980). The rationale for this is that some peptides present in gliadin have opioid activity which could, if they enter the circulatory system as a result of gluten-induced damage to the intestinal mucosa, act at narcotic-sensitive sites in the brain and induce behavioural change (Huebner *et al.* 1984).

However, examination of the effect of either a gluten-free diet or gluten challenge in small groups of schizophrenic people has yielded conflicting results; some studies appear to show a deleterious effect of gluten (Dohan and Grasberger 1973; Singh and Kay 1976) while others show no effect (Potkin *et al.* 1981; Storms *et al.* 1982). The consensus of current opinion is that a gluten-free diet should only be implemented in cases of clinically diagnosed coeliac disease confirmed by biopsy (Reichelt *et al.* 1996).

Nevertheless, it is important that dietitians are aware of the fact that relatives and patients may well come across books and magazines suggesting the benefits of a gluten-free diet for people with schizophrenia and that such a regimen is quite likely to be adopted as an 'alternative' form of treatment. This is undesirable for a number of reasons. The diet will probably have been implemented without the benefit of any qualified dietetic advice and so may well be restricted in terms of food choice and nutrition-

ally unbalanced. The cost of obtaining gluten-free foods (which are not prescribable for schizophrenia) is high and, for those with limited financial means, may result in little money being available to spend on the rest of the diet. There is also a risk that if patients suffer a psychotic episode, the dietary restrictions may suddenly be interpreted as 'punishment' or 'persecution' imposed by their carers.

4.30.2 Care of people with mental illness

Care of people with mental illness has undergone immense change in recent decades. The transition from mainly institutionalized to community care brought both benefits and problems; while many people had the opportunity to lead a better and more normal life, this was not always realized in practice owing to inadequate or inappropriate levels of care support. As a result, the care programme approach (DH 1990) was introduced to ensure that every person with serious mental illness had access to care, treatment and support. The care programme is normally implemented by a multidisciplinary care team which aims to:

- assess the health and social needs of the client
- draw up a care plan in conjunction with the client and carers, together with health, local authority and voluntary sector workers as necessary
- monitor the quality and effectiveness of care
- review progress at regular intervals.

An identified key worker, usually a community mental health nurse or social worker, usually acts as the primary link between the client and the healthcare team.

By the mid-1990s it was suggested that greater co-ordination and integration of mental health services was required in order to provide better quality of care to both clients and their carers (DH 1998). The National Service Framework (NSF) for Mental Health (DH 1999a) sets out how this should be done in order to improve, and reduce variability in, standards of care. Its recommendations focus on five main areas:

- mental health promotion
- primary care and access to services
- effective services for people with severe mental health problems
- carers of people with mental health problems
- action required to reduce suicides.

The NSF endorses the care plan approach and expected that, from April 2000, everyone diagnosed with a severe mental illness should have an integrated assessment and care co-ordinator. However, a major feature of the NSF is that it requires a much greater level of specialist expertise to be available to all service users. Instead of the traditional distinction between primary 'community' care and secondary 'specialist' care, care is much more integrated. Local specialist mental health services provide a comprehensive and expert care service within a particular community, with recourse to specialist secure units serving a wider area as necessary. All dietitians involved in the field of mental health should be aware of the contents of the NSF and its requirements and implications for patient care.

4.30.3 Management of diet-related problems in mental illness

The nutritional requirements of people with mental illness are, in general, no different to those of healthy client groups. Similarly, the principles of correcting identified problems such as undernutrition, dietary imbalance, obesity or constipation remain the same. The differences arise in the way in which these problems are identified and managed in practice.

Providing dietary support for people with mental illness is a specialist area requiring sensitivity and skill. During the acute phase of mental illness such as depression, mania or psychosis, or dementia the client may be, to all practical purposes, as inaccessible as a physically ill, unconscious patient. Attempting to obtain dietary information, and using this as a basis for offering nutritional advice, may be distressing or disturbing to someone whose thought processes, cognitive functions or mood are severely disturbed. Dietary needs and management therefore have to be determined on an individual basis and in close conjunction with other members of the care team.

Dietitians may encounter difficulties with, or even feel threatened by, clients with challenging behaviours and should not hesitate to ask psychologists or other members of the mental health team for guidance and support when this is needed. In some areas, training sessions on this issue are routinely given to new members of a mental health team. The important thing is that dietitians do not try to struggle with such problems in isolation, and work closely with other team members so that they can benefit from their psychiatric knowledge and experience.

Nutritional assessment

The nutritional needs and problems of this client group are often overlooked and dietetic input into a care plan ensures that these issues are addressed.

On receiving a referral for a mentally ill person, it is important that the dietitian ascertains beforehand the nature of the illness and whether that person is well enough to either provide or receive dietary information. If not, medical or nursing notes, or other members of the care team may be able to provide information from which the patient's nutritional status and likely nutritional problems can be ascertained. Important aspects to consider are:

- the nature and duration of the illness
- drug treatment
- socioeconomic circumstances and housing conditions
- physical signs and symptoms of malnutrition, e.g. underweight, dehydration, vitamin deficiencies.

Once mental state improves as a result of treatment, it should be possible to obtain more information directly from the client. Particular aims should be to identify long-term idiosyncrasies and recent changes in the diet, as well as its nutritional adequacy.

Common nutritional problems

Undernutrition

The risk of undernutrition in people with some forms of mental illness is high, particularly if chronic psychotic illness is associated with problems such as low income, poor housing, alcoholism or drug abuse (Scottish Schizophrenia Research Group 2000). General dietary measures to improve energy and nutrient intake and alleviate symptoms impairing food intake are discussed in Section 1.12 (Oral nutritional support). However, the way in which these are applied will depend on the nature of the individual's illness, personal circumstances and care plan.

Dehydration

Acutely mentally ill people may stop eating and drinking and can become severely dehydrated. Dehydration can also be the cause of some acute confusional states, particularly in elderly people (see Section 4.29, Dementias).

Chronic dehydration is a risk in continuing care units (Macdonald *et al.* 1989), usually as a result of the low priority given to monitoring fluid consumption and status. Dehydration may exacerbate problems such as constipation or urinary incontinence secondary to urinary tract infections.

Micronutrient deficiencies

Deficiencies of vitamins, minerals and trace elements may result from distorted eating habits associated with the mental illness, or a consequence of generally poor eating habits associated with lifestyle, socioeconomic problems or inadequate care provision. Whether these problems can be corrected by dietary interventions, or whether supplementation is more appropriate, must be assessed on an individual basis.

Obesity

A large proportion of referrals to dietitians working in the field of mental health are for people requiring weight-reduction advice and support. Factors which increase the likelihood of excessive weight gain in people with mental health problems include:

- poor nutritional knowledge
- reduced skills or motivation for budgeting, shopping and cooking
- lack of activity
- side-effects of medication.

Factors which have led to obesity in a particular individual need to be identified before it can be effectively managed. Conventional weight-reducing guidance may help someone whose obesity is incidental to their mental disorder but is unlikely to be appropriate for a person in whom disordered eating is an integral part of a disorder, such as in depression. In these circumstances, behavioural or other specialist intervention strategies may be necessary to help an individual to regain control over their food intake (Riva *et al.* 1998; Wurtman 1993) (see Sections 4.18, Cognitive–Behavioural therapy in obesity treatment, and 4.19, Eating disorders).

Obesity associated with use of psychotropic medication
Weight gain is a common side-effect of psychotropic medication. The reasons for this remain unclear, but may involve direct effects on metabolic, endocrinological and neurochemical mechanisms, and/or indirect effects on food intake or physical activity (Pijl and Meinders 1996; Ackerman and Nolan 1998).

The potential for weight gain with some of these drugs should not be underestimated. Clozapine, a very successful drug for treatment-resistant schizophrenia, may lead to an increase of 10–20% of usual body weight (Ackerman and Nolan 1998), and similar antipsychotics such as olanzapine, quetiapine and risperidone also tend to increase appetite and body weight, although to a lesser degree. Up to two-thirds of people taking lithium will experience weight gain of at least 5%, and for some the gain will be much greater (Ackerman and Nolan 1998).

Many clients are aware that psychotropic medications can result in weight gain, and the desire to avoid this can sometimes affect compliance with the recommended drug dosage, or even cause people to discontinue the medication altogether (Ackerman and Nolan 1998). If weight gain does occur, this can exacerbate feelings of low self-worth and lack of confidence, and possibly worsen existing mental health problems (Sullivan and Tucker 1999), as well as posing a risk to physical health.

Despite the difficulties, dietetic intervention can help clients to achieve weight loss. In others, weight can be stabilized following a period of rapid gain, and this can be an equally important treatment objective; people can be relieved to discover that it is possible for their weight to be controlled. It is important that all clients understand that the weight increasing effects of psychotopic medication can be offset by appropriate changes in diet and activity; some people wrongly assume that weight gain is inevitable so there is no point in trying to control what they eat.

Suggesting simple positive adjustments that people can make to their eating habits to control their energy intake can be effective, e.g. eat fruit when hungry, use low-calorie soft drinks, double the portion size of vegetables with main meals. Motivational interviewing techniques may be helpful with some clients.

Dietetic support and follow-up are essential. Setting up a patient support group where people experiencing similar problems can share their difficulties and successes can be a useful strategy.

Above all, it is essential that weight problems associated with use of psychotropic drugs are identified and tackled at an early stage (Blackburn 2000). The weight of all clients prescribed such drugs should be recorded at the start of treatment and at regular intervals thereafter, so that emerging problems can receive prompt attention. Prevention is also an important aspect. If every person prescribed a psychotropic drug was, as a matter of routine, also given simple diet and lifestyle guidance (even in the form of an information sheet) to help to prevent unnecessary weight gain, the extent and severity of this problem could be markedly reduced. Closer liaison between dietetic and mental health services may well be needed for this objective to be realized.

Polydipsia Polydipsia is associated with some disorders and types of drug treatment, and may give rise to water intoxication if renal function is impaired (Crammer 1991). Fluid retention may lead to weight gain of up to 0.5 kg/hour, along with a fall in plasma sodium. If 7% or more of early morning weight has been gained, time-limited periods of fluid restriction should be implemented. Twenty four hour fluid restriction will not be tolerated by water-seeking patients, who will search out water from any source (e.g. flower vases), but who may agree to a shorter period of fluid restriction on a daily basis.

Polydispia may also be a factor in drug-related weight gain, e.g. if sugar containing drinks are frequently consumed, and the possibility of a significant energy intake in liquid form should be borne in mind.

Text revised by: Briony Thomas

Acknowledgements: Jane Calow, Karen Lake, Deborah Lazarus, Sheila Merriman and the British Dietetic Association's Mental Health Group.

Useful addresses

British Dietetic Association's Mental Health Group (MHG)
c/o The British Dietetic Association, 5th Floor, Charles House, 148–9 Great Charles Street, Birmingham B3 3HT

The National Schizophrenia Fellowship
28 Castle Street, Kingston-upon-Thames, Surrey KT1 1SS
Tel: 020 8547 3937
National adviceline: 020 8974 6814

MIND (National Association for Mental Health)
15–19 Broadway, London E15 4BQ
Tel: 020 8522 1728
Helpline: 0345 660 0163

Further reading

Gregory GE, Gregory LK. Nutritional aspects of psychiatric disorders. *Journal of the American Dietetic Association* 1989; **89**: 1492–1498.
Perkin RE, Repper JM. *Working Alongside People with Long-Term Mental Health Problems*. London: Chapman and Hall, 1996.

References

Ackerman S, Nolan LJ. Bodyweight gain induced by psychotropic drugs – incidence, mechanisms and management. *CNS Drugs* 1998; 9: 135–151.
American Psychiatric Association. *Diagnostic and Statistical Manual of Mental Disorders*, 4th edn (DSM-IV). Washington, DC: APA, 1994.
Benton D, Donohue RT. The effect of nutrients on mood. *Public Health Nutrition* 1999; **2** (3A): 403–409.

Blackburn GL. Weight gain and antipsychotic medication. *Journal of Clinical Psychiatry* 2000; **61** (Suppl 8): 36–41.

Christiansen L, Somers S. Comparison of nutrient intake among depressed and nondepressed individuals. *International Journal of Eating Disorders* 1996; **20**: 105–109.

Clinical Standards Advisory Group (CSAG). *Schizophrenia*. London: HMSO, 1995.

Crammer JL . Drinking, thirst and water intoxication. *British Journal of Psychiatry* 1991; **159**: 83–89.

Department of Health/Social Services Inspectorate. *The Health of the Nation: Key Area Handbook – Mental Illness*. London: HMSO, 1993.

Department of Health. *Modernising Mental Health Services – Safe, Sound, Supportive*. London, 1998.

Department of Health. *National Service Framework for Mental Health*. London: DH, 1999a.

Department of Health. *Saving Lives: Our Healthier Nation*. London: DH, 1999b.

Department of Health. *Caring for People: The Care Programme Approach for People with Mental Illness Referred to Specialist Psychiatric Services*. Joint Circular HC (90) 23/LASSL (90) 11. London: HMSO, 1990.

Dohan PC. Wartime changes in hospital admissions for schizophrenia and other syndromes in six countries in World War II. *Acta Psychiatrica* 1966; **42**: 1–22.

Dohan PC. Hypothesis: Genes and neuroactive peptides from food as the cause of schizophrenia. In Costa E, Trabucci M (Eds) *Neural Peptides and Neuronal Communication*. New York: Raven Press, 1980.

Dohan PC, Grasberger JC. Relapsed schizophrenics, earlier discharge from hospital after cereal-free, milk-free diet. *American Journal of Psychiatry* 1973; **130**: 685–688.

Edwards R, Peet M, Shay J, Horrobin D. Omega-3 polyunsaturated fatty acid levels in the diet and in red blood cell membranes of depressed patients. *Journal of Affective Disorders* 1998; **48**: 149–155.

Fernstrom JD. Dietary amino acids and brain function. *Journal of the American Dietetic Association* 1994; **94**: 71–77.

Huebner PR, Weberman KW, Rubino RP, Wall JS. Demonstration of high opioid like activity in isolated peptides from wheat protein hydrolysates. *Peptides* 1984; **5**: 1139–1147.

Kazes M, Danjon JM, Grange D *et al*. Eating behaviour and depression before and after antidepressant treatment: a prospective, naturalistic study. *Journal of Affective Disorders* 1994; **30**: 193–207.

McDonald C, Murray RM. Early and late environmental risk factors for schizophrenia. *Brain Research Reviews* 2000; **31**: 130–137.

Macdonald NJ, NcConnell KN, Stephen MR, Dunnigan MG. Hypernatraemic dehydration in patients in a large hospital for the mentally handicapped. *British Medical Journal* 1989; **299**: 1426–1429.

Maes M, Christophe A, Delanghe J *et al*. Lowered omega-3 polyunsaturated fatty acids in serum phospholipids and cholestyl esters of depressed patients. *Psychiatry Research* 1999; **85**: 275–291.

Markus CR, Panhuysen G, Tuiten A *et al*. Does carbohydrate-rich, protein-poor food prevent a deterioration of mood and cognitive performance of stress-prone subjects when subjected to a stressful task? *Appetite* 1998; **31**: 49–65.

Musante GJ, Costanzo PR, Friedman KE. The comorbidity of depression and eating dysregulation processes in a diet-seeking obese population: a matter of gender specificity. *International Journal of Eating Disorders* 1998; **23**: 65–75.

Pijl H, Meinders AE. Bodyweight change as an adverse effect of drug treatment – mechanisms and management. *Drug Safety* 1996; **14**: 329–342.

Potkin SG, Weinberger D, Kleinman J *et al*. Wheat challenge in schizophrenia patients. *American Journal of Psychiatry* 1981; **138**: 1208–1221.

Reichelt KL, Seim AR, Reichelt WH. Could schizophrenia be reasonably explained by Dohan's hypothesis on genetic interaction with a dietary peptide overload? *Progress in Neuropsychopharmacology, Biology and Psychiatry* 1996; **20**: 1083–1114.

Riva G, Ragazzoni P, Molinari E. Obesity, psychopathology and eating attitudes: are they related? *Eating and Weight Disorders* 1998; **3**: 78–83.

Rosenthal NE, Sack DA, Gillin JC *et al*. Seasonal affective disorder: a description of the syndrome and preliminary findings with light therapy. *Archives of General Psychiatry* 1984; **41**: 72–80.

SANE. *Schizophrenia: The Forgotten Illness*. SANE Mental Health Series No. 1. London: SANE Publications, 1993.

Sclare PD. Psychiatric disorder among the homeless in Aberdeen. *Scottish Medical Journal* 1997; **42**: 173–177.

Scottish Schizophrenia Research Group. Smoking habits and plasma lipid peroxide and vitamin E levels in never-treated first episode patients with schizophrenia. *British Journal of Psychiatry* 2000; **176**: 290–293.

Singh MM, Kay SR. Wheat gluten as a pathogenic factor in schizophrenia. *Science* 1976; **191**: 401–402.

Storms LH, Jamie M, Clopton MS *et al*. Effects of gluten on schizophrenics. *Archives of General Psychiatry* 1982; **39**: 323–327.

Sullivan A, Tucker R. Meeting the nutritional needs of people with mental health problems. *Nursing Standard* 1999; **13** (47): 48–53.

Vlissides DN, Venulet A, Jenner FA. A double-blind gluten-free/gluten-load controlled trial in a secure ward population. *British Journal of Psychiatry* 1986; **148**: 447–452.

Ward PE, Sutherland J, Glen EM, Glen AI. Niacin skin flush in schizophrenia: a preliminary report. *Schizophrenia Research* 1998; **29**: 269–274.

World Health Organisation. *The International Classification of Diseases*, 10th edn (ICD-10). Geneva: WHO, 1992.

Wurtman JJ. Depression and weight gain: the serotonin connection. *Journal of Affective Disorders* 1993; **29**: 183–192.

Wurtman RJ, Wurtman JJ. Brain serotonin, carbohydrate-craving, obesity and depression. *Obesity Research* 1995; **3** (Suppl 4): 477S–480S.

Young SN. The 1989 Borden Award Lecture. Some effects of dietary components (amino acids, carbohydrate, folic acid) on brain serotonin synthesis, mood and behaviour. *Canadian Journal of Physiology and Pharmacology* 1991; **69**: 893–903.

Young SN. The use of diet and dietary components in the study of factors controlling affect in humans: a review. *Journal of Psychiatry and Neurosciences* 1993; **18**: 235–244.

4.31 Osteoporosis

Osteoporosis has been defined as 'a systemic skeletal disease characterized by low bone mass and micro-architectural deterioration of bone tissue, with a consequent increase in bone fragility and susceptibility to fracture' (Consensus Development Conference 1993). The problem with this definition is that it does not allow the condition to be recognized until a fracture has occurred. The World Health Organization has therefore proposed an alternative definition, related to bone mass. WHO defined osteoporosis as having a bone mineral content (BMC) or bone mineral density (BMD) of more than 2.5 SD (standard deviations) below the young normal mean (WHO 1994). This definition allows the condition to be diagnosed before clinical consequences are apparent, but in reality it is not feasible to measure BMD routinely. It does, however, with knowledge of the natural progression of bone loss with age, allow a prediction of the prevalence of the disease. Osteoporosis is far more common in women and at the age of 50 years the incidence is likely to be 15%, rising to 40% by the age of 80 years (Kanis *et al.* 1994). It has been estimated that more than one-third of women and one-sixth of men will suffer an osteoporotic fracture during their life (RCP 1999) and therefore osteoporosis can be considered a major public health problem. Not only do fractures cause a great deal of pain but, especially in the elderly, they can lead to a loss of independence by reducing mobility (Keene *et al.* 1993). The cost to the National Health Service (NHS) has been estimated at nearly £750 million/annum for women alone, and if the cost of treating male fractures is included this rises to £942 million/annum (Dolan and Togerson 1998). The majority of fractures occur in the elderly, so with predictions that by 2030 elderly people will account for 1 in 4 of the UK population and that the incidence of fractures worldwide will rise from 1.66 million in 1990 to 6.26 million by 2050, the health and economic impact of osteoporosis is likely to be phenomenal (WHO 1994).

The most effective mechanisms to reduce the risk of developing osteoporosis are to acquire optimal peak bone mass, maintain bone health in early adulthood and reduce the rate of bone loss in later life.

4.31.1 Bone and peak bone mass

The main function of bone is to provide skeletal support for the body and protect body organs. The majority of both red and white blood cells are produced in the bone marrow. The hard bone tissue known as hydroxyapatite con-sists mainly of calcium and phosphate, and 99% of the body content of calcium is stored in bone (NDC 1999).

The most important and active cells are the osteoblasts and osteoclasts which both originate in the bone marrow. Osteoblasts play a role in bone formation by facilitating the creation of osteoid (uncalcified pre-bone tissue) and its subsequent calcification. Osteoclasts are phagocytotic cells which are responsible for the removal of bone. The balanced activity of osteoblasts and osteoclasts allows repair to bone and changes in its architecture in response to mechanical stress, as well as rapid release and resorption of calcium ions.

Bone plays a vital role in calcium homoeostasis. It is responsible for maintaining the level of the body's calcium not stored in bone, and which is actively involved in a number of metabolic functions. A fall in serum calcium concentration will cause an increase in parathyroid hormone (PTH) secretion. PTH acts in a number of ways to restore serum calcium levels to normal, including a direct effect on bone to increase osteoclast activity, leading to bone resorption and release of calcium into the blood. In response to high serum calcium levels, usually from dietary sources, PTH production is inhibited and calcitonin is released from the parathyroid gland, which increases osteoblast activity and promotes uptake of calcium by bone (DH 1998).

Bone is a dynamic tissue in which BMC and BMD increase from infancy until peak bone mass (PBM) is attained in young adulthood (NDC 1999). The exact age at which this occurs is unknown. It was commonly believed that it was not until the end of the third or even early into the fourth decade (Ott 1990; Recker *et al.* 1992), but more recent studies indicate that there is very little gain in bone mass once the age of 30 years is reached. It has been reported that 99% of peak total body BMD is attained by approximately 22 years of age and 99% of peak total BMC by approximately 26 years of age (Teegarden *et al.* 1995). The findings of several studies suggest that, in girls, the rate of bone growth falls dramatically after the age of 16 years (Theintz *et al.* 1992), with the most rapid increase occurring between 11 and 14 years. In boys this occurs somewhat later between 13 and 17 years (Kroger *et al.* 1993). It is well established that during adolescence approximately 50% of PBM is acquired (Bonjour *et al.* 1991).

Growth in bone length ceases at maturity but growth in bone width continues throughout life, although owing to simultaneous endosteal resorption, the cortex becomes thinner as the bone widens. These processes are termed bone modelling and allow renewal of ageing bone, removal of fatigue fractures, skeletal adaptation to stress caused by physical and load-bearing activity, and the release from bone of ionized calcium as required (DH 1998). Bone remodelling on both internal and external surfaces occurs throughout life and in young adults the rate of bone resorption and of calcification of new osteoid are matched to achieve calcium balance. However, with ageing and especially in women at the time of the menopause, bone resorption far exceeds the rate of bone formation, resulting in an overall loss of bone. Although both the accretion and loss of bone mass are largely determined by genetic factors (Grant *et al*. 1996), there is no doubt that a number of modifiable factors, including nutritional intake, can play a vital role in bone health (New 1999).

4.31.2 Nutritional influences on bone health

Calcium

Recommended intakes of calcium in both the UK and other parts of the world are shown in Table 4.68. It can be seen that, in general, UK recommendations are lower than those of other countries, especially for 11–14 year old females. The UK recommendations have recently been reviewed (DH 1998) but the panel concluded that there was insufficient evidence available to recommend any increase.

Calcium intake and peak bone mass

A number of studies have used either calcium salts or dairy products to supplement the calcium intake of children. In 1992 a double-blind, placebo-controlled trial, lasting for

3 years, was undertaken in 45 pairs of identical twins. Half of the group was prepubertal and one twin of each pair acted as a control. The rate of increase in BMD was increased in the prepubertal, calcium-supplemented group (Johnston *et al*. 1992). Since then, several studies have confirmed that calcium supplementation increases BMD and BMC in prepubertal children (Lee *et al*. 1994, 1995). Using calcium-enriched foods, Bonjour *et al*. (1997) showed that the greatest effect was likely to be seen in those who previously had the lowest calcium intake. In a study using milk as the source of the calcium supplement (Cadogan *et al*. 1997), PBM was enhanced in the group who were supplemented for 18 months. However, since milk provides many nutrients other than calcium and, since the milk supplement was taken with breakfast cereal, further enhancing the supplemented groups' diet in nutrients other than calcium, it has been questioned whether PBM enhancement can be attributed solely to the increase in calcium intake (New *et al*. 1998a). These latter two studies found that the effect persisted 1 year after cessation of the supplement (Bonjour *et al*. 1997), but others have found that differences in BMD between supplemented and control groups are no longer evident 18 months to 2 years after supplement cessation (Slemenda *et al*. 1993; Lee *et al*. 1996). The panel which reviewed the evidence (DH 1998) considered that it suggested that the increase in bone mineral appears early in the supplementation period with little effect thereafter and disappears with withdrawal of the supplement. It considered that there were no data to determine whether the effects of the supplements represent a benefit to growing children and whether they result in an increase in PBM in adulthood (DH 1998).

Table 4.68 International recommended daily amounts of calcium

Population group	Dietary reference values for calcium in different countries (mg/day)				
	UK RNI[1]	EU PRI[2]	Aust/NZ RDI[3]	US RDA[4]	USA/Canada AI[5]
0–6 months	525	No value set	Breast fed 300 Formula fed 500	400	210 Formula fed 375
7–12 months	525	400	550	600	270
1–3 years	350	400	700	800	500
4–6 years	450	400	800	800	800
7–10 years	550	550	(8–11 years) 800 male 900 female	800	(7–8 years) 800 (9-10 years) 1300
11–14 years, male	1000	1000	(12–15 years) 1200	1200	1300
15–18 years, male	1000	1000	(16–18 years) 1000	1200	1300
11–14 years, female	800	800	(12–15 years) 1000	1200	1300
15–18 years, female	800	800	(16–18 years) 800	1200	1300
Pregnancy	No extra	No extra	1200	No extra	+300 (if <18 years only)
Lactation	+550	1200	1200	No extra	+300 (if <18 years only)
19–50 years	700	700	800	1200 (<24 years) 800 (>25 years)	1000
50+ years	700	700	(54+ years) 800 male 1000 female		1200

[1]UK RNI: United Kingdom Reference Nutrient Intake (DH 1991).
[2]EU PRI: European Union population Referene Intake (Commission of the European Communities 1993).
[3]Aust/NZ RDI: Australia and New Zealand Reference Dietary Intake (National Health and Medical Research Council 1991).
[4]US RDA: United States Recommended Dietary Allowance (National Research Council (US) 1989).
[5]USA/Canada AI: USA/Canada Adequate Intake (Institute of Nutrition, Food and Health Board 1997).

It is a matter of concern that with the UK recommendations for schoolchildren and adolescents being amongst the lowest in the world, studies have shown that approximately 5% of boys and 18% of girls consume less than the lower reference mutrient intake (LRNI), which is 450 mg and 480 mg, respectively, for 11–18 year olds (DH 1991). It is particularly worrying that many of the lifestyle habits that are adopted at this age (alcohol consumption, smoking, reduction in physical activity, dieting for weight loss) are also detrimental to bone health.

Calcium intake and bone loss

Although there are no recent data, UK figures suggest that 5–16% of women aged 16–64 years consume less than the LRNI for calcium (400 mg/day) (Gregory *et al.* 1990). Bone mineral loss commences at around the age of 40 years and, since there is evidence that the rate of this loss can be affected by calcium intake (Baran *et al.* 1989), such a low calcium intake is likely to have an adverse effect on bone health.

Male and female hormones exert an anabolic effect on bone and a decline in these hormones is associated with bone loss. This is seen most markedly in women at the time of the menopause, when oestrogen levels fall dramatically. Thus, in women, calcium intake appears to have little effect on the dramatic acceleration of bone loss at the time of menopause and also for the next 5 years (DH 1998). Hormone replacement therapy (see below) has a beneficial effect by reducing the rate of bone loss at this time and there is some evidence that this effect may be enhanced by a simultaneous increase in calcium intake to above 1200 mg/day (Nieves *et al.* 1998).

Postmenopausally, there is considerable evidence that calcium supplementation helps to prevent bone loss (Nordin 1997) and the panel reviewing the dietary reference values (DRVs) for calcium conceded that, in established osteoporosis, supplemental calcium may have a role as one part of a therapeutic regimen (DH 1998).

In older people, studies have shown that calcium intake is likely to be adequate in the majority, apart from elderly women (over 85 years) living in the community in whom approximately 15% have a calcium intake below the LRNI (Finch *et al.* 1998). The intake of those who are living in residential care has been shown to be higher, with only 1% consuming less than LRNI, probably as a result of a higher intake of dairy products (DH 1998).

Calcium intake

The reference nutrient intake (RNI) for calcium can be achieved for the majority of the population by consuming two or three portions of milk or milk products daily. For those who cannot or choose not to consume dairy products, advice should be given on alternative non-milk sources of calcium (Table 4.69 and see also Table 2.13 in Section 2.7, Minerals) and how these can be incorporated in the diet. Dietary misconceptions may need to be corrected; some people avoid dairy products in the mistaken belief that they are all high in fat (NDC 1999), while others are unaware

that low-fat dairy products such as skimmed milk and low-fat yoghurt remain rich sources of calcium (Table 4.70).

In recent years a number of calcium-fortified products such as fruit juices have become available in the UK and these may be useful in some circumstances, e.g. for children who refuse to drink milk. However, it should be borne in mind that the bioavailability of calcium from such products is likely to be less than that from dairy products (Weaver 1996).

Vitamin D

Vitamin D is the generic term for ergocalciferol (vitamin D_2), which is found in plants, and cholecalciferol (vitamin D_3), which is formed by the action of ultraviolet (UV) irradiation on the skin. Both forms are transported via the general circulation to the liver where they are converted to 25-hydroxyvitamin D and then to the kidneys, where further metabolism to form 1,25-dihydroxyvitamin D, the active form, takes place. It is this active form which is involved in calcium homoeostasis.

Table 4.69 Calcium content per portion of a range of commonly consumed foods (Adapted from NDC 1999)

Food/beverage	Weight (g)/volume (ml)	Calcium content (mg)
Whole milk	200	237
Semi-skimmed milk	200	248
Skimmed milk	200	249
Cheddar cheese	30	216
Reduced-fat hard cheese	30	252
Macaroni cheese	220	374
Canned sardines with bones	100	460
Low-fat fruit yoghurt	150	225
Fromage frais	100	86
Milk pudding	200	260
White and brown bread	72	72
Wholemeal bread	72	39
Plain scone	48	86
Muesli	50	55
Spinach, cooked	90	144
Baked beans	150	80
Peanuts	50	30
Lentils, cooked	40	9
Orange	160	75
Dried apricots	56	52
Soya milk	200	26

Table 4.70 Risk factors for osteoporosis

Women with premenopausal amenorrhoea, early menopause or hysterectomy
Hypogonadism in men
Family history of osteoporosis
Previous fragility fracture
Long-term oral corticosteroid therapy
Low body weight for height
Little regular physical activity
High alcohol intake
Smoking

Factors affecting vitamin D status

It is now well established that of the two sources of vitamin D, endogenous production (via skin synthesis) is more important than exogenous (dietary) intake. Nevertheless, dietary intake of vitamin D is still a crucial factor to be considered when assessing vitamin D status, particularly in elderly people. They may, for social reasons, have less opportunity to be exposed to sunlight and the efficiency with which vitamin D is produced in the skin, absorbed and converted by the kidneys to the active form reduces with age (Barragry et al. 1978; Tsai et al. 1984; MacLaughlin and Holick 1985). The amount of melanin in the skin also has an effect on vitamin D synthesis from UV light, which takes longer if the skin is more pigmented. For this reason, some ethnic minority groups living in the UK are likely to be at risk of vitamin D deficiency. This risk is increased if they adhere to their traditional lifestyle and do not go outdoors very often, wear clothes that conceal the majority of their body when they do, and exclude meat and fish from their diet (Henderson et al. 1990; Finch et al. 1992; Matsuoka et al. 1992).

There are relatively few dietary sources of vitamin D, and fortified products including breakfast cereals and spreading fats, as well as pastry products, eggs and oily fish are the major dietary contributors (Gregory et al. 1990). The vitamin D content of meat may also be of greater significance than was previously recognized now that newer analytical methods have highlighted its content of the metabolite 25-hydroxycholecalciferol in addition to cholecalciferol (Lee et al. 1995; Gibson and Ashwell 1997).

There is no RNI for vitamin D for the age groups 4–64 years as evidence suggests that the majority can obtain adequate vitamin D if the face and arms are directly exposed to sunlight daily for approximately 30 minutes/day between April and October (DH 1991). It is well established that UV light of appropriate wavelength is only available in the UK during these months because of its northerly latitude (DH 1998). The effect on vitamin D status of measures taken to reduce the risk of skin cancer, such as seeking protection from the sun's rays by wearing clothes or applying sunscreen preparations, is at present uncertain (DH 1998).

For people of 65 years and over the RNI is 10 μg/d and this may only be achievable with regular use of a vitamin D supplement (DH 1998). The results of studies where vitamin D supplements have been given to elderly subjects suggested that they may be beneficial in reducing fracture rates and improving bone density (Heikinheimo et al. 1992; Ooms et al. 1995).

Vitamin K

Vitamin K may play a role in bone metabolism as several proteins involved in the metabolism of bone, including bone Gla protein and matrix Gla protein, depend on vitamin K for their synthesis (Price 1988). Knapen et al. (1989) showed that the increased urinary calcium and hydroxyproline excretion in osteoporosis is reduced by giving physiological doses of vitamin K. In addition, Gla protein, which has been shown to be undercarboxylated in osteoporotic women, is favourably affected by physiological doses of vitamin K (Douglas et al. 1995). Until recently there has been little information available on the vitamin K content of foods and so few studies have investigated the relationship between vitamin K intake and bone mass, but now that databases have been developed (Price et al. 1996) the effect of dietary vitamin K on bone health can be explored.

Sodium and potassium

If dietary sodium intake is increased, both urinary sodium and calcium excretion are increased and it has been suggested that this may be linked to a reduction in BMD; however, the results are not conclusive (DH 1998). Conversely, there is evidence to suggest that, at least in middle-aged women, a high potassium intake is related to a higher BMD (New et al. 1997). Recommendations for healthy eating include advice to reduce salt intake and the daily consumption of at least five portions of fruit and vegetables (which are rich sources of potassium); these measures may well be beneficial for bone health (DH 1998).

Other micronutrients

Phosphorus in the form of phosphate accounts for approximately half of bone mineral by weight but there is little evidence that dietary phosphate intake is directly linked to bone health (NDC 1999). Phosphate is rarely deficient in the diet and it is likely that the calcium:phosphate ratio is of more importance, with a high ratio favouring calcium retention.

Zinc, copper and manganese may also be important to bone health as they are essential cofactors for enzymes involved in the synthesis of several constituents of bone matrix. Together with vitamin C, they may also function in their antioxidant capacity and thus high intakes may be important if the connective tissue of bone is a target for free radical damage (New 1999). The findings from two recent studies suggest that they may play a significant role in bone health (New et al. 1997, 1998b).

A large-scale, multicentre, prospective trial has recently established that long-term exposure to fluoridated drinking water does not increase the risk of osteoporotic fracture (Phipps et al. 2000).

Protein

Both high and low protein intakes have been considered to have detrimental effects on bone health. However, the reported adverse effects of high protein intake relate to consumption in excess of 90 g/day (Feskanich et al. 1996), a level which is rarely consumed on a regular basis in the UK (Gregory et al. 1990). Although protein consumption leads to an increase in urinary calcium excretion, the body adapts by absorbing more calcium, provided that dietary calcium intake is adequate (Heaney 1998). Adequate protein intake, especially in older people, has been shown to be beneficial for bone health (Schurch *et al.* 1998).

Alcohol and caffeine

Heavy and regular alcohol consumption has been shown to be associated with reduced BMD and an increased risk of fractures (Felson *et al.* 1988). Advice on sensible drinking which is appropriate for the general public may be helpful in promoting bone health.

Studies on the effect of caffeine on bone health have not provided any conclusive evidence but it is suggested that a caffeine intake equivalent to less than eight cups of coffee/day will not have a detrimental effect on bone health (Lloyd *et al.* 1997).

4.31.3 Other factors and bone health

Body weight

Body weight is positively linked to bone mass and therefore a higher body weight is associated with a higher bone mass and reduced risk of osteoporotic fracture (Harris and Dawson-Hughes 1996). Intentional weight loss results in an increased rate of bone loss in healthy premenopausal women (Salamone *et al.* 1999) and this is exacerbated if the weight loss is sufficient to cause low oestrogen levels, as in anorexia nervosa (Bachrach 1993). Maintenance of a body mass index (BMI) within the normal range is advocated to help to achieve optimal bone health (DH 1998).

Physical activity

Appropriate physical activity can aid attainment of peak bone mass, reduce age-related bone loss and reduce the risk of fracture in postmenopausal women. However, excessive strenuous exercise can be detrimental to the bone health of young women if it results in loss of menstrual cycles and therefore reduced oestrogen levels (Wilson 1994). Weight-bearing exercise (running, dancing, climbing stairs and brisk walking) has been shown to have the most beneficial effect, but swimming and cycling and other non-weight bearing activities have a beneficial effect on muscle strength and can help to prevent falls and subsequent fracture (DH 1998).

Smoking

Smoking appears to have little effect as an independent factor on BMD or the risk of hip fracture in premenopausal women, but significantly affects the risk of fracture in postmenopausal women and in men (Law and Hackshaw 1997). Cigarette smoking has been implicated in the aetiology of osteoporosis but reported bone changes could in part be due to other lifestyles factors closely associated with smoking, such as low body weight, alcohol consumption and low micronutrient intake (DH 1998).

4.31.4 Causes of osteoporosis

Postmenopausal women are at high risk of developing osteoporosis owing to oestrogen deficiency and, together with women suffering oestrogen deficiency following oophorectomy or prolonged amenorrhoea, account for a very large majority of cases (Liggett and Reid 1999). Corticosteroid-induced osteoporosis is also common and a small percentage of cases occurs as a secondary effect of other disorders and/or their treatment, such as:

- hyperparathyroidism
- thyrotoxicosis
- multiple myeloma
- malabsorption syndrome
- coeliac disease
- anorexia nervosa
- alcoholism.

A range of clinical factors has been recognized as risk factors for the development of osteoporosis (Table 4.31.3). Those which are potentially modifiable should be ascertained prior to treatment and measures to remedy them incorporated into the treatment programme where possible.

4.31.5 Treatment of osteoporosis

On diagnosis of osteoporosis, an individualized treatment regimen must be planned for each patient. This should be devised on the basis of their individual lifestyle, dietary habits and the likely benefits and side-effects of the available therapies. All women with reduced BMD should receive advice on calcium intake, lifestyle and exercise irrespective of any drug therapy (Liggett and Reid 1999).

Calcium intake

In women who appear unlikely to achieve a regular dietary calcium intake of more than 800 mg/day, calcium supplementation should be considered (see below).

Lifestyle

Since regular heavy consumption of alcohol and smoking are likely to have adverse effects on bone health, guidance on sensible drinking limits and smoking cessation should be given when appropriate.

Exercise

Regular weight bearing exercise and, in older people, muscle strengthening exercises for fall prevention should be undertaken for at least three 20 minute sessions weekly. To be of benefit, these measures need to be sustained since it may take as long as 9 months for the effects to become apparent (Liggett and Reid 1999).

Drug therapy

There are at present five different types of drug therapy available in the UK for the prevention and treatment of osteoporosis. These are:

- bisphosphonates: alendronate and etidronate
- calcium and vitamin D
- activated vitamin D: calcitriol
- parenteral calcitonin
- hormone replacement therapy.

Bisphosphonates

These act as specific anti-resorptive agents and have previously been used extensively in the management of both Paget's disease and tumour-induced hypercalcaemia. Two are licensed in the UK for use in the treatment of osteoporosis:

- *Alendronate* is used for the treatment of osteoporosis in postmenopausal women and is taken continuously. If calcium supplementation has also been prescribed it should be taken at a different time of day.
- *Etidronate* is the only drug available for the prevention and treatment of corticosteroid-induced osteoporosis. It has been shown to be effective in preventing vertebral and hip fractures (van Staa 1998). It is taken for 14 days followed by 76 days of calcium supplementation and the cycle is then repeated. There is no limit on the length of time for which it can be prescribed (Miller *et al.* 1997).

Both drugs are poorly absorbed from the gastrointestinal tract and need to be taken prior to food and with water. Alendronate carries a risk of causing oesophagitis and must be taken whilst sitting upright. Each has been shown to approximately halve the risk of further fracture (Liberman *et al.* 1995; Black *et al.* 1996).

Calcium and vitamin D

The combination of calcium and vitamin D supplementation has been shown to be effective in reducing the risk of hip fractures in the elderly (Chapuy *et al.* 1992) and a daily supplement of 800 IU vitamin D and 1 g calcium has been recommended (Liggett and Reid 1999). Calcium supplementation may also be beneficial in women, 5 years after the menopause, either alone (Reid *et al.* 1995) or in combination with vitamin D (Dawson-Hughes *et al.* 1997), especially in those with low dietary calcium intakes.

Calcitriol

Calcitriol (1,25-dihydroxycholecalciferol) acts by regulating intestinal calcium absorption, and also promotes new bone synthesis via its action on osteoblasts. It is used to treat those with established postmenopausal osteoporosis but may need to be taken for up to 3 years before any effect on fracture risk is seen (Liggett and Reid 1999). It is advised that serum calcium levels are regularly monitored, although the risk of hypercalcaemia is very small.

Calcitonin

Calcitonin has been used for many years in the treatment of osteoporosis but is not a popular form of treatment because, in the UK, it has to be given by subcutaneous injection. In the rest of Europe and the USA it is available as a nasal spray, which has been shown to reduce bone loss in those with established osteoporosis (Overgaard *et al.* 1992).

Hormone-replacement therapy

This is the most effective way of reducing early postmenopausal bone loss and subsequent risk of fracture, benefits which appear to persist for as long as it is taken.

4.31.6 Prevention of osteoporosis

It is clear that in order to achieve and maintain optimal PBM within genetic potential and thus reduce the risk of developing osteoporosis, appropriate eating habits must commence at an early age and continue throughout life. The Department of Health (1998) concluded that the best way of ensuring that calcium and vitamin D are adequate for bone health is to integrate requirements for these nutrients in the patterns for healthy living and eating set out in *Eight Guidelines for a Healthy Diet* (HEA 1997) and the *Balance of Good Health* (HEA 1996). Such patterns will also help to ensure the appropriate intake of other nutrients implicated in bone health.

The concurrent maintenance of other healthy lifestyle behaviours such as taking sufficient physical activity, avoidance of smoking or excessive alcohol consumption, and keeping BMI within the normal range may be no less important preventive measures.

Text revised by: Jacki Bishop and Catherine Collins

Acknowledgement: Sue New.

Useful address

The National Osteoporosis Society
PO Box 10, Radstock, Bath BA3 3YB
Tel: 01761 472721
Website: www.nos.org.uk

References

Bachrach L. Bone mineralization in childhood and adolescence. *Current Opinions in Pediatrics* 1993; **5**: 467–473.

Baran D *et al.* Dietary modification with dairy products for preventing vertebral bone loss in premenopausal women: a three year prospective study. *Journal of Clinical Endocrinology and Metabolism* 1989; **70**: 264–270.

Barragry JM *et al.* Intestinal cholecalciferol absorption in the elderly and in younger adults. *Clinical Science and Molecular Medicine* 1978; **55**: 213–220.

Black DM, Cummings SR, Karpf D *et al.* Randomised trial of the effect of alendronate on risk of fracture in women with existing vertebral fractures. *Lancet* 1996; **348**: 1535–1541.

Bonjour JP *et al.* Critical years and stages of puberty for spinal and femoral bone mass accumulation during adolescence. *Journal of Clinical Endocrinology and Metabolism* 1991; **73**: 555–563.

Bonjour JP, Carrie A-L, Ferrari S *et al.* Calcium-enriched foods and bone mass growth in prepubertal girls: a randomized, double-blind, placebo-controlled trial. *Journal of Clinical Investigation* 1997; **99**: 1287–1294.

Cadogan J, Eastall R, Jones N, Barker M. Milk intake and bone mineral acquisition in adolescent girls: randomised, controlled intervention trial. *British Medical Journal* 1997; **315**: 1255–1260.

Chapuy MC, Arlot ME, Duboeuf F *et al.* Vitamin D and calcium to prevent hip fractures in elderly women. *New England Journal of Medicine* 1992; **327**: 1637–1642.

Commission of the European Communities. *Nutrient and Energy Intakes for the European Community.* Reports of the Scientific Committee for Food, 31st Series. Luxembourg: Office for Official Publications of the European Communities, 1993.

Consensus Development Conference. Diagnosis, prophylaxsis and treatment of osteoporosis. *American Journal of Medicine* 1993; **94**: 646–650.

Dawson-Hughes B, Harris S, Krall EA, Dallal GE. Effect of calcium and vitamin D on bone density in men and women 65 years of age or older. *New England Journal of Medicine* 1997; **337**: 670–776.

Department of Health. *Dietary Reference Values for Energy and Nutrients for the United Kingdom.* Report on Health and Social Subjects 41. London: HMSO, 1991.

Department of Health. *Nutrition and Bone Health.* Report on Health and Social Subjects 49. London: The Stationery Office, 1998.

Dolan P, Torgerson DJ. The costs of treating osteoporotic fractures in the UK female population. *Osteoporosis International* 1998; **8**: 611–617.

Douglas AS, Robins SP, Hutchison JD *et al.* Carboxylation of osteocalcin in postmenopausal osteoporotic women following vitamin K and D supplementation. *Bone* 1995; **17**: 15–20.

Felson DT *et al.* Alcohol consumption and hip fractures: the Framingham study. *American Journal of Epidemiology* 1988; **128**: 1102–1110.

Feskanich D, Willett WC, Stampfer MJ, Colditz GA. Protein consumption and bone fractures in women. *American Journal of Epidemiology* 1996; **143**: 472–479.

Finch PJ, Ang L, Maxwell JD. Clinical and histological spectrum of osteomalacia among Asians in South London. *Quarterly Journal of Medicine* 1992; **302**: 439–448.

Finch S, Doyle W, Lowe C *et al. National Diet and Nutrition Survey: People Aged 65 Years and Over. Vol. 1: Report of the Diet and Nutrition Survey.* London: The Stationery Office, 1998.

Gibson SA, Ashwell M. New vitamin D values for meat and their implication for vitamin D intake in British adults. *Proceedings of the Nutrition Society* 1997; **56**: 116A.

Grant SFA *et al.* Reduced bone density and osteoporosis associated with a polymorphic Sp1 binding site in the collagen type 1 alpha 1 gene. *Nature Genetics* 1996; October: 203–205.

Gregory J, Foster K, Tyler HA, Wiseman M. *The Dietary and Nutritional Survey of British Adults.* London: HMSO, 1990.

Harris SS, Dawson-Hughes B. Weight, body composition and bone density in post menopausal women. *Calcified Tissue International* 1996; **59**: 428–432.

Health Education Authority. *The Balance of Good Health.* London: HEA, 1996.

Health Education Authority. *Eight Guidelines for a Healthy Diet: A Guide for Nutrition Educators.* London: HEA, 1997.

Heaney RP. Excess dietary protein may not adversely affect bone. *Journal of Nutrition* 1998; **128**: 1054–1057.

Heikinheimo RJ *et al.* Annual injection of vitamin D and fractures of aged bones. *Calcified Tissue International* 1992; **51**: 105–110.

Henderson FB, Dunnigan MG, McIntosh WB *et al.* Asian osteomalacia is determined by dietary factors when exposure to ultraviolet radiation is restricted: a risk factor model. *Quarterly Journal of Medicine* 1990; **76**: 923–933.

Institute of Nutrition, Food and Health Board. *Dietary Reference Intakes for Calcium, Phosphorus, Magnesium, Vitamin D, and Fluoride.* Washington, DC: National Academy Press, 1997.

Johnston CC, Miller JZ, Slemenda CW *et al.* Calcium supplementation and increases in bone mineral density in children. *New England Journal of Medicine* 1992; **327**: 82–87.

Kanis JA, Melton LJ, Christiansen C *et al.* The diagnosis of osteoporosis. *Journal of Bone Mineral Research* 1994; **9**: 1137–1141.

Keene GS *et al.* Mortality and morbidity after hip fractures. *British Medical Journal* 1993; **307**: 1248–1250.

Knapen MHJ, Hamulyak K, Vermeer C. The effect of vitamin K supplementation on circulating osteocalcin (bone Gla protein) and urinary calcium excretion. *Annals of Internal Medicine* 1989; **111**: 1001–1005.

Kroger H *et al.* Development of bone mass and bone density of the spine and femoral neck – a prospective study of 65 children and adolescents. *Bone and Mineral* 1993; **23**: 171–182.

Law MR, Hackshaw AK. A meta-analysis of cigarette smoking, bone mineral density and risk of hip fracture: recognition of a major effect. *British Medical Journal* 1997; **315**: 841–846.

Lee SM, Buss DH, Hatton D. Vitamin D activity of meat. *Proceedings of the Nutrition Society* 1995; **54**: 130A.

Lee WTK *et al.* Double-blind controlled calcium supplementation and bone mineral accretion in children accustomed to a low calcium diet. *American Journal of Clinical Nutrition* 1994; **60**: 744–750.

Lee WTK *et al.* A randomised double-blind controlled calcium supplementation trial and bone and height acquisition in children. *British Journal of Nutrition* 1995; **74**: 125–139.

Lee WTK, Leung SSF, Leung DMY, Cheng JCY. A follow-up study on the effects of calcium-supplement withdrawal and puberty on bone acquisition of children. *American Journal of Clinical Nutrition* 1996; **64**: 71–77.

Liberman UA, Weiss SR, Broll J *et al.* Effect of oral alendronate on bone mineral density and the incidence of fractures in postmenopausal osteoporosis. *New England Journal of Medicine* 1995; **333**: 1437–1443.

Liggett NW, Reid DM. Osteoporosis and its management. *Hospital Medicine* 1999; **60**: 238–242.

Lloyd TM, Rollings N, Eggli DF *et al.* Dietary caffeine intake and bone status of postmenopausal women. *American Journal of Clinical Nutrition* 1997; **65**: 1826–1830.

MacLaughlin J, Holick MF. Aging decreases the capacity of human skin to produce vitamin D_3. *Journal of Clinical Investigation* 1985; **76**: 1536–1568.

Matsuoka LY, Wortsman J, Daumenberg MJ *et al.* Clothing prevents ultraviolet-B radiation-dependent photosynthesis of vitamin D_3. *Journal of Clinical Endocrinology and Metabolism* 1992; **79**: 1099–1103.

Miller PD, Watts NB, Licata AA *et al.* Cyclical etidronate in the treatment of postmenopausal osteoporosis. *American Journal of Medicine* 1997; **103**: 468–476.

National Dairy Council. *Diet and Bone Health.* London: NDC, 1999.

National Health and Medical Research Council. *Recommended Dietary Intakes for Use in Australia*. Canberra: Australian Government Publishing Service, 1991.

National Research Council (US). Subcommittee on the Tenth Edition of the RDAs. *Recommended Dietary Allowances*. Food and Nutrition Board, Commission on Life Sciences. National Research Council, 10th edn. Washington, DC: National Academy of Life Sciences, 1989.

New SA. Bone Health: the role of micronutrients. *British Medical Bulletin* 1999; **55**: 619–633.

New SA, Bolton-Smith C, Grubb DA, Reid DM. Nutritional influences on bone mineral density: a cross sectional study in premenopausal women. *American Journal of Clinical Nutrition* 1997; **65**: 1831–1839.

New SA, Ferns G, Starkey B. Milk intake and bone mineral acquisition in adolescent girls – increases in bone density may be result of micronutrients in additional cereal. *British Medical Journal* 1998a; **316**: 1747.

New SA, Robins SP, Reid DM. Fruit and vegetable consumption and bone health: is there a link? In Dawson-Hughes B, Burckhardt P, Heaney RP (Eds) *Challenges of Modern Medicine*, pp. 199–207. Italy: Ares-Sereno Symposia Publications, 1998b.

Nieves JW, Komar L, Cosman F, Lindsay R. Calcium potentiates the effect of oestrogen and calcitonin on bone mass: review and analysis. *American Journal of Clinical Nutrition* 1998; **67**: 18–24.

Nordin BEC. Calcium and osteoporosis. *Nutrition* 1997; **13**: 664–689.

Ooms ME, Roos JC, Bezemer P *et al*. Prevention of bone loss by vitamin D supplementation in elderly women: a randomised double-blind trial. *Journal of Clinical Endocrinology and Metabolism* 1995; **80**: 1052–1058.

Ott SM. Attainment of peak bone mass. *Journal of Clinical Endocrinology and Metabolism* 1990; **71**: 1082A–C.

Overgaard K, Hansen MA, Jensen S, Christiansen C. Effect of salcatonin given intranasally on bone mass and fracture rates in established osteoporosis. *British Medical Journal* 1992; **305**: 556–561.

Phipps KR, Orwoll ES, Mason JD, Cauley JA. Community water fluoridation, bone mineral density and fractures: prospective study of effects in older women. *British Medical Journal* 2000; **321**: 860–864.

Price PA. Role of vitamin-K-dependent proteins in bone metabolism. *Annual Reviews in Nutrition* 1988; **8**: 565–583.

Price RS, Shearer M, Bolton-Smith C. Daily and seasonal variation in phylloquinone (vitamin K1) intact in Scotland. *Proceedings of the Nutrition Society* 1996; **55**: 244A.

Recker RR *et al*. Bone gain in young adult women. *Journal of the American Medical Association* 1992; **268**: 2403–2408.

Reid IR, Ames RW, Evans MC *et al*. Long term effects of calcium supplementation on bone loss and fractures in postmenopausal women. *American Journal of Medicine* 1995; **98**: 331–335.

Royal College of Physicians. *Osteoporosis: Clinical Guidelines to Strategies for Prevention and Treatment*. London: RCP, 1999.

Salamone LM *et al*. Effect of a lifestyle intervention on bone mineral density in premenopausal women: a randomized trial. *American Journal of Clinical Nutrition* 1999; **70**: 97–103.

Schurch MA *et al*. Protein supplements increase serum insulin-like growth factor-I levels and attenuate proximal femur bone loss in patients with recent hip fractures. A randomized, double blind, placebo-controlled trial. *Annals of Internal Medicine* 1998; **128**: 801-809.

Slemenda CW, Reister TK, Peacock M, Johnston CC. Bone growth in children following the cessation of calcium supplementation. *Journal of Bone and Mineral Research* 1993; **8** (Suppl 1): S151.

Teegarden D, Proulx WR, Martin BR *et al*. Peak bone mass in young women. *Journal of Bone and Mineral Research* 1995; **10**: 711–715.

Theintz G, Buchs B, Pizzoli R *et al*. Longitudinal monitoring of bone mass accumulation in healthy adolescents. *Journal of Clinical Endocrinology and Metabolism* 1992; **75**: 1060–1065.

Tsai KS, Heath H III, Kumar R, Riggs BL. Impaired vitamin D metabolism with aging in women. *Journal of Clinical Investigation* 1984; **73**: 1668–1672.

van Staa VP, Abenhaim L, Cooper C. Use of cyclical etidronate and prevention of non-vertebral fractures. *British Journal of Rheumatology* 1998; **37**: 87–94.

Weaver C. Calcium and bone health. In *Focus on Women, Nutrition and Health*. Proceedings of a Conference held on 15th November 1995. London: National Dairy Council, 1996.

Wilson JH. Nutrition, physical activity and bone health in women. *Nutrition Research Reviews* 1994; **7**: 67–91.

World Health Organization. *Assessment of Fracture Risk and its Application to Screening for Postmenopausal Osteoporosis*. Report of a WHO Study Group. WHO Technical Report Series 843. Geneva: WHO, 1994.

4.32 Arthritis

The term arthritis means inflammation of a joint. There are several types of arthritis, of which osteoarthritis and rheumatoid arthritis are the most common. Osteoarthritis is the most prevalent form and the type which is popularly referred to as 'arthritis'. Other types include juvenile arthritis (Still's disease) and ankylosing spondylitis. Gout can also be classified as a form of arthritis as its symptoms result from inflammation caused by the deposition of urate crystals within joints (see Section 4.15.1, Gout).

4.32.1 Osteoarthritis

Osteoarthritis is the major cause of disability in the UK and the primary reason for surgical hip replacement.

It is a chronic disease principally affecting the weight-bearing joints such as the hips, knees and spine, its effects ranging from occasional aches and stiffness to crippling disease. It results from degeneration of the cartilage which cushions the ends of bones, allowing them to rub together causing pain, inflammation and impaired movement. New bone is produced underneath the worn cartilage, sometimes resulting in spurs and outgrowths (osteophytes) which further deform the joint and exacerbate pain and problems with movement.

Osteoarthritis is principally a consequence of the 'wear and tear' associated with ageing and, by the age of 75 years, about 85% of people may be affected to some degree (Sack 1995). It is not, however, inevitable with age, nor is it confined exclusively to elderly people. The process of wear and tear does not explain all of the clinical findings or biochemical changes in osteoarthritic cartilage and other factors such as genetics, hormones and diet may also contribute to its aetiology (Sack 1995). Osteoarthritis can also be a secondary consequence of joint damage.

Management of osteoarthritis

Treatment primarily consists of alleviating pain, usually via analgesics such as paracetamol, sometimes in combination with a low dose non-steroidal anti-inflammatory drug (NSAID). Topical application of a NSAID preparation may also provide pain relief. Injections of corticosteroids directly into the joint are sometimes used to relieve severe local pain and inflammation. In time, drugs which help to preserve joint function by inhibiting the production or activity of chondrolytic enzymes and thus slow cartilage degeneration may become available, but are currently still at the stage of development. Surgical joint replacement is an increasingly successful procedure for relieving the pain and disability resulting from severe osteoarthritis in the hip and knee.

Dietary management of osteoarthritis

Osteoarthritis has no specific dietary indications but people with the disease can be at risk of a number of nutrition-related problems.

Undernutrition

Arthritis may result in many of the problems associated with physical disability in terms of food acquisition and preparation (see Section 3.11.1, Physical disabilities). Elderly people are particularly at risk of poor nutrition for this reason, e.g. relying on sandwiches and biscuits instead of cooked meals, or lacking fresh fruit and vegetables because these are difficult to prepare. Dietary guidance should focus on nutrient dense, and if underweight, energy dense food choices which are easy to prepare (see Sections 1.12, Oral nutritional support, and 3.7, Older adults). Ensuring that available local support services such as meals-on-wheels are utilized where appropriate is also important.

Some undernourished patients may require additional oral nutritional support measures so that they can better withstand the metabolic costs of joint replacement surgery.

Obesity

Every step taken increases the load on the hip or knee joint by some three to five times body weight and hence the physical stresses imposed by excessive body weight are considerable. Since osteoarthritis primarily affects load-bearing joints, obesity will always worsen its symptoms and accelerate its progression.

Many patients diagnosed with osteoarthritis are overweight, and others may become overweight as a result of their decreased mobility and/or an inappropriate dietary intake. Weight reduction is an important measure to minimize stress on the joint, to reduce pain and maintain or improve mobility. It may also be a required measure before surgical joint replacement can be carried out.

Weight loss is not necessarily easy to achieve in those with restricted mobility who cannot significantly increase their level of physical activity. Lack of mobility may also compound problems such as comfort or boredom eating. As with anyone who is overweight, dietary guidance should aim to decrease energy intake via more appropriate food choice. It is, however, important that suggested dietary measures take account of any practical difficulties in terms of food procurement or preparation which a patient with osteoarthritis may have.

Surgery

Patients undergoing joint replacement surgery are at risk of nutritional depletion. Ten days after such surgery, patients were found to have significantly lower levels of haemoglobin, ferritin and albumin and intakes of protein than they had pre-operatively (Haugen *et al.* 1999). These problems are likely to be compounded if nutritional status is poor prior to surgery.

Use of dietary supplements, remedies and elimination diets

The acute symptoms of osteoarthritis notoriously come and go, for reasons which are poorly understood and often attributed to factors such as the weather, dampness or diet. The folklore of remedies for arthritis is vast and many patients will try dietary supplements and complementary therapies advocated via the mass media or recommended by friends.

Products such as cider vinegar, honey and algal extracts, and supplements of vitamins C, E, pantothenic acid, selenium and zinc are commonly tried, but there is no scientific evidence of any benefit. More recently, supplements of glucosamine sulphate and chondroitin, which are alleged to 'rebuild cartilage', have become popular, but any such effects also remain to be established.

Whether supplementary long chain omega-3 fatty acids can provide symptomatic relief is uncertain; although benefits are often anecdotally reported by patients, scientific evidence of this is lacking. While there is some evidence that dietary manipulations can have anti-inflammatory effects in people with rheumatoid arthritis (see below), it cannot be assumed that these will apply to people with osteoarthritis; although osteoarthritis often has secondary inflammatory features, the pathogenesis of the two disorders is very different. In a double-blind, placebo-controlled trial, Stammers *et al.* (1992) found no evidence that cod liver oil supplementation was helpful to patients with osteoarthritis.

Most types of supplements and remedies used to treat arthritis are unlikely to do harm, other than to the finances. More significant adverse nutritional effects may result from self-imposed elimination diets used for reasons of 'detoxification' or supposed 'allergies', often diagnosed by dubious methods. The principle of detoxification has no scientific credibility and there is no evidence of any systematic link between allergy or intolerance and osteoarthritis. If used frequently or for prolonged periods, elimination diets of this type can result in profound nutritional imbalances and should be discouraged.

4.32.2 Rheumatoid arthritis

Rheumatoid arthritis (RA) is an autoimmune disorder which results in joint inflammation together with other systemic effects. It most commonly affects people in their 30s and 40s and is three times more common in women than men. It is estimated to affect about 600 000 people in the UK.

RA usually commences with episodes of swelling, pain and morning stiffness in peripheral joints such as the hands, wrists and feet. The pain can be severe and continuous. Flu-like episodes of feverishness and malaise can occur, followed by prolonged phases of extreme fatigue and depression. Progressive destruction of the joint and the areas surrounding it can result in considerable disability. The disease is characterized by remissions and relapses of varying duration.

Diagnosis is confirmed by a blood test which is seropositive to rheumatoid factor.

Treatment of rheumatoid arthritis

Currently there is no cure for RA. Treatment is aimed at suppressing the disease as much as possible, reducing inflammation and pain, and minimizing joint destruction and deformities. This involves the use of NSAIDs (or sometimes corticosteroids) for immediate symptom relief, possibly in conjunction with second-line drugs which suppress the disease process such as gold, penicillamine or chloroquine, or immunosuppressants such as methotrexate or sulfasalazine.

Advising people to rest sufficiently, avoid stress and consume an appropriate diet is also essential for management. Strenuous exercise is usually contraindicated but regular amounts of gentle exercise or physiotherapy are important to help to maintain muscle mass and mobility.

Dietary management of rheumatoid arthritis

Patients with RA are at risk of poor nutritional status because:

- The pain and malaise associated with acute flare-ups of the illness, sometimes followed by prolonged phases of depression, can markedly impair appetite.
- Pain and joint deformity may result in mobility difficulties and hence problems with purchasing, preparing and consuming food.
- Nutrient intake may be compromised as a result of following a 'self-help' regimen (see Alternative remedies, below).
- Drugs used to control the disease may have nutritional side-effects or increase the risk of nutrient deficiencies.

Several studies have found evidence of poor eating patterns in people with RA (Morgan *et al.* 1997). Kremer and Bigaouette (1996) found that the diet of RA patients contained more fat, especially saturated fat, less monounsaturated fat and less fibre than that of the general population. Intake of micronutrients such as folate, pyridoxine, vitamin E, calcium, magnesium, copper and selenium have also been found to be low (Kremer and

Bigaouette 1996; Stone *et al.* 1997; Goff and Barasi 1999). Many of these nutrients are also those most likely to be affected by interactions with drugs prescribed for RA (Bigaouette *et al.* 1987); the low level of folate consumption found in some patients taking methotrexate (a folate antagonist) is a particular concern (Stone *et al.* 1997). Heliovaara *et al.* (1994) highlighted the possible adverse effects of a low level of antioxidant nutrient protection in people with RA.

There is no evidence that there are any specific nutritional indications for people with RA (Martin 1998). Dietary guidance focuses on achieving good nutritional status via a well balanced diet by identifying and correcting nutritional inadequacies and, where possible, helping to alleviate problems which have led to them. People should be encouraged to consume a varied diet based on healthy eating principles, with particular emphasis on food choices which are good sources of micronutrients, particularly fruit and vegetables, low-fat dairy foods and lean meat, fish and pulses. Supplementation may be indicated in some cases to bring micronutrient intake up to reference nutrient intake (RNI) levels, especially folic acid, vitamin E and zinc, but megadosing should be avoided (Stone *et al.* 1997; Martin 1998).

It should be borne in mind that nutritional requirements may vary within an individual during the course of the disease; phases of active disease may result in impaired appetite, decreased mobility, increased use of drugs and consequently an increased likelihood of nutritional needs not being met.

Nutritional status can be improved if its importance is recognized, and dietary counselling tailored to an individual's needs and circumstances should be an integral component of care. Meals should be nutritionally balanced, easy to prepare and easy to eat. Small, nourishing meals and snacks comprised of nutrient dense foods or beverages may be better tolerated than large meals (see Section 1.12, Oral nutritional support). If physical feeding difficulties are present, an occupational therapist can advise on specially adapted feeding utensils (Section 3.11.1, Physical disabilities).

Common nutrition-related problems associated with RA include:

- *Anaemia*: This is often a consequence of the disease itself as a result of the impaired production of haemoglobin during phases of active inflammation. When drug treatment is successful and the inflammation subsides, haemoglobin levels usually rise. Anaemia may also be exacerbated by the use of NSAIDs, which may cause gastrointestinal bleeding. Low dietary iron intake will also compound the problem and it is important to ensure that RA patients consume sufficient iron (ideally mostly as haem iron) and vitamin C (to ensure adequate absorption of non-haem iron).
- *Side-effects of steroid therapy*: Long-term use of corticosteroids may have a number of nutritional implications. Some may increase urinary excretion of zinc, calcium and nitrogen, increasing the risk of impaired nutritional status. Many result in weight gain and an increased risk of obesity and steroid-induced diabetes.

Manipulation of dietary fatty acid composition

The possible benefits of dietary lipid manipulation in people with chronic inflammatory disorders such as RA have been the subject of speculation for many years, in particular supplementation with omega-3 long-chain polyunsaturated fatty acids found in fish oils (Adam 1995). These fatty acids appear to down regulate production of proinflammatory cytokines such as interleukin (IL)-1-beta, IL-1-alpha and tumour necrosis factor, and modulate the effects of other inflammatory mediators such as *n*6 eicosanoids (Caughey *et al.* 1996; Ariza-Ariza *et al.* 1998). Altering dietary polyunsaturated fatty acid (PUFA) composition in favour of increased intake of omega-3 fatty acids could therefore beneficially reduce or modify the inflammatory process and thus reduce disease activity (Sperling 1995; Calder 1997).

There is some evidence that this is the case. Supplementation with omega-3 fatty acids in patients with RA has been found to reduce levels of inflammatory parameters such as IL-1-beta (Kremer 1996), decrease the global activity of RA (Skoldstam *et al.* 1992), reduce pain and morning joint stiffness (Kremer *et al.* 1995) and lessen NSAID usage (Belch *et al.* 1988; Lau *et al.* 1993; Geusens *et al.* 1994). A meta-analysis by Fortin *et al.* (1995) evaluated 10 randomized, double-blind, placebo-controlled trials in over 400 RA patients and concluded that there was a modest but statistically significant improvement in tender joint count and duration of morning stiffness in patients treated with fish oil supplements over a 3 month period. Recent reviews have also concluded that marine *n*3 PUFA supplements alleviate the symptoms of RA to some extent and may decrease the long-term requirements for NSAIDs (de Deckere *et al.* 1998; Ariza-Ariza *et al.* 1998). However, both also concluded that more research was needed. The improvements in outcome measures are often small and do not result in symptomatic improvement in every patient (Skoldstam *et al.* 1992; James and Cleland 1997). The clinical significance of fish oil supplementation therefore remains to be evaluated.

Alternative and complementary dietary therapies

As in many people with chronic incurable disorders, the use of alternative and complementary dietary strategies is common in patients with RA.

Supplement use is particularly prevalent. Half of the respondents to a questionnaire survey of RA patients took supplements; cod liver oil was the most commonly used but supplements of evening primrose oil, iron, garlic, vitamin C, selenium, B vitamins, calcium, general multivitamins and antioxidant supplements were also frequently cited (Goff and Basari 1999).

Alternative dietary strategies such as vegan and exclusion diets may also be adopted by RA patients.

Vegan diets and fasting

Strict vegan diets comprised mainly of uncooked foods rich in lactobacilli (Nenonen *et al.* 1998), sometimes interspersed with periods of fasting for 7–10 days (Kjeldsen-Kragh 1999), have been reported by patients to improve symptoms but these have not always been substantiated by more objective measures of disease activity (Nenonen *et al.* 1998).

It has been suggested that these effects may result from beneficial changes in faecal microbial flora (Peltonen *et al.* 1997). However, the possibility of the placebo effect of such regimens cannot be ignored; there is some evidence that the psychological characteristics of RA patients who agree to participate in such regimens differ from those who do not, particularly in terms of belief in the benefit of alternative therapies (Kjeldsen-Kragh *et al.* 1994).

Total fasting has been shown to result in symptom relief, possibly as a result of reduced production of the chemical mediators of inflammation (Buchanan *et al.* 1991), but such a practice is also likely to have detrimental effects in terms of micronutrient and other aspects of nutritional status and cannot be recommended (Cleland *et al.* 1995).

Exclusion diets

Food intolerances have been demonstrated in some RA patients, particularly to milk, corn, wheat and azo dyes, but there is no evidence that the prevalence of these is greater than in the general population or systematically linked with RA (Buchanan *et al.* 1991; van de Laar and van der Korst 1992; van de Laar *et al.* 1992; Cleland *et al.* 1995). Many patients self-impose food restrictions; Goff and Barasi (1999) found that 67% of a group of RA patients reported food avoidance, most commonly of citrus fruits, but other foods such as tomatoes, vinegars, pickles, dairy products, red meat and alcohol were also avoided. Most subjects avoided more than one food. Avoidance of many of these foods is likely to have implications in terms of micronutrient intake.

Trials of elemental diets in RA patients have provided little objective evidence of benefit (Haugen *et al.* 1994; Kavanaghi *et al.* 1995). Although symptom improvement is often reported, this tends to be subjective in nature and could have resulted from coincidental remission, weight loss and/or the placebo effect (Kavanaghi *et al.* 1995).

A review by Henderson and Panush (1999) concludes that the purported benefits of alternative regimens rely solely on anecdotal and subjective reports, and with episodes of remission and relapse (which are part of the course of the disease) often taken as evidence of dietary success. Well planned, double-blind studies making objective measurements are lacking and none of these interventions can at present be commended to patients.

It is important that a dietary history taken from patients with arthritis explores any use of dietary regimens and/or supplements. Toxicity of high doses of vitamins and minerals should be considered and appropriate advice given. Patients should be made aware of some of the drawbacks of dietary regimens which are particularly restrictive.

The role of the dietitian regarding the use of complementary and alternative therapies in people with chronic disease is discussed in Section 4.37.3 (Alternative diets and cancer).

Text revised by: Briony Thomas

Useful addresses

Arthritis Research Campaign (formerly the Arthritis and Rheumatism Council).
PO Box 177, Chesterfield, Derbyshire S41 7TQ
Website: www.arc.org.uk

Arthritis Care
18 Stephenson Way, London NW1 2HD
Helpline: 0800 289170

Disabled Living Foundation
380–384 Harrow Road, London W9 2HU
Helpline: 0870 603 9177
Website: www.dlf.org.uk

References

Adam O. Review: anti-inflammatory diet in rheumatic diseases. *European Journal of Clinical Nutrition* 1995; **49**: 703–717.

Ariza-Ariza R, Mestanza-Peralta M, Cardiel MH. Omega-3 fatty acids in rheumatoid arthritis: an overview. *Seminars in Arthritis and Rheumatism* 1998; **27**: 366–370.

Belch JJF, Ansell D, Madhok R *et al.* Effects of altering dietary essential fatty acids on requirements for non-steroidal anti-inflammatory drugs in patients with rheumatoid arthritis: a double blind placebo controlled study. *Annals of the Rheumatic Diseases* 1988; **47**: 96–104.

Bigaouette J, Timchalk MA, Kremer J. Nutritional adequacy of the diet and supplements in patients with rheumatoid arthritis who take medication. *Journal of the American Dietetic Association* 1987; **87**: 1687–1688.

Buchanan HM, Preston PM, Buchanan WW. Is diet important in rheumatoid arthritis? *British Journal of Rheumatology* 1991; **30**: 125–134.

Calder PC. *n*-3 polyunsaturated fatty acids and cytokine production in health and disease. *Annals of Nutrition and Metabolism* 1997; **41**: 203–234.

Caughey GE, Mantzioris E, Gibson RA *et al.* The effects on human tumour necrosis factor (and interleukin-1) production of diets enriched in *n*-3 fatty acids from vegetable oil or fish oil. *American Journal of Clinical Nutrition* 1996; **63**: 116–122.

Cleland LG, Hill CL, James MJ. Diet and arthritis. *Baillieres Clinical Rheumatology* 1995; **9**: 771–785.

de Deckere EAM, Korver O, Verschuren PM, Katan MB. Health aspects of fish and *n*-3 polyunsaturated fatty acids from plant and marine origin. *European Journal of Clinical Nutrition* 1998; **52**: 749–753.

Fortin PR, Lew RA, Liang MH *et al.* Validation of a meta-analysis: the effects of fish oil in rheumatoid arthritis. *Journal of Clinical Epidemiology* 1995; **48**: 1379–1390.

Geusens P, Wouters C, Nijs J *et al*. Long term effects of omega-3 fatty acid supplementation in active rheumatoid arthritis. *Arthritis and Rheumatism* 1994; **37**: 824–829.

Goff LM, Basari M. An assessment of the diets of people with rheumatoid arthritis. *Journal of Human Nutrition and Dietetics* 1999; **12**: 93–101.

Haugen MA, Kjeldsen-Kragh J, Forre O. A pilot study of the effect of an elemental diet in the management of rheumatoid arthritis. *Clinical and Experimental Rheumatology* 1994; **12**: 275–279.

Haugen M, Homme KA, Reigstad A, Teigland J. Assessment of nutritional status in patients with rheumatoid arthritis undergoing joint replacement surgery. *Arthritis Care and Research* 1999; **12**: 26–32.

Heliovaara M, Knekt P, Aho K *et al*. Serum antioxidants and risk of rheumatoid arthritis. *Annals of the Rheumatic Diseases* 1994; **53**: 51–53.

Henderson CJ, Panush RS. Diets, dietary supplements, and nutritional therapies in rheumatic diseases. *Rheumatic Diseases Clinics of North America* 1999; **25**: 937–968, ix.

James MJ, Cleland LG. Dietary n-3 fatty acids and therapy for rheumatoid arthritis. *Seminars in Arthritis and Rheumatism* 1997; **27**: 85–97.

Kavanaghi R, Workman E, Nash P *et al*. The effects of elemental diet and subsequent food reintroduction on rheumatoid arthritis. *British Journal of Rheumatology* 1995; **34**: 270–273.

Kjeldsen-Kragh J. Rheumatoid arthritis treated with vegetarian diets. *American Journal of Clinical Nutrition* 1999; **70** (3 Suppl): 549S–600S.

Kjeldsen-Kragh J, Haugen M, Forre O *et al*. Vegetarian diet for patients with rheumatoid arthritis: can the clinical effects be explained by the psychological characteristics of the patients? *British Journal of Rheumatology* 1994; **33**: 569–575.

Kremer JM. Effects of modulation of inflammatory and immune parameters in patients with rheumatic and inflammatory disease receiving dietary supplements of *n*-3 and *n*-6 fatty acids. *Lipids* 1996; **31**: S243–S247.

Kremer JM, Bigaouette J. Nutrient intake of patients with rheumatoid arthritis is deficient in pyridoxine, zinc, copper and magnesium. *Journal of Rheumatology* 1996; **23**: 990–994.

Kremer JM, Lawrence DA, Petrillo GF *et al*. Effects of high-dose

fish oil on rheumatoid arthritis after stopping nonsteroidal anti-inflammatory drugs. Clinical and immune correlates. *Arthritis and Rheumatism* 1995; **38**: 1107–1114.

Lau CS, Morley KD, Belch JJ. Effects of fish oil supplementation on non-steroidal anti-inflammatory drug requirements in patients with mild rheumatoid arthritis – a double blind placebo controlled study. *British Journal of Rheumatology* 1993; **32**: 982–989.

Martin RH. The role of nutrition and diet in rheumatoid arthritis. *Proceedings of the Nutrition Society* 1998; **57**: 231–234.

Morgan SL, Anderson AM, Hood SM *et al*. Nutrient intake patterns, body mass index and vitamin levels in patients with rheumatoid arthritis. *Arthritis Care and Research* 1997; **10**: 9–17.

Nenonen MT, Helve TA, Rauma AL, Hanninen OO. Uncooked, lactobacilli-rich, vegan food and rheumatoid arthritis. *British Journal of Rheumatology* 1998; **37**: 274–281.

Peltonen R, Nenonen M, Helve T *et al*. Faecal microbial flora and disease activity in rheumatoid arthritis during a vegan diet. *British Journal of Rheumatology* 1997; **36**: 64–68.

Sack KE. Osteoarthritis. A continuing challenge. *Western Journal of Medicine* 1995; **163**: 579–586.

Skoldstam L, Borjesson O, Kjallman A *et al*. *Scandinavian Journal of Rheumatology* 1992; **21**: 178–185.

Sperling RI. Eicosanoids in rheumatoid arthritis. *Rheumatic Diseases Clinics of North America* 1995; **21**: 741–758.

Stammers T, Sibbald B, Freeling P. Efficacy of cod liver oil as an adjunct to non-steroidal anti-inflammatory drug treatment in the management of osteoarthritis in general practice. *Annals of the Rheumatic Diseases* 1992; **51**: 128–129.

Stone J, Doube A, Dudson D, Wallace J. Inadequate calcium, folic acid, vitamin E, zinc and selenium intake in rheumatoid arthritis patients: results of a dietary survey. *Seminars in Arthritis and Rheumatism*. 1997; **27**: 180–185.

van de Laar MA, van der Korst JK. Food intolerance in rheumatoid arthritis. I. A double-blind, controlled trial of the clinical effects of the elimination of milk allergens and azo dyes. *Annals of the Rheumatic Diseases* 1992; **51**: 298–302.

van de Laar MA, Aalbers M, Bruins FG *et al*. Food intolerance in rheumatoid arthritis. II. Clinical and histological aspects. *Annals of the Rheumatic Diseases* 1992; **51**: 303–306.

4.33 Disorders of the skin

4.33.1 Atopic eczema

There are several different types of eczema, the most common of which is atopic eczema (atopic dermatitis). This is a genetically linked condition with an allergic basis, closely associated with other atopic conditions such as asthma and hayfever (Section 4.34, Food allergy and intolerance). Atopic eczema is predominantly, although not exclusively, a disorder of childhood. 75% of cases start within the first year of life and in the majority of children it spontaneously disappears by the age of 10 years. The prevalence of atopic eczema has increased considerably in recent decades and it is currently thought to affect 5–15% of schoolchildren and 2–10% of adults (McHenry *et al*. 1995).

Eczema typically produces dry, red, scaly skin which is intensely itchy. Lesions may occur anywhere but the most common sites are where the skin creases or flexes such as inside the elbows, behind the knees, the fronts of the ankles and around the neck. It also often appears on the cheeks of young children. The constant itching results in constant scratching or rubbing and as a result the skin breaks down, causing leakage of serous fluid and sometimes bleeding. Secondary bacterial infection with streptococci or staphylococci causing pustules and crusting is common. Invasion by the herpes simplex virus may cause the serious skin disorder eczema herpeticum. The continual breakdown and partial healing of skin can result in unsightly scab formation, scarring and thickening.

Acute flare-ups of the condition are usually treated with antihistamines to reduce itching and topical corticosteroids to reduce inflammation and help to heal the skin. Topical or systemic antibiotics may be required if secondary bacterial infection occurs. Once under control, eczema can be minimized by the frequent use of emollients to prevent the skin drying out and by the reduction of exposure to allergens known to exacerbate the condition. House dust mite exposure and pet fur are, as with other atopic disorders, the most common triggering allergens. In some but by no means all cases, food allergy may also play a contributory role.

Diet and atopic eczema

The pathogenesis of atopic eczema is not well understood but appears to results from a combination of genetic, immunological and environmental factors. In infants and young children with a genetic susceptibility, certain food allergens can trigger or exacerbate atopic dermatitis. In contrast, food allergy as a cause of atopic dermatitis in adults is rare (Wuthrich 1998).

The most common dietary trigger is exposure to cow's milk protein in the early months of life. Following weaning, atopic eczema is often associated with immunoglobulin E (IgE) allergies to other foods such as egg, fish, soya, citrus fruits or nuts (Hill *et al*. 1999; Ferguson 1992; Sicherer and Sampson 1999). These coexistent allergies will not always contribute directly to the eczema (e.g. nut allergy has no known influence on eczema symptoms) but some can exacerbate symptoms or hinder a response to withdrawal of cow's milk protein (Sicherer and Sampson 1999).

A clinical and dietary history suggestive of cow's milk protein allergy or intolerance requires trial exclusion of milk for a period of at least 2 weeks to see whether symptoms improve (see Section 4.35.2, Milk exclusion). If there are clear indications of benefit, more prolonged milk exclusion will be required. Because such a measure has considerable nutritional implications in infants and young children and the risk of impaired growth is high (Isolauri *et al*. 1998), expert dietetic supervision is essential. Since many children outgrow milk allergy or intolerance by the age of 3 years, they should be reassessed at intervals to ensure that milk exclusion is not imposed for longer than necessary.

If trial milk exclusion does not improve the patient's eczema despite compliance with the regimen (which should be assessed by a dietitian) and maintenance of topical treatment and other measures (which should be reviewed by a clinician), then it is likely that cow's milk protein is unrelated to eczema in that individual (Przybilla *et al*. 1994). However, the possibility that additional food allergies may be contributing to the eczema must be borne in mind and if the dietary history suggests that other specific allergies (e.g. to soya or citrus fruits) may exist, these too should be investigated by trial exclusion in conjunction with milk avoidance.

In the absence of clinical or dietary pointers to a link between food intake and eczema, the justification for further explorative dietary exclusions requires careful consideration. The imposition of prolonged or extreme regimens such as multiple exclusion or elemental diets can create considerable stress and nutritional problems, possibly with very little ultimate benefit in terms of the eczema. Such 'trawling' dietary investigations can probably only be justified as a last resort strategy in severe cases, when conventional clinical treatment has failed to bring the condition under control (McHenry *et al*. 1995).

Diagnostic tests to investigate the role of food allergies in eczema should be used with caution. Skin prick tests are not always reliable in people with eczema (see Diagnosis of food allergy in Section 4.34.3) and IgE titres or radioallergosorbent tests (RAST) can also be misleading (David 1991). Diagnosis of food-mediated reactions should therefore always be based on a combination of clinical history and the effects of food withdrawal and reintroduction rather than on *in vivo* or *in vitro* tests alone (Przybilla and Ring 1990).

It is important that eczema sufferers, and parents of children with eczema, are aware that, although food allergies can exacerbate the condition in some individuals, this is not inevitably the case. Many people experiment with various dietary exclusion diets in the belief that some sort of food allergy must be responsible, often resulting in diets of dubious nutritional content. Even where food sensitivities can be shown to exist, it may be equally important that exposure to non-dietary triggers of eczema such as house dust mite or pet fur is minimized if the dietary exclusion measures are to be of any benefit.

Evening primrose oil supplementation

Supplementation with evening primrose oil (EPO), which is rich in gamma-linolenic acid, has been reported to be beneficial for patients with moderate or severe eczema (Wright and Burton 1982; Stewart *et al.* 1991), possibly as a result of the influences of essential fatty acids on epidermal lipids and hence epidermal permeability. However, not all trials have found such effects (Bamford *et al.* 1985; Berth-Jones and Graham-Brown 1993) and, while a meta-analysis (Morse *et al.* 1989) concluded that EPO supplementation was effective, the validity of this conclusion has been questioned (Sharpe and Farr 1990). Nevertheless, EPO is currently still prescribable for atopic eczema despite equivocal evidence of its value.

If EPO is tried, it may be important that it is given in sufficiently large doses (e.g. 160–320 mg/day for children aged 1–12 years; 320–480 mg/day for adults) and for a period of at least 3 months. If no improvement occurs after this time, it is unlikely to be helpful (McHenry *et al.* 1995). EPO is contraindicated in infants under 1 year and in people suffering from epilepsy.

Chinese herbal remedies

Studies showing that Chinese herbal remedies could improve symptoms of atopic eczema aroused considerable interest (Sheehan *et al.* 1992; Sheehan and Atherton 1992) but, as a result of concerns about their potential hepatotoxicity (Graham-Brown 1992) and immunosuppressive effects (Russell Jones 1991), their use cannot be advocated until their safety has been established.

Prevention of eczema

In those at high risk of atopic disease (e.g. with a strong family history of the condition), exclusive breast feeding and delayed introduction of allergenic foods until the age of 6 months protect against eczema to some extent, either preventing it altogether or delaying its occurrence (Sampson 1997). However, exclusively breast-fed infants can still develop eczema, possibly as a result of sensitivity to cow's milk proteins in maternal milk or due to exposure to other triggers of atopic disease in their environment (Arshad *et al.* 1992; Kjellman 1993; McHenry *et al.* 1995). The role of diet in the prevention of atopy is discussed in detail in Prevention of food allergy, in Section 4.34.3).

4.33.2 Urticaria (nettle rash, hives)

Acute urticaria

This is an acute and extremely itchy rash comprised of smooth, slightly raised areas of redness, often with a pale, fluid-filled centre. The rash may be localized or completely cover the body surface. Symptoms develop rapidly and usually resolve within 2–3 days. Although acute urticaria can result from an IgE-mediated allergic response, it does not always have an immunological basis; the symptoms more usually result from the direct action of triggers on mast cells, causing local histamine release.

Although relatively common, many cases occur sporadically and the cause can be hard to pinpoint. Although about half of all patients with IgE-mediated food allergy have acute urticarial reactions (Wuthrich 1998), numerically this only represents a small proportion of cases. Zuberbier *et al.* (1996) found that acute urticaria was most commonly associated with upper respiratory tract infections (in about 40% of cases) and the use of analgesic drugs, especially salicylates (9% of cases). Reactions only appeared to be linked to food intake in about 1% of cases, typically to foods such as shellfish, strawberries or others capable of directly triggering histamine release.

Where food is a cause of urticaria, the reaction can occur after direct skin contact (e.g. handling the food) as well as after food ingestion, because lipophilic food triggers can penetrate the skin through the hair follicles or broken areas of skin.

Chronic urticaria

In contrast to acute urticaria, there is some evidence that pharmacologically mediated reactions to natural and synthetic food colourants may play a significant role in the causation and perpetuation of chronic urticaria (Henz and Zuberbier 1998). However, further research in this area is required.

4.33.3 Psoriasis

Psoriasis is a genetically related T-cell autoimmune skin disease of a chronic relapsing–remitting nature which affects about 1 in 50 people (Krueger and Duvic 1994). It may develop at any age but most often commences during adolescence and early adulthood. Psoriasis results in the proliferation of epidermal skin cells, resulting in the build-up of immature cells, followed by formation of erythematous plaques with a silvery scaling surface. The diagnostic feature is the appearance of tiny droplets of blood on the surface of the skin if the scales are removed. Treatment includes emollients to moisten the skin, topical steroids to reduce inflammation and, if severe, other treatments such as phototherapy or immunosuppressive therapy (methotrexate or cyclosporin) (Krueger 1993).

As with many autoimmune disorders, possible benefits from fish oil supplementation have been of interest as a result of the ability of long chain omega-3 fatty acids to modulate the production of inflammatory cytokines and other mediators (see Section 4.32.2, Rheumatoid arthritis). A case–control study (Naldi *et al.* 1996) reported that 50% of psoriatic patients given fish oil supplements reported symptomatic improvement. Collier *et al.* (1993) reported benefits from the regular inclusion of oily fish into the diet of people with psoriasis. However, findings have not always been consistent (Soyland *et al.* 1993) and a recent workshop concluded that, on balance, the evidence of a beneficial effect of fish oils in psoriasis is weak (de Deckere *et al.* 1998).

There is no evidence that food allergy or intolerance affects psoriasis, so dietary exclusion has no place in the routine management of the disease.

4.33.4 Dermatitis herpetiformis

Dermatitis herpetiformis (DH) is characterized by a persistent, itchy blistering skin rash which usually occurs on the knees, elbows, buttocks and back, although it can affect any area of skin. DH results from gluten sensitivity and intestinal biopsy nearly always shows the characteristic flattening of intestinal villi. However, unlike coeliac disease, the gastrointestinal symptoms may be mild and are often not apparent at all. Diagnosis of DH is by biopsy of an unaffected area of skin.

DH is less common than coeliac disease, with a UK incidence of about 1 in 20 000. It is slightly more common in men than women (ratio of 3:2) and most commonly appears between the ages of 15 and 40 years; it is rare in children. As with coeliac disease, there is an inherited tendency to develop the disease, and it can be genetically linked with autoimmune thyroid disease or type I diabetes (Reunala and Collin 1997).

The condition is managed by a gluten-free diet (see Section 4.9, Coeliac disease) and proprietary gluten-free foods are ACBS prescribable for dermatitis herpetiformis. As with coeliac disease, there is evidence that modest amounts of oats (up to 50 g/day) can be included in the diet without detriment (Hardman *et al.* 1999; Reunala *et al.* 1998). Once a gluten-free diet is instituted, it may take several months before the rash improves and nearly 2 years before it disappears completely. The antileprotic drug dapsone may also be used to help suppress the skin lesions.

Many of the long-term implications of coeliac disease are also relevant to patients with DH. Prior to diagnosis, the effects of prolonged subclinical malnutrition result in a high prevalence of anaemia among these patients, and this may be exacerbated if dapsone treatment is used. The long-term risk of developing osteoporosis also appears to be increased in people with DH (Reunala and Collin 1997).

It is therefore important that attention is paid to the overall nutritional content of the diet, particularly in respect of micronutrients, as well as gluten avoidance (see Section 4.9.2 in Coeliac disease).

4.33.5 Acrodermatitis enteropathica

This is a familial condition resulting in an inherited defect in the absorption of zinc from the gastrointestinal tract. It causes severe zinc deficiency and is characterized by dermatological eruptions around the mouth, anus and limb extremities, with accompanying hair loss and diarrhoea (Kumar *et al.* 1997). The onset is usually in early infancy, or may be delayed until after weaning in breast-fed babies. Treatment is by permanent high-dose zinc supplementation.

Since the supplemental dose given is necessarily high, there is a risk that this can impair iron and copper absorption, resulting in anaemia (Hambidge 1977). The haematological status of such patients therefore needs to be monitored.

4.33.6 Rosacea

This causes a florid blush, often accompanied by an acne-like condition, around the nose and cheeks. It results from abnormal dilatation and inflammation of small blood vessels. Papules and pustules may form on the skin and occasionally there may be swelling of the nose and eye involvement. It most commonly occurs in middle age, between ages of 30 and 50 years. About 1 in 8 women may suffer from rosacea at some time, particularly if fair-skinned and if there is a family history.

The pathogenesis is unknown and may result from an underlying vascular disorder. While there is no evidence that dietary factors cause rosacea *per se*, they can trigger facial flushing in some patients. These can often be identified by a diet and symptom diary kept for 2–3 weeks, recording times and details of food consumption and flushing episodes. If any food or beverage appears to trigger flushing within 2 hours of ingestion, trial exclusion may be worthwhile. The most common rosaceal triggers include:

- hot drinks in general, and tea and coffee in particular
- alcohol
- spicy foods
- cheese.

4.33.7 Acne

Acne vulgaris is an extremely common condition during puberty, affecting 70–80% of teenagers (Pochi 1990). It is precipitated by production of the male hormone testosterone, which causes the sebaceous glands to overproduce sebum, an oily substance that helps to lubricate the skin. Blockage of pores, local inflammation and secondary bacterial infection lead to the characteristic formation of sore red spots, blackheads and pustules.

Mild acne can be controlled by topical application of preparations containing benzoyl peroxide or salicylic acid, or topical antibiotics. If these are insufficient, 6 monthly courses of oral antibiotics may be given. More refractory cases of acne may be treated with the vitamin A derivative isotretinoin, which is highly effective. Its use does, however, require careful monitoring to avoid the risk of liver damage. Isotretinoin is also teratogenic and teenagers using the drug should be warned of this contraindication to pregnancy.

Contrary to popular belief, diet has little influence on the development or course of acne. There is no evidence that consumption of high-fat or high-sugar foods such as chips, chocolate or fizzy drinks has any effect on the rate of sebum production (Pochi 1990). While there are many good reasons for encouraging healthy eating among teenagers, it is wrong to pretend that curing acne is one of them.

Text revised by: Briony Thomas

Useful addresses

The Coeliac Society
PO Box 220, High Wycombe, Bucks HP11 2HY
Tel: 01494 437278 Fax: 01494 474349
Website: www.coeliac.co.uk

National Eczema Society
163 Eversholt Street, London NW1 1BU
Tel: 020 7388 4097

Psoriasis Association
7 Milton Street, Northampton NN2 7JG
Tel: 01604 711129

Further reading

Champion RH, Burton JL. *Textbook of Dermatology*. Oxford, Blackwell Science, 1998.

References

Arshad SH, Matthews S, Gant C, Hide D. Effect of allergen avoidance on allergic disorders in infancy. *Lancet* 1992; **339**: 1493–1497.

Bamford JTM, Gibson RW, Renier CM. Atopic eczema unresponsive to evening primrose oil (linolenic and gamma-linolenic acids). *Journal of the American Academy of Dermatology* 1985; **13**: 959–965.

Berth-Jones J, Graham-Brown RAC. Placebo controlled trial of essential fatty acid supplementation in atopic dermatitis. *Lancet* 1993; **341**: 1557–1560.

Collier PM, Ursell A, Zaremba K *et al*. Effect of regular consumption of oily fish compared with white on chronic plaque psoriasis. *European Journal of Clinical Nutrition* 1993; **47**: 251–254.

David TJ. Conventional allergy tests. *Archives of Disease in Childhood* 1991; **66**: 281–282.

de Deckere EAM, Korver O, Verschuren PM, Katan MB. Health aspects of fish and *n*-3 polyunsaturated fatty acids from plant and marine origin. *European Journal of Clinical Nutrition* 1998; **52**: 749–753.

Ferguson A. Definitions and diagnosis of food intolerance and food allergy – consensus and controversy. *Journal of Pediatrics* 1992; **121** (5 Suppl Part 2): S7–S11.

Graham-Brown RAC. Toxicity of Chinese herbal remedies. *Lancet* 1992; **340**: 673.

Hambidge KM. The role of zinc and other trace metals in paediatric nutrition and health. *Paediatric Clinics of North America* 1977; **24**: 95–106.

Hardman C, Fry L, Tatham A, Thomas HJ. Absence of toxicity of avenin in patients with dermatitis herpetiformis. *New England Journal of Medicine* 1999; **340**: 321.

Henz BM, Zuberbier T. Most chronic urticaria is food-dependent, and not idiopathic. *Experimental Dermatology* 1998; **7**: 139–142.

Hill DJ, Hosking CS, Heine RG. Clinical spectrum of food allergy in children in Australia and South East Asia: identification and targets for treatment. *Annals of Medicine* 1999; **31**: 272–281.

Isolauri E, Sutas Y, Salo MK *et al*. Elimination diet in cow's milk allergy: risk for impaired growth in young children. *Journal of Pediatrics* 1998; **132**: 1004–1009.

Kjllman NIM. Is atopy prevention realistic? *Allergy and Clinical Immunology News* 1993; **5**: 37–39

Krueger GG. Psoriasis therapy – observational or rational? *New England Journal of Medicine* 1993; **328**: 1845–1846.

Krueger GG, Duvic M. Epidemiology of psoriasis: clinical issues. *Journal of Investigative Dermatology* 1994; **102**: 14S–18S.

Kumar S, Sehgal VN, Sharma RC. Acrodermatitis enteropathica. *Journal of Dermatology* 1997; **24**: 135–136.

McHenry PM, Williams HC, Bingham EA on behalf of a Joint Workshop of the British Association of Dermatologists and the Research Unit of the Royal College of Physicians of London. Management of atopic eczema. *British Medical Journal* 1995; **310**: 843–847.

Morse PF, Horrobin DF, Manku MS *et al*. Meta-analysis of placebo-controlled studies of the efficacy of Epogam in the treatment of atopic eczema: relationship between plasma essential fatty acid changes and clinical response. *British Journal of Dermatology* 1989; **121**: 75–90.

Naldi L, Parazzini F, Peli L. Dietary factors and the risk of psoriasis. Results of an Italian case–control study. *British Journal of Dermatology* 1996; **134**: 101–106.

Pochi PE. The pathogenesis and treatment of acne. *Annual Review of Medicine* 1990; **41**: 187–198.

Przybilla B, Ring J. Food allergy and atopic eczema. *Seminars in Dermatology* 1990; **9**: 220–225.

Przybilla B, Eberlein-König B, Ruëff F. Practical management of atopic eczema. *Lancet* 1994; **343**: 1342–1346.

Reunala T, Collin P. Diseases associated with dermatitis herpetiformis. *British Journal of Dermatology* 1997; **136**: 315–318

Reunala T, Collin P, Holm K *et al*. Tolerance to oats in dermatitis herpetiformis. *Gut* 1998; **43**: 490–493.

Russell Jones R. Recurrent facial herpes associated with Chinese herbal remedy. *Lancet* 1991; **338**: 55.

Sampson HA. Food sensitivity and the pathogenesis of atopic dermatitis. *Journal of the Royal Society of Medicine* 1997; **90** (Suppl 30): 2–8.

Sharpe GR, Farr PM. Evening primrose oil and eczema. *Lancet* 1990; **335**: 667–668.

Sheehan MP, Atherton DJ. A controlled trial of traditional Chinese medicinal plants in widespread non-exudative atopic eczema. *British Journal of Dermatology* 1992; **126**: 179–184.

Sheehan MP, Rustin MHA, Atherton DJ *et al*. Efficacy of traditional Chinese herbal therapy in adult atopic dermatitis. *Lancet* 1992; **340**: 13–17.

Sicherer SH, Sampson HA. Food hypersensitivity and atopic dermatitis: pathophysiology, epidemiology, diagnosis and management. *Journal of Allergy and Clinical Immunology* 1999; **104**: S114–S122.

Soyland E, Funk J, Rajka G *et al*. Effect of dietary supplementation with very long chain n-3 fatty acids in patients with psoriasis. *New England Journal of Medicine* 1993; **328**: 1812–1816.

Stewart JCM, Morse PF, Moss M *et al*. Treatment of severe and moderately severe atopic dermatitis with evening primrose oil (Epogam): a multi-centre study. *Journal of Nutritional Medicine* 1991; **2**: 9–15.

Wright S, Burton JL. Oral evening primrose seed oil improves atopic eczema. *Lancet* 1982; **ii**: 1120–1122.

Wuthrich B. Food-induced cutaneous adverse reactions. *Allergy* 1998; **53** (46 Suppl): 131–135.

Zuberbier T, Ifflander J, Semmler C, Henz BM. Acute urticaria: clinical aspects and therapeutic responsiveness. *Acta Dermato-Venereologica* 1996; **76**: 295–297.

4.34 Food allergy and intolerance

Food allergy and intolerance remain controversial and poorly researched subjects. Many people believe themselves to be 'allergic' to something they eat, a diagnosis that they have often made themselves. Many of them will not be 'allergic' in the strict sense of the term, although a small minority will be. Some may well be intolerant to certain foods or food components which are causing either acute or chronic ill health which can manifest itself in a variety of ways, and practitioners need to be aware of this possibility. Some will not be intolerant to foods at all – or at least, no evidence of this can be found – although a few will continue to believe that this simply means that the investigating practitioner has not yet found the answer. The dietitian has a key role to play in the process of distinguishing between actuality and belief.

As well as playing an important part in diagnosis, dietetic skills are essential for the effective management of food allergy and intolerance because the sole means of treatment is avoidance of the problem food. Although simple in theory, this may be far from simple in practice since the item in question may be present in a wide range of manufactured foods. The consequent restriction in food choice can increase the risk of overall dietary imbalance. If the problem food is normally a major contributor to nutrient intake, the risk of dietary inadequacy in vulnerable groups is high if measures are not taken to avert this. For these reasons, dietary exclusion should never be imposed without justification or for more prolonged periods than necessary.

This section discusses general aspects of the nature, diagnosis and principles of management of food allergy and intolerance. Practical guidance on particular types of food exclusion can be found in Section 4.35 (Food exclusion in the management of allergy and intolerance).

4.34.1 Definitions of food allergy and intolerance

The term 'food intolerance' was originally suggested as an umbrella term to cover a wide range of physiologically mediated reactions to food (RCP/British Nutrition Foundation 1984). Although still sometimes used in this context, 'food intolerance' is being increasingly used to describe non-immunologically mediated reactions to food, i.e. distinct from those which result from true allergy (RCP 1992; Bindslev-Jensen et al. 1994; COT 2000). This is a useful working definition, although it should be borne in mind that the distinction, is not always clear-cut; for example, some reactions to cow's milk protein appear to be immunologically mediated while others are not (Host et al. 1995), yet all will result in a similar clinical picture and require the same dietetic management. Much remains to be learnt about the mechanisms of adverse reactions to food and how these can be accurately identified.

Nevertheless, for practical purposes, unpleasant and reproducible pathological reactions to food can be divided into:

- *Food allergy*: Specific reactions resulting from an abnormal immunological response to a food and which can be severe and life-threatening. Symptoms may be of rapid onset but can also develop more slowly (e.g. coeliac disease, atopic dermatitis).
- *Non-allergic food intolerance*: Reactions to food which can result from a number of causes, none of which is mediated by the immune system. Such reactions may be due to directly triggered histamine release, pharmacological effects, enzyme deficiencies, irritant and toxic effects. There may also be other factors whose influence is not yet fully understood, such as the effect of foods on the composition of gut flora (MAFF 1997). Because of their variable aetiology, the effects are also diverse. They can be acute and severe (although rarely life threatening) but are more usually chronic and diffuse, and hence often difficult to diagnose. Unlike immunologically mediated reactions, relatively large amounts of a food may need to be ingested for adverse effects to occur.

Reactions to food may also be psychologically rather than physically based, i.e. they result from the emotional response to the thought of eating a particular food. This is termed 'food aversion'. This is not classified as food intolerance and is not discussed further in this section. However, the possibility of food aversion should always be considered when investigations of food intolerance are being made.

Food allergy and non-immunologically mediated food intolerance are primarily distinguished on the basis of clinical and dietary history. Additional *in vitro* and *in vivo* immunological tests can help to diagnose food allergy but have no relevance to non-allergic food intolerance. Some forms of the latter such as lactose intolerance, can be confirmed by a specific diagnostic test (e.g. the breath hydrogen test) but most can only be identified by monitoring the effects of controlled food exclusion and reintroduction.

4.34.2 Prevalence of food allergy and intolerance

The prevalence of adverse reactions to food is hard to determine because the effects are so variable and, in many cases, difficult to diagnose. Immunologically mediated food allergy has been estimated to affect about 1–2% of the general population and between 5 and 8% of children (Pearl 1997; COT 2000). The prevalence of non-allergic food intolerance is almost impossible to estimate because of the variability in its causes and effects, the fact that it is difficult to diagnose and is often misdiagnosed, and because of the different definitions used to classify it. The prevalence of some types of food intolerance also varies within the population; for example, lactose intolerance due to primary lactase deficiency may affect over 50% of people of Indian and African–Caribbean origin but only about 3% of the Caucasian population (see Lactose malabsorption in Section 4.8.2).

What is clear is that the *perceived* prevalence of allergy and intolerance among the general population is much higher than is really the case. Young *et al.* (1994) found that about 20% of adults believed themselves to have a food intolerance, whereas the confirmed prevalence by double-blind placebo-controlled food challenge was less than 2% (although this may be an underestimate as the challenge loads may have been too small to detect some types of intolerance). A similar study in The Netherlands found a reported prevalence of 10% but, following blind challenge, only 2% were found to have reproducible symptoms (Jansen *et al.* 1994). Many people believe that they are intolerant to food additives rather than food itself, but reactions to food additives are even rarer, probably affecting about 1 in 10 000 people (MAFF 1997).

Perceived food intolerance is also common among parents, with many believing their child to have a food intolerance and imposing food restrictions as a result (Kilgannen and Gibney 1996; Foster *et al.* 1997; Brugman *et al.* 1998). Double-blind challenges have shown that fewer than one-third of reported food intolerances in children could be substantiated (Bock 1987).

Adverse reactions to food can appear at any age, but allergy is more likely in infants and small children because the immature gastrointestinal tract is less capable of preventing potential antigens from being absorbed, and the developing immune system is more likely to react to their presence. However, 90% of infants allergic to milk and 50% of those allergic to eggs outgrow their clinical reactivity by the age of 3 years (Bindslev-Jensen 1998). Allergies to foods such as peanuts or fish are more likely to persist (Hourihane *et al.* 1998).

There is a genetic susceptibility to the development of food allergy (Hill *et al.* 1999) and it is more likely to occur where there is a family history of atopy (asthma, eczema or hayfever) (Chandra 1997).

4.34.3 Food allergy

Immunologically mediated food allergy is the most serious form of reaction to food because its effects can be rapid, life-threatening and triggered by minute amounts of the allergen.

Causation of food allergy

As with all types of allergy, food allergy results from a faulty and exaggerated response of the immune system following exposure to a foreign protein (antigen).

The human body has a number of defence mechanisms to protect it from substances which could cause harm. The mucosa of the gastrointestinal tract forms the first line of defence against potential pathogens from food by forming a physical barrier normally preventing large molecules such as proteins from entering the body.

The immune system also contains a wide range of cells which provide additional defence mechanisms. The most important of these cells are:

- *T-cell lymphocytes* which recognize antigens and react by producing cytotoxic substances or triggering inflammatory responses which aim to destroy the antigen.
- *B-cell lymphocytes* which create antibodies (various classes of immunoglobulins) which carry out further defensive reactions (Table 4.71).

Table 4.71 Immunoglobulin classes

Immunoglobulin	Function
IgG	The most abundant immunoglobulin (normally comprising more than 70% of serum immunoglobulins), its main task is to combat bacteria and their toxins
	IgG is the only immunoglobulin known to be transferred across the placenta and this begins at about 20 weeks' gestation. Transferred IgG affords a degree of passive immunity for first 3 months of an infant's life; premature infants are therefore at an immunological disadvantage
IgA	Appears in seromucous secretions defending external body surfaces, including the gastrointestinal tract where it binds with antigens to form a complex which is not readily absorbed
	Secretory immunoglobulin A (sIgA) is the predominant antibody in breast milk
IgM	Activates the complement system (a group of enzymes with cytolytic properties)
IgD	A short-lived immunoglobulin whose function is not well understood
IgE	Usually bound to mast cells and basophils and is only present in low concentrations in serum
	When triggered, IgE activates the degranulation of mast cells, resulting in an inflammatory response
	Hypersensitivity reactions are mediated by IgE antibodies

Normally the body's immune system is able to distinguish between antigens that need to be destroyed (such as bacterial pathogens) and those that do not (such as food proteins), and can mount an appropriate response to protect the body from infection and damage. The immune system learns to do this in the early months of life, a process known as developing tolerance. If this learning process is faulty, an abnormal response to food proteins can occur, particularly to those which are encountered in early life when the immune system is still immature. Ingestion of the antigen triggers the production of inappropriately high titres of antibodies and/or altered T-cell reactivity, with consequent systemic effects. This process may be preceded by sensitization, where initial exposure to an antigen results in no clinical effects but the immune system becomes primed to react to any subsequent encounter with the antigen with an enhanced (and abnormal) response.

The area on a food antigen which provokes the immune response is known as an epitope. Epitopes can be linear or conformational. Linear epitopes are composed of short sequences of amino acids, most of which lie on the surface of the protein but which can also be hidden within the protein molecule, only becoming exposed when the protein is digested (thus being more likely to trigger delayed reactions). Conformational epitopes depend on the three-dimensional structure of the protein and are created by the juxtaposition of peptide loops within the protein. Considerable research is underway to identify the epitopes which interact with immunoglobulins E (IgE) class antibody and trigger type I reactions.

There are four basic types of allergic response, of which the acute type I and the delayed type IV reactions are the most common:

- *Type I*: This is the 'classic', and most common, form of allergy where reactions occur within minutes of exposure to the antigen causing symptoms such as swelling in the mouth and throat, streaming eyes and nose (rhinitis), breathing difficulties or asthmatic attack, often followed by reactions in the skin or gastrointestinal tract. If untreated, these effects can result in asphyxiation and circulatory collapse (anaphylaxis) and be fatal. The reactions result from the interaction of the allergen with specific IgE antibodies bound to receptors on mast cells, triggering the rapid release of mediators such as histamine into the circulation causing vasodilatation, capillary leakage, hypotension, oedema and smooth muscle contraction. Type I allergic reactions are the most serious because of their speed of onset and potential severity, often in response to minute quantities of the triggering antigen.
- *Type II* or 'cytotoxic' reactions are also immediate but are confined to cell membranes. Interaction of the cell-bound antigen with IgG causes membrane damage, and the subsequent activation of the complement system results in cell lysis.
- *Type III* or 'immune complex reactions' occur some hours after exposure to the antigen and are known as 'late' reactions. The combination of IgG and circulating antigen results in activation of the complement system,

which triggers enzyme release. Typical reactions occur in the skin and bronchi.
- *Type IV* or 'cell-mediated reactions' only appear 24–48 hours after exposure and are termed 'delayed' reactions. The T-lymphocyte recognizes antigens bound to foreign cells and causes lysis. The sensitized T-cells can also release lymphokines, which activate non-sensitized cells to destroy antigens. Type IV reactions are probably the second most common form of food-provoked allergic reaction after type I, and are probably responsible for the exacerbation of eczema in children with cow's milk protein allergy, and some types of contact or urticarial dermatitis in adults.

Foods known to cause immunologically mediated reactions (COT 2000) include:

- peanuts
- tree nuts (e.g. Brazil nut, almond, hazelnut)
- milk (cow's goat's, sheep's and others)
- soya (and other legumes such as peas or lentils)
- fish
- shellfish
- eggs
- fruit (especially apples, peaches, plums, cherries, bananas, citrus fruit)
- seeds (especially sesame and caraway)
- herbs and spices (especially mustard, paprika and coriander).

Cow's milk, eggs, peanuts and soya are the foods most commonly responsible for allergic and intolerance reactions in children (Schwartz 1992).

Severe type I anaphylactic reactions are most likely to be provoked by peanuts, tree nuts, fish, shellfish, egg, soya and sesame seeds (MAFF 1997). Anaphylaxis can also be triggered by milk, cereals, fruit and many other foods (COT 2000), although these more commonly produce symptoms which are confined to one or more organ systems (e.g. gastrointestinal, dermatological and/or respiratory effects) rather than having general systemic effects. However, any food capable of provoking an immune response should be regarded as potentially anaphylactic.

Most patients only react clinically to just a single food, or a small group of biologically similar foods. However, cross-reactivity can occur if an antigen in an apparently unrelated food or other source has the same epitope, e.g. people with allergic sensitivity to latex can react to fruits such as banana, papaya, avocado, passion fruit, kiwi fruit, fig, melon, mango, pineapple, peach and chestnut (Brehler *et al.* 1997). There are also examples of cross-reactivity between pollens from silver birch and hazel with various raw fruits and vegetables (e.g. apple and carrot), which can manifest in the form of oral allergy syndrome (Asero 1998).

Diagnosis of food allergy

Factors suggestive of classic type I IgE-mediated food allergy are:

- The symptoms are acute, typical and usually involve more than one organ (e.g. oral swelling, nausea, vomiting, abdominal pain, diarrhoea, asthma, rhinitis, urticaria, angio-oedema, anaphylaxis).
- The offending food is usually readily identified.
- The timing of symptoms is closely associated with food intake.
- The patient has a personal or family history of atopic disorders.

Symptoms resulting from type IV delayed allergic reactions may be more diffuse and often less easy to identify (or distinguish from food intolerance), and the dietary history will need to be more closely explored.

Immunologically mediated allergy can be confirmed by both *in vivo* and *in vitro* tests, although these have a varying degree of accuracy, reliability and reproducibility.

In vivo diagnostic tests

These evaluate the body's response to the controlled administration of particular allergens and include the following tests.

Skin prick testing A drop of standardized allergen solution is placed on the skin of the forearm and a sterile needle used to prick the skin through the allergen solution. The same procedure (using a different needle) is conducted with a control solution (and possibly other allergen solutions). After 15 minutes, the reactions are compared. A positive result is a skin weal >2 mm greater than that observed with the negative control. The size of the weal does not necessarily reflect the degree of sensitivity to the allergen as this can be affected by the concentration of allergen used.

Skin prick tests are a simple and useful way of diagnosing IgE-mediated reactions to respiratory allergens but are less reliable for detecting responses to food allergens because the test solutions are less well standardized than to inhaled allergens such as pollen or animal hair. Their positive predictive accuracy for food allergens is only about 50% (Sampson 1999). However, their negative predictive accuracy is about 95%, so a negative skin test result can be a useful way of *excluding* IgE-mediated allergy (Sampson 1999). Skin prick tests can be unsuitable for many patients with eczema because interpretation of the skin reaction is difficult. They also cannot be performed in patients using systemic or topical antihistamines as these will suppress the weal and flare reaction. They are of no value in identifying food intolerance.

Skin prick tests with respiratory allergens are usually safe but occasional systemic reactions including anaphylaxis have been reported when food allergens are used. Testing with food allergens should therefore only be conducted in settings where adrenaline and staff experienced in treating allergic reactions are available (Ewan 1996).

Patch tests Standardized forms of possible allergens are applied to a healthy area of the patient's skin and the effects evaluated 48–72 hours later. Patch tests are used in the diagnosis of more delayed type IV reactions such as allergic dermatitis and may be a useful adjunct to a skin prick test (Isolauri and Turjanmara 1996). However, specialist evaluation is needed to distinguish between allergic reactions and simple irritant ones. This procedure can also trigger acute flare-up reactions and cause sensitization, thus making the problem worse.

In vitro blood tests

These tests look for the presence of IgE antibodies to specific food allergens in a sample of blood, and are safer for people at risk of anaphylaxis than *in vivo* methods where potential allergens are directly introduced into the body. *In vitro* immunological assays include the following tests.

Radioallergosorbent test (RAST) This is a direct radioimmunoassay for antigen-specific IgE in the patient's blood. Blood serum from the patient is added to a mixture containing chemically bound specific allergens and any specific IgE present will attach to the immobilized allergen. Radioactively labelled anti-IgE is then added, which binds to any IgE–allergen complexes. The amount of radioactivity from the bound complexes provides a measure of the amount of antigen-specific IgE in the patient's serum. A modification of this procedure where the assay is done by fluorescence (the CAP-RAST) has also been developed.

Enzyme-linked immunosorbent assay (ELISA) This is a non-radioactive method which uses the same principle of creating specific allergen–IgE complexes, but which are then identified using enzyme-labelled anti-IgE and subsequently measured via photometric assay.

In vitro tests are highly specific and useful in patients where skin prick tests are contraindicated because of concurrent drug therapy, skin disease or a history of anaphylaxis. However, they are expensive and not without problems in terms of interpretation. Both false-positive and false-negative results can occur; some healthy people have raised IgE titres, whereas others with clinical evidence of atopic disease may not produce positive RAST results (David 1991). An additional problem with the newer highly sensitive tests is that they may detect clinically insignificant serological cross-reactions, e.g. IgE raised against grass pollen may also bind to epitopes (antigenic binding sites) on wheat protein, a finding that may misleadingly imply wheat allergy. The results of allergy tests therefore always need to be interpreted in the context of the patient's history (Bindslev-Jensen and Poulsen 1996).

The problems associated with unorthodox or commercially available 'allergy' tests are discussed in Section 4.34.6, below.

Dietary management of food allergy

Management of food allergy is by identifying and avoiding the offending allergen or allergens. Complete exclusion is imperative because reaction can occur to even trace amounts of allergenic protein, and also because sensitivity to the allergen can increase on repeated exposure: a previously mild reaction could subsequently become a life-threatening one.

Specialist dietetic guidance is essential to ensure that:

- All potential sources of the allergen, both obvious and less obvious, are avoided. This may not be a simple procedure. If the food is a common component of manufactured foods (e.g. nuts, egg, wheat) many foods may need to be avoided and, if the food allergen is often present in trace quantities, its presence may be by no means easy to identify.
- The effects of the exclusion diet on the intake of other nutrients and overall dietary balance are minimized. This is especially important if the patient is an infant or child, as is often the case. If the excluded food is normally a major nutritional contributor to the diet (e.g. milk), alternative sources of nutrients will need to be provided.

In practical terms, patients will require clear, written guidance on:

- foods, or types of foods, which must be avoided
- foods, or types of foods, which may need to be avoided and the extent to which this can be determined from ingredients lists on manufactured foods. With some types of food exclusion, lists of manufactured foods free from specified components may be available
- foods, or types of foods, which can safely be eaten
- dietary measures which should be taken either to lessen the impact of dietary exclusions on normal life or to prevent potential nutritional inadequacies.

If any doubt remains as to which food (or foods) trigger the allergic response, patients should keep a symptom score diary for at least 1 week before starting any dietary manipulations and should maintain this until the next dietetic review.

Guidance on specific types of dietary exclusions is given in Section 4.35.

The management of allergic diseases is now recognized as an area of specialization within the National Health Service (NHS) and should ideally be carried out by a clinical immunology and allergy team which includes medical expertise from the fields of respiratory diseases, dermatology, gastroenterology and immunology, and also specialist skills from dietitians and nurses. Children with allergic disease should be under the overall care of a paediatrician since the progression of allergies in children differs from that in adults (RCP/Royal College of Pathologists 1995). There is evidence that the dietetic resources necessary for the appropriate management of allergy are lacking in many hospitals in the UK (Wolfe 1995).

All patients who have had an anaphylactic type I allergic reaction should carry a preloaded syringe containing adrenaline (e.g. EpiPen) and both they and their relatives, close friends or associates or, in the case of children, school staff, should know how to use it. Many people with proven sensitivity to peanuts and tree nuts may also be prescribed this as a precautionary measure, because reactions can intensify or be provoked by a previously unencountered trigger (e.g. someone with a previously mild reaction to peanut could have an unexpected severe reaction to a particular type of tree nut; see Section 4.35.3, Peanut and nut exclusion). Risk factors for anaphylactic reactions to other types of food allergy remain poorly documented but include a history of a previous severe reaction, evidence of increasingly severe reactions and a history of asthma, especially if it is poorly controlled (Patel *et al.* 1994).

In milder cases of allergy, antihistamine drugs may be used to help control symptoms. Antiallergy drugs such as cromoglycate and glucocorticoids which modify the immune response have been investigated in clinical trials with conflicting results and are not generally regarded as helpful (COT 2000).

Many children with a food allergy will lose their clinical reactivity in time and therefore need to be re-evaluated at intervals, possibly annually, to prevent unnecessarily prolonged dietary exclusion (see Reintroduction, below). The exception to this is peanut/nut allergy, or where there is a history of anaphylaxis, where sensitivity is less likely to remit and the dangers from re-exposure to the allergen are considerable (see Section 4.35.3, Peanut and nut exclusion). Because of the risks associated with the reintroduction of foods (David 1984), all such investigations must be conducted under experienced medical supervision (BDA 1990).

Prevention of food allergy

The extent to which food allergy can be prevented by avoiding exposure to potential allergens *in utero* and in early life remains controversial and poorly understood. Most research has focused on the prevention of atopy (the production of specific IgE in response to common environmental allergens such as house dust mite, grass and pet fur). Being atopic is strongly associated with allergic disease in the form of asthma, hayfever and eczema (although not everyone with atopy develops clinical manifestations) and increases the risk of food allergies. Foods may also directly trigger or exacerbate atopic disorders such as eczema and asthma. However, the extent to which clinical atopy can be prevented by dietary exclusion measures during pregnancy, lactation or infancy is uncertain. A Cochrane review of the combined evidence from four trials (Kramer 1999a) concluded that there was no evidence of a significant protective effect of maternal antigen avoidance during pregnancy on the incidence of atopic eczema or asthma during the first 12–18 months of life. They therefore suggest that such measures are unlikely to be of much benefit. They did, however, find that maternal weight gain was less in those who restricted their diet than in those who did not, suggesting that adverse effects on fetal or maternal nutrition cannot be ruled out. This is a matter of concern, particularly when dietetic resources are in general too scarce to monitor the nutritional adequacy of such a vulnerable group (Wolfe 1995). It is also possible that intrauterine sensitization to such foods may be an important part of the process of developing tolerance, the process by which the body learns to distinguish between harmful and harmless proteins (Host 1997).

There is, however, some evidence that intrauterine exposure to particularly potent allergens such as peanut may increase the risk of peanut allergy in those with genetic susceptibility to the condition or with a strong family history of allergic disorders (see Section 4.35.3, Peanut and nut exclusion). The Department of Health has therefore suggested that peanuts should be avoided during pregnancy in such cases (DH 1998).

In infants, exclusive breast feeding offers some protection against the development of allergies (Halken *et al.* 1992; ESPGAN 1993; Saarinen and Kajosaari 1995). Breast feeding not only lessens the exposure to cow's milk protein but also contains IgA, which helps to block the entry of whole proteins from the baby's immature gut into the bloodstream. Human milk also contains macrophages and other immune factors which may help the infants' immune system to mature more rapidly. Breast feeding has been shown to reduce the risk of eczema triggered by cow's milk protein intolerance (Burr 1983; Miskelly *et al.* 1988), although it does not appear to prevent the later development of inhalant allergies such as asthma (Mallet and Henocq 1992).

Substitution of cow's milk with soya milk in infants considered at risk of atopy does not appear to be protective (Miskelly *et al.* 1988; Witherley 1990; Host 1997). In a 7 year follow-up study, Burr *et al.* (1993) found that soya formula-fed children had the same incidence of wheezing, asthma, eczema and allergic rhinitis as cow's milk formula-fed children. Only breast feeding was protective and even then only in non-atopic infants, i.e. those without a genetic predisposition to develop hypersensitivity to foreign proteins. Hydrolysed whey formula may be a valid alternative to reduce the risk of atopic disease in infants at risk of allergy if they cannot be breast fed (Baumgartner *et al.* 1998).

Allergic disease can still occur in breast-fed infants, possibly as a result of the presence of small amounts of food antigens in maternal milk. For this reason, it has been suggested that where there is a family history of atopy, the protective effects of breast feeding may be enhanced if common allergens are excluded from the maternal diet (Cant *et al.* 1984; DH 1994). However, more recently, the benefits of, and necessity for, such a measure have been questioned (NDC 1998). A Cochrane review (Kramer 1999b) of three trials of maternal antigen avoidance during lactation and subsequent development of atopy in the child concluded that while there was some evidence of a protective effect on the incidence of atopic eczema during the child's first 12–18 months of life, all three trials had methodological shortcomings and that better evidence was needed. In a 10 year follow-up study of children with a family history of atopy, Hattevig *et al.* (1999) compared the outcome in those whose mothers either had, or had not, excluded cow's milk, fish and eggs during the first 3 months of lactation. The only difference found was a slightly lower prevalence of atopic dermatitis at 4 years in the children of the maternal exclusion group, a difference that

had disappeared by the age of 10 years. They concluded that this level of benefit did not justify imposing restrictive exclusion diets as a general measure to prevent atopic disease. However, peanuts may again be the exception; peanut protein has been found in breast milk (Gerrard 1979), and in lactating women with, or a family history of allergic disease, avoidance of peanut sources may be advisable (DH 1998).

It is, however, clear that exposure to large quantities of food allergens in the first few months of life, either via cow's milk-based infant formula or as a result of early weaning, increases the risk of allergy (Host 1997). For this reason, it is recommended (DH 1994) that all infants should be exclusively breast fed for the first 4 months of life, and foods containing wheat, eggs and citrus fruits should not be introduced before the age of 6 months. Whether more prolonged avoidance of these foods is advantageous in high-risk infants is more debatable; although their exclusion until the age of 12 months is advocated by some (Chandra 1997), the delayed exposure to different tastes and textures may have adverse consequences in terms of eating habits, nutritional intake and speech development. However, children considered at risk of peanut allergy or with asymptomatic immunological evidence of peanut sensitivity are advised to avoid sources of peanuts for the first 3 years of life (DH 1998).

The extent to which modification of gut microflora (by use of prebiotics or probiotics) may prevent or ameliorate food allergy by changing the allergenicity of dietary proteins, reducing intestinal permeability or the mucosal inflammatory response, or increasing IgA production is an area of current interest and investigation (Kirjavainen *et al.* 1999).

4.34.4 Non-allergic food intolerance

Causation

Non-immunologically mediated forms of food intolerance can result from the following processes.

Non-immunological activation of mast cells

These are sometimes confused with allergic reactions because they can result in similar and acute symptoms such as vomiting, diarrhoea and rashes, but no immunological mechanism is involved. The effects result from direct activation of mast cells, causing the release of histamine and other mediators. The acute effects can be severe and in some cases, hypotension and anaphylactoid reactions can occur (Bruijnzeel-Koomen *et al.* 1995) The main distinguishing feature from true allergy is that significant amounts of the offending food may be needed to cause a reaction and the severity of the symptoms is more likely to be related to the amount ingested (in contrast to an immunologically mediated reaction where a massive effect can result from minute exposure). However, for practical purposes, this type of food intolerance is managed in the same way as food allergy. Food which commonly provoke this response are shellfish and strawberries.

More benign non-immunological reactions may also be provoked by food constituents and additives such as benzoates, salicylates, sulphites and tartrazine (Wuthrich 1993). High levels of benzoic acid in some citrus fruits may cause a harmless, non-IgE-mediated, immediate flare reaction around the mouth, especially in children. This is often misinterpreted as allergy and a child may be unnecessarily stopped from consuming all citrus fruits (Durham 1998).

Pharmacological reactions

Many foods and beverages contain substances which are pharmacologically active. Large intakes of, or undue sensitivity to, these substances can have neurological effects resulting in symptoms such as tremor, sweating, palpitations, headache or migraine, or psychological effects such as insomnia or anxiety. The most common triggers of pharmacological reactions are given below.

Vasoactive amines Amines such as histamine, tyramine, serotonin and tryptamine are powerful vasoconstrictors capable of producing symptoms such as headache, nausea and giddiness; tyramine can trigger migraine in some people. Foods that are likely to be rich sources of vasoactive amines are:

- cheese, especially if matured
- fermented foods such as blue cheese, sauerkraut, fermented soya products
- yeast extracts
- fish, especially if stale or pickled
- microbially contaminated foods
- chocolate
- red wine
- some fruits, especially citrus fruits, bananas, avocado pears.

Vasoactive amines are normally deactivated in the body by the enzyme monoamine oxidase (MAO). People taking MAO inhibitor antidepressant drugs which suppress the activity of this enzyme must therefore avoid high intakes of vasoactive amines (see Section 2.9.3 in Biologically active dietary constituents).

Caffeine This stimulant, can cause palpitations, sweating, shaking and anxiety. As little as 200 mg of caffeine can trigger a response in some individuals (Astrup *et al.* 1990) (see Section 2.9.2 in Biologically active dietary constituents). Major sources of caffeine are:

- coffee
- tea
- chocolate
- cola drinks
- caffeine-containing analgesics.

Monosodium glutamate (MSG) Commonly used as a flavour enhancer, large amounts of MSG can cause flushing, headache and abdominal symptoms and may even mimic the features of a myocardial infarction, with chest pain radiating to both arms and the back, together with general weakness and palpitations. These effects have been described as Chinese restaurant syndrome (or Kwok's syndrome) because they can be triggered by consuming Chinese food with a high MSG content.

Enzyme deficiency

Partial or total deficiency of one or more enzymes in the digestive tract (e.g. lactase) may result in symptoms of malabsorption when foods containing certain components (e.g. lactose) are consumed. This type of intolerance is discussed in Section 4.8.2.

Irritant effects

Irritant effects on the gastrointestinal tract can be induced by foods containing hot spices such as chili or cayenne pepper.

Toxins

Toxic reactions to foods may result from the presence of natural toxins in food (such as the alkaloid solanine in green potatoes or haemagglutinins in uncooked kidney beans) or its contamination by chemicals or microbial pathogens ('food poisoning').

Other causes

There is growing evidence that the composition of colonic microflora may contribute, either directly or indirectly, to some forms of food intolerance (King *et al.* 1998).

Diagnosis of non-allergic food intolerance

Contrary to popular belief, neither the *in vitro* or *in vivo* methods used to diagnose food allergy nor any of the unorthodox 'allergy tests' (see below) have any role to play in the identification of non-allergic food intolerance. Diagnosis can only be made by means of a combination of clinical history and dietary investigation.

Because of the diffuse and variable nature of non-allergic food intolerance, diagnosis can be time-consuming and difficult. Only immediately provoked reactions such as triggered histamine release reactions are readily identifiable (and since these closely mimic allergy, may even be assumed to be such without further investigation). In most cases of a clinical history which is suggestive of food intolerance, or where links between foods and a particular condition commonly occur, phases of dietary exclusion and reintroduction to see whether symptoms are affected provide the only means of investigation.

Manipulative dietary investigations should not be undertaken lightly. They are time-consuming procedures for both patients and professionals, and should only be attempted if the symptoms are sufficiently debilitating to justify the social disruption (Hathaway and Warner 1983), financial strain (Macdonald and Forsythe 1986) and periods of inadequate nutrient intake (Labib *et al.* 1989). Furthermore, there is no guarantee that the end-result will be relief from symptoms. Nevertheless, for some patients, successful dietary diagnosis and treatment can dramatically improve the quality of life.

The dietary investigative strategy employed depends on the nature of the problem. Following any referral for food intolerance, the following need to be ascertained:

- the clinical diagnosis and its current treatment
- whether the client has any documented allergies (e.g. to aspirin) or history of atopic disease
- the nature of the symptoms, together with their severity and frequency
- whether any foods are suspected of causing symptoms
- whether any dietary measures have already been tried and with what result
- the general dietary history and current eating habits and meal pattern
- relevant anthropometric information, e.g. height and weight in children.

In some cases, particularly where symptoms are intermittent and acute, sufficient information may emerge to suggest an obvious cause for the symptoms, e.g. pharmacologically induced effects. Suitable dietary guidance to avoid the offending item(s) may then be all that is required.

In other cases, the patient's clinical history and dietitian's clinical experience may suggest a possible link between diet and symptoms to be explored. For example, in an adult with irritable bowel syndrome (IBS) who reports that symptoms improve if bread is avoided, the possibility of wheat intolerance might be worth pursuing.

Where symptoms are more chronic and diffuse and no obvious dietary links emerge but remain a possibility, asking the patient to keep a food-symptom record for 2 weeks may be useful. All foods and beverages consumed are recorded in a food diary and the prevalence and severity of symptoms (e.g. on a 0–5 scale) recorded on a formatted record sheet at specified intervals (usually twice daily). This may provide useful pointers; it may also in some instances be sufficient to show that a patient's concerns about food-related symptoms are unfounded.

Some patients will present to a dietitian with preconceived ideas of foods to which they are 'allergic' often on the basis of commercial 'allergy', tests. Some may have already self-imposed a number of food restrictions, resulting in a dietary intake that may be highly unbalanced. In such cases it may be necessary to provide basic healthy eating guidance to restore normal eating habits and provide a baseline from which any genuine intolerances can be identified.

Diagnostic exclusion diets

Foods or food constituents which are suspected of causing intolerance are eliminated from the diet to see whether symptoms improve. There are four main ways in which this can be done.

Single exclusion diet   This excludes all sources of a single food (e.g. milk) because dietary enquiry suggests, or the patient has discovered, that symptoms are linked to this particular item. Although simple in theory, these diets are not always simple in practice. While foods such as strawberries, chocolate and shellfish are relatively easy to

exclude, the sources of items such as wheat or milk are less obvious and their avoidance encompasses a wide range of foods. Patients will require clear but comprehensive information detailing both obvious and less obvious sources of the food, and how the latter can be determined from labelling information. If food avoidance results in exclusion of many staple food items (such as bread and cereals or milk and dairy products) guidance on suitable alternatives or substitutes will also be needed.

Considerable dietetic expertise may be needed to ensure that the nutritional requirements of children are met if foods which normally make a significant contribution to nutrient intake (such as milk and dairy products) are excluded. Practical details of dietary regimens free from milk, egg, wheat, etc., are given in Section 4.35 (Food exclusion in the management of food allergy and intolerance).

Multiple food exclusion diet   A multiple exclusion diet excludes a number of foods at the same time. It is used when a dietary link is suspected but cannot be identified. There are no hard and fast rules governing the choice of foods to be excluded and practice varies between different centres. They usually eliminate combinations of foods most commonly associated with particular types of chronic disorders e.g. the Addenbrooke's exclusion diet used for some patients with IBS (Parker *et al.* 1995). Some general guidance on the types of foods that may be excluded or included is given in Table 4.72.

As well as foods and beverages, non-dietary sources of substances that can provoke reactions may need to be excluded. Colours or preservatives can be encountered via toothpastes, medicines, vitamin and mineral preparations, paints, chalk, crayons and cosmetics, while items such as wheat and yeast can be found in pharmaceutical products.

Table 4.72 General guidance for the composition of a multiple exclusion diet (The choice of foods excluded will depend on the symptoms being investigated and the dietary history)

Foods commonly excluded	Milk and milk products
	Eggs
	Wheat
	Citrus fruit
Foods sometimes excluded	Pork, bacon, liver and offal
	Fish and shellfish
	Barley, oats, corn, rye
	Nuts and pips
	Yeasts
	Potatoes, tomatoes, onions and garlic
	Chocolate
	Coffee/tea
	Food colourings (especially azo dyes)
	Food preservatives (especially benzoates and sulphites)
	Soya
Foods commonly permitted	Beef, lamb, turkey, rabbit
	Rice
	Sugar, treacle, syrup
	Lard
	Vegetables (except for potatoes, tomatoes, onions and garlic)
	Fruit (except for citrus fruit)

A multiple exclusion diet is usually followed for a period of 2–3 weeks, but in conditions where there fluctuations in the disease pattern (e.g. rheumatoid arthritis) it may be necessary to continue for up to 6 weeks. If symptomatic improvement occurs, foods then need to be appropriately reintroduced (see Food reintroduction, below) in order to establish which ones have provoked symptoms. If improvement does not occur, the dietitian must carefully review the patient's food intake to ascertain whether the procedure was followed correctly and, if so, must then decide whether other foods should be excluded or whether a food intolerance is unlikely to exist.

Few Foods diet A Few Foods diet is a much more restrictive regimen than the multiple exclusion diet and now rarely used. Its use tends to be confined to cases when a multiple exclusion diet has failed to relieve symptoms but food intolerance is still suspected. It may also be of some value in patients who present with a self-imposed highly restricted diet but without having established any clear relationship with symptoms.

Unlike the multiple exclusion diet, which excludes a few specific foods, a Few Foods diet only includes a few foods and excludes most. The small number of foods consumed comprises those which rarely provoke sensitivity. There is no fixed definition as to which foods these are, and practice varies between treatment centres. Usually they comprise one or two meats, and a selection of starchy foods, vegetables and some fruits. The choice of foods also depends on individual factors such as the acceptability and frequency of consumption of particular foods. The regimen is socially as well as nutritionally restricting and requires considerable commitment from the patient. It should not be imposed lightly.

A Few Foods diet should not be continued for more than 2–3 weeks. If symptom relief is obtained, foods are then reintroduced singly into the diet at appropriate intervals (see Food reintroduction, below). If no improvement occurs the situation should be reassessed. In some instances it may be considered worthwhile constructing a second Few Foods diet using similar principles but containing none of the foods comprising the first diet. If this also produces no relief, the regimen should be discontinued.

Elemental and protein hydrolysate formula diets This regimen withdraws all food and replaces it with an elemental or protein hydrolysate formula diet which, since protein is supplied in the form of amino acids or low molecular weight peptides, is less likely to be antigenic and provoke symptoms. This strategy has in the past been used to help to identify food-related exacerbation of disorders such as eczema in children or Crohn's disease, although in the latter case it can be difficult to distinguish between the effects of a liquid diet on disease remission–recurrence and genuine food intolerance (see Section 4.10.2).

Elemental and hydrolysate diets are unpalatable, monotonous and expensive, and the imposition of such an extreme regimen can only rarely be justified as a means of identifying food intolerance. Its use should be confined to cases where the symptoms are particularly severe or debilitating. If no improvement in symptoms occurs after 2–3 weeks, the normal diet should be resumed. If symptom remission has occurred, foods should be reintroduced singly and at intervals of a few days (see Food reintroduction, below). If severe reaction occurs, patients should return to the elemental diet until symptoms improve. During the first few weeks of testing, patients will require some elemental diet as a nutritional supplement.

Monitoring progress

Whichever type of exclusion diet is employed, its degree of effectiveness should be closely monitored. Most patients should be asked to keep a daily record of their symptoms on a standard proforma so that appropriate details of frequency and severity are provided. Recording should commence at least 1 week prior to commencing the diet and should continue throughout the elimination and reintroduction period so that alteration in symptoms can be related to any dietary change. If possible, an objective method of monitoring symptoms should be kept over the same period, for example, peak expiratory flow in asthmatics or grip strength in arthritics.

Food reintroduction

Dietary exclusion for diagnostic purposes needs to be followed by phased food reintroduction in order to identify or confirm the suspect foods. Note that this does not apply to dietary exclusions imposed following classic type I allergic symptoms where, if any doubt remains about the diagnosis, this must be confirmed by serological tests or under specialized conditions because of the risk of anaphylaxis.

For the diagnosis of non-allergic food intolerance, foods are reintroduced singly and usually at intervals of a few days. The delay between the consumption of a food and the return of symptoms can vary; there may be an immediate response but, in many chronic disorders, this may take a week or more after daily ingestion of the suspect food (Lessof *et al.* 1980; Sicherer 1999).

There is no universally agreed order in which foods should be reintroduced. This will vary from patient to patient and according to the condition being treated. Foods that are most likely to cause problems should be tested later rather than sooner and interspersed with those that are unlikely to precipitate symptoms. A food reintroduction order should be devised for each patient based on considerations such as the original exclusion diet and individual needs.

The quantity of food reintroduced is a matter of debate. Too small a quantity of food (i.e. less than normally consumed) may be insufficient to provoke symptoms (Carter 1995). However, sensitivity to a food may be heightened after a period of withdrawal, particularly in case of infants and children (David 1984). As a general guideline, foods should be reintroduced in amounts similar to that consumed prior to exclusion. Gradual reintroduction may be more appropriate in children or if reactions may be severe. Local protocols for the management of particular disorders in particular groups of the population should be devised in conjunction with other members of the clinical team.

It is important to give patients clear guidance on the form in which a food should be reintroduced. If testing wheat, for example, a sweet biscuit is an inappropriate source since it may contain other ingredients that may provoke symptoms. Foods should be fresh or frozen single items with no additions. Composite dishes, ready meals and other convenience foods should only be reintroduced into the diet when all likely suspect ingredients have been tested separately. Dietary assessment should be carried out throughout this period to determine whether any nutritional supplementation is required.

The reintroduction process can be very slow, up to 9 months in some cases. Patients need to be highly motivated and will require a lot of support from a dietitian. There is always a conflict between the desire to make the diet more acceptable to the patient and the need to ensure that foods are not introduced so quickly that no conclusions can be drawn. If carried out correctly, the potential rewards from these dietary manipulations are high; the quality of life of patients who have been chronically ill for years may be significantly improved. Conversely, patients who have undergone these procedures without identification of any food-related intolerance should be reassured that the investigation has not 'failed' but simply demonstrated that their symptoms are not diet related.

Confirmation of a diagnosis can be obtained by food challenge (see Section 4.34.5).

Management of non-allergic food intolerance

Once diagnosis is certain, patients require dietary guidance on the practical aspects of the maintenance food exclusion diet, and on any necessary measures to ensure that the overall diet remains nutritionally adequate and well balanced.

The principles of dietary management are the same as for food allergy (see above), although the stringency of the food avoidance is not always so critical. In contrast to immunologically mediated reactions, symptoms of some types of food intolerance are only provoked by significant quantities of foods, or particular forms of the food, and hence may only require a reduction in consumption rather than total exclusion (e.g. primary lactase deficiency or foods which appear to exacerbate irritable bowel symptoms).

Patients, especially children, should undergo periodic review to assess the effectiveness of the maintenance regimen in respect of symptoms and its nutritional adequacy. The possibility of the intolerance having disappeared should also be considered. Whether or not food reintroduction should be attempted is largely a matter of judgement based on the potential risks from food reactions if the intolerance still exists, and the benefits from relaxing dietary and lifestyle constraints if it does not.

4.34.5 Food challenge

Food challenge is a means of confirming a diagnosis or continued existence of a food allergy or intolerance. How-ever, it is neither necessary nor appropriate in every patient. It is clearly hazardous in anyone who has experienced type I allergic reactions involving swelling of the lips, tongue or face, respiratory difficulties or anaphylaxis, and is normally contraindicated in such patients. Non-allergically mediated reactions resulting in acute vomiting, diarrhoea or migraine may have been so obvious that the patient has no wish to repeat them, or a food may have been consumed by mistake and already identified by reaction.

The procedure is primarily of value in cases of non-allergic food intolerance where there is doubt about the diagnosis. It may also be used after a period of time to re-evaluate whether a childhood food sensitivity still exists. Some types of allergy and intolerance spontaneously remit or are outgrown, and if the reaction is to a key dietary component such as milk, it is important that this is not excluded for longer than necessary. However, the potential ability of the procedure to provoke acute, possibly anaphylactoid, reactions should not be underestimated and should always be carried out by experienced personnel with resuscitation facilities on hand.

Practical aspects of food challenge procedures

Because of the power of the placebo effect, a food challenge ideally needs to be administered in blind form, ideally in a cross-over pattern with an inert substance as a control, so that an objective assessment can be made. This is particularly important when the purpose of the challenge is to see whether an intolerance still persists and the patient will be well aware that reactions to a particular food have occurred in the past.

However, in practice, blind challenge can be extremely difficult to achieve (Huijbers *et al*. 1994). In order to reproduce some types of chronic reaction, relatively large amounts of food need to be given for several days and it can be difficult to hide this quantity of food in a way that makes it indistinguishable from the placebo. If insufficient food is given, there is a risk that the procedure will not detect a genuine effect (Carter 1995). There are also difficulties in respect of choice of disguising foods (which need to be those which will not themselves provoke reactions) and test foods (it cannot be assumed that someone who relapses with, for example, fresh cow's milk will have the same response to dried and heat-treated milk). Some chronic diseases, e.g. eczema, also have quiescent phases when the results of a challenge may be different (Carter 1995).

Ways in which blind challenge may be conducted include the following, but each method has its limitations.

Masking with other foods

Some suspect items can be disguised in soups, casseroles, fruit juices, puréed fruits or vegetables, bread, cakes or biscuits. These can be made up as required for inpatients, while outpatients can be given previously prepared frozen products, some with and some without the test material, with instructions for use at home. As far as possible the suspect food should be given in a similar quantity and form to that which is normally consumed. The patient should not be able to distinguish, either by sight, smell, texture or taste, which is the active and which is the placebo challenge, but it can be almost impossible to mask some of the stronger tasting foods such as cheese or fish. Suggestions for disguising some of the most commonly implicated foods are given in Table 4.73. For research studies, it may be possible to enlist the help of a food manufacturer to disguise foods in cans or baked products.

Encapsulation of foods

Encapsulation in opaque gelatine capsules may seem an ideal means of disguise, but the type and amount of food that can be administered are limited and may be too small to produce chronic or delayed forms of food reactions. It also bypasses the oral cavity, where responses to some antigens may be provoked. The main advantage of this method is it can provide an 'off-the-shelf' range of readily available challenges, and is a particularly useful way of testing sensitivity to food additives. Pharmacy departments may be able to assist in the preparation of suitable test materials.

Nasogastric administration

Delivery by nasogastric tube is an effective way of preventing identification of the food by the subject. It is also relatively easy to incorporate commonly suspected foods into an elemental or hydrolysate formula. However, it is an invasive technique for the patient and cannot be justified for either routine investigation or controlled studies. It also bypasses the oral cavity (see above).

More detail on conducting food challenge procedures can be found in Sicherer (1999), Bock *et al.* (1988) and Huijbers *et al.* (1994).

Table 4.73 Ways in which foods may be disguised for blind food challenge

Test food	Suitable base materials for disguise
Cow's milk	Soya formula, mashed potato, puréed lentils, soups, casseroles
Soya formula	Cow's milk, puréed lentils
Egg	Mashed potato, puréed lentils
Wheat	Puréed lentils, oatcakes, flapjacks, gluten-free foods
Corn	Oatcakes, flapjacks, soups, casseroles
Rye	Gluten-free bread, soups, casseroles
Oats	Soups, casseroles
Barley	Soups, casseroles
Orange juice	Carrot juice
Sugar	Carrot juice, 'diet' drinks
Food colours	Carrot juice, orange juice
Preservatives	Orange juice

4.34.6 Unorthodox 'allergy' tests

Many commercial tests supposedly capable of diagnosing allergy and food intolerance are promoted to the general public. Most have no scientific evidence to support their claims, and some are potentially dangerous as they could inadvertently provoke type I allergic reactions (Kay and Lessof 1992; RCP/Royal Collage of Pathologists 1995; Consumers' Association 1998). Those which are commonly used include:

- *Leucocytotoxic food test.* This is based on the premise that leucocytes lyse in the presence of allergens. However, studies suggest that the technique does not give results which are either accurate or consistent; the incorrect diagnosis has been given for blood samples from patients with known allergies (Consumers' Association 1998) and results from duplicate blood samples sent under different names have not matched (Lehman 1980).
- *Hair and nail tests.* Hair and nail samples are incapable of revealing information about allergens or other forms of food intolerance. Their only use is in the assay of minerals, e.g. in cases of heavy metal poisoning.
- *Pulse testing.* This test assumes that the pulse rate rises after ingestion of a food allergen. While this may be true in the case of a severe type I reaction, other symptoms such as orofacial swelling and respiratory distress would be so noticeable as to leave the diagnosis in no doubt (and hence make pulse testing superfluous). It is unlikely that non-type I reactions would affect pulse rate either soon enough or markedly enough for this to be registerable, particularly given the variability of pulse rate in situations of stress, such as undergoing the procedure itself.
- *Sublingual provocative testing.* This technique involves the application of a few drops of an extract of a food under the tongue of an individual who has been deprived of that food for a short period and looking for signs of a reaction. This form of testing carries the risk that a genuine type I response would cause rapid swelling of the tongue and pharynx, leading to asphyxiation, anaphylactic shock and possibly death. Non-allergic forms of food intolerance would not be detected by this method.

Other tests such as Vega testing (an electrodermal test) or kinesiology (based on 'muscle weakness') have similarly little scientific credibility (Kay and Lessof 1992; RCP/Royal College of Pathologists 1995).

As well as the dubious nature of many of these tests and the potential hazards from some of them, their main problem is that they often result in people consuming highly restrictive diets which are usually inappropriate and often nutritionally unsound. In addition, few will realize that non-allergic forms of food intolerance cannot be detected by either these or conventional immunological diagnostic tests.

4.34.7 Links between food allergy and intolerance and specific

Food allergy and intolerance are claimed to play a role in the development of many diseases. With some disorders, there is good evidence that this can be the case, whereas in others no evidence of a *systematic* relationship can be found or remains to be explored. It should, however, be borne in mind that, even if no causal link has been established, someone with a particular disororder may still have a genuine food allergy or intolerance by virtue of coincidence.

Links between food allergy and intolerance and certain diseases are summarized below; some of these are discussed in more depth in other parts of the manual.

Asthma

Asthma is the most serious atopic disease, causing significant morbidity and mortality, and the prevalence of childhood asthma has increased by over 300% since the late 1970s and is continuing to rise; it currently affects 1 in 7 children to some degree (Durham 1998). Management of asthma is primarily by avoidance of known trigger factors and suppression of attacks by inhaled antispasmodics or anti-inflammatory corticosteroids.

Although food sensitivities often exist, they are not always clinically significant asthma triggers. Food avoidance measures are most likely to be of benefit in the management of severe asthma and brittle asthma where identification and elimination of dietary triggers can lead to considerable improvement in asthma symptoms, reduced drug therapy and fewer hospital admissions (Baker and Agnes 2000). A procedure for assessing food intolerance in people with brittle asthma has been described by Baker and Ayres (2000). Food-induced symptoms are most likely to occur in young asthmatic patients who also have cutaneous and/or gastrointestinal symptoms (Onorato *et al.* 1986; Novembre *et al.* 1988). It should be noted that poorly controlled asthma is a risk factor for anaphylactic reactions to food.

However, in milder cases of asthma, while sensitivities to foods such as milk, eggs and fish are often immunologically demonstrable (Wraith and Merret 1979), the significance of imposing food restrictions in an attempt to reduce asthma attacks is questionable because other triggers, particularly house dust mite, are of much greater significance (Durham 1998). In most cases, imposing food restrictions may be of little practical benefit in terms of minimizing attacks and have many drawbacks in terms of potential nutritional inadequacies and further disruption to an already compromised lifestyle.

The exception is where there is sensitivity to the vasoconstrictive action of inhaled (and occasionally ingested) food additives such as sulphites, present in the gas released from fizzy drinks, and also found in red wine and home-brewed wines and beers. Avoidance of such products is an obvious remedy.

Recent speculation that dietary fatty acid composition, particularly a low consumption of omega-3 fatty acids, may influence the susceptibility to asthma and other atopic diseases remains to be substantiated (Black and Sharpe 1997; Kankaanpaa *et al.* 1999). It has also been suggested that suboptimal nutrient intake may enhance asthmatic inflammation, consequently contributing to bronchial hyperactivity (Baker and Ayres 2000), but further studies are needed to confirm this. As yet there is no convincing evidence that supplementation with vitamin C or other antioxidants is beneficial (Beilory and Gandhi 1994).

Eczemas

Atopic eczema is often associated with IgE allergies to foods such as cow's milk, egg, fish or nuts (Hill *et al.* 1999) and in some, but not all, cases dietary exclusion can alleviate symptoms. This is discussed in Section 4.33.1 (in Disorders of the skin).

Crohn's disease

The role of food intolerance in Crohn's disease has been a matter of considerable speculation but is difficult to establish because replacement of food by liquid formula diets is known to induce remission, and this remission is gradually lost following food reintroduction. There are several possible reasons for this, none of which is well understood, but which are not necessarily due to food intolerance (see Section 4.10, Inflammatory bowel disease).

Irritable bowel syndrome

IBS is a multifaceted disorder and almost certainly of multifactorial origin. There is little evidence of a systematic pathological link between food intolerance and IBS although sensitivities to foods undoubtedly exist in some cases. Many IBS patients will also believe themselves to have a food intolerance. Dietitians have an important role to play in identifying genuine intolerances but preventing unnecessary food exclusions as a result of assumed ones. The role of food intolerance in the aetiology and management of IBS is discussed in Section 4.11.3 (in Disorders of the colon).

Migraine

Pharmacologically mediated food intolerance is a known trigger of migraine in many, although not all, sufferers. Food most likely to cause problems are those containing vasoactive amines (listed under Pharmacological reactions, above). Investigation by means of diet–symptom record-keeping is a useful strategy for identifying triggers. If migraine attacks are infrequent, daily record keeping for a period of weeks or months may be impractical; in these circumstances, people should make a recalled record of all food and beverages consumed in the 24 hours prior to an attack.

One difficulty with identifying dietary triggers in migraine is that attacks usually result from a combination of factors being present at the same time. It is therefore possible for a dietary component to trigger an attack in one set of circumstances (e.g. following a period of stress) but not on another occasion. Most migraine sufferers learn to recognize which factors increase the likelihood of an attack and avoidance of known dietary triggers, particularly at times of highest risk, can help to minimize their occurrence.

An additional diet-related factor in many cases of migraine is a fall in blood glucose level as a result of prolonged periods without food or unusual levels of exercise (reactive hypoglycaemia). This is a particularly common trigger of childhood migraine.

A summary of the effects of diet and migraine can be found in COT (2000).

Hyperactivity and behavioural disorders

This remains a controversial and poorly researched subject. There are a few well-documented cases where foods have been shown to be linked with behavioural disturbance (Ferguson 1992), but a detailed review of the literature found no evidence of a systematic relationship between food intolerance and hyperkinetic disorders (Robinson and Ferguson 1992). On the rare occasions when genuine sensitivity can be shown to exist, the mechanism is probably pharmacological rather than immunologically mediated (Ferguson 1992).

Dietary measures have been reported to help some children with attention deficit hyperactivity disorder (ADHD) (Egger *et al.* 1985; Kaplan *et al.* 1989; Carter *et al.* 1993; Boris and Mandel 1994) and the conclusion of COT (2000) is that some dietary changes, but not necessarily the same ones for all children, can reduce problem behaviour in at least a few children. However, there is a need for further investigation. Current evidence of benefit tends to be based on subjective assessment (from parents and teachers) rather than objective measures of behavioural change, a nd does not always take account of the possible influence of factors such as change in the level of attention given to the child or the way in which hyperactive behaviour is handled.

Dietitians should retain an open mind when dealing with families who have a child with ADHD, and have an important role in helping parents to find out whether food plays a role or not.

Chronic disorders

There is no convincing evidence food intolerance is a systematic cause of disorders such as chronic fatigue syndrome, rheumatoid arthritis, depression and otitis media (COT 2000; Durham 1998; Manu *et al.* 1993). However, this does not preclude the possibility that, as in the general population, some people may still have a genuine food intolerance, and any such dietary concern should be taken seriously and properly investigated.

Text revised by: Briony Thomas

Acknowledgements: Sue Thurgood, Christine Carter, Gail Pollard and Christine Baker.

Useful addresses

Anaphylaxis Campaign
PO Box 149, Fleet, Hampshire GU13 9XU
Tel: 01252 542029 Fax: 01252 377140
Website: www.anaphylaxis.org.uk

British Allergy Foundation
Deepdene House, 30 Bellegrove Road, Welling, Kent DA16 3PY
Tel: 020 8303 8525 (general enquiries) or 020 8303 8583 (helpline)
Website: www.allergyfoundation.com

British Society for Allergy and Clinical Immunology
66 Weston Park, Thames Ditton, Surrey KT7 0HL
Tel: 020 8398 9240 (supply list of NHS Allergy Clinics to GPs)

Food Intolerance Databank
Leatherhead Food RA, Randalls Road, Leatherhead, Surrey KT22 7RY
Tel: 01372 376761 (01372 822217 direct line);
Fax: 01372 386228

Medic Alert (medical alert bracelets)
12 Bridge Wharf, 156 Caledonian Road, London N1 9UU
Tel: 020 7833 3034

Migraine Trust
45 Great Ormond Street, London WC1N 3HZ
Tel: 020 7831 4818

National Asthma Campaign
Providence House, Providence Place, London N1 0NT
Tel: 0345 010203

National Eczema Society
163 Eversholt Street, London NW1 1BU
Tel: 020 7388 4097

Further reading

David TJ. *Food and Food Additive Intolerance in Childhood.* Oxford: Blackwell Science, 1993.
Durham S (Ed.). *The ABC of Allergies.* London: BMJ Publications, 1998.
Metcalfe DD, Sampson HA. *Food Allergy. Adverse Rreactions to Food and Food Additives.* Oxford: Blackwell Science, 1997.

References

Asero R. Effects of birch pollen-specific immunotherapy on apple allergy in birch pollen-hypersensitive patients. *Clinical and Experimental Allergy* 1998; **28**: 1368–1373.

Astrup A, Toubro S, Cannon S *et al*. Caffeine: a double-blind, placebo-controlled study of its thermogenic, metabolic and cardiovascular effects in healthy volunteers. *American Journal of Clinical Nutrition* 1990; **51**: 759–767.

Baker JC, Ayres JG. Diet and asthma. *Respiratory Medicine* 2000; **94**: 925–934.

Baumgartner M, Brown CA, Exl BM *et al*. Controlled trials investigating the use of one partially hydrolyzed whey formula for dietary prevention of atopic manifestations until 60 months of age: an overview using meta-analytical techniques. *Nutrition Research* 1998; **18**: 1425–1442.

Bielory L, Gandhi R. Asthma and vitamin C (Review). *Annals of Allergy* 1994; **73**: 89–96.

Bindslev-Jensen C. Food allergy (Clinical review). *British Medical Journal* 1998; **316**: 1299–1302.

Bindslev-Jensen C, Poulsen LK. *In vitro* diagnostic methods in the diagnosis of food sensitivity. In Metcalfe DD, Sampson H, Simon RA (Eds) *Food Allergy: Adverse Reactions to Foods and Food additives*, 2nd edn, pp. 137–150 Oxford: Blackwell Science, 1996.

Bindslev-Jensen C, Skov PS, Madsen F, Polsen LK. Food allergy and food intolerance – what is the difference? *Annals of Allergy* 1994; **72**: 317–320.

Black PN, Sharpe S. Dietary fat and asthma: is there a connection? *European Respiratory Journal* 1997; **10**: 6–12.

Bock SA. Prospective appraisal of complaints of adverse reactions to foods in children during the first three years of life. *Pediatrics* 1987; **79**: 683–688.

Bock SA, Sampson HA, Atkins FM *et al*. Double-blind placebo-controlled food challenge as an office procedure: a manual. *Journal of Allergy and Clinical Immunology* 1988; **82**: 986–997.

Boris M, Mandel FS. Foods and additives are common causes of the attention deficit disorder in children. *Annals of Allergy* 1994; **72**: 462–467.

Brehler R, Theissen U, Mohr C, Luger T. 'Latex-fruit syndrome': frequency of cross-reacting IgE antibodies. *Allergy* 1997; **52**: 404–410.

British Dietetic Association. *Policy Statement: Food Allergy and Intolerance*. Birmingham: BDA, 1990.

Brugman E, Meulmeester KF, Spee-van der Wekke A *et al*. Prevalence of self-reported food hypersensitivity among school children in The Netherlands. *European Journal of Clinical Nutrition* 1998; **52**: 577–581.

Bruijnzeel-Koomen CAFM, Ortolani C, Aas K *et al*. Adverse reactions to foods. European Academy of Allergology and Clinical Immunology Subcommittee. *Allergy* 1995; **50**: 623–636.

Burr ML. Does infant feeding affect the risk of allergy? *Archives of Disease in Childhood* 1983; **58**: 561–563.

Burr ML, Limb ES, Maguire MJ *et al*. Infant feeding, wheezing and allergy: a prospective study. *Archives of Disease in Childhood* 1993; **68**: 724–728.

Cant AJ. Diet and the prevention of childhood allergic disease. *Human Nutrition: Applied Nutrition* 1984; **38A**: 455–468.

Carter C. Double-blind placebo-controlled food challenges: a dietitian's perspective (Comment). *Current Medical Literature-Allergy* 1995; **3**: 95–99.

Carter CM, Urbanowicz M *et al*. Effects of a few food diet of attention deficit disorder. *Archives of Disease in Childhood* 1993; **69**: 564–568.

Chandra RK. Food hypersensitivity and allergic disease: a selective review. *American Journal of Clinical Nutrition* 1997; **66**: 526S–529S.

Committee on Toxicity of Chemicals in Food, Consumer Products and the Environment (COT). *Adverse Reactions to Food and Food Ingredients*. Report of a Working Group on Food Intolerance. London: Food Standards Agency, 2000.

Consumers' Association. Food allergy testing. *Health Which?* 1998; December.

David TJ. Anaphylactic shock during elimination diets for severe atopic eczema. *Archives of Disease in Childhood* 1984; **59**: 983–986.

David TJ. Conventional allergy tests. *Archives of Disease in Childhood* 1991; **66**: 281–282.

de Jong MH, Scharp-van der Linden VTM, Aalberse RC *et al*. Randomised controlled trial of brief neonatal exposure to cow's milk on the development of atopy. *Archives of Disease in Childhood* 1998; **79**: 126–130.

Department of Health. *Weaning and the Weaning Diet*. Report on Health and Social Subjects 45. London: HMSO, 1994.

Department of Health, Committee on Toxicity of Chemicals in Food, Consumer Products and the Environment. *Peanut Allergy*. London: DH, 1998.

Durham S (Ed.). *The ABC of Allergies*. London: BMJ Publications, 1998.

Egger J, Carter C, Graham P *et al*. Controlled trial of oligoantigenic diet in the hyperkinetic syndrome. *Lancet* 1985; **i**: 540–545.

ESPGAN. Comment on antigen-reduced infant formulae. *Acta Paediatrica* 1993; **82**: 314–319.

Ewan PW. Clinical study of peanut and nut allergy in 62 consecutive patients: new features and associations. *British Medical Journal* 1996; **312**: 1074–1078.

Ferguson A. Definitions and diagnosis of food intolerance and food allergy – consensus and controversy. *Journal of Pediatrics* 1992; **121** (5 Suppl Part 2): S7–S11.

Foster K, Lader D, Cheeseborough S. *Infant Feeding: 1995*. London: The Stationery Office, 1997.

Gerrard JW. Allergy in breast fed babies to ingredients in breast milk. *Annals of Allergy* 1979; **42**: 69–72.

Halken S, Host A, Hansen LG, Osterballe O. Effect of an allergy prevention programme on incidence of atopic symptoms in infancy. A prospective study of 159 'high-risk' infants. *Allergy* 1992; **47**: 545–553.

Hathaway MJ, Warner JO. Compliance problems in the dietary management of eczema. *Archives of Disease in Childhood* 1983; **59**: 151–156.

Hattevig G, Sigurs N, Kjellman B. Effects of maternal dietary avoidance during lactation on allergy in children at 10 years of age. *Acta Paediatrica* 1999; **88**: 7–12.

Hill DJ, Hosking CS, Heine RG. Clinical spectrum of food allergy in children in Australia and South East Asia: identification and targets for treatment. *Annals of Medicine* 1999; **31**: 272–281.

Host A. Cows' milk allergy. *Journal of the Royal Society of Medicine* 1997; **90** (Suppl 30): 34–39.

Host A, Jacobsen HP, Halken S, Holmenlund S. The natural history of cow's milk protein allergy/intolerance. *European Journal of Clinical Nutrition* 1995; **49** (Suppl 1): S13–S18.

Hourihane J O'B, Roberts SA, Warner JO. Resolution of peanut allergy: case–control study. *British Medical Journal* 1998; **316**: 1271–1275.

Huijbers GB, Colen AA, Jansen JJ *et al*. Masking foods for food challenge: practical aspects of masking foods for a double-blind, placebo-controlled food challenge. *Journal of the American Dietetic Association* 1994; **94**: 645–649.

Isolauri E, Turjanmara K. Combined skin prick and patch testing enhances identification of food allergy in infants with atopic dermatitis. *Journal of Allergy and Clinical Immunology* 1996; **97**: 9–15.

Jansen JJ, Kardinaal AF, Huijbers G *et al*. Prevalence of food allergy and intolerance in the adult Dutch population. *Journal of Allergy and Clinical Immunology* 1994; **93**: 446–456.

Kankaapaa P, Sutas Y, Salminen S *et al*. Dietary fatty acids and allergy. *Annals of Medicine* 1999; **31**: 282–287.

Kaplan BJ, McNichol J *et al*. Dietary replacement in preschool-aged hyperactive boys. *Pediatrics* 1989; **83**: 7–17.

Kay AB, Lessof MH. Allergy: conventional and alternative concepts. A report of the Royal College of Physicians Committee on Clinical Immunology and Allergy. *Clinical and Experimental Allergy* 1992; **22** (Suppl 3): 1–44.

Kilgallen I, Gibney MJ. Parental perception of food allergy or intolerance in children under 4 years of age. *Journal of Human Nutrition and Dietetics* 1996; **9**: 473–478.

King TS, Elia M, Hunter JO. Abnormal colon fermentation in irritable bowel syndrome. *Lancet* 1998; **352**: 1187–1189.

Kirjavainen PV, Apostolou E, Salminenen SJ, Isolauri E. New aspects of probiotics – a novel approach in the management of food allergy. *Allergy* 1999; **54**: 909–915.

Kramer MS. Maternal antigen avoidance during pregnancy for preventing atopic disease in infants of women at high risk (Cochrane Review). In *The Cochrane Library*, Issue 2. Oxford: Update Software, 1999a.

Kramer MS. Maternal antigen avoidance during lactation for preventing atopic disease in infants of women at high risk (Cochrane Review). In *The Cochrane Library*, Issue 2. Oxford: Update Software, 1999b.

Labib M, Garna R, Wright J *et al*. Dietary maladvice as a cause of hypothyroidism and short stature. *British Medical Journal* 1989; **298**: 232–233.

Lehman CW. The leucocyte food allergy test: a study of its reliability and reproducibility. *Annals of Allergy* 1980; **45**: 150–158.

Lessof MH, Wraith DG, Merrett TG *et al*. Food allergy and intolerance in 100 patients: local and systemic effects. *Quarterly Journal of Medicine* 1980; **49**: 259–271.

Macdonald A, Forsythe WI. The cost of nutrition and diet therapy for low income families. *Human Nutrition: Applied Nutrition* 1986; **40A**: 87–96.

MAFF Food Safety Directorate. *Food Allergy and Other Unpleasant Reactions to Food*. London: MAFF, 1997.

Mallet E, Henocq A. Long-term prevention of allergic diseases by using protein hydrolysate formula in at-risk infants. *Journal of Pediatrics* 1992; **121**: S95–100.

Manu P, Matthews DA, Lane TJ. Food intolerance in patients with chronic fatigue. *International Journal of Eating Disorders* 1993; **13**: 203–209.

Miskelly FG, Burr ML, Vaughan Williams E *et al*. Infant feeding and allergy. *Archives of Disease in Childhood* 1988; **63**: 388–393.

National Dairy Council. *Topical Update 2: Adverse Reactions to Food*. London: NDC, 1998.

Novembre E, de Martino M *et al*. Foods and respiratory allergy. *Journal of Allergy and Clinical Immunology* 1988; **81**: 1059–65.

Onorato J, Merland N *et al*. Placebo-controlled double-blind food challenges in asthma. *Journal of Allergy and Clinical Immunology* 1986; **78**: 1139–46.

Patel L, Radivan FS *et al*. Management of anaphylactic reactions to food. *Archives of Disease in Childhood* 1994; **71**: 370–375.

Parker TJ, Naylor SJ, Riordan AM, Hunter JO. Management of patients with food intolerance in irritable bowel syndrome: the development and use of an exclusion diet. *Journal of Human Nutrition and Dietetics* 1995; **8**: 159–166.

Pearl ER. Food allergy. *Lipincotts Primary Care Practice* 1997; **1**: 154–167.

Robinson J, Ferguson A. Food sensitivity and the nervous system: hyperactivity, addiction and criminal behaviour. *Nutrition Research Reviews* 1992; **5**: 203–223.

Royal College of Physicians of London/British Nutrition Foundation. Food intolerance and food aversion. *Journal of Royal College of Physicians of London* 1984; **18**: 83–123.

Royal College of Physicians, Committee on Clinical Immunology and Allergy. Allergy: conventional and alternative concepts. Summary of a report. *Journal of the Royal College of Physicians of London* 1992; **26**: 260–264.

Royal College of Physicians/Royal College of Pathologists. Good allergy practice – standards of care for providers and purchasers of allergy services within the National Health Service. *Clinical and Experimental Allergy* 1995; **25**: 586–595.

Saarinen UM, Kajosaari M. Breastfeeding as prophylaxis against atopic disease: prospective follow-up study until 17 years old. *Lancet* 1995; **346**: 1065–1069.

Sampson H. Food allergy. Part 2: Diagnosis and management. *Journal of Allergy and Clinical Immunology* 1999; **103**: 981–989.

Schwartz RAH. Allergy, intolerance and other adverse reactions to foods. *Pediatric Annals* 1992; **21**: 654–655, 660–662, 665–674.

Sicherer SH. Food allergy: when and how to perform oral food challenges. *Pediatric Allergy and Immunology* 1999; **10**: 226–234.

Tariq SM, Stevens M, Matthews S *et al*. Cohort study of peanut and tree nut sensitisation by age of 4 years. *British Medical Journal* 1996; **313**: 514–517.

Witherley S. Soya formulas are not hypoallergenic. *American Journal of Clinical Nutrition* 1990; **51**: 705–706.

Wolfe SP. 'Prevention programmes' – a dietetic minefield. *European Journal of Clinical Nutrition* 1995; **49** (Suppl 1): S92–S99.

Wraith DG, Merret TG . Recognition of food-allergic patients and their allergens by the RAST technique and clinical investigation. *Clinical Allergy* 1979; **9**: 25–36.

Wuthrich B. Adverse reactions to food additives. *Annals of Allergy* 1993; **71**: 379–384.

Young E, Stoneham MD, Petruckevitch A *et al*. A population study of food intolerance. *Lancet* 1994; **343**: 1127–1130.

4.35 Food exclusion in the management of allergy and intolerance

4.35.1 General aspects of food exclusion diets

Food exclusion may be necessary to diagnose and treat food allergy or intolerance (see Section 4.34). In some instances, identification of sources of a particular food (e.g. shellfish) is relatively easy. In others, where the item is a ubiquitous ingredient in a wide range of manufactured foods (e.g. nuts, wheat and soya) its complete exclusion can be exceedingly difficult.

The nutritional implications resulting from food avoidance must also be considered. Avoidance of a single food or type of food (such as citrus fruit) will be of little significance if nutritionally similar foods (e.g. other fruit and vegetables) can be eaten instead. However, if food avoidance necessitates excluding most or all of a whole group of foods (e.g. milk and dairy products, or most foods in the bread and cereals group) the nutritional impact will be considerable unless measures are taken to avert this. In addition, exclusion of a food which in itself is not nutritionally significant (such as soya or nut) but which is widely present in manufactured foods, may have a considerable knock-on effect on overall dietary balance as a result of the constraints on food choice.

It is important that food exclusions are never imposed unnecessarily. Food 'allergy' is a fashionable ailment among the general public and self-imposed food restriction, often resulting in highly unbalanced diets, is common (see Section 4.34). When food avoidance is indicated, it is vital that people receive expert dietetic guidance in order to do this effectively and ensure that their nutritional intake is not compromised.

It should also be borne in mind that some types of food intolerance remit with time (e.g. many children grow out of cow's milk protein allergy and some forms of food intolerance in adults are transient). The necessity for dietary exclusion should therefore be reviewed at intervals so that dietary restrictions are not imposed for longer than necessary.

The UK Food Intolerance Databank

Identifying ingredients in manufactured foods is not always easy. Some components may be listed in a form which is not immediately obvious to the consumer, e.g. that 'caseinates' or 'lactoglobulin' are milk derivatives. The food origin of other ingredients may not be declared, e.g. the additive lecithin could be derived from either soya or egg. However, following amendments to the Food Labelling Regulations in 1998, the origin of 'starch' or 'modified starch' (e.g. whether derived from wheat or maize) now has to be declared to assist people with gluten or wheat intolerance. Manufactured foods may also contain hidden food components in the form of compound ingredients. If a compound ingredient (e.g. 'sponge' in a trifle) comprises less than 25% of the finished product, the individual components (e.g. egg, wheat flour) do not have to be listed (only any additives present). This has been a particular problem in the identification of peanut/nut components in foods and, to assist people who need to avoid them, many food manufacturers now voluntarily state on food labels when these are present.

To help to overcome some of the problems in identifying specific components of foods, a UK Food Intolerance Databank was set up in 1987 as a central source of information on manufactured foods. This is co-ordinated by the Leatherhead Food Research Association in conjunction with the Food and Drink Federation and the British Dietetic Association (BDA). The services of the databank are available to all state registered dietitians and hospital physicians. The databank currently compiles information on manufactured foods which are free from:

- cow's milk and milk derivatives
- egg and egg derivatives
- wheat and wheat derivatives
- soya and soya derivatives
- BHA and BHT
- sulphur dioxide
- benzoates
- azo colours.

Lists of manufactured foods free from one or certain combinations of these components are produced annually by the BDA but only made available to state registered dietitians to ensure that they are used in conjunction with appropriate dietary advice. Dietitians may also request unpublished lists of other combinations of the above ingredients directly from the databank.

The databank does have some limitations. Some food manufacturers do not participate because of the costs involved; there are also concerns that the databank is not updated frequently enough to be sufficiently reliable. The databank does not include information on gluten-free manufactured foods, as this is available from the Coeliac Society. Foods free from nuts or peanuts are also not included in the databank at the present time. Additional information on foods free from specified ingredients can often be obtained directly from supermarkets and food manufacturers.

4.35.2 Milk exclusion

Allergy or intolerance to milk can result from a number of causes. Since exclusion of milk has serious nutritional implications, particularly in infants and children, and can be difficult to achieve in practice, such a measure should always be overseen by a dietitian. Although there are common features in the management of milk-intolerant disorders, there are difference in the type, extent and duration of milk exclusion required.

Cow's milk protein allergy/intolerance

Allergy or intolerance to cow's milk protein is characterized by gastrointestinal symptoms such as vomiting, diarrhoea, irritability and general failure to thrive (Host 1994). It is commonly associated with a family history of atopy and can exacerbate atopic symptoms such as eczema, asthma and rhinitis (Host 1997). It usually develops early in infancy when the permeability of the gastrointestinal mucosa is greatest, and soon after exposure to cow's milk infant formula (Host and Halken 1990). Onset after the age of 12 months is rare. The risk is greatly reduced by exclusive breast feeding, but may not prevent it altogether since a minority of infants are capable of reacting to low doses of maternal dietary antigens present in breast milk (Isolauri et al. 1998).

The estimated incidence of the disorder, based on strict diagnostic criteria, has been estimated to be about 2–3% in the general infant population (Host et al. 1995). Unlike other diet-induced enteropathies such as coeliac disease, there is no evidence of a dominant human leucocyte antigen (HLA) type in cow's milk protein sensitivities and it affects all ethnic groups equally.

Despite the frequency and clinical importance of cow's milk-induced disease, much remains to be learnt about its pathological mechanisms. The disorder is often divided into cow's milk protein allergy (CMPA), where there is clear evidence of immunological involvement, and cow's milk protein intolerance (CMPI) where no immunological basis can be found. However, it has become increasingly apparent that immune basis of the disease is complex and that immunologically mediated reactions can involve a number of epitopes on one or more milk proteins, and trigger any of the four main types of allergic reaction (Host 1994; Ortolani and Vighi 1995) (see Sectin 4.34.3). Hill and Hosking (1995) identified three groups with characteristic symptom and laboratory profiles:

- those with clear immunoglobulin E (IgE) involvement, who may exhibit a classic type 1 response to cow's milk featuring cutaneous eruptions and, sometimes, anaphylaxis;
- those with evidence of delayed type III (immune complex) reactions, who develop gastrointestinal symptoms within hours of ingesting moderate amounts of cow's milk;
- those with evidence of type IV (cell-mediated) reactions, who develop gastrointestinal symptoms several hours or

days after ingesting cow's milk, often accompanied by respiratory or eczematous symptoms.

Some of these types may exist in combination.

Other variants of milk intolerance may exist, some of which may have no immunological involvement. However, since commonly performed diagnostic tests such as skin-tests prick or radio allergosorbent tests (RAST) may only identify IgE-mediated reactions, it is likely that some forms of allergic reactions will be missed (Host et al. 1995). In practice this is immaterial since whatever the underlying mechanism, the treatment of cow's milk protein allergy or intolerance is the same, i.e. complete dietary exclusion of cow's milk protein.

Nevertheless, because the imposition of a milk-free diet has many nutritional implications, it is important that CMPA/CMPI is correctly diagnosed, and distinguished from non-milk-related disorders such as infantile colic or reflux, which may produce similar symptoms. Since, at present, laboratory tests are incapable of identifying all forms of cow's milk protein sensitivity, accurate diagnosis and confirmation depend on milk protein elimination and challenge procedures. The withdrawal of cow's milk for a period of up to 3 weeks is followed by its reintroduction to see whether symptoms reappear. Because of the risk of hypersensitivity and immediate reaction in some cases, milk challenges must always be conducted under controlled conditions where there are facilities for resuscitation. In most cases, any reactions will be apparent within 4–7 days (Hill et al. 1995).

If symptoms do not improve this may be because:

- the child's symptoms are unconnected with milk
- the child is intolerant to other foods (or inhalants) as well as milk
- the diet has not been entirely milk free.

The prognosis of CMPA/CMPI is good, with remission rates of about 45–50% at 1 year, 60–75% at 2 years and 85–90% at 3 years (Host 1994). It is most likely to persist in those with a strong family history of atopy, IgE-mediated reactions and other food allergies (such as to eggs, soya, peanuts or citrus fruits) (Schrander et al. 1992; Host et al. 1995; Iacono et al. 1998).

Management of cow's milk protein allergy/intolerance

Treatment is by complete avoidance of cow's milk protein, and in non-breast fed infants a nutritionally complete substitute formula will be required. Since many infants will also be intolerant of soya-based milk substitutes (Host 1997), a hydrolysed milk protein formula is usually prescribed (Merritt et al. 1990; Hide and Gant 1994) (Table 4.74).

A minority of infants who are highly sensitive to cow's milk protein can still react to residual epitopes present in hydrolysed protein formulae or breast milk (Hide and Gant 1994; Maldonado et al. 1998) and will require a more extensively hydrolysed or elemental infant formula (Hill

Table 4.74 Nutritionally complete milk substitutes for use in milk-intolerant disorders

Type of milk-intolerant disorder	Product type	Product name (manufacturer)
Cow's milk protein allergy/intolerance (with or without associated lactose intolerance)	*The choice of product depends on the age of the child, the level of sensitivity to milk and the presence of coexisting allergies. Check compositional details and prescribing indications for suitability*	
	Soya-based formulae	Farley's Soya Formula (Farleys)
		Infasoy (Cow & Gate)
		Isomil (Ross)
		Nutrison Soya (Cow & Gate)
		Prosobee (Mead Johnson)
		Wysoy (Wyeth)
	Casein-hydrolysate formulae	Nutramigen (Bristol-Myers)
		Pregestimil (Bristol-Myers)
	Whey-hydrolysate formulae	Alfare (Nestlé Clinical)
		Pepti Junior (Cow & Gate)
		Pepdite (SHS)
		Pepdite 1+ (SHS)
	Elemental/hypoallergenic formulae	Neocate (SHS)
		Prejomin (Milupa)
Lactose intolerance only	*Some of the above products may also be suitable; check prescribing indications*	
	Infant formulae (not cow's milk protein free)	Enfamil Lactofree (Mead Johnson)
		SMA LF (SMA)
	For older children intolerant to lactose or galactose (not cow's milk protein free)	AL110 (Nestlé)
Congenital disorders	*Some of the above products may also be suitable; check prescribing indications*	
Galactosaemia and galactokinase deficiency	Infant formula	Galactomin 17 (Cow & Gate)
Glucose–galactose intolerance	Infant formula	Galactomin 19 (Cow & Gate)

Data compiled September 2000. Note: other products may be available.
Further details of products currently available and their prescribing indications can be found in the British National Formulary or the Monthly Index of Medical Specialities (MIMS) or obtained directly from the manufacturers (for addresses see Appendix 6.9).

et al. 1995, 1999; McLeish *et al.* 1995). However, these are expensive and have an unpleasant taste so should not be used unnecessarily (MacDonald 1995).

Since CMPI is commonly accompanied by secondary lactose intolerance at the time of diagnosis, such infant formulae are also lactose free. The lactose intolerance usually resolves within a few weeks of withdrawal of cow's milk protein, once villous atrophy has been corrected.

Once solid food is introduced into the diet, care has to be taken that it remains free of cow's milk protein, not only from obvious sources such as dairy products but also from its less obvious presence in many manufactured foods. Parents will require guidance on the types of foods likely to contain milk protein and on how to identify the presence of milk derivatives from food labelling information (Tables 4.75 and 4.76). In children with CMPA/CMPI, common allergens such as eggs, wheat, nuts and citrus fruits should not be introduced into the weaning diet before the age of 6 months (DH 1994) (see Prevention of food allergy in Section 4.34.3).

Table 4.75 General guidance for milk exclusion

Exclude	Examples	Notes
Cow's milk	Liquid whole, semi-skimmed or skimmed milk Evaporated or condensed milk Dried full-fat or skimmed milk powder	Goat's and sheep's milk can be used by some older children and adults intolerant to cow's milk protein. They are unsuitable for people requiring total exclusion of lactose or galactose
Dairy products	Butter Margarine or fat spreads containing milk derivatives Cheese and cheese spreads Yoghurt Fromage frais Crème fraiche Cream	Butter and hard cheeses can be used by people with mild or moderate lactose intolerance
Milk or milk derivatives in manufactured foods; components in manufactured foods	May be described on ingredients lists as: milk, milk solids, non-fat milk solids Milk protein, skimmed milk, skimmed milk powder Casein or caseinates Whey, whey solids, buttermilk *Lactose, milk sugar, whey sugar, whey syrup sweetener	*It may not be necessary to exclude lactose and other milk sugars in all cases of cow's milk protein intolerance but, for practical purposes, their presence is usually taken as indicative of the presence of milk, and foods containing them are excluded

Table 4.76 Types of manufactured foods which are particularly likely to contain milk or milk derivatives (This list is far from exhaustive and all food labels must be checked carefully)

Food type	Examples
Cereal foods	Bread and rolls
	Breakfast cereals
	Cakes
	Biscuits and crackers
	Pizza
	Pasta (both fresh and canned)
Fruit and vegetables	Vegetables canned in sauce (e.g. spaghetti in tomato sauce)
	Instant potato
	Baked beans
Meat, fish and alternatives	Meat and fish products, e.g. beefburgers, fish fingers, sausages, ready meals
Other savoury items	Canned and packet soups
	Instant gravies
	Sauces
	Crisps and savoury snack foods
Desserts	Instant desserts
	Dairy desserts
	Ice-cream
	Custards
Confectionery	Chocolate
	Toffee
	Fudge
	Caramel
Fats and spreads	Margarines and fat spreads
Beverages	Drinking chocolate
	Malted milk drinks
	Coffee whiteners

Annually updated lists of manufactured foods free from milk and milk products (constructed from the UK Food Intolerance Databank) are available to dietitians via the British Dietetic Association.

Young children will continue to need a nutritionally complete cow's milk substitute (Table 4.74). The choice of substitute will depend on the age of the patient, the range of foods included in the diet and the quantity consumed. Casein hydrolysate milks, for example, have a strong taste and smell and may be unacceptable to a young child drinking from an open feeding cup, particularly if the milk intolerance develops after the child has become accustomed to the taste of cow's milk. Soya-based milk substitutes are more palatable but are contraindicated in those with soya allergy.

In older children and adults, goat's or sheep's milk can sometimes be used as an alternative, although some people will also react to the proteins in these milks. These milks have a low folate content and can be microbiologically unsafe (DH 1994). Non-prescribable soya milk substitutes sold in health shops and supermarkets are not nutritionally equivalent to cow's milk. However, for those not allergic to soya, these substitutes for yoghurt and dairy desserts can help to make a milk-free diet more socially acceptable.

The risk of nutritional deficiencies (particularly energy and calcium) as a result of milk avoidance is high (David 1995) and delayed growth in children with CMPA has been reported (Isolauri *et al.* 1998). For this reason, it is important that the need for milk exclusion is clearly established and that it is managed under expert dietetic guidance. In some instances, other food allergies will also develop and particular dietetic skills will be needed to ensure that the additional food exclusions do not compromise nutritional adequacy.

Reintroduction of milk

CMPA/CMPI is usually transitory and it is important that milk is not excluded from a child's diet for longer than necessary. The timing of reintroduction will vary according to the clinical circumstances, but the majority of cases will have resolved by the age of 3 years. However, if previous reactions have been severe type I reactions, or other food allergies have developed, reintroduction should be delayed for longer, and always under medical supervision. Because of the risk of enhanced reaction after a period of withdrawal, ideally all reintroductions should be medically supervised but, in practice, milk reintroduction often happens inadvertently and the dietitian discovers from dietary enquiry that the child has already consumed foods containing small amounts of cow's milk.

Persistence into childhood and adulthood necessitates permanent exclusion of cow's milk.

Lactose-intolerant disorders

Lactose intolerance results from an impaired ability to absorb either lactose or its component monosaccharides, resulting in symptoms of malabsorption (see Lactose malabsorption in Section 4.8.2). It can result from:

- *hereditary alactasia*: an extremely rare disorder characterized by complete absence of the digestive enzyme lactase and necessitating total lactose exclusion;
- *primary lactase deficiency*: a common disorder in particular racial groups where there is a reduction in lactase activity after infancy. Unless there is unusual sensitivity, lactose intake only needs to be reduced to individual levels of tolerance, not excluded altogether;
- *secondary lactase deficiency*: usually a temporary disorder following gastrointestinal infection, damage or resection which results in impaired villous lactase production. It is a common accompaniment to CMPI at the time of diagnosis. Lactose restriction is usually only required for a matter of weeks until either villi have regrown or the body has adapted to a reduced capacity for enzyme production.

If lactose needs to be excluded, food avoidance measures are almost the same as for exclusion of cow's milk protein (see above). The main differences with lactose exclusion regimens are that:

- Sheep's and goat's milk are contraindicated because they contain lactose.
- Sources of lactose in pharmaceutical preparations (e.g. as a filler in tablets) must be avoided if total exclusion if required.

- Dairy foods with a low lactose content such as butter and hard cheeses can usually be consumed by people with primary or secondary lactose intolerence. Yoghurt and other fermented milk products may also be well tolerated.
- Commercially available lactose-reduced milks may be useful for those with temporary or partial lactose intolerance. They are not suitable for those with congenital alactasia.

If total and prolonged (or permanent) lactose exclusion is required, the nutritional implications will also be the same as for cow's milk protein avoidance. Short-term lactose avoidance or reduction in lactose intake does not pose the same level of risk although, if the patient is a child, it is important that the nutritional adequacy of the diet is monitored.

Management of lactose intolerance is discussed in more detail in Section 4.8.2.

Congenital disorders of monosaccharide metabolism

Rare inherited disorders such as galactosaemia and galactokinase deficiency, where the ability to metabolize absorbed galactose is blocked, necessitate total and strict exclusion of dietary lactose, galactose, and in the case of glucose–galactose intolerance, glucose. These conditions require intervention soon after birth in order to prevent life-threatening damage, and require specialist dietetic management. Breast feeding is contraindicated and infant formulae specifically formulated for these disorders will be required. Readers are referred to paediatric texts for further details.

4.35.3 Peanut and nut exclusion

Allergy to peanuts (and other types of nuts and seeds) is the most serious forms of food allergy to emerge in recent years. Sensitivity is often extreme, with minute amounts of the allergen being capable of triggering a rapid and severe type I allergic response causing acute oropharyngeal swelling and systemic circulatory effects which can result in asphyxiation and fatal anaphylaxis. In the UK, about six deaths, usually in young people, occur each year as a result of peanut anaphylaxis and many near-fatal episodes occur (Assem 1990; Ewan 1996).

The prevalence of peanut allergy has increased in recent years and has reported to be in the region of 1.3% (Tariq et al. 1996). The age of onset also appears to be decreasing and it is increasingly being reported during the first year of life (Hourihane et al. 1996; Ewan 1996). The rise in prevalence is probably due to increased exposure, due to widespread use of peanuts in food manufacture. Exposure to peanuts via such foods is also likely to occur at a much earlier age than would have been the case a few decades ago. However, the reason why peanuts and nut derivatives are so allergenic remains unknown.

Although the peanut is botanically a legume (pulse), symptomatic allergy to other pulses such as peas, beans and lentils is rare (probably fewer than 5% of cases; Bernhisel-Broadbent and Sampson 1989). There may, however, be a small but distinct subgroup of peanut-allergic patients who are allergic not only to pulses but to many other fruit and vegetables and to sesame (Ewan 1996).

Peanut allergy is commonly associated with allergy to tree nuts, especially Brazil nuts, almonds, hazelnuts and walnuts (Ewan 1996). Different patterns of sensitization occur; in very young children the allergy is nearly always exclusively to peanuts, whereas multiple nut allergies are more common in older children. Although it is possible to identify individual nut allergies via specific IgE testing, there is always a possibility that a provoking nut allergen may not have been tested or that a new sensitivity has developed (Pumphrey and Stanworth 1996). For this reason, and also because of the risk of inadvertent consumption of a nut allergen via other nut mixtures, in practice, any type of peanut or nut allergy should always be treated by total exclusion of all nuts.

In contrast to most other childhood allergies, peanut allergy is less likely to be outgrown. Whereas the majority of children lose their sensitivity to eggs or cow's milk, only about 10% appear to develop tolerance to peanuts (Hourihane et al. 1998). Age of onset may be an important predictor of its persistence; the condition is much more likely to resolve if it appears before the age of 3 years. It is less likely to resolve if it develops in older children or adults, or if other IgE-mediated food allergies coexist (Hourihane et al. 1998; Bock and Atkins 1989).

Like most true food allergies, peanut allergy has strong genetic links and is more likely to occur in families with a history of atopic conditions such as asthma, eczema or hayfever or other type I allergic reactions. Owing to the severity of the condition, and because sensitization to peanuts may occur *in utero* or via breast feeding, the Department of Health (1998) suggests that:

- Pregnant or breast-feeding women with atopic or other diagnosed allergic disease, or if the father or sibling of the child has a clinical history of such disease, should avoid eating peanuts or peanut-containing products. It is not considered necessary for women with no direct or family history of allergic disease to avoid peanuts.
- Infants in a family with a history of atopy or allergic disease should be exclusively breast fed for the first 4–6 months of life and should not be given peanut-containing products until the age of 3 years. No child under the age of 5 years should be given whole peanuts because of the risk of choking.

However, these are precautionary measures and further research is being conducted to evaluate their effectiveness and necessity.

It has also been suggested that any infant or child found to have peanut-specific IgE antibodies but no overt symptoms should avoid all peanut and nut products for 3–5 years (Sampson 1996). If no reactions to inadvertent ingestion have occurred during this time, the child should be re-evaluated for evidence of peanut- and nut-specific IgE antibodies and clinical reactivity to peanuts.

Because of the dietary constraints, and parental anxiety, which result from a diagnosis of peanut allergy, it has been suggested that children with early-onset peanut allergy, or if there has been any doubt about the diagnosis, should undergo challenge procedures as they approach school age to discover whether the allergy has resolved (Hourihane *et al.* 1998). It is, however, imperative that this is done under controlled conditions in hospital under expert medical supervision, and may not be advisable at all in those who have previously had severe or anaphylactic reactions. It should be borne in mind that the pattern of previous reactions in an individual does not necessarily predict the severity of future reactions, so some risk will always remain.

Management of peanut and nut allergy

Expert dietetic guidance is essential for anyone with peanut and nut allergy because of the widespread use of nut and nut derivatives in manufactured foods and because of the potential consequences of inadvertent consumption. As well as avoiding ingestion of peanut (which in practice means avoiding all types of nuts), sufferers have to take measures to avoid its inhalation (e.g. via peanut particles in the air) or absorption through the skin (via direct contact with peanut-containing foods or some topical creams or ointments). Because the risk of inadvertent exposure is so high, with as many as 25% of patients experiencing an accidental ingestion per year (Sampson 1996), it is vital that all nut-allergic patients and their carers carry and know how to administer adrenaline.

Many manufactured food products contain peanuts or nuts or derivatives, often as part of compound ingredients which may not be separately listed on an ingredients list. Most responsible manufacturers now follow a voluntary code of practice and state when a product contains peanuts or nuts, or may do so as a result of cross-contamination during manufacture. However, the absence of such a declaration cannot be taken as proof that a food is peanut free. Changes to international food labelling legislation are being considered to ensure that the presence of peanut protein in all foods is declared, whatever its concentration.

The suitability of foods containing peanut oil has been a matter of some debate. It now seems clear that refined, deodorized peanut oil does not pose a risk because it does not contain protein particles and does not provoke reactions in peanut-sensitive individuals (Hourihane *et al.* 1997). However, crude or cold-pressed peanut oil can contain sufficient protein to be a risk to a some, although not all, peanut-sensitive individuals (Hourihane *et al.* 1997). In practice, the vast majority of manufactured foods will only contain refined peanut oil (either alone or in combination with other oils and described as 'vegetable oil'). Crude or cold-pressed oils, which have a strong taste and smell, are more likely to be encountered as 'gourmet' oils sold in delicatessen or specialist food outlets, or in restaurants serving food containing such oils, particularly Thai,

Chinese, Indonesian or Indian dishes. In the UK, the refiners of edible oils have instituted a code of practice to ensure that the presence of unrefined oils in manufactured food products (occasionally added to create a peanut flavour) is declared. The absence of such a statement can therefore be taken to mean that the food is safe for people with peanut allergy. However, this will not apply to foods produced or sold abroad.

The food emulsifiers E471 and 472a–e may be derived from peanut oil but are not thought to pose a hazard as they are derived from refined oil. For the same reason, the food additive lecithin is unlikely to contain peanut protein.

Dietary sources of nuts and peanuts are summarized in Table 4.77. *Any* manufactured food should be considered a source of peanuts or nuts until it is known that this is not the case. Nut-allergic patients also require dietary guidance concerning:

- *Eating out and takeaway foods*: Detailed ingredients listing is unlikely to be available and there may also be a risk of cross-contamination as a result of poor food preparation practices in the kitchen (e.g. the same cooking utensils or pans used to prepare peanut-containing and non-peanut containing foods). Particular caution is needed when eating in Oriental restaurants as the use of peanut-containing products is common and the risk of inadvertent consumption is high.
- *Airborne contamination*: Some people can react to airborne peanut particles and this is a particular hazard on aeroplane flights where the peanut dust from, for example, someone opening a packet of peanuts will circulate throughout the cabin. Some airlines no longer serve peanuts for this reason, or will agree not to do so on request.
- *Foreign travel*: Lack of, or different rules regarding, food ingredient declarations plus language difficulties can make it very difficult to identify the presence of peanuts. In addition, some brands of products (particularly confectionery) which are nut free in the UK may not be nut free when produced and purchased in other countries, even if they have the same brand name. In parts of Europe, some infant formulae or vitamin D preparations may contain peanut protein (De Montis *et al.* 1993; Moneret-Vautrin and Kanny 1994;), whereas this is unlikely to be a risk with UK-produced products. Allergy sufferers should be advised to consume foods which are as identifiable as possible and usually known to be safe. Other precautions such as learning the word for 'peanut' or 'nuts' in the relevant foreign language, wearing Medic Alert identification and always carrying anti-anaphylactic equipment are strongly recommended.

The Anaphylaxis Campaign provides useful advice to people with peanut allergy, much of it now available on its website (see Useful addresses at the end of this section).

4.35.4 Soya exclusion

Soya can provoke IgE-mediated reactions (Sampson 1988) and in young children can exacerbate atopic dermatitis (see Section 4.33.1, Atopic eczema).

Table 4.77 Guidance for peanut and nut avoidance

Exclude	Examples	Notes

Peanuts and nuts	Peanut
	Brazil
	Walnut
	Hazelnut
	Almond
	Cashew
	Pistachio
	Pecans
		Some of these may be described as:
		  Ground nuts
		  Monkey nuts
		  Earth nuts
		  Goober nuts

Foods made from peanuts/nuts	Peanut butter
	Nut spreads
	Praline
	Noisette
	Marzipan
	Frangipan
	Amaretto products
	Macaroons
	Bakewell tarts
	Almond essence
	Marron
	Worcester sauce
	Satay sauce
	Hydrolysed vegetable protein
	
	Nut-containing or nut-coated cheeses
	Cold-pressed 'gourmet' oils:
	  Peanut oil
	  Arachis oil
	  Groundnut oil
	  Walnut oil
	  Almond oil
	  Hazelnut oil
		
		Usually made from hazelnuts but mixed nuts can be used
		Contain almonds but cheaper brands may contain
		  peanut flour as an extender
		
		Made from chestnuts but other nuts may be included
		Contains walnuts
		Contains peanuts
		This is most likely to be of soya or wheat origin but can
		  be derived from peanut
		
		Refined oils present in manufactured foods or sold as
		  cooking oils are free from nut protein

Manufactured foods containing traces of peanuts/nuts	This can include almost any food, but particularly:
	  Cakes, biscuits and pastries
	  Ice-cream, desserts and dessert toppings
	  Cereal bars and confectionery
	  Savoury snack foods
	  Breakfast cereals, especially muesli or nut mixtures
	  Meat products, vegetarian products and ready
	    meals containing hydrolysed vegetable protein
	  Oriental (particularly Chinese, Thai, Indonesian)
	    foods (especially curries)
	  Sauces and salad dressings
	  Mixed salads
	  Wild rice
		All manufactured foods should be considered a source
		of peanuts/nuts until it is known that this is not the case

Most people with peanut allergy are advised to avoid all types of nuts because of the risk of contamination with peanut products and because coexisting allergies to tree nuts may not have been identified.

The soya bean is a legume containing about 38% protein and 24% fat (of high polyunsaturated content) and its derivatives are widely used by the food industry. It is commonly used as a binder in the form of a flour, either derived from the whole bean or after extraction of some or all of the fat. Soya protein isolate can also be spun into a product of similar texture to meat (hydrolysed or textured vegetable protein) which is used as a meat extender or replacement for meat in vegetarian dishes. Soya derivatives such as lecithin are commonly used as emulsifiers and stabilizers.

In recent years soya products originating from the Far East such as soya sauce and soya bean curd (tofu) have become more readily available in the UK. Oriental cuisine containing them has also become increasingly popular.

As many as 60% of manufactured foods contain soya and hence its avoidance significantly curtails food choice. Its presence may be indicated as:

• soya beans
• soya flour
• soya protein, gum or starch
• textured (or hydrolysed) vegetable protein
• soya sauces
• soya flavouring
• soya lecithin (E322).

Soya oil or soya shortening need not be excluded from soya-free diets because soya oil used in food manufacturing is refined and deodorized and considered to be free from protein. Soya lecithin derived from such oil is also probably protein free but is still currently classified as a soya ingredient by the UK Food Intolerance Databank. However, cold-pressed soya oil, usually sold from delicatessen counters or health-food shops, can contain soya protein and should be avoided.

Types of foods which are particularly likely to contain soya are vegetarian foods, meat and fish products, ready meals, oriental foods and sauces, bread, cakes and biscuits, desserts, snack foods and confectionery, but its use is ubiquitous so all food labels must be carefully checked.

4.35.5 Wheat exclusion

Wheat may provoke allergic reactions (most commonly a delayed type IV response; see Section 4.34.3) or chronic, diffuse gastrointestinal symptoms of intolerance with no obvious immunological basis. Wheat allergy or severe intolerance will require total wheat exclusion. Partial exclusion may be sufficient in some non-immunologically mediated forms of wheat intolerance; the threshold of sensitivity varies and some people can obtain symptom relief by significant reduction of wheat intake.

In the UK, wheat is a major component of most cereal foods and a common ingredient in many other manufactured foods, ranging from sausages to ice-cream. Wheat exclusion therefore has considerable impact on food choice and nutrient intake. Dietary guidance for wheat exclusion is summarized in Table 4.78.

The need to exclude many of the components of a major food group (bread and cereals) means that the intake of dietary fibre and B vitamins is likely to be low. In addition, wheat exclusion increases the risk of dietary imbalance, with a relatively low proportion of dietary energy derived from carbohydrate and a high proportion from fat and protein.

Commercially produced wheat-free (and gluten-free) products such as bread and pasta are available but these are not prescribable for wheat allergy or intolerance *per se* and hence are expensive. Wheat-free products are only

prescribable for people with coeliac disease who react to wheat starch (which contains minute amounts of gluten) present in many proprietary gluten-free foods. Because of their wheat starch content, gluten-free products are not suitable for people with wheat allergy unless they are specifically labelled as wheat free.

4.35.6 Egg exclusion

Allergy to eggs is relatively common in infancy and can precipitate acute type I reactions (see 4.34.3). In most infants, the allergy will resolve by the age of 5 years but, in about 20% of cases, it will persist into adulthood (Dannaeus and Inganaes 1981).

Eggs and egg derivatives include:

- fresh eggs
- dried eggs
- egg yolk
- egg white (or egg albumen)
- egg lecithin: lecithin used in food manufacture (E322) is more likely to be derived from soya than egg but if this is not specified, the origin needs to be checked with the manufacturer.

Eggs are also a major component of foods such as:

- meringue
- quiche-type flans
- egg custards
- scotch egg
- mayonnaise
- yorkshire pudding, batters and pancakes
- cakes.

However, egg can also be a less obvious ingredient of foods such as pasta, biscuits and desserts. Since acute reactions to eggs can result from ingestion of trace amounts, it is vital that all food labels are carefully scrutinized for its presence.

Table 4.78 Dietary guidance for wheat exclusion

Cereal foods which must be excluded	Other foods which may need to be excluded	Cereal foods which can be included
All types of bread including rolls, malt bread, chappatti, pitta, naan, paratha, croissants and fancy breads	Manufactured foods containing any of the following ingredients:	Rice and rice flour
Breakfast cereals unless derived solely from oat, rice and/or maize (corn)	Wholewheat or wheat grains	Oats and oatmeal
Cakes, biscuits and crackers	Wheat flour	Corn (maize) and cornflour
Flour and all foods containing it, e.g. pastry, pies, batters, pancakes, sauces	Wheat starch (or modified starch)	Barley and barley flour
Bran	Wheat bran	Millet
Pasta	Wheat germ	Arrowroot
Semolina, couscous	Wheat germ oil	Buckwheat
Pizza	Wheat binder	Sago and sago flour
Proprietary gluten-free foods containing wheat starch	Wheat gluten	Proprietary gluten-free, wheat-free foods (only prescribable for coeliac disease, not wheat intolerance *per se*)
	Wheat thickener	
	Raising agent containing wheat starch	
	Hydrolysed wheat protein	
	Cereal filler	
	Rusk	
	Breadcrumbs or bread	

4.35.7 Fish and shellfish exclusion

Fish and shellfish can provoke type I allergic or pharmacologically mediated reactions. They are, however, relatively easy to exclude from the diet because foods and meals containing them are usually obvious.

Less obvious sources can include:

- ingredients such as fish stock, purée or bouillon
- Worcester sauce (which may contain anchovies)
- food served at buffets and banquets where the contents of soups, hors-d'œuvres, vol-au-vents, sauces, etc., may not be apparent.
- Oriental (especially Thai) dishes which often contain seafood as an ingredient
- fish oil supplements
- health food preparations such as green lipped mussel extract (particularly cheaper, less purified products).

4.35.8 Exclusion of food additives

Contrary to popular belief, adverse reaction to food additives is rare. Those which are most likely to cause problems are listed below.

Azo colours

These can trigger behavioural disturbances in rare but well-documented cases (Ferguson 1992). However, their use in food has declined dramatically in recent years and most manufacturers now use alternative forms of colour derived from natural vegetable sources (e.g. beta-carotene as an orange colourant in soft drinks) wherever possible.

The presence of azo colours in a food will always be declared either by name and/or E number on a food label:

- E102 Tartrazine
- E110 Sunset Yellow FCF or Orange Yellow S
- E122 Carmoisine or Azorubine
- E123 Amaranth
- E124 Ponceau 4R or Cochineal Red A
- E128 Red 2G
- E129 Allura Red AC
- E151 Brilliant Black PN or Black PN
- E154 Brown FK
- E155 Brown HT
- E180 Litholrubine BK or Pigment Rubine or Rubine.

Sulphur dioxide and associated preservatives

Sulphur dioxide, and other preservatives which can be broken down to release sulphur dioxide, can trigger asthma is some susceptible individuals. Foods containing the following additives will need to be avoided:

- E220 Sulphur dioxide
- E221 Sodium sulfite
- E222 Sodium hydrogen sulfite (sodium bisulfite)
- E223 Sodium metabisulfite
- E224 Potassium metabisulfite
- E226 Calcium sulfite
- E227 Calcium hydrogen sulfite (calcium bisulfite).

Benzoates

These additives have been reported to exacerbate asthma and urticaria:

- E210 Benzoic acid
- E211 Sodium benzoate
- E212 Potassium benzoate
- E213 Calcium benzoate
- E214 Ethyl 4-hydroxybenzoate (ethyl para-hydroxybenzoate)
- E215 Ethyl 4-hydroxybenzoate, sodium salt (sodium ethyl para-hydroxybenzoate)
- E216 Propyl 4-hydroxybenzoate (propyl para-hydroxybenzoate)
- E217 Propyl 4-hydroxybenzoate, sodium salt (sodium propyl para-hydroxzybenzoate)
- E218 Methyl 4-hydroxybenzoate (methyl para-hydroxybenzoate)
- E219 Methyl 4-hydroxybenzoate, sodium salt (sodium methyl para-hydroxybenzoate).

A complicating factor is that benzoates occur naturally in foods, especially fruits, but compositional data are sparse. The role of benzoates in food intolerant reactions is thus difficult to determine, and their avoidance difficult to achieve in practice.

Text revised by: Briony Thomas

Acknowledgements: Sue Thurgood, Christine Carter, Gail Pollard and Christine Baker.

Useful addresses

See also Useful addresses at the end of Section 4.24, Food allergy and intolerance.

Anaphylaxis Campaign
PO Box 149, Fleet, Hampshire GU13 9XU
Tel: 01252 542029 Fax: 01252 377140
Website: www.anaphylaxis.org.uk

Food Intolerance Databank
Leatherhead Food RA, Randalls Road, Leatherhead, Surrey KT22 7RY
Tel: 01372 376761 (Direct line: 01372 822217);
Fax: 01372 386228

Medic Alert (medical alert bracelets)
12 Bridge Wharf, 156 Caledonian Road, London N1 9UU
Tel: 020 7833 3034

Further reading

British Dietetic Association. *Peanut Allergy. Information for Dietitians*. Birmingham: BDA.

British Dietetic Association's Paediatric Group. *Specialised Formulas for Cow's Milk Intolerance Malabsorption Syndromes.* (Updated at regular intervals.)

David TJ. *Food and Food Additive Intolerance in Children.* Oxford: Blackwell Science, 1993.

National Dairy Council. *Milk – Facts and Fallacies.* Topical Update 9. London: National Dairy Council, 1998.

References

Assem ESK. Anaphylaxis induced by peanuts. *British Medical Journal* 1990; **300**: 1377–1378.

Bernhisel-Broadbent J, Sampson HA. *Journal of Allergy and Clinical Immunology* 1989; **83**: 435–440.

Bock SA, Atkins FM. *Journal of Allergy and Clinical Immunology* 1989; **83**: 900–904.

Dannaeus A, Inganaes M. A follow-up study of children with food allergy. Clinical course in relation to serum IgE and IgG antibody levels to milk, egg and fish. *Clinical Allergy* 1981; **11**: 533–539.

David TJ. Food intolerance. In *Nutrition in Child Health*, p. 172. London: Royal College of Physicians, 1995.

De Montis G, Gendrel D *et al.* Sensitisation to peanut and vitamin D oily preparations (Letter). *Lancet* 1993; **341**: 1411.

Department of Health. *Weaning and the Weaning Diet.* Report of Health and Social Subjects 45. London: HMSO, 1994.

Department of Health. *Peanut Allergy.* Report by a Working Group of the Committee on Toxicity of Chemicals in Food, Consumer Products and the Environment. London: DH, 1998.

Ewan PW. Clinical study of peanut and nut allergy in 62 consecutive patients: new features and associations. *British Medical Journal* 1996; **312**: 1074–1078.

Ferguson A. Definitions and diagnosis of food intolerance and food allergy – consensus and controversy. *Journal of Pediatrics* 1992; **121** (5 Suppl Pt 2): S7–S11.

Hide DW, Gant C. Hypoallergenic formulae – have they a therapeutic role? *Clinical and Experimental Allergy* 1994; **24**: 3–5.

Hill DJ, Hosking CS. The cow milk allergy complex: overlapping disease profiles in infancy. *European Journal of Clinical Nutrition* 1995; **49** (Suppl 1): S1–S12.

Hill DJ, Cameron DJ, Francis DE *et al.* Challenge confirmation of late-onset reactions to extensively hydrolysed formulas in infants with multiple food protein intolerance. *Journal of Allergy and Clinical Immunology* 1995; **96** (3): 386–394.

Hill DJ, Heine RG, Cameron DJ *et al.* The natural history of intolerance to soy and extensively hydrolyzed formula in infants with multiple food protein intolerance. *Journal of Pediatrics* 1999; **135** (1): 118–121.

Host A. Cow's milk protein allergy and intolerance in infancy. Some clinical, epidemiological and immunological aspects. *Pediatric Allergy and Immunology* 1994; **5** (Suppl): 1–36.

Host A. Cow's milk allergy. *Journal of the Royal Society of Medicine* 1997; **90** (Suppl 30): 34–39.

Host A, Halken S. A prospective study of cow's milk allergy in Danish infants during the first 3 years of life. Clinical course in relation to clinical and immunological type of hypersensitivity reaction. *Allergy* 1990; **45**: 587–596.

Host A, Jacobsen HP, Halken S, Holmenlund S. The natural history of cow's milk protein allergy/intolerance. *European Journal of Clinical Nutrition* 1995; **49** (Suppl 1): S13–S18.

Hourihane JO'B, Dean TP, Warner JO. Peanut allergy in relation to heredity, maternal diet, and other atopic diseases: results of a questionnaire survey, skin prick tests and food challenges. *British Medical Journal* 1996; **313**: 518–521.

Hourihane JO'B, Kilburn SA, Dean TP, Warner JO. Clinical characteristics of peanut allergy. *Clinical and Experimental Allergy* 1997; **27**: 634–639.

Hourihane J O'B, Roberts SA, Warner JO. Resolution of peanut allergy: case–control study. *British Medical Journal* 1998; **316**: 1271–1275.

Iacono G, Cavataio F, Montalto G *et al.* Persistent cow's milk protein intolerance in infants: the changing face of the same disease. *Clinical and Experimental Allergy* 1998; **28**: 817–823.

Isolauri E, Sutas Y, Salo MK *et al.* Elimination diet in cow's milk allergy: risk for impaired growth in young children. *Journal of Pediatrics* 1998; **132**: 1004–1009.

MacDonald A. Which formula in cow's milk protein intolerance? The dietitian's dilemma. *European Journal of Clinical Nutrition* 1995; **49** (Suppl 1): S56–S63.

McLeish CM, MacDonald A, Booth IW. Comparison of an elemental with a hydrolysed whey formula in intolerance to cow's milk. *Archives of Disease in Childhood* 1995; **73**: 211–215.

Maldonado J, Gil A, Narbona E, Molina JA. Special formulas in infant nutrition: a review. *Early Human Development* 1998; **53** (Suppl): S23–S32.

Merritt RJ, Carter M, Haight M, Eisenberg LD. Whey protein hydrolysate formula for infants with gastrointestinal intolerance to cow milk and soy protein in infant formulas. *Journal of Pediatric Gastroenterology and Nutrition* 1990; **11**: 78–82.

Moneret-Vautrin HR, Kanny G. Risks of milk formulas containing peanut oils contaminated with peanut allergens in infants with atopic dermatitis. *Pediatric Allergy and Immunology* 1994; **5**: 84–188.

Ortolani C, Vighi G. Definition of adverse reactions to food. *Allergy* 1995; **50** (20 Suppl): 8–13.

Pumphrey RSH, Stanworth SJ. The clinical spectrum of anaphylaxis is north-west England. *Clinical and Experimental Allergy* 1996; **26**: 1364–1370.

Sampson HA. IgE mediated food intolerance. *Journal of Allergy and Clinical Immunology* 1988; **81**: 495–504.

Sampson HA. Managing peanut allergy. *British Medical Journal* 1996; **312**: 1050–1051.

Schrander JJ, Oudsen S, Forget PP, Kuijten RH. Follow up study of cow's milk protein intolerant infants. *European Journal of Pediatrics* 1992; **151**: 783–785.

Tariq SM, Stevens M, Matthews S *et al.* Cohort study of peanut and tree nut sensitisation by age at 4 years. *British Medical Journal* 1996; **313**: 514–517.

4.36 AIDS and HIV disease

The acquired immunodeficiency syndrome (AIDS) is a disorder resulting from profound immunosuppression that renders the body highly susceptible to life-threatening opportunistic infections and tumours. AIDS is the result of infection with the human immunodeficiency virus (HIV).

4.36.1 Prevalence of HIV infection and AIDS

The first cases of AIDS were reported in June 1981. By mid-1996 it was estimated that 21 million people worldwide were living with HIV and that there had been 7 million deaths from AIDS (UNAIDS/WHO 1996). Globally, the picture revealed 42% of those infected were women, with the majority of new infections in 15–24 year olds. Sexual transmission accounted for 75–85% of infections, 3–5% of cases were from the transfusion of blood and blood products and 5–10% from intravenous drug use (UNAIDS/WHO 1996). At that time it was also estimated that in industrialized countries 60% of those infected with HIV would progress to AIDS within 12–13 years. Survival after an AIDS diagnosis was suggested to be about 3 years. However, recent advances in drug therapies may extend survival far beyond this.

The UK picture is summarized in Table 4.79. This highlights a major increase in reported cases of HIV from the early to the late 1990s. There appears to be no decline in the number of reported new cases. This, coupled with extended survival through drug therapies, could mean a much larger population living with HIV in future years.

4.36.2 Immunology

An understanding of the immune system is necessary to understand the effects of HIV and the role of nutrition in this disease.

The body has two lines of defence against invading antigens: non-specific and specific immunity. The non-specific immune response relies on the physical barrier of the skin in combination with protective chemicals such as lysozyme in tears and saliva, and hydrochloric acid in gastric juice. Clot formation by the activated complement system and the phagocytic capacity of the blood also form effective barriers to the entry of foreign antigens.

If an antigen manages to break through these barriers, a second line of defence is provided by specific immune responses. The main components of the specific immune system are the white cells of the blood, particularly the lymphocytes. When lymphocytes of the immune system

Table 4.79 Number of HIV-infected individuals in the UK: 1991 and 1998 (Communicable Disease Report Weekly, 1999a)

Number of cases reported in the UK	At end 1991	At end 1998
Number of cases by risk group		
Sex between men	4297 (79%)	22 714 (61%)
Sex between men and women	443	7952
Intravenous drug use	245	3488
Other[1]	466	3247
Total number of reported cases in the UK	5451	37 401

[1]Other cases include transfusion of blood or blood products, mother-to-infant transmission and those of undetermined origin.

meet an antigen, a series of events occurs resulting in the production of activated T-lymphocytes and antibodies (Fig. 4.13). If successful, these eliminate the antigen. This is known as the cell-mediated immune response.

HIV is a retrovirus which has an affinity for a particular subset of lymphocytes: the T-helper/inducer cells. HIV enters the target cell by binding to a protein receptor (CD4) on the cell surface. The virus then replicates by transcribing its RNA genome to double-stranded DNA (with the aid of an enzyme, reverse transcriptase). This DNA is then integrated into the cell and replicated with it.

CD4 receptors are also found on the surface of monocytes and macrophages. Consequently, these cells can also be infected with HIV. This is important as they are transported to other sites in the body, which may explain some of the diverse effects seen in this disease.

The immune response is influenced by genetic potential, age, number of T- and B-lymphocytes and macrophages, the presence of infection and the nature of the antigen (Chandra 1984). In addition, it has been established that nutrition is an important determinant of immune response (Cunningham-Rundles 1982; Chandra 1991).

Undernutrition has its most profound effects on the cell-mediated immune response. All of the lymphoid organs become atrophied and depleted of lymphocytes, and the proportion and absolute number of T-cells decrease (Chandra 1981). Secondary to the impaired cell-mediated immunity are reductions in complement function, bactericidal activity, reduced secretion of immunoglobulin A (IgA) and impaired cutaneous sensitivity reactions (Chandra 1981).

HIV has its most profound effects on the T-cell-mediated immune responses, resulting in the immune system failing to function effectively even though it remains largely

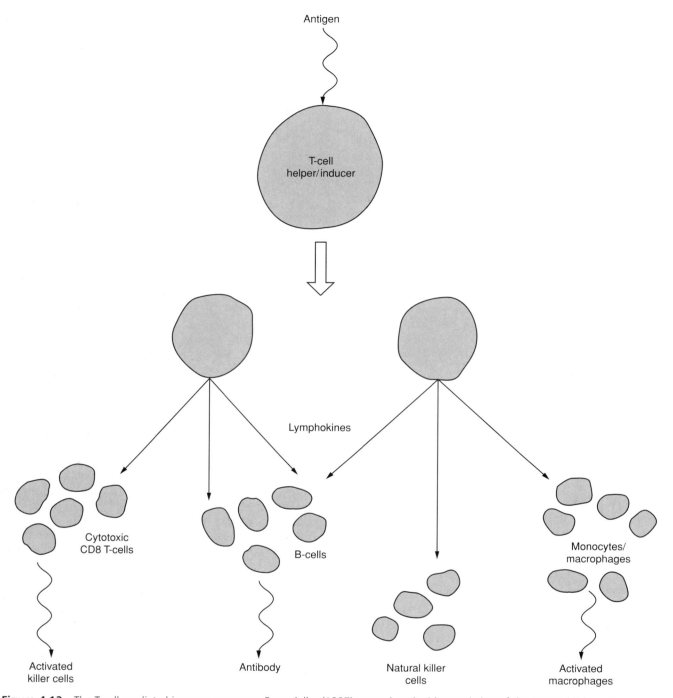

Figure 4.12 The T-cell-mediated immune response. From Adler (1997); reproduced with permission of the BMJ Publishing Group.

intact. This very selective destruction of particular cells within the immune system accounts for the fact that certain rare infections can cause problems in people who are HIV positive.

Although individuals may be HIV antibody positive and healthy for long periods, the disease is characterized by a progressive fall in the number of T-helper/inducer CD4-positive cells. The measurement of CD4-positive cell numbers or the ratio of helper (T4) to suppressor (T8)

lymphocytes is considered a useful indicator of immune status during HIV infection. The normal ratio is 2:1. This ratio changes in HIV disease.

The immunological abnormalities seen in HIV disease and AIDS are very similar to those seen in various nutritional deficiency states. It has been suggested that dietary manipulations might diminish the immune defects seen in HIV infection and enhance resistance to opportunistic infections (Chandra 1984; Moseson *et al.* 1989). However, this remains to be proven. In addition, adverse effects of supplementation have been reported (Beisel *et al.* 1981; Chandra 1984; Moseson *et al.* 1989). Further studies are needed before specific recommendations can be made.

4.36.3 Classification of HIV disease

It is usual to view HIV disease along a spectrum, from infection with HIV to AIDS. The clinical course and time-scale of the disease vary considerably from individual to individual.

Following infection, patients may experience a glandular fever-like or seroconversion illness lasting for a couple of weeks, after which they become asymptomatic or are left with persistent generalized lymphadenopathy (swollen lymph nodes). When a patient is diagnosed with symptomatic HIV disease, conditions such as oral hairy leukoplakia, herpes zoster, pelvic inflammatory disease, recurrent fevers, night sweats and persistent oral candida may exist. The advanced stage of disease is characterized by major infections, including those which would not cause problems in an immunocompetent host (opportunistic infections) and neoplasms. However, it is important to note that many of these infections and neoplasms are treatable and people diagnosed clinically as having AIDS can be physically very well and able to enjoy active and productive lives.

The Centers for Disease Control (CDC) in America have devised a classification system for HIV disease that recognizes three stages (Table 4.80). All patients in categories A3, B3, C1, C2 and C3 are reported as having AIDS.

4.36.4 Modes of transmission

In the UK the main activities by which HIV is transmitted are:

- unprotected sexual intercourse, both vaginal and anal
- the receipt of infected blood products via contaminated needles; usually as a result of sharing injecting equipment among intravenous drug users
- vertical transmission from mother to child during pregnancy, birth or breast feeding.

HIV is also known to be transmitted by:

- contaminated blood products (in the UK all such products are screened for HIV)
- occupational accidents, e.g. needle stick injuries (fewer than 1% of individuals who receive such injuries become infected).

Body fluids from which HIV has been isolated include semen, cervical secretions, lymphocytes, cell-free plasma, cerebrospinal fluid, tears, saliva, urine and breast milk. However, only blood, semen, cervical secretions and breast milk have sufficiently high concentrations of the virus to be infectious.

In the UK, HIV positive mothers are currently advised against breast feeding as safe and adequate alternatives to maternal milk are available. This is not necessarily the case in developing countries.

4.36.5 Nutritional aspects of asymptomatic or weight-stable HIV infection

Being diagnosed with a chronic condition often leaves people feeling out of control. Following the initial shock, strategies for maintaining and promoting health may be sought. Food choice is a facet of management over which a person can exert control. Dietary advice should not threaten that control but aim to optimize food intake and achieve nutritional adequacy.

The rationale for nutritional advice in asymptomatic HIV infection is based on avoiding deficiencies and preventing unintentional weight loss. The relationship between nutrition and the immune system is well documented (Cunningham-Rundles 1982), and it is possible, although unproven, that an adequate intake of all nutrients may delay disease progression. Significant weight loss, although less common with the advent of highly active antiretroviral therapy (HAART), is a feature of advancing HIV disease. Weight and lean tissue loss have been linked to survival (Kotler *et al.* 1989; Palenicek *et al.* 1995) and can also impact negatively on morbidity and quality of life. Early nutritional intervention may minimize complications seen in later stages of disease and provide a contact point for future advice.

The optimum time for nutrition intervention to begin is as soon after a HIV positive diagnosis as possible. For many people this will be early in the course of their disease when they are asymptomatic, but it is important to remember that some people are diagnosed later when there may already have been considerable depletion of nutrient reserves.

For the asymptomatic and weight-stable person, advice is aimed at preserving lean body mass, preventing nutrient deficiencies and optimizing nutritional stores (BDA

Table 4.80 Centers for Disease Control classification system for HIV infection and AIDS (1993)

CD4 count	Symptoms		
	A	B	C
>500	A1	B1	C1
250–520	A2	B2	C2
<200	A3	B3	C3

Symptom category:
A: acute retroviral syndrome, generalized lymphadenopathy, asymptomatic disease.
B: symptoms of AIDS-related complex, candidiasis, mucosal, cervical dysplasia, constitutional symptoms, herpes zoster, idiopathic thrombocytopenic purpura, listeriosis, oral hairy leukoplakia, pelvic inflammatory disease, peripheral neuropathy.
C: AIDS-defining conditions, CD4 count <200, candidiasis, pulmonary or oesophageal, cervical cancer, coccidioidomycosis, cryptosporidiosis, cytomegalovirus infection, herpes oesophagitits, HIV encephalopathy, histoplasmosis, isosporiasis, Kaposi's sarcoma, lymphoma, mycobacterial disease, *Pneumocystis carinii* infection, pneumonia, bacterial, progressive multifocal leucoencephalopenia, salmonellosis.

1995). A baseline nutritional assessment should include a diet history in combination with measurement of height, weight, body mass index and other anthropometric and biochemical indices if possible. Dietary advice should promote a regular, balanced intake of all nutrients in line with current recommendations (DH 1991). The use of food groups with an indication of the number of choices from each group (e.g. *The Balance of Good Health* model; see Section 1.2, Healthy eating), together with ideas on putting together meals and snacks, is a useful way of teaching balanced nutrition.

Precise vitamin and mineral requirements in HIV disease are not known. There is evidence that blood levels of many micronutrients are below normal in both asymptomatic (Beach *et al.* 1992) and symptomatic (Coodley *et al.* 1993) cohorts, and that micronutrient requirements may be higher in HIV infection than in the general population (Baum *et al.* 1994). A daily supplement of a complete vitamin and mineral preparation, at the level of reference nutrient intakes (RNI), is probably appropriate in all patients to cover the possibility of increased needs and is clearly indicated when food intake is compromised. However, the evidence that pharmacological doses of any vitamin or mineral will alter the course of the disease is at present unclear. Patients often wish to self-supplement and it is important to ask about this during the consultation. While dietetic input should be supportive, any potential toxicity should be avoided.

People with HIV disease represent all segments of society with varying socioeconomic circumstances and have varying amounts of nutrition knowledge. Food choice may be complicated by factors such as lack of money, skills, energy, motivation and facilities. Advice must be flexible and practical to accommodate people's varying lifestyles.

4.36.6 Nutritional aspects of symptomatic HIV infection and AIDS
Nutritional problems

The most significant nutritional problem in symptomatic HIV disease is weight loss or wasting. Although its incidence and severity have been greatly reduced through effective combination antiretroviral therapy (Carbonnel *et al.* 1998; Foudraine *et al.* 1998) it remains a problem for some patients, particularly those who cannot or will not take antiretroviral therapy. Malnutrition can increase mortality and morbidity and reduce quality of life. The cause of malnutrition is multifactorial, reflecting the variety of symptoms and infections associated with advanced HIV infection. Whatever the cause, the correct diagnosis and treatment of any underlying condition is of prime importance in reversing the malnutrition (Grunfeld and Kotler 1991).

The main factors precipitating weight loss and wasting in symptomatic HIV disease are:

- reduced food intake
- altered metabolic requirements
- malabsorption.

Reduced food intake

This is the primary cause of weight loss in HIV infection (Grunfeld *et al.* 1992; Macallan *et al.* 1995). It may be due to anorexia, nausea and vomiting, neurological problems, tiredness and depression, sore mouth, swallowing problems or taste changes. The particular cause will depend on the presenting problem (Table 4.81).

Altered metabolic requirements

There is evidence that resting energy expenditure is increased in HIV infection (Melchior *et al.* 1991; Macallan *et al.* 1995; Sharpstone *et al.* 1996). However, weight loss is not clearly correlated to resting metabolic rate. Macallan *et al.* (1995) found that total energy expenditure was actually reduced during periods of HIV-related weight loss, probably from a reduction in voluntary activity. Consequently, the contribution of hypermetabolism to weight loss in HIV infection remains unclear. Altered metabolism may contribute to weight and more specifically lean tissue loss. Although cytokines have been implicated,

Table 4.81 Opportunistic infections and tumours and their potential nutritional implications

Organ affected	Infection	Common nutritional problems
Brain and central nervous system	Cryptococcus	Pyrexia, nausea and vomiting
	Toxoplasmosis ('toxo')	Pyrexia, lethargy, confusion
	HIV encephalopathy	Confusion, appetite loss
Lungs	*Pneumocystis carinii* pneumonia (PCP)	Pyrexia, anorexia, lethargy, and weight loss
	Tuberculosis (TB)	As above
	Kapsosi's sarcoma (KS)	As above
Gastrointestinal tract	Candidiasis (oral/oesophageal)	Sore mouth, altered taste perception, dysphagia
	Cytomegalovirus (CMV)	Dysphagia (if affects oesophagus) diarrhoea, malabsorption, weight loss
	Kaposi's sarcoma (KS)	Sore mouth, dysphagia, abdominal pain, diarrhoea and malabsorption (depending on site affected)
	Mycobacterium avium intracellulare/complex (MAI/MAC)	Pyrexia, anorexia, diarrhoea, malabsorption and weight loss
	Cryptosporidiosis and microsporidiosis and weight loss	Anorexia, nausea, diarrhoea, malabsorption
Eyes	Cytomegalovirus	Blindness/limited vision

their exact role in HIV-related wasting has yet to be elucidated (Grunfeld and Kotler 1992).

Malabsorption

Intestinal absorptive capacity may reduce with advancing disease, particularly in those with chronic diarrhoea (Keating *et al.* 1995). This leads to the possibility of both macronutrient and micronutrient loss in the stool. Diarrhoea and malabsorption are caused by gastrointestinal pathogens and perhaps by HIV itself. The cause of diarrhoea and availability of treatments will determine its effect on absorption and nutritional status. Diarrhoea is also a common side-effect of medication.

Nutritional management of symptomatic HIV infection

The aims of nutritional management are to:

- preserve or increase lean body mass
- provide adequate levels of all nutrients
- achieve or maintain ideal body weight
- provide symptomatic relief.

Basic dietetic principles for nutritional intervention apply. Assessment of nutritional status should be made initially and repeated at regular intervals (see Section 1.8, Assessment of nutritional status). The nutritional requirements of the patient may be altered as a result of co-infections or malignancies and can be assessed using standard methods (see Section 1.10, Estimating nutritional requirements). Vitamin and mineral intake should be at least 100% of the dietary reference value (DRV).

The composition of the diet and most effective route of administration are dependent on the nutritional status, presenting symptoms and stage of disease of the patient. It should be borne in mind that the multifactorial nature of AIDS can produce a different combination of symptoms in each individual. Dietary management during cancer treatment in Section 4.37.2 provides advice on the dietary management of specific nutritional problems which are common to both symptomatic HIV infection and cancer.

Nutritional support

If patients are failing to meet their nutritional needs, a stepwise approach to nutritional support should be adopted (see Section 1.11, Undernutrition and principles of nutritional support). Initially, attempts should be made to improve nutrient intake via nourishing foods, using fortification strategies if appropriate (see Section 1.12, Oral nutritional support). If intake remains inadequate, commercial protein and energy supplements may be helpful.

If a patient still fails to achieve an adequate oral intake, enteral tube feeding should be considered (see Section 1.13, Artificial nutritional support). If support is likely to be required in the short term, for example to aid repletion after an opportunistic infection, nasogastric feeding is usually the route of choice, although this may be diffi-

cult if the patient has nausea and vomiting or a severe *Candida* overgrowth of the oesophagus. This route is also useful to assess the response to feeding prior to the insertion of a gastrostomy.

For long-term artificial nutritional support (>3 months) a percutaneous endoscopic gastrostomy (PEG) should be considered. This has the advantage for the patient of being more discreet and easier to cope with. Care must be taken to minimize infection in this immunocompromised patient group, although several studies have suggested that the rate of infections is no higher than in HIV-negative groups (Suttmann *et al.* 1993; Dowling *et al.* 1996).

Enteral support is usually used as a supplementary rather than total source of nutrition. Most patients, even those with diarrhoea, tolerate a standard low-lactose feed. For a minority of patients with severe gastrointestinal complications and/or malabsorption states, elemental or semielemental feeds may be best tolerated.

Parenteral nutrition (PN) should be reserved for cases when the gastrointestinal tract cannot be used. Home PN may be very difficult to organize in the community in the UK.

Specific considerations when providing artificial nutritional support to HIV patients

Many HIV positive patients receive treatment solely from sexually transmitted disease/HIV clinics and may not have a general practitioner (GP), or may choose not to involve their GP. This raises the question of who prescribes and supplies the product. Hospital prescriptions must be endorsed to be valid outside the hospital pharmacy and home deliveries need a financial code from a hospital source. Dietitians should check with their pharmacy for the correct procedure.

Pharmacological management of weight loss and wasting

A variety of pharmacological agents is available to assist in the treatment of poor appetite and weight loss. Whilst many are still undergoing trials to assess efficacy, treatment with several drugs such as megesterol acetate and testosterone has proved successful to a certain degree. Not all individuals respond to treatment and the benefits often disappear once treatment has stopped.

The drugs most commonly used are considered below. A more detailed review of drug treatments for weight loss and the key findings of the research to date can be found in Balog *et al.* (1998).

Appetite stimulants

Megesterol acetate (MA) This is a progesterone derivative and several studies (reviewed by Balog *et al.* 1998) have demonstrated significant weight gain, increased appetite and improvement in food intake following use of MA. However, body composition studies reveal that weight gained tends to be mainly fat rather than lean body mass (LBM). Some studies have indicated that MA reduces circulating levels of testosterone, possibly preventing repletion of LBM and promoting fat deposition. Trials are in progress to assess the effect of combined MA and testosterone therapy.

The effect of MA appears to be dose related, with the higher doses producing more noticeable effects. Raised blood glucose levels can be a side-effect of MA therapy and the drug should be discontinued if this occurs. MA is contraindicated in people with diabetes mellitus.

Anabolic agents

Testosterone   Low serum testosterone is common in men with HIV-associated weight loss and replacement therapy may help to reverse this. Several small trials of testosterone replacement therapy in male HIV positive subjects have been conducted. Preliminary results indicate that weight gain, primarily as LBM, can occur; however, to date there have been no published controlled studies evaluating testosterone. In addition, it is not known whether appetite or food intake improves in addition to weight. The benefits seem to disappear on cessation of treatment.

Some units have adopted the policy of only offering this therapy if circulating levels of testosterone are low. Testosterone may not be suitable for people with mental health problems, as mood swings and aggression are known side-effects.

Anabolic steroids   Nandrolone decanoate has been investigated in relation to HIV-associated weight loss. In one study (reviewed by Balog *et al.* 1998) intramuscular injections of nandrolone every 2 weeks for a 16 week trial period resulted in significant improvements in weight (both fat and muscle) as well as improvements in mood, energy and libido. The oral anabolic steroid preparation stanozolol is also used by some units in the UK. Adverse effects are associated with anabolic steroids, particularly changes in mood, and in addition exercise may be necessary to promote the anabolic effects of the drugs.

Growth hormone   Several centres in the UK, the USA and elsewhere are investigating the use of human growth hormone (hGH) in HIV infection. Preliminary results are promising and indicate that hGH can promote weight gain and an increase in LBM; however, as with other agents the benefits disappear on treatment cessation. The high cost of administering hGH tends to preclude routine prescription on an individual basis.

Cytokine inhibitors

Thalidomide, cyproheptadine, pentoxifylline and fish oils have been reported to improve weight and appetite, and reduce levels of tumour necrosis factor (TNF) in HIV positive people. However, they are rarely used in clinical practice.

Terminal care

The role of nutritional support in late HIV disease and AIDS is similar to that in terminal oncology patients (see Section 4.39, Terminal illness and palliative care).

4.36.7 HIV disease in children

AIDS was first described in children in 1982. In total, 882 HIV infected children had been reported in the UK, 269 (30%) of whom are known to have died (Communicable Disease Report, 1999b). More than 1600 children acquire HIV infection everyday globally, the majority as a result of mother-to-infant transmission (see www. unaids).

Mode of transmission

Perinatal ('vertical') transmission will account for almost all new cases in countries where the blood supply is screened. In southern Europe, Scotland and Ireland the majority of mothers are intravenous drug users. In northern Europe, including England, most mothers have acquired HIV heterosexually from partners from high-prevalence countries, particularly sub-Saharan Africa. Policy changes and improvements in antenatal testing, perinatal antiretroviral therapy, planned vaginal or elective caesarean birth and safe infant formula feeding have dramatically reduced mother-to-child transmission to less than 2% (Tudor-Williams and Lyall 1999).

Diagnosis

All babies born to infected women will have passively acquired antibodies to HIV. The average time to lose these is 10 months, but may be as late as 18 months. HIV infection can be diagnosed in the majority of infected infants by 1 month of age in non-breast-feeding populations. The optimal diagnostic test in the newborn is a molecular amplification technique such as the polymerase chain reaction (PCR). Children over the age of 18 months can be tested for HIV antibody.

The CDC revised the clinical classification system for HIV infection in children less than 13 years of age in 1994. Table 4.82 summarizes the clinical categories (MMWR 1994).

The clinical presentation in infants and children often differs from that in adults. Recurrent bacterial infections are more common in children, whereas certain opportunistic infections (e.g. toxoplasmosis and cryptococcal meningitis) are infrequent. Kaposi's sarcoma (KS) is also uncommon in children and AIDS-associated malignancies (e.g. lymphomas) are relatively rare compared with adults (Pizzo 1990). Progressive neurological disease due to HIV is more prevalent in children.

Paediatric HIV disease often manifests with failure to thrive or the lack of normal weight gain and growth. Motor development and other skills such as crawling, walking and talking may be delayed.

Nutritional considerations in children with HIV

Nutritional aspects of treatment

There have been considerable advances in the use of HAART in infants and children since 1997. Treatment is

Table 4.82 Centers for Disease Control classification for paediatric HIV infection (Adapted from MMWR 1994)

Clinical category	Symptom severity	Type of symptoms
N	No symptoms	
A	Mildly symptomatic Children with two or more of the following:	Lymphadenopathy; hepatomegaly; splenomegaly; dermatitis; parotitis; recurrent upper respiratory tract infection, sinusitis or otitis media
B	Moderately symptomatic Examples of conditions in clinical category B include:	Anaemia, neutropenia or thrombocytopenia; single serious bacterial infection (e.g. pneumonia, bacteraemia); candidiasis, oropharyngeal (thrush); cardiomyopathy; cytomegalovirus infection; diarrhoea (recurrent or chronic); hepatitis; herpes stomatitis, recurrent; lymphoid interstitial pneumonia (LIP); nephropathy; persistent fever >1 month; varicella zoster (persistent or complicated primary chickenpox or shingles)

C	Severely symptomatic
	Any condition listed in the 1987 surveillance case definition for AIDS, with the exception of LIP
		(1) Serious bacterial infections, multiple or recurrent
		(2) Opportunistic infections:
		    Candidiasis (oesophageal, pulmonary); cytomegalovirus; disease with onset of symptoms at age >1 month; cryptosporidiosis with diarrhoea persisting 1 month; Mycobacterium tuberculosis, disseminated or extrapulmonary; *Mycobacterium avium* complex or *M. kansasii*, disseminated; *Pneumocystis carinii* pneumonia (PCP); progressive multifocal leukoencephalopathy; toxoplasmosis of the brain with onset at age >1 month
		(3) Severe failure to thrive/wasting syndrome
		    Crossing at least two percentile lines on the growth chart (e.g. 90th to 50th, or 50th to 10th) or less than the 3rd percentile and continuing to deviate downwards from it over a 3 month period, or more than 10% loss of body weight in older child *plus*
		    (a) chronic diarrhoea >30 days *or*
		    (b) documented intermittent or constant fever >30 days
		(4) HIV encephalopathy
		    At least one of the following progressive findings for at least 2 months in the absence of a concurrent illness other than HIV infection that could explain the findings:
		    (a) Failure to attain or loss of developmental milestones or loss of intellectual ability, verified by standard developmental scale or neuropsychological tests
		    (b) Impaired brain growth or acquired microcephaly demonstrated by head circumference measurements or by brain atrophy demonstrated by computed tomography or magnetic resonance imaging (serial imaging for children <2 years of age)
		    (c) Acquired symmetric motor deficit manifested by two or more of the following: paresis, pathologic reflexes, ataxia or gait disturbance
		(5) Malignancy

Children are also classified immunologically by age-adjusted CD4 counts.

usually withheld until clinical symptoms develop or there is evidence of declining immune function. Ongoing clinical trials are continuing to define optimal treatment.

As with adults, interactions with foods need to be taken into consideration. Other factors to consider are:

- the formulations available, i.e. liquid, tablet, capsule, powder
- the volume, taste and timing of the medicine
- frequency of administration
- the parents' or carers' own medication needs.

Providing nutrition support to children with HIV is critical for two reasons: it provides the greatest opportunity for normal growth and development, and it supports the optimal functioning of the immune system. (Heller 1997).

When planning nutritional advice for HIV infected children several aspects need to be considered:

- social, e.g. housing, cooking facilities, financial aspects
- physical and mental health of other family members
- confidentiality issues that may prevent families from making use of local health services
- cultural background, including traditional foods.

A multidisciplinary approach to care planning is essential, i.e. close liaison with medical, nursing, occupational therapy, physiotherapy, psychology and social-work specialists. Where possible, links with community specialists should also be made.

Nutritional problems in children with HIV

Nutritional problems in infants and children who are HIV infected are complex. Poor growth and/or weight gain were identified in the 1980s. Long-term survivors with HIV infection are shorter in height than expected, and these changes cannot be explained solely by inadequate nutrition or by endocrine abnormalities. Interactions between a number of factors such as immune function, gastrointestinal tract function (malabsorption of fat, protein and carbohydrate, including lactose, may occur even without diarrhoea), malnutrition, and chronic or recurrent infection have been suggested to contribute to the nutritional deficiencies and problems with growth observed in the HIV-infected child (Winter 1996). Some children also present with obesity, possibly related to low activity levels.

There is also concern about dysregulation of lipid metabolism and the fat redistribution syndrome which may be associated with antiretroviral therapy (see Drugs used in HIV, below).

Nutritional assessment

This should include a history of clinical factors that may affect the mouth and gastrointestinal tract, and an assessment of their growth and development (see Table 4.82). Energy levels, opportunistic infections and fevers should also be considered. Some children present with feeding problems which may affect their nutritional intake. These often include:

- a poor appetite
- limited food preferences
- taking a long time to eat.

Developmental delays may occur and the infant or child's developmental age rather than the actual age should be used to assess the most appropriate textures, feeding position and utensils.

A *diet history* should include the following:

- in infants and young children, intake of milk and solids
- quantity and variety of sources of protein, energy, vitamins and minerals
- textures managed, e.g. puréed, soft, hard foods
- meal pattern and time taken to eat main meals
- type and timing of snacks and drinks
- amount of food eaten outside the home, e.g. at nursery or school.

Parents are often willing to complete a 4–7 day food diary which can be analysed to provide a better estimate the energy, protein, vitamin and mineral intake.

Nutrient requirements

Energy requirements of children with HIV are best estimated to meet 100% of the estimated average requirement (EAR) for age, with adjustments made for mobility, fevers and catch-up growth. The height age (extrapolated from the growth chart, taking the age at which the height is on the 50th centile) may be used as a guideline in children with growth impairment.

Energy supplementation, if required, should begin with ordinary foods, e.g. butter or margarine added to rice, pasta and potatoes; use of full-cream milk. Prescribable energy supplements in the form of glucose or fat polymers (see Appendix 6.7) may be required.

Protein requirements for HIV infected children have been estimated to be 150–200% of the recommended daily allowance (Heller 1997).

Vitamin and mineral requirements of HIV infected children are not known for certain. Supplements are not routinely given (to minimize the drug burden). It would seem prudent to aim for 100% of the RNI for all vitamins and minerals. Following a dietary assessment, if this cannot be met, or improved, by dietary intake alone, vitamin and mineral supplementation in order to reach 100% RNI may be advisable. Various paediatric vitamin and mineral formulations are available either in liquid form or in capsules which can be pin-pricked and the contents mixed with olive or vegetable oil and added to foods at meal times.

If further nutritional support is required, age-appropriate sip feed supplements may be considered. Where long-term nutritional support is predicted, gastrostomy feeding may be considered.

For infants and children with chronic diarrhoea, the possibility of lactose intolerance and the need for a lactose-free or reduced lactose diet should be considered. Semi-elemental or elemental formulae may be temporarily required.

Feeding problems are best approached on a multidisciplinary basis, including advice from a speech and language therapist.

Practical guidance may be helpful in some situations:

- *Poor appetite*: Encourage small meals that the child can easily finish, plus small snacks in between. Identify whether the child is drinking too much before meals, and reduce accordingly.
- *Taking a long time to eat*: Limit meal times to 30 minutes at the most, with manageable portions. Encourage praise on completion and offer extra food if desired.
- *Limited variety*: Offer very small portions of new foods with familiar foods.

Most children enjoy eating with others, so encourage family meal times as often as possible.

Appetite-stimulant drugs, such as cyproheptadine or MA, rarely achieve greater than 10% increase in food intake and, because of the efficacy of HAART, have been largely superseded (Tudor Williams and Pizzo 1994).

Food safety advice should be given where necessary.

4.36.8 Nutrition and intravenous drug misusers

Nutritional status of drug misusers

There have been relatively few studies of nutritional status and dietary intake in drug misusers; however, a recent review of the literature indicates that this group is at risk of both poor nutritional status and food intake, regardless of HIV infection (Noble and McCombie 1997). Low body weight, poor nutrition reserves and inadequate or poor quality dietary intake appear to be the main problems.

Nutritional problems of drug misusers

The nutritional problems faced by the HIV positive intravenous drug misuser (IVDM) are similar to those of the HIV positive non-drug user, but their magnitude tends to be greater as a result of the underlying mental health and social problems and already compromised nutritional status commonly associated with drug misuse. Particularly common nutritional problems among IVDM are:

- *constipation*: as a consequence of opiate drugs, methadone or low intake of dietary fibre
- *anorexia*: associated with opiate drugs, constipation, infections and mental-health problems
- *poor dental hygiene and dental decay*: contributory factors include lack of dental care, high intake of refined carbohydrates and the inhibitory effect of opiates on saliva production. Methadone, used in treatment as a substitute for heroin, has also been considered to be a major contributor to dental caries in IVDM because it contains sugar. However, there is little or no evidence to substantiate this and it seems more likely that the combination of poor dental hygiene and high intake of dietary sugars (in addition to those consumed via methadone) is the principal cause
- *low body weight and poor nutritional reserves*: consequences of a prolonged inadequate dietary intake associated with factors such as poor finances, erratic lifestyle, multidrug use, poor cognition and little nutritional knowledge.

Dietary intake of drug misusers

There have been relatively few nutritional studies in IVDM, but one recent study (Zador *et al.* 1996) suggested that dietary characteristics include:

- high consumption of refined carbohydrates, particularly confectionery, sweetened drinks, cakes and biscuits
- low intake of fruit and vegetables
- high intake of milk: while this usually at a level which would be sufficient to meet protein needs, total energy intake often falls below requirements and hence some of this protein is likely to be diverted to help to meet energy needs.

There is often heavy reliance on high fat takeaway snacks such as pies, pastries and crisps, and little tendency to cook or prepare meals. However, this varies depending on the nature of the drug misuser, and the amount and frequency of the drugs used. Those who are less chaotic or are stabilized in their drug use are more likely to eat regular meals and snacks and to prepare and eat food at home.

Dietary advice to drug misusers

There are very few available data regarding the efficacy of dietary advice in the drug-using population, although one study by Dowling *et al.* (1990) indicated that dietary intervention in a group of predominantly HIV positive drug misusers resulted in a significant increase in the intake of most nutrients measured. As with any individual, however, the advice must be practical and realistic, taking account of social and financial circumstances.

Initially, dietary advice should focus on:

- ensuring that the diet is well balanced
- improving intake of energy-dense foods if body weight is low
- encouraging familiar food
- encouraging easily prepared, inexpensive snacks.

The resulting diet may be one that is high in fat and sugar; however, in the majority of cases the priority is to improve overall energy and nutrient intake in the short term, with a view to improving quality on a longer term basis.

Use of nutritional supplements

There is anecdotal evidence to suggest that there is a misuse of prescribable nutritional supplements (sip feeds) among some of this client group, with some people using them as an easy substitute for meals. The requirement for nutritional supplements needs to be considered on an individual basis with regular review and monitoring of the patient.

4.36.9 HIV infection in multicultural groups

In certain areas of the UK, particularly parts of London, there are considerable numbers of Africans living with HIV infection. In addition to the infection itself, many other factors may affect nutritional intake in this client group. Examples of these factors include:

- cultural and religious beliefs
- availability of traditional foods
- length of time in the host community
- family structure and social networks
- finance.

For those new to the country, knowing where to shop to buy African foods or how to prepare Western alternatives can prove daunting. Not having English as a first language can compound these difficulties. There may be additional problems concerning lack of finance and accommodation and, for some, worries regarding immigration status.

Dietitians need to have knowledge of the dietary habits and beliefs of African communities in their area and provide advice which is culturally and socially appropriate. As Africa is a vast continent, it is beyond the scope of this text to discuss typical diets from each area in detail, but examples of the meal structure and dietary constituents typical of East and West African cuisine can be found in Section 3.9 (People from ethnic minority groups). Other sources of advice about African diets are also available to dietitians. Patients themselves are one of the best resources and are usually happy to discuss traditional eating habits and describe the foods eaten. Local shopkeepers and market traders may also prove useful. The British Dietetic's Association HIV/AIDS group (DHIVA) has produced nutritional information sheets suitable for African clients (see Further reading).

4.36.10 Food and water safety

Intestinal infectious diseases and resulting systemic infections can be threatening to people with HIV disease. The general population acquires most gastrointestinal infections via the faecal–oral route by consuming contaminated food and water. This is probably also true for people with HIV disease. Sexual practices may also contribute to the transmission of infection by this route.

Food safety

As the immune system becomes increasingly compromised, susceptibility to infectious diseases increases. To help to prevent food-borne infection, the HIV patient should be given advice concerning:

- safe handling and cooking of food
- general good food hygiene practices
- avoidance of high risk foods such as raw or undercooked meat and fish, raw or lightly cooked eggs, products containing raw eggs, unpasteurized milk and milk products, soft and blue cheeses, and paté.

The Food Safety booklet produced by MAFF is a useful resource for use with clients (see Further reading).

Water safety

Cryptosporidium has been isolated from tap water. This protozoan can produce severe, chronic diarrhoea in those who are severely immunocompromised. For this reason, patients with a CD4 count below 200 should be advised to use boiled tap water for drinking, tooth brushing and washing fruit, vegetables and salads. It should be noted that:

- Domestic jug filters do not remove *Cryptosporidium* oocysts from water.
- Bottled water cannot be guaranteed to be free from *Crytosporidium* and should not be recommended as an alternative to boiled tap water in the UK.

4.36.11 Drugs used in HIV disease

Drugs used in the management of HIV fall into two broad categories outlined below.

Drugs used to treat or prevent opportunistic infections such as antibacterial, antiviral or antifungal agents

Many of these drugs have side-effects such as nausea and diarrhoea which can impact on nutritional status. Table 4.83 outlines some of the more commonly used drugs and their potential nutritional consequences. In addition to these, a host of anti-emetic and anti-diarrhoeal agents is used for symptom control in HIV. The use of drugs in the management of wasting is discussed in Pharmacological management of weight loss and wasting, above.

Drugs which halt or suppress the replication of HIV itself (antiretroviral agents)

Three main types of antiretroviral agent are currently licensed:

- *Nucleoside analogue reverse transcriptase inhibitors (NRTIs)*: These inhibit the HIV enzyme reverse transcriptase, thus impairing replication of the virus's genetic material.
- *Non-nucleoside reverse transcriptase inhibitors (NNRTIs)*: These also target reverse transcriptase.
- *Protease inhibitors (PIs)*: The viral protease enzyme is involved in the formation of new HIV virions in the cell

Table 4.83 Drugs used in the management of HIV and possible nutritional consequences

Infection	Drug	Side-effects with nutritional implications
Viral:		
Herpes simplex	Acyclovir	Nausea, vomiting, diarrhoea
Cytomegalovirus (CMV)	Ganciclovir	Nausea, vomiting
Fungal infections:		
Candida	Fluconazole	Nausea, diarrhoea
Cryptococcal meningitis	Amphoteracin	Nausea, vomiting, diarrhoea
Protozoan:		
Pneumocystis carinii pneumonia (PCP)	Atovaquone	Nausea, vomiting, diarrhoea
Stevens–Johnson syndrome	Co-trimoxazole	Nausea, diarrhoea,
Toxoplasmosis	Sulphadiazine	Nausea, vomiting
Bacterial:		
Mycobacterium avium intracellulare (MAI)	Clarithromycin	Nausea, vomiting, diarrhoea
Tuberculosis (TB)	Rifabutin	Nausea, vomiting
Cancers:		
Kaposi's sarcoma	Chemotherapy	Nausea, vomiting
	Radiotherapy	Depends on site of radiotherapy

nuclei. PIs block the action of this enzyme, halting the final processing of viral proteins and preventing the production of new infectious viral particles.

Figure 4.13 illustrates how antiretroviral drugs block HIV. A combination of three or more antiretroviral agents has been shown to reduce viral replication, delay disease progression and prolong survival in individuals infected with HIV. The advent of this combination therapy has also led to improvements in nutritional status in these patients (Carbonnel *et al.* 1998).

There are nutritional considerations with some of these drugs:

- *Timing may need to be co-ordinated with food intake to maximize absorption*: A major concern is drug resistance, which can occur if plasma levels of the drug fluctuate. If drug levels fall too low, HIV can mutate to form resistant strains. The absorption of some drugs is inhibited by the presence of food in the gut, whereas others are utilized more efficiently in the presence of fat, protein and carbohydrate. It is important to check whether a drug manufacturer has issued any recommendations concerning diet. In order to time medication correctly and provide minimum disruption to established eating patterns, the dietitian, together with other members of the multidisciplinary team, will often produce food and drug timetables for patients.
- *Side-effects can impact on nutritional status*: Many antiretrovirals have side-effects such as diarrhoea, nausea, mouth ulcers and tiredness, which inevitably affect food intake. Some of these drugs may also increase susceptibility to hyperlipidaemia and diabetes.

- *Fat redistribution syndrome (FRS)*: This is a complication, often linked to antiretrovirals, in which body fat becomes abnormally distributed, with peripheral fat wasting and central redisposition (Shaw *et al.* 1998). Such changes in body shape can be very distressing for patients. While it is unclear how effective dietary manipulation will be in the management of FRS, it seems prudent to follow general healthy eating guidelines for weight loss.

Owing to the number of drugs available and their possible combinations it is beyond the scope of this text to discuss the implications of specific drug therapies in detail. In addition, other drugs not yet formally approved for use in the UK are available through special access schemes and clinical trials. While the problem of drug resistance continues and the lack of a cure for HIV remains, the demand for and development of new drugs will continue to increase. Dietitians need to remain vigilant as to their possible nutritional consequences.

4.36.12 Unproven diet therapies

In common with patients suffering from other incurable diseases, HIV positive clients often seek to take some measure of control over their treatment by following alternative diets. Since there is a wide variety of such regimens in use whose popularity changes with time, it is not appropriate to give exhaustive details of each here. Currently, herbal remedies and the anti-candida diet remain popular with HIV patients. Macrobiotic regimens now seem to be used less frequently than used to be the case.

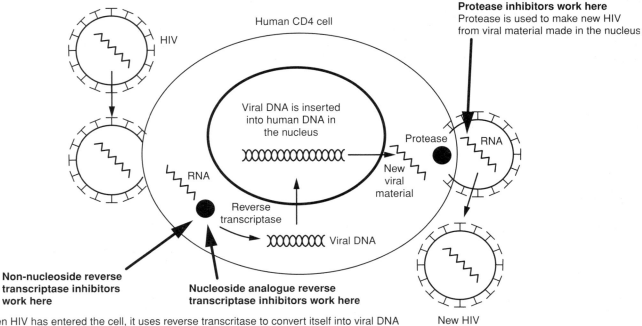

Figure 4.13 Where retrovirals block HIV.
From National AIDS Manual (NAM) Information Series No. 4, *Anti-HIV Drugs*; reproduced with permission from NAM Publications.

Examples of some of these regimens and their implications for the dietitian are discussed elsewhere (see Section 4.37.3, Alternative diets and cancer). However, it is important that dietitians keep up to date with new dietary strategies which come into vogue and consider the implications of these according to individual circumstances.

Megadoses of vitamins and minerals

Patients often decide to self-supplement with a variety of micronutrients, often in doses far in excess of the RNI. As well as the risk of direct toxicity, excessively high intakes of some nutrients are known to have adverse effects on the absorption or metabolism of others (e.g. zinc can inhibit iron absorption) and could potentially have other undesirable consequences such as immunosuppression. At present there are no published guidelines on the use of vitamin and mineral supplements in people with HIV infection. Several studies have examined the role of individual nutrients (Tang *et al.* 1993; Abrams *et al.* 1993), but results remain inconclusive. Dietitians should explore the possibility of supplement use and discourage practices that may be potentially deleterious.

4.36.13 Community care of the HIV patient

The scope of nutrition in the care of HIV positive people in the community is enormous and embraces a wide range of different areas.

Working with non-statutory organizations

Various support services exist for people who are HIV positive, in addition to health and social service provision. Nutritionists can be involved in a number of ways, such as contributing to advice leaflets and newsletters, participating in training sessions with staff and volunteers, providing workshops and one-to-one advice sessions.

Outreach projects and the voluntary sector

There is a role for nutrition incentives and advice in HIV-related projects, e.g. street drug agencies, needle-exchange schemes and health improvement services for the street population.

Nutritional advice needs to be interpreted to reflect the needs of people who may be homeless or suffering financial hardship and who give little priority to food. This may take the form of literature and information, education of other workers and individual advice sessions.

Respite, terminal care and convalescent services

These services, such as hospice care, are often provided by the voluntary sector rather than the National Health Service (NHS). Many hospices had clauses in their constitutions which limited them to accepting only people with cancer for terminal care, but this has changed and, increasingly, non-specialized hospices are accepting people with AIDS. There are a small number of hospices dedicated to caring for people with HIV.

There are a need to work with staff and carers to ensure that people receive good nutritional care.

Home care teams

Many centres offering treatment to people who are HIV positive have established multidisciplinary teams able to provide 24 hour care for people who are no longer able to attend hospital and who wish to remain in their homes.

It may be necessary to provide nutritional support in the home. It is advisable to have policies to cover such provision but they do not need to be HIV specific.

4.36.14 Role of the dietitian in the care of people with HIV disease

Care of the HIV positive person extends far beyond the treatment of a medical problem. People who are HIV positive are often young adults who are frequently well informed about their condition and want to be involved in decisions about their care. They may face periods of poor health, physical changes and premature death. These can impact upon many different areas of their life, ranging from work, finance and housing to family and social support, as well as their ability to feed and care for themselves. A variety of experts working in co-operation with one another is essential to help people to understand their options and make decisions.

Maintaining a good food intake is important throughout the course of the disease. A multidisciplinary team approach to management draws together and co-ordinates all of the service possibilities that can help a person to achieve nutritional goals.

Text revised by: Cathy Hodgson, Jane Butler, Ian Jones, Carole Noble, Alison Thompson and Rachael Donnelly on behalf of the British Dietetic Association's DHIVA (Dietitians in HIV and AIDS) group

Useful addresses

AVERT (AIDS Education and Research Trust)
4 Brighton Road, Horsham, West Sussex RH13 5BA
Tel: 01403 210202   Fax: 01403 211001
E-mail: avert@dial.pipex.com
Has a free information serice available to the general public and health professionals

Terrence Higgins Trust
52–54 Grays Inn Road, London WC1X 8JU
Tel: 020 7831 0330
E-mail: info@tht.org.uk
Information service, library and health-promotion projects.

Provides advice on welfare rights, housing and legal matters for people with HIV. Counselling and family therapy also available.

National AIDS Helpline
Tel: 0800 567123 (A free and confidential 24 hour phoneline)

National AIDS Manual Publications
16a Clapham Common Southside, London SW4 7AB
Tel: 020 7627 3200   Fax: 020 7627 3101
E-mail: admin@ nam.org.uk
Website: www.aidsmap.com

Further reading

DHIVA/Multicultural Group Nutrition Resource Pack (Diet sheets, etc., on African food). Details available from the information and resources officer of DHIVA, c/o The British Dietetic Association.

MAFF. *Food Safety.* Foodsense Booklet No. 1, Ref. No. PB0551. Copies available free of charge from: Foodsense, London SE99 7TT. Tel: 0645 556000.

National AIDS Manual (NAM), Alcom K (Ed.). *AIDS Reference Manual*, 21st ed. London: NAM Publications, 1998/1999.

Pratt R. *AIDS: A Strategy for Nursing Care.* London: Edward Arnold, 1995.

References

Abrams B, Duncan D, Hertz-Picciotto I. A prospective study of dietary intake and acquired immunodeficiency syndrome in HIV – seropositive homosexual men. *Journal of AIDS* 1993; **6**: 949–958.

Adler MW (Ed.). *ABC of AIDS*, 4th edn. London: BMJ Publishing Group, 1997.

Balog DL, Epstein ME, Amodio-Groton MI. HIV wasting syndrome: treatment update. *Annals of Pharmacotherapy* 1998; **32**: 446–458.

Baum M, Cassetti L, Bonvehi P *et al.* Inadequate dietary intake and altered nutritional status in early HIV-1 infection. *Nutrition* 1994; **10**: 16–20.

Beach RS, Mantero-Atienza E, Shor-Posner G *et al.* Specific nutrient abnormalities in asymptomatic HIV-1 infection. *AIDS* 1992; **6**: 701–708.

Beisel WR, Edelman R, Nauss K, Suskind RM. Single nutrient effects on immunological functions. *Journal of the American Medical Association* 1981; **245**, 53–58.

British Dietetic Association. *Nutrition Intervention in Human Immunodeficiency Virus Infection.* Position Paper. Birmingham: BDA, 1995.

Carbonnel F, Maslo C, Beaugerie L *et al.* Effect of Indinavir on HIV related wasting. *AIDS* 1998; **12**: 1777–1784.

Chandra RK. Immunodeficiency in undernutrition and over-nutrition. *Nutrition Reviews* 1981; **39**: 225–231.

Chandra RK. Nutrition and immunology: from basic observations to clinical applications. *Recent Advances in Clinical Nutrition* 1984; **11**: 221–225.

Chandra RK. Nutrition and immunity: lessons from the past and new insights into the future. *American Journal of Clinical Nutrition* 1991; **53**: 1087–1101.

Communicable Disease Report Weekly. Volume 9, No. 9. London: Public Health Laboratory Service, 1999a.

Communicable Disease Report Weekly. Volume 9, No. 18. London: Public Health Laboratory Service, 1999b.

Coodley GO, Coodley MK, Nelson HD, Loveless MO. Micronutrient concentrations in the HIV wasting syndrome. *AIDS* 1993; **7**: 1595–1600.

Cunningham-Rundles S. The effects of nutritional status on immunological function. *American Journal of Clinical Nutrition* 1982; **35**: 1202–1210.

Department of Health. *Dietary Reference Values for Food Energy and Nutrients for the United Kingdom.* Report on Health and Social Subjects 41. HMSO, London, 1991.

Dowling S, Mulcahy F, Gibney MJ. Nutrition in the management of HIV antibody positive patients: a longitudinal study of dietetic out-patient advice. *European Journal of Clinical Nutrition* 1990; **44**: 823–829.

Dowling S, Kane D, Chua A *et al.* An evaluation of percutaneous endoscopic gastrostomy feeding in AIDS. *International Journal of STD and AIDS* 1996; **7**: 106–109.

Foudraine NA, Weverling GJ, van Gool T *et al.* Improvement of chronic diarrhoea in patients with advanced HIV-1 infection during potent antiretroviral therapy. *AIDS* 1998; **12**: 35–41.

Grunfeld C, Kotler DP. The wasting syndrome and nutritional support in AIDS. *Seminars in Gastrointestinal Disease* 1991; **2**: 25–36.

Grunfeld C, Pang M, Shimizu L *et al.* Resting energy expenditure, caloric intake and short term weight change in human immunodeficiency virus infection and the acquired immunodeficiency syndrome. *American Journal of Clinical Nutrition* 1992; **55**: 455–460.

Heller LS. Nutrition support for children with HIV/AIDS. *Journal of the American Dietetic Association* 1997; **97**: 473–475.

Keating J, Bjarnason I, Somasundaram S *et al.* Intestinal absorptive capacity, intestinal permeability and jejunal histology in HIV and their relation to diarrhoea. *Gut* 1995; **37**: 623–629.

Kotler DP, Tierney AR, Wang J, Pierson RN. Magnitude of body cell mass depletion and the timing of death from wasting in AIDS. *American Journal of Clinical Nutrition* 1989; **50**: 444–447.

Macallan DC, Noble C, Baldwin C *et al.* Energy expenditure and wasting in human immunodeficiency virus infection. *New England Journal of Medicine* 1995; **333**: 83–88.

Melchior JC, Salmon D, Rigaud D *et al.* Resting energy expenditure is increased in stable, malnourished HIV infected patients. *American Journal of Clinical Nutrition* 1991; **53**: 437–441.

Morbidity and Mortality Weekly (MMWR). Revised classification system for human immunodeficiency virus infection codes and official guidelines for reporting ICD-9-CM. *Morbidity and Mortality Weekly Report* 1994; **43**: 1–12.

Moseson M, Zeleniuch-Jacquotte A, Belsito DV *et al.* The potential role of nutritional factors in the induction of immunologic abnormalities in HIV positive Homosexual men. *Journal of Aquired Immune Deficiency Syndrome* 1989; **2**: 235–247.

Noble C, McCombie L. Nutritional considerations in intravenous drug misusers: a review of the literature and current issues for dietitians. *Journal of Human Nutrition and Dietetics* 1997; **10**: 181–191.

Palenicek JP, Graham NMH, He YD *et al.* and the Multicenter AIDS Cohort Study Investigators. Weight loss prior to clinical AIDS as a predictor of survival. *Journal of Acquired Immune Deficiency Syndrome* 1995; **10**: 366–373.

Pizzo PA. Paediatric AIDS: problems within problems. *Journal of Infectious Diseases* 1990; **161**: 316–325.

Sharpstone DR, Murray CP, Ross HM *et al.* Energy balance in asymptomatic HIV infection. *AIDS* 1996; **10**: 1377–1384.

Shaw AJ, McLean KA, Evans BA. Disorders of fat distribution in HIV infection. *International Journal of STD and AIDS* 1998; **9**: 595–599.

Suttmann U, Selberg O, Muller MJ *et al.* Home enteral nutrition in patients with acquired immunodeficiency syndrome. *Clinical Nutrition* 1993; **12**: 287–292.

Tang AM, Graham NMH, Kirby A *et al.* Dietary micronutrient intake and risk of progression to acquired immunodeficiency syndrome (AIDS) in human immunodeficiency virus type 1 (HIV-1)-infected homosexual men. *American Journal of Epidemiology* 1993; **138**: 937–951.

Tudor-Williams G, Lyall EGH. Mother to infant transmission of HIV. *Current Opinion in Infectious Diseases* 1999; **12**: 21–26.

Tudor-Williams G, Pizzo PA. Paediatric human-immunodeficiency virus infection. In Steihm RE (Ed.) *Immunological Disorders in Infants and Children*, 4th edn. Philadelphia, PA: WB Saunders & Co., 1994.

UNAIDS/WHO. The HIV/AIDS situation in mid 1996 – global and regional highlights. Press Release 1 July 1996. (http://www.unaids.org/unaids/press/figures.html)

Winter H. Gastrointestinal tract function and malnutrition in HIV-infected children. *Journal of Nutrition* 1996; **126** (10 Suppl): 2620S–2622S.

Zador D, Lyons Wall PM, Webster I. High sugar intake in a group of women on methadone maintenance in South Western Sydney, Australia. *Addiction* 1996; **91**: 1053–1061.

4.37 Cancer

4.37.1 Diet and the causation of cancer

Cancer is a major cause of mortality and morbidity throughout the world. In Britain, about 200 000 new cases occur every year, and cancer has now overtaken heart disease as the leading cause of death in the UK (Mayor 1998).

Cancer will affect about 1 in 3 of the population at sometime in their lives, with more than 70% of cancers occurring in those aged over 65 years. However, it also strikes the population unevenly and there are wide differences in cancer incidence and outcome according to where people live, their socioeconomic circumstances or ethnic origin (DH 1999). It is thought that at least 2 out of 3 cancer-related deaths are preventable, many of them by diet and lifestyle measures. Many cancers are also curable if detected at an early stage. The current UK target is to reduce the death rate from cancer in people under 75 years by at least one-fifth by the year 2010, saving up to 100 000 lives in total (DH 1999).

The term 'cancer' describes a wide range of malignant tumours, classifiable into 81 different types and affecting virtually every organ and tissue in the body. In the UK, the most common cancer sites are those of the lung, colorectum, breast and prostate. Although there is a common underlying aetiology, different factors influence the development of each type of cancer. For this reason, relationships between diet and cancer are complex and variable and dietary factors have a greater influence on some forms of cancers than others.

Development of cancer

Cancer is essentially a consequence of genetic mutations within a cell which result in the production and proliferation of abnormal cells. Some of these genetic mutations are inherited but most simply occur and accumulate over time as the result of lifestyle and environmental factors.

The development of cancer is a complex multistage process which can be summarized as:

1 *Initiation*: Exposure to substances or influences (mutagens) which are capable of initiating genetic mutations. Any DNA damage caused may or may not lead to cancer.
2 *Promotion*: Under the influence of promoters, damaged DNA begins to be expressed resulting in cellular changes. Promoters thus enhance tumour development following exposure to mutagens.
3 *Progression*: A complex process leading to the development of malignant cells which have the capacity to invade other tissues.

A carcinogen is the term for a substance which may influence one or more of these stages. Only a few carcinogens can affect all three.

Cancers spread by invading surrounding tissue until they reach a blood or lymph vessel. Small groups of cells may then break off from the original tumour and be carried to other parts of the body where they may settle and grow (metastases). The new cancers which develop are called secondary cancers (secondaries).

Much remains to be learned about the complex interplay of factors which lead to cancer development, particularly hereditary influences. About 5% of cancer cases are thought to result from inherited genetic mutations, but even the aetiology of this form of cancer is not straightforward; not everyone with a cancer-predisposing genotype develops the disease. Ninety-five per cent of cancer cases are defined as 'sporadic', meaning that they are the unpredictable consequence of a combination of genetics, environment and chance. Since little can be done to alter the influence of genetics and chance, efforts to prevent cancer have to focus on identifying and minimizing the risk from factors which are modifiable, i.e. environmental influences. The main environmental factors implicated in the causation of cancer are:

- *Tobacco*: About one-third of all cancer deaths in the UK are thought to be tobacco related. Cigarette smoking causes 9 out of 10 cases of lung cancer and increases the risk of many other types of cancer, particularly those in tissues most exposed to tobacco carcinogens, i.e. cancers of the mouth, throat, oesophagus, stomach, kidney and bladder.
- *Sunlight*: Most skin cancers are caused by the action of radiation from sunlight on the skin.
- *Diet*: Diet can have either harmful or protective influences on cancer development depending on its composition in terms of foods, nutrients and contaminants (see below).
- *Infection*: Certain viruses can cause genetic mutations which may result in cancer development, e.g. the Epstein–Barr virus is associated with some types of lymphatic cancer and human papilloma virus appears to be closely linked with cancer of the cervix. Infection with the *Helicobacter pylori* bacterium is thought to be a major factor in the development of gastric cancer.
- *Industrial pollutants*: Exposure to toxic substances such as asbestos or vinyl chloride can rapidly lead to cancer. This is more of a problem in developing nations where environmental safety controls are often poor.

- *Ionizing radiation*: Overexposure to X-rays, nuclear emissions or some other sources of radioactivity increases the risk of leukaemias.

Diet and the development of cancer

It has been known for a long time that many components of the diet have carcinogenic potential. Some of these result from food contamination, for example aflatoxin, a potent carcinogen causing liver cancer, is produced by a mould which can grow on grain stored in inappropriate conditions. Other carcinogens such as alkaloids, benzene derivatives or *N*-nitroso compounds occur naturally in foods or are created during cooking or preservation processes.

The human body has many defence systems to protect it from potentially harmful agents in its environment, both dietary and non-dietary, and to a large extent can withstand their continuous onslaught. However, the body's ability to do so depends on factors such as immune competence, integrity of mucosal barriers and levels of detoxifying enzymes. Diet affects all of these. It is therefore not surprising that diet is likely to be one of the factors enhancing or diminishing the risk of cancer.

In 1981 Doll and Peto suggested that about one-third of cancers in Westernized countries may be attributable to dietary factors, and that as many as 70% of cancers in sites such as the large bowel, breast and prostate may be preventable by dietary modification. The evidence for this has since been comprehensively reviewed in two major reports from, firstly, the World Cancer Research Fund in conjunction with the American Institute for Cancer Research (WCRF/AICR 1997) and, secondly, in the UK, by the Working Group on Diet and Cancer of the Committee on Medical Aspects of Food and Nutrition Policy (DH 1998). Their findings are summarized below but readers are referred to these reports for in-depth discussion of this subject.

The reports confirm that there are many links between diet and cancer, both causal and protective. They also make it clear that the relationships are far from simple and, given the quality of the available evidence, difficult to ascertain.

The nature of the evidence for relationships between diet and cancer

Most of the suggested associations between diet and cancer in humans are based on data from epidemiological studies:

- *Cross-sectional studies* compare differences in diet and cancer prevalence, either between or within populations. These observations can provide valuable pointers but are not in themselves evidence of cause and effect as many other relevant factors (e.g. socioeconomic, demographic, genetic, cultural, environmental) will also differ.
- *Case–control studies* look for differences between the diet of people with a particular type of cancer and that

of carefully matched healthy controls. This has the advantage of creating more homogeneous study populations, but at the same time, such homogeneity in terms of age, social class, occupation, etc., also means that dietary differences between the two groups are likely to be small, or not readily detectable given the limitations of dietary assessment methodology. Alternatively, if dietary differences are observed it is difficult to know whether they still existed in the early stages of cancer development, perhaps many years before, or whether they are a consequence of having the disease. Attempting to get round this problem by retrospective dietary assessment is fraught with difficulties; most people cannot remember with any accuracy what they ate 5 or 10 years previously.

- *Prospective (cohort) studies*, where people are followed until cancer develops, thus enabling dietary comparison between those who do or do not develop the disease, are particularly informative. However, because they are also the most difficult and costly studies to carry out, requiring large numbers of subjects to be monitored for 10–20 years or more, relative little information of this type is available.
- *Intervention trials*, where the effects of making dietary change are evaluated in a randomized, controlled prospective trial, can provide the clearest evidence of dietary benefit or risk. However, for reasons of cost they are unlikely to be carried out on a sufficiently large scale, or for long enough, to evaluate the effect of major dietary manipulations (e.g. encouraging a high consumption of fruit and vegetables) on a disease such as cancer. Nor, given the balance of evidence so far, would be it be ethical to do so.

Animal studies are a valuable supplement to human studies to help to explain the mechanisms of carcinogenesis and provide pointers to dietary influences on those mechanisms. Ultimately, however, animal studies cannot predict dietary risk in free-living human populations where many other factors will be operating.

The complexity of the relationship between diet and cancer

The interrelationship between diet and the development of many chronic diseases is known to be complex and multifactorial. Cancer is no exception. However, the relationships between diet and cancer are harder to unravel because of the greater variability of both the disease and the dietary influences on it.

Different cancers are influenced by diet to a different extent. Although all cancers stem from DNA damage, the causes and effects of that damage are very variable. Some cancers (e.g. colorectal) may be strongly linked with diet; others (e.g. leukaemia) have no relationships with diet at all.

Some dietary factors (e.g. non-starch polysaccharide, NSP) may be protective against one type of cancer but have no influence at all on another. Nor do observed dietary relationships always operate in the same direction; energy intake is positively associated with the development of some cancers (e.g. breast and endometrium) but negatively with others (stomach and oesophagus).

A dietary influence may be heightened or diminished by non-dietary factors, for example, a dietary component may only become a risk factor in certain circumstances such as if a person smokes. The risk or benefit from one dietary component may be affected by the presence or absence of other dietary components, for example the level of risk from meat may depend on the level of consumption of protective fruit and vegetables.

For these reasons, attempts to assess whether one particular dietary component is beneficial, harmful or neutral in effect are fraught with difficulty and open to misinterpretation. Few dietary risk factors operate in isolation and it seems increasingly likely that it is the combination of harmful and protective influences from both dietary and non-dietary sources which determines the level of cancer risk.

The relationships between diet and cancer are therefore based on 'best evidence' rather than cast-iron proof. The balance of this evidence is that some dietary components may heighten the risk of some types of cancer while others appear to be protective.

The UK COMA report (DH 1998) concluded that diet-related factors which are most likely to enhance the risk of some cancers are:

- *Obesity*: This may increase the risk of postmenopausal breast cancer and endometrial cancer, possibly as a result of its effects on oestrogen production. Obesity may also enhance the risk of colon cancer. The observed associations between high fat intakes and the development of some cancers, particularly breast and colorectal cancer, probably reflect their contribution to excessive energy intake and obesity rather than a direct relationship with dietary fat per se.

- *High intake of meat and meat products*: There is some evidence that the risk of colorectal cancer is greatest in people with the highest intakes of red and processed meat, possibly as a result of their exposure to carcinogens such as heterocyclic amines created during cooking, or *N*-nitroso compounds formed in the gut. High meat intakes are also associated with some other types of cancer, although there is less evidence that lower meat intakes would be beneficial. A particular problem with assessing the risk from meat is that meat-rich diets are often low in protective fruit and vegetables. It is therefore difficult to establish which is the more important risk factor, or whether it is the combination of both factors that is relevant.

- *Lack of fruit and vegetables*: The level of consumption of fruit and vegetables is strongly and inversely associated with the development of many cancers, particularly colorectal and gastric cancer. The protective effect of these foods is thought to be due to the wide range of antioxidants, vitamins and anticarcinogens that they contain (Johnson 1997). No particular type of fruit or vegetable has been shown to be more beneficial than another; protection is most likely to be achieved by consuming a variety of types.

There is at present no evidence that isolated supplements of vitamins A, C or E or beta-carotene protect against the development of cancers and some evidence that high doses may have adverse effects (ATBC Study Group 1994; Omenn *et al.* 1996). Furthermore, since fruit and vegetables are likely to contain many other protective constituents, some of which have yet to be identified, currently available supplements cannot

Table 4.84 Dietary factors and risk of particular types of cancers (Based on the UK COMA report for which there is 'moderately consistent evidence' of either benefit or risk; DH 1998)

Type of cancer	Higher risk associated with	Lower risk associated with
Oral and pharyngeal cancer	(Smoking) High alcohol intake High consumption of salted fish	
Laryngeal cancer		High intake of fruit and vegetables
Oesophageal cancer		High intake of fruits and vegetables
Gastric cancer	(*Helicobacter pylori* infection) High intake of salted meats and fish High intake of salted and pickled vegetables	High intake of fruit and vegetables High intake of vitamin C High intakes of carotenoids
Pancreatic cancer	High total meat and red meat consumption High levels of coffee consumption	High intake of fruit and vegetables High intake of vitamin C High intake of dietary fibre
Colorectal cancer	High red/processed meat consumption Obesity	High intake of vegetables High intake of fibre
Bladder cancer		High intake of fruit and vegetables
Lung cancer	(Smoking)	High intake of vegetables
Prostate cancer	High red meat consumption	High intake of vegetables, especially raw and salad vegetables
Breast cancer	High meat consumption Obesity (postmenopausally)	High intake of vegetables
Endometrial cancer	Obesity	
Cervical cancer		High intake of folates

Non-dietary factors known to be of key importance are shown in parentheses.

be regarded as an adequate substitute for the foods themselves.

- *Lack of dietary fibre*: High consumption of dietary fibre (NSP) appears to reduce the risk of colorectal and possibly pancreatic cancer. NSP increases the rate at which the remains of food pass along the intestinal tract and hence reduce the time for which the intestinal mucosa is exposed to potentially harmful substances. Anaerobic fermentation in the large bowel also results in the production of short-chain fatty acids, some of which (e.g. butyric) may have antiproliferative properties.

The conclusions of the COMA report for which 'moderately consistent evidence' exists for links between dietary components and particular types of cancer are summarized in Table 4.84. However, it is important not to focus too much on one aspect of a diet and a particular type of cancer unless that form of cancer is of particular importance (e.g. for an individual at high genetic risk). To do so may create dietary imbalances which impair health and may even inadvertently increase the risk of another type of cancer. For the population in general, it is more important to focus on a diet which protects against cancer overall.

Dietary guidelines for the prevention of cancer

The recommendations of the COMA Working Party (DH 1998) are that, in order to reduce the risk from some of the most common types of cancer, people should:

- maintain a healthy body weight within the body mass index (BMI) range 20–25
- consume a wide variety of fruits and vegetables (at least 5 portions/day)
- eat plenty of cereal foods, mainly in an unprocessed form, as a source of NSP
- not exceed the average UK intake of red and processed meat (about 90 g/day or 8–10 portions/week)
- only consume alcohol in moderation (3–4 units/day for men and 2–3 units/day for women)
- not take high-dose supplements of beta-carotene and other micronutrients as a means of cancer protection since it cannot be assumed that they are without risk.

These guidelines should be followed in the context of a balanced diet based on healthy eating principles.

General guidelines for the prevention of cancer based on the European Code Against Cancer (EC 1995) are listed in Table 4.85.

4.37.2 Diet and cancer care

Nutrition is an important aspect of the care of the person with cancer, from diagnosis onwards. Many aspects of cancer can affect nutritional status, and impaired nutritional status can in turn affect the response to treatment, the amount of treatment required and the quality of life (Bruera and Macdonald 1988). Dietitians working in the field of oncology have a vital role to play in ensuring that nutritional aspects of management are an integral component of multidisciplinary care and that all cancer patients receive the dietetic support they need.

Nutritional implications of cancer

People with cancer are at high risk of nutritional depletion because of the physical and psychological effects of both the disease and its treatment:

- Tumour growth increases metabolic rate and hence increases energy requirements (Hyltander *et al.* 1991).
- Physical symptoms (e.g. pain, dysphagia, vomiting, diarrhoea) impair food intake, impair nutrient absorption or increase nutrient losses.
- The psychological effects of a diagnosis of cancer can result in anxiety and/or depression and impaired appetite.
- Cancer treatments often result in pronounced and debilitating side-effects. Gastrointestinal consequences such as anorexia, nausea, vomiting, diarrhoea, bloating, pain or cramping inevitably have an adverse effect on nutritional intake and additional problems such as taste changes, dysphagia, infections and fistulae may further compromise nutritional status.

The risk of weight loss and undernutrition is therefore high. About 40% of cancer patients have been found to have significant protein-energy malnutrition (de Wys 1986; Von-Meyenfeldt *et al.* 1988) and up to 80% may have some degree of malnutrition (Von-Meyenfeldt *et al.* 1988). The adverse consequences of this in terms of postoperative recovery time, prevalence of complications and prognosis are well documented (see Section 1.11, Under-

Table 4.85 General guidelines for cancer prevention (Based on the European Code Against Cancer, EC 1995)

Do not smoke
Only drink alcohol in moderation
Protect yourself from the sun and avoid sunburn, especially in children
Eat a balanced diet containing plenty of fruit and vegetables and high-fibre cereals, and limit intake of saturated fatty acids
Take plenty of exercise and avoid becoming overweight
Observe health and safety instructions on substances which may cause cancer
Participate in recommended screening programmes, e.g. cervical screening, regular mammogram for women over 50 years
Seek early medical advice for any possible early signs of cancer, e.g. a lump, a sore which does not heal, a mole which changes shape, size or colour, or abnormal bleeding. Advice should also be sought for persistent problems such as a persistent cough, hoarseness, change in bowel or urinary habits or unexplained weight loss

nutrition). In cancer patients, undernutrition may also have implications for cancer treatment because radiotherapy dosages are based on body weight and underweight patients may not be given optimum dosages (de Wys *et al.* 1980). The debilitated patient is also less likely to be able to withstand the side-effects of treatment.

Preventing, and correcting, unnecessary nutritional depletion so that physical strength and quality of life can be maintained for as long as possible are therefore important objectives in the cancer patient. The ways in which this is achieved will vary according to the individual clinical circumstances but primarily comprise:

- ensuring that nutritional and hydration needs are met in an acceptable and appropriate way for each individual throughout the course of the disease
- restoring any nutritional inadequacies which occur
- minimizing the nutritional consequences of the symptoms and side-effects of treatment
- instituting additional nutritional support measures if dietary intake is inadequate
- reviewing the effectiveness of nutritional interventions and adjusting them as necessary.

Close interaction with other members of the multidisciplinary team is essential if these objectives are to be achieved (Flowers and Flack 1993).

General aspects of dietary care of cancer patients

Dietary care of cancer patients may range from offering healthy eating guidance for people who have successfully recovered from treatment, to the provision of total artificial nutritional support for those who are critically ill. In practice, most people will require varying degrees of nutritional intervention throughout the treatment and progression of the disease.

Assessment of individual needs and problems is therefore the cornerstone of dietary management and should consider:

- *current nutritional intake*: whether this is sufficient to meet nutritional needs;
- *current nutritional problems*: the extent to which food and fluid intake is impaired by the physical or psychological effects of the disease or its treatment;
- *the degree of any nutritional depletion which exists*: Although to some extent compounded by the cancer process itself, the extent and rapidity of recent weight loss are important indicators of nutritional depletion (see Section 1.8.4 in Assessment of nutritional status). Other markers of nutritional status such as anaemia or poor immune function may also be indicative when considered in conjunction with dietary intake;
- *the likelihood of further (or future) nutritional depletion*: the need for surgery will incur significant metabolic costs as a result of pre-operative and peri-operative starvation and post-operative trauma. Radiotherapy and chemotherapy often result in general disinclination to

eat as well as causing specific problems with eating or swallowing, or exacerbating problems which pre-exist (see below). The risk of nutritional depletion is particularly high in those who are already in a malnourished state;
- *the nutritional implications of specific types of cancer* (e.g. malabsorption resulting from pancreatic cancer) and any consequences of surgical procedures (e.g. dumping syndrome following gastric resection). These are discussed in more detail in other parts of this book.

Even if no nutritional problems are identified, the importance of good nutrition should still be stressed and people encouraged to continue to meet their needs via a healthy, well-balanced diet.

If nutritional intake is inadequate, the dietetic objectives are to:

- increase energy and nutrient intake in ways which are acceptable to the patient
- tackle general and specific problems inhibiting food and fluid intake
- identify when further nutritional support measures are necessary.

In many people, energy, nutrient and fluid intake can be increased by relatively simple dietary measures which increase both the frequency and the energy/nutrient density of foods and beverages consumed (see Section 1.12.1 in Oral nutritional support). Food-enrichment measures (e.g. the addition of milk powder to milk, or adding cheese, butter or cream to foods) can also be an effective way of boosting nutrient intake (see Section 1.12.3).

Remedial measures to help to alleviate treatment side-effects affecting food intake, such as sore mouth, taste changes, nausea, vomiting or diarrhoea, should also be suggested (see Management during cancer treatment, below, and also Section 1.12.2).

If oral intake remains inadequate, additional supplementation in the form of sip feed or other supplements may need to be considered (see Section 1.12.4). Artificial nutritional support (enteral and parenteral nutrition) may be necessary following some types of surgery or in those with severe or worsening malnutrition (see Section 1.13, Artificial nutritional support). If the illness becomes terminal, palliative measures may become the primary consideration (see Section 4.39, Terminal illness and palliative care).

At all stages of the disease, the dietitian has a crucial role to play in identifying when additional support measures are appropriate and what form these should take in order to optimize nutritional status without impairing the quality the life.

Social factors must also not be overlooked. Those who live alone are particularly vulnerable to malnutrition when they are unwell and in pain, and find it an effort to shop, cook and eat food. People should be encouraged to make use of any help offered by friends and neighbours or other support services available in their community.

It is helpful to provide written guidance for patients and carers, together with contact details of a dietitian or other member of the healthcare team. Patients often feel unwell at the time they talk to a dietitian and may find it difficult to remember the advice given, or think of other questions that they wanted to ask later.

Providing appropriate dietetic support and guidance helps patients to feel not only physically better but also often psychologically better equipped to cope with what is inevitably a traumatic phase in their lives. Maintaining nutritional status may improve tolerance to treatment in terms of less medication needed for symptom control, a shorter period of chemotherapy-induced nausea and vomiting, better tolerance of chemotherapy and fewer treatment delays (Bozzetti 1995). All cancer patients should therefore be encouraged to regard 'eating well' as an important component of their medical care, and a positive step that they can take to help to maintain their health.

Specific aspects of dietary management during cancer treatment

Treatment for cancer usually involves surgery, radiotherapy or chemotherapy and sometimes a combination of all three.

Surgery

Surgical removal of a tumour has a number of nutritional implications:

- Preparation for surgery involves a period of nil-by-mouth.
- Surgery incurs a significant metabolic cost as a result of the response to trauma.
- In all cases of surgery, there will be some delay before normal feeding is resumed. If the surgery is major or involves any part of the gastrointestinal tract, there may be considerable delay before feeding is possible via an enteral route. Surgery to the mouth or throat may result in prolonged problems with oral feeding.
- Surgery may result in temporary or permanent side-effects which affect food intake, digestion or absorption (e.g. dumping syndrome, small bowel syndrome, ileostomy).

In addition, some cancer patients will undergo surgery in an already malnourished state and be particularly at risk of severe nutritional depletion. All of these factors need to be taken into account when nutritional care is being planned and will influence:

- whether pre-operative nutritional support is indicated, whether this is feasible and, if so, what form it should take.
- whether peri-surgical and post-surgical nutritional support is likely to be needed, either at an early stage or if there are delays in resumption of oral feeding or complications
- whether nuritional support should be total or partial

- the extent to which the oral route will be accessible
- whether support is likely to be short or long term.

Practical aspects of pre-operative and or post-operative nutritional support can be found in Sections 1.13 (Artificial nutritional support) and 5.6 (Surgery).

As recovery progresses, every effort should be made to restore and maintain good nutritional status, if necessary by means of oral support measures to optimize nutritional intake. Some patients will require specific guidance to alleviate the post-surgical consequences of gastric or intestinal resection such as dumping or short bowel syndrome. The management of these problems is described elsewhere in the Manual.

Arrangements should be made to ensure that, after discharge from hospital, the progress of any nutritionally vulnerable patient, particularly in terms of body weight, is monitored at either the primary or secondary care level.

Radiotherapy

This involves the use of ionizing radiation within a treatment field to destroy cancer cells. Individual radiation treatments, known as fractions (#), are usually given once daily, sometimes more often. The radiation dose is measured in Gray (Gy). The length of treatment can vary from a single fraction to a 7 week course of five fractions per week (Monday to Friday). Radical treatment is given with curative intent, whilst palliative treatment is usually given for symptom control, for example pain or shortness of breath.

Common general side-effects of radiotherapy include:

- anorexia
- nausea
- tiredness
- depression.

Combinations of these, together with travelling for treatment each day, can have a devastating effect on food intake. Some people will find it hard to find the motivation to eat, let alone cope with food purchasing or preparation.

Specific side-effects of radiotherapy to particular areas of the body can further impair food intake. Radiation to the head and neck often affects the ability to eat or swallow, while radiation to the pelvic area often results in abdominal cramps and diarrhoea. If steps are not taken to alleviate them, the nutritional consequences can be severe. The side-effects of radiotherapy may also change during the course of treatment, for example, patients initially experiencing dry mouth may develop a sore mouth at a later stage. Regular dietetic assessment of this patient group is therefore essential to ensure that appropriate and timely advice is given.

Effects of radiation to the mouth, throat, head or neck
This may result in:

- damage to epithelial cells and loss of integrity of the mucosal epithelium, causing:
  - infections of the mouth and throat (e.g. Candida)

- pain and soreness of the mouth due to inflammation (mucositis) or aphthous ulcers
- soreness or burning sensation in the throat;
- damage to the tastebuds, causing:
  - loss of taste
  - changes in taste sensation;
- damage to salivary glands, reducing salivary flow or, if
- the radiation doses are very high, possibly preventing it altogether. This can result in:
  - xerostomia (dry mouth)
  - dysphagia (difficulties with swallowing)
  - difficulties with speaking.

A screening tool to identify nutritional risk in head and neck patients undergoing radiotherapy has been described by Macqueen and Frost (1998). Management of oral problems and measures to alleviate them are discussed further in Section 1.12.2 in Oral nutritional support.

Effects of radiation to the pelvic area Treatment for cancer of the cervix, endometrium and bladder may include a course of radical external beam radiotherapy. This is often given post-operatively and in certain instances, such as some cervical cancers, the treatment may also include intra-cavity caesium. A typical course of treatment will be given each weekday over a minimum period of 4 weeks, either as an inpatient or on an outpatient basis. The target volume of treatment will vary. For example, it will include the whole pelvis for cervical cancer and 1–2 cm around the tumour for bladder cancer.

During pelvic irradiation there is general atrophy of the gut. The villi in the bowel become more cuboidal, and the total epithelial surface and crypt cell mitosis are reduced. During the third and fourth weeks the microvilli are also shortened; however, these return to normal several weeks after completion of treatment. As a result, acute reactions such as nausea, sickness, diarrhoea, abdominal cramps and tenesmus (ineffectual straining to empty the bladder or rectum) commonly occur and may continue for several weeks after completion of treatment. In general, the severity of acute reactions increases with the size of the target dose and target volume required for treatment of the tumour.

Antiemetics and antidiarrhoeal agents may be required to alleviate the acute reactions. It may also be necessary to suspend treatment if the side-effects are severe. Patients with diarrhoea or vomiting or who have a urinary tract infection will require extra fluids.

Most people should be encouraged to eat a normal, well-balanced diet. Various dietary manipulations are sometimes suggested, or self-imposed, to help to alleviate radiation-induced diarrhoea, but there is little evidence that any is universally effective. Such measures may include:

- *Reduction in dietary fibre intake*: Some patients are still routinely advised to consume a low-fibre diet and others will voluntarily reduce their intake of foods such as cereals and fruit juice in an attempt to lessen diarrhoea (Hulshof *et al.* 1987). While the temporary avoidance of foods which appear to exacerbate symptoms may help

individual patients, there is no evidence that routine reduction of fibre intake helps to alleviate the incidence or severity of diarrhoeal symptoms in all patients. Furthermore, untargeted advice to restrict intake of cereals, fruit and vegetables may have significant adverse effects on nutritional intake, especially of micronutrients such as thiamin and vitamin C.

- *Reduction in fat intake*: Pelvic irradiation can impair ileal reabsorption of bile salts, resulting in deconjugated bile acids and fatty acids reaching the colon and triggering diarrhoeal losses of sodium and water. It has been suggested that fat restriction to 40 g/day may help to alleviate these effects (Chary and Thomson 1984), although others have questioned the contribution of bile acid malabsorption to radiation-induced diarrhoea (Schuster *et al.* 1986). Although low-fat diets may assist symptom relief in some patients, the potential detrimental effects on energy intake and body weight, particularly in patients who are already nutritionally depleted, should not be overlooked (Bye *et al.* 1992). The necessity for fat restriction should be determined on an individual basis according to the patient's current level of consumption and symptom severity. If fat intake is already low, further restriction is unlikely to be helpful. If some curtailment appears advisable, this should be achieved by avoidance of high-fat foods to a level of individual tolerance, with any energy deficit being restored via carbohydrate-containing foods or supplements.

- *Reduction in lactose intake*: Impaired lactase production is often assumed to be a contributory cause of radiation-induced diarrhoea and hence lactose restriction, and avoidance of milk and dairy foods, may be advocated. However, since the terminal ileum (where lactase levels are low) usually receives the highest irradiation dose, whereas the mid-jejunum and upper ileum (where lactase levels are highest) are less likely to be affected, there may be little necessity for this measure (Stryker *et al.* 1977; Stryker and Bartholomew 1986). Avoidance of milk and milk products is also likely to have a significant impact on nutritional intake since many patients with poor appetites rely on such easily assimilable foods. If an individual patient's diarrhoeal symptoms appear to be worsened by consumption of milk-containing foods, avoidance of large lactose loads, particularly between meals, may be helpful (see Section 4.8.2 in Malabsorption). However, routine lactose exclusion should not be imposed on all patients.

General signs of malnutrition, either before or during treatment, should be corrected at an early stage, either by dietary means or if necessary with additional supplementation (see Section 1.12, Oral nutritional support). Female patients undergoing pelvic irradiation are more likely to have an impaired food intake than male patients, possibly owing to the higher target doses needed to treat some gynaecological tumours (Hulsof *et al.* 1987). Complete bowel obstruction necessitating parenteral nutrition is an occasional complication of pelvic irradiation.

Chemotherapy

Chemotherapy has a systemic effect, the aim of which is to destroy cancer cells, but which will also affects normal tissue. The consequences, and hence side-effects, are worst in rapidly dividing tissues such as the lining of the mouth and gastrointestinal tract. Administration of chemotherapy can be as:

- oral tablets
- bolus infusion
- continuous infusion
- combinations of the above.

The number of cytotoxic drugs used to treat cancer is continually increasing. Each drug has different side-effects. When drugs are used in combination the aim is to increase toxicity to the cancer cells while minimizing the side-effects for the patient. Nevertheless, side-effects are common and those which may affect appetite and food intake include:

- nausea and vomiting
- taste changes
- stomatitis
- mucositis (resulting in sore or painful mouth)
- oesophagitis
- diarrhoea
- constipation.

In addition to the impact of these on nutritional status, cytotoxic drugs may increase the requirement for certain nutrients as a result of drug–nutrient interactions. For example, methotrexate is a folate antagonist, so its use may be accompanied by 'folinic acid rescue', i.e. the administration of folinic acid to speed recovery from methotrexate-induced mucositis or myelosuppression.

Dietary measures which may help to alleviate effects of chemotherapy such as nausea, taste changes or sore mouth are described in Section 1.12.2 in Oral nutritional support).

Monitoring progress of cancer patients

Nutritional assessment should be an integral part of patient monitoring following cancer treatment. Some patients with severe nutritional problems will be continue to have dietetic follow-up but, for many, continuing care will be provided via primary care or outpatient visits. It is essential that all members of the healthcare team are aware of the need to look for and identify emerging nutritional problems so that they can be rectified at an early stage. Particularly important aspects to consider are:

- weight change
- appetite
- dietary intake and meal pattern
- fluid intake
- difficulties with eating or swallowing
- the impact of symptoms on nutrient intake or requirements.

Appropriate guidance should be given for identified problems or patients referred for dietetic assessment and advice. Patients who are unable to maintain an adequate dietary intake may need nutritional supplementation or artificial nutritional support.

Enteral feeding may be indicated for patients with severe anorexia, dysphagia or mucositis, or who have become nutritionally debilitated. In the short term, this is usually achieved by nasogastric or jejeunostomy tube, sometimes on an overnight basis. In the long term (for 4 weeks or more), it is more likely to be via gastrostomy or jejunostomy.

Parenteral nutrition should only be used when use of the gastrointestinal route is contraindicated, usually for reasons such as bowel obstruction, uncontrollable vomiting or severe malabsorption.

Post-recovery dietary guidance

Patients who have successfully recovered from cancer treatment are usually anxious to consume a diet which minimizes the chance of recurrence. Some may be tempted to follow one of the 'alternative' dietary regimens promoted for cancer sufferers (see below). People should be assured that present evidence suggests that a diet based on the principles of healthy eating, i.e. a well-balanced diet relatively high in starch and fibre and low in fat, will offer the most protection. Particular emphasis should be placed on the importance of plentiful consumption of fruit and vegetables and wholegrain cereal foods. In the UK, *The Balance of Good Health* is an appropriate teaching model. Dietary guidance for cancer protection is summarized in Section 4.37.1. General guidelines for the avoidance of cancer (Table 4.85) may also be helpful.

Palliative care

In some people, cancer cannot be cured and treatment becomes palliative, i.e. focusing on the relief of symptoms rather than on treating their cause.

As the disease progresses, eating and swallowing difficulties become increasingly likely. The patient's food intake is often a great concern to relatives and carers and can even be a source of conflict. Patients become increasingly cachectic and the extent to which nutritional and hydration support should be used to sustain life may eventually need to be discussed. The nutritional care of people who are terminally ill is discussed in Section 4.39 (Terminal illness and palliative care). Some of the ethical issues involved are discussed in Section 1.19 (Healthcare ethics).

4.37.3 Alternative diets and cancer

Many people with cancer are tempted to try unconventional remedies, including alternative and complementary diets, in the hope of cure or remission (Downer *et al.* 1994). The rationale for their doing so is understandable; faced with the prospect of a life-threatening condition, people will try anything which they think might improve their chances of survival. However, no randomized, controlled trials have been carried out to evaluate the benefit of such diets and many healthcare professionals remain sceptical about their value.

The problem with many alternative and complementary diets (Tables 4.86 and 4.87) is that they are more likely to worsen nutritional status than improve it. Such diets tend to share a number of common features such as:

- being vegetarian or vegan
- containing large amounts of raw food
- advocating the use of organic foods
- being low in fat
- being low in sugar, or sugar free
- being low in salt
- restricting intake of dairy products
- avoiding processed foods and beverages containing caffeine
- encouraging the use of vitamin and mineral supplements.

These diets often have a low energy density as a result of their high content of bulky fibrous foods and low content of fat and carbohydrate. People may therefore find it difficult to eat sufficient to meet their needs, particularly if they have eating or swallowing problems associated with the disease or its treatment. Restrictions in food choice may cause dietary imbalances. Megadoses of vitamins and minerals can create other nutritional distortions and may even be hazardous.

Such regimens may also be expensive, unpalatable and time-consuming to prepare. Patients put up with these problems because they have high expectations of a diet's success, but may suffer feelings of anger and frustration if these are

Table 4.86 Definition of complementary and alternative diets

Complementary diet	Any unusual or unorthodox change to a normal diet which claims to benefit people with cancer, followed in association with accepted cancer treatments
Alternative diet	A change to a diet which claims to treat or cure cancer, followed instead of conventional cancer treatment

subsequently not met (Hunter 1991). They may also feel guilty if they have to abandon the diet for any reason.

While there is no evidence that these regimens offer any benefit over conventional therapies, and in some instances make matters worse (Hunter 1988; Cassileth *et al.* 1991), some cancer patients claim to feel better on these diets. The reason for this is unclear but may be associated with 'doing something positive' to take control of their disease and treatment, and also as a result of the, often excellent, psychological support offered along with dietary advice as part of holistic therapy.

It is important that dietitians are aware that patients may be tempted to try, or already be following, alternative or complementary diets. In this situation, the role of the dietitian is not to be judgemental but to equip the patients with the facts which enable them to make an informed choice about the wisdom of this course of action:

- *If patients ask* whether they should try a particular alternative diet, encourage them to find out all they can about the regimen and discuss the potential benefits and hazards openly.

Table 4.87 Examples of alternative and complementary dietary regimens used by cancer patients

Dietary regimen	Philosophy	Main dietary principles
The Bristol Cancer Centre Diet (complementary regimen)	The Centre believes that, as part of a holistic approach, diet and nutritional supplements can be important and may well have an influence on recovery by enhancing the effectiveness and reducing side-effects of cancer treatment, improving well-being and in some cases prolongiong survival	Wholefoods Fresh fruit and vegetables Raw cereals Organically grown foods Organic poultry, eggs, game and fish Beans and pulses Freshly made fruit and vegetable juices Supplements of vitamin C, beta carotene, vitamin B complex, selenium, zinc
Macrobiotics (complementary regimen)	Foods are classified as yin foods, representing feminine, dark and negative principles, and yang foods, representing masculine, light and positive principles. The aim is to balance these for each individual in order to obtain a healthy mind and body	Mainly based on cereal grains Vegetables, sea vegetables (edible seaweeds) and fruit Bean and bean products Nuts and seeds Fish Soup made with vegetables, (edible seaweeds) beans, grains and sea vegetables seasoned with sea salt, soy sauce or miso
Gerson therapy (alternative regimen)	Aim is to stimulate the body's own defence system to overcome cancer. Both the nutritional and detoxification parts of the therapy are required	Vegan Fresh fruit and vegetables Freshly made fruit and vegetable juices Supplements of digestive enzymes, niacin, liver capsules, iodine, thyroid extract, potassium compound and vitamin B_2 injections Coffee enemas

• *If patients are determined to try one of these diets*, encourage them to follow it for a short period such a month and then to return for further assessment and discussion.

• *If an alternative diet is already being followed*, discuss any obvious dietary shortcomings with the patient and suggest positive measures which the patient can take to improve nutritional intake. Some patients may be prepared to compromise and incorporate some aspects of their alternative regimen into a more balanced nutritional programme.

Ultimately, the patient is responsible for making the decision to follow a complementary or alternative dietary regimen. However, it is the responsibility of the dietitian to ensure that the patient has been given sufficient balanced information and advice on which to base that decision. In order to do this, it is important that dietitians keep up to date with the types of diets being promulgated for cancer and their nutritional implications.

The progress and dietary intake of patients following alternative diets should be monitored in order to try and ensure that good nutritional status is maintained.

Text revised by: Briony Thomas

Acknowledgements: Sue Acreman, Julie Ashton, Julie Lees, Julie Nedin, Jane Power, Elizabeth Waters, Jane Wood, Hayley Wordsworth and the British Dietetic Association's Oncology Group.

Useful addresses

BACUP
3 Bath Place, Rivington Street, London EC2A 3JR
Tel: 020 7696 9003
Website: www.cancerbacup.org.uk
BACUP offers support and practical advice to people with cancer and their families and friends.

Cancerlink
11–21 Northdown Street, London N1 9BN
Freephone Cancer Information Helpline: 0800 132905
Freephone Asian Cancer Information Helpline in Bengali, Hindi, Punjabi, Urdu and English: 0800 590415
Provides emotional support and information in response to telephone enquiries and letters on all aspects of cancer to people with cancer, their families, friends, carers and professionals working with them.

Cancer Research Campaign
10 Cambridge Terrace, London NW1 4JL
website: www.crc.org.uk

Macmillan Cancer Relief
Anchor House, 15–19 Britten Street, London SW3 3TZ
Tel: 0845 601 6161

World Cancer Research Fund
105 Park Street, London W1Y 3FB
Tel: 020 7343 4200 Fax: 020 7343 4201

Further reading

Cummings JH, Bingham SA. Diet and the prevention of cancer. *British Medical Journal* 1998; **317**: 1636–1640.

Hill MJ. Meat and colorectal cancer: what does the evidence show? *European Journal of Cancer Prevention* 1997; **6**: 415–417.

La Vecchia C, Tavani A. Fruit and vegetables and human cancer. *European Journal of Cancer Prevention* 1998; 7: 3–8.

Kohlmeier L, Mendez M. Controversies surrounding diet and breast cancer. *Proceedings of the Nutrition Society* 1997; **56**: 369–382.

Willett WC. Diet, nutrition and avoidable cancer. *Environmental Health Perspectives* 1995; **103** (Suppl 8): 165–170.

References

Alpha-Tocopherol, Beta-Carotene Cancer Prevention Study Group (ATBC). The effect of vitamin E and beta-carotene on the incidence of lung cancer and other cancers in male smokers. *New England Journal of Medicine* 1994; **330**: 1029–1035.

Bozzetti F. Nutrition support in patients with cancer. In Payne-James J, Grimble G, Silk D (Eds) *Artificial Nutritional Support in Clinical Practice*. London: Edward Arnold, 1995.

Bruera E, MacDonald RN. Nutrition in cancer patients: an update and review of our experience. *Journal of Pain and Symptom Management* 1988; **3**: 133–140.

Bye A *et al.* The influence of low fat, low lactose diet on diarrhoea during pelvic radiotherapy. *Clinical Nutrition* 1992; **11**: 147–153.

Cassileth BR *et al.* Survival and quality of life among patients receiving unproven as compared with conventional cancer therapy. *New England Journal of Medicine* 1991; **324**: 1180–1185.

Chary S, Thomson DH. A clinical trial evaluating cholestyramine to prevent diarrhea in patients maintained on low-fat diets during pelvic irradiation therapy. *International Journal of Radiation Oncology, Biology, Physics* 1984; **10**: 1885–1890.

Department of Health. Report of the Working Group on Diet and Cancer of the Committee on Medical Aspects of Food and Nutrition Policy. *Nutritional Aspects of the Development of Cancer*. Report on Health and Social Subjects 48. London: The Stationery Office, 1998.

Department of Health. *Saving Lives: Our Healthier Nation*. London: DH, 1999.

De Wys WD. Weight loss and nutritional abnormalities in cancer patients: incidence, severity and significance. *Clinics in Oncology* 1986; **5**: 251–261.

De Wys WD, Begg C, Lavin PT *et al.* Prognostic effect of weight loss prior to chemotherapy in cancer patients. *American Journal of Medicine* 1980; **69**: 491–497.

Doll R, Peto R. The causes of cancer; quantitative estimates of avoidable risks of cancer in the United States today. *Journal of the National Cancer Institute* 1981; **66**: 1192–1308.

Downer SM, Cody MM, McClusky P *et al.* Pursuit and practice of complentary therapies by cancer patients receiving conventional treatment. *British Medical Journal* 1994; **309**: 86–89.

European Community. *The European Code against Cancer*. Brussels: EC, 1995.

Flowers M, Flack S. Improving nutritional status requires team effort. *Nursing Times* 1993; **89**: 61–64.

Hulshof KFAM, Gooskens AC, Wedel M, Bruning PF. Food intake

in three groups of cancer patients. *Human Nutrition: Applied Nutrition* 1987; **41A**: 23–27.

Hunter M. Unproven dietary methods of treatment of oncology patients. In *Recent Results in Cancer Research*, Vol. 108. Berlin: Springer, 1988.

Hunter M. Dietary therapies for cancer: challenging the alternatives. *European Journal of Cancer Care* 1991; **1**: 1.

Hyltander A, Drott C, Korner U *et al.* Elevated energy expenditure in cancer patients with solid tumours. *European Journal of Cancer* 1991; **27**: 9–15.

Johnson IT. Plant anticarcinogens. *European Journal of Cancer Prevention* 1997; **6**: 515–517.

Macqueen CE, Frost G. Visual analogue scales: a screening tool for assessing nutritional need in head and neck radiotherapy patients. *Journal of Human Nutrition and Dietetics* 1998; **11**: 115–124.

Mayor S. Cancer is main cause of death in Britain. *British Medical Journal* 1998; **316**: 571.

Omenn GS, Goodman GE, Thornqvist MD *et al.* Effects of a combination of beta-carotene and vitamin A on lung cancer and cardiovascular disease. *New England Journal of Medicine* 1996; **334**: 1150–1155.

Schuster JJ, Strylker JA, Demers LM, Mortel R. Absence of bile acid malsborption as a late effect of pelvic irradiation. *International Journal of Radiation Oncology, Biology, Physics* 1986; **12**: 1605–1610.

Stryker JA, Bartholomew M. Failure of lactose-restricted diets to prevent radiation-induced diarrhea in patients undergoing whole pelvis irradiation. *International Journal of Radiation Oncology, Biology, Physics* 1986; **12**: 789–792.

Stryker JA, Mortel R, Hepner GW. The effect of pelvic irradiation on ileal function. *Radiology* 1977; **124**: 213–216.

Von-Meyenfeldt MF, Fredrix EWHM, Haagh WAJJM *et al.* The aetiology and management of weight loss and malnutrition in cancer patients. *Bailliere's Clinical Gastroenterology*, 1988; **2**,: 869–885.

World Cancer Research Fund/American Institute for Cancer Research (WRCF/AICR). *Food, Nutrition and the Prevention of Cancer: A Global Perspective*. London: World Cancer Research Fund, 1997.

4.38 Immunosuppressed states

Treatment of leukaemias and other haematological malignancies often involves destruction of bone marrow by chemotherapy and/or radiotherapy prior to bone marrow transplant or peripheral blood stem-cell transplant. Following this, patients will be neutropenic (have a low white blood cell count) and immunosuppressed, and as a result are very susceptible to infection. Immunosuppressed states may also occur in organ transplant patients, people with the acquired immunodeficiency syndrome (AIDS) (Khan 1990) and some patients treated with chemotherapy for other types of cancer.

In order to reduce the risk of infection, the profoundly immunosuppressed patient has traditionally been protected from the external environment by means of a plastic tent or laminar air-flow room, given high doses of antibiotics to make the gastrointestinal tract sterile, and only given sterile foods. Recently, there have been doubts over the benefits of, and need for, such a high level of protection, and these measures are now used much less often, or for shorter periods (Pryke and Taylor 1995). However, the provision of a 'clean' diet (i.e. one with a low microbial content) is still necessary for immunosuppressed patients at high risk of infection.

4.38.1 Sterile diets

Complete sterilization of food is difficult, labour intensive and hence expensive, and results in an extremely limited and unpalatable diet. Sterile foods are defined as those which are free from fungal and bacterial growth 7 days after treatment (Pryke and Taylor 1995).

Foods can be sterilized by:

- *Autoclaving*: This markedly impairs taste and texture and is generally only suitable for liquid and semiliquid food.
- *Irradiation*: Gamma irradiation is an effective way of sterilizing food and usually results in fewer organoleptic changes. To achieve sterility, foods have to be irradiated at two to three times the level used commercially for food preservation and this can result in problems such as accelerated lipid oxidation and amino acid breakdown causing 'off flavours' in particular types of food (particularly high fat milk products). However, recent advances in technology have overcome many of these problems (Pryke and Taylor 1995).

It should be noted that microwaving does not sterilize food, as is sometimes mistakenly assumed (Bibbington 1993). Most canned food can, however, be regarded as sterile.

Sterility also needs to be maintained when the foods are prepared for the patient. To avoid recontamination, this requires their being opened in a laminar air-flow cabinet, heated in special foil-closed containers, double wrapped in sterile paper bags and taken straight to the patient. People preparing the food also need to wear sterile gowns and observe strict hygiene procedures.

With increasing doubt over the need for sterile diets, their use is now becoming rare in UK hospitals. However, some units still use irradiation to sterilize foods normally contraindicated in a low microbe diet, such as herbs, spices, poultry and salads, thus increasing the choice of foods available to patients (Pryke and Taylor 1995).

4.38.2 'Clean' diets

A 'clean' food regimen is a more practical alternative to a sterile diet (Pattison 1993). It aims to provide a nutritionally adequate, palatable diet comprised of foods which either are well-cooked or have a minimum number of potential pathogen-forming units and which therefore minimize the risk to the patient (Pizzo *et al.* 1982).

Choice of foods for a 'clean' food diet

In general, foods which are contraindicated are those which are uncooked or have been exposed to the air and hence likely to be contaminated with bacteria or fungi. Foods which pose the greatest risk to immunosuppressed patients include:

- raw or undercooked animal foods such as eggs or unpasteurized milk or dairy products
- raw vegetables and salads
- fish, particularly shellfish
- meat, especially if inappropriately thawed or undercooked, or if raw meat juices contaminate other foods during food storage or preparation
- foods in opened containers or used communally (e.g. large cartons of ice-cream, the domestic butter dish or tubs of fat spread, jars of jam or marmalade, bottled sauces).
- foods which are stale or near their 'use by' date.

Suitable and unsuitable foods for a 'clean' food diet are summarized in Table 4.88.

Care must also be taken with choice of beverages (see also Table 4.88). Tap water should be boiled before use and

Table 4.88 Suitable and unsuitable foods in a 'clean' diet

Type of food	Suitable choices	Unsuitable choices
Meat	Well-cooked beef, lamb, pork, bacon, poultry Well-cooked sausages and hamburgers Tinned meat	Raw or undercooked meat or poultry Bought precooked cold meats (e.g. ham, sliced chicken or turkey) Salami or similar precooked sausage; paté
Fish	Freshly cooked fish, fish fingers, fish cakes Tinned fish (except for shellfish and fish in cans which have to be opened with a key)	Bought precooked fish (e.g. smoked mackerel, smoked salmon) Fish paté or other delicatessen fish products Shellfish (e.g. prawns, mussels)
Soups	Canned soups Packet soups made with boiled water Freshly prepared home-made soups using permitted ingredients	Reheated canned or home-made soup
Ready meals	Fresh or frozen ready meals which need to be cooked (e.g. shepherd's pie, fish pie, pizza, pasta dishes)	Chilled or fresh products which do not need further cooking (e.g. ready-to-eat poultry, flans and quiches, precooked pizza)
Milk	Sterilized milk UHT milk and milkshakes Pasteurized milk if bought from a shop with a fast turnover, kept refrigerated both before and after purchase, and used within 24 hours Milkshake powder	Unpasteurized milk Products made from unpasteurized milk Syrup-type milkshake mixes Milkshakes from takeaway outlets
Cream	Sterilized, UHT or pasteurized cream	Unpasteurized cream Cream squirted from cans or dispensers
Yoghurt	Smooth pasteurized yoghurt Pasteurized fromage frais	Pasteurized yoghurt containing nuts, muesli or other large food particles Unpasteurized, 'live' or 'bio' yoghurt
Cheese	Processed cheese triangles Individually wrapped processed cheese slices Vacuum-packed hard cheese (e.g. Cheddar, Edam) if used within 2–3 days of opening	Blue-veined cheeses Soft cheeses (e.g. Brie, Camembert, cream cheese, cottage cheese, paneer). Cheese with rind or mould coating
Eggs	Only if extremely well cooked whole eggs should be boiled for 10 minutes Pasteurized egg can be used for cooking	Raw or undercooked eggs Products containing raw egg (e.g. mayonnaise, lemon curd, mousses)
Butter and fat spreads	In the hospital setting, these should be individualized portions At home, the smallest sized tubs should be purchased and only a clean knife allowed to come into contact with the contents	Unwrapped or communally used butter, margarine, spreads or ghee
Bread	Wrapped bread Packaged rolls, muffins, crumpets, chapati, etc. All must either be used within 24 hours, or frozen and used as required	Unwrapped bread and rolls, etc. Bread or burger buns containing or coated with nuts and seeds (e.g. sesame or poppy seeds, fruit breads) Granary and garlic breads
Breakfast cereals	Plain cereals without nuts or dried fruit	Muesli Fruit and/or nut cereals
Cakes and biscuits	Prewrapped cakes Plain biscuits from a small or newly opened packet (once opened keep in a sealed container)	Unwrapped cakes or pastries Cakes with cream, dried fruit, nuts or coconut Cereal or muesli bars
Rice and pasta	Dried or canned rice Dried or canned pasta Pot rice and noodles	Rice salads Fresh pasta Pasta salads
Fruit	Well-washed and peeled fresh fruit Canned and frozen fruit (except for berry fruits)	Unwashed and unpeeled fruit Damaged fruit Dried fruit Berry fruits (e.g. strawberries, raspberries, blackberries) Grapes, unless peeled
Vegetables	All cooked, peeled and washed fresh vegetables Cooked frozen vegetables Canned vegetables Dried potato (made with boiled water) Frozen chips, waffles or croquettes Jacket potatoes if skin is removed	Raw vegetables Salad vegetables Prepared vegetables and salads (e.g. coleslaw, potato salad, herb salads) Dried pulses (e.g. beans, chick peas and lentils)
Beverages	Cooled boiled water or sterile water Tea bags or instant tea Instant coffee Individual cartons of fruit juice or other soft drinks (larger ones should be used within 24 hours)	Ground fresh coffee Bottled water or spring/mineral water

Table 4.88 Continued

Type of food	Suitable choices	Unsuitable choices
Beverages	Cans or small bottles of fizzy drinks (larger sizes should always be used within 24 hours) Sachets of instant drinks Cans of beer or lager (if alcohol is permitted)	
Snack foods	Individual bags of crisps or savoury snacks Wrapped bars of plain or milk chocolate Wrapped sweets	Dried fruit or nuts Unwrapped sweets or chocolate Chocolate containing fruit or nuts Mithai (Indian sweets) Chevda (Bombay mix)
Puddings and desserts	All canned products Milk puddings made with newly opened pasteurized milk UHT desserts Jelly Individually wrapped ice-cream bars	Purchased unwrapped desserts (e.g. trifle, gateau, cheesecake) Desserts containing raw egg (e.g. soufflé, mousse) Desserts containing dried fruit or nuts Purchased desserts containing cream Ice-cream from mobile vans Ice-cream from communally used large tubs
Sugar and preserves	In the hospital setting, individual portions of sugar, jam, marmalade or honey At home, these should be kept in small-sized containers and dispensed with clean cutlery	Communally used sugar, jam, marmalade or honey. Raw or unpasteurized honey Lemon curd Peanut butter Marzipan
Seasonings and sauces	Salt, tomato ketchup, salad cream, yeast extracts: as for sugar, jam, etc. above Pepper: in the hospital setting this should be irradiated Herbs and spices: if added before, not after, cooking Gravy granules	Herbs and spices should not be sprinkled on food after cooking

most types of bottled or spring/mineral water are contraindicated. Previously boiled tap water should be used for cleaning the teeth.

Cooking methods for a 'clean' food diet

Safe cooking methods include:

- *Conventional gas and electric ovens*: The oven should always be preheated to ensure that the food cooks rapidly. The cooking time should be sufficient to achieve a core temperature of 70°C in the food. If necessary, this can be checked using a thermometer with a probe on a *duplicate* food sample; the probe must not be used on food to be eaten by the patient.
- *Boiling on the hob*: Food should be put into rapidly boiling water and brought back to boiling point as soon as possible.
- *Pressure cooking and steaming*: Either a domestic-sized pressure cooker or large-scale catering steamer may be used.

Unsuitable cooking methods are:

- *Microwave ovens*: Although convenient, these are not suitable for cooking foods for 'clean' diets. Microwaves heat food unevenly and, if applied for insufficient time, parts of the food may not have reached the temperature required to kill micro-organisms. It can be difficult to gauge the necessary cooking time as much depends on the size and power of the oven, the volume of the food (especially its uniformity of shape and thickness), its

water, fat and ion content (Dealler and Lacey 1990), and observation of the recommended 'standing times' after cooking.

Microwave ovens can be used for heating canned foods (e.g. baked beans) or for defrosting frozen foods or meals. However, the latter must then be cooked in a conventional oven.

- *Cook–chill systems*: Food preparation involving cooking, chilling, storage and reheating exposes the food to unsuitable temperatures, an unacceptable amount of food handling and many opportunities for contamination. It is therefore not a safe food production system for patients with impaired immunity.

Food preparation and service

Scrupulous attention to food hygiene procedures is essential.

For patients in hospital, food preparation and service should be carried out in a kitchen within the unit where patients are treated. This has several advantages (Gauvreau-Stern *et al.* 1989):

- Food preparation is more easily controlled and there is less risk of food contamination.
- Food can be provided as needed rather than at fixed meal times, thus encouraging more frequent consumption of foods and liquids and hence better nutrient intake.
- Food intake is more easily monitored.

In the hospital setting, cutlery and plates should prefer-

Table 4.89 Food safety guidelines for immunosuppressed patients

---

Buying food

Always check 'use by' dates. Avoid buying food near its 'use by' date and never consume it after this date
Do not buy foods in damaged packaging, e.g. dented cans or torn or crushed packets

Storing food

Store raw and cooked food separately. Keep raw meat, fish and eggs in containers at the bottom of the fridge.
Check fridge and freezer are at the correct temperature. The fridge should be below 5°C; the freezer below 18°C)

Preparing and cooking food

Wash hands thoroughly in hot, soapy water before and after handling food. It is also important to wash hands between handling raw food and cooked food
Keep kitchen surfaces and equipment scrupulously clean. Make sure that any item which comes into contact with food (knives, spoons, chopping boards, etc.) is as clean as possible and free from cracks or food encrustation. Metal spoons and ceramic chopping boards are preferable to wooden ones.
Ensure that canned food is clean. Wash cans before opening and also wash the can opener in hot, soapy water before use. Ring-pull cans are suitable but do not use cans which have to be opened with a key.
Do not use a microwave oven for cooking food. It can be used for heating canned food (e.g. baked beans) or defrosting (but not cooking) frozen food.
Keep cold foods cold and hot foods hot. Cold foods should be kept in a fridge until needed. Hot foods should be served as soon as they are cooked. Always follow the manufacturer's cooking instructions
Never reheat food which has already been heated
Never refreeze thawed frozen food
Avoid using food used communally, e.g. tubs of butter or spread, large cartons of ice-cream, or jars of jam or marmalade. Keep small supplies separately for your own use.

Eating out

It is safer to avoid eating and drinking outside the home while on a 'clean' food diet, as there is always a risk that strict food hygiene measures may not have been observed. If eating out is unavoidable ensure that you:

Never eat foods (or food components) listed as unsuitable, e.g. salads, shellfish. Note that some types of fast foods, e.g. burger buns with seeds, are not suitable.
Only consume foods from reputable restaurants or outlets, not street traders
Never eat barbecued food

---

ably be disposable. Reusable plastic cutlery and crockery should be kept in Milton solution and designated for the sole use of a particular patient.

Following discharge from hospital, patients will need to observe 'clean' food measures for 3–6 months, or until the while cell count is at a level which provides sufficient immunocompetence. All will require written guidance on suitable and unsuitable food choices and general food safety advice to minimize the risk of food poisoning (Tables 4.88 and 4.89).

When 'clean' food measures are no longer necessary, it is usually advisable for patients to avoid high-risk foods such as unpasteurised milks, blue-veined or soft cheeses, live yoghurts, paté and shellfish for a further month after discontinuing the diet.

4.38.3 General dietary considerations in immunosuppressed patients

Many immunosuppressed patients will feel extremely ill as a result of their illness or its treatment. As a result, they are often nutritionally debilitated, and at high risk of further depletion. Chemotherapy and radiotherapy may have resulted in side-effects such as nausea, loss of appetite, sore mouth or taste changes. Chewing or swallowing may have become difficult because of mucositis or oesophagitis. Following some types of transplant, graft-versus-host disease (GVHD) may develop. This occurs when immunological-

ly competent cells from the donor source recognize the host tissues as 'foreign' and mount an attack against them. GVHD affecting the gastrointestinal tract may cause temporary lactose and/or gluten intolerance, with resultant diarrhoea or steatorrhoea and malabsorption.

These problems require active dietetic intervention to ameliorate their effects (see Section 1.12.2 in Oral nutritional support and the relevant parts of Section 4 relating to disease management). Other oral nutritional support measures may also be necessary (see Section 1.12).

It is important that dietary guidance to minimize the risk of microbial exposure takes account of individual preferences in terms of palatability, food texture and food choice in order to optimize nutrient and energy intake.

Text revised by: Briony Thomas

Acknowledgements: Carole Middleton and the dietitians of the Leeds Teaching Hospitals.

References

Bibbington A. Grey areas in 'clean diets' for BMT patients. *Clinical Nutrition Update* 1993; **3**: 3.

Dealler SF, Lacey RW. Superficial microwave heating (Letter). *Nature* 1990; **344**: 496.

Gauvreau-Stern JM, Cheney CL, Aker SN, Lenssen P. Food intake patterns and food-service requirements on a marrow transplant unit. *Journal of the American Dietetic Association* 1989; **89**: 367–372.

Khan P. Food safety in an era of immune suppression: is it a problem in the food processing environment? *Nutrition Today* 1990; **25**: 16–20.

Pattison AJ. Review of current practice in 'clean' diets in the UK. *Journal of Human Nutrition and Dietetics* 1993; **6**: 3–11.

Pizzo PA, Purvis DS, Waters C. Microbiological evaluation of food items. *Journal of the American Dietetic Association* 1982; **81**: 272.

Pryke DC, Taylor RR. The use of irradiated food for immunosuppressed hospital patients in the United Kingdom. *Journal of Human Nutrition and Dietetics* 1995; **8**: 411–416.

4.39 Terminal illness and palliative care

Palliative care aims to optimize the quality of life for people with advanced or incurable disease. Even if nothing more can be done to halt disease progression, much can often be done to make the patient more comfortable, both physically (by controlling pain and other symptoms) and psychologically (by meeting social, spiritual and emotional needs).

The pioneering work of the hospice movement has led to the development of palliative care as a specialist branch of medicine, and one which is increasingly being applied in a range of care settings via palliative care liaison staff and cancer care nurses. Palliative or terminal care can now be given to people at home, in day-care centres, nursing homes and hospitals, as well as within a hospice or palliative care unit.

4.39.1 The role of the dietitian in the palliative care team

Palliative care usually involves a multidisciplinary care team which may include doctors, ward nurses, liaison nurses, district nurses, Macmillan and Marie Curie nurses, dietitians, physiotherapists, occupational therapists, social workers and members of charitable and voluntary organizations. Although palliative care is focused on the patient, it is not always confined to that individual alone; providing support to the patient's relatives and carers is now recognized as being an integral part of care (Higginson *et al.* 1990).

The role of the dietitian within the care team is to help to identify and alleviate any nutritional factors which are impairing a patient's physical and psychological well-being. The primary nutritional objective is to improve the quality of life for that individual. This may involve:

- assessing the nutritional needs and problems of the patient
- advising on ways in which the nutritional requirements of the patient may be met, and when nutritional support measures may be appropriate
- suggesting ways in which nutrition-related problems caused by the physical or psychological effects of the disease or its treatment may be alleviated
- providing advice and guidance for carers
- providing training and support for professional colleagues.

Dietitians working in the field of palliative care require good listening and counselling skills in order to create an empathic relationship with patients and carers. The ability to communicate and interact effectively with other members of the care team is also essential.

4.39.2 Effect of terminal illness on nutritional status

Terminal illness can affect nutritional status in a number of ways:

- The psychological effect of being diagnosed with an incurable and progressive illness is profound, particularly if the diagnosis is unexpected. The consequent anxiety and/or depression, and perhaps an attitude of 'what's the point?', can markedly impair food intake.
- Worsening symptoms of the disease, particularly if of a dysphagic or gastrointestinal nature, may make food consumption physically difficult or associated with discomfort.
- Medication may cause side-effects such as nausea, vomiting or diarrhoea which reduce food intake. Drowsiness induced by sedation or pain relief such as opioids or narcotics may also result in disinclination to eat.
- If treatments such as chemotherapy or radiotherapy are given, their side-effects can markedly affect food intake and increase the likelihood of nutritional inadequacies (see General aspects of Dietary care of cancer patients, in Section 4.37.2).
- Nutritional requirements may be increased by the physiological effects of the illness (e.g. pyrexia, secondary infection, increasing tumour mass) or by nutrient losses (e.g. malabsorption).
- As the final phase of the illness develops, physiological functions such as gastric emptying, digestion and absorption, and peristalsis decline. Both appetite and the ability to tolerate food will decrease.

If nutritional steps are not taken to alleviate these effects at an early stage, patients may enter the terminal phases of their illness in a seriously nutritionally depleted state.

4.39.3 Nutritional objectives in palliative care

The principal objectives are to maximize food enjoyment and minimize food-related discomfort. It is also important to prevent or treat avoidable and unnecessary malnutrition since this can affect both physical and psychological well-being. However, it is equally important that nutritional support measures are not so invasive or unacceptable to the patient that they impair the quality of life.

The way in which these objectives are achieved will vary according to individual needs, problems and clinical circumstances, but will primarily follow a stepwise process of:

- assessing the patient's eating habits and current nutritional status
- identifying any nutrition-related problems or barriers to food and fluid intake, and evaluating their physical and psychological impact
- exploring any nutritional concerns of the patient's family or carers
- discussing with patients and carers dietary goals which are appropriate and achievable.
- integrating these goals into the care plan in a way which is compatible with medical and nursing objectives
- regularly reviewing progress, evaluating the effectiveness of any measures implemented and modifying them as necessary.

As a result of these measures, a patient is more likely to be able to:

- retain the ability to derive pleasure from food and the social aspects of eating
- retain physical strength long enough to fulfil final wishes and ambitions
- have sufficient physical strength to obtain benefit from physiotherapy and occupational therapy rehabilitation
- retain some control over the disease process through attention to nutrition
- die with some dignity and not as a result of starvation.

4.39.4 Practical aspects of dietary guidance

Maintaining good nutrition

Patients should be encouraged to retain an interest in food, and to regard good nutrition as a positive step which can be taken to help to maintain strength and improve well-being. Practical guidance on sensible eating may be welcomed but, while nutrient intake is adequate, the emphasis should be on maintenance of preferred eating habits and continued enjoyment of food.

If nutrient needs are not being met, suggestions to improve nutrient intake by increasing food consumption frequency, and choosing foods of greater nutrient density are a useful first step. Fortification strategies to boost energy intake can be useful and if these prove inadequate, or at times when food intake is particularly poor, oral supplements may be helpful (see Section 1.12, Oral nutritional support).

An important role of the dietitian is to educate other healthcare professionals concerning the means by which good nutrition can be achieved. There is a common belief among the medical and nursing profession that poor nutritional intake always indicates a need for proprietary oral supplements. As a result, there is considerable overpre-scribing of products such as sip feeds, which is both cost-ly to the National Health Service (NHS) and unnecessary (McCombie 1999). While such products play a valuable role in some circumstances, simple nutritional support measures using ordinary foods and fluids should always be considered first.

Maintaining good hydration

Good hydration is important for well-being but it is important that adequate fluid provision is not achieved in such a way that it impairs appetite and compromises nutrient intake from food (e.g. by the overuse of high-volume, low-energy beverages such as soups and soft drinks). If food intake is generally poor, nutrient-rich sources of fluids should be encouraged.

Alleviating problems affecting food intake

Remedial measures for many of the symptoms that commonly impair food intake can be found in Section 1.12 (Oral nutritional support). Guidance that may be particularly helpful for people with terminal illness is summarized below.

Poor appetite

The effects of pain, discomfort, sedation and drug- or treatment-related side-effects commonly result in a reduced appetite. Useful guidance may be to:

- eat small, frequent, attractively presented foods
- eat favourite foods or those which are fancied
- consume fluids after, rather than with, meals to maximize food intake
- ensure that posture helps rather than hinders eating
- eat in surroundings which are as pleasant as possible
- eat in the company of others.

Oral problems

Problems such a sore mouth, dry mouth and taste changes may make eating painful, difficult or unpleasant. As a result, food intake may be impaired or lacking in variety and nutrient intake compromised. Remedial measures are discussed in Section 1.12.2 (in Oral nutritional support), but may include:

- *Sore mouth*: Salty, spicy or acidic foods may be replaced with blander, less astringent alternatives.
- *Dry mouth (xerostomia)*: Measures such as taking frequent small sips of water, sucking ice cubes, ice lollies or citrus-flavoured boiled sweets, chewing fruit-flavoured sweets may help to stimulate salivary flow. Meals should be moist in texture.
- *Taste changes*: Problematic foods should be substituted with nutritionally similar alternatives, e.g. poultry or fish instead of red meat, soft drinks or milk instead of tea or coffee, boiled sweets or pastilles instead of chocolate. The use of herbs and spices in cooking may be helpful for those suffering from loss of taste.

Dysphagia

This requires expert assessment and management in order to provide food of an appropriate consistency while also maintaining nutrient intake (see Section 4.3, Dysphagia). In some nursing homes, there is still a tendency to liquidize everything for a person with swallowing problems and over-reliance on soups or drinks of low nutrient density.

Early satiety or gastrointestinal discomfort following eating

Food should be consumed in smaller amounts but more frequently. The use of nutrient-dense food choices should be encouraged.

Belching and/or flatulence

This is a common manifestation of gastric disturbance and can be very distressing for the patient. Some alleviation may be possible by:

* avoiding foods and drinks which exacerbate gas production, such as carbonated beverages, beer, and vegetables such as brassicas (broccoli, spinach, cauliflower, Brussels sprouts), peas, beans, sweetcorn, onion and radish;
* reducing the amount of ingested air by eating slowly, keeping the mouth shut when chewing and swallowing, and avoiding sucking drinks through a straw.

Constipation

This is a common problem as a result of reduced dietary intake, immobility and the use of pain-relieving medication. Relief of constipation by medical means should be followed by dietetic attempts to prevent its recurrence. Increasing fluid intake is an important remedial measure, but this needs to be achieved in a way which does not compromise nutrient intake. While some increase in fibre intake may be appropriate, excessive fibre intakes should be avoided by people with small appetites and are contraindicated in those at risk of intestinal obstruction or with existing dehydration (see Section 4.11.1, Constipation).

Diarrhoea

This can have a number of causes, the most common being impaired gastrointestinal function and drug side-effects. Foods which seem to be particularly poorly tolerated may need to be avoided but in general the diet should aim to include as wide a variety of foods as possible to minimize dietary imbalance and food fatigue.

Hypercalcaemia

No attempt should be made to reduce or restrict dietary sources of calcium, as this is ineffective in alleviating hypercalcaemia. The consumption of carbonated beverages containing phosphoric acid may be beneficial if the patient finds them palatable.

4.39.5 Guidance for carers

Simple measures to encourage someone to eat who, for a variety of reasons, may not feel much like eating, can often make an enormous difference to nutrient intake. One feature of hospices is that the quality and presentation of food offered is usually exceptionally good: the menus are tempting, snacks can be provided at any time and food is always attractively served. This is possible because hospices usually have a high level of volunteer staff who have time to administer to individual needs and wishes. Hospitals and nursing homes rarely have this luxury, but dietitians can often suggest simple measures which can improve the quality and availability of food service (e.g. suitable snacks which can be kept available in a ward kitchen).

Useful guidance for carers is to:

* feed the patient when hungry, at any time of day or night. Patients may well have altered sleep patterns which render them wakeful during the night and asleep during the day
* serve small portions of food
* set an attractive table, tray or plate
* encourage gently, never nag
* help the patient to get some fresh air before a meal by taking the person outside or opening a window
* remove bedpans, vomit bowls and other waste receptacles from the eating area.

When people are cared for in the domestic setting, food may become a source of tension and conflict. The giving and receiving of nourishment is a means of showing love and affection, and consequently food refusal can cause offence and create barriers within the family unit. Involving carers in discussions about the nutritional needs and difficulties of the patient can help to defuse problems. Carers usually welcome guidance on how better food intake may be achieved. Most find it helpful to be given written material providing ideas for good choices of nutrient-dense foods or drinks, food fortification strategies and tips on the size and presentation of meals.

Dietitians should also be aware of the needs and problems of the carers themselves and ensure that they are aware of the support available to those who care for someone with chronic illness (see Section 4.29.7 in Dementias).

4.39.6 Nutritional issues in the latter stages of terminal illness

Artificial nutritional support

As a result of increasing debility or dysphagia, a point may be reached when adequate nutrition can only be maintained by nasogastric or gastrostomy feeding. This raises a number of ethical questions (Boyd and Beeken 1994). For some patients, artificial nutritional support may be a beneficial step; for others, it may not be appropriate. The likely effect of nutritional support on the quality of life must always be borne in mind (Grindel et al. 1996). It is vital that each patient is considered individually, the goals

Table 4.90 Artificial hydration for people who are terminally ill
Summary of recommendations prepared by a Joint Working Party between the National Council for Hospice and Specialist Palliative Care Services and the Ethics Committee of the Association for Palliative Care Medicine of Great Britain and Ireland, 1997; Reproduced with permission of the National Council for Hospice and Specialist Palliative Care Services

1 A blanket policy of artificial hydration, or of no artificial hydration, is ethically indefensible.
2 Towards death, a person's desire for food and drink lessens. Study evidence is limited but suggests that artificial hydration in imminently dying patients influences neither survival nor symptom control. As such, it may constitute an unnecessary intrusion.
3 Thirst or dry mouth in people who are terminally ill may frequently be caused by medication. In such circumstances artificial hydration is unlikely to alleviate the symptom. Good mouth care and reassessment of medication become the most appropriate interventions.
4 Appropriate palliative care will involve consideration of the option of artificial hydration, where dehydration results from a potentially correctable cause (e.g. overtreatment with diuretics and sedation, recurrent vomiting, diarrhoea and hypercalcaemia).
5 It is a responsibility of the clinical team to make assessments concerning the relevance of hydration to the experience of individual patients. The appropriateness of artificial hydration should be judged on a day-to-day basis, weighing up the potential harms and benefits. The practicalities of appropriate provision will vary according to setting, but good practice will require that patients needing artificial hydration are transferred to a unit equipped to provide such care.
6 Relatives at the bedside of dying patients frequently express concern about lack of fluid or nutrient intake. Healthcare professionals may not subordinate the interests of patients to the anxieties of relatives but should, nevertheless, strive to address those anxieties.

The appropriateness of artificial hydration continues to depend on regular assessment of the likely benefits and burdens of such intervention

of care are clear, and the resulting decision is a joint one involving both the care team and the patient. The patient's wishes are paramount and the regimen must be regularly reviewed and adjusted according to changes in condition and circumstances (Lennard-Jones 1998). Some of the ethical issues concerning feeding in terminally ill people are discussed in Section 1.19 (Healthcare ethics).

Artificial hydration

In the last few days of life, people may be too weak to take oral foods and fluids, partly as a result of declining physical function but often as a result of a reduced level of consciousness due to the use of sedative and pain-relieving drugs. Whether intravenous hydration should be given at this stage has been a matter of debate and raises ethical issues (Dunphy *et al.* 1995)

The extent to which intravenous fluids offer symptomatic relief to such patients is unknown (Dunphy *et al.* 1995). Some have argued that artificial rehydration is necessary to satisfy thirst and other symptoms due to lack of fluid intake (Craig 1994, 1996). Others consider that simpler measures such as attention to oral hygiene are sufficient to prevent discomfort, and that intravenous hydration at this stage is unnecessarily invasive and can cause a physical barrier between the patient and their family at an important time (Dunphy *et al.* 1995).

A summary of the issues and guidelines on the use of artificial hydration in terminally ill people has been produced by a joint working party between the National Council for Hospice and Specialist Palliative Care Services and the Ethics Committee of the Association for Palliative Medicine of Great Britain and Ireland (1997). Their recommendations are summarized in Table 4.90. The principal conclusion is that a blanket policy of 'artificial hydration' or 'no artificial hydration' is ethically indefensible; decision as to what is appropriate for each case must be decided on an individual basis according to the likely benefits and burdens of such intervention.

The recommendations also emphasize that good practice regarding decisions on artificial hydration should involve a multidisciplinary team, the patient, and relatives and carers. While the senior doctor has ultimate responsibility for the decision, a competent patient has the right to refuse artificial hydration even if it may be considered of clinical benefit. Incompetent patients retain this right through a valid advance refusal.

The primary goal of treatment in terminal care is the comfort of the patient, and the decision of whether or not to rehydrate must be made on this basis.

Text revised by: Briony Thomas and Sue Acreman

Useful addresses

Cruse Bereavement Care
Cruse House, 126 Sheen Road, Richmond, Surrey TW9 1UR.
Tel: 020 8940 4818

Hospice Information Service
St Christopher's Hospice, 51–59 Lawrie Park Road, Sydenham, London SE26 6DZ
Tel: 020 8778 9252
Publishes a directory of hospice and palliative care services

Macmillan Cancer Relief
Anchor House, 15–19 Britten Street, London SW3 3TZ
Tel: 0845 601 6161

National Council for Hospice and Specialist Palliative Care Service.
7th Floor, 1 Great Cumberland Place, London W1H 7AL
Tel: 020 7723 1639 Fax: 020 7723 5380

Further reading

Dunphy K, Randall F. Ethical decision-making in palliative care. *European Journal of Palliative Care* 1997; 4: 126–128.

Holmes S. The challenge of providing nutrition support to the dying. *International Journal of Palliative Medicine* 1998; **4**: 26–31.

Penson J, Fisher R. *Palliative Care for People with Cancer*. London: Edward Arnold, 1994.

Shaw C, Hunter M. Using the potential of the dietetic team. *Nursing Standard* 1990; **4**: 34–35.

Randall FM. Ethical issues in palliative care. *Acta Anaesthesiologica Scandinavica* 1999; **43**: 954–956.

Tchekmedyian N, Zehyna D, Halpert C. Clinical aspects of nutrition in advanced cancer. *Oncology* 1992; **49** (Suppl 2): 3–7.

References

Boyd K, Beeken L. Tube feeding in palliative care: benefits and problems. *Palliative Medicine* 1994; **8**: 156–158.

Craig G. On withholding nutrition and hydration in the terminally ill: has palliative medicine gone too far? *Journal of Medical Ethics* 1994; **20**: 139–143.

Craig G. On withholding nutrition and hydration from terminally ill sedated patients: the debate continues. *Journal of Medical Ethics* 1996; **22**: 147–153.

Dunphy K, Finlay I, Rathbone G *et al.* Rehydration in palliative and terminal care: if not – why not? *Palliative Medicine* 1995; **9**: 221–228.

Grindel C, Whitmer K, Barsevick A. Quality of life and nutritional support in patients with cancer. *Cancer Practice* 1996; **4**: 81–87.

Higginson I, Wade A, McCarthy M. Palliative care: views of patients and their families. *British Medical Journal* 1990; **301**: 227–281.

Lennard-Jones J. *Ethical and Legal Aspects of Clinical Hydration and Nutrition Support*. Maidenhead: BAPEN, 1998.

McCombie L. Sip feed prescribing in primary care: an audit of current practice in Greater Glasgow Health Board, Glasgow, UK. *Journal of Human Nutrition and Dietetics* 1999; **12**: 210–212.

National Council for Hospice and Specialist Palliative Care Services. *Ethical Decision-making in Palliative Care: Artificial Hydration for People who are Terminally Ill*. Paper prepared by a Joint Working Party between the National Council for Hospice and Specialist Care Services and the Ethics Committee of the Association for Palliative Medicine of Great Britain and Ireland, April 1997.

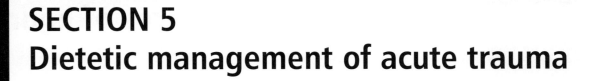

SECTION 5
Dietetic management of acute trauma

5.1 Metabolic consequences of injury

5.1.1 Differences between the effects of starvation and injury

The effects of starvation

Inadequate nutrient provision induces the adaptive process of starvation, to allow the body to survive for periods with insufficient or no food. Adaptive processes include the mobilization of glycogen stores from the liver and muscle tissue, with subsequent gluconeogenesis from glucogenic amino acid release from muscle and visceral tissue into the plasma. Mobilization of amino acids serves a dual purpose of maintaining plasma levels for utilization elsewhere, and reducing muscle mass and therefore energy expenditure, thus permitting the body to survive for longer on the limited energy intake.

In the absence of sepsis, fatty acid mobilization produces ketone bodies, an energy source for the brain and red blood cells. Semi-starvation frequently occurs on wards, with hydration taking precedence over nutritional support. The 400 kcal provided by 2 litres of dextrose-saline daily may be sufficient to prevent ketogenesis, but absence of exogenous protein supply enhances catabolism. Reduction in tissue protein adversely affects muscle function and immune function.

Iatrogenic starvation occurs when patients require prolonged fasting periods for tests, or if feeding access is difficult to establish. It is the dietitian's role to act as advocate for the patient and suggest potentially successful feeding routes.

The effects of injury, trauma and sepsis

The changes that occur following injury are different to starvation, being designed to mobilize tissues for defence and repair. This mechanism takes priority even in the presence of starvation.

The metabolic response to injury traditionally has three phases, although each can be moderated by modern pharmacology:

1 the 'ebb' phase
2 the catabolic or 'flow' phase
3 the anabolic phase.

The ebb phase

This lasts for only a few hours; there is a depression of metabolic function and a reduction in energy expenditure.

The flow phase

Metabolic rate increases and energy reserves from fat are mobilized. Visceral and muscle tissue provide amino acids that can be used for gluconeogenesis, providing glucose for brain and red blood cells, and wound-healing mechanisms.

This response is moderated by the use of antibiotics and analgesia, such that the catabolic process is strongly downgraded.

Severe or prolonged injury, in tandem with sepsis or other ongoing inflammatory processes, can progress to multiple organ failure (MOF). The provision of adequate nutritional support in the presence of a severe inflammatory stimulus only attenuates the gluconeogenic process, with the breakdown of lean tissue continuing. Provision of adequate protein stimulates protein synthesis, but it also stimulates breakdown (Campbell 1999).

Achievement of energy balance (non-protein or total energy) fails to alleviate catabolism in critically ill patients. Provision of caloric intake to match energy expenditure seems unnecessary during the acute phase of post-traumatic catabolic illness (Frankenfield *et al.* 1997).

Nitrogen balance is a poor marker of dietary adequacy in sepsis, but other markers are available to discriminate between malnutrition and the metabolic effect of stress. Blood levels of the acute-phase proteins prealbumin (PRA), retinol-binding protein (RBP) and C-reactive protein (CRP) measured sequentially in intensive care unit patients requiring parenteral nutrition (PN), demonstrated a progressive increase in the rapid-turnover proteins RBP and PRA that significantly correlated with improvement in nitrogen balance, whilst plasma concentrations of CRP remained unchanged in the presence of persistent inflammation (Casati *et al.* 1998). This suggests that monitoring of RBP and PRA could complement the clinical evaluation of nutritional therapy of critically ill patients.

In sepsis or trauma, provision of glucose reduces but does not abolish gluconeogenesis, and fat oxidation increases, with a concomitant reduction in glucose oxidation. Exogenous fat emulsions are adequately oxidized in both starvation and sepsis.

The metabolic changes following injury are proportional to the severity of the injury and are most extreme following burn injuries (Wilmore 1978) (see Section 5.5, Burn injury). Nutritional losses can be attenuated during this time with judicial use of sedation and pain relief. Nutritional repletion is associated with significant improvements in skeletal muscle function that occurs after only a few days of feeding and are independent of changes in body protein stores. This may reflect repletion of intracellular phosphates or possibly a consequence of restoration of type II muscle fibres in association with changes in certain enzymes of glycolysis and the tricarboxylic acid cycle.

Both malnutrition and starvation alter cognitive function, contributing to depression, apathy and malaise. These changes are all reversible with nutritional support.

The anabolic phase

Eventually, catabolism declines and the flow phase passes into the anabolic phase. This is usually coupled with an increase in appetite and ambulation. Nutritional therapy should now aim to restore muscle mass and increase protein synthesis.

Attempts to restore body mass and nutritional status rapidly may induce adverse metabolic consequences (Klein *et al*. 1998). Underweight and overweight people and the elderly population are particularly vulnerable to overfeeding, because of the difficulties in assessing true requirements. Overfeeding protein can cause uraemia, hypertonic dehydration and metabolic acidosis. Excessive carbohydrate infusion has resulted in hyperglycaemia and hypertriglyceridaemia, with associated pancreatitis and hepatic steatosis. High fat infusions have caused hypertriglyceridaemia and fat-overload syndrome. Hypercapnia and the 'refeeding syndrome' are also caused by aggressive overfeeding.

Routine oral or enteral supplementation seems to improve the nutritional indices of adult patients, but there are insufficient data to be certain whether mortality is reduced (Potter *et al*. 1998). The reader is directed to the sections on nutritional support (Sections 1.11–1.13) for further information.

Comparative effects of injury and starvation

The major effects of starvation and injury are summarized in Table 5.1. The clinical picture is often complicated, as patients seldom fall simply into one category or the other. They may be injured after a period of undernutrition, or underfed for some time after an injury.

5.1.2 Nutritional implications of the effects of injury

The application of current knowledge of nutritional pharmacology and effective pain relief can modify the metabolic response and reduce the clinical consequences.

An exaggerated inflammatory response and generation of free oxygen radicals lead to tissue hypoxia, subsequent damage and ultimately MOF, with its high mortality. Maintenance of tissue oxygenation, control of infection and provision of early nutritional support all have a role to play in minimizing the inflammatory response (Singer 1998).

Researchers have tried to attenuate the loss of lean body mass during the acute-phase response by using hormones or drugs in addition to nutritional support. Such drugs include anabolic effectors such as insulin and recombinant human growth hormone (hGH). Insulin has an anabolic effect on protein kinetics, yet administration of exogenous insulin in conjunction with feed to a group of trauma patients failed to demonstrate any beneficial effect (Clements *et al*. 1999). Administration of hGH is controversial, with some patient groups demonstrating a physiological benefit with its use, whilst others fail to improve.

Early feeding

Early initiation (within 12 hours) of enteral feeding in the critically ill reduces predicted mortality by half (Bower *et al*. 1996).

Enteral versus parenteral route

Feeding route may influence both the risk of development and the degree of severity of sepsis. Much of the inflammatory response is thought to be due to migration of gut bacteria across the gut wall ('bacterial translocation'), causing septicaemia and attendant consequences. This may be due in part to intestinal atrophy, or poor perfusion of the gut during periods of dehydration or anaemia post-surgery. The restoration of blood supply to hypoxic tissue leads to a surge in oxygen free radical species, which cause local damage and subsequent 'reperfusion injury' which reduces the gut defences.

Provision of enteral nutrition support hypothetically maintains gut integrity and ensures adequate blood supply, thus minimizing septic complications in post-surgical patients. In major trauma and burns, enteral nutrition significantly decreases the acute-phase response and incidence of septic complications when compared with PN.

In acute pancreatitis (one of the major causes of MOF),

Table 5.1 Comparison of the effects of starvation and injury (After Woolfson 1978)

	Starvation	Injury
Metabolic rate	Decreased	Increased
Weight	Slow loss, almost all from fat stores	Rapid loss, 80% from fat stores, remainder from body protein
Nitrogen	Losses reduced	Losses increased
Hormones	Early small increases in catecholamines, cortisol, hGH; then slow fall in glucagon and cortisol	Increases catecholamines, glucagon, cortisol, hGH
	Insulin decreased	Insulin increased but relative insulin deficiency.
Water and sodium	Initial loss	Retention

hGH: human growth hormone.

enteral nutrition improves outcome by moderating the inflammatory response, and reduces sepsis, possibly by maintaining gut integrity (Windsor *et al.* 1998). This is in contrast to PN, which increases both the levels of free radicals and markers of cell damage.

Modified nutrients

Glutamine is an important metabolic fuel for intestinal enterocytes, lymphocytes and macrophages, and for metabolic precursors such as purines and pyrimidines. Glutamine is a conditionally essential amino acid during periods of stress, and is essential for maintaining intestinal function, immune response and amino acid homeostasis. Normally abundant in plasma, low plasma and tissue levels of glutamine in the critically ill suggest that demand may exceed endogenous supply.

Clinical trials in metabolically stressed patients demonstrate the role of glutamine in improving nitrogen balance, increased cellular proliferation, decreased incidence of infection and shortened length of stay (Sacks 1999). In a prospective, randomized, controlled trial of critically ill patients requiring PN, 6-month survival was significantly improved in the group supplemented with glutamine compared with the isonitrogenous, isocaloric control group (Griffiths 1997).

Lipids also are of clinical interest. Supplementation of PN with oral or enteral fish oil (1.8 g/day eicosapentaenoic acid) in oesophagectomy patients significantly reduced post-operative interleukin-6 production and improved cell-mediated immunity, which continued throughout subsequent chemoradiation therapy (Tashiro *et al.* 1998).

However, further research into the inclusion of these substrates in products formulated for nutritional support is required before they gain widespread acceptance in clinical nutrition.

Text revised by: Catherine Collins

References

Bower RH, Cerra FB, Bershadsky B *et al*. Early enteral administration of a formula (Impact) supplemented with arginine, nucleotides and fish oil in intensive care unit patients: results of a multicenter, prospective, randomized clinical trial. *Critical Care Medicine* 1995; **23**: 436–449.

Campbell IT. Limitations of nutrient intake. The effect of stressors: trauma, sepsis and multiple organ failure. *European Journal of Clinical Nutrition* 1999; **53** (Suppl 1): S143–S147.

Casati A, Muttini S, Leggieri C *et al*. Rapid turnover proteins in critically ill ICU patients. Negative acute phase proteins or nutritional indicators? *Minerva Anestesiologica* 1998; **64**: 345–350.

Clements RH, Hayes CA, Gibbs ER *et al*. Insulin's anabolic effect is influenced by route of administration of nutrients. *Archives of Surgery* 1999; **134**: 274–277.

Frankenfield DC, Smith JS, Cooney RN. Accelerated nitrogen loss after traumatic injury is not attenuated by achievement of energy balance. *Journal of Parenteral and Enteral Nutrition* 1997; **21**: 324–329.

Griffiths RD. Outcome of critically ill patients after supplementation with glutamine. *Nutrition* 1997; **13**: 752–754.

Klein CJ, Stanek GS, Wiles CE. Overfeeding macronutrients to critically ill adults: metabolic complications. *Journal of the American Dietetic Association* 1998; **98**: 795–806.

Potter J, Langhorne P, Roberts M. Routine protein energy supplementation in adults: systematic review. *British Medical Journal* 1998; **317**: 495–501.

Sacks GS. Glutamine supplementation in catabolic patients. *Annals of Pharmacology* 1999; **33**: 348–354.

Singer M. Management of multiple organ failure: guidelines but no hard-and-fast rules. *Journal of Antimicrobial Chemotherapy* 1998; **41** (Suppl A): 103–112.

Tashiro T, Yamamori H, Takagi K *et al*. *n*-3 versus *n*-6 polyunsaturated fatty acids in critical illness. *Journal of the Japanese Surgical Society* 1998; **99**: 256–263.

Wilmore DW. *Metabolic Management of the Critically Ill*. New York: Plenum Press, 1978.

Windsor AC, Kanwar S, Li AG *et al*. Compared with parenteral nutrition, enteral feeding attenuates the acute phase response and improves disease severity in acute pancreatitis. *Gut* 1998; **42**: 431–435.

Woolfson AMJ. Metabolic considerations in nutritional support. In Johnson IDFA, Lee HA (Eds) *Developments in Clinical Nutrition*. Proceedings of a Symposium held at the Royal College of Physicians, London, October 1978, pp. 35–47. Tunbridge Wells:, MCS Consultants, 1978.

5.2 Intensive care

Intensive care is a branch of medicine primarily concerned with the management of patients with acute life-threatening disorders. Such patients are normally cared for within designated intensive care units (ICU). The immediate objective of care is to preserve life and to prevent, minimize or reverse damage to vital organs. The objectives of nutritional support are the same.

Department of Health guidelines suggest that 1–2% of acute beds in a general hospital should be designated ICU beds, and that this number be greater when there are specialist units (e.g. those performing cardiac or major vascular surgery, or neurosurgery).

Common causes for admission to an ICU include:

- major trauma including head injury and road traffic accidents
- post-operative care: cardiac, abdominal, transplantation or major vascular surgery
- respiratory failure
- post-cardiopulmonary resuscitation
- pre-operative stabilization, termed 'optimization'.

Most ICUs use an admission scoring system to predict a patient's severity of illness and the chance of survival. The most commonly used score is the APACHE II (Acute Physiology and Chronic Health Evaluation) score which uses age, the Glasgow Coma Scale score, 12 current physiological variables and the patient's chronic health status to predict mortality risk (Knaus *et al.* 1986). However, the APACHE II score has poor outcome predictors; below 10 there are few deaths, beyond 25 there are few survivors. The updated APACHE III score failed to demonstrate greater accuracy in predicting outcome and so remains less used (Beck *et al.* 1997). Other forms of patient assessment include TISS (Tissue Injury Scoring System) and SAPS (Simplified Acute Physiology Score) (Bertolini *et al.* 1998).

ICU patients present with, or are at risk of developing, more than one organ failure. Multiple organ failure syndrome (MOFS) is the most common cause of death in the ICU. Precipitating factors including sepsis, trauma or pancreatitis causing an exaggerated inflammatory response leading to organ dysfunction and tissue damage. Management revolves around support of organ function and prevention of iatrogenic complications until recovery occurs. An increasing emphasis is being placed on prevention of organ dysfunction, including maintenance of tissue oxygenation, nutrition and infection control (Singer 1998).

Nutritional intervention in patients with organ failure can influence outcome. Nutritional support has become a standard component of managing critically ill patients (Heyland 1998), and plays an important role in the provision of nutrition and modulation of the immune response (Heys *et al.* 1999). Dietitians working in the field of critical care should take time to familiarize themselves with the equipment and treatment procedures if appropriate dietary advice is to be given.

A shortcut in clinical appraisal is rather like writing a pocket reference on dismantling bombs: cutting corners can be disastrous! Nutritional support should be carefully tailored to the patient's clinical condition and treatment schedules, and should be based on current dietary principles. Current developments appear to herald the development of a new discipline in dietetics related to nutrition pharmacology.

5.2.1 Intensive care unit data

Information regarding the patient on an ICU is to be found in a variety of locations. Medical notes provide the usual background health evaluation, and indicate the current reason for admission. Doctors' notes written during an ICU stay may be kept in this folder or in a separate folder at the patient's bed.

ICU patients have a single, daily record sheet for temperature, blood pressure, cardiac monitoring, fluid balance, blood gases and serum electrolytes, which may be computed hourly. Daily biochemistry and haematology results are often recorded on an accumulative flow chart Twenty four hours is a long time in ICU, and so blood results from 3 days ago may be of little help in assessing the current picture (Runcie and Dougall 1990).

Serial biochemistry results should be used to interpret the impact of nutritional support in the context of the clinical picture. Iatrogenic and medication changes also impact on nutrition therapy.

5.2.2 Intensive care unit equipment

Each piece of equipment surrounding the ICU patient is there to support a failing organ. A brief review of equipment not usually found on a general ward is discussed below.

Artificial ventilator (life-support machine)

The artificial ventilator controls the breathing pattern of patients with acute breathing problems (respiratory failure with worsening blood gases, or neuromuscular problems, e.g. Guillain–Barré syndrome). The ventilator delivers an inspired oxygen supply varying from 21% oxygen (room air) to 100% oxygen, and is adjusted to maintain arterial oxygenation (PaO$_2$) between 10 and 14 kPa partial pressure (Table 5.2).

The patient is ventilated via an endotracheal tube passed through the mouth or the nose into the trachea. Tracheostomy is considered for long-term ventilation, or paradoxically if a patient fails to 'wean' from ventilation because they gag or become agitated when awoken with the endotracheal tube *in situ*. A 'cuffed' endotracheal tube or tracheostomy may be a risk factor for the insertion of a fine bore enteral feeding tube, guiding the tube towards the lung (Carey and Holcombe 1991). Endotracheal tubes can cause problems with temporary dysphagia and inability to co-ordinate swallowing (especially with liquids) once an oral diet is initiated. The presence of a gag reflex does not necessarily protect against aspiration of pharyngeal contents (DeVita and Spierer-Rundback 1990).

A background positive (i.e. greater than atmospheric) pressure maintained during entire ventilation prevents lung collapse and improves gas exchange. This positive end-expiratory pressure (PEEP) improves arterial oxygenation but may compromise venous return, which is dependent on a negative pressure in the chest wall. PEEP greater than 8 cmH$_2$O pressure reduces renal perfusion by impairing venous return. Renal initiation of the renin – angiotensin – aldosterone mechanism causes fluid and sodium retention, further compromising lung function. An energy-dense feed may be required to minimize fluid retention. Artificial ventilation using high airways pressures can induce a cytokine response, helping to perpetuate the acute-phase response (Ranieri *et al.* 1999).

Metabolism of high fat feeds produces less carbon dioxide by altering respiratory quotient (RQ) and may benefit patients with previously good lung function who are hypercapnic, or patients with chronic obstructive airways disease (COAD) who have an arterial carbon dioxide tension (PaCO$_2$) above tolerable levels (Al-Saady *et al.* 1989) (Table 5.2).

Overfeeding should be avoided, as it negates any potential benefit of high fat feeds by producing a disproportionately large production of carbon dioxide, enhances the inflammatory response and increases the risk of 'refeeding syndrome' (Klein *et al.* 1998).

Intra-aortic balloon pump (IABP) and left ventricular assist device (LVAD)

These control cardiac function in the presence of a failing heart by providing cardiac support post-operatively, or maintaining the patient with severe heart failure awaiting transplantation (Holzum 1990). One-quarter of patients are likely to develop *Candida* spp. infection, and the device biomaterial adversely affects T-cell response (Ankersmit *et al.* 1999). Anticlotting therapy is required, and achieved with heparin rather than warfarin.

Table 5.2 Arterial blood gases

	Normal values	Acute respiratory failure
Pa$_{CO_2}$	4.7–6.0 kPa (35–45 mmHg)	>6.0 kPa (>45 mmHg)
Pa$_{O_2}$	9.3–14.0 kPa (70–100 mmHg) Saturation: 95–100%	<8.0 kPa (<60 mmHg)
Base excess	−2 to +2	
Saturation	>95% arterial saturation	

PaCO$_2$: arterial carbon dioxide tension; PaO$_2$: arterial oxygen saturation.

Swan–Ganz or pulmonary artery catheters

Cardiac output and hydration status are difficult to determine in patients with rapidly changing haemodynamics, especially in those with impaired myocardial function or respiratory disease. Pulmonary artery catheters (PAC) can be used to measure haemodynamic status.

These double- or triple-lumen catheters are advanced via a central vein through the heart into the pulmonary artery, where the tip of the catheter rests. Catheters to measure cardiac output incorporate a thermistor near the catheter tip, and a hub for connection to a cardiac monitor. Cardiac output is calculated by thermodilution, which involves injecting 10 ml of ice-cold 5% dextrose through the CVP lumen into the right atrium, and the subsequent measurement of the blood cooling curve obtained in the pulmonary artery. The fluid requirement for cardiac output measurement is unlikely to exceed 50 ml day, and so can be ignored in fluid-balance equations.

The inflatable balloon at the tip of a Swan–Ganz PAC can be temporarily inflated to occlude the pulmonary artery and measure the pulmonary artery ('wedge') pressure, giving an indication of cardiac function and fluid status.

Air-fluidized beds

These reduce the incidence of pressure sores and enhance the healing process. Air drawn through the base of the bed is warmed and filtered, and then rises through the silicon-coated glass beads to form a 'fluidized' mattress. The minimum temperature differential is 6°C above room temperature, but this can be varied from 28 to 36°C, while humidity is fixed at 35–40%.

Increased insensible skin losses and an inability to measure accurately body fluids lost into the bed often create a negative fluid balance. The localized ambient temperature reduces nitrogen turnover and energy expenditure (Ryan and Clague 1990).

Continuous arteriovenous haemofiltration/haemodiafiltration (CAVHF, CAVHDF)

Acute renal failure is a common problem in the ICU patient, occurring in isolation or combined with other organ failures. These continuous renal-replacement therapies (CRRTs) allow for clearance of low molecular weight solutes and large volumes of water, and allow aggressive nutrition and fluid support in critically ill patients.

In addition, CRRTs have additional advantages in critically ill patients, including haemodynamic stability, prevention of cerebral oedema and a possible anti-inflammatory effect in septic patients (Bellomo and Ronco 1998).

The glucose content of the dialysate solution contributes to energy intake. Increasing dialysate glucose concentration or flow rate increases glucose uptake. Up to 50% of dialysate glucose can potentially be extracted during continuous arteriovenous haemodiafiltration (CAVHDF), so nutritional support should be tailored accordingly. Nitrogen losses can amount to 24 g/day, with a mean negative nitrogen balance during feeding of 3.6 g N/24 hours. Urea N comprises 60–70% of total urinary excretion, the remaining being non-urea nitrogen. Lipid homeostasis is unaffected by CAVHD (Bellomo *et al*. 1991).

5.2.3 Practical aspects of feeding patients on the intensive care unit

Choice of feeding route

Enteral, rather than parenteral, feeding is the nutritional support route of choice in European ICUs (Vincent 1999), as few patients can take an oral diet. Enteral feeding requires a functioning intestine and a relatively stable haemodynamic state, with a potential reduction in subsequent morbidity and mortality the earlier the patient is fed (Sax 1996; Cerra *et al*. 1997; Kudsk 1998). Delay in initiating enteral feeding beyond 24 hours is associated with increased intestinal permeability and severity of ensuing MOFS (Rombeau and Takala 1997; Kompan *et al*. 1999).

Enteral nutrition can prevent stress ulceration (Raff *et al*. 1997), maintain gut integrity, enhance biliary immunoglobulin A secretion and reduce the production of acute-phase proteins. Duodenal feeding is associated with an increased delivery of nutrients and reduced aspiration risk (Kortbeek *et al*. 1999).

Parenteral nutrition (PN) is reserved for those with a non-functioning gut or severe ileus and can be given through a triple-lumen or pulmonary artery catheter already *in situ* to monitor haemodynamics (Horowitz *et al*. 1990). PN does not reduce mortality, although it may reduce morbidity in malnourished patients (Heyland *et al*. 1998). The complications associated with catheter insertion, increased infection risk (particularly for *Candida* spp. septicaemia) and PN-enhanced free-radical activity may worsen the clinical outcome in patients with acute respiratory distress syndrome (ARDS) or MOFS (Chuang and Chuang 1991; Borzotta and Beardsley 1999; Basu *et al*. 1999).

Assessment of nutritional status is predominantly based on clinical and biochemical parameters rather than on functional, anthropometric or immunological data management of patients (Preiser *et al*. 1999), as no single indicator is of consistent value in the nutritional assessment of critically ill patients (Manning and Shenkin 1995).

PN is discussed in greater detail in Section 1.15. The remaining text in this section is concerned with the use of enteral feeding in the critically ill patient.

Feeding tubes

Fine-bore enteral feeding tubes are impractical in the ICU setting as many medications are administered nasogastrically, and mechanical obstruction of such tubes often follows administration of crushed tablets or drug suspensions (Abernathy *et al*. 1989). Fine-bore feeding tubes offer little benefit in preventing aspiration (Sands 1991) and tend to reduce checking of residual gastric volumes (Metheny *et al*. 1999). Rapid decompression of the stomach to prevent aspiration also necessitates the use of a wider bore tube.

Continuous feeding versus intermittent bolus techniques

Continuous feeding minimizes potentially adverse metabolic effects on cardiac, respiratory and renal function (Heymsfield and Casper 1989), and diminishes the thermogenic response by 10–15% of total daily resting energy expenditure (REE) (Heymsfield *et al*. 1987). In practice, continuous feeds usually run for 20 hours a day, to allow a significant rest period to catch up on delayed feeds, or to allow intragastric pH to fall to a bacteriostatic acidity. The normal cyclical diurnal variation of basal energy expenditure is abolished in ventilated patients (van Lanschot *et al*. 1988), and so there are few metabolic problems associated with continuous enteral feeding.

Gastric emptying

Anaesthesia, sedatives and muscle relaxants can all reduce small bowel motility. Absence of bowel sounds alone is not an indication of ileus, and should not prevent trial of enteral feeding.

Gastric emptying rates are variable throughout the day (Tarling *et al*. 1997) and during feed initiation, with maximum gastric residues occurring around 2 hours after feed commencement (Kleibeuker and Ek 1991). Hyperosmolar and high-fat feeds (Paraskevopoulos *et al*. 1988) and the use of morphine (Bosscha *et al*. 1998) also retard gastric emptying.

Gastric stasis can be overcome by the regular administration of prokinetic agents such as metoclopromide or erythromycin (at half the standard antibiotic dose). The prokinetic Cisapride improves gastric emptying in mechanically ventilated, critically ill patients but has been barred from use by the Committee on Safety of Medicines owing to its potential side-effect of bradycardia.

Feed aspiration

Feed aspiration (i.e. feed entering the lungs) is a serious complication, leading to respiratory distress, respiratory arrest and subsequent ischaemic cardiac arrest if not promptly corrected (dePaso 1991). The presence of an endotracheal tube or tracheostomy fails to protect the lungs, as feed can easily leak around the high-volume, low-pressure tracheal cuff. The risk of pulmonary aspiration in the ICU patient has a probability of 0.9%, compared with 4.9% on medical/surgical wards (Mullan *et al*. 1992), and appears to be related to staffing intensity.

Subclinical aspiration of feed and subsequent pneumonia may occur in up to 20% of ventilated patients (Kingston *et al*. 1991). Testing endotracheal aspirates with a glucose oxidase reagent strip for the presence of glucose from the enteral feed using can help to identify those at risk of aspiration pneumonia (Metheny *et al*. 1999).

Preventive measures to minimize the risk include elevation of the head of the bed, the use of gastric motility agents and the frequent checking of residual gastric volumes. A single, high-residual volume (>200 ml) should not cause immediate cessation of an enteral feed, as subsequent residual volumes may well decrease (McClave *et al*. 1992).

Transpyloric–duodenal feeds significantly reduce the time required to achieve targeted enteric nutrition (Kortbeek *et al*. 1999) and are well tolerated immediately post-surgery (Grahm *et al*. 1989). Jejunal feeding with simultaneous gastric decompression may prove useful in patients with high gastric aspirate (Shang *et al*. 1999).

Diarrhoea

Nosocomial (hospital acquired) diarrhoea is a major problem in the ICU. Non-infectious causes include feed malabsorption, faecal impaction and hypoalbuminaemia, but these are not major risk factors for the development of diarrhoea (Patterson *et al*. 1990; Pesola *et al*. 1990). Drugs containing sorbitol or magnesium salts can induce diarrhoea (Edes *et al*. 1990; Fine *et al*. 1991).

Long-term antibiotics are also associated with the decimation of commensile gut flora, colonization by antibiotic-resistant bowel pathogens and possible pseudomembranous colitis. Stool cultures should be taken to exclude the gut pathogen *Clostridium difficile*, a spore-forming organism causing diarrhoea, which is capable of prolonged survival in the hospital setting (Cunha 1998).

Fibre-containing feeds appear of little clinical benefit in alleviating diarrhoea in the ICU patient (Dobb and Towler 1990), although probiotics such as live yoghurt may help to recolonize the gut following antibiotic therapy (Siitonen *et al*. 1990). Prophylactic administration of probiotics may also be useful (Bleichner *et al*. 1997) but should be avoided in immunocompromised patients. Predigested feeds should be considered if malabsorption is suspected.

Interruptions to feed

With the exception of magnetic resonance imaging (MRI) or computed tomography (CT) scans, diagnostic procedures such as X-ray or endoscopy are performed on the ICU. Feed infusion can continue throughout most physiotherapy techniques. Some antibiotics and anti-rejection drugs are incompatible with enteral feeds, and so the advice of the ward pharmacist should be sought regarding concurrent feed and drug administrations (Power *et al*. 1998). In practice, it is rare for all of the daily feed prescribed to be delivered. A recent study indicated that an average 78% of feed prescribed was delivered, with two-thirds of the feed interruptions attributable to avoidable causes (McClave *et al*. 1999) (Table 5.3).

Interaction between nutritional support and drug therapy

Enteral feeds provide around 1 mg vitamin K/kg body weight, which is sufficient to antagonize warfarin therapy (Martin and Lutomski 1989). INR (International Normalized Ratio) and prothrombin time should be monitored during feeding. If feeding is halted for interventive therapy (e.g. if the patient is to have a tracheostomy) then warfarin dose should be reviewed, otherwise surgery may be delayed because the clotting time is prolonged. Heparin may also be used as an anticoagulant and this is not affected by the enteral feed.

Physical incompatibility of oral medications with enteral feeds is common. In extreme cases, inadequate tube flushing permits the development of a solidified mass of feed and drug (a bezoar) around the feeding tube, causing oesophageal obstruction (Garcia-Luna *et al*. 1999).

The bioavailability of drugs may be reduced if given concurrently with feed (Engle and Hannawa 1999).

Table 5.3 Reasons for discontinuation of enteral feed on the intensive care unit (From McClave *et al*. 1999)

Category	Examples	Frequency of occurrence	Considered potentially avoidable
Residual volumes	Volumes >200 ml , even though commonly isolated events	45%	70%
Tube displacement	Patient or staff removal	41%	66%
Procedures	Bronchoscopy, tracheostomy, transoesophageal echo, endoscopy, surgical intervention	39%	80%
Diagnostic tests	Chest X-ray, CT or MRI scan, fistulogram, ultrasound	27%	52%
Nursing care	Patient baths, changing bedding, tracheostomy care	30%	99%
Other	Haemodynamic instability, nausea, vomiting, ileus	32%	52%

CT: computed tomography; MRI: magnetic resonance imaging.

Phenytoin, carbemazepine, ciprofloxacin, rifampicin, tacrolimus, warfarin and sucralfate all have altered absorption kinetics if administered concurrently with enteral feeds (Fleisher *et al.* 1990; Cohn *et al.* 1996).

5.2.4 Nutritional aspects of feeding patients on the intensive care unit

Macronutrient supply should be considered for its impact on specific organ failures. The dietetic prescription should clearly state energy, protein, fluid and the main electrolyte content of the feed (sodium, potassium and phosphate).

An introduction regimen, optimum feeding rate and total fluid volume provided at full rate should be recorded, along with any potential drug interactions.

Energy requirements

Patients can be broadly distinguished into two categories (Apovian *et al.* 1990):

- nutritionally depleted patients with resolving medical problems (who can safely be fed to repletion)
- stressed or unstable patients (who will derive most benefit from 'maintenance' support until the clinical condition is stabilized).

The latter form the majority of ICU patients.

The primary dietetic consideration should be to feed to estimated requirements (Brandi *et al.* 1997). The REE of the ICU patient is variable, influenced by the impact of the illness and its treatment, but requirements rarely exceed 2000 kcal/day (Cerra *et al.* 1997). Accurate prediction of the REE in the critically ill is difficult, but indirect calorimetry remains the gold standard, despite its limitations (Flancbaum *et al.* 1999). This method has been utilized in both general situations (Table 5.4) and specific disease states.

Aggressive overfeeding can have metabolic consequences (Klein *et al.* 1998), including the 'refeeding syndrome'.

Non-feed energy sources should be included in dietary considerations. Vaso-irritant drugs (such as the anaesthetic Propofol and the benzodiazepines) are administered in a lipid base (Intralipid) contributing 1.1 kcal/ml. Intravenous 5% dextrose provides 200 kcal/l and additional glucose is absorbed from dialysis solutions (see above).

Resting metabolic rate using the Ireton–Jones equations

The Schofield and Harris–Benedict equations are widely used to predict energy expenditure in hospitalized populations (see Section 1.10, Estimating nutritional requirements), but their use is limited in ICU patients. The Ireton-Jones formulae were developed from indirect calorimetry measurements of ICU patients, and so are more appropriate to use for predicting energy requirements in this group (Ireton-Jones and Jones 1998).

Ireton-Jones formula for spontaneously breathing ICU patients:

$$EEE = 629 - 11 (A) + 25 (W) - 609 (O).$$

Ireton-Jones formula for ventilator-dependent ICU patients:

$$EEE = 1784 - 11 (A) + 5 (W) + 244 (G) + 239 (T) + 804 (B),$$

Where: EEE = estimated energy expenditure, O = presence of obesity (score 0 if absent, 1 if present), G = gender (score 0 if female, 1 if male), B = burns (score 0 if absent, 1 if present), A = age in years, and W = weight in kg.

Dietary carbohydrate

Insulin resistance and hyperglycaemia are well documented in sepsis (Jeevanandam *et al.* 1990a), often secondary to raised endogenous production or exogenous provision of insulin antagonists, e.g. noradrenaline, adrenaline, cortisol and glucagon. Chronic sepsis reduces mitochondrial pyruvate dehydrogenase complex, which converts pyruvate into acetyl coenzyme A, and so limits the oxidation of glucose (Seigal *et al.* 1989). Carbohydrate overload results in hyperglycaemia, hypertriglyceridaemia, hypercapnia and fatty liver (Hawker 1991).

Hyperglycaemia delays wound healing, increases fibrinogen levels, and reduces erythrocyte lifespan and total lymphocyte count (Schumann 1990). Maximum glucose utilization is approximately 3–5 g/kg per day. Sliding-scale insulin is a standard treatment and it may be of benefit to consider a feed with a higher fat profile.

Dietary fat

Fat provides an energy source of low respiratory quotient, thus reducing the carbon dioxide load to be excreted, but fatty acids also influence the immune response. Fat is a preferential energy source in trauma, injury and burns (Wolfe 1999), and is efficiently metabolized at intakes up to 6.5 g/kg body weight per day in critically ill septic patients (Druml *et al.* 1998). Excess lipid can impair the reticuloendothelial system, causing immunosuppression. Altering the fat composition of parenteral nutrition can

Table 5.4 Estimated energy requirements in general situations

Requirements (kcal/kg per day)	Group	Reference
22	Healthy young men at rest	Jeevanandam (1990a)
24	Septic patients, ICU	
35	'Flow' phase of severe trauma	Jeevanandam (1990b)
25–35	General requirements	Cerra (1987) Hunter *et al.* (1988)
30 ± 5	Multiple organ failure	Forsberg *et al.* (1991)
25 ± 4	Acute pancreatitis	Dickerson *et al.* (1991)
26 ± 4	Pancreatitis with sepsis	Dickerson *et al.* (1991)

influence the fat content of red cell membranes within a week (Planas *et al.* 1999).

Dietary fats are integral components of the cell membrane, and are responsible for structural and functional integrity. Cell membrane omega-6 polyunsaturated fatty acids (*n*-6 PUFA) increase production of macrophage-derived dienoic prostaglandins (such as prostaglandin E_2) and cytokines such as interleukin-1 (IL-1), IL-6 and tumour necrosis factor (TNF), which potentiate the inflammatory response to trauma and sepsis (Chambrier *et al.* 1999).

Substitution of *n*3 PUFA for *n*6 PUFA is associated with less MOFS and a reduced ICU stay (Gadek *et al.* 1999). Monounsaturates and medium-chain triglycerides (MCT) appear neutral in these inflammatory processes. However, non-nutritional factors may also influence the severity of the inflammatory response in the ventilated patient. Artificial ventilation with high airways and end-expiratory pressures can induce a cytokine response that may be attenuated by a strategy to minimize overexpansion and recruitment/de-recruitment of the lung (Hirvela 2000).

Nitrogen requirements

Patients are unlikely to achieve a positive nitrogen balance whilst critically ill (Wolfe 1999). Protein dynamics are influenced by both severity of trauma and underlying nutritional status.

With mild injury (e.g elective surgery) there is a normal or slightly depressed rate of protein synthesis, but with severe injury both protein synthesis and breakdown rates are increased (Tashiro *et al.* 1991). This may be a teleological (i.e. physiologically beneficial) response to mobilize amino acids from skeletal muscle for utilization by the liver and other tissues (Fischer and Hasselgren 1991), with muscle restored slowly, or not at all in the elderly population (Wernerman *et al.* 1996).

Hypoalbuminaemia is common in the ICU patient, reflecting the relative unimportance of albumin versus acute-phase proteins in the stressed, infective or traumatized patient. A fall in plasma albumin and transferrin is associated with a concurrent rise in the acute-phase proteins, e.g. C-reactive protein (CRP), haptoglobulin, caeruloplasmin and fibrinogen, mediated in part by IL-1 and other cytokines (Gabay and Kushner 1999). Hypoalbuminaemia with normal or low CRP indicates malnutrition; a low albumin with raised CRP levels indicates the acute-phase response. Replacement of serum albumin in critically ill patients has no clinical benefit on morbidity or mortality (Blackburn and Driscoll 1992; Cochrane Injuries Group Albumin Reviewers 1998).

Retinol binding protein and prealbumin levels may complement the clinical evaluation of nutritional therapy in ICU patients with ongoing inflammation (Casati *et al.* 1998).

Provision of protein at levels of 0.7–1.8 g/kg body weight per day is sufficient. Excess protein contributes to uraemia, hypertonic dehydration and metabolic acidosis, and may necessitate earlier renal-replacement therapy. Protein intake above 2 g/kg per day is not recommended owing to excessive stimulation of the ventilatory drive. Peptide feeds may restore constituent serum proteins more quickly than whole protein feeds (Heimburger *et al.* 1997).

Assessment of nitrogen balance is impossible in the ICU patient. Urea production is influenced by hepatic function, dietary adequacy, stress, sepsis and urine volume, the latter influenced by renal function, fluid balance or diuretic therapy. As urinary urea nitrogen is not a constant proportion of total urinary nitrogen, using this method to assess adequacy of nutrition support is grossly flawed (Konstantinides *et al.* 1991).

Glutamine

Glutamine, a non-essential amino acid abundant in the bloodstream, can be used as a protein or energy source for inflammatory cells and enterocytes (Wilmore and Shabert 1998). Small bowel enterocytes contain a large quantity of glutaminase enzyme to utilize both luminal and circulating glutamine for energy.

Starvation, immunosuppression, chemotherapy, injury, infection and PN combined with bowel rest are associated with reduced glutamine bioavailability and a breakdown in the barrier function of the gut, increasing the risk of septicaemia through bacterial translocation (van der Hulst *et al.* 1996). However, administration of 20 g glutamine daily to PN feeds failed to demonstrate a reduction in infective complications or length of hospital stay compared with those receiving standard PN, although inclusion in surgical patient was associated with a significant reduction in length of stay (Powell-Tuck *et al.* 1999).

In a group of 78 ICU patients with an APACHE II score of >11, those receiving a glutamine-supplemented enteral feed had a statistically significant reduction in median post-intervention ICU and hospital patient costs (US\$23 000), compared with those fed an isonitrogenous, unsupplemented enteral feed (\$30 900), although mortality rates in both groups were unchanged (Jones *et al.* 1999). Similarly, glutamine-supplemented PN significantly improved 6-month survival rates compared with controls fed an isonitrogenous, isocaloric regimen (Griffiths 1997).

Arginine

Arginine is a semiessential amino acid required for growth and in post-traumatic states. Supplements of 25 g L-arginine per day enhance or preserve immune function in high-risk surgical patients (Daly *et al.* 1990a). Arginine is the only nitrogen moiety containing two nitrogen atoms, and can be metabolized to nitric oxide (NO) at a cellular level. This potent vasodilator mimics the effect of inhaled NO in producing selective pulmonary vasodilatation, improving blood flow, tissue oxygenation and clinical outcome (Camsookai 1997).

Peri-operative administration of an arginine-supplemented immune feed significantly reduced plasma CRP levels, raised serum NO levels, and improved intestinal microperfusion and gut oxygen metabolism parameters post-operatively compared with patients given a standard feed (Braga *et al.* 1996). However, NO can be converted to the free radicals NO_2/NO_3, with raised levels of the latter worsening the severity and prognosis of critically injured patients (Hayashi *et al.* 1999).

Fluid requirements

Fluid requirements are highly variable, and the recommended intake is 1 ml/kcal energy expenditure (Kleiner 1999). Normal fluid requirements in the adult patient are 20–50 ml/kg per day. Patients in renal and respiratory failure may require fluid restriction, and critically ill patients are easily fluid overloaded, precipitating pulmonary and peripheral oedema.

Insensible water loss is influenced by environment, increasing with high temperatures, high altitude and low humidity. The increased fluid loss through nursing on air-fluidized beds requires compensation as a result of increased dermal losses. Humidified ventilation reduces insensible water losses via the lungs by 50% (some 500–900 ml).

Head-injured patients are often diuresed with intravenous mannitol to reduce cerebral swelling and limit further brain damage.

Fluid balance is recorded hourly, and records of the previous 2–3 days are useful to establish fluid balance. The drug chart and daily spreadsheet will indicate the minimum fluid contribution from drugs and intravenous line flushing.

Urine output is influenced by renal perfusion adequacy, diuretic therapy and the use of inotropes (e.g. adrenaline) and vasodilators that improve renal blood supply.

Large, intermittent boluses of feed or fluid could adversely affect cardiac and haemodynamic instability, hence continuous feed administration is preferred. Additional fluid can be added to the feed as sterile water, to ensure a constant hourly nutrition and fluid load to the patient. Factors increasing fluid requirements are outlined in Table 5.5.

Sodium requirements

Sodium is an extracellular ion, with normal requirements around 70–120 mmol/day. Salt and water overload should be avoided in patients in the early stages of refeeding who suffer from cardiopulmonary disorders.

Hypernatraemia is common in the critically ill patient, caused by excessive sodium administration, inadequate

Table 5.5 Factors increasing fluid requirements in patients on the intensive care unit

Pyrexia
Aspiration losses
Hyperventilation with inadequate humidity
Diuretic therapy
Osmotic diuresis (hyperglycaemia)
Diabetes insipidus (head injury)
Fistulae or wound drain losses
Gastrointestinal stoma losses
Diarrhoea
Nursing at ambient temperature

water intake, excessive water loss or a combination of these (Oh and Carroll 1992). Sodium retention may occur in acute renal failure, or as stress-induced syndrome of inappropriate antidiuretic hormone (SiADH). A 24-hour urine collection for urinary urea, electrolytes and osmolality can identify the cause of hypernatraemia.

Hypernatraemia with raised urinary sodium excretion indicates sodium overload. This is difficult to achieve by enteral feeding alone, but may be caused by:

- high levels of sodium in parenteral nutrition
- the use of normal saline (containing 150 mmol/l) instead of dextrose saline (30 mmol/l)
- magnesium-containing antacids
- sodium salts of antibiotics (e.g. ampicillin)
- administration of Gaviscon (6 mmol per 10 ml) or sodium bicarbonate to correct a metabolic acidosis.

Standard feeds are sufficiently low in sodium to maintain a gradual improvement in biochemistry, but low-sodium, energy-dense feed may be necessary if fluid restriction is required (Appendix 6.7).

Hyponatraemia is commonly due to fluid overload, with or without inadequate sodium intake, or associated with hepatic failure (Arieff 1991). Fluid restriction to raise serum sodium levels is the first-line treatment, but sodium supplementation may be necessary (Ayus and Arieff 1999).

Desired changes in serum sodium should not exceed 6–10 mmol/24 hours, as more rapid repletion and dehydration is associated with damage to the pontine area of the brain.

Potassium requirements

Potassium is an intracellular cation, with extracellular concentrations of 3.5–5.0 mmol/l. Dietary requirements are in the region of 80–120 mmol/day.

Hyperkalaemia may be iatrogenic, associated with excessive use of potassium-sparing diuretics, potassium supplements (often administered intravenously), catabolic states such as rhabdomyolysis (where tissue destruction releases intracellular potassium) or the metabolic acidosis of progressive renal failure.

Hypokalaemia is associated with the use of steroids, diuretics, continuous haemofiltration, haemodialysis or SiADH resulting in increased urinary losses of potassium. Hypokalaemia secondary to cellular uptake of glucose is more pronounced with insulin therapy. The body has no known potassium-retaining hormone, so increased urinary or gastrointestinal losses may also induce hypokalaemia.

Anabolic states may significantly deplete serum potassium, phosphate and magnesium, a process termed 'cellular steal' or 'refeeding syndrome'. The fall in serum potassium levels is most dramatic 2–3 days after initiation of feeding following a period of starvation (Marik and Bedigan 1996).

Magnesium requirements

Hypokalaemia and hypophosphataemia are associated risk

factors for hypomagnesaemia; 60–65% of surgical ICU patients have low serum magnesium (Chernow *et al.* 1989). Factors which reduce serum magnesium include:

- clinical conditions such as hypothermia, burns, gastro-intestinal, renal losses and refeeding syndrome
- drugs such as aminoglycosides, mannitol, diuretics, digitalis, cisplatin and cyclosporin.

The clinical manifestations of magnesium depletion include cardiac dysrrhythmias and neurotoxicity (muscle weakness). Requirements are in the region of 15–20 mmol/day.

Phosphate requirements

Hypophosphataemia (<0.8 mmol/l) is common on the ICU, causing depletion of tissue ATP (a major phosphate compound required for cell function) and red blood cell 2,3-diphosphoglycerate (thus reducing the affinity of oxygen to haemoglobin, causing tissue hypoxia), resulting in respiratory insufficiency, muscle weakness and anorexia. Hypophosphataemia impairs skeletal muscle strength and delays weaning the ventilated patient (Conti *et al.* 1990).

Phosphate is lost by increased renal and gastrointestinal losses, respiratory alkalosis, excessive use of aluminium-containing antacids and fat-free PN solutions. Administration of 0.5 mmol phosphate/kg body weight per day will prevent a fall in the serum level (Daly *et al.* 1990b).

Refeeding hypophosphatemia occurs commonly in critically ill patients in the ICU, and is more common in those with prior poor nutritional status. Serum phosphate should be closely monitored and supplemented as required.

Calcium requirements

Hypocalcaemia has many causes, including sepsis, hypomagnesaemia, rhabdomyolysis, renal disease, and primary or secondary hypoparathyroidism. Most patients with an ionized calcium concentration >0.8 mmol/l are asymptomatic and do not require intervention unless they become symptomatic. Conservative treatment is preferred, as calcium supplementation can be harmful during ischaemic and septic states. If necessary, calcium repletion is usually commenced with intravenous calcium, and once the serum levels have stabilized the enteral route can be used. Most patients require 1–4 g/day, administered as a continuous infusion or in divided doses (Zaloga 1992).

Additions of electrolytes to enteral feeds

Electrolytes can be added to feeds to maintain an adequate serum level as a constant infusion. Ampoules of electrolytes intended for injection are more compatible with enteral feeds than oral versions and provide a defined dose in a small volume (Hamill *et al.* 1991). Suitable ampoules to use include:

NaCl 30% w/v = 50 mmol Na/10 ml

KCl 20% w/v = 27 mmol/10 ml or KCl 15% w/v = 20 mmol/10 ml

$CaCl_2$ = 5 mmol/10 ml

Addiphos = 30 mmol K, 30 mmol Na, 40 mmol PO_4 in 20 ml vial.

One-off ('stat') doses of electrolytes are best confirmed on the drug chart rather than on the feed protocol to avoid duplicate prescribing.

Addition of electrolytes should be based on the previous day's requirements, less any contribution from feed. Interim addition of 1–2 × 10ml ampoule(s) per 10–12 hours (approximately 1 litre) of feed can be used, and titred according to the blood results. Potassium infusions should be infused at a maximum rate of 10 mmol K/hour.

Vitamin and mineral requirements

The impact of the clinical disease and its treatment influence markers such as plasma protein carriers and trace element levels (Singh *et al.* 1991), making them unreliable nutritional markers in critical illness (Phang and Aeberhardt 1996).

Plasma levels of alpha-tocopherol, ascorbate, beta-carotene and selenium are decreased in patients with ARDS, with increased oxidative stress demonstrated by elevated plasma levels of malondialdehyde (a marker of lipid peroxidation), and reduced neutrophil antioxidant enzyme capability (Metnitz *et al.* 1999). The minimal changes in activity of the antioxidative enzymes catalase, superoxide dismutase and glutathione peroxidase demonstrate that these enzymes can continue to function adequately even in the presence of inadequate micronutrient levels.

Plasma ferritin is unreliable in patients with inflammation or liver disease. Transferrin levels fall and caeruloplasmin levels rise with sepsis. Haemoglobin levels reflect recent blood transfusion, or anaemia secondary to acute or chronic blood loss.

The reference nutrient intake (RNI) should be the minimum aim, bearing in mind that excessive amounts of trace elements may compromise the response to infection. If considered necessary, trace elements and vitamins, e.g. Seravit (SHS), can be used to supplement a feed without an additional load of sodium or potassium.

5.2.5 Nutritional pharmacology

Current nutritional support techniques aim to influence morbidity and mortality by preventing generalized or specific nutrient deficiency. However, specific components to the diet can influence organ-specific functions, and nutrients are now considered to have as much potential for modifying the immune response as pharmacological agents (Ward and Lentsch 1999). This is a rapidly developing area and current research is not sufficient to make absolute recommendations regarding the amount and use of specific micronutrients and macronutrients in the diet.

A meta-analysis of the provision of nutritional support supplemented with key nutrients to patients with critical illness demonstrated a reduction in infectious complications and overall hospital stay compared with patients receiving standard nutritional support, although mortality was unaffected (Heys *et al.* 1999). However, most studies have methodological problems which may negate the outcome (Zaloga 1998).

The efficacy of certain disease-specific enteral formulae has been demonstrated in clinical practice, but cost–benefit analyses remain to be determined (Chan *et al.* 1999).

Text revised by: Catherine Collins

Further reading

Hinds CJ. *Intensive Care: A Concise Textbook*. London: Baillière-Tindall, 1988.
Park GR, Manara AR. *Intensive Care–Pocket Reference*. Tunbridge Wells: Castle House Publications, 1988.

Journals

Critical Care Medicine. Williams and Wilkins.
Intensive Care Medicine. Springer

References

Abernathy GB, Heizer WD, Holcombe BJ *et al.* Efficacy of tube feeding in supplying energy requirements of hospitalized patients. *Journal of Parenteral and Enteral Nutrition* 1989; **13**: 387–391.

Al-Saady NM, Blackmore CM, Bennett ED. High fat, low carbohydrate enteral feeding lowers $PaCO_2$ and reduces the period of ventilation in artificially ventilated patients. *Critical Care Medicine* 1989; **15**: 290–295.

Ankersmit HJ, Tugulea S, Spanier T *et al.* Activation-induced T-cell death and immune dysfunction after implantation of left-ventricular assist device. *Lancet* 1999; **354**: 550–555.

Apovian CM, McMahon M, Bistrian B. Guidelines for refeeding the marasmic patient. *Critical Care Medicine* 1990; **18**: 1030–1033.

Arieff AI. Treatment of symptomatic hyponatremia. *Critical Care Medicine* 1991; **19**: 748–751.

Ayus JC, Arieff AI. Chronic hyponatremic encephalopathy in postmenopausal women: association of therapies with morbidity and mortality. *Journal of the American Medican Association* 1999; **281**: 2299–2304.

Basu R, Muller DP, Papp E *et al.* Free radical formation in infants: the effect of critical illness, parenteral nutrition, and enteral feeding. *Surgery* 1999; **34**: 1091–1095.

Beck DH, Taylor BL *et al.* Prediction of outcome from intensive care: a prospective cohort study comparing Acute Physiology and Chronic Health Evaluation II and III prognostic systems in a United Kingdom intensive care unit. *Critical Care Medicine* 1997; **25**: 9–15.

Bellomo R, Ronco C. Continuous renal replacement therapy: continuous blood purification in the intensive care unit. *Annals of the Academy of Medicine, Singapore* 1998; **27**: 426–429.

Bellomo R, Martin H, Parkin G *et al.* Continuous arteriovenous haemodiafiltration in the critically ill: influence on major nutrient balance. *Intensive Care Medicine* 1991; **17**: 399–402.

Bertolini G, D'Amico R, Apolone G *et al.* Predicting outcome in the intensive care unit using scoring systems: is new better? A comparison of SAPS and SAPS II in a cohort of 1,393 patients. *Medical Care* 1998; **36**: 1371–1382.

Blackburn GL, Driscoll DF. Time to abandon routine albumin supplementation. *Critical Care Medicine* 1992; **20**: 157–158.

Bleichner G, Blehaut H, Mentec H, Moyse D. *Saccharomyces boulardii* prevents diarrhea in critically ill tube-fed patients. A multicenter, randomized, double-blind placebo-controlled trial. *Intensive Care Medicine* 1997; **23**: 517–523.

Borzotta AP, Beardsley K. Candida infections in critically ill trauma patients: a retrospective case–control study. *Archives of Surgery* 1999; **134**: 657–664.

Bosscha K, Nieuwenhuijs VB, Vos A *et al.* Gastrointestinal motility and gastric tube feeding in mechanically ventilated patients. *Critical Care Medicine* 1998; **26**: 1510–1517.

Braga M, Gianotti L, Cestari A *et al.* Gut function and immune and inflammatory responses in patients perioperatively fed with supplemented enteral formulas. *Archives of Surgery* 1996; **131**: 1257–1264.

Brandi LS, Bertolini R, Calafa M. Indirect calorimetry in critically ill patients: clinical applications and practical advice. *Nutrition* 1997; **13**: 349–358.

Camsooksai J. Inhaled nitric oxide: a possible therapy for ARDS. *Nursing in Critical Care* 1997; **2**: 251–254.

Carey TS, Holcombe BJ. Endotracheal intubation as a risk factor for the complications of nasoenteric tube insertion. *Critical Care Medicine* 1991; **19**: 427–429.

Casati A, Muttini S, Leggieri C *et al.* Rapid turnover proteins in critically ill ICU patients. Negative acute phase proteins or nutritional indicators? *Minerva Anestesiologica* 1998; **64**: 345–350.

Cerra FB. Hypermetabolism, organ failure and metabolic support. *Surgery* 1987; **101**: 1–8.

Cerra FB, Benitez MR, Blackburn GL *et al.* Applied nutrition in ITU patients. A consensus statement of the American College of Chest Physicians. *Chest* 1997; **111**: 769–778.

Chambrier C, Guiraud M, Gibault JP *et al.* Medium- and long-chain triacylglycerols in postoperative patients: structured lipids versus a physical mixture. *Nutrition* 1999; **15**: 274–277.

Chan S, McCowen KC, Blackburn GL. Nutrition management in the ITU. *Chest* 1999; **115** (5 Suppl): 145S–148S.

Chernow B, Bamberger S, Stoiko M *et al.* Hypomagnesaemia in patients in post-operative intensive care. *Chest* 1989; **95**: 391–397.

Chuang JH, Chuang S-F. Implication of a distant septic focus in parenteral nutrition. *Journal of Parenteral and Enteral Nutrition* 1991; **15**: 173–175.

Cochrane Injuries Group Albumin Reviewers. Human albumin administration in critically ill patients: systematic review of randomised controlled trials. *British Medical Journal* 1998; **317**: 235–240.

Cohn SM, Sawyer MD, Burns GA *et al.* Enteric absorption of ciprofloxacin during tube feeding in the critically ill. *Journal of Antimicrobial Chemotherapy* 1996; **38**: 871–876.

Conti G, Rocco M, Gasparetto A. Acute hypophosphataemia. Update. In *Intensive Care and Emergency Medicine*, VCl. 10, pp. 792–797. Vienna: Springer, 1990.

Cunha BA. Nosocomial diarrhea. *Critical Care Clinics* 1998; **14**: 329–338.

Daly JM, Reynolds J, Sigal *et al.* Effect of dietary protein and amino acids on immune function. *Critical Care Medicine* 1990a; **18**: S86–S93.

Daly WH, Tonneson AS, Allen SJ. Hypophosphatemia–incidence,

etiology and prevention in the trauma patient. *Critical Care Medicine* 1990b; **18**: 1210–1214.

DePaso WJ. Aspiration pneumonia. *Clinical Chest Medicine* 1991; **12**: 269–284.

DeVita MA, Spierer-Rundbeck L. Swallowing disorders in patients with prolonged orotracheal intubation or tracheostomy tubes. *Critical Care Medicine* 1990; **18**: 1328–1330.

Dickerson RN, Vehe KL, Mullen JL, Feurer ID. Resting energy expenditure in patients with pancreatitis. *Critical Care Medicine* 1991; **19**: 484–490.

Dobb GJ, Towler SC. Diarrhoea during enteral feeding in the critically ill: a comparison of feeds with and without fibre. *Intensive Care Medicine* 1990; **16**: 252–255.

Druml W, Fischer M, Ratheiser K. Use of intravenous lipids in critically ill patients with sepsis without and with hepatic failure. *Journal of Parenteral and Enteral Nutrition* 1998; **22**: 217–223.

Edes TE, Walk BE, Austin JL. Diarrhea in tube fed patients: feeding formula not necessarily the cause. *American Journal of Medicine* 1990; **88**: 91–93.

Engle KK, Hannawa TE. Techniques for administering oral medications to critical care patients receiving continuous enteral feed. *American Journal of Health-System Pharmacy* 1999; **56**: 1441–1444.

Fine KD, Santa Ana CA, Fordtran JS. Diagnosis of magnesium induced diarrhoea. *New England Journal of Medicine* 1991; **324**: 1012–1017.

Fischer JE, Hasselgren P-O. Cytokines and glucocorticoids in the regulation of the 'hepato-skeletal muscle axis' in sepsis. *American Journal of Surgery* 1991; **161**: 266–271.

Flancbaum L, Choban PS, Sambucco S *et al*. Comparison of indirect calorimetry, the Fick method, and prediction equations in estimating the energy requirements of critically ill patients. *American Journal of Clinical Nutrition* 1999; **69**: 461–466.

Fleisher D, Sheth N, Kou JH. Phenytoin interactions with enteral feedings administered through nasogastric tubes. *Journal of Parenteral and Enteral Nutrition* 1990; **14**: 513–516.

Forsberg E, Soop M, Thorne A. Energy expenditure and outcome in patients with multiple organ failure following abdominal surgery. *Intensive Care Medicine* 1991; **17**: 403–409.

Gabay C, Kushner I. Acute-phase proteins and other systemic responses to inflammation. *New England Journal of Medicine* 1999; **340**: 448–454.

Gadek JE, DeMichele SJ, Karlstad MD *et al*. Enteral Nutrition in ARDS Study Group. Effect of enteral feeding with eicosapentaenoic acid, gamma-linolenic acid, and antioxidants in patients with acute respiratory distress syndrome. *Critical Care Medicine* 1999; **27**: 1409–1420.

Garcia-Luna PP, Garcia E, Pereira-JL *et al*. Esophageal obstruction by solidification of the enteral feed: a complication to be prevented. *Intensive Care Medicine* 1999; **23**: 790–792.

Grahm TW, Zadrozny RN, Harrington T. The benefits of early jejunal hyperalimentation in the head-injured patient. *Neurosurgery* 1989; **25**: 729–735.

Griffiths RD. Outcome of critically ill patients after supplementation with glutamine. *Nutrition* 1997; **13**: 752–754.

Hamill RJ, Robinson LM, Wexler HR, Monte C. Efficacy and safety of potassium infusion therapy in hypokalaemic critically ill patients. *Critical Care Medicine* 1991; **19**: 694–699.

Hawker F. Liver dysfunction in critical illness. *Anaesthesia and Intensive Care* 1991; **19**: 165–181.

Hayashi N, Utagawa A, Kinoshita K, Izumi T. Application of a novel technique for clinical evaluation of nitric oxide-induced free radical reactions in ICU patients. *Cellular and Molecular Neurobiology* 1999; **19**: 3–17.

Heimburger DC, Geels VJ, Bilbrey J *et al*. Effects of small-peptide and whole-protein enteral feedings on serum proteins and diarrhea in critically ill patients: a randomized trial. *Journal of Parenteral and Enteral Nutrition* 1997; **21**: 162–167.

Heyland DK. Nutritional support in the critically ill patients. A critical review of the evidence. *Critical Care Clinics* 1998; **14**: 423–440.

Heyland DK, MacDonald S, Keefe L, Drover JW. Total parenteral nutrition in the critically ill patient: a meta-analysis. *Journal of the American Medical Association* 1998; **280**: 2013–2019.

Heymsfield SB, Casper K. Congestive heart failure: clinical management by use of continuous nasoenterie feeding. *American Journal of Clinical Nutrition* 1989; **50**: 539–544.

Heymsfield SB, Casper K, Grossman GD. Bioenergetic and metabolic response to continuous intermittent nasoenteric feeding. *Metabolism* 1987; **36**: 570–575.

Heys SD, Walker LG, Smith I, Eremin O. Enteral nutritional supplementation with key nutrients in patients with critical illness and cancer: a meta-analysis of randomized controlled clinical trials. *Annals of Surgery* 1999; **229**: 467–477.

Hirvela ER. Advances in the management of Acute Respiratory Distress Syndrome: protective ventilation. *Archives of Surgery* 2000; **135**: 126–135.

Holzum D. Intrapulmonary artery balloon pumping after CABG surgery. *Critical Care Nurse* 1990; **10**: 48–53.

Horowitz HW, Dworkin BM, Savino JA *et al*. Central catheter-related infections: comparison of pulmonary artery catheters and triple lumen catheters in a critical care setting. *Journal of Parenteral and Enteral Nutrition* 1990; **14**: 588–592.

Hunter DC, Jaksic T, Lewis D *et al*. Resting energy expenditure in the critically ill: estimations versus measurement. *British Journal of Surgery* 1988; **75**: 875–878.

Ireton-Jones CS, Jones JD. Should predictive equations or indirect calorimetry be used to design nutrition support regimens? *Nutrition in Clinical Practice* 1998; **13**: 141–145.

Jeevanandam M, Grote-Holman E, Chikenji T *et al*. Effects of glucose on fuel utilization and glycerol turnover in normal and injured man. *Critical Care Medicine* 1990a; **18**: 125–137.

Jeevanandam M, Young DII, Schiller WR. Influence of parenteral nutrition on rates of net substrate oxidation in severe trauma patients. *Critical Care Medicine* 1990b; **18**: 467–73.

Jones C, Palmer TE, Griffiths RD. Randomized clinical outcome study of critically ill patients given glutamine-supplemented enteral nutrition. *Nutrition* 1999; **15**: 108–115.

Kingston GW, Phang PT, Leathley MJ. Increased incidence of nosocomial pneumonia in mechanically ventilated patients with subclinical aspiration. *American Journal of Surgery* 1991; **161**: 589–592.

Kleibeuker JH, Ek B-V. Acute effects of continuous nasogastric tube feeding on gastric function: comparison of a polymeric and a non-polymeric formula. *Journal of Parenteral and Enteral Nutrition* 1991; **15**: 80–84.

Klein CJ, Stanek GS, Wiles CE III. Overfeeding macronutrients to critically ill adults: metabolic complications. *Journal of the American Dietetic Association* 1998; **98**: 795–806.

Kleiner S. Water: an essential but overlooked nutrient. *Journal of the American Dietetic Association* 1999; **99**: 200–206.

Knaus WA, Draper EA, Wagner DP, Zimmerman JE. An evaluation of outcome from intensive care in major medical centers. *Annals of Internal Medicine* 1986; **104**: 410–418.

Kompan L, Kremzar B, Gadzijev E. Prosek M. Effects of early enteral nutrition on intestinal permeability and the development of multiple organ failure after multiple injury. *Intensive Care Medicine* 1999; **25**: 157–161.

Konstantinides FN, Konstantinides NN, Li JC *et al*. Urinary urea nitrogen: too insensitive for calculating nitrogen balance studies in surgical clinical nutrition. *Journal of Parenteral and Enteral Nutrition* 1991; **15**: 189–193.

Kortbeek JB, Haigh PI, Doig C. Duodenal versus gastric feeding in ventilated blunt trauma patients: a randomized controlled trial. *Journal of Trauma* 1999; **46**: 992–996.

Kudsk KA. Early enteral nutrition in surgical patients. *Nutrition* 1998; **14**: 541–544.

McClave SA, Snider HL, Lowen CC *et al*. Use of residual volume as a marker for enteral feeding intolerance: prospective blinded comparison with physical examination and radiographic findings. *Journal of Parenteral and Enteral Nutrition* 1992; **16**: 99–105.

McClave SA, Sexton LK, Spain DA *et al*. Enteral tube feeding in the intensive care unit: factors impeding adequate delivery. *Intensive Care Medicine* 1999; **27**: 1252–1256.

Manning EM, Shenkin A. Nutritional assessment in the critically ill. *Critical Care Clinics* 1995; **11**: 603–634.

Marik PE, Bedigan MK. Refeeding hypophosphatemia in critically ill patients in an intensive care unit. *Archives of Surgery* 1996; **131**: 1043–1047.

Martin JE, Lutomski DM. Warfarin resistance and enteral feedings. *Journal of Parenteral and Enteral Nutrition* 1989; **13**: 206–208.

Metheny NA, Aud MA, Wunderlich RJ. A survey of bedside methods used to detect pulmonary aspiration of enteral formula in intubated tube-fed patients. *American Journal of Critical Care* 1999; **8**: 160–167.

Metnitz PG, Bartens C, Fischer M *et al*. Antioxidant status in patients with acute respiratory distress syndrome. *Intensive Care Medicine* 1999; **25**: 180–185.

Mullan H, Roubenoff RA, Roubenoff R. Risk of pulmonary aspiration among patients receiving enteral nutrition support. *Journal of Parenteral and Enteral Nutrition* 1992; **16**: 160–164.

Oh MS, Carroll IU. Disorders of sodium metabolism: hypernatremia and hyponatremia. *Critical Care Medicine* 1992; **20**: 94–103.

Paraskevopoulos JA, Houghton LA, Eyre-Brooke I *et al*. Effect of composition of gastric contents on resistance to emptying of liquids from stomach in humans. *Digestive Diseases and Sciences* 1988; **33**: 914–918.

Patterson ML, Dominguez JM, Lyman B *et al*. Enteral feeding in the hypoalbuminemic patient. *Journal of Parenteral and Enteral Nutrition* 1990; **14**: 362–365.

Pesola GR, Hogg JE, Eissa N *et al*. Hypertonic nasogastric tube feedings: do they cause diarrhea? *Critical Care Medicine* 1990; **18**: 1378–1382.

Phang PT, Aeberhardt LE. Effect of nutritional support on routine nutrition assessment parameters and body composition in intensive care unit patients. *Canadian Journal of Surgery* 1996; **39**: 212–219.

Planas M, Porta I, Sagrista ML *et al*. Fatty acid composition of platelet membrane lipids after administration of two different fat emulsions in critically ill patients. *Intensive Care Medicine* 1999; **25**: 395–398.

Powell-Tuck J, Jamieson CP, Bettany GE *et al*. A double blind, randomised, controlled trial of glutamine supplementation in parenteral nutrition. *Gut* 1999; **45**: 82–88.

Power BM, Forbes AM, van Heerden PV, Ilett KF. Pharmacokinetics of drugs used in critically ill adults. *Clinical Pharmacokinetics* 1998; **34**: 25–56.

Preiser JC, Berre J, Carpentier Y *et al*. Management of nutrition in European intensive care units: results of a questionnaire. Working Group on Metabolism and Nutrition of the European Society of Intensive Care Medicine. *Intensive Care Medicine* 1999; **25**: 95–101.

Raff T, Germann G, Hartmann B. The value of early enteral nutrition in the prophylaxis of stress ulceration in the severely burned patient. *Burns* 1997; **23**: 313–318.

Ranieri VM, Suter PM, Tortorella C *et al*. Effect of mechanical ventilation on inflammatory mediators in patients with acute respiratory distress syndrome. *Journal of the American Medical Association* 1999; **282**: 54–61.

Rombeau JL, Takala J. Summary of round table conference: gut dysfunction in critical illness. *Intensive Care Medicine* 1997; **23**: 476–479.

Runcie CJ, Dougall JR. Assessment of the critically ill patient. *British Journal of Hospital Medicine* 1990; **43**: 74–76.

Ryan DW, Clague MB. Nitrogen sparing and the catabolic hormones in patients nursed at an ambient temperature following major surgery. *Intensive Care Medicine* 1990; **16**: 287–290.

Sands JA. Incidence of pulmonary aspiration in intubated patients receiving enteral nutrition through wide- and narrow-bore nasogastric feeding tubes. *Heart and Lung* 1991; **20**: 75–80.

Sax HC. Early nutritional support in critical illness is important. *Critical Care Clinics* 1996; **12**: 661–666.

Schumann D. Post-operative hyperglycaemia: clinical benefits of insulin therapy. *Heart Lung* 1990; **19**: 165–173.

Seigal JH, Vary TC, Rivkind A *et al*. Abnormal metabolic control in the septic multiple organ failure syndrome: pharmacotherapy for altered fuel control mechanisms. *Second Vienna Shock Forum*, pp. 535–554, 1989.

Shang E, Kahler G, Meier-Hellmann A, Scheele J. Advantages of endoscopic therapy of gastrojejunal dissociation in critical care patients. *Intensive Care Medicine* 1999; **25**: 162–165.

Siitonen S, Vapaatalo H, Salminen S *et al*. Effect of *Lactobacillus GG* yoghurt in prevention of antibiotic associated diarrhoea. *Annals of Medicine* 1990; **22**: 57–59.

Singer M. Management of multiple organ failure: guidelines but no hard-and-fast rules. *Journal of Antimicrobial Chemotherapy* 1998; **41** (Suppl A): 103–112.

Singh A, Smoak B, Patterson KY *et al*. Biochemical indices of selected trace elements in man: effect of stress. *American Journal of Clinical Nutrition* 1991; **53**: 126–131.

Tarling MM, Toner CC, Withington PS *et al*. A model of gastric emptying using paracetamol absorption in intensive care patients. *Intensive Care Medicine* 1997; **23**: 256–260.

Tashiro T, Mashima Y, Yamamori H *et al*. Alteration of whole-body protein kinetics according to severity of surgical trauma in patients receiving total parenteral nutrition. *Journal of Parenteral and Enteral Nutrition* 1990; **15**: 169–172.

van der Hulst RR, von Meyenfeldt MF, Soeters PB. Glutamine: an essential amino acid for the gut. *Nutrition* 1996; **12** (Suppl): S78–S81.

Van Lanschot JJB, Feenstra B, Vermeij CG, Bruining HA. Accuracy of intermittent metabolic gas exchange recordings extrapolated for diurnal variation. *Critical Care Medicine* 1988; **16**: 737–742.

Vincent JL. Management of nutrition in European intensive care units: results of a questionnaire. Working Group on Metabolism and Nutrition of the European Society of Intensive Care Medicine. *Intensive Care Medicine* 1999; **25**: 95–101.

Ward PA, Lentsch AB. The acute inflammatory response and its regulation. *Archives of Surgery* 1999; **134**: 666–669.

Wernerman J, Hammarqvist F, Gamrin L, Essen P. Protein metabolism in critical illness. *Baillieres Clinical Endocrinology and Metabolism* 1996; **10**: 603–615.

Wilmore DW, Shabert JK. Role of glutamine in immunologic responses. *Nutrition* 1998: **14**: 618–626.

Wolfe RR. Sepsis as a modulator of adaptation to low and high carbohydrate and low and high fat intakes. *European Journal of Clinical Nutrition* 1999; **53** (Suppl 1): S136–S142.

Zaloga GP. Hypocalcemia in critically ill patients. *Critical Care Medicine* 1992; **20**: 251–262.

Zaloga GP. Immune-enhancing enteral diets: where's the beef? *Critical Care Medicine* 1998; **26**: 1143–1146.

5.3 Head injury

It is possible to injure the head without causing damage to the brain, but in this section the term 'head injury' is taken to mean externally induced brain injury. 'Brain injury' is an all-encompassing term which includes damage induced both internally (e.g. as a result of stroke) and externally (as a result of trauma). Although there are many similarities in the rehabilitation of all brain-injured patients whatever the cause, and some long-term consequences may be the same, there are differences in the nutritional management of patients with externally induced brain injury, particularly in the acute post-injury phase.

In the UK, head injury accounts for about 10% of admissions to accident and emergency departments and results in 300 per 100 000 of the population per year being admitted to hospital (Lindsay et al. 1991). Every year about 5000 people die from head injury. Many of these people are young; head injury is a leading cause of death in people under 30 years old, and the most common cause of death in children between 1 and 15 years of age (Morris and Malt 1994). Those who survive serious head injury have a high incidence of morbidity, and externally induced brain injury (i.e. distinct from brain injury resulting from stroke or neurological disease) is one of the most common causes of serious disability in young adults, particularly men between the ages of 15 and 35 years. Those who do recover mobility and speech may still suffer personality changes or impaired intellectual function, with consequent effects on employment prospects, social skills and personal relationships.

The principal causes of head injury include road traffic accidents, falls, assaults, and injuries occurring at work, in the home and during sports. The relative frequency of each cause varies between different age groups and by region in the country. Head injuries from road traffic accidents are most common in young males and alcohol is frequently involved. Road traffic accidents, although only constituting 25% of all patients with head injury, result in more serious injuries; they cause 60% of deaths from head injury, half of which occur before reaching hospital.

5.3.1 Consequences of head injury

Head injury may result in diffuse and local brain damage. Diffuse neuronal damage is due to rotatory shearing movements, with the clinical severity varying from concussion to dementia. Local damage is caused by compression of the brain by skull fracture or haematoma. Secondary brain injury results from swelling, due to axonal damage and haematoma, both of which may raise intracranial pressure (ICP). Ultimately, compression of the medulla (coning) can result in bradycardia and cardiorespiratory arrest.

The extent of initial and secondary brain injury is assessed by a combination of procedures, the most important of which are the Glasgow Coma Scale (GCS) (Teasdale and Jennett 1974), pupillary reaction and computed tomographic (CT) scan. These measures, considered in conjunction with a person's age, give an indication of prognosis. A combination of low GCS (i.e. poor motor, verbal and eye function), fixed dilated pupils (often indicative of cerebral oedema) and haematoma (identified by CT scan) in someone of advanced age is indicative of poor prognosis. A younger person with a similarly low GCS may achieve a much better outcome (Table 5.6).

The long-term consequences of head injury depend on the degree of permanent damage to the brain and the extent to which rehabilitation can overcome or mitigate some of the consequences. Some head-injured patients will in time make a full recovery; others suffer effects ranging from mild cognitive impairment to persistent vegetative state (PVS).

Table 5.6 Outcome after acute head injury in relation to age and initial parameters of brain injury (After Bullock and Teasdale 1990)

Parameters 24 hours after injury		Outcome at 6 months after head injury	
		% dead or vegetative state	% with moderate disability or good recovery
Age	0–29 years	39	50
	30–59 years	49	34
	≥ 60 years	81	11
Best coma score	3–5	84	11
	6–7	56	29
	8–10	28	58
	11–15	16	72
Best pupil reaction	Both fixed	86	6
	One or both reacting	16	72

5.3.2 Management of head injury

Once a head injury has occurred, nothing can alter the primary damage. The aim of head injury management is to minimize damage arising from secondary complications.

Increasingly, patients with brain injury are managed by a multidisciplinary neurological rehabilitation team of which dietetic expertise is an integral part. Rehabilitation is considered to start from the moment the patient is admitted to hospital.

Management of brain injury can be divided into four phases:

1 very acute post-injury
2 acute post-injury
3 rehabilitation
4 continuing rehabilitation.

Very acute post-injury phase

The aim of treatment in this period is to achieve haemodynamic stabilization and prevent complications resulting from the injury, principally increased ICP and infection.

Baseline observations start as soon as possible in order to detect any change in ICP. Neurological state is assessed by the GCS and pupillary reaction (Price and Knill-Jones 1979). Patients with a GCS <8 usually undergo a CT scan within 1 hour of admission, with immediate craniotomy for those with mass lesions. Craniotomy is performed to debride the wounds, elevate skull fractures or remove haematoma within the first 24 hours after injury. Controlling ICP and central perfusion pressure is a central aspect of management.

Fluid and electrolyte balance may be disrupted following brain injury and careful monitoring of fluid and electrolyte balance is essential. Some degree of fluid restriction may be imposed to minimize cerebral oedema, although the efficacy of this has been questioned (Smith 1996) and local practice may vary. The primary aim is to normalize circulating blood volume and cerebral perfusion pressure.

Hypernatraemia may occur if synthesis of antidiuretic hormone (ADH) is reduced as a result of damage to the hypothalamus or if insufficient fluid is provided. Alternatively, persistent release of ADH will result in high sodium losses via urine. Both hyponatraemia and hypernatraemia may have deleterious effects on the level of consciousness or coma (Parobek and Alamo 1996; Smith 1996).

Acute post-injury phase

Within 2–3 days, the metabolic response to injury induces hypermetabolism and hypercatabolism, effects which are likely to persist for several weeks (see Section 5.1). The nutritional priorities in the acute post-injury phase are to:

- assess nutritional requirements, which may be considerably increased as a result of the metabolic response to injury
- instigate appropriate nutritional support measures to ensure that these needs are met.

Assessing nutritional requirements

Energy Head injury induces a hypermetabolic state which is roughly proportionate to the severity of injury (Robertson *et al.* 1984) and persists for 4–6 weeks (Borzotta *et al.* 1994). Typically, measured resting energy expenditure (REE) has been found to be between 135–146% (Bruder *et al.* 1991) and 130–135% (Weeks and Elia 1996) above basal metabolic rate (BMR), with considerable interindividual variation. For this reason, individual energy requirements are difficult to predict.

Factors which tend to reduce energy expenditure are:

- *loss of body weight* during the post-injury period
- *sedation*: heavy sedation (e.g. use of drugs such as midazolam, propofol or thiopentone) slows metabolism, inhibits motor activity and has been shown to reduce energy expenditure from 138% of the BMR to 89% (Clifton *et al.* 1984). Curarization has been reported to produce a 42% reduction in REE (Clifton *et al.* 1986).

Factors which tend to increase energy expenditure are:

- *Weaning from mechanical ventilation*: This may play a role in the increase in energy expenditure occurring from day 4 to 18 (Bruder *et al.* 1991).
- *Decerebrate rigidity*: This results in limbs being in a state of extension and neck muscles being retracted.
- *Increased activity level*: REE has been shown to remain constant for up to 28 days after injury in patients who remained unchanged neurologically, but to increase as patients improve from responding only to painful stimuli to showing spontaneous activity (Robertson *et al.* 1984).
- *Nursing procedures*: Airway suction and physiotherapy increase energy expenditure (and reduce blood flow to the gastrointestinal tract).

Energy expenditure may also be influenced by the extent to which patients are fed; dietary-induced thermogenesis will be less in those who are fasted or fed less than their energy requirements (Weeks and Elia 1996).

Energy requirements are thus likely to be highest immediately after the injury, fall to some extent as the injury resolves, but increase again as recovery progresses and activity level increases. It is therefore important to consider the energy needs of each patient on an individual and continuous basis. Prediction equations may be used to help to assess energy requirements (see Section 1.10), but it important that the estimates obtained are not regarded as definitive but merely as a starting point for adjustment in the light of further evaluation, monitoring and empirical evidence (e.g. nitrogen balance or body weight). No specific prediction equations have been devised for use on head-injured patients.

Nitrogen Head injury induces a hypercatabolic state resulting in high nitrogen losses, typically in the region of 0.35 g/kg per day (Rapp *et al.* 1983). Nitrogen excretion peaks during the second week post-injury and remains elevated for a considerable period of time (Borzotta *et al.* 1994; Clifton *et al.* 1984; Robertson *et al.* 1984; Young *et al.* 1985). Nitrogen balance is likely to remain negative in head-injured patients for the first 2–3 weeks after injury, irrespective of nitrogen intake (Haider *et al.* 1975; Rapp *et al.* 1983; Gadisseux *et al.* 1984; Clifton *et al.* 1986).

Protein is preferentially utilized as a fuel by the body in the first weeks after injury, and nitrogen losses are rarely balanced by nitrogen intake, although an intake of 0.35g/kg per day is more effective than 0.24 g/kg per day (Twyman *et al.* 1985; Cerra *et al.* 1987). Because of the individual variability in nitrogen excretion (ranging between 0.29 and 0.73 g/kg per day; Borzotta *et al.* 1994), nitrogen requirements are best estimated by empirical measurement of nitrogen loss.

Nitrogen requirements of head-injured patients are thus high but, during the catabolic phase, losses can only be minimized, not prevented.

Nutritional support

Tolerance of enteral feeding has been shown to be inversely related to increased ICP and the severity of the brain injury (Norton *et al.* 1988). Enteral feeding either via the nasogastric route or by percutaneous gastrostomy (PEG) is likely to be contraindicated for at least 72 hours in the initial post-injury phase owing to delayed gastric emptying (Ott *et al.* 1991) and the increased risk of aspiration pneumonia (Saxe *et al.* 1994). However, enteral nutrition can be introduced via the jejunal route as soon as the patient has been resuscitated (usually within 12 hours of injury) (Grahm *et al.* 1989).

There is evidence that commencement of early and adequate feeding improves neurological recovery and the outcome of brain injury (Young *et al.* 1987; Godbole *et al.* 1991). It is therefore imperative that sufficient nutritional support is provided at the earliest possible stage. The level of nutritional support associated with improved clinical outcome is between 60 and 100% of estimated energy and nitrogen requirements within 48 hours of injury (Taylor *et al.* 1999). The optimal level of nutritional delivery has not been precisely determined. Early parenteral nutrition has been associated with patients reaching their ultimate neurological state more quickly, but the efficacy of early enteral versus parenteral nutrition has not been tested.

Nutritional intake is often inadequate following head injury owing to the combination of high nutritional requirements and lack of nutritional support during the post-injury period. In two groups of patients with a peak GCS of 4–10 in the first 24 hours, nutritional intake via nasogastric feeding was found to be inadequate for a mean of 11.5 days (Norton *et al.* 1988). Even when tube feeding commenced by the second day post-injury, 35% did not reach the target of 150% of REE until the second week post-injury (Ott *et al.* 1991). Similar findings have been reported elsewhere (Kempner *et al.* 1992).

Recent research (Taylor and Fettes 1998; Taylor *et al.* 1999) suggests that 'enhanced enteral nutrition' (where patients are given their full nutritional requirements either nasogastrically or nasojejunally as soon as possible post-injury) produces a more appropriate level of nutritional support than standard nasogastric feeding practice (a gradual increase in the feed rate as determined by gastric residuals). Patients receiving enhanced enteral nutrition tolerated 60–70% of their estimated energy and nitrogen requirements from day 2 post-injury, compared with 25% in controls. The likelihood of nutritional and fluid requirements being met was increased partly because of the higher initial feeding rate, but also because best use was made of available feeding time (e.g. overnight feeding when fewer interruptions occur).

In long-term follow-up of patients given either enhanced enteral nutrition or standard feeding, neurological outcome at 6 months was similar between groups but there was a tendency for the intervention patients to have a better neurological outcome at 3 months (61% compared with 39% of control patients) (Taylor *et al.* 1999). Compared with controls, fewer intervention patients had an infective complication (61% versus 85%) or more than one total complication (37% versus 61%). Enhanced enteral nutrition was associated with a reduction in the ratio of serum concentration of C-reactive protein:albumin up to day 6 post-injury. Enhanced enteral nutrition may therefore accelerate neurological recovery and reduce the inflammatory response, possibly secondary to a reduction in the incidence of major complications.

There is some evidence that the composition of feed may alter the cytokine response (Meydani 1990) and that it may be possible to manipulate feed formulation in order to maximize its beneficial effects and minimize the detrimental effects of catabolism. However, this area of research requires further investigation before any practical recommendations can be made (see Section 5.2, Intensive care).

Rehabilitation

Many patients will enter the phase of rehabilitation in a malnourished state. Brooke *et al.* (1989) found that about 60% of brain-injured patients commenced rehabilitation below 90% of their ideal body weight; the average weight loss between admission and rehabilitation was 13.2 kg. Similar findings have been reported by others (Haynes 1992; Finestone *et al.* 1995; Molyneux 1996), suggesting it to be a widespread problem. The greater the extent of the brain injury, the greater the risk and extent of malnutrition.

Identifying and correcting nutritional depletion is an early priority during the rehabilitation phase (see Section 4.28, Neurorehabilitation). Poor nutritional status exacerbates problems such as muscle weakness and fatigue, thus hampering the rehabilitation process (Haynes 1992). Rehabilitation will be unnecessarily prolonged if the individual is unable to cope with the physical demands involved.

Continuing rehabilitation

The process of recovery from brain injury is variable and improvements can both start and stop unexpectedly. Although damaged brain tissue cannot be regenerated, recovery can occur to some extent as a result of 'plasticity', i.e. when one region of the brain is destroyed another region may be able to take over some or all of its function. The extent to which this can happen depends on the location and extent of the original injury, and the functions which this area performed.

Neurological damage can have profound effects on an individual's physical and mental capabilities including effects on eating behaviour and the ability to consume food. As a result, brain injury may have many long-term nutritional consequences (see Section 4.28, Neurorehabilitation). Some of these may result in poor food intake and undernutrition, but other problems such as disordered eating patterns or obesity are also likely to occur (Henson *et al.* 1993). Dietitians have a key role in the neurorehabilitation team in assessing the nature of individual dietary problems and helping people to overcome or mitigate their difficulties.

Text revised by: Briony Thomas, Helen Molyneux and Stephen Taylor

Acknowledgement: The British Dietetic Association's Dietitians in Neurological Therapy (DINT) group.

Useful address

Headway (National Head Injuries Association)
7 King Edward Court, King Edward Street, Nottingham NG1 1EW

Further reading

Headway booklets (for address see above). A series of booklets covering various aspects of the effects and management of head injury which are helpful for patients, carers and health professionals.

Muir-Giles G, Clark-Wilson J. *Brain Injury Rehabilitation: A Neurological Approach*. London: Chapman and Hall, 1993.

Rose FD, Johnson DA. *Brain Injury and After*. Chichester: John Wiley and Sons, 1996.

References

Borzotta AP, Pennings J, Papasadero B *et al*. Enteral versus parenteral nutrition after severe closed head injury. *Journal of Trauma* 1994; **37**: 359–368.

Brooke MM, Barbour PG, Cording LG *et al*. Nutritional status during rehabilitation after injury. *Journal of Neurological Rehabilitation* 1989; **3**: 27–33.

Bruder N, Dumont JC, Francois G. Evolution of energy expenditure and nitrogen excretion in severe head-injured patients. *Critical Care Medicine* 1991; **19**: 43-48.

Bullock R, Teasdale G. ABC of major trauma. Head injuries – I and II. *British Medical Journal* 1990; **300**: 1515–1518, 1576–1579.

Cerra F, Blackburn G, Hirsch J *et al*. The effect of stress level amino acid formula, and nitrogen dose nitrogen retention in traumatic and septic stress. *Annals of Surgery* 1987; **205**: 282–287.

Clifton GL, Robertson CS, Grossman RG *et al*. The metabolic response to severe head injury. *Journal of Neurosurgery* 1984; **60**: 687–696.

Clifton GL, Robertson CS, Choi SC. Assessment of nutritional requirements of head-injured patients. *Journal of Neurosurgery* 1986; **64**: 895–901.

Finestone HM, Greene-Finestone LS, Wilson ES, Teasell RW. Malnutrition in stroke patients on the rehabilitation service and at follow-up: prevalence and predictors. *Archives of Physical Medicine Rehabilitation* 1995; **76**: 310–316.

Gadisseux P, Ward JD, Young HF, Becker DP. Nutrition and the neurosurgical patient. *Journal of Neurosurgery* 1984; **60**: 219–232.

Godbole KB, Berbiglia VA, Goddard L. A head injury patient: caloric needs, clinical progress and nursing care principles. *Journal of Neuroscience Nursing* 1991; **23**: 290–294.

Grahm TW, Zadrozny DB, Harrington T. The benefits of early jejunal hyperalimentation in the head-injured patient. *Neurosurgery* 1989; **25**: 729–735.

Haider W, Lackner F, Schlick W. Metabolic changes in the course of severe acute brain damage. *European Journal of Intensive Care Medicine* 1975; **1**: 19–26.

Haynes MKM. Nutrition in the severely head-injured patient. *Clinical Rehabilitation* 1992; **6**: 153–158.

Henson MB, De Castro JM, Stringer AY, Johnson C. Food intake by brain-injured humans who are in the chronic phase of recovery. *Brain Injury* 1993; **7**: 169–178.

Kempner M, Critt C, Weissman C, Hyman AI. Caloric requirements and supply in critically ill surgical patients. *Critical Care Medicine* 1992; **20**: 344–348.

Lindsay K, Bone I, Callander R. Head injury. In *Neurology and Neurosurgery Illustrated*, pp. 214–232. Edinburgh: Churchill Livingstone, 1991.

Meydani JK. Dietary manipulation of cytokine production and biological functions. *Nutrition Reviews* 1990; **48**: 361–369.

Molyneux HJ. Malnutrition following brain injury. *European Journal of Neurology* 1996; **3** (Suppl 2): 43.

Morris PJ, Malt RA. Head injuries. In *Oxford Textbook of Surgery*, Vol. 22, pp. 2145–2153. Oxford: Oxford University Press, 1994.

Norton JA, Ott LG, McClain C *et al*. Intolerance to enteral feeding in the brain-injured patient. *Journal of Neurosurgery* 1988; **68**: 62–66.

Ott L, Young B, Phillips R *et al*. Altered gastric emptying in the head-injured patient: relationship to feeding intolerance. *Journal of Neurosurgery* 1991; **74**: 738–742.

Parobek V, Alaimo I. Fluid and electrolyte management in the neurologically impaired patient. *Journal of Neuroscience Nursing* 1996; **28**: 322–328.

Price D, Knill-Jones R. The prediction of outcome of patients admitted following head injury in coma with bilateral fixed pupils. *Acta Neurochurgica* 1979; **28** (Suppl): 179–182.

Rapp RP, Young B, Twyman D. The favouirable effect of early parenteral feeding on survival in head injured patients. *Journal of Neurosurgery* 1983; **58**: 906–912.

Robertson CS, Clifton GL, Grossman RG. Oxygen utilization and cardiovascular function in head-injured patients. *Neurosurgery* 1984; **15**: 307–314.

Saxe J, Ledgerwood A, Lucas C, Lucas W. Lower oesophageal sphincter dysfunction precludes gastric feeding after head injury. *Journal of Trauma* 1994; **37**: 581–586.

Smith M. Acute care. In Rose FD, Johnson DA (Eds) *Brain Injury and After*. Chichester: John Wiley and Sons, 1996.

Taylor SJ, Fettes SB. Enhanced enteral nutrition in head injury: effect on the efficacy of nutritional delivery, nitrogen balance, gastric residuals and risk of pneumonia. *Journal of Human Nutrition and Dietetics* 1998; **11**: 391–401.

Taylor SJ, Fettes SB, Jewkes C, Nelson RJ. Prospective randomised controlled trial to determine the effect of early enhanced enteral nutrition on clinical outcome in mechanically ventilated patients suffering head injury. *Critical Care Medicine* 1999; **27**: 2525–2531.

Teasdale G, Jennett B. Assessment of coma and impaired consciousness: a practical scale. *Lancet* 1974; **ii**: 81–86.

Twyman D, Young AB, Ott L *et al*. High protein enteral feedings: a means of achieving positive nitrogen balance in head injured patients. *Journal of Parenteral and Enteral Nutrition* 1985; **9**: 679–684.

Weeks E, Elia M. Observations on the patterns of 24-hour energy expenditure changes in body composition and gastric emptying in head injured patients receiving nasogastric tube feeding. *Journal of Parenteral and Enteral Nutrition* 1996; **20**: 31–37.

Young B, Ott L, Norton J *et al*. The metabolic and nutritional sequela of the nonsteroid treated injury patient. *Neurosurgery* 1985; **17**: 784–791.

Young B, Ott L, Twyman D *et al*. The effect of nutritional support on outcome from severe head injury. *Journal of Neurosurgery* 1987; **67**: 668–676.

5.4 Spinal cord injury

Accurate figures are not available, but about 500 people each year sustain an injury sufficiently serious to require admission to a spinal unit in the UK. Most patients are young and male, the most common cause of spinal injury being road traffic accidents (Table 5.7). A high proportion of new admissions are tetraplegic. Other injuries such as head and chest injury may complicate management and rehabilitation.

The UK has 11 spinal injury units with a total of about 350 beds for the rehabilitation of patients who have a spinal injury (Fig. 5.1). The first UK unit was opened in 1944 (Stoke Mandeville) and the newest unit in 1992 (Glasgow).

The metabolic response to injury is well documented (see Section 5.1) and the prevalence of malnutrition and its effects on the patient with spinal cord injury (SCI) have been recognized since the time of Hippocrates (Guttmann 1973). Prior to World War II few SCI patients survived for more than 2 years. Nowadays, life expectancy ranges between 70 and 92% of normal, depending on the level and completeness of injury (Yeo *et al.* 1998).

As with any patient suffering acute injury necessitating subsequent rehabilitation, dietetic care should be an integral part of management. In the past, this has often been overlooked. The variability in dietetic cover in UK spinal injury units in mid-1999 is shown in Table 5.8.

5.4.1 Consequences of spinal cord injury

The effects of SCI depend on which segments of the spinal cord are damaged (Fig. 5.2). Figure 5.3 shows the likely consequences of spinal injury on sensory dermatomes (areas of skin supplied with afferent nerve fibres by a single posterior spinal root). These may include:

- *Complete and incomplete lesions*: In the former, all neurological function is lost below the level of the lesion. In incomplete lesions there is partial preservation of neurological function and any combination of motor, sensory or autonomic function may be spared.
- *Paraplegia*: function of the lower limbs is lost as a result of damage to the thoracic, lumbar or, to a lesser extent, sacral cord segments.
- *Quadriplegia (tetraplegia)* results from damage to cervical segments causing loss of function of all four limbs.

    In both paraplegia and quadriplegia there is impairment of autonomic function, including bladder and bowel control.

Table 5.7 Causes of spinal injury (Estimated figures for 1992 from the Spinal Injury Association, reproduced with permission)

Causes of spinal cord injury	Percentage of spinal injury cases
(A) *Road traffic accidents*	39%
Motorcycle	19%
Car	15%
Pedestrian	3%
Cyclist	2%
(B) *Domestic and industrial accidents*	24%
Domestic fall	17%
Accident at work	7%
(C) *Sporting accidents*	17%
Diving into shallow water	8%
Horse riding	4%
Other (skiing, judo, gym, hang-gliding, water skiing etc.)	3%
(D) *Non-traumatic* (medical, surgical, viral, neurological, vascular)	16%
(E) *Self-harm and physical assault* (Falls, stabbings etc)	4%

Table 5.8 Dietetic cover to UK spinal injury units in mid-1999

Spinal cord injury units (bed complement)	Dietetic cover (hours/week)
Belfast (15)	2
Cardiff (20)	18.25
Glasgow (42)	18.25
Hexham (19)	8.3
Oswestry (44)	10
Salisbury (54)	10
Sheffield (54)	18.45
Southport (38)	2–4
Stanmore (24)	As required
Stoke Mandeville (115)	11
Wakefield (30)	2–4

Dietetic cover was mostly at Senior I level or above.
All SCI units except for one have scales for weighing wheelchairs, but only three have bed weighing scales.

- *Muscle wasting*: Muscle mass above the level of injury has the potential to be entirely normal. At the level of the lesion there is a band of denervation and consequent muscle atrophy. Although loss of muscle is observed above and below the lesion, it is difficult to assess how much is due to denervation or malnutrition. Post-injury muscle wasting results in a reduction of lean body mass and in the longer term, a sedentary lifestyle

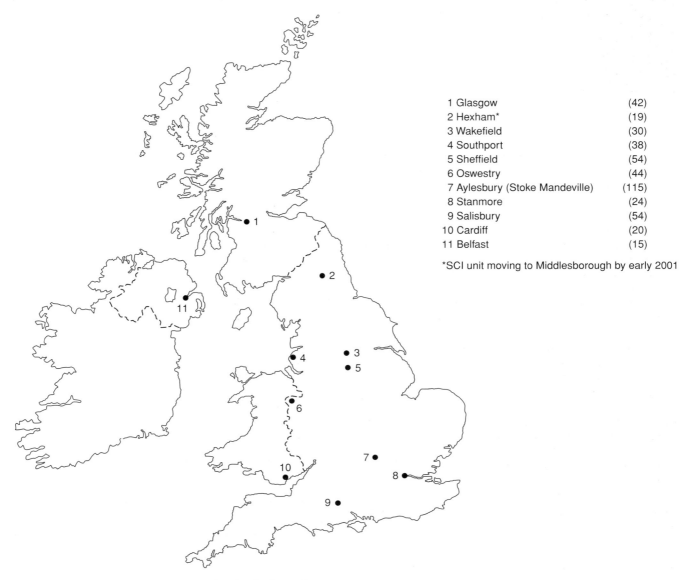

1 Glasgow   (42)
2 Hexham*   (19)
3 Wakefield   (30)
4 Southport   (38)
5 Sheffield   (54)
6 Oswestry   (44)
7 Aylesbury (Stoke Mandeville)   (115)
8 Stanmore   (24)
9 Salisbury   (54)
10 Cardiff   (20)
11 Belfast   (15)

*SCI unit moving to Middlesborough by early 2001

Fig. 5.1 Map of UK spinal injury units showing bed complement.

encourages an increase in total body fat (Greenway *et al*. 1970; Shizgal *et al*. 1986; Rasmann Nuhlicek *et al*. 1988).

5.4.2 Management of spinal cord injury

Initial post-injury period (within the first week of injury)

Complex physiological changes occur following SCI and these vary with the level of the lesion, the Frankel classification (extent of damage to the spinal cord), presence of concomitant injury or illness and the time elapsed since injury, resulting in a dynamic metabolic state which may adversely affect the nutritional status at any time (Worthington *et al*. 1993). The requirements for energy and nitrogen will be increased, but the presence of delayed gastric emptying and paralytic ileus often precludes enteral feeding.

At this stage, priorities in clinical care may result in neglect of nutritional needs; weighing the patient is often impossible and interpretation of anthropometry difficult. It is now usual, however, for SCI patients to transfer from general hospital into spinal injury units having had at least some nutritional assessment or support, unless transfer occurs very quickly.

The initial nutritional needs of SCI patients are far from clear and some studies have shown energy requirements to be as low as 1500 kcal/6.25 MJ per day, while others suggest that requirements may exceed those of burns patients (Clarke 1966; Kearns *et al*. 1982, 1992; Cox *et al*. 1985; Kaufman *et al*. 1985; Mollinger *et al*. 1985; Rodriguez 1997). Current research is indicating, surprisingly, energy requirements to be in the region of 34 kcal/kg

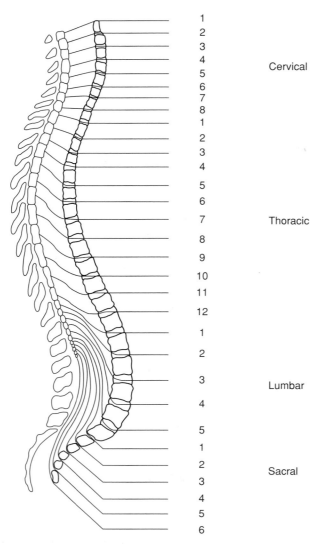

1	
2	
3	
4	Cervical
5	
6	
7	
8	
1	
2	
3	
4	
5	
6	
7	Thoracic
8	
9	
10	
11	
12	
1	
2	
3	Lumbar
4	
5	
1	
2	Sacral
3	
4	
5	
6	

Fig. 5.2 The spinal cord.

Nutritional status is adversely affected by SCI, particularly during the first 2–4 weeks (Laven *et al.* 1989), and nutritional depletion resulting from the initial metabolic response to trauma may be severe. Positive nitrogen balance is unlikely to be achieved within this period. Gastrointestinal problems arise in both the acute and long-term setting, with paralytic ileus and gastric ulcers commonly found during the first 4 weeks of injury and lower tract dysfunction thereafter (Frost 1998).

General guidelines for the nutritional assessment of patients at this phase of rehabilitation can be found in Section 4.28 (Neurorehabilitation), but particular aspects which are relevant to those with spinal injuries are discussed below.

Assessing the degree of weight loss

The degree of weight loss since the injury is an important indicator of nutritional depletion and most SCI patients will be able to recall their pre-morbid weight (unlike many patients with brain injury who will have problems with memory, speech or cognition). However, obtaining measurement of current weight may be even more difficult in patients with SCI than in those with brain injury unless they are in a bed with integral weight scales. In some cases, estimate of weight loss will have to be done visually, although it should be borne in mind that muscle wasting may to some extent have resulted from denervation resulting from the injury rather than nutritional depletion.

Other anthropometric assessments

Estimates of muscle mass by measurements such as mid-arm muscle circumference are likely to be distorted by the effects of the spinal injury and consequent paraplegia. Estimates of adiposity by means of the body mass index (BMI) will be dependent on the ability to obtain a meaningful estimate of current body weight. While direct measurement of height is likely to be impossible, an estimate of height can usually be supplied by the patient.

Assessing current nutrient intake

Although it is often possible to obtain estimates of previous and current dietary intake from SCI patients, records of food and fluid intake and changes in appetite noted by care staff should also be taken into account. People with quadriplegia and incomplete injuries appear to be more likely to be underfed within the first 4 weeks (unpublished data from Glasgow SCI Unit, June 1999).

Assessing factors likely to reduce nutritional intake

- *Neurogenic factors*: level of injury, extent of damage to spinal cord, pain and delayed spinal stabilization.
- *Psychological consequences of having suffered the injury*: many patients will be depressed and disinterested in eating. Refusal to eat and/or drink may also occur as a result of anger or attention-seeking behaviour. Some patients may be confused or have a decreased level of consciousness.
- *Infections* of the urinary tract or bladder, chest or infect-

body weight for complete injuries and 29 kcal/kg body weight for incomplete injuries (unpublished data from Kerr, Glasgow SCI Unit, 2000). Nutritional status in SCI patients has been discussed by Levine *et al.* (1992) and Worthington *et al.* (1993).

Subsequent post-injury period (within the first 12 weeks following injury)

All patients with SCI are transferred as soon as possible to one of the UK spinal injury units. In these units the importance of nutritional assessment, identification of those at nutritional risk and appropriate nutritional support are being increasingly recognized. It is essential that dietitians working in this area have a clear understanding of the extent of the patient's injuries (see Fig. 5.2 and 5.3), the profound psychological effects of those injuries and the practical difficulties of nutritional assessment and support.

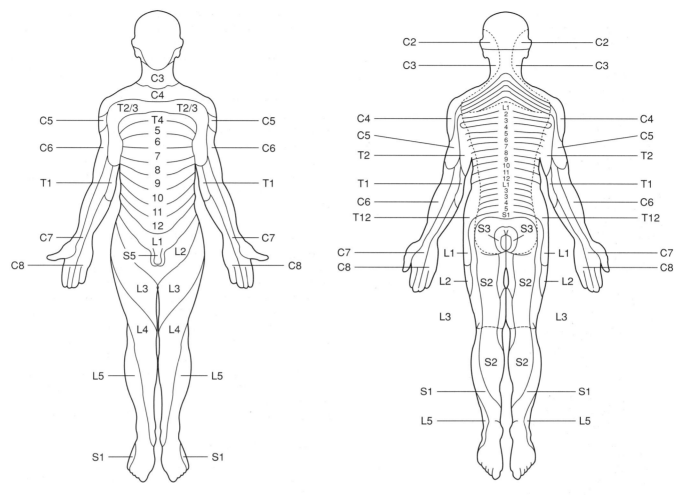

Fig. 5.3 Sensory dermatomes.

ed pressure sores will increase nutritional requirements and may also reduce nutrient intake.

- *Drug treatment*: nausea, vomiting or diarrhoea are common side-effects and inevitably impair nutrient intake.
- *Physical difficulties with eating or drinking* as a result of lying flat: patients may object to being fed or feel reluctant to bother busy nursing staff.
- *Respiratory factors*: ventilator support >72 hours and tracheostomy.
- *Gastrointestinal factors*: dysphagia, ileus, nausea and vomiting, gastrointestinal bleed, diarrhoea or constipation, early satiety, pancreatitis and abdominal injuries.
- *Social factors*: drug or alcohol abuse, stress and lack of social support.

Assessing factors likely to increase nutritional requirements

- *Associated injuries*: long-bone fractures, head injuries and burns.
- *Pressure sores*.
- *Fever, infection, sepsis*.
- *Steroid use*.

Nutritional support may be required at any stage to offset catabolic losses and commence the process of nutritional repletion.

Continuing rehabilitation (after the first 12 weeks following injury)

The aim of rehabilitation is to enable patients to develop the maximum potential possible for their disability (see Section 4.28, Neurorehabilitation).

For the patient who has lost weight during the acute post-injury period, weight regain and restoration of muscle mass are priorities so that the patient is able to derive maximum benefit from physiotherapy and occupational therapy sessions.

Nutritional supplements in the form of sip feed drinks and high-energy snacks may help to boost energy intake. Where patients are still unable to meet their needs by oral intake alone, overnight nasogastric feeding may be a useful method of nutritional support as this strategy does not interfere with daytime therapy sessions.

At this stage of rehabilitation, it is usually easier to measure and monitor the patient's weight, and some of the

Table 5.9 Guide to weighing patients with spinal injuries

Degree of patient mobility	Suitable weighing method
Fully mobile patient:	
(a) with good balance	Standing scales, i.e. platform/bathroom type
(b) with poor balance	Chair scales, e.g. Avery
Wheelchair-dependent patient:	
(a) able to transfer and can hold legs free from the floor	Chair scales, e.g. Avery
(b) unable or inconvenient to transfer in wheelchair	Platform scales
	Platform scales (sunken into floor or with ramp), e.g. Avery
	Electronic scales
	Marsden wheelchair
	Ramp or weighbridge sited near or in the unit, e.g. Avery
(c) able to transfer but cannot hold legs free from the chair	Platform scales or weighbridge
Patient in or on bed/trolley and patient can be lifted by hoist	Hoist scale with sling or stretcher attachment, e.g. Arjo electronic box on hoist
Patient bed-bound and bed can be moved easily	Weighbridge sited in or near unit, e.g. Avery
Patient bed-bound, bed cannot be moved	Electronic scales with jack that can raise bed on to sensitive weighing pads, e.g. Seca
Patient bed-bound, bed has internal weighing device or it can be attached	The Egerton Paragon 9000 Turning Bed

Addresses for manufacturers of this equipment are given at the end of this section.

ways in which this can be done are listed in Table 5.9. Because of the muscle wasting associated with paraplegia and tetraplegia, suitable weight targets for SCI patients may be about 4.5–6.5 kg below those for comparable able-bodied people (Greenway *et al.* 1970; Pfeiffer *et al.* 1981).

As rehabilitation progresses, becoming overweight is an increasing risk as appetite and food intake return to, or even exceed, pre-injury levels but energy expenditure remains reduced as a consequence of paralysis (Monroe *et al.* 1998; Steven *et al.* 1990). Regular monitoring of body weight, and dietary guidance to ensure that energy intake is appropriate, are essential.

Other problems which may arise include:

- *Pressure sores*: Pressure sores are a high risk in SCI patients because of the loss of sensation of pressure, ischaemia of the skin, incontinence and the patient's inability or reluctance to change position. Being either underweight or overweight increases the likelihood of pressure-sore development. Pressure sores can increase nutritional requirements as they leak protein-rich exudate and also expose tissue to infection. Antibiotic treatment of pressure sores may also reduce food intake as a result of associated side-effects. The prevention and management of pressure sores are discussed in Section 5.8 (Wound healing and tissue viability).
- *Renal calculi*: SCI patients have a greater tendency to the formation of renal calculi, primarily as a result of recurrent bladder infections and immobility. To help to prevent bladder infections at least 2 litres of fluid per day is normally recommended and some centres encourage daily intake of cranberry juice (Avorn *et al.* 1994). Dietary restriction of calcium, however, is not indicated.
- *Constipation*: This is a common and by no means trivial problem in SCI. In a study of 127 SCI patients, Stone *et al.* (1990) found that one in 5 still had difficulty with evacuation five or more years after the injury. In people

with SCI, seemingly benign gastrointestinal problems such as this often impair the quality of life and can even lead to life-threatening complications.

Neurogenic bowel dysfunction (NBD) is one of the many impairments that result from SCI. According to Stiens *et al.* (1997) there are two patterns of NBD which occur post-SCI: the upper motor neurone (UMN) bowel syndrome (from cervical and thoracic injury) and the lower motor neurone (LMN) bowel syndrome. The UMN bowel syndrome includes constipation with faecal retention behind a spastic anal sphincter. The LMN bowel syndrome produces constipation with a high risk of frequent incontinence through a lax external sphincter mechanism.

The effects of dietary fibre on colonic function after SCI are not yet known. In one small study (Cameron *et al.* 1996), a mean increase of 6 g insoluble fibre/day for 3 weeks was associated with increased colonic transit time, but stool weight and mouth to anus times remained unchanged. Further research is needed to determine the optimal dietary fibre intake in SCI patients. In the meantime, individualized advice on a high-fibre intake is still recommended for most people with SCI. Weingarden (1992) suggests an intake of 30 g fibre/day.

Text revised by: Anthony Twist, Tanya Wright and Nicola Kerr

Useful addresses

General
MASCIP (The Multidisciplinary Association of Spinal Cord Injury Professionals)
The Duke of Cornwall Spinal Treatment Centre, Salisbury District Hospital, Odstock Road, Salisbury SP2 8BJ
Tel: 01722 336 262

Scottish Spinal Cord Injury Association (SSCIA)
The Festival Business Centre
150 Brand Street, Glasgow G51 1DH

Spinal Injuries Association (UK)
76 St James Lane, London N10 3DF
Tel: 020 8444 2121

Spinal Injury Units in the UK
Belfast:
Spinal Cord Injuries Unit, Musgrove Park Hospital, Stockman's Lane, Balmoral, Belfast BT9 7JB

Cardiff (Rookwood):
Rookwood Spinal Injuries Rehabilitation Unit, Rookwood Hospital, Fairwater Road, Cardiff CF5 2YN

Glasgow:
Queen Elizabeth Spinal Injuries Unit, Southern General Hospital, 1345 Govan Road, Glasgow G51 4TF

Hexham:
Regional Spinal Injuries Unit, Hexham General Hospital, Hexham NE46 1QJ

Middlesborough:
South Cleveland Hospital, Martin Road, Middlesborough TF4 3BW

Oswestry:
The Midland Centre for Spinal Injury, The Robert Jones & Agnes Hunt Orthopaedic Hospital, Oswestry, Shropshire SY10 7AG

Salisbury:
The Duke of Cornwall Spinal Treatment Centre, Salisbury District Hospital, Odstock Road, Salisbury SP2 8BJ

Sheffield:
The Princess Royal Spinal Injuries Unit, Northern General Hospital, Osbourne Building, Herries Road, Sheffield S5 7AU

Southport:
Regional Spinal Injuries Centre, Southport and Formby General Hospital, Town Lane, Kew, Southport PR8 6NJ

Stanmore:
The London Spinal Unit, Royal National Orthopaedic Hospital, Brockley Hill, Stanmore HA7 4LP

Stoke Mandeville:
National Spinal Injuries Centre, Stoke Mandeville Hospital, Mandeville Road, Aylesbury, Bucks HP21 8AL

Wakefield:
Yorkshire Regional Spinal Unit, Pinderfields General Hospital, Aberford Road, Wakefield WF1 4DG

Addresses for manufacturers of weighing equipment
Arjo Ltd
St Catherine's Street, Gloucester GR1 2SL
Tel: 08702 430430

Avery Ltd
Foundry Lane, Smethwick, Warley, West Midlands B66 2LP
Tel: 0121 625 1112

Marsden Weighing Machine Group Ltd
Unit 16, Suttons Business Park, Reading RG6 1AZ
Tel: 0118 935 1655

Pegasus-Egerton
Waterbury Drive, Waterlooville, Hampshire PO7 7XX
Tel: 01689 827062

Seca Ltd
Seca House, 40 Barn Street, Digbeth, Birmingham BS SQB
Tel: 0121 643 9349

Further reading

Burke DC, Murray DD. *Handbook of Spinal Cord Medicine*. London: Macmillan Education, 1988.
Grundy D, Swain A. *The ABC of Spinal Cord Injury*. London: BMJ Publications, 1996.
Frost RA *et al*. The role of percutaneous endoscopic gastrostomy in spinal cord injured patients. *Paraplegia* 1995; **33**: 416–418.
Rice HB, Poinchera-Mulcare JA, Glaser RM. Nutrition and the spinal cord injured individual. *Clinical Kinesiology* 1995; Spring: 21–27.
Spinal Injuries Association. *Moving Forward. The Guide to Living with Spinal Cord Injury*. London: SIA, 1998.
Spinal Injuries Association. *People with Spinal Injuries, Treatment and Care*, Vol. 1. London: SIA, 1980 (revision due 2000).
Useful website on Spinal Cord Injury: www.spinalcord.uab.edu

References

Avorn J, Monane M, Gurwitz JH *et al*. Reduction of bacteria and pyuria after ingestion of cranberry juice. *Journal of the American Medical Association* 1994; **271**: 751–754.
Cameron KJ, Nyulasi IB, Collier GR, Brown DJ. Assessment of the effect of increased dietary fibre intake on bowel function in patients with spinal cord injury. *Spinal Cord* 1996; **34**: 277–283.
Clarke KS. Caloric costs of activity in paraplegic persons. *Archives of Physical Medicine and Rehabilitation* 1966; **47**: 427–435.
Cox SAR, Weiss SM, Posuniak EA *et al*. Energy expenditure after spinal cord injury: an evaluation of stable rehabilitating patients. *Journal of Trauma* 1985; **25**: 419–423.
Frost FS. Spinal cord injury: gastrointestinal implications and management. *Topics in Spinal Cord Injury Rehabilitation* 1998; **4**: 56–80.
Greenway RM, Houser H, Lindan O, Weir DR. Long term changes in gross body composition of paraplegic and quadriplegic patients. *Paraplegia* 1970; **7**: 301–318.
Guttmann L. *Spinal Cord Injuries: Comprehensive Management and Research*. Oxford: Blackwell Scientific Publications, 1973.
Kaufman H, Rowlands BJ, Stein DK *et al*. General metabolism in

patients with acute paraplegia and quadriplegia. *Neurosurgery* 1985; **16**: 309–313.

Kearns PJ, Pipp TL, Quirk M, Campolo M. Nutritional requirements in quadriplegics. *Journal of Parenteral and Enteral Nutrition* 1982; **6**: 577.

Kearns PJ, Thompson JD, Werner PC *et al*. Nutritional and metabolic response to acute spinal cord injury. *Journal of Parenteral and Enteral Nutrition* 1992; **16**: 11–15.

Laven GT, Huang CT, DeVivo MJ *et al*. Nutritional status during the acute stage of spinal cord injury. *Archives of Physical Medicine and Rehabilitation* 1989; **70**: 277–282.

Levine AM, Nash MS, Green BA *et al*. An examination of dietary intakes and nutritional status of chronic healthy spinal cord injured individuals. *Paraplegia* 1992; **30**: 880–889.

Mollinger LA, Spurr GB, Elghatit AZ *et al*. Daily energy expenditure and basal metabolic rates of patients with spinal cord injury. *Archives of Physical Medicine and Rehabilitation* 1985; **66**: 420–426.

Monroe MB, Tataranni PA, Pratley R *et al*. Lower daily expenditure as measured by a respiratory chamber in subjects with spinal cord injury compared with control subjects. *American Journal of Clinical Nutrition* 1998; **68**: 1223–1227.

Pfeiffer SC, Blust P, Leyson JFJ. Nutritional assessment of the spinal cord injured patient. *Perspectives in Practice* 1981; **78**: 501–505.

Rasmann Nuhlicek DN, Spurr GB, Barboriak JJ *et al*. Body composition of patients with spinal cord injury. *European Journal of Clinical Nutrition* 1988; **42**: 765–773.

Rodriguez DJ, Benzel EC, Clevenger FW. The metabolic response to spinal cord injury. *Spinal Cord* 1997; **35**: 599–604.

Shizgal HM, Roza A, Leduc B *et al*. Body composition in quadriplegic patients. *Journal of Parenteral and Enteral Nutrition* 1986; **10**: 364–368.

Steven FG, Greasey GH, Couser AE. Nutritional status of a Scottish spinal injury population. *Journal of Human Nutrition and Dietetics* 1990; **3**: 371–372.

Stiens SA, Bergman SB, Goetz LL. Neurogenic bowel dysfunction after spinal cord injury: clinical evaluation and rehabilitative management. *Archives of Physical Medicine and Rehabilitation* 1997; **78** (3 Suppl): S86–S101.

Stone JM, Wolfe VA, Nino Murcia M, Perkash I. Chronic gastrointestinal problems in spinal cord injury patients: a prospective analysis. *American Journal of Gastoenterology* 1990; **85**: 1114–1119.

Weingarden SI. The gastrointestinal system and spinal cord injury. *Physical Medicine and Rehabilitation Clinics of North America* 1992; **3**: 765–781.

Worthington P, Crowe MA, Armenti V. Nutritional support for patients with spinal cord injury. *Trauma Quarterly* 1993; **9**: 82–92.

Yeo JD, Walsh J, Rutkowski S *et al*. Mortality following spinal cord injury. *Spinal Cord* 1998; **36**: 329–336.

5.5 Burn injury

Extensive thermal injury elicits the most pronounced response to stress that the human body is capable of generating. Resting energy expenditure (REE) increases as hormone-induced breakdown of body protein and fat occurs at greatly accelerated rates. Weight loss of 1.5 kg/day is possible. The patient is almost certain to die if weight loss approaches 30% of the pre-burn weight (Davenport 1979).

Nutritional therapy must provide sufficient nutrients to prevent weight loss, or in practice to restrict weight loss to less than 10% of the admission weight. The aims are to preserve lean body mass, promote maximal wound healing and skin graft take, and maintain immunocompetence. In order to maintain or restore lean body mass, Molnar *et al.* (1983) recommend that aggressive nutritional therapy is undertaken in burn patients with the following features or complications:

- >20% full-thickness burn
- pre-injury malnutrition
- septic complications
- associated injury, including pulmonary involvement
- threat of >10% weight loss.

Ideally, all new burn admissions should be assessed by a dietitian within 24–48 hours of injury, and nutritional support be initiated promptly. Other groups at risk on admission include those with hand and facial burns, all children and those on existing therapeutic diets.

5.5.1 Fatal burn injuries

As a rule of thumb, a patient with a percentage body surface area (BSA) burn (Fig. 5.4) and an age which when totalled together exceed 100 is unlikely to survive, for example:

86 year old with 30% burn = 116   (survival unlikely)
13 year old with 55% burn = 68   (survival likely).

This formula does not apply to children under 10 years old. More sophisticated formulae also exist for predicting mortality (Tobiasen *et al.* 1982).

In cases of non-survivable injury, the patient should be kept well hydrated and given adequate analgesia, but no nutritional therapy attempted; the patient usually succumbs to the injury within a few days.

5.5.2 Minor burn injuries

Small burn injuries (i.e. <15% BSA burn in adults; <10%

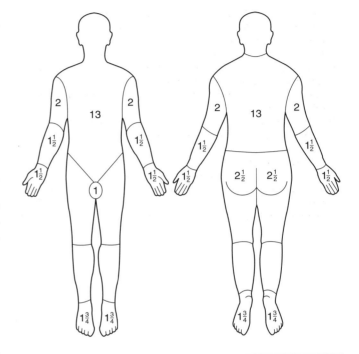

Age	Age (years)					
	0	1	5	10	15	Adult
Head and neck	21	19	15	13	11	9
Thigh	$5\frac{1}{2}$	$6\frac{1}{2}$	8	9	9	$9\frac{1}{2}$
Calf	5	5	$5\frac{1}{2}$	6	$6\frac{1}{2}$	7

Fig. 5.4 Percentage of different parts of the body at different ages. From Harvey Kemble and Lamb (1984); reproduced with permission.

BSA burn in children) do not require resuscitation with intravenous fluids. REE is only mildly elevated and weight can usually be maintained on a high-protein – high-energy diet supplemented with palatable high-energy and/or high-protein drinks (see Section 1.12, Oral nutritional support). Oral diet and fluids should be encouraged as soon as possible after admission. However, intake of foods and fluids may be compromised by 'nil by mouth' regimens for change of dressings or theatre procedures requiring anaesthesia, or impaired by factors such as sedation and analgesia, fear, pain or foul-smelling dressings, all of which may reduce appetite. Patients cannot be forced to eat to order, so flexibility in catering arrangements and feeding regimens is an advantage.

5.5.3 Major burn injuries or 'shock burns'
Metabolic response to burn injury

Ebb phase

Immediately post-burn, fluid moves from the circulation into the tissues. Plasma and other fluids are given parenterally to preserve blood volume and urine output. Burn patients become hypercatabolic within hours of injury. Traditional clinical teaching restricts oral and enteral tube feeding at this time because of the risk of paralytic ileus developing, secondary to reduced blood flow to the gut (Dobb 1996). However, research has shown that feeding within several hours of burn injury can prevent the development of ileus (Raff *et al.* 1997), prevent gut vasoconstriction (Inoue *et al.* 1989), blunt the hypermetabolic response and maintain gut integrity (Mochizuki *et al.* 1984; Saito *et al.* 1986), thereby reducing the risk of gut-origin sepsis secondary to bacterial translocation (Epstein *et al.* 1992). Most UK burns units have an early-feeding policy and commence enteral tube feeding within 4–6 hours of injury with a low incidence of paralytic ileus. Nasoduodenal or nasojejunal feeding early post-burn may have some advantages over nasogastric feeding as provision of nutrients directly into the small intestine may reduce the incidence of abdominal distension, aspiration and nausea observed as a consequence of delayed gastric emptying, and permits more of the prescribed volume of feed to be delivered (La Hausse-Brown *et al.* 1997).

Flow phase

This will be well underway by the end of the resuscitation period and its duration will be determined by the depth of the burn (Table 5.10) and the time taken to achieve skin coverage, along with inevitable episodes of septicaemia. Increased production of catabolic hormones (adrenaline, noradrenaline, glucagon and the corticosteroids) leads to hypermetabolism, accelerated protein and fat breakdown and altered carbohydrate metabolism (see Section 5.1, Metabolic consequences of injury).

The abnormalities of carbohydrate metabolism include elevated glucose levels, increased gluconeogenesis and profound insulin resistance. All are attributable to the hormonal imbalance which suppresses the influence of insulin on peripheral tissues (Davies 1977; Richards 1977;

Wilmore and McDougal 1977). Septicaemia will further accentuate post-injury glucose intolerance, necessitating an insulin infusion. This requirement resolves on successful treatment of the underlying sepsis (Woolfson *et al.* 1977). It is important to treat the hyperglycaemia with insulin and not restrict the nutrient intake, but it may be worth rechecking calculations to see whether an overestimation of energy requirements has been made.

The maximum catabolic response usually occurs 5–10 days post-burn. Thereafter, healing of partial-thickness burns and early excision and grafting of deep burns reduces wound size and thus the exogenous demand for nutrients. However, donor sites should also be taken into consideration before reducing nutrient intake.

Anabolic phase

Soroff *et al.* (1961) showed that patients with major burn injuries were entering an anabolic phase by 30 days post-burn and, provided that weight loss has not occurred, nutrient intake can return to normal levels as healing progresses. It should, however, be noted that synthesis of lean body mass may require extra vitamin and mineral supplementation.

Water and nutrient losses

Nitrogen

Losses occur via:

- *Urine*: Increased urinary urea is the principal route of nitrogen loss. Trace element and electrolyte losses may also be elevated.
- *Exudate*: Fluid loss from a burn wound may be considerable and can contain 4–6 g protein/100 ml, representing 25–50% of total nitrogen loss (Molnar *et al.* 1983). Exudate losses vary between patients and from day to day, and cannot be measured routinely in burn units so have to be estimated. In a review of the literature, Davies (1977) suggested nitrogen losses to be 0.2 g N/% BSA burn daily for the first week post-burn. Subsequently, the losses decrease as healing progresses. The exudate nitrogen loss from partial-thickness burns rapidly decreases to 0.1 g N/% BSA burn daily. When the burns are extensive and of full thickness, so that virtually no healing occurs, the exudate losses continue at 0.2 g N/% BSA burn daily until the eschar (burned layer of skin) separates to reveal granulating tissue.
- *Faecal*: Nitrogen losses via faeces are 1–3 g N/day (Davies

Table 5.10 Burn injuries

	Severity of burn injury			
	Superficial	Partial thickness		Full thickness
Depth of burn	Epidermis only	Some of dermis		All of dermis
Healing time	3–10 days	10–14 days		Many months or never
Scarring	No	Deep burns likely to produce scarring and contractures		Contractures unless grafted
Skin grafting	No	Deep burns may need grafting		Large areas need grafting

Pressure or infection may convert a partial-thickness burn into a full-thickness burn.

1977) and relatively small compared with urine and exudate losses. Losses will increase if the patient has diarrhoea.

Fluid

In addition to fluid losses via urine, exudate and faeces (see above), considerable amounts may be lost via evaporation. Burn patients lack the water-impermeable barrier of the skin over large areas of their body. Evaporation losses are therefore high, despite attempts to reduce energy losses as heat by nursing in a warm, dry environment. Wilmore and McDougal (1977) estimate the evaporative water loss using the formula:

$$(25 + \% \text{ burn}) \times \text{body surface area in m}^2 = \text{ml water lost/hour.}$$

This formula is in agreement with the finding of Micheels and Sorenson (1983) that a healthy non-burned volunteer on a Clinitron (air-fluidized) bed lost 63.5 ml/m^2 per hour. With burn injury the loss may be increased to 3 litres/day.

Electrolytes

Large losses of electrolytes can occur via exudate, urine and as a result of pyrexia, diarrhoea and/or vomiting. Additional oral or parenteral supplementation may be required and should be based on biochemical parameters.

Vitamins and minerals

With loss of skin, increased muscle breakdown and increased fluid throughput, vitamin and mineral losses are likely to exceed dietary reference values for non-stressed individuals. However, there are no firm recommendations for replacement in burn patients (Molnar *et al.* 1983). The following should be borne in mind:

- Vitamin C has a known role in collagen synthesis. Recommendations suggest total daily intakes of 300–1000 mg/day.
- Requirements for B group vitamins increase proportionately to energy requirements because of their roles in oxidative pathways.
- Vitamin A deficiency may play a role in causing stress

ulcers due to thinning of the gut epithelium (Molnar *et al.* 1983; Gottschlich 1989).

- Iron supplements are often given in an attempt to increase haemoglobin levels.
- Trace elements are vital cofactors in enzyme systems, immune function and wound healing, and as antioxidants (Table 5.11). About 5–10% of body zinc and 20–40% of body copper may be lost via burn exudate in the first week post-injury. Losses via urine, eschar, diarrhoea and vomiting also occur and reduced intake further adds to the risk of deficiency.

The Burns Interest Group of the BDA (1999) recommends giving no more than twice the dietary reference value (DRV) of the remaining vitamins and minerals to avoid any potential problems with overdose. Most enteral feeds suitable for major burns provide approximately this level in 2 litres of feed and often contain more than twice the DRV of the nutrients listed above. The Burns Interest Group considers that, with the possible exceptions of vitamin C and trace elements, additional supplementation is unnecessary and may result in competition for absorption, e.g. between copper and zinc. Where micronutrient supplementation is required, administration of preparations at different times can help to reduce this effect.

Additional contributions to vitamin and mineral intake from diet, sip and supplementary tube feeds should not be overlooked.

Estimating nutritional requirements

Many formulae have been devised to assess the amount of energy and protein required to prevent weight loss in burns (Davies 1977). None takes into account all of the factors that affect requirements, i.e. weight, gender, height, BSA burn, burn depth, donor sites, respiratory involvement, activity level, infection and other injuries. Estimations of requirements must be regarded only as a starting point for nutritional support and must be tailored for each individual patient through regular monitoring (see Section 1.10, Estimating nutritional requirements).

However, even with extensive burns it is rare for a

Table 5.11 Trace elements: roles in enzyme systems (From Burns Interest Group of the British Dietetic Association 1999)

Element	Normal serum level	Metalloenzyme	Clinical symptoms of deficiency
Copper	0.7–1.7 µg/l 13–22 µmol/l	Lysyloxidase L-Amino levulinate Cytochrome oxidase Ceruloplasmin	Hypochromic anaemia Neutropenia
Selenium	0.8–1.6 µmol/l 70–139 ng/ml	Glutathione peroxidase	Cardiomyopathy
Zinc	0.15–0.23 mmol/l	Carbonic anhydrase Alkaline phosphatase Collagenases – various Poor wound healing	Skin rash Diarrhoea Taste impairment
Magnesium	0.7–0.96 mmol/l	ATPases DNA replication RNA synthesis Enzymes active in anaerobic glycolysis	Muscle weakness Ataxia Depression

patient's REE to exceed twice basal metabolic rate (BMR) as this seems to be the limit set by the cardiovascular and respiratory systems (Wilmore 1976). The energy needs of burns patients have reduced during the 1990s as a result of advances in overall burn care, including early excision and grafting, occlusive dressings, nursing in a thermoneutral environment, improved analgesia and antibiotic regimens. As a result, some predictive formulae for burns patients (e.g. the Sutherland formula 1987) have become invalid as they tend to overestimate energy and nitrogen needs.

For adults, the Burns Interest Group of the BDA recommends using Schofield (1985) to predict BMR and Elia (1990) to account for activity and burn depth. For example, for a 70 kg male, with 30% BSA burn, aged 25 years:

BMR (18–30 years) = 15 × 70 kg + 690 = 1740 kcal
Adjust BMR for 'stress' + 30%
Adjust for being 'bed bound but mobile' + 15%
Total = 1740 + 45% = 2523 kcal

Actual measurements of energy expenditure (by indirect calorimetry) usually reveal a lower total than that derived from predictive formulae.

Nasoenteric feeding of burn patients

The general lack of randomized controlled trials of the treatment of burns patients means that clinical practice in this area is not always evidence based, and uncertainties include the optimal method of enteral feeding in these patients (Childs 1998). The following points should be considered when selecting a feed for hypercatabolic burns patients.

Protein

Burn-injured patients use protein to provide around 20% of their energy requirements, so a suitable feed must meet this by having an energy:nitrogen ratio of 100–120:1 for shock burn cases, and 120–150:1 in non-shock cases (Matsuda *et al.* 1983).

Whole protein formulae are more advantageous than either parenteral or enteral amino acid based or peptide-based feeds, as well as being considerably cheaper (Alexander and Gottschlich 1990). There is no place for the routine use of elemental feeds in burn therapy (Wilmore and McDougal 1977).

There is currently much interest in 'pharmaconutrients' and the theory that the addition of certain amino acids to whole protein feeds may improve the response to nutrition. For example, glutamine has been suggested to enhance the immune system (Newsholme and Parry-Billings 1990), maintain gut mucosal integrity (Souba *et al.* 1990) and improve nitrogen balance (Furst 1990). Arginine is also of interest and is thought to enhance the immune system (Kirk and Barbul 1990). However, their application to human patients, in particular those with burns, remains to be established (see Section 5.2, Intensive care).

Lipid

The lipid component of feeds is often supplied by either corn or sunflower oil, both of which are high in linoleic acid, an omega-6 (*n*6) essential fatty acid. There are some indications that *n*3 fatty acids such as eicosapentaenoic acid found in fish oil may be capable of reducing the hypermetabolic response and boosting immunocompetence, in contrast to *n*6 fatty acids which may be immunosuppressive (Alexander *et al.* 1986; Gottschlich *et al.* 1989). Low fat feeds have been reported to reduce infectious morbidity in burns patients compared with higher fat formulations (Garrel *et al.* 1995).

It has been suggested that feeds containing a greater proportion of medium-chain triglycerides (MCT) may confer the advantage of preferential usage in stress-adapted metabolism (Cerra *et al.* 1980), having carnitine-independent entry into the mitochondria. Artificially structured lipids of MCT/fish oil may also reduce the metabolic response to burns compared with conventional lipid (Teo *et al.* 1989), as do MCT/long-chain triglyceride structured lipids (DeMichele *et al.* 1989), and future burn feed formulations may include such developments. However, caution should be applied in view of the potential adverse effects of increased lipid peroxide generation in critically ill patients given *n*3 fatty acids (O'Leary and Coakley 1996).

Carbohydrate

Carbohydrate is an important fuel for aerobic glycolysis, resulting in protein sparing through inhibition of gluconeogenesis. A feed providing a lipid–carbohydrate mixture has been suggested to have a better protein-sparing effect than glucose alone (Jeejeebhoy 1981) because there is a limit to the amount of glucose that can be used before hyperglycaemia or respiratory problems develop.

Other considerations

Enteral tube feeds should ideally be administered by pump infusion, using undiluted formula to permit the maximum infusion volume to be reached rapidly. Diluting the feed does not reduce the incidence of nausea and diarrhoea but does reduce nutrient intake at a vital time; it also increases the risk of microbial contamination.

Enteral tube feeding should continue until only small areas are left to heal or a patient is able to maintain an adequate oral intake. Overnight tube feeding is often useful in the transition period. If problems such as extensive weight loss, slowly healing wounds or graft rejection occur, enteral feeding should continue.

Constipation may occur as a result of side-effects of analgesia or lack of dietary fibre in the enteral feed formula. Long-term enteral feeding with no oral or enteral intake of dietary fibre can lead to diarrhoea, constipation or faecal impaction with 'overflow' diarrhoea. Many commercially available feeds now contain soluble and/or insoluble fibre and may help to alleviate these problems.

Table 5.12 Minimum to maximum glucose oxidation rates for a 70 kg male

Rate of glucose oxidation (mg/kg per minute per day)	Minimum amount of glucose (mg) that can be metabolized in 24 hours [rate x body weight (kg) $\times$ 60 minutes $\times$ 24 hours)
4–7	Worked example using the above equation: $4 \times 70 \times 60 \times 24 = 403\ 200$ mg $= 403$ g carbohydrate ($\times$ 4 to convert to kcal) $= 1612$ kcal from carbohydrate/24 hours

Note: Always use lower value as a starting point for glucose administration.

Parenteral feeding of burns patients

Parenteral nutrition is undesirable in burned patients because of the risk of septicaemia, and because gaining suitable venous access can be problematic owing to the burn distribution and peripheral shutdown. Delayed gastric emptying and large aspirates, particularly in the ventilated patient, are the usual reasons for failing to establish nasogastric feeding. These can be overcome by placement of a nasojejunal tube, ideally one with a double lumen which will permit simultaneously gastric decompression and feeding. In the case of prolonged paralytic ileus, there may be no choice other than to feed parenterally.

The same nutritional principles should apply to parental nutrition as to enteral feeding. Lipid-free regimens should be discouraged as the burns patient cannot oxidize glucose at as great a rate as healthy individuals. If glucose intake exceeds the maximal oxidation rate (Table 5.12), fat is synthesized. This is an energy-consuming process and large volumes of CO_2 are produced, raising the respiratory quotient, which may be dangerous to patients with pulmonary insufficiency. Overfeeding is known to increase metabolic rates in both normal and hypermetabolic humans. It has been suggested that the extremely high energy intakes of 8000–10 000 kcal (33–42 MJ)/day given to burns patients in the past may have contributed in part to the high measured metabolic rates (Molnar *et al.* 1983).

Vitamin and mineral preparations in parenteral solutions often provide basal requirements only for healthy adults, not for catabolic patients. Doses should be adjusted and monitored closely.

Monitoring progress

Morath *et al.* (1983) reviewed the problems of monitoring nutritional therapy in burns patients and concluded that no single parameter indicates short-term nutritional status but that regular repeated measurements can indicate trends (Table 5.13). Important aspects to monitor are as follows.

Body weight

Ideally, patients should be weighed immediately on admission without dressings, as the burn oedema which develops during the resuscitation period increases body weight by at least 10%. 'Dry weight' occurs some 14 days post-burn, so weight measured before 14 days is distorted by oedema. Thereafter, accurate repeated measurements of body weight help to assess nutritional therapy. Exudate-soaked dressings invalidate daily weighing: to obtain a more accurate reading the patient is weighed in dressings, the discarded dressings are then collected in a plastic bag and weighed, and the difference between the two provides an accurate body weight.

Food intake and fluid balance charts

Food and drinks consumed should be recorded by nursing staff, patients and/or relatives. Total intake can be calculated from oral, enteral and parenteral records and compared with predicted requirements. Fluid balance charts should be monitored to ensure that patients receive the prescribed volume of feed. Administered blood products are not usually included in nutrient totals.

Serum proteins

Serum albumin decreases very quickly post-burn and is slow to reflect improvement in nutritional status owing to its long half-life (20 days). It is also affected by infusions of blood and blood products, sepsis, surgery and other factors. C-reactive protein (CRP) is an acute-phase protein with a short half-life which can be used to help to interpret albumin levels. Hypoalbuminaemia with normal or low CRP indicates malnutrition; a low albumin with raised CRP levels indicates the acute-phase response (see Section 5.2, Intensive care).

Urinary urea

Urinary urea is the yardstick used to estimate stress. Twenty-four hour urinary urea nitrogen indicates internal

Table 5.13 Postburn nutritional monitoring

Parameter	Frequency
24 hour urine collection	Daily during first week
Maximum body temperature	Daily
Nutrient record (food and fluid balance)	Daily
Body weight	When dressings are changed
Serum urea and electrolytes	Daily during first week, then twice weekly
Blood glucose	4 hourly during the first 24 hours; thereafter as indicated
C-reactive protein	Twice weekly
Liver function tests	Twice weekly
Calcium and phosphate	Twice weekly
Haemoglobin and white cell count	Twice weekly
Trace elements	Weekly

nitrogen metabolism (Lee and Hartley 1975). However, nitrogen output depends on both nitrogen intake and nitrogen retention, and the latter is influenced by the magnitude of catabolic stress. The catabolic index (Bistrian 1979) indicates the magnitude of this stress.

> Catabolic index = urinary urea nitrogen − (0.5 × dietary nitrogen + 3 g)
> <0 indicates no stress
> 0–5 indicates moderate stress
> >5 indicates severe stress.

This assumes that 50% of ingested protein is catabolized via gluconeogenesis. The constant (3 g) added for non-urea nitrogen loss will almost always underestimate true losses in burns due to exudate; nonetheless, the catabolic index usefully indicates the change from stressed to non-stressed status.

It should also be noted that this assumes normal renal function and a complete 24 hour collection of urine.

Daily maximum body temperature

Body temperature is easily measured and available on all burns units. It helps to indicate the extent of hypermetabolism at any given time secondary to sepsis. Persistent pyrexia will necessitate recalculation of requirements for energy, nitrogen, fluid and electrolytes.

Clinical condition

This should be reassessed daily to take into account the effects of activity, graft take, ventilation, etc., which are likely to influence the patient's metabolic requirements.

Body surface area burn

This should be reassessed by experienced nursing/medical staff at each dressing change to permit re-estimation of nutritional requirements. Grafted areas should not be regarded as healed for the first month, and donor sites will contribute to the area left to heal.

5.5.4 Electrical burns

Care must be taken with the nutrition of patients with high-voltage electrical injury. In addition to surface burn injury (entry and exit points), conduction through the body causes destruction of the underlying nerves, blood vessels, muscles, bones, tendons and visceral coverings. The more resistant the tissue, the more heat is generated as current flows through it (Diamond et al. 1982); thus, muscle close to bone may be necrosed. A high urinary urea output in these patients indicates that severe damage has occurred (Balogh and Bauer 1982). Burns feeding formulae based on percentage burn will underestimate the amount of nutrients required by these patients.

5.5.5 Burn injury in children

All children are at nutritional risk on admission as, in addition to the burn injury, normal growth and development need to be maintained.

Children have a higher BMR than adults and a greater requirement for protein per kilogram of body weight. Burn injury does not raise REE proportionally as much in children as in adults, and when normally active children are confined to bed by burn injury, this saving in energy output partially offsets the increase in REE (Goran et al. 1990; Childs 1994, 1995). Weight maintenance can normally be achieved by providing the estimated average requirement (EAR) for a non-burned child. For example:

> 2-year-old female, 30% scald, 12.5 kg (50th percentile)
> EAR for energy = (95 kcal × 12.5) = 1180 kcal.

Protein requirements are less well established. The Burns Interest Group of the BDA is presently addressing this problem and currently advises giving 1.5–2.0 times the reference nutrient intake (RNI) for protein. For example:

> RNI for protein = (1.1 × 12.5) × 2 = 27.5 g.

The Sutherland formula (1987) for children is no longer used as it overestimates requirements.

Enteral feeding of children aged 1–6 years with large burns can be successfully carried out using commercially available tube feeds which are modified in micronutrient and macronutrient composition to meet the developmental needs of this age group. For children under 1 year old, it is suggested that they are maintained on their usual infant formula.

Enteral feeding should be considered for all burns >10% BSA but can often be avoided in smaller burns provided the child will drink juice or milk-based supplements. Milk can be fortified with dried milk powder (30 g added to 500 ml) to boost protein intake in burned children.

Text revised by: Carole Glencorse and the British Dietetic Association's Burns Interest Group

Useful address

The Burns Interest Group of the British Dietetic Association
c/o British Dietetic Association, 5th Floor, Elizabeth House, 22 Suffolk Street, Queensway, Birmingham B1 1LS
Tel: 0121 616 4900
Website: www.bda.uk.com

References

Alexander JW, Gottschlich MM Nutritional immunomodulation in burn patients. *Critical Care Medicine* 1990; **18**: S149–S153.

Alexander JW, Saito H, Ogle CK, Trocki O. The importance of lipid type in the diet after burn injury. *Annals of Surgery* 1986; **204**: 1–8.

Balogh D, Bauer M. Determination of catabolism in the burns patient. *Chirurgia Plastica* 1982; **7**: 67–74.

Bistrian BR. A simple technique to estimate the severity of stress. *Surgery, Gynaecology and Obstetrics* 1979; **148**: 675–678.

Burns Interest Group of the British Dietetic Association. *Feeding Guidelines for Adult Burned Patients*, 2nd edn. Birmingham: BDA, 1999.

Cerra FB, Siegel JH, Coleman B *et al*. Septic autocannibalism. A failure to provide exogenous nutritional support. *Annals of Surgery* 1980; **192**: 570–579.

Childs C. Studies in children provide a model to re-examine the metabolic response to burn injury in patients treated by contemporary burn protocols. *Burns* 1994; **20**: 291–300.

Childs C. Feeding the burned patient. Energy requirements, timing and effects of dietary intake. *British Journal of Intensive Care* 1995; 157–164.

Childs C. Is there an evidence-based practice for burns? *Burns* 1998; **24**: 29–33.

Davenport PJ. Nutritional support in severe burns. *Res Clin Forums* 1979; **1**: 79–82.

Davies JWL. The nutrition of patients with burns. In Richards JR, Kinney JM (Eds) *Nutritional Aspects of Care of the Critically Ill*, pp. 595–623. Edinburgh: Churchill Livingstone, 1977.

DeMichele SJ, Karlstaad MD, Bistrian BR *et al*. Enteral nutrition with structured lipids: effect on protein metabolism in thermal injury. *American Journal of Clinical Nutrition* 1989; **50**: 1295–1302.

Diamond TH, Twomey A, Myburgh DF. High voltage electrical injury. *South African Medical Journal* 1982; **27**: 318–321.

Dobb GJ. The role of the gut in critical illness. *Current Anaesthesia and Critical Care* 1996; **7**: 62–68.

Elia M. Artificial nutritional support. *Medicine International* 1990; **82**: 3392–3396.

Epstein MD, Banducci DR, Manders EK. The role of the gastrointestinal tract in the development of burn sepsis. *Plastic and Reconstructive Surgery* 1992; **90**: 524–531.

Furst P. Peptides in clinical nutrition. *Clinical Nutrition* 1990; **10** (Suppl): 19–24.

Garrel DR, Razi M, Lariviere F *et al*. Improved clinical status and length of care with low fat nutrition support in burn patients. *Journal of Parenteral and Enteral Nutrition* 1995; **19**: 482–491.

Goran MI, Peters EJ, Herndon DN *et al*. Total energy expenditure in burned children using the doubly labelled water technique. *American Journal of Physiology* 1990; **259**: E576–E585.

Gottschlich MM. Micronutrients. In Slipper A (Ed.) *Dietitian's Handbook of Enteral and Parenteral Nutrition*. New York: ASPEN Publishers Inc, 1989.

Gottschlich MM, Jenkins M, Warden GD *et al*. Differential effects of three enteral dietary regimens on selected outcome variables in burn patients. *Journal of Parenteral and Enteral Nutrition* 1989; **14**: 225–236.

Harvey Kemble JV, Lamb BE. *Plastic Surgical and Burns Nursing (Current Nursing Practice)*. Eastbourne: Bailliere Tindall, 1984.

Inoue S, Lukes S, Alexander JW *et al*. Increased gut blood flow with early enteral feeding in burned guinea-pigs. *Journal of Burn Care and Rehabilitation* 1989; **10**: 300–308.

Jeejeebhoy KN. Protein nutrition in clinical practice. *British Medical Bulletin* 1981; **37**: 11–17.

Kirk SJ, Barbul A. Role of arginine in trauma, sepsis and immunity. *Journal of Parenteral and Enteral Nutrition* 1990; **14**: 226S–229S.

La Hausse-Brown TP, Stephenson AJ, Glencorse C, Freedlander E. Nasojejunal feeding in burns patients. *Proceedings of the British Burn Association*, 9–11 April 1997.

Lee HA, Hartley TF. A method of determining daily nitrogen requirements. *Postgraduate Medical Journal* 1975; **51**: 441–445.

Matsuda T, Kagan RJ, Hanumadass M, Jonasson O. The importance of burn wound size in determining the optimal calorie:nitrogen ratio. *Surgery* 1983; **94**: 562–568.

Micheels J, Sorensen B. The physiology of a healthy normal person in the air-fluidised bed. *Burns* 1983; **9**: 158–168.

Mochizuki H, Trocki O, Dominoni L *et al*. Mechanism of prevention of postburn hypermetabolism and catabolism by early enteral feeding. *Annals of Surgery* 1984; **200**: 297–308.

Molnar JA, Wolfe RR, Burke JF. Burns: metabolism and nutritional therapy in thermal injury. In Schneider HA, Anderson CE, Cousin DB (Eds) *Nutritional Support of Medical Practice*, 2nd edn, pp. 260–281. Philadelphia, PA: Harper & Row, 1983.

Morath MA, Miller SF, Finley RK, Jones LM. Interpretation of nutritional parameters in burns patients. *Journal of Burn Care and Rehabilitation* 1983; **4**: 361–366.

Newsholme EA, Parry-Billings M. Properties of glutamine release from muscle and its importance for the immune system. *Journal of Parenteral and Enteral Nutrition* 1990; **14**: 63S–67S.

O'Leary MJ, Coakley JH. Nutrition and immunonutrition. *British Journal of Anaesthesia* 1996; **77**: 118–127.

Raff T, Hartmann B, Germann G. Early intragastric feeding seriously burned and long-term ventilated patients: a review of 55 patients. *Burns* 1997; **23**: 19–25.

Richards JR. Metabolic responses to injury and starvation. An overview. In Richards JR, Kinney JM (Eds) *Nutritional Aspects of Care in the Critically Ill*, pp. 273–302. Edinburgh: Churchill Livingstone, 1977.

Saito H, Trocki O, Alexander JW *et al*. The effect of route of nutrient administration on the nutritional state, catabolic hormone secretion, and gut mucosal integrity after burn injury. *Journal of Parenteral and Enteral Nutrition* 1986; **11**: 1–7.

Schofield WN. Predicting basal metabolic rate, new standards and review of previous work. *Human Nutrition: Clinical Nutrition* 1985; **39** (Suppl 1): 5–41.

Soroff HS, Pearson E, Artz CP. An estimation of the nitrogen requirements for equilibrium in burned patients. *Surgery, Gynaecology and Obstetrics* 1961; **112**: 159–172.

Souba WW, Klimberg VS, Plumley DA *et al*. The role of glutamine in maintaining a healthy gut and supporting the metabolic response to injury and infection. *Journal of Surgical Research* 1990; **48**: 383–391.

Sutherland AB. Nutrition of the burn patient. *Clinical Anaesthesiology* 1987; **1**: 663–671.

Teo TC, DeMichele SJ, Selleck KM *et al*. Administration of structural lipid composed of MCT and fish oil reduces net protein catabolism in enterally fed burned rats. *Annals of Surgery* 1989; **210**: 100–107.

Tobiason J, Hiebert JM, Edlich RF. A practical burn severity index. *Journal of Burn Care and Rehabilitation* 1982; **3**: 229–232.

Wilmore DW. Hormonal responses and their effect on metabolism. *Surgical Clinics of North America* 1976; **56**: 999–1018.

Wilmore DW, McDougal WS. Nutrition in burns. In Richards JR, Kinney JM (Eds) *Nutritional Aspects of Care in the Critically Ill*, pp. 583–594. Edinburgh: Churchill Livingstone, 1977.

Woolfson AMJ, Heatley RV, Allison SP. Significance of insulin in the metabolic response to injury. In Richards JR, Kinney JM (Eds) *Nutritional Aspects of Care in the Critically Ill*, pp. 367–388. Edinburgh: Churchill Livingstone, 1977.

5.6 Surgery

Undernutrition in hospitals is a widespread problem (see Section 1.11, Undernutrition) but is particularly prevalent among surgical patients, as is the failure to identify and correct it. Common themes include failure to recognize malnourished or underweight individuals on admission to hospital, random provision of nutrition support which fails to meet requirements or is discontinued before the patient can consume sufficient without it, and failure to record even the simplest of assessment parameters such as body weight on admission (Bruun *et al.* 1999).

5.6.1 Pre-operative undernutrition

Evidence demonstrates that about 40% of patients are malnourished on hospital admission, yet many do not have any nutrition information documented (Rasmussen *et al.* 1999). Mean weight loss at discharge is greatest in those most undernourished, yet can be reversed in those given appropriate nutrition support (McWhirter and Pennington 1994). Mean length of stay in moderately malnourished patients has been shown to be twice that of those considered well nourished on admission (Potter and Luxton 1999). The longer the duration of hospital stay, the greater the risk of weight loss.

Within the hospital setting, undernutrition often continues. The causes are multifactorial, but include:

- lack of familiarity with, or acceptability of, hospital foods
- inappropriate dietary restrictions (such as a low fat diet for acute cholecystitis)
- nil-by-mouth for tests that may be delayed or cancelled
- prolonged use of a 'free fluid' regimen without consideration of the use of nutritional supplements
- increased requirements for healing following major surgery.

Physical difficulty with eating, pain, nausea and diarrhoea will also affect a patient's ability to consume an adequate diet, whilst the increased levels of cytokines associated with stress prevent anabolism from taking place.

Many patients presenting for surgery may be malnourished as a consequence of underlying pathology (cancer-related cachexia, nausea or vomiting) or associated symptoms (such as malabsorption with small bowel affected Crohn's disease). Excessive nutrient losses and increased metabolic needs also influence nutritional status presentation.

Increasing age is an independent risk factor for adverse surgical outcomes. Age-related decrease in energy requirement due to a reduction in lean body mass compromises micronutrient intake. The SENECA Study on European elderly people found evidence of biochemical vitamin deficiency in 47% of people for vitamin D, 23.3% for vitamin B_6, 2.7% for vitamin B_{12} and 1.1% for vitamin E (Haller 1999).

Undernutrition and involuntary weight loss continue to be prevalent among hospitalized and long-term care patients, particularly those who are elderly, despite studies correlating poor nutritional status and low body weight with impaired wound healing. Chronic, non-healing wounds are particularly difficult to treat and contribute to significant morbidity, mortality and hospitalizations (Himes 1999).

Many patients admitted for surgery present with wasting and cachexia associated with severe physiological, psychological and immunological consequences, regardless of the underlying causes. Cachexia has been associated with infections, decubitus ulcers and increased mortality risk (Yeh and Schuster 1999). Drugs that promote appetite stimulation and weight gain, such as progestational agents, cyproheptadines, pentoxifylline and thalidomide, may work by down-regulating these proinflammatory cytokines

All patients will have a minimal requirement for energy and protein daily, which can be assessed from the prediction formulae described in Section 1.10 (Estimating nutritional requirements). For most, this will mean an intake of some 1600–2300 kcal/day, with 45–80 g protein to prevent endogenous catabolism and match nitrogen losses. Standard hydration therapy of 2 litres of dextrose-saline or 5% dextrose daily will provide a maximum of 375 kcal/day, i.e. less than 20% of estimated energy requirements. If 1 litre of normal saline replaces one of the dextrose bags, the energy provision falls to less than 200 kcal/day. The resultant weekly deficit of nearly 10 600 kcal would represent around 1.2 kg of adipose tissue or 10 kg of lean tissue.

5.6.2 Post-operative undernutrition

The energy requirements post-surgery will vary according to the degree of trauma and concurrent clinical factors. After minor surgical procedures, energy expenditure will hardly change, whereas major procedures with resultant sepsis and high-output stoma or drain losses will greatly increase energy and protein requirements.

Nutritional support via the gastrointestinal tract reduces septic morbidity in severely injured patients (Kudsk

1998), yet early enteral feeding post-surgery has failed to demonstrate a clinical advantage, despite a higher energy and protein intake in the enterally fed group (Heslin *et al.* 1997). In a study of patients with upper gastrointestinal cancer, immediate post-operative jejunal feeding was associated with impaired respiratory mechanics and post-operative mobility, and did not influence the loss of muscle strength or the increase in fatigue that occurred after major surgery. For this reason, immediate post-operative enteral feeding is unnecessary in well-nourished patients at low risk of nutrition-related complications (Watters *et al.* 1997).

The historic classification of malnourished surgical patients into four groups – depleted, hypercatabolic, hypercatabolic and depleted, or chronic malabsorption (Elwyn 1980) – is of limited use today, as earlier nutritional support and more aggressive management of pain control through medication reduce the predicted catabolic response to surgical injury.

5.6.3 Identification of at-risk patients

Routine pre-operative nutritional assessment and continued monitoring (at least weekly) should be undertaken on all surgical patients by nursing and dietetic staff and include the following observations (Goulet 1998):

- record of body weight: on admission and regular intervals. Involuntary weight loss over a 3-month period is of concern
- symptoms associated with nutritional implications: nausea, vomiting, diarrhoea, infection, fever, oedema or dehydration, decubitus ulcer or dysphagia
- biochemistry associated with undernutrition: hypoglycaemia, low serum urea or creatinine, low haemoglobin
- diet history: to include a brief account of any eating problems and loss of appetite
- need for supervised meal selection and assistance with eating if required
- observation of food and fluids consumed: keeping an accurate record of nutritional intake if requested.

These simple measures can help to identify at an early stage those patients in need of nutritional support.

Nutritional risk assessment is discussed in greater detail in Section 1.9.

5.6.4 The role of nutrition in surgical patients

The objectives of nutritional support in surgical patients are to:

- enhance wound healing
- reduce post-operative complications
- shorten the period of convalescence
- prevent or correct further deterioration in the nutritional state.

The value of pre-operative and peri-operative nutrition support

Some controversy exists regarding the benefit of pre-operative and post-operative nutritional support and its effect on morbidity and mortality. Protein-energy malnutrition in hospital patients is associated with impaired cell-mediated immunity (Beier-Holgersen and Brandstrup 1999) and prolonged post-operative recovery. It may also reduce pulmonary function and increase the risk of the surgical procedure.

Malnutrition has been recognized as a poor prognostic indicator for cancer treatment-related morbidity and mortality in general, affecting 30–50% of all patients with head and neck cancer. Apart from the well-known clinical prognostic parameters, pre-operative weight loss and major post-operative complications were predictive of higher early mortality in patients undergoing surgery for advanced head and neck cancer (van Bokhorst-de van der Schuer *et al.* 1999).

Pre-operative feeding

Pre-operative nutritional status has a significant impact on surgical outcome. In a prospective study of patients undergoing arthroplasty, low levels of serum albumin pre-operatively correlated with increased resource utilization, length of stay and operative time in patients undergoing joint-replacement surgery, independent of age and severity of presenting illness (Lavernia *et al.* 1999). Allowing a patient's nutritional state to deteriorate through the peri-operative period adversely affects measurable outcome related to nosocomial infection, multiple organ dysfunction, wound healing and functional recovery.

Combining chemotherapy and nutrition support pre-operatively for malnourished patients with gastrointestinal cancer improves short-term nutritional status without increasing the proliferation of tumour cells and prevents the post-operative complications that occur when such patients are given chemotherapy without nutrition support. The results also suggest, but do not prove, that parenteral nutrition may increase the effectiveness of chemotherapy in malnourished patients (Jin *et al.* 1999).

Peri-operative feeding

Peri-operative nutritional support significantly reduces the incidence of wound infections (Williams *et al.* 1977) and improves the rate of wound healing (Moghissi *et al.* 1977). It also improves both surgical outcome in malnourished patients (Torosian 1999), and long-term morbidity and mortality risks (McClave *et al.* 1999). Enteral rather than parenteral is the preferred route of artificial nutrition support (Duerksen *et al.* 1998).

Post-operative feeding

An early post-operative jejunostomy feeding protocol commenced within 12 hours post-surgery for patients undergoing bowel resection resulted in significant cost savings per success in the fed group (Hedberg *et al.* 1999), and is associated with earlier discharge (Barb *et al.* 1999).

Controversial areas of feeding

Early post-surgery

Immediate post-operative enteral feeding in patients undergoing intestinal resection appears to be safe, prevents an increase in gut mucosal permeability and produces a positive nitrogen balance (Carr *et al.* 1996). Early enteral feeding may help to prevent stress haemorrhage in the upper gastrointestinal tract secondary to burn injury (Raff *et al.* 1997) and is a suitable alternative to parenteral nutrition after major pancreatic and gastric surgery (Braga *et al.* 1998).

Pancreatitis

Clinical conditions such as pancreatitis have increasing evidence to support the role of jejunal feeding in maintaining nutritional status (Wyncoll 1999).

Aggressive replacement of fluid losses to correct the circulating volume, correction of electrolyte and glucose abnormalities, and respiratory, cardiovascular and renal support should be given as necessary. Patients with pancreatic infections, necrosis or deteriorating organ failure require surgery. Patients with sterile necrosis should receive a broad-spectrum prophylactic antibiotic to penetrate pancreatic tissue. Due attention should also be paid to nutritional support, for which a jejunal feeding tube with enteral nutrition is recommended as early as is achievable.

Intestinal fistulae

The high mortality (35%) of enterocutaneous fistulae is attributed to malnutrition, electrolyte imbalances and sepsis, especially in high-output fistulae. Parenteral nutrition may substantially improve the prognosis of such patients by increasing the rate of spontaneous closure and improving the nutritional status of patients requiring repeat operations. Enteral feeding with predigested formula may also be successful if a somatostatin analogue (octreotide) is given to reduce gastrointestinal secretions. Moreover, other studies have shown that nutritional support decreases or modifies the composition of the gastrointestinal secretions and is thus considered to play a primary therapeutic role in the management of fistula patients (Dudrick *et al.* 1999).

Risk of anastamotic breakdown

In a study of almost 3000 patients undergoing surgery from the oesophagus to the colon, the risk of anastamotic dehiscence was approximately 2% and its development could not be predicted from standard risk stratifiers (Pickleman *et al.* 1999). Continuous enteral nutrition may enhance gastrointestinal integrity and reduce the risk of wound dehiscence (Frileux *et al.* 1999).

Presence of chylothorax

Surgery to the chest may result in damage to the thoracic duct, and subsequent chylothorax. An oral or enteral very low fat diet can be used for conservative management, in preference to parenteral nutrition (see Section 5.7, Chyle leakage).

Presence of obesity

Gross obesity is associated with increased anaesthetic and surgical risks in elective surgery. The patient should be advised to reduce weight sensibly whilst on the waiting list for admission, rather than by short-term crash dieting.

Obesity can mask underlying malnutrition and is not a reason for withholding nutritional support in surgical patients if post-operative complications arise, or if anthropometric and biochemical nutritional indices demonstrate nutritional inadequacies or malnutrition. The obesity should be treated at a later stage when the patient has fully recovered.

Introduction of post-operative oral fluids and diet

After a general anaesthetic, gastric motility is reduced and gastric emptying delayed. It is common practice, but without clinical evidence to support it, to withhold oral fluids and food until bowel sounds are heard. Bowel sounds reflect the movement of gas along the digestive tract, but in the prolonged absence of food and decompression of the bowel at surgery, bowel sounds are likely to be absent. The patient should be encouraged to take initial fluids as instinct dictates, as research suggests that patients can best assess their own gastric tolerance. Delayed reintroduction of oral intake may necessitate intravenous fluids of saline and/or dextrose-saline, which maintain hydration but not nutritional needs (2 litres of 5% dextrose provides a mere 400 kcal; see above). Enteral feeding should be considered at an early stage if oral intake is slow to become established.

Immunonutrients such as arginine, glutamine, nucleotides and omega-3 fatty acids reduce septic complications in trauma patients post-surgery compared with those fed an isonitrogenous, isocaloric standard enteral feed, with unfed patients having the highest complication rate (Kudsk *et al.* 1996), and may be beneficial in conditions associated with high cytokine production such as pancreatitis (Barber *et al.* 1999; von Meyenfeldt 1999). Meta-analysis of immune-enhancing enteral feeds demonstrated a significant reduction in the risk of infectious complications, and reduced overall hospital stay in critically ill patients and those with gastrointestinal cancer, with little influence on mortality (Heys *et al.* 1999).

In a study of head and neck cancer patients undergoing surgery, peri-operative nutritional supplementation with an immunomodulatory feed significantly reduced the incidence of infectious complications. The length of hospitalization was significantly prolonged in patients with post-operative infections, suggesting potential cost savings with the use of immune-enhancing formulae (Snyderman *et al.* 1999). Conversely, parenteral nutrition containing fat emulsion administered during the early post-injury period increased susceptibility to infection, prolonged pulmonary failure and delayed recovery in critically injured patients (Battistella *et al.* 1997).

Factors complicating nutritional monitoring

Regular monitoring of the patient's fluid intake and output, body weight, haematology, and serum and urinary biochemistry should be carried out throughout the hospital stay. It is common for deranged biochemistry in surgical patients not to be corrected as quickly as on the medical wards. The dietitian should ensure that appropriate treatment and intervention are obtained for patients with hyperglycaemia, disordered electrolyte levels or post-surgical acute renal failure (see Sections 1.10, Estimating nutritional requirements, and 5.2, Intensive care).

Common plasma proteins levels are altered in the presence of the acute-phase response to injury or infection. Serum albumin is not a marker of nutritional status (Klein 1990), but can predict an increased likelihood of post-operative organ dysfunction, nosocomial infections, prolonged mechanical ventilation and mortality risk (Rady *et al.* 1997). In many patients, the most important part of the assessment continues to be the clinical and dietary history, together with a careful physical examination (Shenkin 1997).

Nitrogen balance can be used as a crude marker of protein turnover. Direct measurement of *total* urinary nitrogen is preferred, although nitrogen excretion often is derived from 24 hour urinary *urea* measurement, which is simpler but less accurate. Measurement of serum biochemistry for minerals and trace elements is often distorted during the acute-phase response, is expensive and often requires external laboratory analysis, contributing to a time delay. The most widely used measures of nutritional state are nitrogen balance and secretory protein concentrations, and these indices improve when sick patients recover (Manning and Shenkin 1995).

Most patients are discharged home before their natural appetite fully returns, and dietetic advice and supervision should continue in the community and at follow-up clinics whenever possible.

Text revised by: Catherine Collins

References

Barb MD, Kasper K, Sutton GP. Early postoperative feeding following major abdominal gynecologic surgery reduced the length of hospitalisation. *Gynecologic Oncology* 1999; **74**: 152.

Barber MD, Ross JA, Preston T *et al.* Fish oil-enriched nutritional supplement attenuates progression of the acute-phase response in weight-losing patients with advanced pancreatic cancer. *Journal of Nutrition* 1999; **129**: 1120–1125.

Battistella FD, Widergren JT, Anderson *et al.* A prospective, randomized trial of intravenous fat emulsion administration in trauma victims requiring total parenteral nutrition. *Journal of Trauma* 1997; **43**: 52–58.

Beier-Holgersen R, Brandstrup B. Influence of early postoperative enteral nutrition versus placebo on cell-mediated immunity, as measured with the Multitest CMI. Scandinavian *Journal of Gastroenterology* 1999; **34**: 98–102.

Braga M, Gianotti L, Vignali A *et al.* Artificial nutrition after major abdominal surgery: impact of route of administration and composition of the diet. *Critical Care Medicine* 1998; **26**: 24–30.

Bruun LI, Bosaeus I, Bergstad I, Nygaard K. Prevalence of malnutrition in surgical patients: evaluation of nutritional support and documentation. *Clinical Nutrition* 1999; **18**: 141–147.

Carr CS, Ling KD *et al.* Randomised trial of safety and efficacy of immediate postoperative enteral feeding in patients undergoing gastrointestinal resection. *British Medical Journal* 1996; **312**: 869–871.

Dudrick SJ, Maharaj AR, McKelvey AA. Artificial nutritional support in patients with gastrointestinal fistulas. *World Journal of Surgery* 1999; **23**: 570–576.

Duerksen DR, Nehra V, Bistrian BR, Blackburn GL. Appropriate nutritional support in acute and complicated Crohn's disease. *Nutrition* 1998; **14**: 462–465.

Elwyn DH. Nutritional requirements of adult surgical patients. *Critical Care Medicine* 1980; **8**: 9–20.

Frileux P, Attal E, Sarkis R, Parc R. Anastomic dehiscence and severe peritonitis. *Infection* 1999; **27**: 67–70.

Goulet O. Assessment of nutritional status in clinical practice. *Baillieres Clinical Gastroenterology* 1998; **12**: 647–669.

Haller J. The vitamin status and its adequacy in the elderly: an international overview. *International Journal for Vitamin and Nutrition Research* 1999; **69**: 160–168.

Hedberg AM, Lairson DR, Aday LA *et al.* Economic implications of an early postoperative enteral feeding protocol. *Journal of the American Dietetic Association* 1999; **99**: 802–807.

Heslin MJ, Latkany L, Leung D *et al.* A prospective, randomized trial of early enteral feeding after resection of upper gastrointestinal malignancy. *Annals of Surgery* 1997; **226**: 567–577.

Heys SD, Walker LG, Smith I, Eremin O. Enteral nutritional supplementation with key nutrients in patients with critical illness and cancer: a meta-analysis of randomized controlled clinical trials. *Annals of Surgery* 1999; **229**: 467–477.

Himes D. Protein-calorie malnutrition and involuntary weight loss: the role of aggressive nutritional intervention in wound healing. *Ostomy Wound Management* 1999; **45**: 46–51, 54–55.

Jin D, Phillips M, Byles JE. Effects of parenteral nutrition support and chemotherapy on the phasic composition of tumor cells in gastrointestinal cancer. *Journal of Parenteral and Enteral Nutrition* 1999; **23**: 237–241.

Klein S. The myth of serum albumin as a measure of nutritional status. *Gastroenterology* 1990; **99**: 1845–1846.

Kudsk KA. Early enteral nutrition in surgical patients (Abstract). *Nutrition* 1998; **14**: 541–544.

Kudsk KA, Minard G, Croce MA *et al.* A randomized trial of isonitrogenous enteral diets after severe trauma. An immune-enhancing diet reduces septic complications. *Annals of Surgery* 1996; **224**: 531–540.

Lavernia CJ, Sierra RJ, Baerga L. Nutritional parameters and short term outcome in arthroplasty. *Journal of the American College of Nutrition* 1999; **18**: 274–278.

McClave SA, Snider HL, Spain DA. Preoperative issues in clinical nutrition. *Chest* 1999; **115**: 64S–70S.

McWhirter JP, Pennington CR. Incidence and recognition of malnutrition in hospital. *British Medical Journal* 1994; **308**: 945–948.

Manning EM, Shenkin A. Nutritional assessment in the critically ill. *Critical Care Medicine* 1995; **11**: 603–634.

Moghissi K, Hornshaw J, Teasdale PR, Dawes EA. Parenteral nutrition in carcinoma of the oesophagus treated by surgery: nitrogen balance and clinical studies. *British Journal of Surgery* 1977; **64**: 125–128.

Pickleman J, Watson W, Cunningham J *et al.* The failed gastrointestinal anastomosis: an inevitable catastrophe? *Journal of the American College of Surgery* 1999; **188**: 473–482.

Potter MA, Luxton G. Prealbumin measurement as a screening tool for protein calorie malnutrition in emergency hospital admissions: a pilot study. *Clinical and Investigational Medicine* 1999; **22**: 44–52.

Rady MY, Ryan T, Starr NJ. Clinical characteristics of preoperative hypoalbuminemia predict outcome of cardiovascular surgery. *Journal of Parenteral and Enteral Nutrition* 1997; **21**: 81–90.

Raff T, Germann G, Hartmann B. The value of early enteral nutrition in the prophylaxis of stress ulceration in the severely burned patient. *Burns* 1997; **23**: 313–318.

Rasmussen HH, Kondrup J, Ladefoged K, Staun M. Clinical nutrition in Danish hospitals: a questionnaire-based investigation among doctors and nurses. *Clinical Nutrition* 1999; **18**: 153–158.

Shenkin A. Impact of disease on markers of macronutrient status. *Proceedings of the Nutrition Society* 1997; **56** (1B): 433–441.

Snyderman CH, Kachman K, Molseed L *et al.* Reduced postoperative infections with an immune-enhancing nutritional supplement. *Laryngoscope* 1999; **109**: 915–921.

Torosian MH. Perioperative nutrition support for patients undergoing gastrointestinal surgery: critical analysis and recommendations. *World Journal of Surgery* 1999; **23**: 565–569.

van Bokhorst-de van der Schuer, van Leeuwen PA, Kuik DJ *et al.* The impact of nutritional status on the prognoses of patients with advanced head and neck cancer. *Cancer* 1999; **86**: 519–527.

von Meyenfeldt MF. Nutritional support during treatment of biliopancreatic malignancy. *Annals of Oncology* 1999; **4** (10 Suppl): 273–277.

Watters JM, Kirkpatrick SM, Norris SB *et al.* Immediate postoperative enteral feeding results in impaired respiratory mechanics and decreased mobility. *Annals of Surgery* 1997; **226**: 369–377.

Williams RHP, Heatley RV, Lewis MH, Hughes LE. In Baxter DH, Jackson GM (Eds) *Clinical Parenteral Nutrition*, p. 52. Chester: Geistlich Education, 1977.

Wyncoll DL. The management of severe acute necrotising pancreatitis: an evidence-based review of the literature. *International Care Medicine* 1999; **25**: 146–156.

Yeh SS, Schuster MW. Geriatric cachexia: the role of cytokines. *American Journal of Clinical Nutrition* 1999; **70**: 183–197.

5.7 Chyle leakage

Chyle leakage is variously described in the literature as chylothorax, chylous fistula, chylous ascites and chyloretroperitoneum; the nomenclature relates to the area of the body into which the chyle is draining.

Untreated chyle leakage rapidly leads to hypovolaemia, hyponatraemia, hypochloraemia and lymphopenia, and may result in significant morbidity and contribute to mortality.

5.7.1 Background

In order to understand the implications and management of chyle leakage, it is necessary to be familiar with the physiology and terminology of fat digestion.

Fat digestion

Chylomicrons produced from fat digestion pass from intestinal epithelial cells into interstitial fluid and are then absorbed by the lacteals (lymph-system capillaries which extend into the villi of the small intestine). However, medium-chain triglycerides (MCT) pass into the gut mucosal cells and then directly into the systemic circulation. Most other products of digestion are likewise absorbed directly into the bloodstream from the gut and pass via the hepatic portal vein to the liver.

The lymphatic system

The lymphatic system functions as an accessory to the cardiovascular system. It returns interstitial fluid and protein to the blood, and transports fat from the gut back to the systemic circulation. Seventy-five per cent of lymph drains into the left subclavian vein via the thoracic duct (Fig. 5.5).

Chyle (the fat-rich lymph fluid) also contains quantities of protein (e.g. albumin), lymphocytes and antibodies, and has an electrolyte composition similar to that of plasma. Chyle flow is reduced by fasting and increased by administration of enteral fat. Oral fluids increase chyle flow, whereas intravenous fluids have no effect (Nguyen *et al.* 1995).

5.7.2 Aetiology

The cause of chyle leakage may be:

- iatrogenic (e.g. thoracic or head and neck surgery)
- traumatic (e.g. road traffic accident)
- obstructive (e.g. secondary to malignancy)
- congenital
- idiopathic (occasionally), e.g pregnancy (Zoran *et al.* 1997).

Pseudochylothorax may occur secondary to tuberculosis or rheumatoid arthritis (Garcia-Zamalloa *et al.* 1998). Despite its numerous potential causes it remains a rare condition.

5.7.3 Management options

Chyle production can be halted conservatively by dietary manipulation or inhaled nitric oxide therapy at 20 ppm (Berkenbosch and Withington 1999), or by surgical closure of the fistula.

Conservative management

Certain types of chyle leakage (chyloretroperitoneum and chylous ascites following abdominal surgery, and chylous fistula following radical neck dissection) appear to respond well to conservative management (Martin *et al.* 1993). In contrast, poor outcomes are associated with chyle leakage due to malignancy, such as lymphoma (Pabst *et al.* 1993). Mixed outcomes have been reported regarding chyle leakage caused by cardiothoracic surgery (Terzi *et al.* 1994).

Conservative management to minimize enteral fat intake and/or bypass the enteral feeding route reduces chyle flow, combined with a medical procedure such as drainage to encourage spontaneous healing of the fistula (Sauvanet *et al.* 1998). The literature lacks consensus about the indications for either option (Meurer and Cohen 1990).

Nutritional management
This may take the form of:

- parenteral nutrition (PN)
- minimal-fat diet with or without MCT
- low fat/MCT-based enteral feed.

Parenteral nutrition   In some respects this can be considered to be the most effective form of conservative management because even the ingestion of water orally can increase the flow of chyle. However, the inherent risks of PN, plus those incurred by insertion of a central line into a patient with altered thoracic physiology, must be taken into consideration. An initial trial of a minimal-fat diet or enteral feed (which or without MCT) is generally preferable.

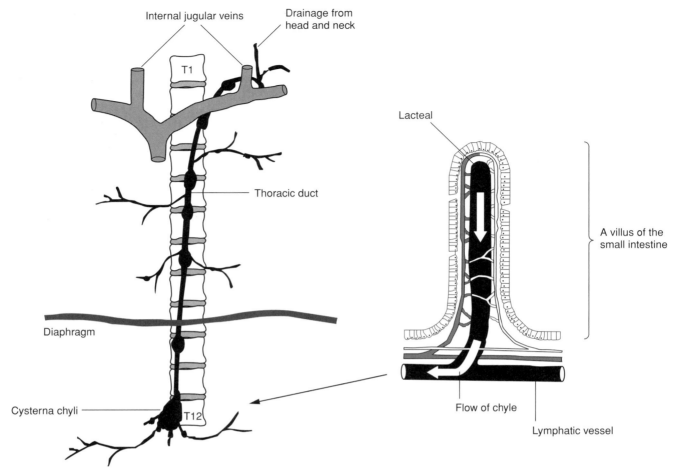

Fig. 5.5 Schematic diagram demonstrating the flow of chyle from the small intestine to the systemic circulation.

Minimal-fat diet There is a lack of specific guidelines on appropriate fat intake in the management of chyle leakage (Bonner and Warren 1998). However, given that any dietary fat (long-chain triglycerides) increases chyle production, a virtually fat-free diet is required. An intake of 5–10 g/day is the lowest level practically achievable, unless the patient is managed solely on a modular feed based on skimmed milk powder or on fat-free nutritional supplements.

Proprietary modular carbohydrate supplements such as Maxijul (SHS), Polycal (Nutricia) or Caloreen (Nestlé Clinical Nutrition) can be given either alone or in combination with fat-free liquid supplements such as Enlive (Ross Laboratories), Fortijuce (Nutricia) or Provide Ultra (Fresenius) (see Appendix 6.7). Energy supplement powders such as Build Up (Nestlé Clinical Nutrition) are fat-free if reconstituted with skimmed milk.

MCT oils (Mead-Johnson, SHS) can be used for cooking but, with their low flash point, should not be used for roasting.

Low-fat/MCT-based enteral feed Inadequate oral intake may require enteral feeding. Feeds should preferably be very low fat or contain the majority of their fat source as MCT, such as Peptamen (Nestlé Clinical Nutrition).

Surgical management

Chylous drainage of more than 2.5 litres/day despite conservative management is associated with increased morbidity, hospital stay, operative mortality and the need for surgical intervention (Alexiou *et al.* 1998). Surgical management of the leak is by ligation of the thoracic duct or pleural shunt formation (Fogli *et al.* 1993). Pleurodesis and the use of fibrin glue are alternative techniques, with thoracoscopy offering a less invasive means of access for these procedures (Terzi *et al.* 1994). A high-fat feed and/or methylene blue given pre-operatively may aid in the location of the leak (Ramzy *et al.* 1982).

Text written by: Janet Warren, Gillian Bonner and Catherine Collins

References

Alexiou C, Watson M, Beggs D *et al.* Chylothorax following oesophagogastrectomy for malignant disease. *European Journal of Cardiothoracic Surgery* 1998; **14**: 460–466.

Berkenbosch JW, Withington DE. Management of postoperative chylothorax with nitric oxide: a case report. *Critical Care Medicine* 1999; **27**: 1022–1024.

Bonner GM, Warren J. A review of the nutritional management of chyle leakage in adults. *Journal of Human Nutrition and Dietetics* 1998; **11**: 105–114.

Fogli L, Gorini P, Belcastro S. Conservative management of traumatic chylothorax: a case report. *International Care Medicine* 1993; **19**: 176–177.

Garcia-Zamalloa A, Ruiz-Irastorza G, Aguayo FJ *et al.* Pseudochylothorax. Report of 2 cases and review of the literature. *Annals of Thoracic Surgery* 1998; **66**: 1845–1846.

Martin IC, Marinho LH, Brown AE, McRobbie D. Medium chain triglycerides in the management of chylous fistulae following neck dissection. *British Journal of Oral and Maxillofacial Surgery* 1993; **31**: 236–238.

Meurer MF, Cohen DJ. Current treatment of chylothorax: a case series and literature review. *Texas Medicine* 1990; **86**: 82–85.

Nguyen DM, Shum Tim D, Dobell AR, Tchervenkov CI. The management of chylothorax/chylopericardium following paediatric cardiac surgery: a 10-year experience. *Journal of Cardiac Surgery* 1995; **10**: 302–308.

Pabst TS, McIntyre KE Jr, Schilling JD *et al.* Management of chyloperitoneum after abdominal aortic surgery. *American Journal of Surgery* 1993; **166**: 194–198.

Ramzy AI, Rodriguez A, Cowley RA. Pitfalls in the management of traumatic chylothorax. *Journal of Trauma* 1982; **22**: 513–515.

Sauvanet A, Baltar J, Le Mee J, Belghiti J. Diagnosis and conservative management of intrathoracic leakage after oesophagectomy. *British Journal of Surgery* 1998; **85**: 1446–1449.

Terzi A, Furlan G, Magnanelli G *et al.* Chylothorax after pleuropulmonary surgery: a rare but unavoidable complication. *Thoracic and Cardiovascular Surgery* 1994; **42**: 81–84.

Zoran A, Biserka K, Miroslav D *et al.* Ideopathic chylothorax in a 25 year old pregnant woman. *Chest* 1997; **112** (Suppl): 3S.

5.8 Wound healing and tissue viability

Many nutrients affect tissue viability and play a crucial role in wound healing (Collins 1996). Malnutrition and specific nutrient deficiencies can delay wound healing and increase susceptibility to wound or systemic infection (Ondrey and Hom 1994). This, in turn, can have significant effects in terms of increased morbidity and mortality (Lennard-Jones 1992). Nutritional adequacy is therefore an important aspect of wound care and the prevention and management of pressure sores and leg ulcers.

5.8.1 Nutrition and wound healing

Nutritional factors which can influence wound healing are summarized in Table 5.14. The following aspects may be of particular importance.

Dietary energy insufficiency

This can affect tissue viability and wound healing in a num-

Table 5.14 Role of dietary factors in tissue viability and wound healing

Nutrient	Function	Effects of deficiency
Protein	Required for synthesis of new tissue	Slow wound healing exacerbating loss of protein via exudate from wound site Tissue of poor tensile strength Oedema
Fat and carbohydrate	Required to prevent dietary or tissue protein being used as an energy source Fatty acids play a key role in cell-membrane synthesis	Loss of fat stores providing padding between bone and skin Impaired immunocompetence
Vitamin A	Improves cell-mediated immunity Antioxidant (beta-carotene) Fibroplasia and epithelialization Improves collagen synthesis/cross-linkage	Increased wound infections Decreased epithelialization Decreased collagen synthesis/cross linking
Vitamin B complex	Coenzymes for energy metabolism Cofactor for collagen deposition/cross-linkage White blood cell/antibody formation	Impaired immunity
Vitamin C	Protection of metalloenzymes from oxidation Neutrophil superoxide production Proline and lysine hydroxylation Collagen synthesis Collagen cross-linkage Angiogenesis	Decreased neutrophil/monocyte chemotaxis Impaired local bacteriocidal activity Increased capillary fragility Wound dehiscence
Vitamin E	Quenches free-radical production Prevents oxidation of membrane polyunsaturated fatty acids	(Excessive amounts may be detrimental to wound healing and increase fibrosis and the risk of haemorrhage)
Vitamin K	Coagulation	Coagulopathies Increased haemorrhage risk Increased haematoma formation
Iron	Prevents anaemia Optimizes tissue perfusion Promotes collagen synthesis	Tissue ischaemia Impaired collagen cross-linking Reduced tensile wound strength
Zinc	Cofactor in enzyme systems for: Cell proliferation Membrane stabilization Protein synthesis Protein, fat and carbohydrate metabolism	Decreased epithelialization rate Reduced collagen synthesis Impaired wound strength Reduced retinol binding protein synthesis
Copper	Covalent cross-linkage of collagen fibrils (wound maturation)	(Unlikely)
Manganese	Cofactor in metalloenzymes	(Magnesium can substitute if manganese status poor)
Selenium	Incorporated in glutathione peroxidase enzyme to protect cell from hydrogen peroxide damage	Impaired macrophage function

ber of ways. Loss of the protective cushioning effect of fat stores increases the likelihood of pressure injuries. Once the body's fat stores are diminished, lean tissue will be used to meet energy needs, resulting in further loss of body mass. In conditions of low energy intake, dietary protein will be used to help to meet energy needs, exacerbating a state of protein depletion with effects such as impaired immune function. Low energy intake is also usually associated with low intake of micronutrients and any resultant deficiencies may, in turn, impact on wound healing.

Protein depletion

Protein inadequacy adversely affects wound healing by blunting the fibroblastic response, neoangiogenesis, collagen synthesis and wound-remodelling processes. The presence of oedema, particularly where oedematous tissue extends through the wound opening, may aggravate protein losses. A large wound may lose 90–100 g protein/day in this way.

Sufficient dietary protein optimizes wound-healing rates, but excessive protein fails to alleviate catabolism (Meyer *et al.* 1994). During wound healing, protein requirements may rise to between 1.2 and 2.0 g/kg body weight per day in order to provide the protein necessary for protein synthesis and to achieve a positive nitrogen balance. Calculations should be based on actual body weight and exclude any weight increase due to the presence of oedema, taking into account the risk of renal dysfunction, especially in the older patient.

Specific amino acids may modify the healing process. Arginine appears to influence wound healing favourably by effecting microvascular and haemodynamic changes (Rodeberg *et al.* 1995) and by enhancing collagen production (Kirk *et al.* 1993).

Fatty acid intake

Fatty acids are an essential component of cell membranes, and dietary deficiency will inhibit tissue repair and wound healing. Diets rich in omega-3 fatty acid inhibit platelet aggregation by altering the haemostatic response, and may reduce wound-healing strength by affecting the fibroblastic and maturation phases of the healing response (Albina *et al.* 1993).

Micronutrient intake

Micronutrients with the ability to prevent or attenuate peroxidative damage can potentially enhance wound healing. These include vitamins A, C and E, zinc, selenium and magnesium (Dickerson 1993: DeBiasse and Wilmore 1994). The role of other micronutrients in wound healing is summarized in Table 5.14 (Collins 1996). Care should be taken with the interpretation of measured serum micronutrient status, as low levels may reflect a teleological response rather than a clinical deficiency.

The relationship between malnutrition and wound healing is, however, difficult to evaluate because nutrition is not the sole factor affecting tissue repair (Albina 1994). Non-nutritional factors such as the quality of nursing care will also have a considerable effect. Furthermore, even in patients with significant weight loss and malnutrition, the body's metabolic response to trauma will still ensure that sufficient substrate is mobilized via lipolysis and other mechanisms to enable wound healing to occur.

The extent to which nutritional supplementation can accelerate the wound-healing response is also poorly researched and complicated by the fact that any benefits from supplementation depend on the nature and extent of the nutritional depletion in a particular individual, and this may not be accurately identified.

It is, however, clear that nutrition can influence, either directly or indirectly, the development and/or healing of some types of tissue injury, and that nutritional inadequacies should be identified and corrected at an early stage in order to minimize the complications and costs associated with them.

5.8.2 Pressure sores

Pressure sores (decubitus ulcers) are a serious and costly problem. They can cause great pain and distress to the patient, may significantly extend the length of a hospital stay and, if severe, may lead to life-threatening complications such as septicaemia. Allcock *et al.* (1994) found that almost 20% of patients in a UK hospital had significant pressure sores. Incident pressure ulcers are associated with a two- to three-fold increase in hospital costs and length of stay (Ilman *et al.* 1999).

Aetiology of pressure sores

Pressure sores are caused primarily by unrelieved pressure. Sustained external pressure, without periodic relief, causes damage to the local microcirculation, leading to hypoxia and tissue necrosis (Fig. 5.6). Other factors, predominantly shearing forces, friction and moisture, contribute to pressure sore development by providing indirect pressure, increased friction and breakdown of the skin's integrity (Bergstrom 1997), predisposing to skin and soft tissue infections (Smith *et al* 1999). Secondary factors have also been identified (Table 5.15) and their relative contribution to the development of sores will vary according to individual circumstances.

Areas of the body where skin lies over a bony prominence, and which are not adapted for weight bearing over prolonged periods, are most susceptible to pressure sore development. These include the back of the head, the spines of the scapulae, the sides of the ankles (malleoli), the great trochanters, elbows, heels and the lower sacrum (Fig. 5.7).

Individuals who are particularly at risk are those who:

- are unconscious and/or immobile, e.g. head- and spinal injury patients

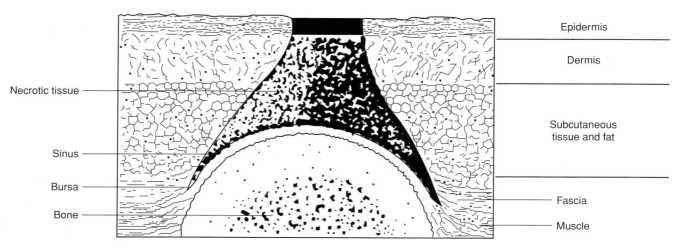

Figure 5.6 Diagram of a necrotic pressure sore showing deep tissue destruction.

- have impaired mobility, e.g. stroke patients, orthopaedic patients, people with a physical disability
- are elderly
- have diabetes
- have a chronic illness.

Pressure sores can be classified into five grades according to their developmental stage (Waterlow 1977) (Table 5.16).

Nutritional aspects of pressure sore development

Prolonged malnutrition increases an individual's suscep-

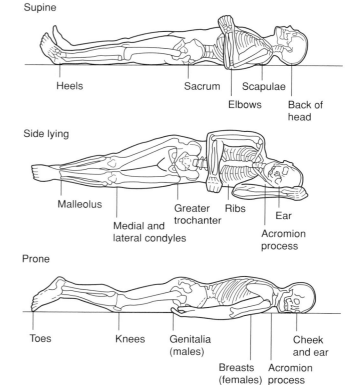

Figure 5.7 Pressure points in various positions.
From Gruis and Innes (1976); reproduced with permission.

Table 5.15 Factors involved in the aetiology of pressure sores

Primary factors	Secondary factors
Pressure	Low or high body weight
Shearing forces	Nutritional status
Moisture	Anaemia
Friction	Immobility, and its duration
	Neurological changes (e.g. loss of pain sensation)
	Infection
	Medication
	Dehydration
	Age
	Chronic illness
	Iatrogenic (e.g. poor turning technique, prolonged lying on hard surfaces)

Table 5.16 Classification of pressure sore development (Waterlow 1977)

Stage	Characteristic features
1	Skin discoloration with persistent erythema after pressure is released. (Blanching with light finger pressure indicates that the microcirculation is still intact.) A blister may be forming
2	Oedema, blistering, epidermal skin loss, with exposure of the dermis. Pain is present. Often results from abrasion
3	Loss of tissue through the dermis. The edge of the pressure sore is distinct and is surrounded by erythema and induration
4	Lesions extend into the subcutaneous tissue and may penetrate into the deep fascia and muscle. This presents initially as an area of bluish-black discoloration which turns into a black scar. After a few days this separates to reveal an underlying cavity formed by pressure destruction of deep tissue
5	Joints and body cavities may become involved, multiple sores may merge together. Infection and septicaemia can occur

tibility to pressure sore development, primarily as a result of the loss of cushioning from fat stores. Associated nutrient deficiencies may increase tissue fragility and hinder tissue repair. Impaired immune function may increase the likelihood of pressure sore infection and, if pyrexia and anorexia result, nutritional status may deteriorate further, thus exacerbating the situation (Stotts and Hunt 1997). Malnourished stroke patients have been shown to have an increased frequency of infections and pressure sores in comparison with an appropriately nourished group (Davalos *et al.* 1996).

However, it should not be overlooked that nutrition is only one of the factors influencing pressure sore development and that nutritional adequacy alone is not sufficient to prevent them (McLaren 1992; Pinchcofsky-Devin 1994). In a study of elderly patients undergoing hip surgery, two-thirds developed pressure sores during their hospital stay, irrespective of the quantity and quality of diet, as assessed by a food frequency questionnaire (Lewis 1998). Supplementary feeding of elderly people has not been shown to reduce the incidence or rate of healing of pressure sores (Bourdel-Marchasson *et al.* 1997; Hartgrink *et al.* 1998). Patient age and Norton score appear to be the strongest risk factors for pressure ulcers, with reduced appetite sufficient to warrant enteral feeding a further risk (Perneger *et al.* 1998).

Nutritional aspects of pressure sore management

Nutritional considerations should be an integral part of pressure-sore management (Thomas 1997). Estimated nutritional requirements should take account of factors such as:

- age
- body weight and weight loss
- reason for admission or underlying clinical condition
- grade of pressure sore
- losses from wound site
- pyrexia
- mobility
- pain
- current nutritional intake.

The following nutritional aspects are particularly important in pressure sore management.

Energy intake

Adequate energy intake is important to help to restore, or prevent further loss of fat stores which provide cushioning against pressure. Energy sufficiency is also important to prevent dietary and tissue protein being used as a source of energy. Food-fortification measures or energy supplements may be necessary in some patients to help to achieve this. In cases of extreme nutritional depletion, additional nutritional support measures such as overnight enteral feeding may be necessary. However, excessive energy intakes are unnecessary as requirements are likely to be lowered by reduced mobility. Energy surplus must also be avoided in patients who are, or are at risk of becoming overweight, as this will also increase the risk of pressure sore development.

Protein

Protein intakes should be sufficient to ensure healing and to cover exudative losses.

Fatty acids

The role of fatty acids in skin synthesis may be particularly relevant to pressure sore development. Topical application of 20 ml omega-6-rich PUFA to high-risk skin areas three times daily has been shown to be associated with a significant reduction in pressure sore development, and increased skin hydration and elasticity (Declair 1997).

Micronutrients

Vitamin C Low concentrations of leucocyte vitamin C have been shown to be associated with the development of pressure sores (Goode *et al.* 1992) and, in the presence of clear evidence of deficiency, supplementation is justified. However, there is no evidence that routine vitamin C supplementation (which is commonly advocated for pressure sore patients) is either necessary or beneficial. When dietary intake of vitamin C is unrestricted and tissue levels are normal, wounds heal quite rapidly. It is, however, important that patients consume sufficient vitamin C (probably a minimum of 60 mg vitamin C daily), preferably via dietary sources and/or with the use of additional drinks such as fresh fruit juice or fortified blackcurrant drinks. Multivitamin preparations containing supplementation at this level may be useful if requirements cannot be met by diet alone. Megadoses of vitamin C exceeding 1 g/day have been advocated to promote wound healing, but since tissue saturation is reached at an intake of 200 mg/day (Levine *et al.* 1999) any excess above this level is likely to be unnecessary and may increase the risk of renal stone formation and rebound scurvy on discontinuation of the supplement (Tyrrell 1974).

Zinc Zinc deficiency has been associated with delayed wound healing (Andews and Gallagher-Allred 1999) and dietary zinc adequacy may be important in patients with pressure sores. For this reason, zinc supplementation is often advocated, although the need for, and effectiveness of, this measure are difficult to evaluate; biochemical zinc levels are rarely available and are not in any case a reliable indicator of zinc status during infection (Shanbogue and Paterson 1990). Indication for zinc supplementation therefore has to be based on assessment of current dietary intake and the likelihood of any inadequacy not being met by dietary means. This is primarily a clinical decision but should always be a consideration in patients with severe sores or those which are slow to heal. When necessary, supplements of 200–220 mg zinc sulphate are usually administered one to three times per day.

Iron Low haemoglobin levels are often seen in those with established pressure sores. Healing cannot occur until this is corrected, since an adequate blood flow for tissue oxygenation is essential at the wound site (McClemont *et al.* 1984). Blood transfusions may be indicated if haemoglobin levels fall below 8 mg/l, particularly when surgery is contemplated; otherwise, iron supplements should be given. Clinical anaemia is usually treated with 200 mg ferrous sulphate, two to three times daily.

Oversupplementation of any one mineral should be avoided since this may affect absorptive or metabolic interactions between zinc, iron and copper, and impair nutritional status.

Fluid Dehydrated skin becomes inelastic, fragile and more susceptible to breakdown. The fluid intake of patients with, or at risk of, pressure sores is therefore an important consideration. Older, debilitated patients are particularly vulnerable to dehydration, and may voluntarily decrease fluid intake to control urinary incontinence, thus increasing their risk of pressure sore formation (Natow 1983). It is important that fluid status is routinely monitored, and if necessary corrected, as part of nursing procedures.

Prevention of pressure sores

The early identification of at-risk patients is vital for the prevention of pressure sores. A variety of risk assessment charts is available for identifying such patients at an early stage, and some commonly examples are given in Fig. 5.8. One of these assessments should ideally be carried out by nursing staff within 1 hour of a patient's admission. Reassessment should occur whenever there is a significant change in the patient's condition, e.g. the level of consciousness or degree of mobility.

While the importance of some factors such as good skin care are usually recognized by the health-care team, the benefits of good nutritional status are often overlooked. Educational programmes, aimed at reducing the incidence of pressure sores, should ensure that staff are aware of the vital role of nutrition and know how to identify individuals with nutritional difficulties (Culley 1998). The primary aim should be to increase awareness at the ward level and ensure the prompt early referral of patients to the dietitian, ideally before the development of sores. The provision of nutritional risk assessment charts which enable nursing staff to assess dietary adequacy and identify those who may benefit from dietetic advice is a useful way in which to achieve this (see Section 1.9, Assessment of nutritional risk). Some of the dietary aspects which could be incorporated into risk assessment for pressure sore development are shown in Table 5.17.

5.8.3 Leg ulcers

A leg ulcer is a loss of skin below the knee or foot which takes more than 6 weeks to heal. Ulcers can result in severe pain and can significantly reduce mobility and the quality of life, especially in elderly people.

The most common causes of leg ulceration are:

- chronic venous insufficiency
- arterial disease
- rheumatoid arthritis
- diabetes.

Less common causes include:

- physical trauma
- infection
- contact dermatitis
- haematological disease
- neoplasm.

Table 5.17 Nutritional aspects of pressure sore risk assessment.

Nutritional factors which may enhance pressure sore risk	Dietary aspect to consider	Categories of increasing risk	Other factors to consider
Inadequate energy intake	Ability to eat	Able to eat independently Requires help with eating Needs to be fed Dysphagic/unable to consume normal foods	Use of proprietary energy/protein supplements Assess level of usage
	Appetite	Good: clears plate Moderate: only eats small amounts Poor: often refuses food/drink	
Zinc inadequacy	Consumption of meat/dairy products/fish/eggs	Daily 2–3 times/week <2 times/week	Use of zinc or multivitamin supplements Assess level of intake
Vitamin C inadequacy	Consumption of citrus fruits, fruit juice or blackcurrant drinks	Daily 2–3 times/week 1 or 0 times/week	Use of vitamin C or multivitamin supplements Assess level of intake
Existing malnutrition	Body weight	Normal Overweight Underweight/recent weight loss Cachectic	Nutritional support measures already implemented

5.8 Wound healing and tissue viability

(a)

The Douglas pressure sore risk calculator
Score 18 or less = 'at risk'

Nutritional status		Activity		Incontinence	
Well balanced diet	4	Fully mobile	4	Continent	4
Inadequate diet	3	Walk with difficulty	3	Occasionally	3
Fluids only	2	Chairbound	2	Urine	2
Peripheral-parenteral feeding	1	Bedfast	1	Doubly	1
Low haemoglobin (<10)	1				

Pain		Skin state		Mental state	
Pain free	4	Intact	4	Alert	4
Fear of pain	3	Dry/red/thin	3	Apathetic	3
Periodic	2	Superficial break	2	Stuporous	2
Pain on movement	1	Full tissue		Unco-operative	1
Continual discomfort	0	thickness/cavity	1	Comatose	0

Special risks: Deduct 2 for each of the following:
Steroid therapy, diabetes, cytotoxic therapy, dyspnoea

(b)

Waterlow risk assessment card

Ring scores in table, add total
several scores per category can be used

Build/weight for height	*	Risk areas visual skin type	*	Sex Age	*	Special risks	*
						Tissue malnutrition	*
Average	0	Healthy	0	Male	1	E.G. terminal cachexia	8
Above average	1	Tissue paper	1	Female	2	Cardiac failure	5
Obese	2	Dry	2	14–49	1	Peripheral vascular failure	5
Below average	3	Oedematous	3	50–64	2	Anaemia	2
		Clammy	4	65–74	3	Smoking	1
Continence	*	Discoloured	5	75–80	4	Neurological deficit	*
		Broken/spot	6	81+	5		
Complete/ catheterized	0					E.G. diabetes, CVA	
Occasion incon.	1	Mobility	*	Appetite	*	M.S. paraplegia	4–6
Cath/incontinent of faeces	2	Fully	1	Average	0	Motor sensory	
Doubly incont.	3	Restless/fidgity	2	Poor	1	Major surgery/ trauma	*
		Apathetic	3	N.G. tube/fluids	2		
		Restricted	4	NBM/anorexic	3	Orthopaedic- below waist, spinal	5
		Inert/traction bound	5			On table > 2 hours	5
		Chairbound	6			Medication	*
						Steroids, cytotoxics, anti-inflamatory	4

Score:	10 + at risk	15 + high risk	20 + very high risk

(c)

Norton scale
Score 14 or below – 'at risk'

A Physical condition*		B Mental		C Activity		D Mobility		E Incontinence	
Good	4	Alert	4	Walks	4	Full	4	Does not have	4
Fair	3	Apathetic	3	Walks with help	3	Slightly limited	3	Has occasionally	3
Poor	2	Confused	2	Chairbound	2	Very limited	2	Usually urinary	2
Very bad	1	Stuporous	1	Bedfast	1	Immobile	1	Double	1

Figure 5.8 Examples of pressure-sore risk-assessment cards.
(a) Douglas pressure-sore indicator; (b) Waterlow pressure-sore prevention/treatment policy; (c) Norton scale.

Management of leg ulcers will vary according to the underlying cause and it is important that this is correctly identified to avoid ineffective or possibly hazardous treatment (Cornwall *et al.* 1986).

Venous ulcers

These require correction of the abnormally high blood pressure in the superficial veins and improvement in leg drainage by raising the affected limb above heart level. Bed rest may be necessary to achieve this. Compression bandaging is necessary to prevent pooling of blood in the capillaries and leakage of fluid into the surrounding tissues. About 75% of venous ulcers will heal within 3 months if correct treatment is applied at an early stage.

Ischaemic (arterial) ulcers

These are treated by effective wound management designed to prevent secondary infection; compression bandaging is contraindicated (Moffatt 1992).

There has been little research on the relationship between nutrition and leg ulcers but, as with any significant wound, the importance of adequate nutrition to promote healing and prevent recurrence should not be overlooked. Nutritional inadequacies in terms of intake of energy, zinc, vitamin C, iron and protein have been found in elderly people with venous ulceration of the leg (Agren *et al.* 1986; Lewis *et al.* 1993), suggesting that such patients may commonly be nutritionally at risk.

Nutritional aspects of the underlying cause of the ulceration may also need to be addressed, for example, dietary measures to improve diabetic control or reduce cardiovascular risk.

Text revised by: Catherine Collins and Briony Thomas

Useful address

The Tissue Viability Society
Website: www.tvs.org.uk

References

Agren MS, Stromberg HE, Rindby A, Hallmans G. Selenium, zinc, iron and copper levels in serum of patients with arterial and venous leg ulcers. *Acta Dermato-Venereologica* 1986; **66**: 237–240.

Albina JE. Nutrition and wound healing. *Journal of Parenteral and Enteral Nutrition* 1994; **8**: 367–376.

Albina JE, Gladden P, Walsh WR. Detrimental effects of an omega-3 fatty acid-enriched diet on wound healing. *Journal of Parenteral and Enteral Nutrition* 1993; **17**: 519–521.

Allcock N, Wharrad H, Nicolson A. Interpretation of pressure sore prevalence. *Journal of Advanced Nursing* 1994; **20**: 37–45.

Andrews M, Gallagher-Allred C. The role of zinc in wound healing. *Advances in Wound Care* 1999; **12**: 137–138.

Bergstrom NI. Strategies for preventing pressure ulcers. *Clinics in Geriatric Medicine* 1997; **13**: 437–454.

Bourdel-Marchasson I, Dumas F, Pinganaud G *et al.* Audit of percutaneous endoscopic gastrostomy in long-term enteral feeding in a nursing home. *International Journal for Quality in Health Care* 1997; **9**: 297–302.

Collins C. Nutrition and wound healing. *Care of the Critically Ill* 1996; **12**: 87–90.

Cornwall JV, Dore CJ, Lewis JD. Legs ulcers: epidemiology and aetiology. *British Journal of Surgery* 1986; **73**: 693–696.

Culley F. Nursing aspects of pressure sore prevention and therapy. *British Journal of Nursing* 1998; **7**: 879–882.

Davalos A, Ricart W, Gonzalez-Huix F *et al.* Effect of malnutrition after acute stroke on clinical outcome. *Stroke* 1996; **27**: 1028–1032.

DeBiasse MA, Wilmore DW. What is optimal nutrition support? *New Horizons* 1994; **2**: 122–130

Declair V. The usefulness of topical application of essential fatty acids (EFA) to prevent pressure ulcers. *Ostomy Wound Management* 1997; **43**: 48–54.

Dickerson JWT. Ascorbic acid, zinc and wound healing. *Journal of Wound Care* 1993; **2**: 350–353.

Goode HF, Burns E, Walker BE. Vitamin C depletion and pressure sores in elderly patients with femoral neck fracture. *British Medical Journal* 1992; **305**: 925–927.

Gruis M, Innes B. Assessment: essential to prevent pressure sores. *American Journal of Nursing* 1976; **76**: 1762–1764.

Hartgrink HH, Wille J *et al.* Pressure sores and tube feeding inpatients with a fracture of the hip: a randomized controlled trial. *Clinical Nutrition* 1998; **17**: 287–292.

Ilman RM, Goode PS, Burst N *et al.* Pressure ulcers, hospital complications, and disease severity: impact on hospital costs and length of stay. *Advances in Wound Care* 1999; **12**: 22–30.

Kirk SJ, Hurson M, Regan MC *et al.* Arginine stimulates wound healing and immune function in elderly human beings. *Surgery* 1993; **108**: 155–160.

Lennard-Jones JE. *A positive Approach to Nutrition as a Treatment*. London: King's Fund Centre, 1992.

Levine M, Rumsey SC, Daruwala R *et al.* Criteria and recommendations for vitamin C intake. *Journal of the American Medical Association* 1999; **281**: 1415–1423.

Lewis BK. Nutrient intake and the risk of pressure sore development in older patients. *Journal of Wound Care* 1998; **7**: 31–35.

Lewis BK, Hitchings H, Bale S, Harding KG. Nutritional status of elderly patients with venous ulceration of the leg – report of a pilot study. *Journal of Human Nutrition and Dietetics* 1993; **6**: 509–515.

McClemont EJW, Archibald RM, Ratnsay BM. Pressure sores. *Nursing* 1984; Suppl, Series 2 (21): 1046.

McLaren S. Nutrition and wound healing. *Journal of Wound Care* 1992; **1** (3): 45–55.

Meyer MA, Muller MJ, Herndon DN. Nutrient support of the healing wound. *New Horizons* 1994; **2**: 202–214.

Moffat C. Compression bandaging, the state of the art. *Journal of Wound Care* 1992; **1**: 945–950.

Natow AB. Nutrition in the prevention and treatment of decubitus ulcers. *Topics in Clinical Nursing* 1983; **5**: 39–44.

Ondrey FG, Hom DB. Effects of nutrition on wound healing. *Otolaryngology – Head and Neck Surgery* 1994; **110**: 557–559.

Perneger TV, Heliot C, Rae AC *et al.* Hospital-acquired pressure ulcers: risk factors and use of preventive devices. *Archives of Internal Medicine* 1998; **158**: 1940–1945.

Pinchcofsky-Devin G. Nutrition and wound healing. *Journal of Wound Care* 1994; **3**: 231–234.

Rodeberg DA, Chaet MS, Bass RC *et al*. Nitric oxide: an overview. *American Journal of Surgery* 1995; **170**: 292–303.

Shanbogue LK, Paterson N. Effect of sepsis and surgery on trace elements. *Journal of Parenteral and Enteral Nutrition* 1990; **14**: 287–289.

Smith PW, Black JM, Black SB. Infected pressure ulcers in the long-term-care facility. *Infection Control and Hospital Epidemiology* 1999; **20**: 358–361.

Stotts NA, Hunt TK. Pressure ulcers. Managing bacterial colonization and infection. *Clinics in Geriatric Medicine* 1997; **13**: 565–573.

Thomas DR. The role of nutrition in prevention and healing of pressure ulcers. *Clinics in Geriatric Medicine* 1997; **13**: 497–511.

Tyrrell DAJ. Vitamin C and the common cold. *Prescribers Journal* 1974; **14**: 21–24.

Waterlow J. Waterlow card for prevention and management of pressure sores – towards a pocket policy. *Care Science and Practitioner* 1977; **6**: 80–86.

Waterlow JA. A risk assessment card. *Nursing Times* 1985; **89**: 49–51.

SECTION 6
Appendices

6.1 Weights and measures reference data

6.1.1 Height/length

1 inch	= 2.54 cm
1 foot (12 inches)	= 30.48 cm (0.305 m)
1 yard (36 inches)	= 91.44 cm
1 cm	= 0.394 inch
1 m	= 39.37 inches

To convert height in feet and inches to metres
(e.g. a client who is 5 feet 5 inches)
1 Convert to inches by multiplying feet by 12 and adding the additional inches
(e.g. $5 \times 12 = 60$; $+5 = 65$ inches)
2 Convert to centimetres by multiplying inches by 2.54
(e.g. $65 \times 2.54 = 165.1$ cm)
3 Convert to metres by dividing by 100
(e.g. $165.1/100 = 1.651$ m)

6.1.2 Weight/mass

1 ounce	= 28.35 g (in round figures, 28 g)
1 pound (16 oz)	= 454 g or 0.45 kg
1 stone (14 lb)	= 6.35 kg
1 kg (1000 g)	= 2.2 lb

To convert weight in stones and pounds to kilograms
(e.g. a client who is 11 stone 6 lb)
1 Convert to pounds by multiplying stones by 14, and adding the additional pounds
(e.g. $11 \times 14 = 154$; $+ 6 = 160$ lb)
2 Convert pounds to kilograms by dividing by 2.2
(e.g. $160/2.2 = 72.7$ kg)

To convert kilograms to stones and pounds
(e.g. a client who is 55 kg)
1 Multiply by 2.2
(e.g. $55 \times 2.2 = 121$ lb)
2 Divide by 14 to derive stones
(e.g. $121/14 = 8.643$ stone)
3 Multiply the fraction by 14 to derive pounds
(e.g. $0.643 \times 14 = 9.0$ lb. Imperial weight is therefore 8 stone 9 lb)

Table 6.1 Inches/centimetres conversion table

Inches to centimetres		Centimetres to inches	
Inches	cm	cm	Inches
1	2.54	1	0.39
2	5.08	2	0.79
3	7.62	3	1.18
4	10.16	4	1.57
5	12.70	5	1.97
6	15.25	6	2.36
7	17.78	7	2.76
8	20.32	8	3.15
9	22.86	9	3.54
10	25.40	10	3.94
20	50.8	20	7.87
30	76.2	30	11.81
40	101.6	40	15.75
50	127.0	50	19.69
60	152.4	60	23.62
70	177.8	70	27.56
80	203.2	80	31.50
90	228.6	90	35.43
100	254.0	100	39.37

6.1.3 Volume

1 fluid ounce	= 28.41 ml
1 pint (20 fl oz)	= 568.3 ml (or 0.568 litres)
1 litre (1000 ml)	= 1.76 pints

Table 6.2 Height conversion table (feet and inches to metres)

Feet	Inches	m	Feet	Inches	m
4	0	1.22	5	3	1.60
4	0½	1.23	5	3½	1.61
4	1	1.24	5	4	1.63
4	1½	1.26	5	4½	1.64
4	2	1.27	5	5	1.65
4	2½	1.28	5	5½	1.66
4	3	1.29	5	6	1.68
4	3½	1.31	5	6½	1.69
4	4	1.32	5	7	1.70
4	4½	1.33	5	7½	1.71
4	5	1.35	5	8	1.73
4	5½	1.36	5	8½	1.74
4	6	1.37	5	9	1.75
4	6½	1.38	5	9½	1.76
4	7	1.40	5	10	1.78
4	7½	1.41	5	10½	1.79
4	8	1.42	5	11	1.80
4	8½	1.43	5	11½	1.82
4	9	1.45	6	0	1.83
4	9½	1.46	6	½	1.84
4	10	1.47	6	1	1.85
4	10½	1.49	6	1½	1.87
4	11	1.50	6	2	1.88
4	11½	1.51	6	2½	1.89
			6	3	1.90
5	0	1.52	6	3½	1.92
5	0½	1.54	6	4	1.93
5	1	1.55	6	4½	1.94
5	1½	1.56	6	5	1.96
5	2	1.57	6	5½	1.97
5	2½	1.59	6	6	1.98

Table 6.3 Ounces/grams conversion table (approximate rounded figures)

Ounces to grams			Grams to ounces	
oz	g	(approximate conversion)	g	oz (approximate conversion)
1	28	(25–30)	10	0.35 (⅓ oz)
2	57	(50–60)	15	0.53 (½ oz)
3	85	(75–90)	20	0.71 (¾ oz)
4 (¼ lb)	113	(100–120)	30	1.06 (1 oz)
5	142	(150)	40	1.41
6	170	(175)	50	1.76 (1¾ oz)
7	198	(200)	60	2.12 (2 oz)
8 (½ lb)	227	(225)	70	2.47
9	255	(250)	80	2.82
10	284	(300)	90	3.17
11	312	(325)	100	3.53 (3½ oz)
12 (¾ lb)	340	(350)	110	3.88
13	368	(375)	120	4.23
14	397	(400)	130	4.58
15	425	(425)	140	4.94
16 (1 lb)	454	(450)	150	5.29
			175	6.31
			200	7.05
			225	7.94 (8 oz/½ lb)
			250	8.82
			300	10.58
			350	12.34 (12 oz/¾ lb)
			400	14.1
			450	15.9 (16 oz/1 lb)
			500	17.6
			1000	35.27 (2.2 lb)

Table 6.4 Body weight conversion table (stones and pounds to kilograms)

Stones	lb	kg	Stones	lb	kg	Stones	lb	kg	Stones	lb	kg	Stones	lb	kg
0	1	0.45	6	5	40.37	9	13	63.05	13	7	85.73	17	1	108.41
	2	0.90		6	40.82	10	0	63.50		8	86.18		2	108.86
	3	1.36		7	41.28		1	63.96		9	86.64		3	109.32
	4	1.81		8	41.73		2	64.41		10	87.09		4	109.77
	5	2.27		9	42.18		3	64.86		11	87.54		5	110.22
	6	2.72		10	42.64		4	65.32		12	88.00		6	110.68
	7	3.17		11	43.09		5	65.77		13	88.45		7	111.13
	8	3.63		12	43.55		6	66.23	14	0	88.91		8	111.59
	9	4.08		13	44.00		7	66.68		1	89.36		9	112.04
	10	4.54	7	0	44.45		8	67.13		2	89.81		10	112.49
	11	4.99		1	44.91		9	67.59		3	90.27		11	112.95
	12	5.44		2	45.36		10	68.04		4	90.72		12	113.40
	13	5.90		3	45.81		11	68.49		5	91.17		13	113.85
				4	46.27		12	68.95		6	91.63	18	0	114.31
1	0	6.35		5	46.72		13	69.40		7	92.08		1	114.76
2	0	12.70		6	47.17	11	0	69.85		8	92.53		2	115.21
3	0	19.05		7	47.63		1	70.31		9	92.98		3	115.67
4	0	25.40		8	48.08		2	70.76		10	93.44		4	116.12
	1	25.86		9	48.54		3	71.22		11	93.90		5	116.58
	2	26.31		10	48.99		4	71.67		12	94.35		6	117.03
	3	26.76		11	49.44		5	72.12		13	94.80		7	117.48
	4	27.22		12	49.90		6	72.58	15	0	95.26		8	117.94
	5	27.67		13	50.35		7	73.03		1	95.71		9	118.39
	6	28.12	8	0	50.80		8	73.48		2	96.16		10	118.84
	7	28.57		1	51.26		9	73.94		3	96.62		11	119.30
	8	29.03		2	51.71		10	74.39		4	97.07		12	119.75
	9	29.48		3	52.16		11	74.84		5	97.52		13	120.20
	10	29.93		4	52.62		12	75.30		6	97.98	19	0	120.66
	11	30.39		5	53.07		13	75.75		7	98.43		1	121.11
	12	30.84		6	53.52	12	0	76.20		8	98.88		2	121.56
	13	31.30		7	53.98		1	76.66		9	99.34		3	122.02
5	0	31.75		8	54.43		2	77.11		10	99.79		4	122.47
	1	32.21		9	54.89		3	77.57		11	100.24		5	122.93
	2	32.66		10	55.34		4	78.02		12	100.70		6	123.38
	3	33.11		11	55.79		5	78.47		13	101.15		7	123.83
	4	33.57		12	56.25		6	78.93	16	0	101.61		8	124.29
	5	34.02		13	56.70		7	79.38		1	102.06		9	124.74
	6	34.47	9	0	57.15		8	79.83		2	102.51		10	125.19
	7	34.93		1	57.61		9	80.29		3	102.97		11	125.65
	8	35.38		2	58.06		10	80.74		4	103.42		12	126.10
	9	35.83		3	58.51		11	81.19		5	103.87		13	126.55
	10	36.29		4	58.97		12	81.65		6	104.33	20	0	127.27
	11	36.74		5	59.42		13	82.10		7	104.79		7	130.45
	12	37.19		6	59.88	13	0	82.55		8	105.24	21	0	133.64
	13	37.65		7	60.33		1	83.01		9	105.69		7	136.82
6	0	38.10		8	60.78		2	83.46		10	106.14	22	0	140.00
	1	38.56		9	61.24		3	83.92		11	106.60		7	143.18
	2	39.01		10	61.69		4	84.37		12	107.04	23	0	146.36
	3	39.46		11	62.14		5	84.82		13	107.50	24	0	152.73
	4	39.92		12	62.60		6	85.28	17	0	107.96	25	0	159.09

Table 6.5 Pints/litres conversion table

fl oz/pints	ml/litres	(Approximate measure)	ml/litres	fl oz/pints
1 fl oz	28	(25)	50 ml	1.75 fl oz
1/4 pint (5 fl oz)	142	(150)	100 ml	3.5 fl oz
1/2 pint (10 fl oz)	284	(275)	200 ml	7 fl oz
3/4 pint (15 fl oz)	426	(425)	250 ml	8.8 fl oz
1 pint	568	(550)	500 ml	17.6 fl oz
2 pints	1.1 litres		750 ml	26.4 fl oz
3 pints	1.7 litres		1000 ml (1 litre)	1.76 pints (1 3/4 pints)
4 pints	2.3 litres			
5 pints	2.8 litres			

6.2 Dietary reference data

6.2.1 Conversion factors

Energy

Conversion factors for kilocalories to kilojoules/megajoules

1 kilocalorie (kcal)	= 4.184 kilojoules (kJ)
1000 kcal	= 4.184 megajoules (MJ)
1 kilojoule	= 0.239 kcal
1 megajoule (1000 kJ)	= 239 kcal

For converting the energy content of diets of normal composition, a conversion factor of 1 kcal = 4.2 kJ can be used

To convert:

kcal to kJ	Multiply by 4.2
kcal to MJ	Multiply by 4.2/1000
	or
	Divide by 239
kJ to kcal	Divide by 4.2
MJ to kcal	Divide by 4.2 × 1000
	or
	Multiply by 239

Protein/nitrogen

Protein g = Nitrogen g × 6.25*
Nitrogen g = Protein g/6.25*

*This conversion factor is only appropriate for a mixture of foods. For milk or cereals alone, the factors 6.4 or 5.7, respectively, should be used.

Nitrogen balance

Nitrogen input g	= Protein g taken in 24 hours/6.25
Nitrogen output g	= Nitrogen g lost in urine + 2–4 g (obligatory nitrogen losses in skin and faeces)
Nitrogen balance	= Nitrogen input – nitrogen output

(See Section 1.10.2 in Estimating nutritional requirements.)

Table 6.6 Energy yields

Nutrient	Energy yield per gram	
	kcal	kJ
Protein	4	17
Fat	9	37
Carbohydrate	3.75	16
Alcohol	7	29
Medium-chain triglyceride (MCT)	8.4	35

Vitamin A

The active vitamin A content of the diet is usually expressed in retinol equivalents:

1 μg retinol equivalent	= 1 μg retinol or 6 μg beta-carotene equivalents
μg retinol equivalents	= μg retinol + (μg beta-carotene equivalents/6)

Occasionally the vitamin A content of foods is still expressed in international units (IU)
1 IU = 0.3 μg retinol (or 0.6 μg carotene equivalents)

Vitamin D

1 μg vitamin D = 40 IU
1 IU = 0.025 μg vitamin D

To convert:

μg vitamin D to IU:	Multiply by 40
IU vitamin D to μg:	Divide by 40

Nicotinic acid/tryptophan

1 mg nicotinic acid can be produced from 60 mg tryptophan.

Nicotinic acid mg equivalents = Nicotinic acid mg + (Tryptophan mg/60)

6.2.2 Dietary reference values

Table 6.7 Estimated average requirements (EARs) for energy

	EAR (kcal/day)	
Age	Males	Females
0–3 months	545	515
4–6 months	690	645
7–9 months	825	765
10–12 months	920	865
1–3 years	1230	1165
4–6 years	1715	1545
7–10 years	1970	1740
11–14 years	2220	1845
15–18 years	2755	2110
19–50 years	2550	1940
51–59 years	2550	1900
60–64 years	2380	1900
65–74 years	2330	1900
75+ years	2100	1810
Pregnancy		+200[1]
Lactation:		
1 month		+450
2 months		+530
3 months		+570
4–6 months (group 1)[2]		+480
4–6 months (group 2)		+570
>6 months (group 1)		+240
>6 months (group 2)		+550

[1]Last trimester only
[2]Group 1: Women who practise exclusive or almost exclusive breast feeding until the baby is 3–4 months old. Group 2: Women whose intention is that breast milk should provide the primary source of nourishment for the baby for 6 months or more.
Source: Department of Health. *Dietary Reference Values for Food Energy and Nutrients for the United Kingdom*. Report on Health and Social Subjects 41. London: HMSO, 1991.
Crown copyright material is reproduced with the permission of the Controller of Her Majesty's Stationery Office.

Table 6.8 Reference nutrient intakes (RNIs) for protein

Age	RNI[1] (g/day)
0–3 months	12.5[2]
4–6 months	12.7
7–9 months	13.7
10–12 months	14.9
1–3 years	14.5
4–6 years	19.7
7–10 years	28.3
Males	
11–14 years	42.1
15–18 years	55.2
19–50 years	55.5
50+ years	53.3
Females	
11–14 years	41.2
15–18 years	45.0
19–50 years	45.0
50+ years	46.5
Pregnancy[3]	+6
Lactation[3]	
0–4 months	+11
4+ months	+8

[1]These figures, based on egg and milk protein, assume complete digestibility.
[2]No values for infants 0–3 months are given by WHO. The RNI is calculated from the recommendations of COMA.
[3]To be added to adult requirement through all stages of pregnancy and lactation.
Source: Department of Health. *Dietary Reference Values for Food Energy and Nutrients for the United Kingdom*. Report on Health and Social Subjects 41. London: HMSO, 1991.
Crown copyright material is reproduced with the permission of the Controller of Her Majesty's Stationery Office.

Table 6.9 Reference nutrient intakes (RNIs) for vitamins

Age	Thiamin (mg/day)	Riboflavin (mg/day)	Niacin[1] (mg/day)	Vitamin B_6[2] (mg/day)	Vitamin B_{12} (μg/day)	Folate (μg/day)	Vitamin C (mg/day)	Vitamin A (μg/day)	Vitamin D (μg/day)
0–3 months	0.2	0.4	3	0.2	0.3	50	25	350	8.5
4–6 months	0.2	0.4	3	0.2	0.3	50	25	350	8.5
7–9 months	0.2	0.4	4	0.3	0.4	50	25	350	7
10–12 months	0.3	0.4	5	0.4	0.4	50	25	350	7
1–3 years	0.5	0.6	8	0.7	0.5	70	30	400	7
4–6 years	0.7	0.8	11	0.9	0.8	100	30	500	–
7–10 years	0.7	1.0	12	1.0	1.0	150	30	500	–
Males									
11–14 years	0.9	1.2	15	1.2	1.2	200	35	600	–
15–18 years	1.1	1.3	18	1.5	1.5	200	40	700	–
19–50 years	1.0	1.3	17	1.4	1.5	200	40	700	–[3]
50+ years	0.9	1.3	16	1.4	1.5	200	40	700	[3]
Females									
11–14 years	0.7	1.1	12	1.0	1.2	200	35	600	–
15–18 years	0.8	1.1	14	1.2	1.5	200	40	600	–
19–50 years	0.8	1.1	13	1.2	1.5	200	40	600	–[3]
50+ years	0.8	1.1	12	1.2	1.5	200	40	600	[3]
Pregnancy	+0.1[4]	+0.3	[5]	[5]	[5]	+100	+10	+100	10
Lactation									
0–4 months	+0.2	+0.5	+2	[5]	+0.5	+60	+30	+350	10
4+ months	+0.2	+0.5	+2	[5]	+0.5	+60	+30	+350	10

[1]Nicotinic acid equivalent.
[2]Based on protein providing 14.7% of the estimated average requirement (EAR) for energy.
[3]After the age of 65 years the RNI is 10 μg/day for men and women.
[4]For the last trimester only.
[5]No increment.
Source: Department of Health. *Dietary Reference Values for Food Energy and Nutrients for the United Kingdom*. Report on Health and Social Subjects 41. London: HMSO, 1991. Crown copyright material is reproduced with the permission of the Controller of Her Majesty's Stationery Office.

Table 6.10 Reference nutrient intakes (RNIs) for minerals

Age	Calcium (mg/day)	Phosphorus[1] (mg/day)	Magnesium (mg/day)	Sodium[2] (mg/day)	Potassium[3] (mg/day)	Chloride[4] (mg/day)	Iron (mg/day)	Zinc (mg/day)	Copper (mg/day)	Selenium (µg/day)	Iodine (µg/day)
0–3 months	525	400	55	210	800	320	1.7	4.0	0.2	10	50
4–6 months	525	400	60	280	850	400	4.3	4.0	0.3	13	60
7–9 months	525	400	75	320	700	500	7.8	5.0	0.3	10	60
10–12 months	525	400	80	350	700	500	7.8	5.0	0.3	10	60
1–3 years	350	270	85	500	800	800	6.9	5.0	0.4	15	70
4–6 years	450	350	120	700	1100	1100	6.1	6.5	0.6	20	100
7–10 years	550	450	200	1200	2000	1800	8.7	7.0	0.7	30	110
Males											
11–14 years	1000	775	280	1600	3100	2500	11.3	9.0	0.8	45	130
15–18 years	1000	775	300	1600	3500	2500	11.3	9.5	1.0	70	140
19–50 years	700	550	300	1600	3500	2500	8.7	9.5	1.2	75	140
50+ years	700	550	300	1600	3500	2500	8.7	9.5	1.2	75	140
Females											
11–14 years	800	625	280	1600	3100	2500	14.8[5]	9.0	0.8	45	130
15–18 years	800	625	300	1600	3500	2500	14.8[5]	7.0	1.0	60	140
19–50 years	700	550	270	1600	3500	2500	14.8[5]	7.0	1.2	60	140
50+ years	700	550	270	1600	3500	2500	8.7	7.0	1.2	60	140
Pregnancy	–*	–*	–*	–*	–*	–*	–*	–*	–*	–*	–*
Lactation											
0–4 months	+550	+440	+50	–*	–*	–*	–*	+6.0	+0.3	+15	–*
4+ months	+550	+440	+50	–*j719	–*	–*	–*				

6.2.3 Nutrient content of food portions

Table 6.11 Food portions containing approximately 6 g or 2 g protein

Food	Portion size	Protein/portion (g)	Approximate energy/portion (kcal)
Milk	180 ml	6	115 (full-fat) 85 (semi-skimmed) 60 (skimmed)
Cheddar cheese	25 g	6	100
Yoghurt	125 g	6	125
Egg	50 g (1 small egg)	6	70
Meat/poultry; lean, cooked	25 g	6	40
White fish	35 g	6	30
Baked beans	120 g	6	100
Peas	100 g	6	70
Bread (1 large thin slice)	25 g	2	50
Pasta (boiled)	50 g	2	50
Rice (boiled)	100 g	2	140
Most breakfast cereals	25 g	2	90
Digestive biscuits	15 g (1 biscuit)	2	70
Potatoes	140 g	2	100
Crisps	30 g	2	160

Table 6.12 Food portions containing approximately 10 g carbohydrate

Food	Portion providing about 10 g carbohydrate	Approximate energy content (kcal)
White bread	20 g (1 large thin slice)	50
Wholemeal bread	25 g (1 small thin slice)	50
Wholewheat breakfast cereal	20 g (5 tablespoons)	50
Cornflakes/plain breakfast cereal	10 g (5 tablespoons)	40
Muesli	15 g (2 tablespoons)	50
Rice (cooked)	30 g (1 tablespoon)	40
Pasta (cooked)	50 g (2 tablespoons)	50
Baked beans	70 g (3 tablespoons)	60
Potato (boiled)	50 g (1 egg-sized)	40
Potato (chips)	25 g (4 large chips)	65
Milk	200 ml	130 (full-fat) 90 (semi-skimmed) 65 (skimmed)
Fresh fruit	120–150g (1 medium-sized piece of fruit or serving)	50
Dried fruit	15 g (1 tablespoon)	40
Unsweetened fruit juice	100 ml (1 wine glass)	40
Digestive biscuits	15 g (1 biscuit)	70
Plain/semi-sweet biscuits	15 g (2 biscuits)	60
Sponge cake	20 g	90
Fruit cake	16 g	60
Sugar-containing soft drinks (squash/fizzy)	100 ml (1 small glass)	40
Pastry	15 g	80
Flour	10 g	40

Table 6.13 Food portions containing approximately 4 mmol potassium

Food	Portion size providing about 4 mmol potassium	Food	Portion size providing about 4 mmol potassium
Milk	100 ml	Wholemeal bread	70 g
Yoghurt	60 g	Apple	125 g
Cheddar cheese	130 g	Orange with skin	100 g
Egg	100 g (2 small eggs)	Grapes/orange without skin	50 g
Meat/fish	50 g	Potato boiled	50 g
White flour	120 g	Orange juice	100 ml
Wholemeal flour	45 g	Tomato juice	60 ml
White bread	160 g		

6.2.4 E number classification system

(See Section 2.11.5 in Food and nutrition labelling.)

Summary of E number classification

E 100–180	Colours
E 200–283	Preservatives
E 300–321	Antioxidants
E 322–495	Emulsifiers, stabilizers, acidity regulators, thickeners
E 950–969	Artificial sweeteners

Table 6.14 Commonly used additives

Type of additive	E number	Chemical name	Type of additive	E number	Chemical name
Colours				E227	Calcium hydrogen sulphite (calcium bisulphite)
Natural/nature-identical colours	E101	Riboflavin (yellow)	Nitrites and nitrates	E249	Potassium nitrite
	E100	Curcumin (yellow)		E250	Sodium nitrite
	E120	Cochineal (red)		E251	Sodium nitrate
	E140	Chlorophyll (green)		E252	Potassium nitrate
	E150a	Plain caramel (brown/black)	Acetic, lactic and propionic acid derivatives	E260–E263	Acetic acid and acetates
	E153	Carbon (black)		E270	Lactic acid
	E160a	Alpha-, beta- and gamma-carotene (yellow/orange)		E280–E283	Propionic acid and propionates
	E160b	Annatto (yellow/red)	**Antioxidants**		
	E160c	Capsanthin (paprika extract) (red/orange)	Ascorbic acid and derivatives	E300	Ascorbic acid (vitamin C)
	E160d	Lycopene (red extract from tomatoes)		E301–E304	Ascorbates and ascorbyl palmitate
	E162	Beetroot red (betanin) (purple/red)	Tocopherols	E306	Vitamin E
	E163	Anthocyanins (red/blue/violet)		E307–E309	Synthetic tocopherols
Synthetic colours	E102	Tartrazine[1] (yellow)	Gallates	E310–E312	Propyl, octyl and dodecyl gallates
	E104	Quinoline Yellow[1]	BHA/BHT	E320	Butylated hydroxyanisole (BHA)
	E110	Sunset Yellow FCF[1]			
	E122	Carmoisine (Azorubine)[1] (red)		E321	Butylated hydroxytoluene (BHT)
	E123	Amaranth[1] (purple/red)			
	E124	Ponceau 4R[1] (red)	**Emulsifiers and stabilizers**		
	E127	Erythrosine[1] (pink/red)	Emulsifier	E322	Lecithins
	E128	Red 2G[1]	Acidity regulators, buffers, stabilizers	E325–E327	Sodium, potassium and calcium lactate
	E129	Allura Red AC[1]			
	E132	Indigo carmine (Indigotine)[1] (blue)		E330–E333	Citric acid; sodium, potassium and calcium citrates
	E142	Green S[1]		E334–E337	Tartaric acid; sodium and potassium tartrates
	E150b–d	Caustic sulphite caramel; ammonia caramel; sulphite ammonia caramel (brown/black)		E338–E341	Phosphoric acid; sodium, potassium and calcium phosphates and orthophosphates
	E151	Black PN[1]			
	E154	Brown FK[1]		E350–E352	Sodium, potassium and calcium malates
	E155	Brown HT[1]			
	E180	Litholrubine BK (Pigment Rubine; Rubine)[1]	Gelling agents	E401–E405	Sodium, ammonium, potassium and calcium alginates
Preservatives					
Sorbic acid and derivatives	E200	Sorbic acid		E406	Agar
	E201–E203	Sodium, potassium and calcium sorbates		E407	Carrageenan
Benzoic acid and derivatives	E210	Benzoic acid	Gums	E410	Locust bean gum
	E211–E213	Sodium, potassium and calcium benzoates		E412	Guar gum
	E214–E219	Ethyl, methyl or propyl hydroxybenzoates		E413	Tragacanth
				E414	Gum arabic
				E415	Xanthan gum
Sulphur dioxide and derivatives	E220	Sulphur dioxide	Emulsifiers and stabilizers	E471–E477	Esters and glycerides of fatty acids (e.g. monoglycerides and diglycerides of fatty acids or glyceryl monostearate and distearate)
	E221	Sodium sulphite			
	E222	Sodium hydrogen sulphite (sodium bisulphite)			
	E223	Sodium metabisulphite			
	E224	Potassium metabisulphite			
	E226	Calcium sulphite			

[1]Azo dye (see Section 4.35.8 in Food Exclusion in the management of allergy and intolerance).

6.3 Body mass index reference data

$$\text{Body mass index (BMI)} = \frac{\text{weight kg}}{(\text{height m})^2}$$

Interpretation of BMI
<16   Severely underweight
16–19   Underweight
20–25   Normal range
26–30   Overweight
31–40   Obese
>40   Morbidly obese
(but see Section 1.8.4 in Assessment of nutritional status)

An accompanying waist circumference >94 cm (37 inches) in men and >80 cm (32 inches) in women is indicative of central obesity.

Table 6.15 Body mass index (BMI) ready reference table

	BMI	Weight (kg)																						
Morbidly obese (BMI >40)	45	102	104	107	110	113	116	119	121	124	127	131	134	137	140	143	146	150	153	156	159	163	170	173
	44	99	102	105	108	110	113	116	119	122	125	128	131	134	137	140	143	146	149	153	156	159	166	169
	43	97	100	102	105	108	111	113	116	119	122	125	128	131	134	137	140	143	146	149	152	156	162	166
	42	95	97	100	103	105	108	111	113	116	119	122	125	128	131	134	137	140	143	146	149	152	159	162
	41	93	95	98	100	103	105	108	111	113	116	119	122	125	127	130	133	136	139	142	145	148	155	158
Obese (BMI 31–40)	40	90	93	95	98	100	103	105	108	111	113	116	119	122	124	127	130	133	136	139	142	145	151	154
	39	88	91	93	95	98	100	103	105	108	111	113	116	119	121	124	127	130	132	135	138	141	147	150
	38	86	88	91	93	95	98	100	103	105	108	110	113	115	118	121	124	126	129	132	135	138	143	146
	37	84	86	88	90	93	95	98	100	102	105	107	110	112	115	118	120	123	126	128	131	134	140	143
	36	81	84	86	88	90	93	95	97	100	102	104	107	109	112	115	117	120	122	125	128	130	136	139
	35	79	81	83	86	88	90	92	95	97	99	102	104	106	109	111	114	116	119	122	124	127	132	135
	34	77	79	81	83	85	87	90	92	94	96	99	101	103	106	108	111	113	116	118	121	123	128	131
	33	75	77	79	81	83	85	87	89	91	94	96	98	100	103	105	107	110	112	115	117	120	125	127
	32	72	74	76	78	80	82	84	87	89	91	93	95	97	100	102	104	106	109	111	114	116	121	123
	31	70	72	74	76	78	80	82	84	86	88	90	92	94	96	99	101	103	105	108	110	112	117	120
Overweight (BMI 26–30)	30	68	70	72	73	75	77	79	81	83	85	87	89	91	93	96	98	100	102	104	106	109	113	116
	29	66	67	69	71	73	75	77	78	80	82	84	86	88	90	92	94	97	99	101	103	105	110	112
	28	63	65	67	69	70	72	74	76	78	79	81	83	85	87	89	91	93	95	97	99	102	106	108
	27	61	63	64	66	68	70	71	73	75	77	78	80	82	84	86	88	90	92	94	96	98	102	104
	26	59	61	62	64	65	67	69	70	72	74	76	77	79	81	83	85	87	88	90	92	94	98	100
Normal weight (BMI 20–25)	25	57	58	60	61	63	64	66	68	69	71	73	74	76	78	80	81	83	85	87	89	91	95	96
	24	54	56	57	59	60	62	63	65	67	68	70	71	73	75	76	78	80	82	83	85	87	91	93
	23	52	54	55	56	58	59	61	62	64	65	67	68	70	72	73	75	77	78	80	82	83	87	89
	22	50	51	53	54	55	57	58	60	61	63	64	66	67	69	70	72	73	75	77	78	80	83	85
	21	48	49	50	52	53	54	56	57	58	60	61	63	64	65	67	68	70	72	73	75	76	79	81
	20	45	47	48	49	50	52	53	54	56	57	58	60	61	62	64	65	67	68	70	71	73	76	77
Underweight (BMI 16–19)	19	43	44	46	47	48	49	50	52	53	54	55	57	58	59	61	62	63	65	66	68	69	72	73
	18	41	42	43	44	45	47	48	49	50	51	52	54	55	56	57	59	60	61	63	64	65	68	70
	17	39	40	41	42	43	44	45	46	47	48	50	51	52	53	54	56	57	58	59	61	62	64	66
	16	36	37	38	39	40	41	42	43	45	46	47	48	49	50	51	52	53	55	56	57	58	61	62
Severely under-weight (BMI <16)	15	34	35	36	37	38	39	40	41	42	43	44	45	46	47	48	49	50	51	52	53	55	57	58
	14	32	33	34	35	35	36	37	38	39	40	41	42	43	44	45	46	47	48	49	50	51	53	54
	13	30	30	31	32	33	34	35	35	36	37	38	39	40	41	42	43	44	44	45	46	47	49	50
	12	27	28	29	30	30	31	32	33	34	34	35	36	37	38	38	39	40	41	42	43	44	46	47
	11	25	26	27	27	28	29	29	30	31	31	32	33	34	35	35	36	37	38	39	39	40	42	43
	10	23	24	24	25	25	26	27	27	28	29	29	30	31	31	32	33	34	34	35	36	37	38	39
Height (m)		1.5	1.52	1.54	1.56	1.58	1.6	1.62	1.64	1.66	1.68	1.7	1.72	1.74	1.76	1.78	1.8	1.82	1.84	1.86	1.88	1.9	1.94	1.96
Height (feet inches)		4 11	5 0	5 1	5 1½	5 2¼	5 3	5 3¼	5 4½	5 5½	5 6	5 7	5 7¼	5 8½	5 9¼	5 10	5 11	5 11¾	6 0½	6 1¼	6 2	6 3	6 4½	6 5½

6.4 Anthropometric reference data

6.4.1 Demiquet and Mindex

These can be used as an index of adiposity in elderly people (see Section 1.8.4 in Assessment of nutritional status).

$$\text{Demiquet} = \frac{\text{Weight kg}}{(\text{Demispan m})^2}$$

$$\text{Mindex} = \frac{\text{Weight kg}}{\text{Demispan m}}$$

6.4.2 Upper arm anthropometry

For measurement techniques and discussion see Section 1.8.4 in Assessment of nutritional status.

References

Bishop CW *et al. American Journal of Clinical Nutrition* 1981; **34**: 2530–2539.
Griffith CDM, Clark RG. *Clinical Nutrition* 1984; **3**: 147–151.
Klidjian AM *et al. British Medical Journal* 1980; **281**: 899–901.
Lehmann AB *et al. Clinical Nutrition* 1991; **1**: 18–23.

Table 6.16 Distribution of Demiquet and Mindex in a normal population over the age 65 years (Data derived from Lehmann *et al.* 1991)

	Percentile						Percentile				
	10th	30th	50th	70th	90th		10th	30th	50th	70th	90th
Men (Demiquet kg/m^2)						Women (Mindex kg/m)					
64–74 years	87.6	99.6	106.7	117.1	130.7	64–74 years	68.3	77.8	84.8	92.3	110.6
75+ years	84.5	98.9	106.3	113.4	125.0	75+ years	63.1	73.6	81.7	88.4	102.2

Table 6.17 Triceps skinfold thickness (TSF) (Data derived from Bishop *et al.* 1981)

Men		Centile						
Age (years)	Mean (mm)	5th	10th	25th	50th	75th	90th	95th
18–74	12.0	4.5	6.0	8.0	11.0	15.0	20.0	23.0
18–24	11.2	4.0	5.0	7.0	9.5	14.0	20.0	23.0
25–34	12.6	4.5	5.5	8.0	12.0	16.0	21.5	24.0
35–44	12.4	5.0	6.0	8.5	12.0	15.5	20.0	23.0
45–54	12.4	5.0	6.0	8.0	11.0	15.0	20.0	25.5
55–64	11.6	5.0	6.0	8.0	11.0	14.0	18.0	21.5
65–74	11.8	4.5	5.5	8.0	11.0	15.0	19.0	22.0

Women		Centile						
Age (years)	Mean (mm)	5th	10th	25th	50th	75th	90th	95th
18–74	23.0	11.0	13.0	17.0	22.0	28.0	34.0	37.5
18–24	19.4	9.4	11.0	14.0	18.0	24.0	30.0	34.0
25–34	21.9	10.5	12.0	16.0	21.0	26.5	33.5	37.0
35–44	24.0	12.0	14.0	18.0	23.0	29.5	35.5	39.0
45–54	25.4	13.0	15.0	20.0	25.0	30.0	36.0	40.0
55–64	24.9	11.0	14.0	19.0	25.0	30.5	35.0	39.0
65–74	23.3	11.5	14.0	18.0	23.0	28.0	33.0	36.0

Table 6.18 Mid-arm circumference (MAC) (Data derived from Bishop *et al.* 1981).

Men		Centile						
Age (years)	Mean (cm)	5th	10th	25th	50th	75th	90th	95th
18–74	31.8	26.4	27.6	29.6	31.7	33.9	36.0	37.3
18–24	30.9	25.7	27.1	28.7	30.7	32.9	35.5	37.4
25–34	30.5	25.3	26.5	28.5	30.7	32.4	34.4	35.5
35–44	32.3	27.0	28.2	30.0	32.0	34.4	36.5	37.6
45–54	32.7	27.8	28.7	30.7	32.7	34.8	36.3	37.1
55–64	32.1	26.7	27.8	30.0	32.0	34.2	36.2	37.6
65–74	31.5	25.6	27.3	29.6	31.7	33.4	35.2	36.6
Women		Centile						
Age (years)	Mean (cm)	5th	10th	25th	50th	75th	90th	95th
18–74	29.4	23.2	24.3	26.2	28.7	31.9	35.2	37.8
18–24	27.0	22.1	23.0	24.5	26.4	28.8	31.7	34.3
25–34	28.6	23.3	24.2	25.7	27.8	30.4	34.1	37.2
35–44	30.0	24.1	25.2	26.8	29.2	32.2	36.2	38.5
45–54	30.7	24.3	25.7	27.5	30.3	32.9	36.8	39.3
55–64	30.7	23.9	25.1	27.7	30.2	33.3	36.3	38.2
65–74	30.1	23.8	25.2	27.4	29.9	32.5	35.3	37.2

Table 6.19 Mid-arm muscle circumference (MAMC)
MAMC cm = MAC cm − (TSF mm × 0.314)
(Data derived from Bishop *et al.* 1981)

Men		Centile						
Age (years)	Mean (cm)	5th	10th	25th	50th	75th	90th	95th
18–74	28.0	23.8	24.8	26.3	27.9	29.6	31.4	32.5
18–24	27.4	23.5	24.4	25.8	27.2	28.9	30.8	32.3
25–34	28.3	24.2	25.3	26.5	28.0	30.0	31.7	32.9
35–44	28.8	25.0	25.6	27.1	28.7	30.3	32.1	33.0
45–54	28.2	24.0	24.9	26.5	28.1	29.8	31.5	32.6
55–64	27.8	22.8	24.4	26.2	27.9	29.6	31.0	31.8
65–74	26.8	22.5	23.7	25.3	26.9	28.5	29.9	30.7
Women		Centile						
Age (years)	Mean (cm)	5th	10th	25th	50th	75th	90th	95th
18–74	22.2	18.4	19.0	20.2	21.8	23.6	25.8	27.4
18–24	20.9	17.7	18.5	19.4	20.6	22.1	23.6	24.9
25–34	21.7	18.3	18.9	20.0	21.4	22.9	24.9	26.6
35–44	22.5	18.5	19.2	20.6	22.0	24.0	26.1	27.4
45–54	22.7	18.8	19.5	20.7	22.2	24.3	26.6	27.8
55–64	22.8	18.6	19.5	20.8	22.6	24.4	26.3	28.1
65–74	22.8	18.6	19.5	20.8	22.5	24.4	26.5	28.1

Table 6.20 Dynamometry (grip strength) (Data derived from Klidjian *et al.* 1980; Griffith and Clark 1984)

Age (years)	Normal values (kg)	85% of normal[1] (kg)	Age (years)	Normal values (kg)	85% of normal[1] (kg)
Men			Women		
18–69	40.0	34.0	18–69	27.5	23.0
70–79	32.5	27.5	70–79	25.0	21.0
80+	22.5	19.0	80+	20.0	17.0

[1]Values at or below this level are indicative of protein malnutrition.

To estimate energy requirements in clinical situations based on Schofield equations (see Section 1.10.1 in Estimating nutritional requirements):

1 Estimate basal metabolic rate (BMR) for healthy adults.
2 Adjust for stress using the Elia nomogram
3 Add a combined factor for activity and dietary-induced thermogenesis:

    Bedbound, immobile   + 10%
    Bedbound, mobile or sitting + 15–20%
    Mobile, on ward   + 25%

Table 6.21 enables the BMR (kcal/24 hours) of a healthy individual to be predicted from weight and age.

The Elia nomogram (Fig. 6.1) provides a guide to the required adjustment in BMR for the level of metabolic stress.

Reference

Elia M. Artificial nutritional support, *Medicine* 1990; **82**: 3394.

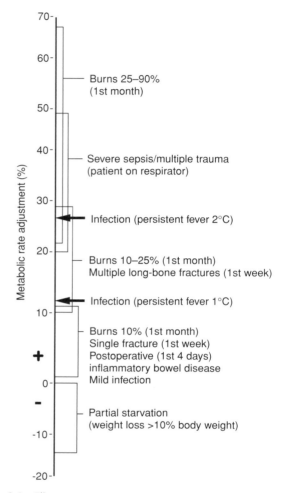

Fig. 6.1 Elia nomogram
From Elia (1990); reproduced with permission.

6.5 Energy prediction reference data

Table 6.21 Basal metabolic rate (BMR) ready reference table

Age (years) Weight (kg)	Men					Women				
	10–17	18–29	30–59	60–74	74+	10–17	18–29	30–59	60–74	74+
25	1100	1070	1161	998	1031	1027	857	1054	917	869
26	1117	1085	1172	1009	1039	1040	872	1062	926	879
27	1135	1100	1184	1021	1048	1054	887	1070	935	889
28	1153	1115	1195	1033	1056	1067	901	1078	945	898
29	1170	1130	1207	1045	1065	1081	916	1087	954	908
30	1188	1145	1218	1057	1073	1094	931	1095	963	918
31	1206	1160	1230	1069	1081	1107	946	1103	972	928
32	1223	1175	1241	1081	1090	1121	961	1112	981	938
33	1241	1190	1253	1093	1098	1134	975	1120	991	947
34	1259	1205	1264	1105	1107	1148	990	1128	1000	957
35	1277	1221	1276	1117	1115	1161	1005	1137	1009	967
36	1294	1236	1287	1128	1123	1174	1020	1145	1018	977
37	1312	1251	1299	1140	1132	1188	1035	1153	1027	987
38	1330	1266	1310	1152	1140	1201	1049	1161	1037	996
39	1347	1281	1322	1164	1149	1215	1064	1170	1046	1006
40	1365	1296	1333	1176	1157	1228	1079	1178	1055	1016
41	1383	1311	1345	1188	1165	1241	1094	1186	1064	1026
42	1400	1326	1356	1200	1174	1255	1109	1195	1073	1036
43	1418	1341	1368	1212	1182	1268	1123	1203	1083	1045
44	1436	1356	1379	1224	1191	1282	1138	1211	1092	1055
45	1454	1372	1391	1236	1199	1295	1153	1220	1101	1065
46	1471	1387	1402	1247	1207	1308	1168	1228	1110	1075
47	1489	1402	1414	1259	1216	1322	1183	1236	1119	1085
48	1507	1417	1425	1271	1224	1335	1197	1244	1129	1094
49	1524	1432	1437	1283	1233	1349	1212	1253	1138	1104
50	1542	1447	1448	1295	1241	1362	1227	1261	1147	1114
51	1560	1462	1460	1307	1249	1375	1242	1269	1156	1124
52	1577	1477	1471	1319	1258	1389	1257	1278	1165	1134
53	1595	1492	1483	1331	1266	1402	1271	1286	1175	1143
54	1613	1507	1494	1343	1275	1416	1286	1294	1184	1153
55	1631	1523	1506	1355	1283	1429	1301	1303	1193	1163
56	1648	1538	1517	1366	1291	1442	1316	1311	1202	1173
57	1666	1553	1529	1378	1300	1456	1331	1319	1211	1183
58	1684	1568	1540	1390	1308	1469	1345	1327	1221	1192
59	1701	1583	1552	1402	1317	1483	1360	1336	1230	1202
60	1719	1598	1563	1414	1325	1496	1375	1344	1239	1212
61	1737	1613	1575	1426	1333	1509	1390	1352	1248	1222
62	1754	1628	1586	1438	1342	1523	1405	1361	1257	1232
63	1772	1643	1598	1450	1350	1536	1419	1369	1267	1241
64	1790	1658	1609	1462	1359	1550	1434	1377	1276	1251
65	1808	1674	1621	1474	1367	1563	1449	1386	1285	1261
66	1825	1689	1632	1485	1375	1576	1464	1394	1294	1271
67	1843	1704	1644	1497	1384	1590	1479	1402	1303	1281
68	1861	1719	1655	1509	1392	1603	1493	1410	1313	1290
69	1878	1734	1667	1521	1401	1617	1508	1419	1322	1300
70	1896	1749	1678	1533	1409	1630	1523	1427	1331	1310
71	1914	1764	1690	1545	1417	1643	1538	1435	1340	1320
72	1931	1779	1701	1557	1426	1657	1553	1444	1349	1330
73	1949	1794	1713	1569	1434	1670	1567	1452	1359	1339
74	1967	1809	1724	1581	1443	1684	1582	1460	1368	1349
75	1985	1825	1736	1593	1451	1697	1597	1469	1377	1359
76	2002	1840	1747	1604	1459	1710	1612	1477	1386	1369
77	2020	1855	1759	1616	1468	1724	1627	1485	1395	1379
78	2038	1870	1770	1628	1476	1737	1641	1493	1405	1388
79	2055	1885	1782	1640	1485	1751	1656	1502	1414	1398
80	2073	1900	1793	1652	1493	1764	1671	1510	1423	1408
81	2091	1915	1805	1664	1501	1777	1686	1518	1432	1418
82	2108	1930	1816	1676	1510	1791	1701	1527	1441	1428
83	2126	1945	1828	1688	1518	1804	1715	1535	1451	1437
84	2144	1960	1839	1700	1527	1818	1730	1543	1460	1447
85	2162	1976	1851	1712	1535	1831	1745	1552	1469	1457
86	2179	1991	1862	1723	1543	1844	1760	1560	1478	1467
87	2197	2006	1874	1735	1552	1858	1775	1568	1487	1477
88	2215	2021	1885	1747	1560	1871	1789	1576	1497	1486

Table 6.21   Continued

Age (years) Weight (kg)	Men					Women				
	10–17	18–29	30–59	60–74	74+	10–17	18–29	30–59	60–74	74+
89	2232	2036	1897	1759	1569	1885	1804	1585	1506	1496
90	2250	2051	1908	1771	1577	1898	1819	1593	1515	1506
91	2268	2066	1920	1783	1585	1911	1834	1601	1524	1516
92	2285	2081	1931	1795	1594	1925	1849	1610	1533	1526
93	2303	2096	1943	1807	1602	1938	1863	1618	1543	1535
94	2321	2111	1954	1819	1611	1952	1878	1626	1552	1545
95	2339	2127	1966	1831	1619	1965	1893	1635	1561	1555
96	2356	2142	1977	1842	1627	1978	1908	1643	1570	1565
97	2374	2157	1989	1854	1636	1992	1923	1651	1579	1575
98	2392	2172	2000	1866	1644	2005	1937	1659	1589	1584
99	2409	2187	2012	1878	1653	2019	1952	1668	1598	1594

Data are kcal/24 hours.
The deviation from the predicted value may be greater at the extremes of body composition. There are limited data on the BMR of individuals with body weights greater than 80 kg.
   Discussion on the use of these tables is given in Section 1.10.1.

6.6 Clinical chemistry reference data

6.6.1 Millimoles, milligrams and milliequivalents

Millimoles

1 millimole (mmol) = atomic weight in mg

To convert:

mg to mmol — Divide mg by the atomic weight
mmol to mg — Multiply mmol by the atomic weight

Milliequivalents

1 milliequivalent (mEq) = atomic weight in mg divided by the valency

To convert:

mg to mEq — (mg × valency)/atomic weight
mEq to mg — (mEq × atomic weight)/valency

For minerals with a valency of 1, mEq = mmol
For minerals with a valency of 2, mEq = mmol × 2

6.6.2 Osmolarity and osmolality

Osmolality is the number of osmotically active particles (milliosmoles) in a *kilogram* of *solvent*. Osmolarity is the number of osmotically active particles in a *litre* of *solution* (i.e. solvent + solute).

In body fluids, there is only a small difference between the two. However, in commercially prepared feeds, osmolality is always much higher than osmolarity. Osmolality is therefore the preferred term for comparing the potential hypertonic effect of liquid diets (although, in practice, it is often osmolarity which is stated).

The osmolality of a liquid feed is considerably influenced by the content of amino acids and electrolytes such as sodium and potassium. Carbohydrates with a small particle size (e.g. simple sugars) increase osmolality more than complex carbohydrates with a higher molecular weight. Fats do not increase the osmolality of solutions because of their insolubility in water.

The osmolality of plasma is normally in the range of 280–300 mosmol/kg and the body attempts to keep the osmolality of the contents of the stomach and intestine at an isotonic level. It does this by producing intestinal secretions which dilute a concentrated meal or drink. If enteral

Table 6.22 Atomic weights and valencies of some minerals and trace elements

Mineral	Atomic weight	Valency
Sodium	23.0	1
Potassium	39.0	1
Phosphorus	31.0	2
Calcium	40.0	2
Magnesium	24.3	2
Chlorine	35.4	1
Sulphur	32.0	2
Zinc	65.4	2

Table 6.23 Mineral content of compounds and solutions

Solution/compound	Mineral content	
1 g sodium chloride	393 mg Na	(17.1 mmol Na^+)
1 g sodium bicarbonate	274 mg Na	(12 mmol Na^+)
1 g potassium bicarbonate	390 mg K	(10 mmol K^+)
1 g calcium chloride (dihydrate)	273 mg Ca	(6.8 mmol Ca^{2+})
1 g calcium carbonate	400 mg Ca	(10 mmol Ca^{2+})
1 g calcium gluconate	89 mg Ca	(2.2 mmol Ca^{2+})
1 litre normal saline	3450 mg Na	(150 mmol Na^+)

Table 6.24 Conversion factors for millimoles, milligrams and milliequivalents

Mineral	mg/mmol		mg/mEq		mmol/mEq	
	mg =	mmol =	mg =	mEq =	mmol =	mEq =
Sodium	mmol × 23	mg ÷ 23	mEq x 23	mg ÷ 23	mEq	mmol
Potassium	mmol × 29	mg ÷ 39	mEq × 39	mg ÷ 39	mEq	mmol
Phosphorus	mmol × 31	mg ÷ 31	mEq × 15.5	mg ÷ 15.5	mEq ÷ 2	mmol × 2
Calcium	mmol × 40	mg ÷ 40	mEq × 20	mg ÷ 20	mEq ÷ 2	mmol × 2
Magnesium	mmol × 24.3	mg ÷ 24.3	mEq × 12.15	mg ÷ 12.15	mEq ÷ 2	mmol × 2
Chlorine	mmol × 35.4	mg ÷ 35.4	mEq × 35.4	mg ÷ 35.4	mEq	mmol
Sulphur	mmol × 32	mg ÷ 32	mEq × 16	mg ÷ 16	mEq ÷ 2	mmol × 2
Zinc	mmol × 65.4	mg ÷ 65.4	mEq × 32.7	mg ÷ 32.7	mEq ÷ 2	mmol × 2

feeds with a high osmolality are administered, large quantities of intestinal secretions will be produced rapidly in order to reduce the osmolality. In order to avoid diarrhoea, it is therefore important to administer such feeds slowly; the number of mosmoles given per unit of time is more important than the number of mosmoles per unit of volume.

6.6.3 Biochemical and haematological reference ranges

The results of laboratory tests are interpreted by comparison to reference or normal ranges. These are usually defined as the mean ±2 SD (standard deviation), which assumes a Gaussian or normal (symmetrical) type distribution (Fig. 6.2). Unfortunately, most biological data have a skewed rather than a symmetrical distribution and more complex statistical calculations are required to define the reference ranges.

The reference ranges as defined usually include approximately 95% of the normal 'healthy' population; consequently, 5% of this population will have values outside the reference range but cannot be said to be abnormal. The use of reference ranges may be illustrated by taking the reference range of blood urea as 3.3–6.7 mmol/l. Approximately 95% of the normal 'healthy' population would come within these limits. However, it would be wrong to interpret a value of 6.4 mmol/l as normal while assuming a value of 7.0 mmol/l to be abnormal. Nature 'abhors abrupt transitions', so there is no clear-cut division between 'normal' and abnormal'. This applies equally well to body weight and height and also to measurements undertaken in the laboratory.

The majority of the normal 'healthy' population will have results close to the mean value for the population as a whole and all values will be distributed around that mean. Therefore, the probability that a value is abnormal increases the further it is from the mean value (Fig. 6.3).

A variety of factors can cause variation in the biochemical and haematological constituents present within the blood. These can be conveniently divided into factors causing variation within an individual and those causing variation between groups of individuals.

Variations within individuals

The following factors can cause significant variation in clinical biochemical and haematological data and should be considered when interpreting individual results.

Diet
Variation in diet can affect the levels of triglycerides, cholesterol, glucose, urea and other blood constituents.

Drugs
These can have significant effects on a number of biochemical determinations, often resulting from secondary effects on sensitive organs, e.g. liver, kidney and endocrine glands. Steroids, including oral contraceptives, can cause variations in a number of biochemical and haematological parameters, including a reduction in albumin, increases in several carrier proteins, e.g. transcortin, thyroxine binding globulin, caeruloplasmin and transferrin, as well as increases in coagulation factors, e.g. fibrinogen, factor VII and factor X.

Menstrual cycle
Several biochemical constituents show marked variations

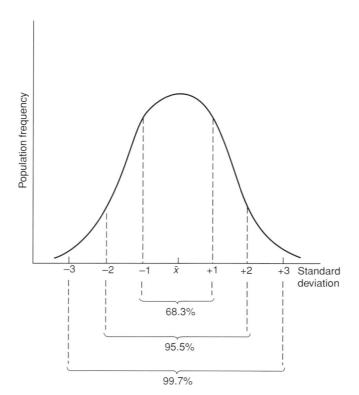

Fig. 6.2 Normal or Gaussian distribution curve.

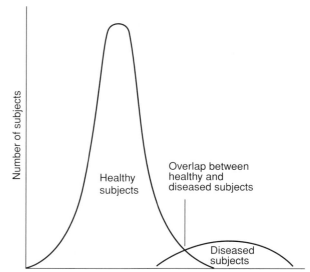

Fig. 6.3 Theoretical distribution of results from healthy and diseased subjects.

with the phase of the cycle; these include the pituitary gonadotrophins, ovarian steroids and their metabolites. There is also a marked fall in plasma iron just before and during menstruation. This is probably caused by hormonal changes rather than blood loss.

Muscular exercise

Moderate exercise can cause increases in levels of potassium, together with a number of enzymes including aspartate transferase, lactate dehydrogenase, creatine kinase and hydroxybutyrate dehydrogenase.

Posture

Significant differences in the concentration of many blood constituents may be obtained by collecting blood samples from ambulant compared with recumbent individuals. The red cell and white cell counts, together with the concentration of proteins (e.g. albumin, immunoglobulins) and protein-bound substances (e.g. calcium, cholesterol, T_4, cortisol), may decrease by up to 15% following 30 minutes of recumbency. This is probably due to fluid redistribution within the body. Hospitalized patients usually have their blood samples collected early in the morning following overnight recumbency, and consequently have significantly lower values than the normal ambulant (outpatient) population.

Stress

Both emotional and physical stress can alter circulating biochemical constituents, causing increases in the levels of pituitary hormones [e.g. adrenocorticotropic hormone (ACTH, prolactin, growth hormone] and adrenal steroids (cortisol).

Time of day

Some substances exhibit a marked circadian (diurnal) variation which is independent of meals or other activities, e.g. serum cortisol, iron and the amino acids tyrosine, phenylalanine and tryptophan. Cortisol levels are at their highest in the morning (9 am) and at their lowest levels at midnight, while iron concentration may decrease by 50% between the morning and evening. Plasma phenylalanine levels are at their lowest after midnight and reach their highest concentrations between 8.30 and 10.30 am.

Variations between groups of individuals

Several factors influence the reference values quoted for individuals. These include age, sex and race.

Age

The blood levels of many biochemical and haematological constituents are age related; these include haemoglobin, total leucocyte count, creatinine, urea, inorganic phosphate and many enzymes, e.g. alkaline phosphatase, creatine kinase and γ-glutamyl transferase. Haemoglobin levels and total leucocyte counts are highest in the newborn and gradually decrease through childhood, reaching

the adult reference range at puberty. As creatinine is related to muscle mass, paediatric reference ranges are lower than those of adults. Urea levels rise slightly with age but this may well indicate impaired renal function. Alkaline phosphatase activity and inorganic phosphate levels are at their highest during childhood, reaching peak levels at puberty.

Gender

Many biochemical and haematological parameters show concentration differences which are sex dependent, including creatinine, iron, urea, urea and the various sex hormones. Ferritin, haemoglobin and red cell counts are slightly higher in males than in females. Creatinine and urea levels are 15–20% lower in premenopausal females than in males. Premenopausal females also have lower serum iron levels than males, but after the menopause iron levels are similar in both sexes.

Race

Racial differences have been reported in some biochemical constituents, including cholesterol and protein. The reference ranges for cholesterol are higher in Europeans than in similar groups of Japanese. Similarly, the Bantu Africans have higher serum globulins than corresponding Europeans. African and Middle-Eastern individuals have lower total leucocyte and neutrophil counts than other races. Some of these racial differences are probably genetic in origin, although the environment and diet may also be contributory factors.

Laboratory variations

Methods of analysis and standardizations vary considerably from laboratory to laboratory. These differences will influence the quoted reference ranges, and therefore readers are advised to use only those quoted by their local laboratory. Local reference ranges may be at variance with the levels quoted in the following tables.

Correction of serum calcium for low albumin

Corrected serum calcium level (mmol/l)
$$= \begin{matrix} \text{Measured serum} \\ \text{calcium (mmol/l)} \end{matrix} + \left(\frac{40 - \text{measured albumin}}{40} \right)$$

An alternative (and possibly more accurate) formula is:

Corrected serum calcium level (mmol/l)
$$= \begin{matrix} \text{Measured serum} \\ \text{calcium (mmol/l)} \end{matrix} + \left[\left(\begin{matrix} 40 - \text{measured} \\ \text{albumin} \end{matrix} \right) \times 0.02 \right]$$

To be even more accurate, the serum protein level should be considered as well

Corrected serum calcium level (mmol/l)
$$= \begin{matrix} \text{Measured serum} \\ \text{calcium (mmol/l)} \end{matrix} + \left[\left(\begin{matrix} 72 - \text{measured} \\ \text{protein} \end{matrix} \right) \times 0.02 \right]$$

This corrected calcium value should be added to that

obtained from the correction for low albumin, and a mean of the two levels obtained, calculated to two decimal places.

Table 6.25 Serum/plasma levels: general biochemistry

Blood constituent	Gender	Range	Units
Albumim		35–45	g/l
Bicarbonate		22–32	mmol/l
Bilirubin		<17	μmol/l
Calcium		2.25–2.65	mmol/l
Chloride		95–105	mmol/l
Cholesterol		3.5–7.8	mmol/l
Creatinine		40–130	μmol/l
Glucose (fasting)		3.0–5.0	mmol/l
Inorganic phosphate		0.8–1.4	mmol/l
Magnesium		0.7–1.0	mmol/l
Osmolality		278–305	mosmol/kg
Potassium		3.5–5.0	mmol/l
Sodium		135–150	mmol/l
Total protein		60–80	g/l
Triglycerides		0.7–1.8	mmol/l
Urate	Male	0.25–0.45	mmol/l
	Female	0.15–0.35	mmol/l
Urea		3.3–6.7	mmol/l

Table 6.26 Urine constituents

Constituent	Range	Units
Calcium	<7.5	mmol/24 hours
Creatinine	9–18	mmol/24 hours
Inorganic phosphate	15–50	mmol/24 hours
Osmolality	50–1500	mosmol/24 hours
Potassium	40–120	mmol/24 hours
Protein	<0.50	g/24 hours
Sodium	100–250	mmol/24 hours
Urate	<3.0	mmol/24 hours
Urea	250–600	mmol/24 hours

Table 6.27 Faeces constituents

Constituent	Range	Units
Faecal fat	<18	mmol/24 hours
Nitrogen	70–140	mmol/24 hours

Table 6.28 Red cells

Parameter	Age/Sex	Range	Units
Haemoglobin	Male	13.5–17.5	g/dl
	Female	11.5–15.5	g/dl
	Newborn	15–21	g/dl
	3 months	9.5–12.5	g/dl
Haematocrit (Packed cell volume; PCV)	Male	40–52	%
	Female	36–48	%
Red cell count	Male	4.5–6.3	10^{12}/l
	Female	4.2–5.4	10^{12}/l
Mean cell haemoglobin (MCH)		27–32	pg
Mean cell volume (MCV)		80–95	fl
Mean cell haemoglobin concentration (MCHC)		32–36	g/dl

6.7 Nutritional supplements and enteral feeds

Tables 6.29–6.34 provide a guide to the range of proprietary supplements, feeds and other nutritional support products currently available in the UK. It should be noted that the composition of products within a particular category will differ, and some products may be more appropriate than others in particular clinical circumstances. It should also be borne in mind that, with the passage of time, the availability and composition of some products may change and new products will appear. The information given here is therefore for guidance only, and all details should be checked before clinical usage.

Many of these products are prescribable in specified clinical circumstances and these are defined by the Advisory Committee on Borderline Substances (ACBS). Such products are termed 'ACBS prescribable' and must only be prescribed in accordance with these conditions.

Details of the current availability, composition and prescribing indications of products can be found in the British National Formulary or the Monthly Index of Medical Specialities (MIMS), or obtained directly from the manufacturers (for addresses see Appendix 6.9).

Table 6.29 Modular nutritional supplements

	Principal nutrient component(s)			
	CHO	Fat + CHO	Fat	Protein
Powdered products	Caloreen (Nestlé Clinical Nutrition) Maxijul LE Powder (SHS) (low Na, K, P and Cl) Maxijul Super Soluble Powder (SHS) Polycal Powder (Nutricia Clinical Care) Polycose (Ross)	MCT Duocal Powder (SHS) Super Soluble Duocal Powder (SHS) QuickCal (Vitaflo)		Casilan 90 (Heinz) (90% protein) Dialamine (SHS) (25% protein; 65% CHO) Maxipro Super Soluble (SHS) (80% protein) ProMod (Ross) (75% protein) Protifar (Nutricia Clinical Care) (89% protein) Renapro (Syner-Med) (>90% protein) Forceval Protein Powder (Unigreg) (55% protein + CHO) Pro-Cal (Vitaflo) (Protein /energy supplement: 13% protein + fat +CHO)
Solid products		Duobar (SHS)		
Liquid products	Maxijul Liquid (SHS) Polycal Liquid (Nutricia Clinical Care)	Duocal Liquid (SHS)	Calogen (SHS) Liquigen (SHS) (MCT emulsion) MCT Oil (Bristol-Myers; SHS) Solagen (SHS)	

Data compiled February 2001.
CHO: carbohydrate, MCT: medium-chain triglyceride.

Table 6.30 Prescribable liquid (sip feed) supplements
Note: Many sip feed supplements are available in a variety of flavours to offset taste fatigue. Some, but not all, are nutritionally complete: check compositional details before use. Some products can also be used for tube feeding.

Type of product	Product name (manufacturer)	Notes
Standard energy (1 kcal/ml)	Clinutren Iso (Nestlé Clinical Nutrition) Complan (Heinz) Ensure (Ross) Fresubin Original (Fresenius Kabi)	In cup, not carton Also available as a non-prescribable powder which can be made up with milk
Juice-type (low fat)	Clinutren Fruit (Nestlé Clinical Nutrition) Enlive (Ross) Fortijuce (Nutricia Clinical Care) Provide Xtra (Fresenius Kabi)	1.25 kcal/ml 1.25 kcal/ml 1.5 kcal/ml 1.25 kcal/ml
Fibre enriched	Enrich (Ross) Enrich Plus (Ross) Fresubin Energy Fibre (Fresenius Kabi) Resource Fibre (Novartis Consumer Health) Fortisip Multifibre (Nutricia Clinical Care)	1.25 kcal/ml 1.5 kcal/ml 1.5 kcal/ml 1.7 kcal/ml 1.5 kcal/ml
High energy	Clinutren 1.5 (Nestlé Clinical Nutrition) Ensure Plus (Ross) Fresubin Energy (Fresenius Kabi) Fortifresh (Nutricia Clinical Care) Fortisip (Nutricia Clinical Care) Resource Shake (Novartis Consumer Health) Calshake Powder (Fresenius Kabi) Scandishake (SHS) Vitasavoury (Vitaflo)	1.5 kcal/ml 1.5 kcal/ml 1.5 kcal/ml 1.55 kcal/ml (yoghurt taste) 1.5 kcal/ml 1.7 kcal/ml 2 kcal/ml when made up with milk 2 kcal/ml when made up with milk 2 kcal/ml in powdered form made up with water
High protein	Fortimel (Nutricia Clinical Care) Resource Protein Extra (Novartis Consumer Health)	1 kcal/ml; low fat 1.25 kcal/ml; low sodium and potassium

Data compiled February 2001.

Table 6.31 Prescribable solid/semi-solid supplements

Type of product	Product name (manufacturer)	Notes
Solid/semi-solid desserts	Clinutren Dessert (Nestlé Clinical Nutrition) Formance (Ross) Forticreme (Nutricia Clinical Care) Maxisorb (SHS) Resource Dessert Energy (Novartis Consumer Health)	 Powder reconstituted with water or milk to make dessert; high protein
Bar	Ensure bar (Ross)	

Data compiled February 2001.

Table 6.32 Non-prescribable liquid supplements
These products can be purchased by patients from supermarkets and chemists and are useful at times when dietary intake is poor. None is nutritionally complete.

Product name (manufacturer)	Notes
Build-up (Nestlé Clinical Nutrition) Complan Powder (Heinz) Recovery (Boots)	Made up with milk or water Made up with water A nutritionally complete ready-to-drink version is ACBS prescribable; see above Made up with water or milk

Data compiled February 2001.

Table 6.33 Enteral feeds: standard indications

Type of product	Product name (manufacturer)	Notes
Standard Energy	Ensure (Ross)	1 kcal/ml
	Fresubin Original (Fresenius Kabi)	1 kcal/ml
	Isosource Standard (Novartis Consumer Health)	1 kcal/ml
	Nutrison Standard (Nutricia Clinical Care)	1 kcal/ml
	Nutrison Soya (Nutricia Clinical Care)	1 kcal/ml; milk-free
	Osmolite (Ross)	1 kcal/ml
	Osmolite Plus (Ross)	1.2 kcal/ml
	Sondalis Iso (Nestlé Clinical Nutrition)	1 kcal/ml; 44% of fat as MCT
Fibre enriched	Enrich (Ross)	1 kcal/ml
	Fresenius 1000 Complete (Fresenius Kabi)	1 kcal/ml. Nutritionally complete in 1000 kcal/1000 ml
	Fresenius 1200 Complete (Fresenius Kabi)	0.8 kcal/ml. Nutritionally complete in 1200 kcal/1500 ml
	Fresubin Energy Fibre (Fresenius Kabi)	1.5 kcal/ml
	Fresubin Original Fibre (Fresenius Kabi)	1 kcal/ml
	Isosource Fibre (Novartis Consumer Health)	1 kcal/ml
	Jevity (Ross)	1 kcal/ml
	Jevity Plus (Ross)	1.2 kcal/ml
	Nutrison Multifibre (Nutricia Clinical Care)	1 kcal/ml
	Novasource Forte (Novartis Consumer Health)	1.5 kcal/ml
	Novasource GI Control (Novartis Consumer Health)	1 kcal/ml
	Sondalis Fibre (Nestlé Clinical Nutrition)	1 kcal/ml; 49% of fat as MCT
High energy	Ensure Plus (Ross)	1.5 kcal/ml
	Fresubin Energy (Fresenius Kabi)	1.5 kcal/ml
	Isosource Energy (Novartis Consumer Health)	1.6 kcal/ml
	Nutrison Energy (Nutricia Clinical Care)	1.5 kcal/ml
	Sondalis 1.5 (Nestlé Clinical Nutrition)	1.5 kcal/ml; 48% of fat as MCT
	Sonadalis HP (Nestlé Clinical Nutrition)	1.33 kcal/ml, 6.7 g protein/100 ml, 48% fat as MCT
Introduction/half strength	Introlite (Ross)	0.5 kcal/ml
	Novasource Start (Novartis Consumer Health)	0.75 kcal/ml
	Nutrison Pre (Nutricia Clinical Care)	0.5 kcal/ml

Data compiled February 2001. MCT: medium-chain triglyceride.

Table 6.34 Specialist indication enteral feeds and supplements

Type of product	Product name (manufacturer)	Notes
Elemental/semi-elemental	Elemental 028 (SHS)	Elemental powder
	E028 Extra/E028 Extra Liquid (SHS)	Elemental powder or liquid (0.86 kcal/ml)
	Emsogen (SHS)	Elemental powder; most fat as MCT
	Novasource peptide (Novartis Consumer Health)	
	Nutrison Pepti (Nutricia Clinical Care)	Semi-elemental liquid (1kcal/ml) and powder; low fat
	Pepdite 1+ (SHS)	Semi-elemental powder
	Peptamen (Nestlé Clinical Nutrition)	Semi-elemental liquid (1 kcal/ml); 70% fat as MCT
	Peptisorb (Nutricia Clinical Care)	1 kcal/ml. Semi-elemental liquid
	Perative (Ross)	Semi-elemental liquid (1.3 kcal /ml); with added arginine, beta-carotene and omega-3 fatty acids
	Survimed OPD (Fresenius Kabi)	Semi-elemental liquid (1 kcal/ml)
MCT as main fat source	Fresubin HP Energy (Fresenius Kabi)	1.5 kcal/ml
	Monogen (SHS)	0.74 kcal/ml, 93% MCT
	Nutrison MCT (Nutricia Clinical Care)	1 kcal/ml
Low sodium	Nutrison Low Sodium (Nutricia Clinical Care)	1 kcal/ml
Low electrolytes/high energy	Nepro (Ross)	2 kcal/ml
	Nutrison Concentrated LE (Nutricia Clinical Care)	2 kcal/ml
Low protein/high energy	Nutrison Low Protein/Low Mineral (Nutricia Clinical Care)	2 kcal/ml; low in calcium and phosphate
	Suplena (Ross)	2 kcal/ml
Low phosphate/high energy	Renamil (Kimal)	Powder
Low fat/high energy	Advera (Ross)	1.25 kcal/ml; low fat. Formulated for HIV/AIDS
Crohn's disease	Modulen IBD (Nestlé Clinical Nutrition)	Powder. Rich in TGFβ$_2$
Impaired respiratory function	Pulmocare (Ross)	1.5 kcal/ml; high fat; low CHO
	Oxepa (Ross)	High fat; contains EPA and GLA
Catabolic states	TwoCal HN (Ross)	2 kcal/ml
Critical care (Enriched with e.g. glutamine and arginine)	Alitraq (Ross)	1 kcal/ml
	Impact (Novartis Consumer Health)	1 kcal/ml
	Reconvan (Fresenius Kabi)	1 kcal/ml
	Stresson (Nutricia Clinical Care)	1.25 kcal/ml

Data compiled February 2001. MCT: medium-chain triglyceride; HIV: human immunodeficiency virus; AIDS: acquired immunodeficiency syndrome; CHO: carbohydrate; EPA: eicosapentaenoic acid; GLA: gamma-linolenic acid.

AA	Amino acid *or*	BMD	Bone mineral density
	Arachidonic acid	BMI	Body mass index
ABW	Actual body weight	BMR	Basal metabolic rate
ABV	Alcohol by volume	BNF	British National Formulary *or*
ACBS	Advisory Committee on Borderline		British Nutrition Foundation
	Substances	BNO	Bowels not open
ACE	Angiotensin-converting enzyme	BOR	Bowels open regularly
ACMSF	Advisory Committee on the Microbiological	BP	Blood pressure
	Safety of Food	BPA	British Paediatric Association
ACNFP	Advisory Committee on Novel Foods and	BS	Bowel sounds *or*
	Processes		Breath sounds *or*
ADA	American Dietetic Association		Blood sugar
ADH	Antidiuretic hormone	BSA	Body surface area
ADHD	Attention deficit hyperactivity disorder	BSG	British Society of Gastroenterology
ADI	Acceptable daily intake	BT	Bedtime *or*
adm	Admitted		Brain tumour *or*
ADP	Adenosine diphosphate		Breast tumour
AF	Atrial fibrillation	BUN	Blood urea nitrogen
AHCPR	Agency for Health Care Policy and Research	BW	Body weight
AICR	American Institute for Cancer Research	Bx	Biopsy
AIDS	Acquired immunodeficiency syndrome	c	With
AIO	All-in-one	Ca	Carcinoma
AOAC	Association of Official Analytical Chemists	CABG	Coronary artery bypass graft
AP	anterior/posterior (position)	CAPD	Continuous ambulatory peritoneal dialysis
APA	American Psychiatric Association	CAT	Computerized axial tomography *or*
APACHE II	Acute Physiology and Chronic Health		Catalase (antioxidative enzyme)
	Evaluation Score	CAVHDF	Continuous arteriovenous
APD	Automated peritoneal dialysis		haemodiafiltration
ARDS	Acute respiratory distress syndrome	CAVH	Continuous arteriovenous haemofiltration
ARF	Acute renal failure	CBT	Cognitive behavioural therapy
ARMS	Action for Research for Multiple Sclerosis	CCF	Congestive cardiac failure
ARR	Absolute risk reduction	CCK	Cholecystokinin
ATP	Adenosine triphosphate	CCU	Coronary care unit
A+W	Alive and well	CD	Crohn's disease
AXR	Abdominal X-ray	CDC	Centres for Disease Control
BAPEN	British Association for Parenteral and	CF	Cystic fibrosis
	Enteral Nutrition	CFTR	Cystic fibrosis transmembrane regulator
BBB (L/R)	Bundle branch block (left/right)	CHC	Community health council
BCAA	Branched-chain amino acid	CHD	Coronary heart disease
bd	Twice a day	CHF	Congestive heart failure
BDA	British Dietetic Association (or the British	CHImp	Commission for Health Improvement
	Diabetic Association; the former name of	CJD	Creutzfeldt–Jakob disease
	Diabetes UK)	CLD	Chronic lung disease
BEE	Basal energy expenditure	CMO	Chief Medical Officer
BIA	Bioelectrical impedance analysis	CMPA	Cow's milk protein allergy
BID	Brought in dead	CMPI	Cow's milk protein intolerance
BM	Bowel movement	CNG	Community Nutrition Group
BMA	British Medical Association	CNO	Chief Nursing Officer
BMC	Bone mineral content	CNS	Central nervous system

C/O	Complains of
CO	Cardiac output
COAD	Chronic obstructive airways disease
CoC	Committee on Carcinogenicity of Chemicals in Food, Consumer Products and the Environment
CoM	Committee on Mutagenicity of Chemicals in Food, Consumer Products and the Environment
COMA	Committee on Medical Aspects of Food Policy
COPD	Chronic obstructive pulmonary disease
COT	Committee on Toxicity of Chemical in Food, Consumer Products and the Environment
CPD	Continuing professional development
CPK	Creatine phosphokinase
CPR	Cardiopulmonary resuscitation
CPSM	Council for Professions Supplementary to Medicine
Cr III	Trivalent chromium (Cr^{3+})
Cr VI	Hexavalent chromium
CRF	Chronic renal failure
CRP	C-Reactive protein (acute-phase protein)
CRRT	Continuous renal replacement therapy
CSAG	Clinical Standards Advisory Group
CSF	Cerebrospinal fluid
CT	Computed tomography
CVA	Cardiovascular accident (stroke)
CVC	Central venous catheter
CVD	Cardiovascular disease
CVP	Central venous pressure
CVS	Cardiovascular system
CVVH	Continuous veno-venous haemofiltration
CXR	Chest X-ray
d/c	Decrease or Discharge or Discontinue
D&C	Dilatation and curettage
DEXA	Dual-energy X-ray absorptiometry
DfEE	Department for Education and Employment
DH	Department of Health or Dermatitis herpetiformis
DHA	Docosahexaenoic acid
DHHS	Department of Health and Human Services (USA)
DHIVA	Dietitians in HIV and AIDS
DHSS	Department of Health and Social Security (now replaced by the DH and the DSS)
DINT	Dietitians in Neurological Therapy
DIOS	Distal intestinal obstructive syndrome
DM	Diabetes mellitus
DMF	Decayed, missing, filled (teeth)
DNA	Did not attend
DOA	Dead on arrival
DOE	Dyspnoea on exertion
DRV	Dietary reference value
DSM	Diagnostic and Statistical Manual (American Psychiatric Association)

DSS	Department of Social Security
DU	Duodenal ulcer
D+V	Diarrhoea and vomiting
DVT	Deep vein thrombosis
DXA	Dual-energy X-ray absorptiometry
DXT	Deep X-ray therapy
EAR	Estimated average requirement
EATCL	Enteropathy-associated T-cell lymphoma
EBM	Evidence-based medicine or Expressed breast milk
EBRT	External beam radiation therapy
EC	European Community
ECG	Electrocardiogram
ECT	Electroconvulsive therapy
EDD	Expected date of delivery
EEE	Estimated energy expenditure
EEG	Electroencephalogram
EFA	Essential fatty acid
EGCG	Epigallocatechin gallate
ELBW	Extremely low birthweight
EMA	Endomysial antibody
ENT	Ear, nose and throat
EPA	Eicosapentaenoic acid
EPAP	Ethical and Professional Advisory Panel (of the British Dietetic Association)
EPO	Erythropoietin or Evening primrose oil
ERCP	Endoscopic retrograde cholangiopancreatography
ESPGAN	European Society of Paediatric Gastroenterology and Nutrition
ESR	Erythrocyte sedimentation rate
ESRF	End-stage renal failure
ET	Endotracheal tube
EU	European Union
EVM	Expert Group on Vitamins and Minerals
FAC	Food Advisory Committee
FAE	Fetal alcohol effect
FAO	Food and Agriculture Organization
FAP	Familial adenomatous polyposis
FAS	Fetal alcohol syndrome
FB	Fasting blood sugar or Finger breadth or Foreign body
FBC	Full blood count
FCH	Familial combined hyperlipidaemia
FFM	Fat-free mass
FFQ	Food-frequency questionnaire
FG	French gauge
FH	Familial hypercholesterolaemia or Family history
FHP	Fulminant hepatic failure
FMF	Food Manufacturers' Federation
FOS	Fructo-oligosaccharide
FRS	Fat redistribution syndrome
FSA	Food Standards Agency
FUO	Fever of unknown origin
GABA	Gamma-aminobutyric acid
GB	Gall bladder

GCS	Glasgow Coma Scale
GDA	Guideline daily amount
GFR	Glomerular filtration rate
GI	Gastrointestinal or Glycaemic index
GLA	Gamma-linolenic acid
GM	Genetically modified
GTN	Glyceryl trinitrate
GTT	Glucose tolerance test
GU	Genitourinary
GVHD	Graft-versus-host disease
Gy	Gray
HAART	Highly active antiretroviral therapy
Hb	Haemoglobin
HbA$_{Ic}$	Glycosylated haemoglobin A$_{Ic}$
HBV	High biological value
HDA	Health Development Agency
HDL	High-density lipoprotein
HDU	High-dependency unit
HEA	Health Education Authority
HETF	Home enteral tube feeding
hGH	Recombinant growth hormone
HIV	Human immunodeficiency virus
HLA	Histocompatibility locus antigen
HMGCoA	Hydroxymethlyglutaryl coenzyme A
HNPCC	Hereditary non-polyposis colorectal cancer
HO	House officer
HoN	*Health of the Nation* strategy
HPC	History of present condition
HPN	Home parenteral nutrition
Hx	History
IABP	Intra-aortic balloon pump
IBD	Inflammatory bowel disease
IBS	Irritable bowel syndrome
IBW	Ideal body weight
ICD	International Classification of Diseases (WHO)
ICP	Intracranial pressure
ICU	Intensive care unit
i.d.	Intradermal
IDDM	Insulin-dependent diabetes mellitus (now called type 1 diabetes)
IDL	Intermediate-density lipoprotein
IDPN	Intradialytic parenteral nutrition
IEFS	Institute of European Food Studies
IFG	Impaired fasting glycaemia
Ig	Immunoglobulin
IGD	Institute of Grocery Distribution
IGT	Impaired glucose tolerance
IL-1	Interleukin-1
IL-6	Interleukin-6
i.m.	Intramuscular
INR	International normalized ratio
I/O	Intake and output
IOM	Institute of Medicine
i.p.	Intraperitoneal
IPAA	Ileal pouch – anal anastomosis
IPD	Intermittent peritoneal dialysis
IPII	Implantable insulin infusion

ITU	Intensive therapy unit
IU/iu	International units
IUGR	Intrauterine growth retarded
i.v.	Intravascular or Intravenous
IVDM	Intravenous drug misuser
J	Jaundice
kcal	Kilocalorie
kJ	Kilojoule
KS	Kaposi's sarcoma or Kidney/spleen
l	Litre
LBM	Lean body mass
LBV	Low biological value
LBW	Low birthweight
LCP or LCPUFA	Long-chain polyunsaturated fatty acid
LCT	Long-chain triglyceride
LD	Lethal dose
LDL	Low-density lipoprotein
LDSAG	Local Diabetes Services Advisory Group
LFT	Liver function tests
LK	Liver/kidney
LLL	Left lower lobe (lung)
LLQ	Left lower quadrant (abdomen)
LMI	Likelihood of Malnutrition Index
LMN	Lower motor neurone
LMP	Last menstrual period
LP	Lumbar puncture
LRNI	Lower reference nutrient intake
LUQ	Left upper quadrant (abdomen)
LVAD	Left ventricular assist device
LVF	Left ventricular failure
LVH	Left ventricular hypertrophy
m	Metre
MA	Megesterol acetate
MAC	Mid-arm circumference or Methacrylic acid copolymer
MAFF	Ministry of Agriculture, Fisheries and Food
MAMC	Mid-arm muscle circumference
MAOI	Monoamine oxidase inhibitor
MCH	Mean corpuscular haemoglobin
MCHC	Mean corpuscular haemoglobin concentration
MCT	Medium-chain triglyceride
MCV	Mean corpuscular volume
MDA	Malondialdehyde
MDRD	Modification of Diet in Renal Disease
MDT	Multidisciplinary team
mEq	Milliequivalent
mg	Milligram
MHG	Mental Health Group
MI	Motivational interviewing or Myocardial infarction
MID	Multi-infarct dementia
MIMS	Monthly Index of Medical Specialities
MJ	Megajoule
ml	Millilitre
MMC	Migratory motor complex

mmHg	Millimetre of mercury
mmol	Millimole
MND	Motor neurone disease
MOF	Multiple organ failure
MOFS	Multiple organ failure syndrome
m.osmol	Milliosmole
MRI	Magnetic resonance imaging
MS	Mitral stenosis *or*
	Multiple sclerosis
MSG	Monosodium glutamate
MSU	Midstream urine
MUFA	Monounsaturated fatty acid
N	Nitrogen *or*
	Normal
*n*3	Omega-3 (fatty acids)
*n*6	Omega-6 (fatty acids)
NACNE	National Advisory Committee of Nutrition Education
NAD	Nothing abnormal detected
NADP	Nicotinamide adenine dinucleotide
NAGE	Nutrition Advisory Group for Elderly People
NAS	National Academy of Sciences *or* No added salt
NBD	Neurogenic bowel dysfunction
NBM	Nil by mouth
NCH	National Children's Home
NCJ	Needle catheter jejunostomy
NDC	National Dairy Council
NDNS	National Diet and Nutrition Survey
NEC	Necrotizing enterocolitis
NEPDF	Nutrient-enriched postdischarge formula
NFS	National Food Survey
NG	Nasogastric
NHDC	Neohesperidine DC
NHS	National Health Service
NICE	National Institute for Clinical Excellence
NIDDM	Non-insulin-dependent diabetes mellitus (now called type 2 diabetes)
NIH	National Institute of Health (USA)
NMES	Non-milk extrinsic sugars
NMR	Nuclear magnetic resonance
NNRTI	Non-nucleoside reverse transcriptase inhibitor
NNT	Number needed to treat
NO	Nitric oxide
NOF	Fractured neck of femur
NPN	Non-protein nitrogen
NRTI	Nucleoside analogue reverse transcriptase inhibitor
NSAID	Non-steroidal anti-inflammatory drug
NSF	National Service Framework
NSP	Non-starch polysaccharide
NTF	Nutrition Task Force
NTD	Neural tube defect
N+V	Nausea and vomiting
OA	On admission *or* Osteoarthritis
od	Every day/once a day

OE	On examination
OGTT	Oral glucose tolerance test
OHN	*Our Healthier Nation*
ONS	Office of National Statistics
OOB	Out of bed
OPA	Outpatient appointment
OPCS	Office of Population Censuses and Statistics
PAC	Pulmonary artery catheter
PaCO$_2$	Arterial carbon dioxide
PAI	Platelet activator inhibitor
PAL	Physical activity level
PaO$_2$	Arterial oxygen
PAR	Physical activity ratio
PARNUTS	(Foods for) particular nutritional uses
PBC	Primary biliary cirrhosis
PBM	Peak bone mass
PBP	Progressive bulbar palsy
pc	After meals
PCB	Polychlorinated biphenyl
PCR	Polymerase chain reaction *or* Protein catabolic rate
PCV	Packed cell volume
PD	Peritoneal dialysis
PDCAAS	Protein digestibility corrected amino acid score
PDUO	Previous day's urinary output
PE	Physical examination
PE	Pulmonary embolism
PEEP	Positive end-expiratory pressure
PEG	Percutaneous endoscopic gastrostomy
PEJ	Percutaneous endoscopic jejunostomy
PEM	Protein-energy malnutrition
PENG	Parenteral and Enteral Nutrition Group
PERT	Pancreatic enzyme replacement therapy
PET	Pre-eclampsia toxaemia
PF	Peak flow
PI	Protease inhibitor
PICC	Peripherally inserted central catheter
PID	Pelvic inflammatory disease
PKU	Phenylketonuria
PM	Post mortem
PMA	Progressive muscular atrophy
PMH	Past medical history
PMS	Premenstrual syndrome
PN	Parenteral nutrition (or total parenteral nutrition, TPN)
PNI	Prognostic Nutritional Index
PO	Per os (by mouth)
POMC	Pro-opiomelaninocortin
PPF	Plasma protein fraction
PPH	Postpartum haemorrhage
PR	Per rectum
PRA	Prealbumin (acute-phase protein)
prn	When required
PSE	Portal systemic encephalopathy
PT	Prothrombin time
PTH	Parathyroid hormone
PU	Peptic ulcer
PUFA	Polyunsaturated fatty acid

PUO	Pyrexia of unknown origin	SGA	Small for gestational age *or* Subjective global assessment
PV	Per vagina	SH	Social history
PVD	Peripheral vascular disease	SiADH	Stress-induced syndrome of inappropriate antidiuretic hormone
PVS	Persistent vegetative state		
PWS	Prader–Willi syndrome	SIGN	Scottish Intercollegiate Guidelines Network
PZI	Protamine zinc insulin		
qd	Every day	SLE	Systemic lupus erythematosus
qds	Four times a day	SLT	Speech and language therapist
qh	Every hour	SNAG	School Nutrition Action Group
QUID	Quantitative ingredients declaration	SNS	Sympathetic nervous system
RA	Rheumatoid arthritis	SOA	Swelling of ankles
RAST	Radioallergosorbent test	SOB	Shortness of breath
RBC	Red blood cell/count	SOD	Superoxide dismutase (antioxidative enzyme)
RBP	Retinol-binding protein (acute-phase protein)		
		SOS	Swedish obese subjects
RBS	Random blood sugar	SRD	State-registered dietitian
RCN	Royal College of Nursing	STAT	Immediately
RCOG	Royal College of Obstetricians and Gynaecologists	STD	Sexually transmitted disease
		T_3	Triiodothyronine
RCP	Royal College of Physicians	T_4	Thyroxine
RCPath	Royal College of Pathologists	TAH	Total abdominal hysterectomy
RCT	Randomized controlled trial	TB	Tuberculosis
RDA	Recommended daily amount/recommended dietary allowance	TBW	Total body water
		TCA	To come/call again
RDI	Reference daily intake	TCI	To come in
REE	Resting energy expenditure	tds	Three times a day
RES	Reticuloendothelial system	TDS	Total Diet Study
RFT	Respiratory function tests	TDT	Transitional dietary therapy
RLE	Right lower extremity	TIA	Transient ischaemic attack
RLL	Right lower lobe	TIBC	Total iron-binding capacity
RLQ	Right lower quadrant	TISS	Tissue Injury Scoring System
RMR	Resting metabolic rate	TLC	Tender loving care
RNI	Reference nutrient intake	TNF	Tumour necrosis factor
ROS	Reactive oxygen species *or* Review of symptoms	TOP	Termination of pregnancy
		tPA	Tissue plasminogen activator
RQ	Respiratory quotient	TPN	Total parenteral nutrition (now called PN)
RRT	Renal replacement therapy	TSF	Triceps skinfold thickness
RS	Respiratory system	TSH	Thyroid-stimulating hormone
RSC	Royal Society of Chemistry	TTO	To take out/to take home
RSO	Resident surgical officer	Tx	Treatment/therapy
RTA	Renal tubular acidosis	UA	Urinalysis
RUQ	Right upper quadrant	UC	Ulcerative colitis
Rx	Treatment/prescribed drugs	U+E	Urea and electrolytes
s	Without	UKM	Urea kinetic modelling
SACN	Scientific Advisory Committee on Nutrition (formerly COMA)	UKPDS	United Kingdom Prospective Diabetes Study Group
SAPS	Simplified Acute Physiology Score		
SALT	Speech and language therapist	UMN	Upper motor neurone
s/b	Seen by	UO	Urinary output
SBE	Subacute bacterial endocarditis	UPD	Uniparental disomy
s/c	Subclavian *or* Subcutaneous	URR	Urea reduction ratio
		U/S	Ultrasound
SCFA	Short-chain fatty acid	UTI	Urinary tract infection
SCI	Spinal cord injury	UUN	Urinary urea nitrogen
SCII	Subcutaneous insulin infusion	VLBW	Very low birthweight
SDAG	Scottish Diet Action Group	VLCD	Very low calorie diet
SEAC	Spongiform Encephalopathy Advisory Committee	VLDL	Very low-density lipoprotein
		VO_2max	Maximum oxygen uptake
SFA	Saturated fatty acid	VOICES	Voluntary Organisations Involved in Caring in the Elderly Sectors

WHO	World Health Organization	<	Less than
WRCF	World Cancer Research Fund	>	Greater than
WTE	Whole-time equivalent	°	Absent/not detected
μg	Microgram	#	Fracture
5-HT	5-Hydroxytryptamine (serotonin)	Δ	Diagnosis

Action for Blind People
14–16 Verney Road, London SE16 3DZ
Tel: 020 7732 8771

Age Concern England
1268 London Road, London SW16 4ER

Alzheimer's Disease Society
Gordon House, 10 Greencoat Place, London SW1P 1PH
Tel: 020 7306 0606

Anaphylaxis Campaign
PO Box 149, Fleet, Hampshire GU13 9XU
Tel: 01252 542029 Fax: 01252 377140
Website: www.anaphylaxis.org.uk

Arthritis Care
18 Stephenson Way, London NW1 2HD
Helpline: 0800 289170

Arthritis Research Campaign (formerly the Arthritis and
Rheumatism Council)
PO Box 177, Chesterfield, Derbyshire S41 7TQ
Website: www.arc.org.uk

Association of Breastfeeding Mothers
26 Hearnshaw Close, London SE26 4T11

Association for Spina Bifida and Hydrocephalus (ASBAH)
ASBAH House, 42 Park Road, Peterborough,
Cambridgeshire PE1 2UQ
Tel: 01733 555988

Association of Palliative Medicine
11 Westwood Road, Southampton SO17 1DL
Tel: 01703 672888

AVERT (AIDS Education and Research Trust)
4 Brighton Road, Horsham, West Sussex RH13 5BA
Tel: 01403 210202   Fax: 01403 211001
E-mail: avert@dial.pipex.com

BACUP
3 Bath Place, Rivington Street, London EC2A 3JR
Tel: 020 7696 9003
Website: www.cancerbacup.org.uk

Boots Company plc
Thane Road, Nottingham NG2 3AA

Brewhurst Health Food Supplies Ltd
Abbot Close, Oyster Lane, Byfleet, Surrey KT14 7JP
Tel: 01932 334501

Bristol-Myers
Bristol-Myers Squibb Pharmaceuticals Ltd,
141–149 Staines Road, Hounslow, Middlesex TW3 3JA
Tel: 0800 7311 736   Fax: 020 8754 3677

British Allergy Foundation
Deepdene House, 30 Bellegrove Road, Welling,
Kent DA16 3PY
Tel: 020 8303 8525 (general enquiries) or
020 8303 8583 (helpline)
Website: www.allergyfoundation.com

British Association for Parenteral and Enteral Nutrition
(BAPEN)
PO Box 922, Maidenhead, Berks SL6 4SH

British Cardiac Society
9 Fitzroy Square, London W1P 5AH
Tel: 020 7383 3887
Website: www.cardiac.org.uk

British Diabetic Association. See Diabetes UK

British Dietetic Association
5th Floor Charles House, 148–149 Great Charles Street,
Birmingham B3 3HT
Tel: 0121 200 8080   Fax: 0121 200 8081
E-mail: info@bda.uk.com
Website: www.bda.uk.com

British Digestive Foundation
3 St Andrew's Place, London NW1 4LB
Tel: 020 7486 0341
Website: www.bdf.org.uk

British Geriatric Society
1 St Andrew's Place, London NW1 4LB
Tel: 020 7935 4004

British Heart Foundation
14 Fitzhardinge Street, London W1H 4DH
Website: www.bhf.org.uk

British Liver Trust
Ransomes Europark, Ipswich IP3 9QG

Tel: 0808 800 1000 (information line)
E-mail: info@britishlivertrust.org.uk
Website: www.britishlivertrust.org.uk

British Nutrition Foundation
High Holborn House, 52–54 High Holborn, London
WC1V 6RQ
Tel: 020 7404 6504
Website: www.nutrition.org.uk

British Society for Allergy and Clinical Immunology
66 Weston Park, Thames Ditton, Surrey KT7 0HL
Tel: 020 8398 9240

British Society of Gastroenterology
3 St Andrews Place, Regent's Park, London NW1 4LB
Tel: 020 7935 2815
Website: www.bsg.org.uk

Cancerlink
11–21 Northdown Street, London N1 9BN
Freephone Cancer Information Helpline: 0800 132905
Freephone Asian Cancer Information Helpline in
Bengali, Hindi, Punjabi, Urdu and English:
0800 590415

Cancer Research Campaign
10 Cambridge Terrace, London NW1 4JL
website: www.crc.org.uk

Carers National Association
20–25 Glasshouse Yard, London EC1A 4JS

Caroline Walker Trust (publications)
22 Kindersley Way, Abbots Langley, Herts WD5 0DQ
Tel: 01923 269902
Website: www.cwt.org.uk

Centre for Evidence Based Medicine
University of Oxford, Nuffield Department of Clinical
Medicine, Level 5, The Oxford Radcliffe NHS Trust,
Headley Way, Headington, Oxford OX3 9DU
Tel: 01865 221321
Website: cebm.jr2.ox.ac.uk

Centre for Policy on Ageing
25–31 Ironmonger Row, London EC1V 3QP
Tel: 020 7253 1787

Child Growth Foundation
2 Mayfield Avenue, London W4 1PW

CJD Support Network
E-mail: cjdnet@alzheimers.org.uk

Cleft Lip and Palate Association (CLAPA)
235–237 Finchley Road, London NW3 6LS
Tel: 020 7431 0033
Website: www.clapa.cwc.net

Cochrane Library
Update Software Ltd, Summertown Pavilion, Middle Way,
Summertown, Oxford OX2 7LG
Tel: 01865 513902
Website: www.update-software.co.uk or www.cochrane.
org/cochrane/cdsr.htm

Coeliac Society
PO Box 220, High Wycombe, Bucks HP11 2HY
Tel: 01494 437278 Fax: 01494 474349
Website: www.coeliac.co.uk

Coronary Prevention Group
102 Gloucester Place, London W1H 3DA
Tel: 020 7935 2889

Cow & Gate. See Nutricia Clinical Care

Cruse Bereavement Care
Cruse House, 126 Sheen Road, Richmond, Surrey
TW9 1UR
Tel: 020 8940 4818

Cystic Fibrosis Trust
11 London Road, Bromley, Kent BR1 1BY
Tel: 020 8464 7211

Deafblind UK
100 Bridge Street, Peterborough, Cambridgeshire PE1
1DY
Tel: 01733 358100
Helpline: 0800 132 320

Department for Education and Employment (DfEE)
DfEE Publications Centre
Tel: 0845 60 22260
Website: www.dfee.gov.uk

Department of Health (DH)
Richmond House, 79 Whitehall, London SW1A 2NL
Tel: 0207 210 4850
E-mail: dhmail@doh.gsi.gov.uk
Website: www.doh.gov.uk

Diabetes UK
10 Queen Anne Street, London W1M 0BD
Tel: 0207 323 1531
Careline: 020 7636 6112
Website: www.diabetes.org.uk

**Digestive Disorders Foundation (formerly the British
Digestive Foundation)**
3 St Andrew's Place, London NW1 4LB
Tel: 020 7486 0341
Website: www.digestivedisorders.org.uk

Disabled Living Foundation
380–384 Harrow Road, London W9 2HU
Helpline: 0870 603 9177
Website: www.dlf.org.uk

Down's Syndrome Association
153–155 Mitcham Road, London SW17 9PG
Tel: 020 8682 4001

Eating Disorders Association
1st Floor, Wensum House, 103 Prince of Wales Road,
Norwich NR1 1DW
Tel: 01603 621414

Family Heart Association
7 North Road, Maidenhead SL6 1PL
Tel: 01628 522177

Farley Health Products
Mint Bridge Road, Kendal LA9 6NL
Tel: 01539 797204
Website for health-care professionals: www.farleys-heinz-hcp.co.uk

Federation of Multiple Sclerosis Therapy Centres
Bradbury House, 155 Barkers Lane, Bedford MK41 9RX
Tel: 01234 325781

Food Intolerance Databank
Leatherhead Food RA, Randalls Road, Leatherhead,
Surrey KT22 7RY
Tel: 01372 376761 (Direct line 01372 822217)
Fax: 01372 386228

Food Standards Agency (FSA)
England: Room 6/21, Hannibal House, PO Box 30080,
London SE1 6YA
Fax: 020 7238 6330
E-mail: helpline@foodstandards.gsi.gov.uk
Website: www.foodstandards.gov.uk
Scotland: St Magnus House, 6th Floor, 25 Guild Street,
Aberdeen AB11 6NJ
Fax: 01224 28516
Wales: 1st Floor, Southgate House, Wood Street, Cardiff
CF10 1EW
Fax: 029 2067 8918/9
Northern Ireland: 10B and 10C Clarendon Quay,
Clarendon Dock, Clarendon Road, Belfast BT1 3BW
Fax: 028 9041 7726

Fresenius Kabi
Building C, Hampton Court, Tudor Road, Manor Park,
Runcorn, Cheshire WA7 1UF
Tel: 01928 594200

General Dietary Ltd
PO Box 38, Kingston upon Thames, Surrey KT2 7YP
Tel: 020 8336 2323

Gluten Free Foods Ltd
Unit 270, Centennial Park, Centennial Avenue, Elstree,
Borehamwood, Herts WD6 3SS
Tel: 020 8953 4444
Website: www.glutenfree-foods.co.uk

Headway (National Head Injuries Association)
7 King Edward Court, King Edward Street, Nottingham
NG1 1EW

Health Development Agency (formerly the Health
Education Authority)
Trevelyan House, 30 Great Peter Street, London
SW1 2HW
Tel: 020 7222 5300
Website: www.hda-online.org.uk

Health Promotion England
50 Eastbourne Terrace, London W2 3QR
Website: www.hpe.org.uk

HJ Heinz Co. Ltd
Kitt Green, Wigan, Lancs WN5 0JL
Website for health-care professionals: www.farleys-heinz-hcp.co.uk

Help the Aged
St James Walk, Clerkenwell Green, London EC1R 0BE
Tel: 020 7253 0253

Hospice Information Service
St Christopher's Hospice, 51–59 Lawrie Park Road,
Sydenham, London SE26 6DZ
Tel: 020 8778 9252

IA (formerly the Ileostomy Association, now the
Ileostomy and Internal Pouch Support Group)
PO Box 132, Scunthorpe DN15 9YW
Tel: 01724 720150
Helpline: 0800 018 4724
Website: www.ileostomypouch.demon.co.uk

Institute of Grocery Distribution (IGD)
Grange Lane, Letchmore Heath, Watford, Herts WD2
8DQ
Tel: 01923 857141

Jacobs Bakery
PO Box 1, Long Lane, Liverpool L9 7BQ
Tel: 0151 525 3661

Joint Breastfeeding Initiative
Department of Health, Skipton House, 80 London Road,
London SE1 6LW
Tel: 020 7972 2000

King's Fund Centre
11–13 Cavendish Square, London W1M 0AN

La Leche League
PO Box BM 3424, London WC1N 3XX
Website: www.lalecheleague.org

Macmillan Cancer Relief
Anchor House, 15–19 Britten Street, London SW3 3TZ
Tel: 0845 601 6161

MAFF Publications
Admail 6000, London SW1A 2XX
Telephone orders (for free publications): 08459 556000

Maternity Alliance
5th Floor, 45 Beech Street, London EC2P 2LX
Tel: 020 7588 8583/020 7588 8582

Mead Johnson Nutritionals. See Bristol-Myers
Customer service line: 020 8754 3764
E-mail: mjn.customerservices@bms.com

Medic Alert (medical alert bracelets)
12 Bridge Wharf, 156 Caledonian Road, London N1 9UU
Tel: 020 7833 3034

MENCAP (Royal Society for Mentally Handicapped Children and Adults)
117–123 Golden Lane, London EC1Y 0RT
Tel: 020 7454 0454

Migraine Trust
45 Great Ormond Street, London WC1N 3HZ
Tel: 020 7831 4818

MIND (National Association for Mental Health)
15–19 Broadway, London E15 4BQ
Tel: 020 8522 1728
Helpline: 0345 660 0163

Ministry of Agriculture, Fisheries and Food (MAFF)
3–8 Whitehall Place, London SW1A 2HH
Helpline: 0645 335577
Fax: 020 7270 8419
E-mail: helpline@maff.gsi.gov.uk
Website: www.maff.gov.uk
MAFF Publications, Admail 6000, London SW1A 2XX
Tel: 0645 556000

Motor Neurone Disease (MND) Association
PO Box 246, Northampton NN1 2PR
Tel: 01604 250505

Multidisciplinary Association of Spinal Cord Injury Professionals (MASCIP)
The Duke of Cornwall Spinal Treatment Centre, Salisbury District Hospital, Odstock Road, Salisbury SP2 8BJ
Tel: 01722 336 262

Multiple Sclerosis Society
25 Effie Road, Fulham, London SW6 1EE
Tel: 020 7736 9861
Helpline: 0808 800 8000
Website: www.mssociety.org.uk

Muscular Dystrophy Group
7–11 Prescott Place, Clapham, London SW4 6BS
Tel: 020 7720 8055

National AIDS Helpline
Tel: 0800 567123

National Association for Colitis and Crohn's Disease (NACC)
4 Beaumont House, Sutton Road, St Albans, Herts AL1 5HH
Tel: 01727 830038

National Asthma Campaign
Providence House, Providence Place, London N1 0NT
Tel: 0345 010203

National Autistic Society (NAS)
393 City Road, London EC1V 1NE
Tel: 020 7833 2299
NAS Information Service: 020 7903 3599

National Childbirth Trust
Alexander House, Oldham Terrace, Acton, London W3 6NH
Tel: 020 8992 8637
Website: www.nct-online.org

National CJD Surveillance Unit, Edinburgh
Website: www.cjd.ed.ac.uk

National Eczema Society
163 Eversholt Street, London NW1 1BU
Tel: 020 7388 4097

National Coaching Foundation
114 Cardigan Road, Headingley, Leeds LS6 3BJ
Tel: 0113 274 4802

National Council for Hospice and Specialist Palliative Care Service
7th Floor, 1 Great Cumberland Place, London W1H 7AL
Tel: 0202 7723 1639 Fax: 020 7723 5380

National Institute for Clinical Excellence (NICE)
11 Strand, London WC2N 5HR
Tel: 020 7766 9191
Website: www.nice.org.uk

National Osteoporosis Society
PO Box 10, Radstock, Bath BA3 3YB
Tel: 01761 472721
Website: www.nos.org.uk

National Schizophrenia Fellowship
28 Castle Street, Kingston-upon-Thames, Surrey KT1 1SS
Tel: 020 8547 3937
National adviceline: 020 8974 6814

Nestlé Clinical Nutrition
St Georges House, Croydon, Surrey CR9 1NR
Tel: 020 8667 5130

NHS Centre for Reviews and Dissemination
University of York, Helsington, York YO1 5DD
Tel: 01904 433634
Website: www.york.ac.uk/inst/crd

Novartis Consumer Health UK Ltd
Wimblehurst Road, Horsham, West Sussex RH12 5AB
Tel: 01403 324135

Nuffield Trust
59 New Cavendish Street, London W1M 7RD

Nutricia Clinical Care/Nutricia Dietary Care
Nutricia Ltd, White Horse Business Park, Trowbridge,
Wilts BA14 0XQ
Tel: 01225 711677

Nutrition Point Ltd
13 Taurus Park, Westbrook, Warrington WA5 5ZT
Tel: 07041 544044

Oesophageal Patients Association
16 Whitefields Crescent, Solihull, West Midlands
B91 3NU
Tel: 0121 704 9860

Parkinson's Disease Scottish Resource
10 Claremont Terrace, Glasgow G3 7XR
Tel/Fax: 0141 332 3343

Parkinson's Disease Society of the United Kingdom
United Scientific House, 215 Vauxhall Bridge Road,
London SW1V IEJ
Tel: 020 7931 8080   Fax: 020 7233 9908
Helpline: 020 7233 5373
Website: http://glaxocentre.merseyside.org/pds.html
E-mail: mailbox@pdsuk.demon.co.uk

Patients Association
PO Box 935, Harrow, Middlesex HA1 3YJ
Tel: 020 8423 9111
Website: www.patients-association.com

Prader–Willi Syndrome Association (UK)
33 Leopold Street, Derby DE1 2HF
Website: www.pwsa-uk.demon.co.uk

Psoriasis Association
7 Milton Street, Northampton NN2 7JG
Tel: 01604 711129

Realeat Survey Office
Howard Way, Newport Pagnell, Bucks BK16 9PY
Tel: 01908 211311

Research into Ageing
Braid House, 15–17 St Cross St, London EC1N 8UN

Ross Products Division
A Division of Abbott Laboratories Limited,
Abbott House, Norden Road, Maidenhead, Berks
SL6 4XE
Tel: 01628 773355
Nutrition helpline: 0800 252882

Royal Association for Disability and Rehabilitation
(RADAR)
12 City Forum, 250 City Road, London EC1V 8AF
Tel: 020 7250 3222

Royal National Institute for the Blind (RNIB)
224 Great Portland Street, London W1N 6AA
Tel: 020 7388 1266
Helpline: 0845 766 9999

Royal National Institute for Deaf People (RNID)
19–23 Featherstone Street, London EC1Y 8SL
Tel: 020 7296 8000
Helpline: 0808 808 0123/0808 808 9000

Schär
PO Box 126, Worcester WR5 2ZN
Tel: 0808 100 0483
Website: www.schaer.com

Scottish Down's Association
158–160 Balgreen Road, Edinburgh EH11 3AU
Tel: 0131 313 4225

Scottish Intercollegiate Guidelines Network (SIGN)
SIGN Secretariat, Royal College of Physicians, 9 Queen
St, Edinburgh EH2 1JQ
Tel: 0131 225 7324
Website: www.show.scot.nhs.uk/sign/home.htm

Scottish Spinal Cord Injury Association (SSCIA)
The Festival Business Centre, 150 Brand Street, Glasgow
G51 1DH

SHS International Ltd
100 Wavertree Boulevard, Liverpool L7 9PT
Tel: 0151 228 8161
www.shsweb.co.uk

SMA Nutrition
Huntercombe Lane South, Taplow, Maidenhead, Berks
SL6 0PH
Tel: 0845 776 2900

Spinal Injuries Association (UK)
76 St James Lane, London N10 3DF
Tel: 020 8444 2121

The Stationery Office
Website: www.tsonline.co.uk

Stroke Association
CHSA House, Whitecross Street, London EC1Y 8JJ
Tel: 020 7490 7999

Sutherland Health Ltd
Unit 1, Rivermead, Pipers Way, Thatcham, Berks RG19
4EP
Tel: 01635 874488

Syner-Med
Airport House, Purley Way, Croydon, Surrey CR0 0XZ
Tel: 020 8410 6400

Terrence Higgins Trust
52–54 Grays Inn Road, London WC1X 8JU
Tel: 020 7831 0330
E-mail: info@tht.org.uk

Trufree
PO Box 99, Trowbridge, Wiltshire BA14 0YN
Tel: 01225 711801

Ultrapharm Ltd
Centenary Business Park, Henley-on-Thames,
Oxfordshire RG9 1DS
Tel: 01491 578016
Website: www.glutenfree.co.uk

Unigreg Ltd
Enterprise House, 181–189 Garth Road, Morden, Surrey
SM4 4LL
Tel: 020 8330 1421

United Kingdom Drug Information Pharmacists Group
(UKDIPG)
Website: www.ukdipg.org.uk

Vegan Society
7 Battle Road, St Leonards-on-Sea, East Sussex
TN37 7AA
Tel: 01424 427 393

Vegetarian Society
Parkdale, Denham Road, Altrincham, Cheshire
WA14 4QG
Tel: 0161 928 0793

Vitaflo Ltd
11 Century Building, Tower Street, Brunswick Business
Park, Liverpool L3 4BL
Tel: 0151 709 9020
E-mail: vitaflo@vitaflo.co.uk

VOICES (Voluntary Organisations Involved in Caring in
the Elderly Sector)
c/o Association of Charity Officers, Beechwood House,
Wyllyotts Close, Potters Bar, Herts EN6 2HN

World Cancer Research Fund
105 Park Street, London W1Y 3FB
Tel: 020 7343 4200 Fax: 020 7343 4201

Index

The page numbers of sections are shown in **bold**